Care of the
Gynecologic/Obstetric Patient

SERIES EDITOR

Fred F. Ferri, M.D., F.A.C.P.

Clinical Associate Professor
Brown University School of Medicine
Chief, Division of Internal Medicine
St. Joseph's Hospital and Fatima Hospital
Providence, Rhode Island

OTHER HANDBOOKS IN THE "PRACTICAL GUIDE TO THE CARE OF" SERIES

Ambulatory Patient

Critically Ill Patient

Geriatric Patient

Medical Patient

Pediatric Patient

Psychiatric Patient

Surgical Patient

Practical Guide to the Care of the Gynecologic/Obstetric Patient

George T. Danakas, M.D., F.A.C.O.G.
Clinical Assistant Professor
Department of Obstetrics and Gynecology
State University of New York
Buffalo, New York

Marcello Pietrantoni, M.D.
Associate Professor
Department of Obstetrics and Gynecology
Division of Maternal-Fetal Medicine
University of Louisville School of Medicine
Louisville, Kentucky

with 131 *illustrations*

Mosby
An Imprint of Elsevier Science
St. Louis London Philadelphia Sydney Toronto

Mosby
An Imprint of Elsevier Science

Vice President and Publisher: Anne S. Patterson
Editor: Emma D. Underdown
Developmental Editor: Christy Wells
Project Manager: Linda McKinley
Production Editor: Paul J. Stoecklein
Design Coordinator: Liz Fett
Manufacturing Manager: Linda Ierardi
Cover Illustration: David Zielinski

Printed in the United States of America

Mosby, Inc.
11830 Westline Industrial Drive
St. Louis, Missouri 63146

ISBN 0-8151-2316-7

02 03 04 / 9 8 7 6 5 4 3

Contributors

Philip J. Aliotta, M.D., M.S.H.A., F.A.C.S.

Director, Urogynecology Section-Urologist
Attending Urologist
Department of Obstetrics and Gynecology
Sisters of Charity Hospital
Buffalo, New York

Brad Angle, M.D.

Assistant Professor
Department of Pediatrics
University of Louisville
Louisville, Kentucky

JoAnne Arnold, M.D.

Clinical Instructor
Department of Gynecology and Obstetrics
State University of New York School of Medicine
Buffalo, New York

Ronald E. Batt, M.D.

Professor of Clinical Gynecology
Department of Gynecology-Obstetrics
School of Medicine and Biomedical Sciences
State University of New York
Buffalo, New York

John R. Barton, M.D.

Director of Maternal-Fetal Medicine
Department of Obstetrics and Gynecology
Central Baptist Hospital
Lexington, Kentucky

Harold Bays, M.D., F.A.C.P.

Director
Lipid Center
Columbia/HCA Audubon Hospital
Louisville, Kentucky

Germaine M. Buck, Ph.D.

Associate Professor
Department of Social and Preventive Medicine
School of Medicine and Biomedical Sciences
State University of New York at Buffalo
Buffalo, New York

Beth Buehler, M.S., C.G.C.

Director, Genetic Counseling
The Prenatal Center
Palm Beach Gardens, Florida

Stephen J. Carlan, B.S., M.D.

Director, Department of Obstetrics and Gynecology
Arnold Palmer Hospital for Children and Women
Orlando, Florida

Harold C. Castilone, M.D.

Clinical Associate Professor
Department of Gynecology and Obstetrics
State University of New York at Buffalo School of Medicine
Buffalo, New York
Clinical Chief, Department of Gynecology and Obstetrics
Millard Fillmore Surgery Center
Williamsville, New York

Vernon Cook, M.D.

Assistant Professor
Department of Obstetrics and Gynecology
University of Louisville School of Medicine
Louisville, Kentucky

Maria A. Corigliano, M.D., F.A.C.O.G.

Clinical Assistant Professor
Department of Obstetrics and Gynecology
State University of New York at Buffalo
Buffalo, New York
Department of Obstetrics and Gynecology
Millard Fillmore Suburban Hospital
Williamsville, New York

Bryan J. DeMarco, M.D.

Department of Obstetrics and Gynecology
Promina NW Health System
Austell, Georgia

Carolyn M. Doherty, M.D.

Assistant Clinical Professor
Department of Gynecology and Obstetrics
University of Nebraska Medical Center
Director
Nebraska Methodist Reproductive Endocrinology and Assisted Reproductive Technologies Laboratory
Nebraska Methodist Hospital
Omaha, Nebraska

Ivan D'Souza, M.D., F.R.C.S., F.A.C.O.G.

Clinical Assistant Professor
Department of Obstetrics and Gynecology
State University of New York at Buffalo School of Medicine
Buffalo, New York

Tamara S. Evans, Pharm.D., B.C.P.S.

Clinical Instructor Department of Pharmacy Practice
Clinical Pharmacy Coordinator
Department of Pharmacology
Buffalo General Hospital
Buffalo, New York

Barb Fingar, R.Ph.

Clinical Coordinator
Department of Pharmacy
Norton Hospital
Louisville, Kentucky

J. Kevin Fitzpatrick, M.D.

Clinical Instructor
Department of Obstetrics and Gynecology
State University of New York at Buffalo
Buffalo, New York

Armando Fuentes, M.D.

Clinical Instructor
Department of Obstetrics and Gynecology
Division of Maternal-Fetal Medicine
Arnold Palmer Hospital for Children and Women
Orlando, Florida

Stanley A. Gall, M.D.

Professor and Chairman
Department of Obstetrics and Gynecology
University of Louisville School of Medicine
Louisville, Kentucky

Jeffery R. Graves, M.D.

Staff Anesthesiologist
Department of Anesthesiology
Naval Medical Center
Portsmouth, Virginia

Lawrence J. Gugino, M.D.

Clinical Assistant Professor
Department of Obstetrics and Gynecology
State University of New York at Buffalo School of Medicine
Children's Hospital of Buffalo
Buffalo, New York

Patricia Harris, R.N., R.D., L.D.

Senior Nutritionist, Department of Obstetrics and Gynecology
University of Louisville School of Medicine
Louisville, Kentucky

E. Nigel Harris, M.D., D.M.

Dean and Senior Vice President for Academic Affairs
Morehouse School of Medicine
Atlanta, Georgia

Joseph Hersh, M.D.

Professor
Department of Pediatrics
Child Evaluation Center
University of Louisville School of Medicine
Louisville, Kentucky

Karen Houck, M.D.

Clinical Instructor
Department of Gynecology and Obstetrics
State University of New York at Buffalo
School of Medicine
Buffalo, New York

Helen Y. How, M.D.

Assistant Professor
Department of Obstetrics and Gynecology
Marshall University School of Medicine
Department of Obstetrics and Gynecology
Cabell Huntington Hospital
Huntington, West Virginia

Anna K. Huang, M.D.

Assistant Professor
Department of Infectious Diseases
University of Louisville School of Medicine
Louisville, Kentucky

Mushtaque Juneja, M.D.

Director of Obstetric Anesthesia
Norton Hospital
Associate Professor of Anesthesiology
University of Louisville School of Medicine
Louisville, Kentucky

Milan Kos, M.D.

Asim Kurjak, M.D.

Professor and Chairman
Department of Obstetrics and Gynecology
Bolnica Sveti DVH
Zagreb, Croatia

Shashikant Lele, M.D.

Clinical Professor
Department of Gynecology and Obstetrics
State University of New York at Buffalo
Buffalo, New York

Luanne Lettieri, M.D.

Assistant Professor
Director of Maternal-Fetal Medicine
Department of Obstetrics and Gynecology
Texas Tech University Health Science Center
Odessa, Texas

Susan J. Littler, M.D., Ph.D.

Attending Physician
Department of Gynecology and Obstetrics
Georgetown Hospital
Georgetown, South Carolina

Michael P. Marcotte, M.D.

Fellow
Department of Obstetrics and Gynecology
Medical College of Ohio
Toledo, Ohio

David L. Marchetti, M.D.

Assistant Professor
Department of Gynecology/Obstetrics
Division of Gynecologic Oncology
State University of New York at Buffalo
Buffalo, New York

John M. O'Brien, M.D.

Director, Perinatal Diagnostic Center
Maternal-Fetal Medicine
Central Baptist Hospital
Lexington, Kentucky

Dennis M. O'Connor, M.D.

Associate Professor
Department of Obstetrics and Gynecology and Pathology
University of Louisville School of Medicine
Staff Physician
Department of Obstetrics and Gynecology and Pathology
University of Louisville Hospital
Louisville, Kentucky

Michael Parsons, M.D.

Associate Professor
Department of Obstetrics and Gynecology
University of South Florida
Tampa General Hospital
Tampa, Florida

Kathleen B. Porter, M.D.

Associate Professor
Department of Obstetrics and Gynecology
University of South Florida
Tampa General Hospital
Tampa, Florida

Ronald L. Richardson, M.D.

Assistant Clinical Professor of Medicine
University of Louisville School of Medicine
Active Staff, Norton Hospital
Louisville, Kentucky

Bruce D. Rodgers, M.D.

Director, Division of Maternal-Fetal Medicine
Department of Obstetrics and Gynecology
State University of New York at Buffalo School of Medicine
Attending and Consultant, Maternal-Fetal Medicine
Department of Obstetrics and Gynecology
Children's Hospital at Buffalo
Buffalo, New York

Dilara E. Samadi, M.D.

Clinical Instructor
Department of Gynecology and Obstetrics
State University of New York at Buffalo School of Medicine
Attending Physician
Department of Gynecology and Obstetrics
Buffalo General Hospital
Buffalo, New York

Shirley K. Sawai, M.D.

Department of Obstetrics and Gynecology
Division of Maternal-Fetal Medicine
Good Samaritan Hospital
Phoenix, Arizona

Mary Self, M.D.

Catherine Sewell, M.D.

Baha M. Sibai, M.D.

Avi Sklar, M.D., F.A.C.O.G., F.A.C.S., F.R.C.S.C.

Assistant Clinical Professor
Department of Gynecology and Obstetrics
State University of New York at Buffalo School of Medicine
Buffalo, New York

Maria Elena Soler, M.D.

Department of Obstetrics and Gynecology
State University of New York at Buffalo School of Medicine
Buffalo, New York

Joseph A. Spinnato II, M.D.

Professor and Director
Maternal-Fetal Medicine Division
University of Louisville School of Medicine
Department of Obstetrics and Gynecology
University of Louisville Hospital
Louisville, Kentucky

Salvador M. Udagawa, M.D.

Section of Colon and Rectal Surgery
Department of Surgery
Sisters of Charity Hospital
Buffalo, New York

Deward Voss, M.D.

Assistant Professor
Department of Obstetrics and Gynecology
Division of Maternal-Fetal Medicine
University of Louisville School of Medicine
Louisville, Kentucky

Stephanie Walton, M.D.

Instructor
Department of Medicine
Division of Rheumatology
University of Louisville School of Medicine
Louisville, Kentucky

Jonathan W. Weeks, M.D.

Assistant Professor
Department of Obstetrics and Gynecology
Division of Maternal-Fetal Medicine
University of Louisville
Louisville, Kentucky

Dennis M. Weppner, M.D.

Clinical Assistant Professor
Department of Obstetrics and Gynecology and Medicine
State University of New York at Buffalo School of Medicine
Clinical Chief
Department of Obstetrics and Gynecology
Buffalo General Hospital
Buffalo, New York

Louis Weinstein, M.D.

Professor and Chairman
Department of Obstetrics and Gynecology
Medical College of Ohio
Toledo, Ohio

Gail Williams, M.D.

Mark Williams, M.D.

Assistant Professor
Department of Obstetrics and Gynecology
University of South Florida
Tampa General Hospital
Tampa, Florida

Scott J. Zuccala, D.O.

Clinical Assistant Professor
Department of Gynecology-Obstetrics
School of Medicine and Biomedical Sciences
State University of New York at Buffalo
Buffalo, New York

This book is dedicated to the women in our lives, Maria and Doreen, two wonderful wives for all their love and support and our daughters, Rose, Alexandra, Dina, Bianca, and Olivia for all the time taken away from them.

Preface

Practical Guide to the Care of the Gynecologic/Obstetric Patient is a concise and portable source to aid practitioners in both inpatient and outpatient treatment of their female patients. The book is divided into two sections: first gynecology and then obstetrics. Also, there is a detailed medications chapter and laboratory interpretation chapter for quick reference.

We hope this manual will be helpful to anyone involved in women's healthcare: practicing gynecologists, family physicians, internists, nurse practitioners, residents, and medical students.

The book follows an outline format and, although complete, is not meant to be used as a replacement of standard textbooks in the fields of obstetrics and gynecology. References have been included for the readers who desire more information.

We would like to acknowledge all the contributors of this text. We also wish to acknowledge Mary Danakas, Sheila Datzler, Heather McShane, and Sandy Nevitt for all the typing in preparing the manuscript.

We are grateful for the help of our editors at Mosby, Emma Underdown, Christy Wells, and their assistants, artists, and copy editors.

And special thanks to a good friend and collegue, Dr. Fred Ferri, for his guidance and encouragement, which made a dream a reality.

George T. Danakas
Marcello Pietrantoni

Contents

Key Telephone Numbers

1

This chapter is a listing of the phone numbers of departments and individuals in the hospital who might be needed for immediate consultation.

Department

Admissions	________
Ambulatory surgery	________
Antenatal testing	________
CCU	________
ECG/ECHO	________
ER	________
Gynecology clinic	________
ICU—medical	________
ICU—surgical	________
Information	________
IV team	________
Intensive care nursery	________
Laboratory—blood gas lab	________
central lab	________
chemistry	________
hematology	________
microbiology	________
cytology	________
other	________
Library	________
Labor wing	________
Medical records	________

Recovery room
Respiratory therapy
Radiation therapy
Surgery—scheduling
nurse coordinator
holding area
Security
Social service
Sonography
Urodynamics
Other

Nursing stations

House staff

Attending staff

2 Medical Record Abbreviations

a.a. of each
abd abdomen
ABG arterial blood gases
a.c. before meals
A/C anterior chamber
Ac acute
ACBG aortocoronary bypass graft
ACD automatic cardiac defibrillator
ACL anterior cruciate ligament
ADA American Diabetic Association
ADL activities of daily living
AF atrial fibrillation
AFB acid fast bacillus
AFP alphafeto protein
AI aortic insufficiency
AIDS acquired immune deficiency syndrome
AKA above knee amputation
alb albumin
ALL acute lymphocytic leukemia
alt alternate
Alt H alternate hours
ALTP argon laser trabeculoplasty
AM in the morning
AMA against medical advice
amb ambulation
AMI acute myocardial infarction
angio angiogram
ant anterior
AODM adult onset diabetes mellitus
AP apical pulse
A+P anterior and posterior
approx approximately
appt. appointment
A.P.S. Adult Protection Service
ARA alcohol rehabilitation assistance
ARC AIDS-related complex
ARDS acute respiratory distress syndrome
AROM artificial rupture of membranes
AS aortic stenosis
ASA aspirin
ASCAD arteriosclerotic coronary artery disease
ASCVD arteriosclerotic cardiovascular disease
ASD atrial septal defect
ASHD arteriosclerotic heart disease
asst assistance
as tol as tolerated
ASU ambulatory surgery unit
AT applanation tonometry
ATC around the clock
At. Fib. atrial fibrillation
AV arteriovenous fistula
avg average
AVR/MVR aortic valve repair/mitral valve repair
A+W alive and well
A/W alive and well

BBB bundle branch block
BC Blue Cross
BCM birth control method
BD base down
B.E. barium enema
B/F black female
BI base in
bid twice a day
bil bilateral
biw twice weekly
B-K below knee amputation
BLE both lower extremities
B/M black male
BM bowel movement
BMR basal metabolism rate
BO base out
BP base pressure

BPD biparietal diameter
BPH benign prostatic hypertrophy
BPP biophysical profile
BS bowel sounds
B/S breath sounds
BSE breast self examination
BSI body substance isolation
BSO bilateral salpingo-oophorectomy
BU base up
BUN blood urea nitrogen
BW bite-wing radiograph
B/W twice weekly
Bx biopsy

c with
CA carcinoma
CABG coronary artery bypass graft
CAD coronary artery disease
cal calorie
cap capsule
CAPD continued ambulatory peritoneal dialysis
C.A.S. Client Advocacy Service
CAT creative arts therapy
CATT computerized axial tomography
C+B crown and bridge
CBC complete blood count
CC chief complaint
c c with correction
CCPD continuous cycling peritoneal dialysis
CCU coronary care unit
C/D cup to disc ratio
CDC Centers for Disease Control and Prevention
CF count fingers
CFU colony forming units
CHB complete heart block
CHF congestive heart failure
cho carbohydrate
chr chronic
CIC certified infection control
circ circumcision
cl clear
CLL chronic lymphocytic leukemia
cl liq clear liquids
CMT cervical motion tenderness
CNS central nervous system
CO- cardiac output
con't. continued
COPD chronic obstructive pulmonary disease
CPL criminal procedure law
CPM continued passive motion
CPR cardiopulmonary resuscitation
C.P.S. Child Protective Service
CPT chest physiotherapy
CRF chronic renal failure
C+S culture and sensitivity
C/S cesarean section
CSF cerebrospinal fluid
CVA cerebral vascular accident
CVC central venous catheter
CVP central venous pressure
cx cervix
Cysto cystoscopy

D distal
Day. Tx. day treatment
dbl disabled
D/C discontinue
D&C dilation and curettage
defib defibrillation
dept department
DES diethystilbesterol
diff differential
Dil dilute
DIP distal interphalangeal joint
DM diabetes mellitus
DN dermal nevus
DNR do not resuscitate
DNS did not show
d/o disorder
DOA dead on arrival
DOB date of birth
DOE dyspnea on exertion
DOS day of surgery
DP dorsalis pedis pulse
DPD pacemaker (type of)
DPT diphtheria/pertussis/tetanus
drng drainage
drsg dressing
DTR deep tendon reflex
DTs delirium tremens
DUB dysfunctional uterine bleeding
DVT deep vein thrombosis
DX diagnosis
D_5W dextrose 5% in water

E esophoria
ECCE extracapsular cataract extraction
ECG electrocardiogram
ECHO echocardiography
ECT electroconvulsive therapy
ED emergency department
E.D. eligibility determination
Ed. education
EEG electroencephalogram

EENT eyes, ears, nose, and throat
EGA estimated gestational age
EGD esophageal gastroduodenoscopy
EKG electrocardiogram
EMG electromyogram
ENDO endodontic
ENT ears, nose, and throat
EO extraoral
EOM extraocular movements
EPID epidural
EPIS episiotomy
EPS electrophysiology studies
EPT electric pulp test
ER emergency room
ERCP endoscopic retrograde cholangiopancreatography
ESRD end stage renal disease
est estimated
ESWL extracorporeal shock wave lithotripsy
ET endotracheal tube
ETOH ethyl alcohol
ETP elective termination of pregnancy
ETT endotracheal tube
ex exercise
EXO exodontia
exp exploratory

F.A. functional assessment
FBS fasting blood sugar
FCC full cast crown
F.D. functional disability
FEP fibroepithelial polyp
FEN fluid/electrolyte nutrition
FGC full gold crown
FHR fetal heart rate
fib fibrillation
FL fluoride
FOB father of baby
FPD fixed partial denture
freq frequency
FS finger stick
FT finger tension
FTG full thickness graft
FUO fever of unknown etiology
FWB full weight bearing
Fx fracture

GA general anesthesia
GB gallbladder
Gc gonorrhea
GI gastrointestinal
gluc tol glucose tolerance
gm gram
GN glomerulonephritis
grav gravida
gtt. drop
GTT glucose tolerance test
GU genitourinary
GXT graded exercise test
Gyn gynecology

H hyperphoria
H.A. headache
Hb hemoglobin
HBP high blood pressure
HBSAg hepatitis B surface antigen
HCVD hypertensive cardiovascular disease
HD hemodialysis
HDL high-density lipoprotein
HEENT head, eyes, ears, nose, throat
hemi hemiplegia
Hep hepatitis
Hgt height
HHN handheld nebulizer
HIV human immune virus
H&N head and neck
HM hand movements
H/O history of
HO hot packs
HO house officer
HOB head of bed
HP hot packs
H&P history and physical
HPV human papillomavirus
hr hour
HR heart rate
Ht height
HT hypertropia
HTN hypertension
HV home visit
Hx history

IABP intraaortic balloon pump
IBW ideal body weight
IBWR ideal body weight range
IC Intercare
ICC inner cannula care
ICCE intracapsular cataract extraction
ICP intracranial pressure
ICU intensive care unit
I&D incision and drainage
IM intramuscularly
IMA internal mammary artery
IMF intermaxillary fixation
inc incontinent
incm income
indep independent
inf infection

inj. injection
INS insurance
instru instructions
int internal
invol involuntary
I&O intake and output
IOP intraocular pressure
IPD intermittent peritoneal dialysis
IPPB intermittent positive pressure breathing
IQ intelligence quotient
IR inferior rectus
IRM intermittent restorative material
IS incentive spirometer
isol isolation
IU international unit
IUD intrauterine device
IUFD intrauterine fetal death
IUGR intrauterine growth retardation
IUP intrauterine pregnancy
IVF *in vitro* fertilization
IVP intravenous pyelogram

JN junctional nevus
JODM juvenile onset diabetes mellitus
jt joint
JVD jugular venous distention

K potassium
KA keratoacanthoma
kg kilogram
kid kidney
KP keratitic precipitates
KUB flat film of kidney, ureters, bladder
KVO keep vein open

l liter
L lingual
Lab laboratory
Lac laceration
LAD left anterior descending
Lang language
lat lateral
LBBB left bundle branch block
LBP low back pain
LBW low birth weight
LDL low-density lipoprotein
LE lower extremity
LFT liver function test
lg large
Liq liquid
LLB long leg brace
LLC long leg cast
LLE left lower extremity
LLL left lower lobe
LLQ left lower quadrant
LML left medial lateral
LMP last menstrual period
LNMP last normal menstrual period
LOA left occiput anterior
LOC loss of consciousness
LOP left occiput posterior
LOT left occiput transverse
LP lumbar puncture
LP c P light perception with projection
LPM liters per minute
LPN licensed practical nurse
LR lactated Ringer's
LRG long-range goals
LS lumbosacral
L/S lecithin/sphingomyelin ratio
L.S.S.P. lumbosacral spine and pelvis
lt left
LTG long-term goals
LUE left upper extremity
LUL left upper lobe
LUQ left upper quadrant
LV left ventricle
LVF left ventricular failure
LVH left ventricular hypertrophy
LWOC leave without consent
Lytes electrolytes

m murmur
MA mental age
MAE moving all extremities
mand mandibular
MAP mean arterial pressure
MAX maxillary
max maximal
mcg microgram
MCP metacarpal interphalangeal joint
M.D. medical doctor
MDI manic depressive illness
mech mechanical
med medicine
Med. ER medical emergency room
mEq milliequivalent
met/mets metastasis
mg milligram
MGF maternal grandfather
MGM maternal grandmother
MGP maternal grandparents
MH medical history
MHR maximum heart rate
MHTA mental hygiene therapy aide
MI myocardial infarction
MICU medical intensive care unit
min minimal

ml milliliter
MM malignant melanoma
MMF maxillomandibular fixation
MMPI Minnesota Multiphasic Personality Inventory
MMT manual muscle test
mod moderate
mono mononucleosis
MOV/M multiple oral vitamins/mineral
MOV multiple oral vitamin
MPD myofacial pain dysfunction
MR medial rectus
MRI magnetic resonance imaging
MS multiple sclerosis
M.S.E. mental status examination
MSW master social work
M/T maintain
mult multiple
MV mitral valve
MVP mitral valve prolapse
MVR mitral valve replacement

N_2O nitrous oxide
N normal
NaF sodium fluoride
N/A not applicable
NA nursing assistant
N/B newborn
NB note well
neg negative
NG nasogastric
NIDDM noninsulin dependent diabetes mellitus
NKA no known allergies
NKDA no known drug allergies
nl normal
NLP no light perception
NNMP next normal menstrual period
noct night
NP nurse practitioner
NPC near point of convergence
NPO nothing by mouth
NR nonreactive
NS normal saline
NSR normal sinus rhythm
NST non-stress test
N&V nausea and vomiting
NVD normal vaginal delivery
NWB non-weight bearing

O occlusal
O_2 oxygen
OB obstetrics
OC oral contraceptives
OCT oxytocin challenge test
OD right eye
OE oral examination
OHI oral hygiene instruction
OHS open heart surgery
OOB out of bed
OOC out of chair
OOD out of district
OP outpatient
Op operative
OPD outpatient department
OPS outpatient surgery
OR operating room
ORIF open reduction with internal fixation
Ortho no strabismus
OS left eye
OT occupational therapy
O.U. both eyes

P pulse
pa public assistance
PA periapical radiograph
P&A percussion and auscultation
PAC premature atrial contractions
Pan panorex radiograph
PAP papanicolaou smear
PAPD pulmonary artery diastolic pressure
para paraplegia
PARR postanesthesia recovery room
PAS peripheral anterior synechia
PAT preadmission testing
PAWP pulmonary artery wedge pressure
2 PC two physicians' certificates
p.c. after meals
P&C post and core
PCA patient controlled analgesia
P.C.C. patient care coordinator
PCC patient care conference
PCD pacer cardioverter defibrillator
PCG primary care giver
P.C. IOL posterior chamber IOL
PCM protein calorie malnutrition
PCWP pulmonary capillary wedge pressure
PD peritoneal dialysis
PD/P postural drainage and percussion
P.E. physical examination
PE pulmonary embolism
PEEP positive end expiratory pressure
per by
PERRLA pupils equal, round, reactive to light and accommodation

PFM porcelain fused metal crown
PFT pulmonary function test
PGF paternal grandfather
PGM paternal grandmother
PGP paternal grandparents
PH past history
PHx past history
phy ther physical therapy
PI peripheral iridectomy
PID pelvic inflammatory disease
PIF peak inspiratory force
PIP proximal interphalangeal
PIV peripheral intravenous
PJC porcelain jacket crown
PK penetrating keratoplasty
PKU phenylketonuria
PM in the evening
PMD private physician
PMH past medical history
PMI point of maximal impulse
PMP previous menstrual period
PND postnasal drip
P.O. postoperative
POI postoperative instructions
Pos or + positive
Post posterior
PP postpartum
PPD purified protein derivatives
PPH previous psychiatric history
PPHA private proprietary home for adults
PRBC packed red blood cells
preg pregnancy
prep prepare for
prog program
PROM premature rupture of membranes
prophy prophylaxis
PRP panretinal photocoagulation
PS posterior synechia
PSA posterior superior alveolar
PSC postsubcapsular cataract
PSH past social history
PSVT paroxysmal supraventricular tachycardia
Psy. psychologist
Psych ER psychiatric emergency room
pt. patient
Pt. patient
PT physical therapy
PTA prior to admission
PTCA percutaneous transluminal coronary angioplasty
PVC premature ventricular contractions
PVD peripheral vascular disease
PWB partial weight bearing

q__h every__hours
qad quadriplegia
q.n.s. insufficient quantity
q.s. sufficient quantity

RBP resting blood pressure
RCU respiratory care unit
RD retinal detachment
RDS respiratory distress syndrome
ref refused
rehab. rehabilitation
Resp respiratory
RF rheumatic fever
RHD rheumatic heart disease
RLE right lower extremity
RLL right lower lobe
RLQ right lower quadrant
RML right middle lobe
RN registered nurse
R/O rule out
ROA right occiput anterior
ROM range of motion
ROP right occiput posterior
ROS review of systems
ROT right occiput transverse
RPD removal partial denture
R&R release and reapply—restraints
RROM resisted range of motion
RRR regular rate and rhythm
RSR regular sinus rhythm
rt right
RT radiation therapy
RTC return to clinic
Ru retrograde urogram
RUE right upper extremity
RUL right upper lobe
RUQ right upper quadrant
R/V revisit
Rv retroverted
RV right ventricle

s soft
S1 first heart sound
S2 second heart sound
S3 third heart sound
S4 fourth heart sound
SAH subarachnoid hemorrhage
SB sinus bradycardia
SBE subacute bacterial endocarditis
S.B.F.T. small bowel follow through
s c without correction
Sc subcutaneous
SCC squamous cell carcinoma

Schiz. schizophrenia
sed rate erythrocyte sedimentation rate
sev severe
SG specific gravity
SGA small for gestational age
SGOT serum glutamic oxaloacetic transaminase
SGPT serum glutamic pyuric transaminase
SICU surgical intensive care unit
sig. directions
SK seborrheic keratosis
skel skeletal
SL sublingual
SLB short leg brace
SLC short leg cast
SLE systemic lupus erythematosus
SLR straight leg raising
SN student nurse
SNF skilled nursing facility
SO superior oblique
SOAP: S subjective
O objective
A assessment
P plan
SOB shortness of breath
SOM serous otitis media
sono sonogram
S/P status post
SP soft palate
SpAB spontaneous abortion
spec specimen
spon spontaneous
SQ subcutaneous
SR superior rectus
SROM spontaneous rupture of membranes
S&S swish and swallow
SS stainless steel
SSA Social Security Administration
SSC stainless steel crown
SSD social security disability
SSE soap suds enema
SSI supplemental security income
SSW Stepping Stones Workshop
ST Schiotz tonometry
STC Stone Treatment Center
STD sexually transmitted disease
STG short-term goals
STSG split thickness skin graft
Surg surgery
SVR systemic vascular resistance
SW social worker
Sx signs and symptoms

T&A tonsillectomy/adenoidectomy
TAB therapeutic abortion
tab. tablet
tach tachycardia
TAH total abdominal hysterectomy
TBW total body weight
TD tardive dyskinesia
TDWB touch down weight bearing
TF tube feeding
THR total hip replacement
TIA transient ischemic attack
tiw three times a week
TKR total knee replacement
TLC total lymphocyte count
TM tympanic membrane
TMJ temporomandibular joint
T.O. telephone order
TOC test of cure
tol tolerated
T&P turn and position
TPA tissue plasminogen activator
TPN total parenteral nutrition
TPR temperature, pulse, respiration
Trach tracheotomy
Trans transfusion
TUR transurethral resection
TURP transurethral resection prostate
TX transplant

U/A urinalysis
UE upper extremity
UGI upper gastrointestinal
U&L upper and lower
u.o. urine output
urethral dil urethral dilation
URI upper respiratory infection
Urol urology
US ultrasound
USN ultrasonic nebulizer
UTI urinary tract infection

VA visual acuity
VA c C visual acuity with correction
VA s C visual acuity without correction
vag vaginal
VC vital capacity
vd void
vent ventricular
VF ventricular fibrillation
VNA Visiting Nurses Association
Voc vocational
VS vital signs
VSAP Volunteer Advocacy Support Program

V.S.S. vital signs stable
VT ventricular tachycardia
VT tidal volume

WAIS Wechsler Adult Intelligence Scale
WASS Wassermann
WBAT weight bearing as tolerated
WBC white blood count
W/D well developed
W/F white female
WFL within functional limits
WHC Woman's Health Center
WIC Women/Infants/Children
W/M white male
W/N well nourished
W/U work-up

x times
X exophoria
xfer transfer
X/R x-ray
XT exotropia
xylo xylocaine

y.o. year old

1° first degree
2° second degree
2° secondary
3° third degree
L left
R right
0 none
c with
s without
— change
pounds
m murmur
.. therefore
p after
♀ female
♂ male
> greater than
< less than
≥ greater than or equal to
≤ less than or equal to
+ positive
− negative
↑ increased
↓ decreased

3 Charting

George T. Danakas, M.D.

3.1 HISTORY AND PHYSICAL EXAMINATION

1. Chief complaint: reason patient has come to see you; should be in her own words (Why have you come in to see me today?)
2. Present illness: The patient describes each presenting problem in detail. When did the problem begin (onset)? Is this a new problem or a recurrence? If the problem is pain, describe: location (localized or does it radiate), quality (deep, sharp, dull, throbbing, achy), severity, timing in relation to menstrual cycle, duration (how long it lasts), aggravating or relieving factors, relationship to eating, any associated gastrointestinal (GI) or genitourinary (GU) symptoms, and prior treatment.
3. Medical history
   a. Pediatric and adult illnesses: mumps, measles, chicken pox, rheumatic fever, arthritis, rheumatism, chorea, scarlet fever, pneumonia, tuberculosis, diabetes mellitus, heart disease, renal disease, hypertension, jaundice
   b. Immunizations:
   c. Hospitalizations (medical and surgical):
   d. Trauma:
   e. Transfusions:
   f. Current medications:
   g. Allergies: drugs (describe reaction):
      food:
   h. Habits (drugs, alcohol, tobacco, exercise, diet):
4. Family history (diagram pedigree if indicated): diabetes mellitus, tuberculosis, cancer, stroke, hypertension, renal disease, deafness, gout or arthritis, anemia, heart disease, osteoporosis
5. Patient profile
   a. Birthplace:
   b. Occupation:
   c. Education:
   d. Marital status:
   e. Religion:
   f. Home situation (local environment):
   g. Availability of family:

h. Hobbies or special interests:
i. Behavior during assessment:
j. Ability to communicate and understand:
k. Additional comments:

6. Systems review
   a. General: weakness, fatigue, change in weight, appetite, sleeping habits, chills, fever, night sweats
   b. Integument: color changes, pruritus, nevus, infections, tumor (benign or malignant), dermatosis, hair changes, nail changes
   c. Hematopoietic: anemia, abnormal bleeding, adenopathy, excessive bruising
   d. Central nervous system
      (1) General: syncope, loss of consciousness, convulsions, meningitis, encephalitis, stroke
      (2) Mentative: speech disorders, emotional status, orientation, memory disorders, change in sleep pattern, history of nervous breakdown
      (3) Motor: tremor, weakness, paralysis, clumsiness of movement
      (4) Sensory: radicular or neuralgic pain (head, neck, trunk, extremities), paresthesias, anesthesias
   e. Eyes: vision, glasses or contact lenses, date of last eye examination, scotomata, pain, excessive tearing
   f. Ears: tinnitus, deafness, other
   g. Nose, throat, and sinuses: epistaxis, discharge, sinusitis, hoarseness
   h. Dentition: caries, pyorrhea, dentures
   i. Breasts: masses, discharge, pain, family history of breast cancer, any past problems
      (1) Self breast examination: yes or no
      (2) How frequent (should be monthly):
   j. Respiratory: cough (productive or nonproductive), change in cough, amount and characteristic of sputum, duration of sputum production, smoking, number of packs a day, years of tobacco use, wheezing, hemoptysis, recurrent respiratory tract infections, positive tuberculin test
   k. Cardiovascular: chest pain, typical angina pectoris, dyspnea on exertion, orthopnea, paroxysmal nocturnal dyspnea, peripheral edema, murmur, palpitation, varicosities, thrombophlebitis, claudication, Raynaud's phenomenon, syncope, near syncope
   l. GI: nausea, vomiting, diarrhea, constipation, melena, hematemesis, rectal bleeding, change in bowel habits, hemorrhoids, dysphagia, food intolerance, excessive gas or indigestion, abdominal pain, jaundice, use of antacids, use of laxatives
   m. Urinary tract: renal colic, frequency of urination, nocturia, polyuria, dysuria, micturition (retention, hesitancy, urgency, dysuria, narrowing of stream, dribbling incontinence), hematuria, albuminuria, pyuria, kidney disease, renal stones, cystoscopy
   n. Genitoreproductive system
      (1) Gynecologic history: age of menarche, last menstrual period, age at menopause, postmenopausal bleeding, abnormal menses, amount of bleeding, intermenstrual bleeding, postco-

ital bleeding, leukorrhea, pruritus, history of venereal disease, serology, last Papanicolaou smear and results; menopausal symptoms, hormone replacement therapy history
- (a) Dysmenorrhea (onset, duration, severity)
- (b) Cycle interval, amount of flow (light, moderate, heavy)
- (c) Vaginal discharge (onset, color, odor, itching, burning, or pain)

(2) Obstetric history
- (a) G __ P __ __ __ __
- (b) Gravida (number of pregnancies)
- (c) Parity (full term, preterm, abortion, living children)
- (d) Complications of pregnancies, infertility (Has the patient ever had difficulty becoming pregnant? Was she ever evaluated or treated for this problem? If yes, describe in detail.), libido
- (e) Description of each pregnancy
  - *i.* Date
  - *ii.* Vaginal, vacuum, forceps, or cesarean delivery
  - *iii.* Weight and sex of each baby
  - *iv.* Hours in labor
  - *v.* Complications (antenatal, during labor and delivery or postpartum)

(3) Methods of contraception
- (a) Present
- (b) Past

(4) Sexual history
- (a) Age of first coitus, number of partners
- (b) Orgasmic—yes or no
- (c) Dyspareunia—superficial or deep
- (d) Any problems, complaints, questions

o. Musculoskeletal system
- (1) Joints: pain, edema, heart rubor, stiffness, deformity
- (2) Muscles: myalgias

p. Endocrine system: goiter, heat intolerance, cold intolerance, change in voice, polyuria, polydipsia, polyphagia

q. Psychiatric: hyperventilation, nervousness, depression, insomnia, nightmares, memory loss

r. Additional historical data

7. Physical examination

a. Vital signs
- (1) Pulse ______ reg/irreg. Respirations ______
- (2) Temp ______ oral/rectal
- (3) Blood pressure:
  - (a) Supine R arm ______ L arm ______
  - (b) Sitting R arm ______ standing R arm ______
- (4) Weight

b. General

c. Integument: turgor, texture, pigmentation, cyanosis, telangiectasis, petechiae, purpura, ecchymosis, infection, lesions, hair, nails, mucous membranes

d. Lymph nodes: cervical, postauricular, supraclavicular, axillary, inguinal, epitrochlear
e. Skull: trauma, bruits, other
f. Eyes: lacrimal glands, cornea, lids, sclerae, conjunctivae, exophthalmos, lid lag
g. Fundi: discs, arteries, veins, hemorrhages, exudates, microaneurysm
h. Ears: tophi, tympanic membranes, external canal, hearing
i. Mouth, nose, and throat: dentition, gingiva, tongue, tonsils, pharynx, nasal mucosa, nasal septum, sinuses
j. Neck: mobility, scars, masses, thyroid, bruit, salivary glands, tracheal shift
k. Breasts: masses, discharge, nipples, asymmetry, skin retraction, axillary adenopathy
l. Chest
   (1) Respiratory rate: ___/min; amplitude: shallow/deep/normal
   (2) Respiratory rhythm: regular, irregular, periodical
   (3) Chest wall
      (a) Deformities
      (b) Motion
      (c) Lateral motion: good, fair, absent
      (d) Use of accessory muscles: yes or no
   (4) Auscultation
      (a) Rales, wheezes, rhonchi
      (b) Breath sounds: increased, decreased, normal, other

   (Diagram location of abnormal breath sounds, transmitted voice, or abnormal percussion.)
m. Cardiovascular system
   (1) First heart sound (S1):
   (2) Second heart sound (S2):
   (3) Gallops:
   (4) Systolic murmur:
   (5) Diastolic murmur:
   (6) Other:
n. Peripheral pulses
   (1) Carotid, brachial, radial, aorta, femoral, Popliteal, dorsalis pedis (DP)
      (a) Right
      (b) Left
      (c) Classifications: *O*, absent; *1+*, thready; *2+*, decreased; *3+*, normal; *4+*, hyperactive
o. Extremities: edema, cyanosis, stasis, ulceration, hair distribution, clubbing
p. Abdomen: obesity, contour, scars, tenderness, cerebral vascular accident (CVA) tenderness, masses, rebound, rigidity, fluid wave, shifting dullness, frank ascites, bruits, hernia, venous collaterals
   (1) Bowel sounds: normal, absent, hyperactive, hypoactive, obstructive
   (2) Organomegaly: liver, spleen, kidneys, bladder, gallbladder
      (a) Liver size _____ cm (total dullness)

(b) Liver tenderness: absent, increased
(c) Liver edge: smooth, irregular, nodular

q. Genitoreproductive system
(1) External genitalia: labia, clitoris, introitus, urethra, perineum, document any lesions
(2) Internal genitalia: vagina, cervix, adnexa, cul-de-sac, discharge
(3) Papanicolaou smear: done, omitted
(4) Rectal: hemorrhoids, sphincter tone, bleeding, masses
(5) Stool for occult blood
(6) External genitalia: hair pattern, labia majora and minora, clitoris, urethral Bartholin, periurethral and Skene's glands
(7) Speculum examination: Choose the appropriate-size speculum (either a medium Graves, a Smith-Anderson, or a pediatric) and insert it into the vagina. The speculum may be moistened with warm water, if necessary, but no other kinds of lubrication should be used because they can affect cultures and cytology. Spread the labia and insert the speculum vertically through the introitus and then rotate horizontally. Open the blades of the speculum and visualize the cervix. Note any lesions on the cervix, if present. Obtain a Papanicolaou smear—insert a cytobrush or cotton swab into the endocervical canal, rotate, and smear the specimen on a slide. Next obtain a specimen from the vaginal portio using a wooden Ayer spatula and apply on slide. Apply fixative. Next obtain cervical cultures for chlamydia, gonorrhea, human papillomavirus (HPV) if clinically warranted.
(a) Vagina: discharge?
(8) Bimanual examination: Palpate vagina, cervix, uterus, adnexa, and cul-de-sac. Insert the index and middle fingers of the examining hand into the vagina. The abdominal hand brings down the organs to the examining hand in the vagina. Specifically note the following:
(a) Cervix: position, consistency, pain with cervical motion
(b) Uterus: size, shape (normal, globular, irregular), position (anterior, posterior, midline), tenderness on motion
(c) Adnexa: masses or tenderness
(9) Rectovaginal examination: With the index finger in the vagina and the middle finger in the rectum, palpate rectovaginal septum, uterosacral ligaments, cardinal ligaments, cul-de-sac, looking for masses or tenderness.

r. Joints: deformity, rubor, calor, tenderness, edema
(1) Range of motion: fingers, wrists, elbow, shoulder, hips, knees, ankles
(2) Spine: deformity (kyphosis, lordosis, scoliosis), thoracic excursion

s. Neurologic system
(1) Cerebral function: alert wakefulness, lethargic, obtunded, stuporous, semicomatose, comatose
(a) Mental status:
(b) Orientation:
(c) Cranial nerves:

t. Reflexes

	Bi	Tri	Br	F	K	A	Plantar	Abdomen	Snout	Grasp	Jaw	Suck
R												
L												

0, Absent with facilitation; *tr*, trace; *1+*, decreased; *2+*, normal; *3+*, hyperactive; *4+*, sustained clonus. *Bi*, Biceps; *Tr*, triceps; *Br*, brachical; *F*, flexor carpiradialis; *K*, knee; *A*, ankle.

3.2 PROGRESS NOTES

Use mnemonic SOAP:

S (Subjective):	Patient complaints
O (Objective):	Physical findings, laboratory results, x-ray, or any other testing is recorded
A (Assessment):	Diagnosis (What do you think the diagnosis is based on your assessment of subjective and objective findings?)
P (Plan):	Diagnostic studies and therapeutic regimen

3.3 ADMISSION ORDERS

Use the mnemonic ABC-David:

A Admit:	Indicate floor to which patient is being admitted and to whose service (name of attending physician)
B Because:	Diagnosis
C Condition:	Stable, fair, poor, critical
D Diet:	NPO, clear liquids, regular house diet, diabetic diet
A Allergies:	Medications and food
Activity:	Bedrest, bathroom privileges, ad lib
V Vital signs:	Frequency (e.g., q1h, every shift)
I IV Fluids:	IV solution and rate
D Diagnostic tests:	Laboratories X-rays
Drugs:	medications, dose, frequency, rate of administration (e.g., Motrin 800 mg q8h PO prn for pain)

3.4 PREOPERATIVE EVALUATION

1. Medical history and physical examination
   a. Significant medical history or illnesses that may complicate anesthesia or recovery
   b. Current medications: prescription and nonprescription
   c. Allergies
   d. Previous surgery
      (1) Review operative reports from previous pelvic surgery especially if patient has had surgery for pelvic inflammatory disease (PID), endometriosis, pelvic abscess, or malignancy.

   e. Family history: excessive bleeding, malignant hyperthermia
   f. General review of systems, especially GI and GU
2. Laboratory evaluation
   a. Complete blood count (CBC)
   b. Serum chemistry with liver function tests (LFTs)
   c. CXR, electrocardiogram (EKG) if over 40 (if under 40 only if medical history warrants these studies)
   d. Intravenous pyelogram (IVP), barium enema, upper GI with small bowel follow-through, CT if felt necessary
3. Obtain consent
   Informed consent is not merely getting the patient to sign the hospital consent form. A detailed discussion with the patient, her significant other, and any other family member she thinks necessary should be undertaken before surgery. The discussion should include the following:
   a. Risks of proposed surgery
   b. Complications of proposed surgery
   c. Postoperative recovery period
   d. Long-term effects of the surgery (i.e., menopausal symptoms and consequences after bilateral salpingo-oophorectomy [BSO]) or if surgery not done
   e. The nature and extent of the disease process
   f. Benefits of surgery
   g. Alternative methods of therapy along with the risks and benefits of these other methods of therapy
   h. Failure rates of procedure (i.e., sterilization)
   i. Type of anesthesia planned: Questions should be addressed to the anesthesiologist. If the patient has preexisting medical condition that could complicate anesthesia, a presurgical consult with the anesthesia department would be a good idea.
   j. Expected length of surgery
   k. Description of the surgical procedure: Use pictures if felt necessary; is procedure only diagnostic or is it therapeutic?
      (1) Intraoperative and postoperative bleeding; postoperative infection; venous thrombosis; and injury to bowel, bladder, ureter
   l. Time for the patient and family members to ask questions
4. Bowel preparation should be performed in patients with pelvic mass, endometriosis, cancer, multiple previous abdominal surgeries, or previous bowel surgery.
5. Antibiotic prophylaxis
   a. It is generally accepted to use preoperative antibiotics 30 minutes before initial incision.
   b. Prophylactic antibiotics should not be used for more than 24 hours. I prefer only a single dose because there is no definitive proof that continuing antibiotics × 24 hours is any more effective. First-generation cephalosporin is adequate (1 g).
6. Thromboembolic prophylaxis
   a. Needs to be considered in patients at risk for thromboembolic event after surgery (i.e., previous thromboembolic disease,

venous insufficiency, obesity, anticipation of prolonged immobility)

b. Low-dose heparin, 5000 units subcutaneously 2 hours preoperative, followed by 5000 units q12h until ambulatory well

3.5 PREOPERATIVE NOTE

1. Brief summary of history and physical (only significant facts listed)
2. Proposed surgery
3. Indication for proposed surgery
4. Consent reviewed and signed
5. Lab results, x-ray reports, EKG (if done)
6. Patient allergies
7. If major surgery, whether or not blood typed and crossed

Operating Room (OR) Note

Preoperative diagnosis:
Postoperative diagnosis:
Procedure:
Anesthesia:
Surgeon:
Assistants:
Findings:
Transferred to recovery room in ________________ condition.

3.6 POSTOPERATIVE ORDERS

1. Admit: to recovery room and then to _____ floor
2. Diagnosis: status post (S/P) total abdominal hysterectomy (TAH) for endometrial carcinoma
3. Condition:
4. Diet:
5. Activity:
6. Fluids:
7. Graphics: vitals, weights, urine output, etc.
8. Allergies:
9. Nursing instructions: Foley, nasogastric, spirometry, drains
10. Labs
11. Medication: pain, antibiotics, sleeper
12. Call house officer for ________________________

3.7 DISCHARGE SUMMARY

Patient name: ________________________________

Discharge date: ________________________________

Medical records number: ________________________

Admitting diagnosis: ______________________________

Statement of history and physical findings: ______________________________

____

Significant findings (x-rays film, laboratory results, consults, etc.): ______

____

Course in hospital (complications, progress of patient, etc.): __________

____

____

Condition on discharge:

Instructions to patient and family

1. Diet
2. Level of activity
3. Medications
4. Follow-up instructions

Principal diagnosis: ______________________________

Secondary diagnosis: ______________________________

Procedures: ______________________________

Gynecologic Anatomy

4

David L. Marchetti, M.D.

The anatomic study of the female reproductive tract and related anatomy is a necessary adjunct to proper diagnosis and treatment of gynecologic disease. Such knowledge is a prerequisite of advanced surgical technique. This chapter presents this information from both a surgical and an anatomic perspective.

4.1 ANTERIOR LATERAL ABDOMINAL WALL

Anatomic study of the abdomen includes the abdomen proper and the pelvis. The perineum is continuous with the anterior abdominal wall and is located at the outlet of the pelvis. For descriptive purposes, the abdomen can be divided into nine regions by two horizontal and two vertical planes (Fig. 4-1).

Superficial fascia

The superficial fascia of the anterior abdominal wall is composed of Camper's fascia, which is the superficial fatty layer (Fig. 4-2). It is continuous over the inguinal ligament with the similar corresponding layer of the thigh and medially continues into the labia majora.

Deep layer

The deep layer of the membranous subcutaneous fascia is identified as Scarpa's fascia and is a membranous sheath containing little or no adipose tissue (see Fig. 4-2). It forms a continuous sheath across the midline, where it attaches to the linea alba. Inferiorly it passes over the inguinal ligament and is securely attached to either the ligament itself or to the fascia lata just beyond it. Inferior to the ligament, the corresponding layer is called the fascia cribrosa as it covers and fills the fossa ovalis. At the medial end of the inguinal ligament, it passes over the external inguinal ring without attachment and continues along the groove between the labia majora and thigh into the perineum where it is called the fascia of Colles. These attachments of Scarpa's fascia form a gutter that empties into the superficial perineal pouch. The abdomen and perineum communicate through the abdominal labial opening posterior to the fascia of Scarpa and Colles. Hemorrhage of the anterior abdominal wall may be associated with extravasation into the perineum.

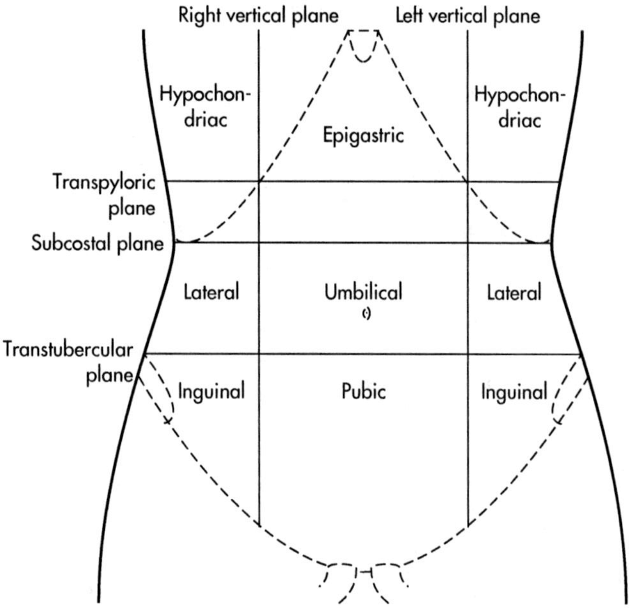

Figure 4-1
Anatomical subdivisions of the anterior abdominal wall.

Deep fascia

The deep fascia (Gallaudet's fascia) is identified easily in the lateral portion of the anterior abdominal wall, where it covers the fleshy fibers of the external oblique muscle. It is continuous with the fascia of the latissimus dorsi and the pectoralis major. More medially, it is indistinguishable from the muscular fascia of the external abdominal oblique muscle, and it is thickened in the midline to form the suspensory ligament of the clitoris.

In the superficial fascia of Camper, the superficial circumflex iliac artery, the superficial epigastric artery, and the superficial external pudendal artery are seen as inguinal branches of the femoral artery, whereas the corresponding venous tributaries drain into the great saphenous vein.

4.2 MUSCLES AND FASCIA OF THE ANTERIOR LATERAL ABDOMINAL WALL

At each side of the abdomen there are three flat muscles: the external oblique, the internal oblique, and the transversus abdominis. There is one vertical muscle, the rectus abdominis.

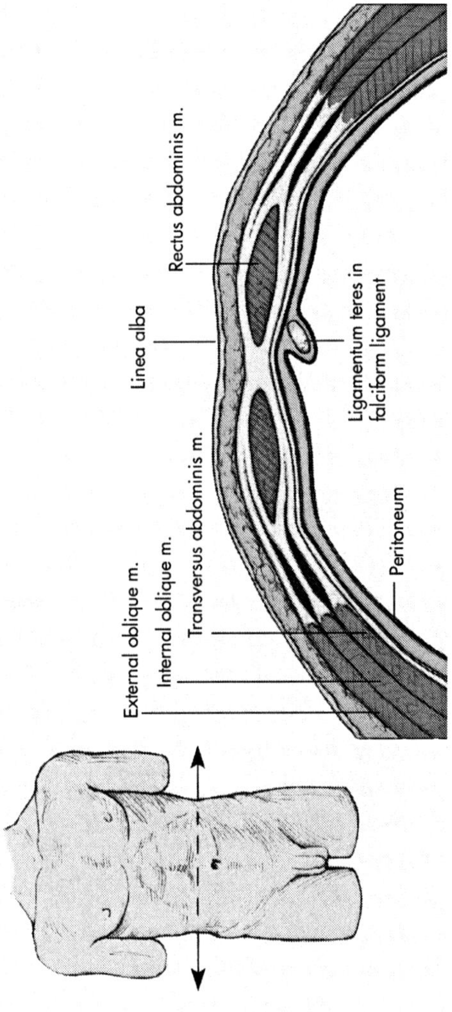

Figure 4-2
Fascial and muscular layers of the anterior abdominal wall and the inguinal and subinguinal regions. (From *C.L.A.S.S. principles*, St Louis, 1995, Mosby.)

External oblique muscle

The external oblique muscle arises from the lower eight ribs to insert at the outer lip of the anterior half of the iliac crest. The fibers of the muscle continue anteriorly as a thin but dense aponeurosis to decussate with those of the opposite side at the linea alba (Fig. 4-3). The linea alba represents the insertion of the muscles of the anterior abdominal wall at the midline. Below, it attaches with the pubic tubercle medially and the anterior superior iliac spine laterally, with the free lower border of the aponeurosis folding inward to become the inguinal ligament. Short of the pubic tubercle, the fibers form the triangular lacunar ligament, whereas those fibers that extend along the pectineal line form the pectineal ligament of Cooper. Fibers attaching to the pubic tubercle constitute the lateral crus of the superficial inguinal ring, whereas the fibers extending to the front of the pubis form its medial crus.

Internal oblique muscle

The internal abdominal oblique arises from the anterior two thirds of the intermediate lip of the iliac crest and the lateral two thirds of the inguinal ligament. Most of the fibers are directed upward and forward at a right angle to those of the external oblique muscle and continue as the aponeurosis. Posterior fibers ascend vertically to insert in the lower four ribs, whereas the lowest fibers run horizontally and inferiorly.

Linea arcuata

The linea arcuata is a tendinous band in the posterior rectus sheath located at the approximate midpoint between the umbilicus and the pubic symphysis. Above the arcuate line, the aponeurosis of the internal oblique splits at the lateral border of the rectus muscle (linea semilunares) into anterior and posterior layers. These participate in the formation of the rectus sheath and decussate with the opposite muscle at the linea alba. Below the arcuate line, the aponeurosis does not split but joins totally the anterior lamina of the rectus sheath.

Transversus abdominus muscle

The transversus abdominus muscle arises from the thoracolumbar fascia, the inner surface of the lower six costal cartilages, the inner lip of the anterior two thirds of the iliac crest, and the lateral one third of the inguinal ligament. Its fibers course transversely forward and continue as the aponeurosis, joining the posterior lamina of the rectus sheath above the arcuate line and the anterior lamina below the arcuate line.

Fascia transversalis

The fascia transversalis is thin and is part of the endoabdominal fascia and forms the posterior wall of the rectus sheath below the arcuate line. When fat is absent, the fascia transversalis adheres to the peritoneum as a single layer.

Thoracolumbar fascia

The thoracolumbar fascia consists of three layers arising from the vertebral spines, the tips of the transverse processes, and the anterior portion of the transverse processes, respectively. Layers join laterally to provide origin for the internal oblique and transversus muscles.

Rectus sheath

The rectus sheath contains the rectus abdominus muscle, which arises by a tendon from the pubic bone medial to the tubercle. The muscle inserts into the fifth and seventh costal cartilages and the xiphoid process. The pyramidalis muscle is present in front of the lower part of the rectus muscle, rising from the pubis below the origin of the rectus, and inserts into the linea alba. In addition to these two muscular structures, the rectus sheath contains the anterior cutaneous branches of the seventh through twelfth thoracic nerves and the superior and inferior epigastric vessels, which lie posterior to the muscle bed. The superior epigastric artery is a terminal branch of the internal thoracic, whereas the inferior is a branch of the external iliac artery. As described previously, the rectus sheath is formed by the aponeuroses of the external oblique, internal oblique, and transversus muscles. Fibers of the right and left sheaths decussate at the midline to form the linea alba. The anterior lamina of the sheath (see Fig. 4-3) is composed of all the aponeuroses below the level of the arcuate line but only of the external oblique and anterior layer of the internal oblique above the arcuate line. The posterior lamina above the arcuate line is formed by the aponeurosis of the transversus muscle and the posterior lamina of the internal oblique aponeurosis.

Group actions

Group actions of the abdominal wall muscles include constriction of the cavity, assisting in the noble function of parturition and the more servile functions of defecation, urination, and emesis. They also assist in flexion of the thorax or pelvis as well as in rotation of the trunk. They can also assist in expiration.

4.3 EXTERNAL GENITALIA

The female urogenital triangle (Fig. 4-4) is separated into right and left halves by the pudendal cleft, which is bounded by the two labia majora. The labia majora emerge in front of the pubic symphysis and form the mons pubis. Inside the pudendal cleft are skin folds identified as the labia minora, which are devoid of hair and subcutaneous fat. The labia minora join to form the prepuce of the clitoris superiorly and the frenulum of the clitoris inferiorly. The clitoris, which consists of the glans, a body, and two crura, is connected to the pubic symphysis by the suspensory ligament of the clitoris. The space between the two labia minora is designated the vestibule and opens into the vagina posteriorly and the urethra anteriorly. The ostia of the major vestibular glands (of Bartholin) are located between the vaginal orifice and labia minora. The opening of the vagina is partially closed by the hymen.

4.4 THE PERINEUM

Boundaries of the perineum (Fig. 4-5) are anteriorly, the pubic symphysis; posteriorly, the coccyx; anterolaterally, the pubic arch and ischiotuberosity; and posterolaterally, the sacrotuberous ligament. The floor of the perineum is the skin and the roof is the pelvic diaphragm (levator ani and coccygeus muscles). The perineum can be divided into a posterior anal triangle and an anterior urogenital triangle.

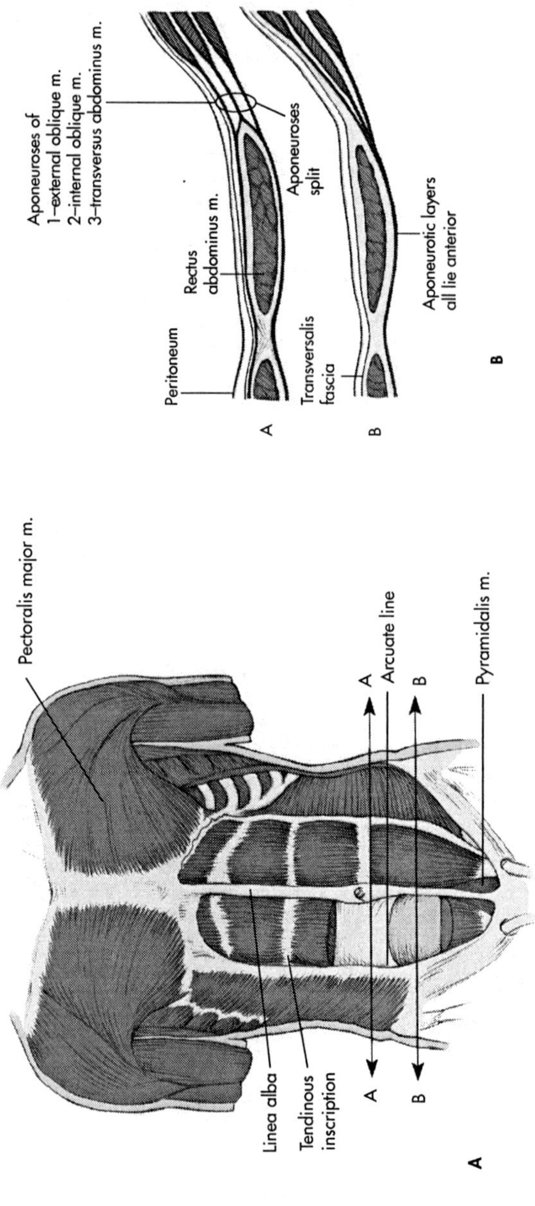
Pectoralis major m.
Linea alba
Tendinous inscription
A
B
A
Arcuate line
B
Pyramidalis m.
A
Aponeuroses of
1—external oblique m.
2—internal oblique m.
3—transversus abdominus m.
Peritoneum
Rectus abdominus m.
Aponeuroses split
Transversalis fascia
Aponeurotic layers all lie anterior
A
B
B

Figure 4-3

The rectus abdominis muscle. **A,** The anterior abdominal wall is made up on each side of three layers of flattened muscle and a pair of elongated vertical muscles, each known as rectus abdominis. The rectus muscle has two or three transverse whitish bands, the tendinous inscriptions, between the level of the umbilicus and the xiphoid. In cross-section *A-A,* just inferior to the umbilicus, the external oblique aponeurosis lies anterior to the rectus; the aponeurosis of the internal oblique muscle splits pass both in front of and behind the rectus, and the aponeurosis of the transversus abdominus muscle passes posterior to the rectus. In cross-section *B-B,* all three of these aponeurotic layers lie anterior to the rectus; only the transversalis fascia and peritoneum lie posterior. **B,** A portion of the rectus muscle has been removed to reveal the arrangement of aponeuroses derived from the more lateral abdominal muscles. The gently curved aponeurotic edge, the arcuate line, represents the point at which all the aponeurotic layers first lie anterior to the rectus. Viewed from the interior, the arcuate line marks the point at which the inferior epigastric vessels enter and lie in the transversalis fascia posterior to the rectus. The small pyramidalis muscle lies anterior to the lower end of the rectus abdominis muscle.

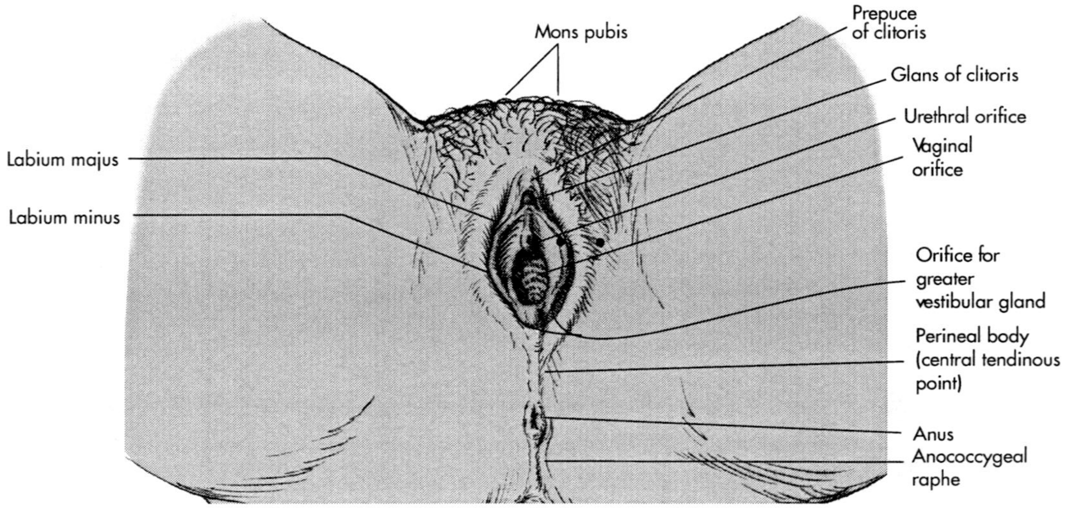

Figure 4-4
External genitalia of the female. The labia majora flank the labia minora, and the urethral and vaginal orifices are seen between the labia minora. (From *C.L.A.S.S. principles,* St Louis, 1995, Mosby.)

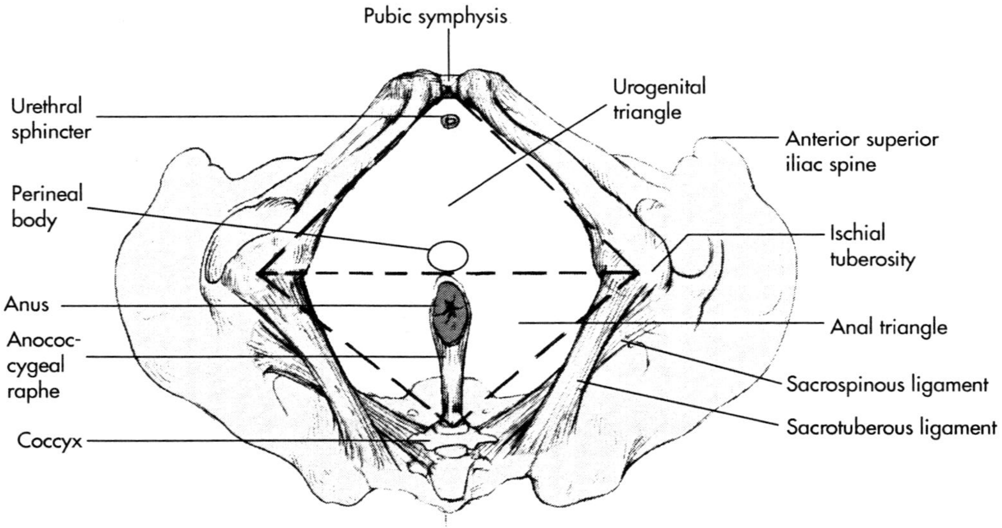

Figure 4-5
Urogenital and anal triangles. The perineum is a diamond-shaped region. It is bordered by the two ischiopubic rami and the two sacrotuberous ligaments. (Some authors define the posterior margins of this region to be imaginary lines on each side extending from the ischial tuberosity to the coccyx.) A horizontal line connecting the two ischial tuberosities divides the perineum into the anterior urogenital triangle and the posterior anal triangle. At the midpoint of this line is found the perineal body, just anterior to the anal canal. (From *C.L.A.S.S. principles,* St Louis, 1995, Mosby.)

Anal triangle

The anal triangle consists of a central anal canal and the lateral ischiorectal fossae. The sphincter ani externus muscle has three parts: subcutaneous, superficial, and deep. Muscle fibers are attached to the perineal body anteriorly and to the anococcygeal ligament posteriorly. The muscle is supplied by the inferior rectal nerve and vessels.

The ischiorectal fossae occupy the lateral portion of the anal triangle. The medial boundaries are the sphincter ani externus muscle and anal canal, the levator ani and coccygeus muscles, and their fasciae. The obturator internus muscle identifies the lateral wall. The posterior wall is the sacrotuberous ligament, covered by the gluteus maximus muscle. The anterior wall is the superficial and deep spaces of the urogenital triangle. The superior roof of the fossa is formed by the obturator internus and levator ani muscles. The skin and superficial fascia form the base of the fossa.

The contents of the ischiorectal fossae include the inferior rectal nerve, which is a branch of the pudendal nerve, supplying the levator ani and sphincter ani externus muscles; the inferior rectal artery, which is a branch of the internal pudendal artery; and the inferior rectal vein, which drains to the internal pudendal vein. All these structures then communicate with the pudendal nerve and internal pudendal artery and vein, which are located in the pudendal canal. The canal is formed by the obturator internus fascia and is located in the lateral wall of the ischiorectal fossa.

Urogenital triangle

The urogenital triangle consists of three layers of fasciae that separate the superficial and deep perineal spaces (Figs. 4-6 and 4-7). They consist of the superficial fascia, which is attached laterally to the pubic arch and posterosuperiorly to the perineal membrane. As in the abdomen, there are two layers. There is a superficial fatty layer and a deeper membranous layer, referred to as the fascia of Colles instead of Scarpa. Anteriorly, the deep layer of the superficial fascia is continuous with Scarpa's fascia in the abdomen. The fusion of this superficial perineal fascia and the perineal membrane forms the posterior boundary of the superficial perineal space. The middle fascial layer is the perineal membrane (inferior fascia of the urogenital diaphragm), which is also attached laterally to the pubic arch. In the middle of the line of fusion between the anus and the vagina is the central perineal tendon or perineum. The perineal membrane is fused posteriorly with the deeper superior fascia of the urogenital diaphragm to form the deep perineal space.

Superficial perineal pouch

1. The contents of the superficial perineal pouch are as follows:
   a. The posterior labial nerve is a branch of the pudendal nerve.
   b. The posterior labial artery is a branch of the internal pudendal artery.
   c. The superficial transverse perineal muscles form the posterior boundary of the superficial pouch. These muscles arise from the ischiotuberosities and insert into the perineal body. Their function is to stabilize the perineum.

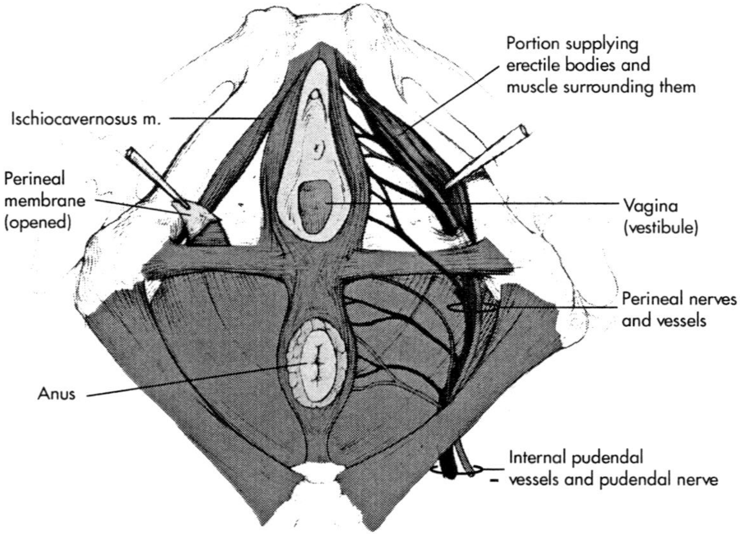

Figure 4-6
Female perineum, superficial dissection. Here the female perineum is partially dissected to show the inferior layer of the fascia of the urogenital diaphragm, otherwise known as the perineal membrane, and on the opposite side the course and distribution of pudendal vessels and nerves in the perineal region. (From *C.L.A.S.S. principles,* St Louis, 1995, Mosby.)

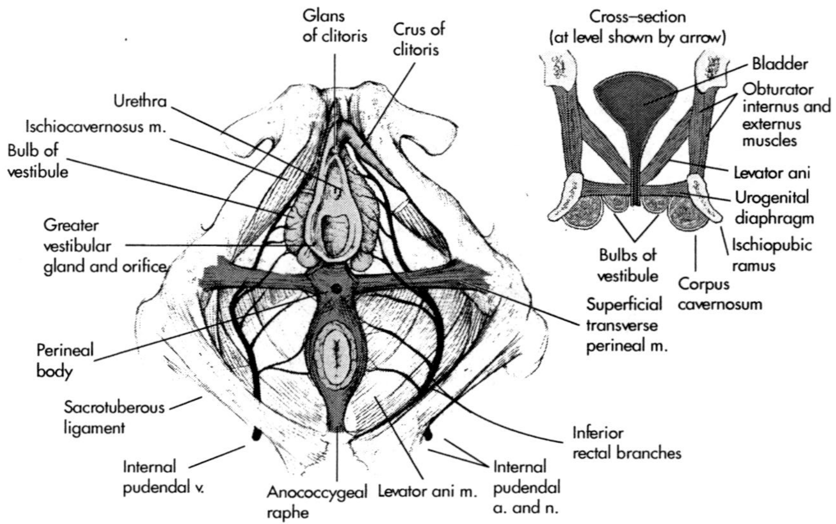

Figure 4-7
Female perineum, deeper dissection. Erectile bodies are present in the superficial pouch. The pudendal arteries and veins are shown, each on one side of the perineum. The glans and frenulum of the clitoris are also shown here. The striated ischiocavernosus muscle surrounds the proximal part of each corpora cavernosa, where they are attached firmly to the medial sides of the ischiopubic rami. (From *C.L.A.S.S. principles,* St Louis, 1995, Mosby.)

d. The bulbospongiosis muscles are exposed by cutting away the labia minora, and they cover the bulb of the vestibule. They arise from the perineal body and insert into the dorsum of the clitoris. Their function is to close the vaginal orifice.
e. The vestibular bulbs consist of erectile tissue that lies on each side of the vaginal orifice and are attached to the perineal membrane overlapping the greater vestibular glands (of Bartholin) posteriorly. The bulbs are united anteriorly by a plexus of veins (the commissure) between the urethra and the clitoris. The commissure is attached to the glans of the clitoris by a thin strip of erectile tissue.
f. The ischiocavernosus muscles cover the two crura of the clitoris and arise from the ischial ramus and insert into the crura of the clitoris. They cause erection of the clitoris. The clitoris itself has a free glans and a fixed body composed of two corpora cavernosa, which attach to the ischial pubic rami by two crura.

Deep perineal pouch

1. The deep perineal pouch is bounded by the perineal membrane inferiorly and the superior fascia of the urogenital diaphragm superiorly (Figs. 4-7 and 4-8). The perineal membrane or inferior fascia of the urogenital diaphragm is a layer of dense fibrous tissue. The membrane separates the superficial and deep perineal pouches. Its attachments laterally are the pubic arch, whereas anteriorly it is

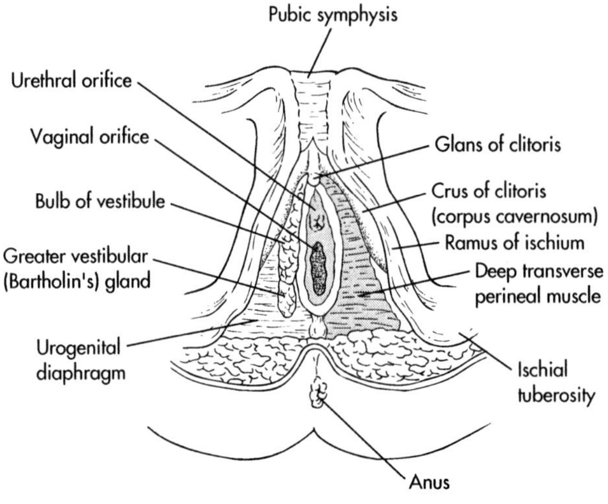

Figure 4-8
The female urogenital diaphragm seen from below. Also illustrated are the swelling bodies or cavernosus bodies. On the right side, the urogenital diaphragm is cut to show the major vestibular gland. (From Hafferl A: *Lehrbuch der topographischen Anatomie,* Berlin, 1957, Springer-Verlag.)

thickened to form the transverse perineal ligament. Between this ligament and the inferior pubic ligament, the deep dorsal vein of the clitoris passes. The contents of the deep perineal pouch include the following:

a. The urethra
b. The vagina
c. The sphincter urethrae muscle is thin and divisible into a central and a peripheral portion. The central circular fibers surround the urethra, whereas the peripheral, transverse fibers attach to the pubic arch and the perineal membrane. These fibers run anterior and posterior to the urethra. This muscle functions to constrict the urethra and is supplied by the deep perineal nerve. The posterior fibers of the sphincter urethrae muscle are continuous with the deep transverse perineal muscle, which together form the urogenital diaphragm.
d. The deep transverse perineal muscles arise from the ischial rami and perineal membrane. They insert into the perineal body. Their function is to stabilize the perineum, and their nerve supply arises from the deep perineal nerve. The muscles of the urogenital diaphragm also function to constrict the urethra.
e. The internal pudendal artery enters the deep perineal pouch posteriorly after leaving the pudendal canal and courses along the pubic arch, terminating as the deep and dorsal arteries of the clitoris. There is also a branch distributed to the bulbocavernosus.
f. The pudendal nerve terminates as the dorsal nerve of the clitoris, entering the deep perineal pouch on the lateral sides of the internal pudendal artery, which is medial to the pubic arch. It functions as a sensory nerve supplying the erectile tissue of the clitoris. The deep perineal nerve, representing a second terminal branch of the pudendal nerve, gives off the posterior labial nerve from the anterior part of the pudendal canal along with several muscular branches to supply all the muscles of the superficial and deep perineal pouches.

Lymphatic drainage

Lymphatic drainage from the inferior perineal structures, which include the inferior anal canal, lower vagina, and distal urethra, drains to the medial superficial inguinal lymph nodes. Superiorly, lymphatic flow is directed to the pelvic lymph nodes.

4.5 PELVIC DIAPHRAGM, OBTURATOR, AND PIRIFORMIS MUSCLES

Muscles of the pelvic diaphragm are the levator ani and coccygeus muscles. These muscles are both the roof of the perineum and the floor of the pelvis (Figs. 4-9 and 4-10).

Levator ani muscle

The levator ani muscle originates anteriorly from the body of the pubis, the tendinous arch, and the ischial spines. The four components of this muscle are listed in Table 4-1.

The nerve supply includes branches of the third, fourth, and fifth sacral nerves, and the inferior rectal nerves. The function is to elevate the pelvic

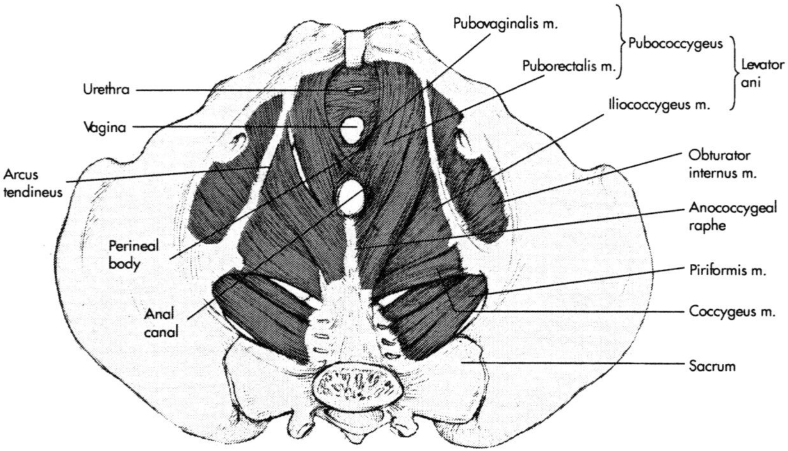

Figure 4-9

Pelvic diaphragm, superior view, female. All of the viscera have been removed to reveal the muscles forming the pelvic floor, with apertures for the rectum/anus, vagina, and urethra. The most medial and largest muscle in this area is the pubococcygeus, with its subdivisions puborectalis and pubovaginalis shown as well. Further posterior, on each side, is the iliococcygeus muscle. The posterior margin of this muscle is at the level of the sacrospinous ligament, with which the coccygeus muscle is often blended. The iliococcygeus muscle is also unique in originating from the ischial spine and along the fibrous arcus tendineus, on the medial surface of the obturator internus muscle. The piriformis muscle appears to "fill in" the gap between the posterior edge of the coccygeus and the sacrum but is not a true pelvic floor muscle. (From *C.L.A.S.S. principles,* St Louis, 1995, Mosby.)

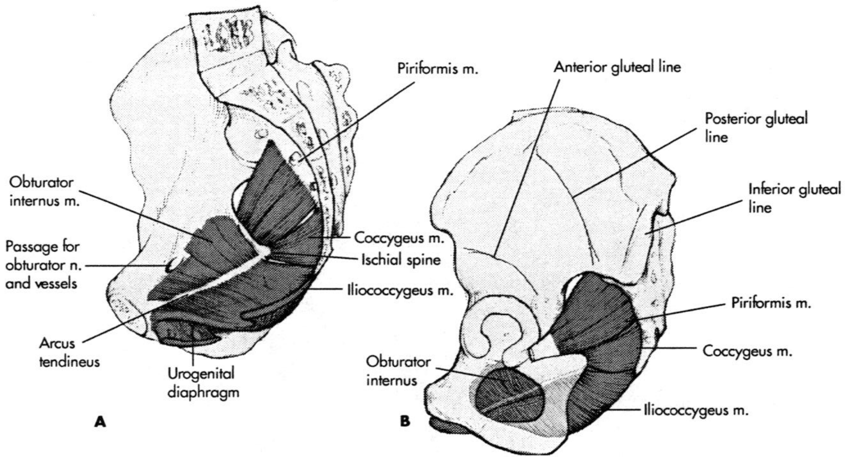

Figure 4-10
Pelvic and urogenital diaphragms. Internal view of the right hemipelvis and an external view of the left hemipelvis. It is as though the intact pelvis had been split in the midsagittal plane and the two halves separated. **A,** In the internal view, the piriformis, obturator internus, and obturator foramen are labeled. Note the arcus tendineus, extending from the inner surface of the pubic symphysis anteriorly to the ischial spine posteriorly. Anteriorly, note the deep transverse perineal muscle, and the anterior recess of the ischiorectal fossa that lies between it and the iliococcygeus. **B,** On the lateral or external view, the posterior half of the bony ring surrounding the obturator foramen has been removed. The portion of the obturator internus inferior to the arcus tendineus has also been removed to reveal the inferior surface of the iliococcygeus muscle. (From *C.L.A.S.S. principles,* St Louis, 1995, Mosby.)

Table 4-1 Components of the levator ani muscle

Muscle	Origin	Insertion	Function
Pubovaginalis	Pubic bone	Perineal body	Constriction of the vagina
Puborectalis	Pubic bone	Posterior rectum	Sphincter of anal canal
Pubococcygeus	Tendon of obturator fascia	Anococcygeal ligament	Constriction of the anal canal
Iliococcygeus	Tendon of obturator fascia	Anococcygeal ligament	Constriction of the anal canal

floor, increase intrabdominal pressure during forced respiration, and assist in defecation and vomiting.

Coccygeus

The coccygeus originates from the ischial spine and inserts into the lower border of the sacrum and coccyx. This muscle tends to be fibrous and is incorporated in the sacrospinous ligament. It is supplied by the fifth sacral nerve and has no significant function.

Obturator internus

The obturator internus arises from the medial, inferior, and lateral margins of the obturator foramen and inserts into the medial side of the greater trochanter of the femur. It is covered by the obturator fascia, which is thickened to form the tendinous arch for the attachment of the levator ani muscle. The fascia, as previously mentioned, forms the pudendal canal. Its function is the same as that of the piriformis muscle.

Piriformis

The piriformis originates from the second, third, and fourth segments of the sacrum, leaving the pelvis through the greater sciatic foramen, and is inserted into the upper border of the greater trochanter of the femur. It laterally rotates and abducts the hip.

4.6 THE PELVIC VISCERA

The ovaries are intraperitoneal structures measuring approximately $3 \times 1.5 \times 1$ cm. The ovary lies in the lateral wall of the pelvic cavity between the ureter, medially, and the external iliac vein, laterally. The uterine tube lies anteriorly. The distal portion of the tube curves around the lateral end of the ovary and is attached by one or more fimbriae. The ovary is attached to the superior surface of the broad ligament by the mesovarium and is attached to the uterus by the ligament of the ovary. The ovarian artery arises from the aorta below the renal artery and ascends along the posterior abdominal wall, crossing the external iliac artery, and entering the lateral part of the broad ligament via the suspensory ligament of the ovary or infidulopelvic ligament. The peritoneum covering the uterine tube forms the broad ligament that extends from both sides of the uterus to the lateral walls of the pelvis. The broad ligament can be divided into the mesovarium, mesosalpinx, and mesometrium (Fig. 4-11). The ovarian ligament proper connects the ovary to the uterus. The round ligament extends from the uterus to the labia majora. The uterine tube has three parts, the medial isthmus, middle ampula, and distal infundibulum, leading to the internal ostia and outer fimbria of the tube, respectively. The uterus is a fibromuscular organ, the dimensions of which vary considerably in premenopausal and postmenopausal women. This is a function of estrogenic stimulation and parturition. The uterus is composed of the upper muscular corpus and the lower cervix. The portion of the corpus above the fallopian tubes is identified as the fundus. The isthmus of the uterus is located between the body and the cervix. The uterine corpus is lined by the endometrium, which is composed of epithelium, forming glands, and also contains a specialized stroma. The portion of the cervix protruding into the vagina is identified as the portio vaginalis. The cervix consists of predominant fibrous connective tissue with a small amount of smooth muscle. The border of the cervical canal, where the canal widens into the endometrial cavity, is termed the internal os. The lower portion of the canal is the external os (Fig. 4-12). The uterine artery, which is a branch of the internal iliac artery, joins the uterus above the junction of the cervix and isthmus, where it communicates with the marginal artery along the lateral wall of the uterus. The marginal artery also communicates with the ovarian artery.

4.7 SPACES

Paravesical space

The anterior leaf of the broad ligament forms the roof of the paravesical space, blending with the bladder peritoneum medially and the parietal peritoneum laterally. The space is composed of connective tissue and fat. The bladder occupies the medial border, and the obturator internus muscle forms the lateral border. The posterior limit of the space is formed by the cardinal ligament, and the floor is composed of the levator ani muscle. The anterior leaf of the broad ligament should be opened at the midportion of the round ligament (Fig. 4-13). The incision extends laterally to expose the pelvic vessels and medially to reflect the bladder peritoneum. The space is entered on the lateral side of the obliterated hypogastric artery, and blunt dissection is carried to the level of the levator ani muscle.

Pararectal space

The pararectal space lies beneath the pelvic peritoneum. Its borders include the cardinal ligament anterolaterally and the uterosacral ligament medially. The sacrum forms the posteromedial margin of the space and the ureter is attached to the peritoneum, forming the roof of the space. The hypogastric artery and vein are located in the pararectal space, and entry should be cautious, with medial displacement of the ureter and its attached peritoneum. Surgical entry is accomplished by cephalad extension of the previous incision for the paravesical space along the lateral border of the infundibulopelvic ligament.

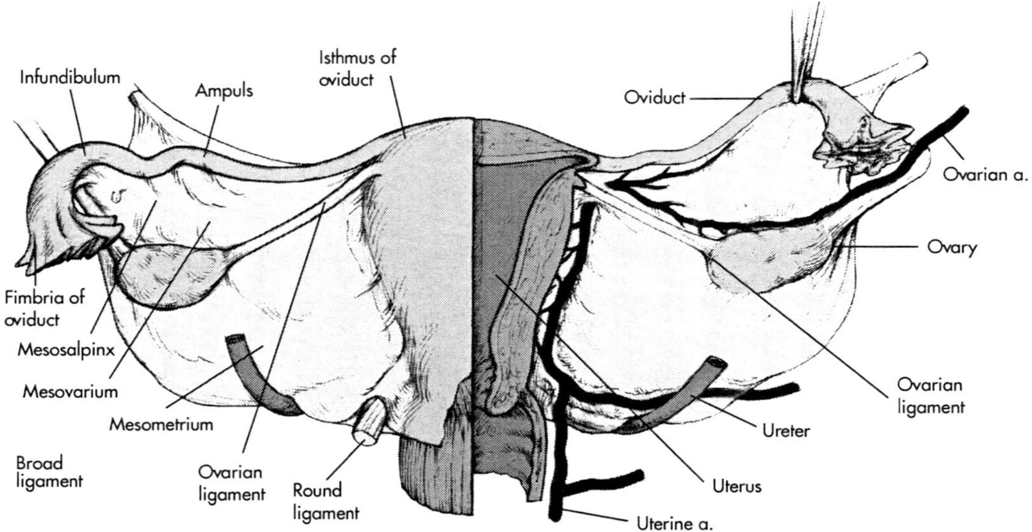

Figure 4-11

Female internal genitalia. Viewing the ovaries and uterus from the posterior aspect, the structures that lie lateral to the uterus can be seen enclosed within the two layers of the broad ligament. The structures are shown intact on the left side and are revealed by removing the posterior leaflet of the broad ligament on the right. (From *C.L.A.S.S. principles,* St Louis, 1995, Mosby.)

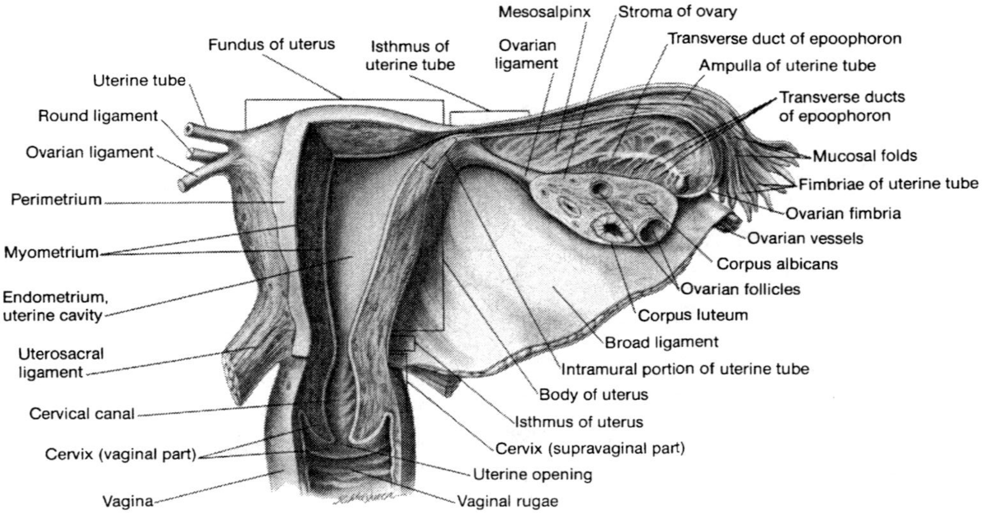

Figure 4-12

A schematic drawing of a posterior view of the cervix, uterus, fallopian tube, and ovary. Note that the cervix is divided by the vaginal attachment into an external portio segment and a supravaginal segment. Note that the uterus is composed of the dome-shaped fundus, the muscular body, and the narrow isthmus. Note the fimbria ovarica, or ovarian fimbria, attaching the oviduct to the ovary. (From Droegemueller W: *Comprehensive gynecology,* ed 2, St Louis, 1987, Mosby.)

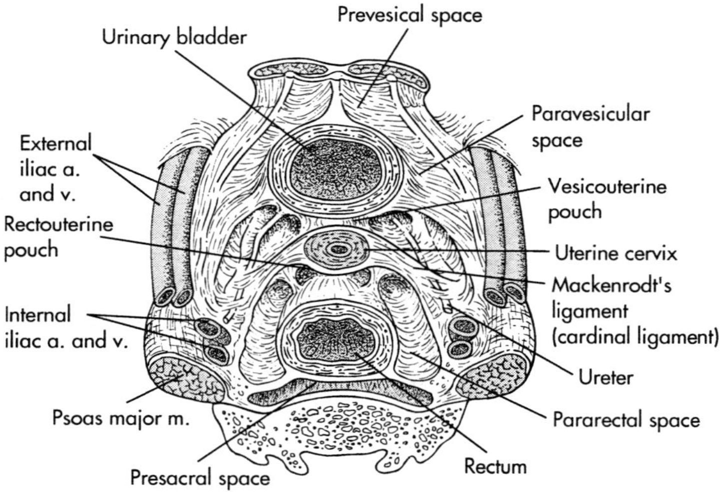

Figure 4-13
Schematic sectional drawing of the pelvis shows the firm connective tissue and the paraspaces (Amreich). The bladder, cervix, and rectum are surrounded by a connective tissue covering. The Mackenrodt ligament extends from the lateral cervix to the lateral abdominal pelvic wall. The vesicouterine ligament originating from the anterior edge of the Mackenrodt ligament leads to the covering of the bladder on the posterior side. The sagittal rectum column spreads both to the connective tissue of the rectum and to the sacral vertebrae closely nestled against the back of the Mackenrodt ligament and lateral pelvic wall. Between the firm connective tissue bundles there is loose connective tissue (paraspaces). (From Von Peham H, Amreich JA: *Gynaekologische operationslehre,* Berlin, 1930, S Karger.)

Retropubic space

The retropubic space is developed anterior to the peritoneum and bladder by posteriorly retracting the bladder to expose the retropubic space. The space is filled with loose fatty tissue and is bordered anteriorly by the pubic symphysis and superiorly by the anterior abdominal wall between the two obliterated umbilical arteries. The posterior border is the rectovesical fascia, which encloses the ureter and blood vessels of the posterolateral border of the bladder. The lateral structures include the pubic bone, the obturator internis and levator ani muscles, the obliterated umbilical artery, and the obturator nerve. The inferolateral surface of the bladder is the medial border. The floor of the space includes two thickened fascial cords that represent the pubovesical ligament. This ligament extends from the neck of the bladder to the inferior border of the pubic symphysis.

4.8 PELVIC PERITONEUM

The structure of the pelvic floor forms the sigmoid mesocolon and pararectal and paravesical fossa. The uterus divides the peritoneal cavity into a rectouterine fossa (pouch of Douglas) bounded laterally by the rectouterine folds and an anterior vesicouterine fossa. The peritoneum covering the folds also forms the broad ligament. The pelvic viscera are connected to the pelvic wall by their adventitial layers. Between these attachments are cleavage planes separating one organ from the other. These planes include the vesicovaginal space, the rectovaginal space, the retrorectal space, and the pararectal and paravesical spaces previously mentioned.

4.9 CARDINAL AND UTEROSACRAL LIGAMENTS

The cardinal ligaments are fibromuscular bands embedded in the adipose tissue of the lower portion of the broad ligaments. These bands extend from the lower portion of the cervix and upper portion of the vagina across the pelvic floor as a deeper continuation of the broad ligament. As the ligaments reach the lateral pelvic diaphragm, their ventral and dorsal extensions attach to the deep fascia on the inner surface of the levator ani, coccygeus, and piriformis muscles. This forms a white line 2 cm below the arcus tendineus of the levator ani, which is called the arcus tendineus of the pelvic fascia. Ventral extension is continuous with the supporting tissue of the bladder, whereas the dorsal extension blends with the uterosacral ligaments.

The uterosacral ligaments are the prominent fibrous bands extending from the cervix to the sacrum. They are attached to the periosteum and fascia of the sacrum. The peritoneum surrounding the ligaments create the rectouterine folds that enclose the pouch of Douglas.

4.10 THE VAGINA

The vagina is approximately 9 cm long posteriorly and approximately 7 cm long anteriorly. It forms an angle with the uterus that is greater than 90° (Fig. 4-14). The recess posterior to the cervix is the posterior fornix, and there are similar but smaller recesses anteriorly and laterally. The posterior surface of the vagina is separated from the upper rectum by the rectouterine fossa. The

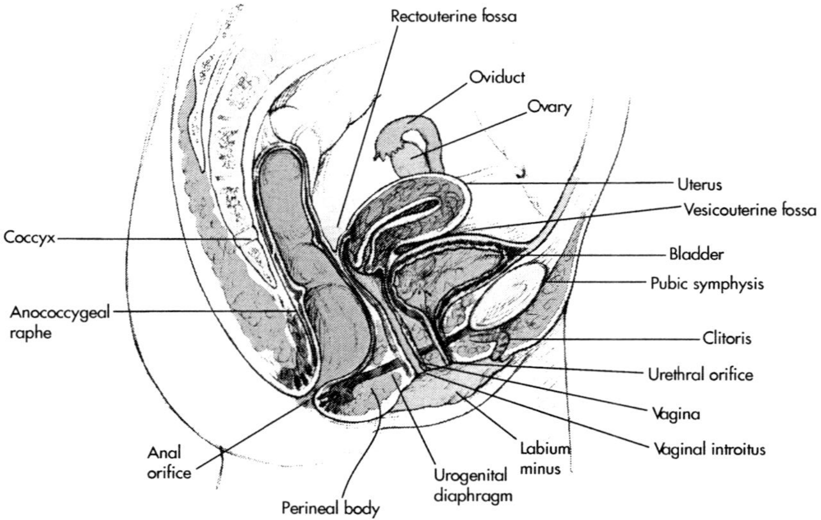

Figure 4-14

Female pelvic floor, midsagittal view. The anterior limit of the perineal area is the pubic symphysis, and the posterior limit the coccyx. Just anterior to the anal canal is the perineal body, an important landmark and point of attachment for several perineal muscles, ligaments, and organs. The anterior parts of the two corpora cavernosa are seen as the clitoris, lying just inferior to the pubic symphysis. Note that the urethral orifice is about halfway between the clitoris and the vaginal opening. The peritoneal membrane, covering the superior surfaces of the organs located in the pelvis, forms two special areas, the vesicouterine fossa and the rectouterine fossa (or pouch of Douglas). (From *C.L.A.S.S. principles,* St Louis, 1995, Mosby.)

middle portion of the rectum is separated from the vagina by the rectovaginal fascia (of Denonvillier), and the lower fourth is separated from the anal canal by the perineal body.

4.11 THE URINARY TRACT

The abdominal ureter is a muscular tube, approximately 25 cm long and 5 mm wide, extending from a slight constriction at its junction with the pelvis of the kidney and descending vertically in a line parallel with the tips of the lumbar transverse processes to the midpoint of the ureter. This midpoint lies at the origin of the external iliac artery, where the ureter then enters the lesser pelvis. The blood supply of the ureter includes small branches from the renal and ovarian arteries, as well as the aorta and the common, internal iliac, uterine, and superior vesical arteries. These branches form longitudinal anastomoses that lie on the surface of the ureter. Because of this anastomotic network, branches can be divided without interfering with the blood supply.

The pelvic ureter runs posteroinferiorly anterior to the internal iliac artery and deep to the peritoneum of the lateral wall of the pelvis (Fig. 4-15). It travels along the lateral fornix of the vagina inferior to the broad ligament and uterine artery turning superiorly into the broad ligament. It enters the bladder wall to open into the superolateral angle of the trigone of the bladder.

The internal surface of the bladder is ridged by folds of mucous membrane, whereas on the posterior wall there is a smooth triangular area previously mentioned as the trigone of the bladder. The median internal urethral orifice is located at the inferior angle of the triangle. Fibrous bundles between the anteroinferior part of the pubic symphysis and the urethra represent the pubourethral ligament, which stabilizes the urethra and forms the inferior boundary of the retropubic space.

4.12 BLOOD SUPPLY OF THE PELVIS (FIGS. 4-16 AND 4-17)

Ovarian arteries

The ovarian arteries arise from the aorta just below the renal arteries. They pass distally under the peritoneum, resting on the psoas major muscle. On entering the pelvis, the arteries are enclosed in the layers of the suspensory ligament of the ovary.

Superior rectal artery

The superior rectal artery is the continuation of the inferior mesenteric artery and descends between the layers of the mesentery of the sigmoid colon crossing the left common iliac artery. Opposite the distal portion of the sacrum the artery divides into two branches that descend on either side of the rectum.

Middle sacral artery

The middle sacral artery arises from the distal portion of the aorta posteriorly, descending behind the left common iliac vein and anterior to the fifth lumbar vertebra and the sacrum. The corresponding vein drains into the left common iliac vein.

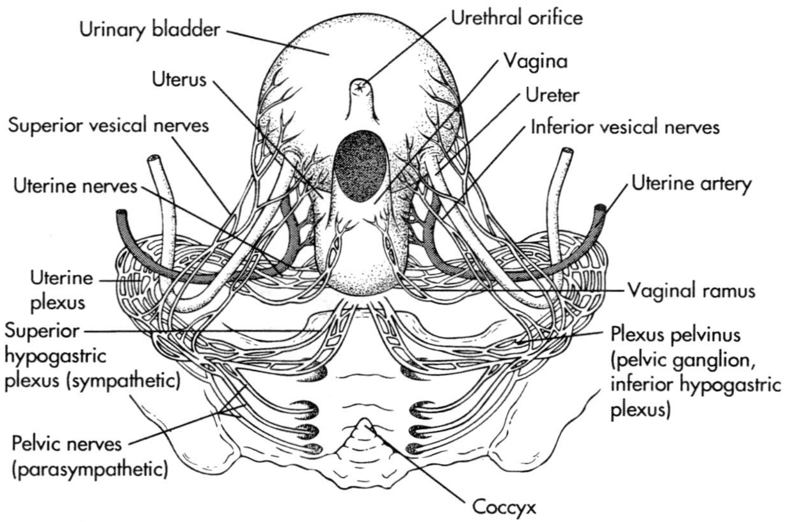

Figure 4-15

Innervation of uterus, bladder, and vagina, viewed from the perineum. *1,* Inferior vesical nerves; *2,* superior vesical nerves; *3,* uterine artery; *4,* uterine plexus (uterovaginal); *5,* plexus pelvinus (pelvic ganglion, inferior hypogastric plexus); *6,* pelvic nerves (parasympathetic); *7,* superior hypogastric plexus (sympathetic); *8,* vaginal ramus; *9,* uterine nerves; *10,* vagina; *11,* uterus; *12,* ureter; *13,* urinary bladder. (From Reiffenstuhl G, Platzer W: *Die vaginalen operationen. Chirug anatomie u operationslehre,* Berlin, 1974, Urban-Schwarzenberg.)

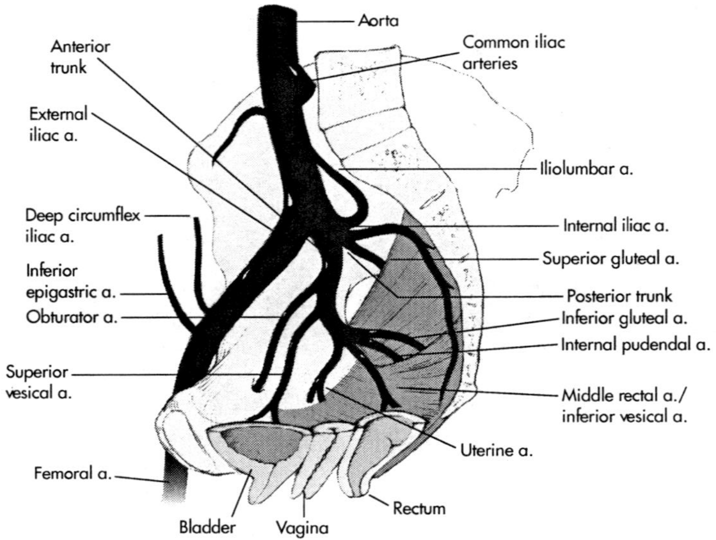

Figure 4-16

Branches of the common iliac artery. The common iliac artery divides into an internal and an external branch. The internal iliac artery supplies the gluteal and internal pelvic structures, whereas the external iliac artery continues inferiorly as the femoral artery, the major blood supply to the entire lower limb. (From *C.L.A.S.S. principles*, St Louis, 1995, Mosby.)

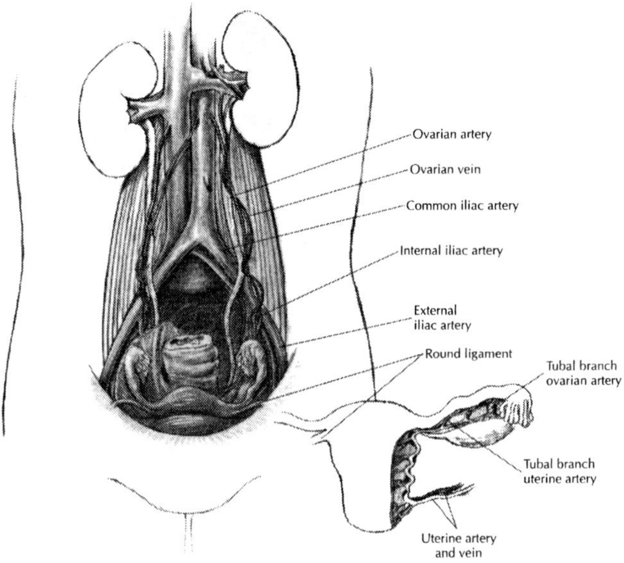

Figure 4-17
Pelvic blood supply. (From Davis JH et al, editors: *Surgery,* ed 2, St Louis, 1995, Mosby.)

Common iliac arteries

The common iliac arteries descend obliquely from the fourth lumbar vertebra to the pelvic brim. The vessels bifurcate into the external and internal iliac arteries opposite the lumbosacral joint. There are accompanying common iliac veins that unite to form the inferior vena cava. These vessels are slightly posterior and a portion of the right common iliac vein is lateral to the right common iliac artery, whereas the left common iliac is always medial. Each common iliac vein receives the iliolumbar and sometimes the lateral sacral veins. As stated previously, the left common iliac vein receives the middle sacral vein as well.

External iliac artery

The external iliac artery passes laterally along the medial border of the psoas major muscle to a midpoint beneath the inguinal ligament between the anterior superior iliac spine and the pubic symphysis. It enters the thigh and becomes the femoral artery.

Internal iliac artery

The internal iliac artery is the main arterial supply of the pelvis. It enters the pelvis behind the ureter and anterior to the internal iliac vein in the sacroiliac joint. The artery divides into anterior and posterior trunks at the upper border of the greater sciatic foramen. The anterior trunk has three somatic branches and four visceral branches.

Anterior trunk

1. Anterior trunk of the internal iliac artery.
   a. The umbilical artery is the intrapelvic portion of the fetal umbilical artery. It retains its lumen for a short distance from the internal iliac and gives off the superior vesical artery. Distally it forms a fibrous cord running beside the bladder to the umbilicus as the lateral umbilical ligament or the obliterated hypogastric artery.
   b. The obturator artery courses along the lateral wall of the pelvis to the obturator canal. Superior to the artery is the obturator nerve, and the vein is inferior. There is a pubic branch communicating with the pelvic surface of the pubic bone and anastomosing with a similar branch from the inferior epigastric artery. This anastomosis may replace the more common course of the obturator artery originating from the internal iliac and is called the abnormal obturator artery.
   c. The uterine artery runs forward to the base of the broad ligament, where it crosses the ureter anteriorly and ascends along the lateral border of the uterus. It forms an anastomosis with the ovarian and vaginal arteries.
   d. The vaginal artery corresponds to the inferior vesical artery in the male; it supplies the vagina, the uterus, and the inferior portion of the bladder.
   e. The middle rectal artery arises from a common trunk with the vaginal artery. It communicates with the superior and inferior rectal arteries.
   f. The internal pudendal artery leaves the pelvis through the greater sciatic foramen and reenters at the lesser sciatic foramen, where it goes forward to the pudendal canal.
   g. The inferior gluteal artery also leaves the pelvis through the greater sciatic foramen and passes to the gluteal region. It is located posterior to the internal pudendal artery.

Posterior trunk

1. Posterior trunk of the internal iliac artery.
   a. The iliolumbar artery passes posteriorly and laterally between the fourth and fifth lumbar nerves, passing behind the psoas major muscle and proximal portion of the obturator nerve. Its vein terminates in the common iliac vein.
   b. The lateral sacral artery has a superior and an inferior branch that may have separate or common origins. The superior branch enters the vertebral canal between the upper two anterior sacral foramina, and the inferior branch is directed to the lower two foramina and the coccyx.
   c. The superior gluteal artery runs posteriorly between the fourth and fifth lumbar nerves or between the lumbosacral trunk and the first

sacral nerve. It travels through the greater sciatic foramen to the gluteal region.

Collateral circulation

Collateral circulation between the branches of the internal iliac artery and the systemic circulation is clinically significant. The lumbar branch of the iliolumbar artery communicates with the lumbar arteries of the systemic circulation. The lateral sacral artery communicates with the median sacral artery. The middle rectal artery communicates with the inferior and superior rectal arteries.

4.13 LYMPHATIC DRAINAGE OF THE PELVIS

External iliac lymph nodes

The external iliac lymph nodes receive lymphatic drainage from the bladder, the isthmus of the uterus, and deep inguinal nodes.

Internal iliac lymph nodes

The internal iliac lymph nodes receive drainage from the pelvic viscera, the gluteal region, and the deep perineum. They do not receive drainage from the ovaries or uterine tubes.

Sacral group

The sacral group is located along the median and lateral sacral arteries, and these nodes receive drainage from the posterior pelvic wall, the rectum, and the isthmus of the uterus.

Lower paraaortic nodes

The lower paraaortic nodes communicate with lymphatics from the ovaries and uterine tubes.

4.14 PELVIC JOINTS

Lumbosacral

The lumbosacral is located between the fifth lumbar vertebra and the upper end of the sacrum.

Sacroiliac

The sacroiliac connects the auricular surfaces of the sacrum and the ilium.

Pubic symphysis

The pubic symphysis is joined by the interpubic disc of fibrocartilage, which is strengthened by the anterior, posterior, superior, and inferior (arcuate) ligaments.

Sacrococcygeal and coccygeal joints

The sacrococcygeal and coccygeal joints are miniatures of intervertebral joints.

4.15 LIGAMENTS

Sacrotuberous ligament

The sacrotuberous ligament (Fig. 4-18) originates from the dorsal surface of the sacrum and coccyx and from the posterior and inferior iliac spine, passing inferiorly and laterally to the medial surface of the ischiotuberosity. It helps form the medial margin of the greater and lesser sciatic foramen.

Sacrospinous ligament

The sacrospinous ligament (see Fig. 4-18) originates from the lateral margin of the coccyx and the lowermost portion of the sacrum and attaches to the ischial spine. The greater and lesser sciatic foramina are located superiorly and inferiorly to the sacrospinous ligament. The greater sciatic foramen is superior to the pelvic diaphragm, whereas the lesser is located inferiorly. As a result, structures passing to the perineum and ischiorectal fossa initially travel through the greater sciatic foramen and reemerge through the lesser. The pudendal nerve and artery are dorsal and posterior to the sacrospinous ligament and are seen just medial to the ischial spine. The sciatic nerve is similarly located but is lateral to the ischial spine. It is for this reason that surgical fixation of the vagina to the sacrospinous ligament is performed approximately 2 to 3 cm medial to the ischial spine. The coccygeus muscle is located anterior to the sacrospinous ligament and the fibers of both structures are intimately adherent.

4.16 NERVES OF THE LESSER PELVIS (FIG. 4-19)

Lumbosacral trunk

The lumbosacral trunk (L4, L5) is a thick nerve formed from the entire ventral ramus of the fifth lumbar nerve and the descending portion of the fourth. It descends distally anterior to the sacral ala posterior to the pelvic fascia and joins the ventral rami of the sacral nerves anterior to the piriformis muscle.

Sacral plexus

The sacral plexus (L4, L5, and S1 through S4) is formed by the ventral rami of the fifth lumbar vertebra, the first three sacral rami, and a portion of the fourth lumbar and fourth sacral rami. The lumbosacral trunk unites with the first sacroventral ramus and, together with the second, third, and part of the fourth sacral ramus, forms the solid triangular sacral plexus. The plexus is located between the piriformis and the pelvic fascia.

Sciatic nerve

The sciatic nerve (L4, L5, S1, S2, and S3), as a terminal branch of the sacral plexus, is composed of fibers from the fourth and fifth lumbar nerves and the first through third sacral nerves. The sciatic nerve later splits into the common peroneal and tibial nerves.

Pudendal nerve

The pudendal nerve (S2, S3, S4) is composed of sacral branches from the second, third, and fourth sacral nerves and leaves the pelvis through the

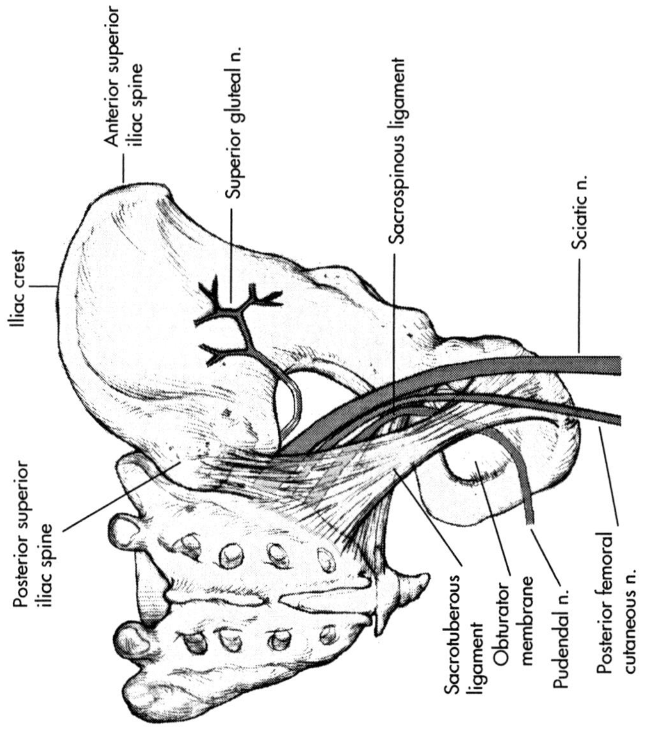

Figure 4-18
Pelvic ligaments, external view from posterior. Visible are the sacrotuberous and sacrospinous ligaments, as well as the sciatic, superior gluteal, posterior femoral cutaneous, and pudendal nerves. (From *C.L.A.S.S. principles*, St Louis, 1995, Mosby.)

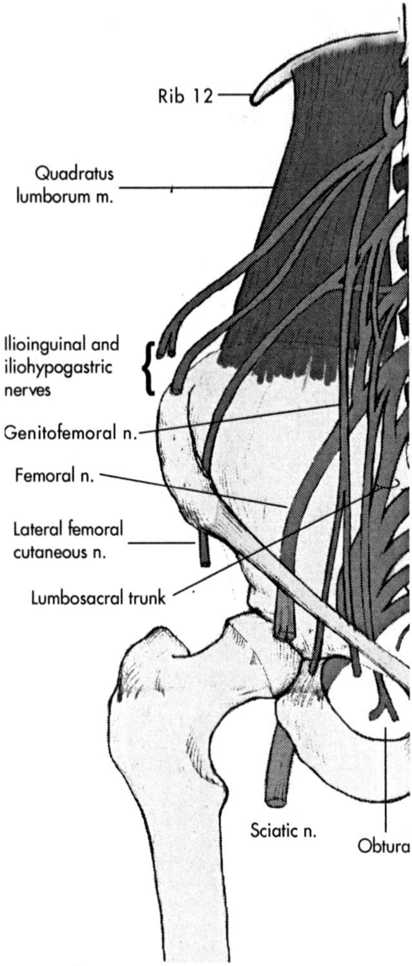

A

Figure 4-19
Lumbosacral plexus. **A,** The lumbar and sacral plexuses are shown here as a continuum of nerve fibers emerging from vertebral levels L1 to S5. The lumbar plexus is directed at innervation of the lower anterolateral abdominal wall and the inguinal canal. The sacral plexus innervates pelvic organs and continues outside the pelvis to supply the posterior thigh and nearly all of the lower limb below the knee.

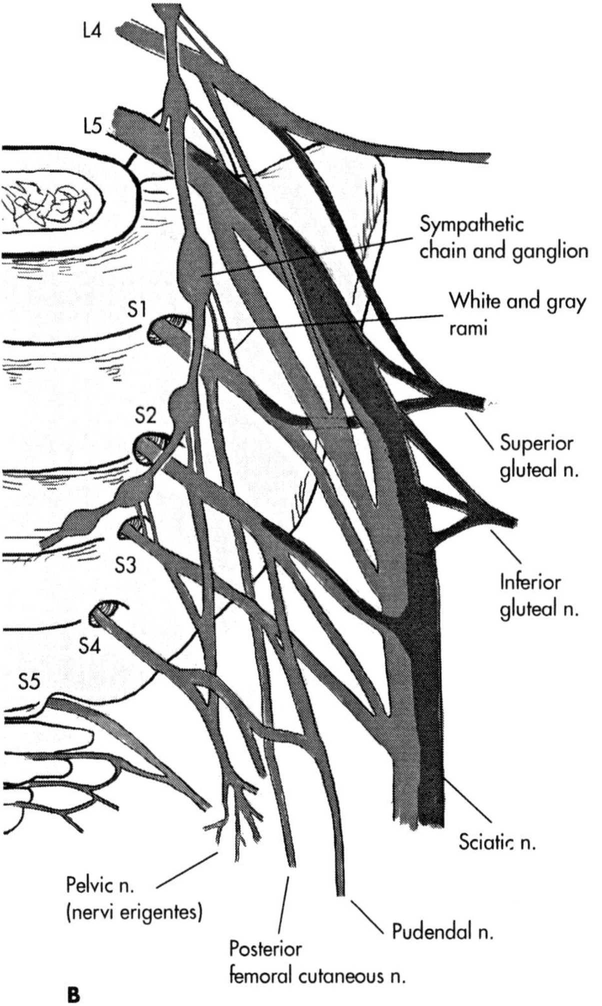

Figure 4-19, cont'd

B, This schematic drawing of the sacral plexus illustrates formation of its major branches and the distribution of anterior and posterior division branches in them. (From *C.L.A.S.S. principles,* St Louis, 1995, Mosby.)

greater sciatic foramen and, as mentioned previously, reenters through the lesser sciatic foramen to enter the pudendal canal.

Coccygeal plexus

The coccygeal plexus (S4, S5) is formed from ventral rami of the fourth and fifth sacral nerves, as well as the coccygeal nerve, innervating the pelvic diaphragm and the skin posterior to the coccyx.

Lumbar plexus

The lumbar plexus is formed by the ventral rami of the first three and the greater part of the fourth lumbar nerves. It is located dorsal to or within the fasciculi of the psoas major muscle. Although these fibers emerge from the posterior abdominal wall, many traverse the pelvis en route to their site of innervation. The branches of the lumbar plexus are listed in Table 4-2.

Iliohypogastric nerve

1. The iliohypogastric nerve emerges from the upper part of the lateral border of the psoas major muscle, penetrates the posterior part of the transversus abdominus muscle near the crest of the ilium, and divides into a lateral and an anterior cutaneous branch.
   a. The lateral cutaneous branch is distributed to the skin of the gluteal region.
   b. The anterior cutaneous branch continues on a course between the internal oblique and transversus muscles and penetrates the aponeurosis of the external oblique 2 cm above the external inguinal ring, where it is distributed to the skin of the hypogastric region.

Ilioinguinal nerve

1. The ilioinguinal nerve arises just caudal to the iliohypogastric nerve, traversing posteriorly to the crest of the ilium. It penetrates the internal oblique muscle, travels through the external inguinal ring, and is distributed to the skin of the mons pubis and labia majora.

Genitofemoral nerve

1. The genitofemoral nerve passes distally through the substance of the psoas major muscle, emerging at the level of the fourth lumbar vertebra, where it is covered by peritoneum.

Table 4-2 Branches of the lumbar plexus

Branch	Level
Iliohypogastric	L1, T12
Ilioinguinal	L1
Genitofemoral	L1, L2
Lateral femoral cutaneous	L2, L3
Obturator	L2, L3, L4
Femoral	L2, L3, L4

a. The genital branch progresses to the inguinal ligament, where it accompanies the round ligament of the uterus. It provides sensory fibers to the round ligament and the labia majora.
b. The femoral branch, which is lateral to the genital branch, passes under the inguinal ligament with the external iliac artery and enters the femoral sheath, penetrating the fascia lata to supply the skin of the proximal anterior thigh.

Lateral femoral cutaneous nerve

1. The lateral femoral cutaneous nerve emerges from the lateral portion of the psoas major, where it passes under the inguinal ligament and over the sartorius muscle, dividing into an anterior and posterior branch.
   a. The anterior branch innervates the skin of the lateral and anterior thigh as far distally as the knee.
   b. The posterior branch innervates the lateral and posterior surfaces of the thigh. This innervation extends from the level of the greater trochanter to the midportion of the thigh.

Obturator nerve

1. The obturator nerve provides motor innervation to the adductor muscles of the thigh. It emerges from the medial border of the psoas near the pelvic brim posterior to the common iliac vessels. It continues distally lateral to the internal iliac vessels and the ureter, then runs along the lateral wall of the pelvis to enter the obturator foramen with the obturator artery and vein.

Femoral nerve

1. The femoral nerve represents the largest branch of the lumbar plexus and is the principal motor innervation of the anterior thigh. It originates in the pelvis within the fibers of the psoas major, emerging from the psoas below the iliac crest. It descends between the psoas and iliacus muscles covered by the fascia. It passes underneath the inguinal ligament and remains lateral to the femoral sheath. Besides its motor function, it has sensory cutaneous function. The cutaneous branches penetrate the fascia lata of the thigh approximately 7 to 8 cm distal to the inguinal ligament, dividing into an anterior and a medial branch.

4.17 THE AUTONOMIC NERVOUS SYSTEM

The autonomic nervous system (Figs. 4-20 and 4-21) affecting the pelvic viscera can by divided into a sympathetic (thoracolumbar) system and a parasympathetic (craniosacral) system. The neurotransmitter for the sympathetic nervous system is adrenergic, whereas the parasympathetic is cholinergic. In general, adrenergic stimulation favors storage and cholinergic stimulation favors evacuation.

Sympathetic pathway

The sympathetic pathway from the spinal cord to the viscera always involves two neurons. The synapse occurs either in the paravertebral ganglia of the

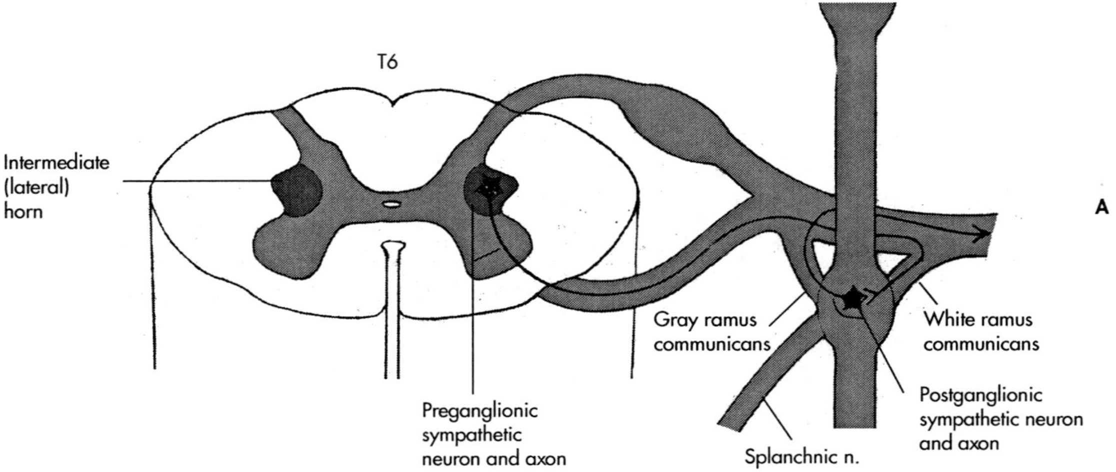

Figure 4-20
Sympathetic nerves at different vertebral levels. **A,** At vertebral levels T1 to L2, preganglionic sympathetic neuron cell bodies are located in the intermediate horn, and their axons travel in the ventral root to reach the sympathetic chain. The axons then traverse the white ramus communicans to enter the sympathetic ganglion and, as shown here, synapse in a neuron in that ganglion (other options would be to enter the splanchnic nerve or to ascend or descend in the sympathetic chain). When they synapse in the sympathetic ganglion, the postganglionic axon then traverse the gray ramus communicans to reenter the spinal nerve.

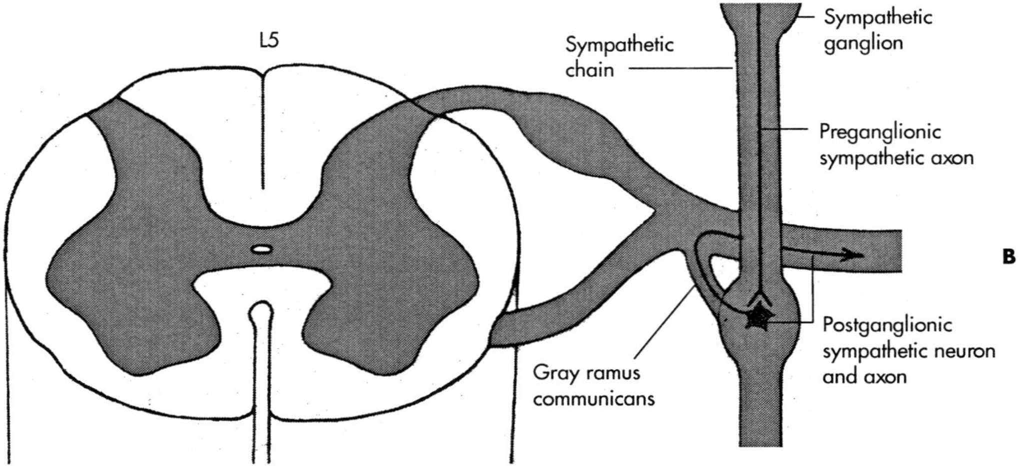

Figure 4-20, cont'd

B, At a level where no lateral horn exists, the sympathetic ganglion receives preganglionic input through the sympathetic chain. The postganglionic axons traverse the gray ramus to enter the spinal nerve for that level. (From *C.L.A.S.S. principles,* St Louis, 1995, Mosby.)

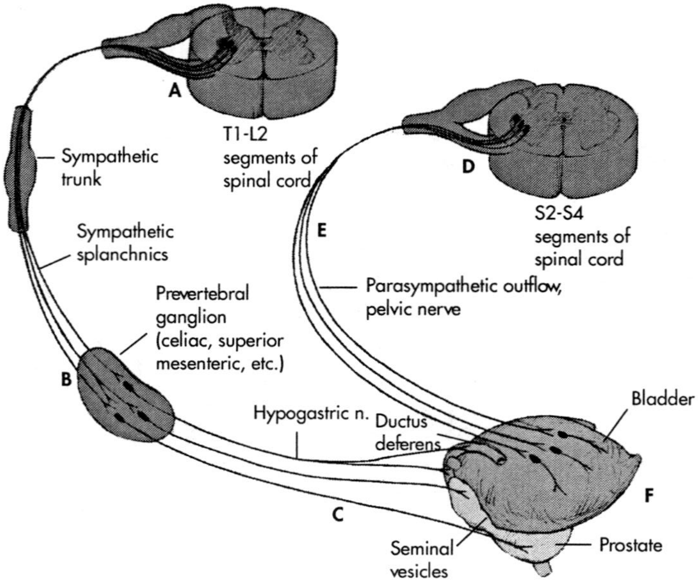

Figure 4-21

Autonomic innervation of the bladder. The sympathetic innervation begins with preganglionic axons arising in the lower thoracic spinal cord **(A)** in the intermediolateral cell column. These axons must synapse in a peripheral ganglion, and it is from the neurons of those ganglia that the axons actually innervating the intended target tissues arise. For pelvic viscera, preganglionic axons travel as part of the group of splanchnic nerves (greater, lesser, and least) that separate from the segmental thoracic nerves and descend along the posterior thoracic wall to enter the abdomen. Here they synapse in one of the large prevertebral ganglia **(B)** along the aorta (e.g., the celiac, superior mesenteric, renal, etc.). Postganglionic axons arising in these ganglia distribute themselves along the arterial branches of the abdominal aorta, and, in addition, a portion of them continues inferiorly to descend from the bifurcation of the aorta into the pelvis and the hypogastric nerve (or plexus) **(C).** Parasympathetic innervation begins with preganglionic axons arising in spinal cord segments S2 to S4 **(D).** These axons travel in the pelvic nerve **(E)** to small groups of neurons embedded in the walls of target organs. Here the preganglionic axons synapse, and the small neurons give rise to postganglionic axons **(F),** which actually innervate the muscle or glands in that organ. (From *C.L.A.S.S. principles,* St Louis, 1995, Mosby.)

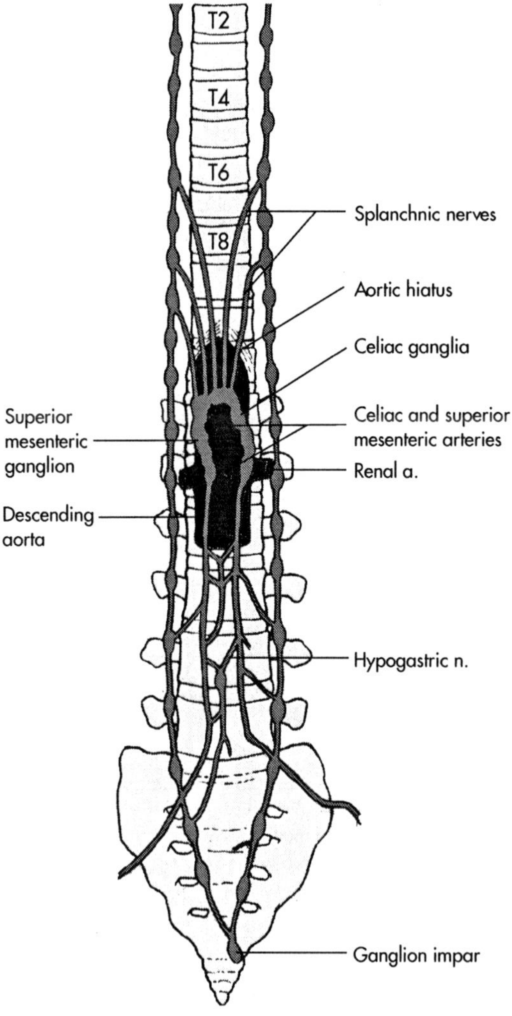

Figure 4-22
Sympathetic chains and splanchnic nerves. The sympathetic chains emit medial branches from the T6 to T12 levels (the splanchnic nerves). These synapse in ganglia positioned at the origin of branches of the abdominal aorta, especially the celiac ganglion. The sympathetic chains continue inferiorly in the abdomen and eventually meet in the midline, anterior to the coccyx (the ganglion impar). (From *C.L.A.S.S. principles,* St Louis, 1995, Mosby.)

sympathetic trunk or in prevertebral ganglia (i.e., the inferior mesenteric ganglion). Preganglionic sympathetic fibers supplying the pelvic organs originate from the white rami of the upper two lumbar nerves and from the lowest thoracic nerve. These fibers pass through the corresponding ganglia of the sympathetic trunk (paravertebral ganglia) terminating in the inferior mesenteric ganglia (prevertebral). Postganglionic fibers or axons are then sent by way of the superior hypogastric and inferior hypogastric plexi to the pelvic viscera. Each spinal nerve receives grey rami communicantes from the sympathetic trunk. The grey ramus consists of postganglionic sympathetic fibers, which innervate blood vessels, hair, and glands of the body wall. The four pairs of ganglia of the sympathetic trunk anterior to the sacrum contribute branches from the first two ganglia to the inferior hypogastric plexus, whereas the last two supply the rectum directly.

Parasympathetic system

The parasympathetic system consists of preganglionic fibers that originate from the second, third, and fourth sacral nerves forming the pelvic nerve (also termed nervi erigentes) and terminate in the ganglia of the pelvic plexi. Postganglionic fibers from these plexi supply the effectors of the pelvic organs, including the urinary bladder, the descending colon, the rectum, and the reproductive organs.

Anatomically (Fig. 4-22), the two sympathetic trunks descend into the pelvis along the medial side of the anterior sacral foramina and end as a single ganglion impar anterior to the coccyx. Each trunk usually has four ganglia, which send grey rami to the sacral and the coccygeal nerves. The superior hypogastric plexus lies in front of the fifth lumbar vertebra, the sacral promontory, and the ventral surface of the lower aorta. This plexus also receives important pain fibers from the pelvic viscera. From the superior hypogastric plexus descend two hypogastric nerves along the course of the internal iliac vessels. These nerves terminate as the inferior hypogastric plexus.

The inferior hypogastric plexus consists of the uterovaginal plexus along the medial surface of the uterine vessels lateral to the uterosacral ligament. In addition, extensions of the inferior hypogastric plexi are located on the walls of the pelvic viscera. This includes the rectal plexus and the vesical plexus.

Suggested reading

Anderson J: *Grant's atlas of anatomy,* ed 8, Baltimore, 1983, Williams & Wilkins.
Gray H: *Gray's anatomy,* ed 37, New York, 1989, Churchill Livingstone.
Mathers LH et al: *Clinical anatomy principles,* St Louis, 1996, Mosby.
Nichols DH: *Gynecologic and obstetric surgery,* St Louis, 1993, Mosby.
Romanes G: *Cunningham's manual of practical anatomy,* vol 1, *Upper and lower limbs,* New York, 1993, Oxford University Press.
Romanes G: *Cunningham's manual of practical anatomy,* vol 2, *Thorax and abdomen,* New York, 1992, Oxford University Press.

Diagnostic Studies

5

5.1 PAPANICOLAOU SMEAR

George T. Danakas, M.D., and Karen Houck, M.D.

The usefulness of a Papanicolaou smear as a screening test depends on obtaining an adequate, well-presented, and well-preserved sample. The basic procedure for obtaining a Papanicolaou smear is explained here. It should be kept in mind that various institutions have different protocols for obtaining, preparing, fixing, and labeling samples, and one should be aware of the institution's requirements.

Patient preparation

The patient should be instructed to avoid douching or using vaginal creams for at least 24 hours before her examination. As well, Papanicolaou smears should not be obtained during menstruation because the red blood cells may obscure the sample. Sampling should be done before a bimanual pelvic examination, and the use of lubrication should be avoided if possible. However, water used to warm the speculum will not affect the sample. After the patient is positioned in the dorsal lithotomy position, choose a speculum that allows visualization of the entire cervix. Note any abnormalities of the cervix at this time.

Sampling

The choice of sampling devices depends on personal preference as well as on instrument availability. It will be necessary to sample both the endocervix and the ectocervix. Some physicians advocate sampling the posterior fornix to obtain desquamated cells from the cervix and endometrial cavity; however, a well-sampled endocervix and ectocervix generally provide an adequate smear. With an Ayre spatula or a similar device, the entire transition zone is sampled by rotating the spatula 360° around the cervix. The specimen can be left on the spatula until all sampling is completed or it can be smeared onto a slide that is then immediately fixed. The endocervix is sampled with a cotton-tipped applicator or cervical brush. The latter should generally be avoided in pregnancy. Insert the cotton-tipped applicator or cervical brush into the os and gently rotate. One half turn is usually sufficient to sample the endocervix.

Preparing and fixing the smear

The samples should be spread thinly and evenly onto the glass slide. One or two slides may be used. The ectocervical spatula should be smeared across the slide, and both sides of the spatula should be sampled. The endocervical sample is placed by rolling the applicator across the slide using gentle pressure; rubbing the applicator back and forth results in a less desirable specimen. After the slide is prepared, it must quickly be fixed because even brief exposure to air can cause distortion of the cells. The slides can be fixed either by immersion in ethyl alcohol or by flooding with spray fixative. Once the slide has been adequately fixed, it can be sent to the laboratory for processing. The slide must be properly labeled and the requisition must contain all pertinent patient and clinical data.

Grading of the smear

Table 5-1 lists the classification of Papanicolaou smears.

5.2 COLPOSCOPY

George T. Danakas, M.D., and Karen Houck, M.D.

A colposcope is a binocular microscope with magnification from 6× to 40× and a variable intensity light source to allow visualization of the lower genital tract. The box on page 63 lists the common terms in colposcopy.

Table 5-1 Classification of Papanicolaou smears

Bethesda System	WHO System	CIN System	Class
Within normal limits	Normal	Normal	I
Infection/reactive and reparative changes	Inflammatory atypia		II
Squamous cell Abnormalities Atypical squamous cells of undetermined significance (ASCUS)	Squamous atypia	Cervical intraepithelial neoplasia (CIN)	
Squamous intraepithelial Lesion	Dysplasia		III
Low grade SIL:HPV	Mild	CIN I	
High grade SIL	Moderate	CIN II	
	Severe	CIN III	IV
	Carcinoma in situ	CIN IV	
Squamous cell cancer	Squamous cell cancer	Squamous cell cancer	V

SIL, Squamous intraepithelial lesion; *HPV*, human papillomavirus; *CIN*, cervical intraepithelial neoplasia.

Patient preparation and procedure

1. The patient is placed in the lithotomy position, and the largest speculum that can comfortably be inserted is used to visualize the cervix and upper vagina.
2. Any excess mucus is gently removed with a cotton swab.
3. The entire cervix and transition zone must be clearly visualized. Inability to visualize the entire squamocolumnar junction results in an unsatisfactory colposcopy.
4. A green filter and high magnification may be used to allow improved visualization of the subepithelial angioarchitecture and to help identify abnormal vasculature.
5. Acetic acid (3% to 5%) is gently applied to the cervix with a cotton swab. Acetic acid reacts with nuclear protein, causing the tissue to swell, which prevents light from passing through it. Abnormal or dysplastic lesions have a large amount of nuclear protein; they therefore have a strong reaction to acetic acid and appear white (acetowhite).
6. Once abnormal tissue has been identified, colposcopic biopsy can be performed using a cervical biopsy punch. If needed, multiple biopsies can be obtained. Each biopsy should be sent separately and labeled as to its location of origin. Any bleeding from the biopsy site can be controlled with Monsel's solution or a silver nitrate stick.
7. An endocervical curettage (ECC) allows sampling of the endocervical canal above the squamocolumnar junction.
8. It is necessary to make a carefully diagrammed picture of the findings in the chart as well as to document plans for follow-up.

Colposcopic Terminology

1. Acetowhite epithelium (modification of epithelium after application of 5% acetic acid solution).
   Grade 1: pale, pinkish appearance of underlying stroma still visible
   Grade 2: whiter epithelium, increased thickness
   Grade 3: very opaque, irregular surface
2. Punctation: set of vascular red dots disseminated in acetowhite lesion. Regularity and coarseness vary with severity of lesion.
3. Mosaic: surface vessels arranged in a mosaic pattern. Density and irregularity of epithelial paving vary with grade of lesion.
4. Hyperkeratosis: white epithelial lesion present before acetic acid application representing surface keratin.
5. Abnormal vessels: abnormal forms of surface vessels described as commas, corkscrews, or spaghetti-like. These vessels are signs of invasive disease.

From Alexander Meisels, Carol Morin: *Cytopathology of the uterine cervix*, p. 196. © 1991 by the American Society of Clinical Pathologists.

5.3 HYSTEROSCOPY

Harold C. Castelone, M.D.

As more physicians become aware of the inadequacy of the dilation and curettage (D&C) in the diagnosis and treatment of abnormal uterine bleeding, hysteroscopy is gaining in popularity because of the greater amount of information it provides.

Indications

1. Abnormal uterine bleeding
2. Postmenopausal bleeding
3. Infertility
4. Lost intrauterine device (IUD)
5. Abnormal hysterosalpingogram
6. Repeated pregnancy loss

Contraindications

1. Infection of cervix or vagina
2. Cervical cancer
3. Pregnancy
4. Profuse bleeding

Equipment

1. Rigid hysteroscopes—optics 0°, 12°, 30° (most common)
    a. Diagnostic
        (1) 5 mm, inflow only
        (2) 5.5 mm, continuous flow
    b. Operative
        (1) 9 mm (can be used for diagnosis)
2. Flexible hysteroscopes (less brightness and color resolution)
    a. 3.6 mm, 0° optics
    b. 4.9 mm, 0° optics
3. Light source
    a. Halogen cold light
    b. Xenon for photography and camera
4. Video camera and monitor (optional for office work)
5. Carbon dioxide (CO_2) insufflator (office)
6. Solutions for uterine distension
    a. High viscosity, Hyskon (32% dextran)
    b. Low viscosity
        (1) Nonelectrolyte
            (a) 3% sorbitol
            (b) 1½% glycine
        (2) Electrolyte
            (a) Saline
            (b) Ringer's lactate
7. Photographic equipment for recording of findings

Locations for diagnostic hysteroscopy

1. Office
2. Hospital or surgery center

Procedure

1. Do in proliferative phase when possible.
2. Achieve adequate anesthesia.
   a. General
   b. Basal and local
   c. Local only with preoperative analgesic
3. Ascertain position of uterus.
4. Place tenaculum on cervix.
5. Attempt to pass scope with fluid or CO_2 running.
6. If unable to pass scope, dilate cervix, avoiding passage of dilator beyond internal os.
7. Pass scope to fundus under direct visualization.
8. Observe shape of cavity, ostia, thickness of endometrium, presence or absence of septa, adhesions, myomas, polyps, and irregular surface contour.
9. Observe all surfaces of uterus.
10. Photograph salient features.
11. Observe cervical canal as scope is slowly withdrawn.
12. Avoid intrauterine pressure > 100 mm Hg (uterine distension is achieved at 75 mm Hg) by gauge if using CO_2 or by hanging fluids 1½ m above patient.

Benefits

1. Diagnosis and localization of polyps, myomas, septa, adhesions, adenomyosis, polypoid endometrial hyperplasia, carcinoma, and IUDs
2. Directed tissue sampling

Complications

1. Infection
2. Bleeding
3. Uterine perforation
4. Interruption of early pregnancy
5. Cervical laceration (by tenaculum or dilator)
6. NOTE: D&C has the same complications but also results in a missed diagnosis 10% to 35% of the time.

Practical tips

1. Do procedure in proliferative phase so endometrium is thinner.
2. Always attempt to insert the hysteroscope before any other instrument.
3. Advance scope to fundus under direct vision.
4. If using a 30° lens, rotate the scope to view tubal ostia and all surfaces of the uterus by grasping the light cord with the dominant hand.
5. Hold the video camera with the nondominant hand to prevent rotation of the camera using the third, fourth, and fifth fingers.

6. Focus camera as necessary with the thumb and index finger.
7. If necessary to clear blood, do the following:
   a. Remove and reinsert scope.
   b. Dilate cervix more to allow egress of fluid.
   c. Use catheter in uterus to drain blood and wash out with saline.
8. Document findings with photographs.
9. Do not allow the camera to rotate. This is a common mistake, and it destroys the orientation.
10. Do not insert any instrument into the uterus before the scope. This causes bleeding or partial tearing of the endometrium, making visualization difficult.

5.4 ABDOMINAL-PELVIC DIAGNOSTIC LAPAROSCOPY

Scott J. Zuccala, D.O., Germaine M. Buck, Ph.D., and
Ronald E. Batt, M.D.

Preadmission preparation

Dictate a problem-oriented preoperative note summarizing all previous operative reports, consultations, history, and physical and laboratory findings. Read this note 5 minutes before surgery to focus on the patient's problems.

Obtain an operative consent in the office as part of the process of informed consent. Discuss risks, benefits, and alternatives to the procedure.

Advise the patient not to take any nonsteroidal antiinflammatory drugs (NSAIDs) for 2 weeks before surgery.

Order mechanical cleansing of bowel and betadine douche the night before surgery.

Operating room preparation for a right-handed surgeon (Fig. 5-1)

1. Lower genital tract instruments
   a. Straight catheter in urinary bladder
   b. Uterine dilator in uterus for manipulation
   c. Rectal probe available for manipulation
2. Instruments for open laparoscopy
   a. Toothed forceps
   b. No. 15 scalpel
   c. (2) narrow S retractors
   d. (2) short, straight Kocher clamps
   e. (2) tonsil clamps (Varco Clamps)
   f. Metzenbaum scissors
   g. 2-0 Vicryl suture on urology needle for fascia
   h. Hasson laparoscopic cannula
   i. 10-mm 180° laparoscope
   j. Video camera
   k. (2) Video monitors, one with photographic printer
   l. (2) Short, screw-type 5-mm trochars (Apple Company)
   m. Laser suction irrigator with lactated Ringer's solution
   n. Calibrated probe

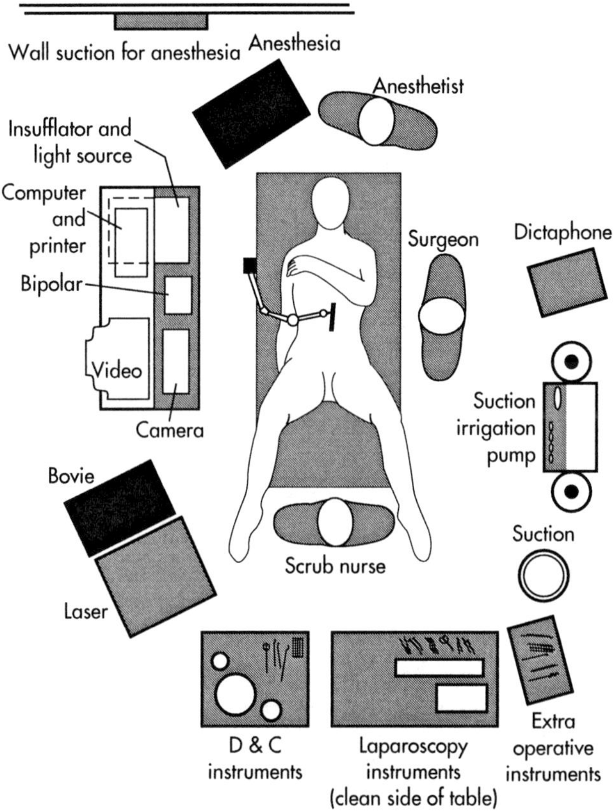

Figure 5-1
Layout of the operating room. The operating theater should be comfortable and efficient, with all instrumentation and personnel available. (From Hunt RB: *Atlas of female infertility surgery,* ed 2, St Louis, 1992, Mosby.)

o. Ovarian biopsy forceps to grasp and palpate lesions
p. Bipolar forceps
q. 10-mm 30° laparoscope (available)
r. 5-mm laparoscope (available)

3. Instruments for laparoscopic surgery
   a. 10-mm laser-operating laparoscope with coupler
   b. Hot water, to warm laparoscope to body temperature
   c. Superpulse carbon dioxide laser or KTP laser
   d. Sharp scissors (available)
   e. (2) Atraumatic grasping forceps
   f. Monopolar dissecting needle and generator

4. Allen stirrups: While awake, the patient is placed in the low thigh dorsal lithotomy position to ensure comfort to back, hips, and lower extremities.
5. Left arm: The left armboard should be avoided. The patient's left arm should be tucked across the chest to increase the right-handed surgeon's access to the operative field. Comfort reduces fatigue.
6. Right arm: The right arm is extended on an armboard to receive the intravenous fluids.
7. General anesthesia: The patient is anesthetized with an intratracheal tube and a warming unit for the upper half of the body to prevent hypothermia during surgery.
8. Examination under anesthesia: Betadine preparation and sterile draping; bladder emptied by straight metal catheter. Examine the pelvis thoroughly. Determine the position of the uterus. Insert and fix an intrauterine dilator or HUMI catheter to control uterine movement during the operation. Place straight catheter to drainage in anticipation of an operative laparoscopic surgery.
9. Height of operating table for laparoscopy: Height should be adjusted to the comfort of the tallest surgeon; shorter members of the operating team should stand on stools as needed for comfort.
10. One surgeon controls the operation: Both diagnostic and operative laparoscopy should be performed by one surgeon. The assistant should assist, not attempt to perform the surgery. The assistant should be still, maintain surgical exposure, and hold the video camera for the surgeon if requested.

Examination procedure

1. Placement of Hasson cannula

   Note: The patient should remain supine with no degree of Trendelenberg before the insertion of all trocars to prevent injury to the aorta, the vena cava, and the iliac vessels.

   a. Umbilicus: The depths of the umbilicus must be thoroughly cleaned with cotton swabs and betadine to remove all lint and powder.
   b. Vertical infraumbilical skin incision: The surgeon elevates the skin of umbilicus at 6 o'clock with a toothed forceps, while the assistant spreads the umbilicus open with a tonsil clamp. The surgeon makes a vertical incision through the skin starting near the base of the umbilicus. The surgeon spreads the subcutaneous tissues with tonsil clamps to identify the white anterior fascia.
   c. Vertical fascial incision: Using two S clamps, the assistant separates the subcutaneous tissue and exposes the fascia. The surgeon identifies, grasps, and elevates the white anterior fascia with two straight Kocher clamps and incises in the midline with scalpel. The surgeon spreads the incision with the tonsil clamp. The rectus muscles should be visible. The surgeon places two stay sutures through the fascia for later fixation of the Hasson cannula.
   d. Vertical incision in posterior sheath: Using two S clamps, the assistant separates the areolar tissue to expose the posterior sheath. The surgeon identifies, grasps, and elevates the white posterior sheath with two tonsil clamps. The surgeon carefully incises the posterior sheath with scissors. (Occasionally the peritoneum is incised at the same time.)

e. Vertical incision in peritoneum: Using two S clamps, the assistant separates the areolar tissue to expose the peritoneum. The surgeon identifies, grasps, and elevates the white peritoneum with two tonsil clamps, being observant for underlying bowel adhesions. The surgeon incises the peritoneum vertically with scissors. In obese patients, the peritoneum may be entered bluntly with the index finger. Neither technique guarantees prevention of bowel injury.
f. Insertion of Hasson cannula: With confirmation of intraabdominal entry, an S retractor is placed thorough the opening and the Hasson cannula is inserted using the retractor as a guide. Insufflate the abdomen with CO_2 to a pressure of 18 mm Hg, not to exceed 20 mm Hg. Insert the laparoscope and check for bleeding.
g. Depth adjustment of Hasson cannula: Withdraw the laparoscope into the cannula. Loosen the screw and, holding the acorn tip snugly against the abdomen, withdraw the cannula until the edge of the peritoneum comes into view; then insert the cannula inward 0.5 cm, tighten the screw, and fix the stay sutures.

2. Placement of trochars lateral to deep epigastric vessels
   a. Identify deep epigastric vessels: On the video screen, the surgeon identifies the right, deep epigastric vessels. The deep epigastric vessels are marked with the surgeon's left hand, and the anterior superior iliac spine is marked with the index finger of the surgeon's left hand. The abdominal wall is transilluminated between the deep epigastric vessels and the anterior superior iliac spine to identify superficial blood vessels. The skin is incised in a clear area.
   b. The surgeon inserts the 5-mm trochar through the fascia and peritoneum, keeping the sharp point under constant visual control. The trochar is directed toward the uterus. *The trochar is never directed laterally or inferiorly toward the iliac vessels.* The sharp stylet is removed, and the calibrated probe is inserted.
   c. The procedure is repeated for the left lower quadrant trochar with the deep epigastric vessels marked with the index finger of the surgeon's left hand and the left anterior superior iliac spine marked with the thumb of the surgeon's left hand. The laser-suction irrigator is inserted.
3. Bipolar forceps test
   a. The surgeon identifies a fine, superficial blood vessel on the bladder peritoneum and tests the bipolar forceps.
4. Three-step laparoscopic examination
   a. Step I: abdominal examination in supine position
      (1) The gall bladder, liver, diaphragms, stomach, omentum, spleen, splenic flexure, transverse colon, hepatic flexure, ascending colon, cecum, and vermiform appendix are examined. Endometriosis, adhesions, malrotation of the bowel, or inflammatory disease are looked for.
      (2) A calibrated probe is placed through the right lower quadrant portal to elevate the liver for examination of the gall bladder. The suction irrigator is placed through the left lower quadrant portal to lift the liver to examine the stomach. The omentum is moved to examine the spleen, splenic flexure of the colon, transverse colon, and hepatic flexure of the colon. The left lower quadrant suction irrigator is lain in the right colic gutter,

and the cecum is gently lifted and rotated medially. The mobility of the right colon and the status of the vermiform appendix are ascertained.

(3) Where detailed examination of the transverse colon and jejunum is required, the surgeon should stand between the patient's legs and use two atraumatic instruments to run the bowel.

b. Step 2: examination of small bowel and left colon

(1) With the patient in the steep Trendelenberg position, the surgeon examines the distal 150 cm of ileum, descending colon, sigmoid colon, rectum, rectovaginal pouch of Douglas, and uterosacral ligaments. The ileum is checked for endometriosis, Crohn's disease, adhesions, and Meckel's diverticulum. The surgeon examines the descending colon, sigmoid colon, and rectum for endometriosis, malignancy, diverticulitis, and adhesive disease, and the rectovaginal pouch and uterosacral ligaments for endometriosis.

(2) Starting at the ileal–cecal junction, the surgeon uses two instruments to gently elevate the loops of small bowel out of the pelvis to a position above the sacral promontory.

(3) With the uterus anteverted, the surgeon uses two instruments to elevate the sigmoid colon out of the pelvis and put the rectum on stretch for examination. The rectum points like an arrow to any deep rectal endometriosis adherent to the uterosacral ligaments or uterus.

(4) The surgeon examines the rectovaginal pouch for endometriosis. The rectal probe may be used with advantage to differentiate between an open, partially obliterated, and obliterated rectovaginal pouch, and between rectal and pararectal endometriosis. Rectal lesions can be palpated between the rectal and abdominal probes. Deep peritoneal endometriosis can be grasped with a pair of toothed ovarian biopsy forceps, elevated and evaluated for size and depth of invasion.

c. Step 3: alpha sequence examination of the pelvis

(1) Alpha sequence: The surgeon examines the anterior abdominal wall, round ligaments, bladder, anterior uterus, posterior uterus, and uterosacral ligaments; then the *left* anterior broad ligament, fallopian tube, ovary, ureter, and posterior broad ligament; and last, the *right* anterior broad ligament, fallopian tube, ovary, ureter, and posterior broad ligament.

(2) The surgeon examines for endometriosis, malignancy, fibroids, salpingitis isthmica nodosa, hydrosalpinx, pelvic adhesions, and congenital anomalies: inguinal hernias, peritoneal pockets, deep recesses in the lateral pelvic wall(s), medial displacement of the ureter(s), and pelvic kidney.

(3) With the uterus retroverted into the rectovaginal pouch, the surgeon examines the anterior abdominal wall, round ligaments, bladder, anterior uterus, and uterine fundus.

(4) With the uterus anteverted, the surgeon examines the posterior uterus, the uterosacral ligaments, and the rectovaginal pouch for a second time.

(5) Then the surgeon examines the left fallopian tube from the cornual angle laterally. The left ovary is examined on all surfaces, elevating it with the contralateral instrument and holding it with the ipsilateral instrument. Still holding the ovary and tube, the surgeon lifts the sigmoid colon medially with the right lower quadrant instrument and examines the left pelvic wall and posterior broad ligament. The surgeon locates the pulsations of the hypogastric artery. Usually the ureter runs lateral to the hypogastric artery in the posterior pelvis. The relation of the ureter to the hypogastric artery, the infundibulopelvic ligament, and the uterosacral ligament should be noted.

(6) The surgeon examines the right fallopian tube, the right ovary, the right pelvic wall and broad ligament, the right hypogastric artery, and the ureter in same sequence.

5. Proceed to laparoscopic surgery

Hemostasis

The surgeon checks for complete hemostasis; all trochars are withdrawn under direct visualization and the pneumoperitoneum is decompressed. Fascial sutures are tied on all 10-mm incisions. The skin is closed with inverted 5-0 vicryl subcuticular sutures or with interrupted nylon skin sutures.

Operative report

The laparoscopic photographs, preadmission note, and the American Fertility Society Revised Classification form are assembled. The surgeon dictates the operative report immediately in the same sequence as the three-step abdominal–pelvic laparoscopic examination.

Suggested Reading

Batt RE, Wheeler JM: Endometriosis: advanced diagnostic laparoscopy. In Hunt RB, editor: *Atlas of female infertility surgery,* ed 2, St Louis, 1992, Mosby, pp. 422-435.

Batt RE, Wheeler JM: Endometriosis: advanced laparoscopic surgery. In Hunt RB, editor: *Atlas of female infertility surgery,* ed 2, St Louis, 1992, Mosby, pp. 436-453.

Hasson HM: Open techniques for equipment insertion. In Martin DC, editor: *Manual of endoscopy,* Sante Fe Springs, Calif, 1990, American Association of Gynecologic Laparoscopists, pp. 23-29.

Hulka JF, Reich H: *Textbook of laparoscopy,* ed 2, Philadelphia, 1994, WB Saunders.

Soderstom RM: *Operative laparoscopy: the masters' techniques,* New York, 1993, Raven Press.

5.5 BOWEL INJURY

Salvador M. Udagawa, M.D., Germaine M. Buck, Ph.D., and
Ronald E. Batt, M.D.

Small intestine

Injury to the small intestine may occur during difficult operations; this is especially true of operations in the pelvis for neoplastic or inflammatory diseases, in endometriosis, or when there have been previous multiple surgeries. Injuries vary from partial to through-and-through small or large lacerations, perforations, monopolar or bipolar burn injuries, and avulsion injuries to the mesentery and hemorrhages. Success in management of these complications depends on their immediate recognition and treatment. Failure or delay in identifying these injuries may lead to other more serious complications.[1,2]

1. Laceration injury to small bowel
    a. After proper local hemostasis, irrigation, and debridement, the bowel may be closed safely with interrupted nonabsorbable sutures. It is closed transversely according to the Heineke-Mikulicz principle.
    b. Large lacerations or multiple small lacerations in the same segment are treated with a limited resection and an end-to-end anastomosis.
    c. Lacerations to the mesenteric border, unless they are quite small, are difficult to repair and may be associated with vascular impairment. When in doubt of the vascular integrity, a resection should be undertaken. Antibiotic coverage should be used accordingly in relation to the degree and duration of local contamination.
2. Perforation injury to small bowel
    a. Sharp and small perforations, such as those inflicted by the Veress needle used in laparoscopy, are self-limited and may require a small pursestring closure if leakage is confirmed.
    b. Sharp and large perforations such as those inflicted by primary and secondary laparoscopic trochars need a careful local assessment and immediate primary closure using interrupted, nonabsorbable suture material. As in all penetrating or stab wounds of the bowel, ideally the trochar or sleeve should not be removed to facilitate location and repair of single, through-and-through and multiple puncture injuries to the bowel.
3. Thermal injury to small bowel
    a. The most serious injury is the one caused by monopolar energy with necrosis of the bowel wall beyond the area of actual perforation. If a persistent blanched area or a blanched area around a perforation is found, resect at least 5 cm of bowel on either side of the injury.[3] Examine minutely for active bleeding from the wound edges after debridement or resection before local repair or bowel anastomosis is done. Active bleeding from the wound edges indicates healthy blood supply that is nesscary for optimal healing.
    b. Wound resection adequate to reach viable tissue is less extensive after a bipolar or a laser energy burn to the bowel. Nevertheless, the surgeon is encouraged to resect and debride the injury until there is active bleeding from the wound edges before proceeding to local repair or bowel anastomosis as needed.
4. Avulsion injury to mesentery
    a. Avulsion injuries usually occur from undue traction exerted on the mesentery. Copious bleeding is the most troublesome. Safe control of the hemorrhage requires adequate exposure and visualization. The surgeon can confidently and deliberately control the exact bleeding point without resorting to the use of mass suture ligatures or thermocoagulation. It is better to provide local tamponage, for a few minutes, with steady finger pressure to the bleeding area or by means of a small pack. The bleeding will have ceased and individual ligation of lacerated blood vessels

can be done. Repair of large and important veins may be necessary.

Colon and rectum

The morbidity and mortality from injuries to the colon have been significantly reduced by an aggressive surgical approach. Sepsis is the most formidable added risk when dealing with colonic injury.

Specific care should be directed by the type, location, and extent of injury as well as the condition of the colon, whether or not it is obstructed and distended or is simply filled with fecal content. Also the anatomic location of the injury is important: whereas injuries to the *intraperitoneal* right, transverse, and sigmoid colon do not require drainage, injuries to the *retroperitoneal* descending colon and rectum require that the suture line be protected by retroperitoneal drainage and/or fecal diversion by colostomy.

It is important that the time from injury to definitive operation be as short as possible. It is similarly important to avoid, by all means, fecal soilage or contamination. Antimicrobials are not a substitute for surgical technique. However, antibiotics should be used judiciously preoperatively and postoperatively.

1. Diagnosis
   a. A sudden smell of fecal odor during an abdominal or laparoscopic procedure, even in the absence of visible extravasation of stool, indicates an entrance into the colon or rectum. Careful inspection leads to the recognition of the injury and a complete repair.
   b. Plain film of the abdomen should be employed if there is a perforated colon with leakage of air into the free peritoneal cavity following laparotomy. This examination is of limited value after laparoscopic procedures. Sigmoidoscopy or colonoscopy can be used in the examination of patients suspected of colonic perforation after surgery. CT scan of the abdomen and pelvis may be helpful in selected cases. Barium contrast material should not be used because of the high morbidity and mortality associated with leakage of barium and feces into the free peritoneal cavity. Aqueous opaque media such as Gastrografin are preferable when penetration of the colon is suspected.
2. Treatment
   a. An incision capable of an easy extension is used because operation on the colon often requires wide mobilization of at least two flexures. Incisional infections are discouraged by protecting the wound with moist pads or 7-in. ring plastic wound protectors (Vidrape, 3M Corporation).
   b. First the peritoneal cavity should be carefully explored and close examination of the lesion itself reserved for last. The strategy of the operation is planned, and the procedure is conducted with the avoidance of contamination or bleeding.

References

1. Levy BS, Soderstrom RM, Dail DH: Bowel injuries during laparoscopy: gross anatomy and histology, *J Reprod Med* 30:168-179, 1985.
2. Soderstrom RM: Bowel injury litigation after laparoscopy, *J Am Assoc Gynecol Laparoscopists* 1:74-77, 1993.

3. Soderstom RM: *Operative laparoscopy: the masters' techniques,* New York, 1993, Raven Press, p. 195.

5.6 URETERAL DISSECTION

Ronald E. Batt, M.D., and Germaine M. Buck, Ph.D.

Precise localization of the ureters is recommended before all operative interventions. Ureteral dissection and displacement from harm is recommended whenever the possibility of ureteral injury exists. Placement of ureteral catheters preoperatively is recommended in patients with extensive pelvic disease that distorts the pelvic anatomy.

Indication for ureteral dissection

1. When operating near the ureter, it is safer and faster to dissect and expose the ureter to clear view than to stop repeatedly and check its position or perform the dissection under emergency circumstances.
2. Ureteral dissection is recommended in the following instances:
   a. Obliteration of rectovaginal pouch by deep fibrotic endometriosis
   b. Medial displacement of ureter near uterosacral ligaments
   c. Excision of deep fibrotic endometriosis from vaginal cuff and uterosacral ligaments, status posthysterectomy
   d. Deep endometriosis adherent to or partially obstructing the ureter
   e. Left-frozen-pelvis from endometriosis
   f. Ovary, oviduct, or sigmoid colon adherent to ureter
   g. Extensive chronic salpingo-oophoritis.
   h. Laparoscopically assisted vaginal hysterectomy (LAVH) for endometriosis
   i. Extraperitoneal lymphadenectomy for malignancy
   j. To isolate and ligate retracted bleeding uterine artery
   k. Salpingo-oophorectomy

Topograpohical anatomy

1. Anatomic divisions of the ureter
   a. The iliopectineal line divides the ureter into abdominal and pelvic portions. The pelvic ureter is divided into the following three parts:
      (1) The pars posterior, which runs from the sacroiliac joint along the lateral pelvic wall to the entrance of the preformed tunnel in the cardinal ligament
      (2) The pars intermedia, which runs within the broad ligament to the vesicouterine ligament
      (3) The pars anterior, which runs from the entrance into the vesicouterine ligament to the ureteral orifice of the bladder
   b. The left ureter may be identified above the iliopectineal line at the apex of the intersigmoid fossa by displacing the left adnexa anterolaterally and the sigmoid colon medially and cephalad. In difficult cases, the ureter may be located near the pelvic brim, lateral to the pulsations of the hypogastric artery. Normal peristalsis should be observed. When the ureter lies close to the infundibulopelvic ligament, the infundibulopelvic ligament must be displaced laterally. This maneuver compresses the peritoneum over the ureter and facilitates identification.

   c. The right ureter crosses the iliac vessels at the bifurcation of the common iliac artery and is easier to locate than the left ureter. Near the pelvic brim, it lies lateral to the pulsations of the hypogastric artery.
2. Congenital anomalies: medial displacement of one or both ureters occurs in the following ways[1]:
   a. As an isolated congenital anomaly
   b. In association with peritoneal pockets in the posterior pelvis
   c. As the medial border of a large broad ligament recess
3. The sigmoid colon traps menstrual detritis against the left ureter, increasing the risk of endometriosis. It may also envelop the left tube and ovary in dense obliterative adhesions in response to repeated ruptures of an ovarian endometrioma.

Operative procedures for ureteral dissection

1. Preoperative preparation
   a. The surgeon examines old operative reports.
   b. An intravenous pyelogram (IVP) is recommended when there is severe and extensive endometriosis and selectively in other situations.
   c. Cleansing enemas or a formal bowel preparation are recommended the day before surgery.
2. Excision of endometriosis at the level of the left ovary[3]: Endometriotic plaques overlying or invading the ureter are often associated with endometriomas of the ovary.
   a. The course of the left ureter must be explored and defined before adhesiolysis is attempted.
   b. The surgeon elevates the peritoneum lateral to the ureter with a toothed forceps and incises (with scissors or CO_2 laser) for a distance of 2 cm to expose the ureter and the endometriosis.
   c. The surgeon separates the ureter from surrounding tissues, using blunt aquadissection and perpendicular and parallel spreading with a blunt dissecting forceps.
   d. With the ureter exposed, the ovarian adhesions are placed on tension and the initial incision is made with scissors or a CO_2 laser. Gentle blunt aquadissection with the suction irrigator usually completes the ovariolysis.
   e. The ovarian endometrioma(s) is excised to improve surgical exposure.
   f. The peritoneal incision is extended lateral to the endometriotic plaque.
   g. The surgeon grasps the lateral margin of the endometriotic plaque with a pair of toothed forceps and reflects it medially.
   h. The endometriotic plaque is dissected with aquadissection and blunt spreading forceps, cutting the peritoneum and dense adhesion bands to the muscularis of the ureter with scissors or a CO_2 laser.
   i. Caution must be exercised so that the dense adhesion bands do not tent the ureter. This dissection may be tedious and time consuming. The surgeon should be gentle and persistent, avoiding impulsive moves and rough dissection.

j. Hemoclips or fine bipolar forceps can be used for hemostasis. The surgeon excises the endometriosis.
k. The surgeon examines the ureter. Additional ureterolysis is performed if needed.
l. The peritoneal wounds are left open to heal.

3. Excision of endometriosis at level of the left uterosacral ligaments[3]: Medial displacement of the ureter adjacent to the uterosacral ligament may occur as a congenital anomaly or from contraction of deep fibrotic endometriosis in the uterosacral or broad ligament. Dissection of the ureter must be performed very carefully to avoid brisk bleeding from the extensive venous network in the cardinal ligament and from the uterine artery. The retroperitoneal approach is recommended.[5]
   a. The peritoneum is incised lateral to the ureter 2 cm from the cardinal ligament, and the incision is extended caudally.
   b. The ureter is dissected free with aquadissection and perpendicular and parallel spreading with a blunt dissecting forceps, until it can be displaced laterally with a blunt probe.
   c. Hemostasis is applied with clips or bipolar coagulation. If bipolar coagulation is necessary to control bleeding, the power density must be kept low to prevent the lateral spread of thermal energy, but it must be sufficient for hemostasis.
   d. With the ureter displaced laterally, the surgeon grasps the endometriosis with a pair of toothed forceps and maintains constant medial traction.
   e. Excision with hemostasis is facilitated by use of the CO_2 or KTP laser. Scissors dissection may require hemostasis with hemoclips or bipolar electrocoagulation.
   f. To prevent or control bleeding or hematoma formation in the broad ligament, the uterine artery must be ligated. The paravesical and pararectal spaces must be opened and developed. The surgeon identifies the external iliac vein and artery, the internal iliac artery, the uterine artery, and the ureter. The surgeon displaces the ureter medially out of harm's way and ligates the uterine artery with clips, bipolar electrocoagulation, or ligature.[5]
4. Dissection of left-frozen-pelvis: In some cases of extensive endometriosis (greater than RAFS stage IV-70), the left tube and ovary are irrecoverably damaged, trapped by obliterative, adhesive disease between the sigmoid colon and the pelvic wall. The left-frozen-pelvis may be a complication of previous conservative surgery. The ureter is particularly at risk for ligation or transection. The experienced pelvic endosurgeon may attempt retroperitoneal dissection and left salpingo-oophorectomy; however, the prudent course in most cases is to gain access to the pelvis by laparotomy.[2]
5. Dissection of frozen pelvis and frozen ureter: When the pelvic anatomy is totally distorted by obliterative endometriotic disease and the ureters are firmly embedded in endometriosis, laparotomy is recommended as the only mode of access. The surgical team (gynecologist, colorectal surgeon, and urologist) should be prepared for bowel resection as well as resection of the ureter(s) and implantation into the bladder.

Preoperative ureteral catheters

Surgery for severe and extensive endometriosis is often more challenging than surgery for malignancy. Deeply invasive disease combined with dense, obliterative adhesions so distort pelvic anatomy that dissection is long, tedious, and bloody. Ureteral catheters facilitate identification of the ureters and should be used in such cases. This gives the urologist an opportunity to meet the patient, read the detailed preoperative note, and perform a cystoscopy and insert the ureteral catheters. If a urologic problem arises, the urologist comes to the operating table prepared.

Ureteral injuries

A detailed discussion of detection and intraoperative repair of ureteral injuries, as well as the diagnosis and treatment of unrecognized ureteral injuries and unsuccessful ureteral repairs, is beyond the scope of this chapter. Detailed information is readily available.[4]

References

1. Batt RE et al: A case-series study of peritoneal pockets and endometriosis: rudimentary duplications of the mullerian system, *Adolesc Pediatr Gynecol* 2:47, 1989.
2. Batt RE, Udagawa SM, Wheeler JM: Endometriosis: microconservative surgery. In Hunt RB, editor: *Atlas of female infertility surgery,* ed 2, St Louis, 1992, Mosby, pp. 454-481.
3. Batt RE, Wheeler JM: Endometriosis: advanced laparoscopic surgery. In Hunt RB, editor: *Atlas of female infertility surgery,* ed 2, St Louis, 1992, Mosby, pp. 436-453.
4. Hurt WG, Jones CM III: Intraoperative ureteral injuries and urinary diversion. In Nichols DH, editor: *Gynecologic and obstetric surgery,* St Louis, 1993, Mosby, pp. 900-910.
5. Kadar N: An operative technique for laparoscopic hysterectomy using a retroperitoneal approach, *J Am Assoc Gynecol Laparoscopists* 1:365-377, 1994.

5.7 URODYNAMIC STUDIES

Philip J. Aliotta, M.D., M.S.H.A., F.A.C.S.

Definition

Urodynamics is the study of the changing parameters of bladder filling, storage, and emptying, dealing with the interaction of the bladder with its urethra.[15]

Steps in the micturition process

1. Voluntary relaxation of the external sphincter
2. Reduced sympathetic nervous system outflow
3. Smooth muscle relaxation with resultant funneling of the bladder neck and opening of urethra
4. Bladder contraction with evacuation of the bladder's contents

Urodynamic evaluation of the female patient

1. History (focuses on)
   a. Existing systemic disorders
   b. Congenital disorders
   c. Psychosocial factors

   d. Existing neurologic disorders
   e. Disorders specific to the urologic tract
2. Physical examination
   a. General examination
   b. Evaluation of estrogen status
   c. Examination of the vagina and periurethral area for signs of fistula, abscess, and diverticula
   d. Examination for cystocele, rectocele, and enterocele
   e. Rectal examination to assess sphincter tone and the bulbocavernosus reflex
   f. Neurologic examination
      (1) Mental status assessment
      (2) Assessment of cranial nerves II through XII
      (3) Cerebellar testing for truncal ataxia, gait ataxia, finger–nose test, heel–shin test
         (a) Clinically, cerebellar lesions produce spontaneous, high-amplitude detrusor reflex contractions
         (b) Poor hand coordination makes clean intermittent catheterization impractical
      (4) Deep tendon reflexes
         (a) Supranuclear lesions: hyperreflexia
         (b) Cauda equina lesions: diminished or absent reflex
         (c) Peripheral neuropathy: diminished or absent reflex
      (5) Sensory assessment
         (a) Pain and temperature awareness
         (b) Position, vibration, light, and crude touch
3. Frequency/volume voiding diary: an investigational record of fluid intake, output, and other voiding characteristics occuring in a 24 hour period that includes the following:
   a. Daily intake and output
   b. Frequency of micturition
   c. Time interval between voidings
   d. Volume voided
   e. Urgency
   f. Incontinence
   g. Number of continence pads used per day
4. Urinalysis and culture
   a. Treatment for existing infections
   b. Hematuria work-up
5. Radiographic evaluation
   a. Plain film of abdomen: to rule out bony abnormalities of the vertebral column and pelvis
   b. Intravenous pyelogram to assess the following:
      (1) Upper tract anatomy and anomalies
      (2) Ureters: ureteral ectopy and duplication
      (3) Bladder configuration and abnormalities of contour and position
      (4) Postvoid residual
      (5) Vesicovaginal fistula
   c. Video cystourethrography combines voiding cystourethrography

(VCUG), fluroscopy, and pressure recordings of the bladder and abdomen along with urinary flow rates

6. Urethroscopy
   a. Under direct visualization, the urethra is examined using a 0°, 5°, or 30° lens.
   b. Gas urethroscopy allows measurement of urethral opening pressure, which in a normal patient is between 70 and 90 cm of water.[13]
   c. Water urethroscopy does not allow for urethral opening pressures.
   d. The interior of the urethra is examined for any obstructing lesions, discharge from periurethral glands, diverticuli, or an ectopic ureter. The normal urethra has a pink epithelium.
   e. The bladder is entered, and the urethrovesical junction is examined during bladder filling. The urethrovesical junction is normally described as round and symmetric. The trigone, located on the floor of the bladder, is pale pink. The ureteral orifices appear as slitlike openings on the floor of the bladder and should be observed for expulsion of urine.
   f. The following changes are seen with bladder filling[13]:
      (1) The urethrovesical junction closes.
      (2) The periurethral striated muscles tighten (Table 5-2).
7. Residual urine
   a. Integrates the activity of the bladder and outlet during the emptying phase of micturition[18]
   b. Defined as the volume of fluid remaining in the bladder immediately following the completion of micturition[12]
   c. Estimated by using the following:
      (1) Catheter
      (2) Cystoscopy
      (3) Intravenous urogram (IVP)
      (4) VCUG
      (5) Radioisotope studies
   d. Findings
      (1) Increased residual (> 100 cc): failure to empty
      Possible causes include the following:
         (a) Anxiety (if suspected, repeat test)
         (b) Increased outlet resistance
         (c) Decreased bladder contractility
         (d) Combination of all of the above
      (2) No residual of significance (< 100 cc)
      Possible causes include the following:
         (a) Normal function
         (b) Increased bladder contractility
         (c) Incompetent sphincter
8. Uroflow studies: defined as the volume of fluid expelled from the urethra per unit time expressed in ml/sec.[18] It expresses the combined activity of the detrusor and urethra. The box on p. 80 lists the terminology of the International Continence Society relating to the urodynamic description of urinary flow. The flow pattern in Fig. 5-2 is normal. Minimum acceptable urine flow rates are listed in Table 5-3. Volumes under 150 cc should be interpreted with caution.[5]

Urine Flow Rate Parameters

Flow time: time over which measurable flow occurs
Time to maximum flow: time elapsed from the onset of flow to maximum rate
Maximum flow rate: the maximal rate of flow
Voided volume: the total volume expelled by way of the urethra
Average flow rate: the voided volume divided by flow time
Voiding time: the total duration of micturition, including interruptions
Flow pattern: may be continuous, interrupted, or specifically described

Table 5-2 Urethroscopy of normal and abnormal patients

Dynamic Function of the Urethrovesical Junction during	Normal	Genuine Stress Incontinence	Unstable Bladder
Empty bladder	Closed	Closed	Closed
Partially filled bladder	Closed	Slowly opens	Closed if no vesical contraction
Full bladder	Closed	Slowly opens	Closed if no vesical contraction
Holding	Closes	Sluggish closure	Closes
Straining	Remains closed	Opens	Remains closed if no vesical contraction
Coughing	Remains closed	Opens	Remains closed if no vesical contraction
Vesical contraction	Opens, then closes, with suppression		Opens and remains open due to inability to suppress
Ability to suppress a vesical contraction	Present	Present	Absent

Modified from Robertson JR: Dynamic urethroscopy. In Ostergard DR, Bent AE, editors: *Urogynecology and urodynamics–theory and practice,* Baltimore, 1991, Williams & Wilkins.

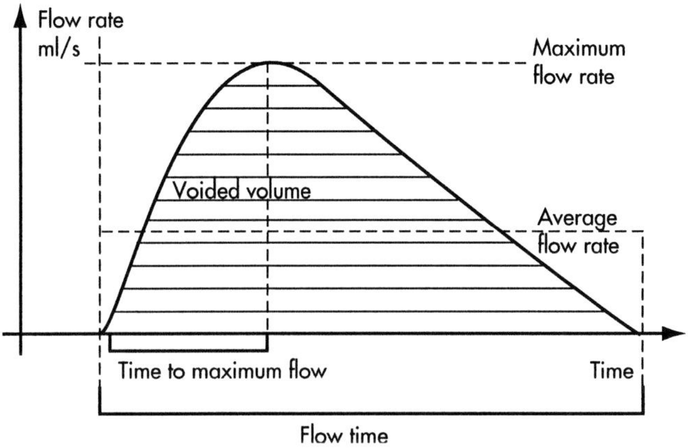

Figure 5-2
Terminology of the International Continence Society as it applies to a normal flow pattern (see also the box on p. 80). (From Wein AJ, English WS, Whitmore KE: *Urol Clin North Am* 15:621, 1988.)

Table 5-3 Minimum acceptable urine flow rates

Age (yr)	Minimum Voided Volume (ml)	Flow Rates (ml/sec)	
		Males	Females
4-7	100	10	10
8-13	100	12	15
14-45	200	21	18
46-55	200	22	15
56-80	200	9	10

From Abrams P: The urethral pressure profile measurement. In Mundy AR et al, editors: *Urodynamics: principles, practice, and application,* Edinburgh, 1984, Churchill Livingstone.

9. Urethral Pressure Profile
   a. Allows for the measurement of the active and passive tone of the urethra[15]
   b. Measures urethral pressure with the patient lying down, the bladder at rest, and the urethra closed
   c. Uses a specially designed catheter with multiple side holes and an occluded tip (Fluid infused along the catheter escapes through the side holes and the urethral pressure profile measures the resistance of the urethral walls to distension by the escaping fluid.)
   d. Nomenclature for the urethral pressure profile
      (1) Maximum urethral pressure: the maximum pressure of the profile

(2) Maximum urethral closing pressure: the difference between the maximum urethral pressure and bladder pressure
(3) Functional profile length: the length of the urethra along which the pressure exceeds bladder pressure
(4) Total urethral length: functional length plus the additional length to reach atmospheric pressure

e. Types of urethral pressure profile
(1) Static: measures urethral pressure with the patient lying down, the bladder at rest, and the urethra closed
(2) Perfusion: using saline or gas perfusion through a motorized syringe pump
(3) Stress: while the catheter is withdrawn from the bladder through the urethra at a rate of 0.1 cm/sec, the patient is asked to cough. In patients with genuine stress urinary incontinence, there is a failure of pressure transmission to the proximal two thirds of the urethra. Normal patients demonstrate intraabdominal pressure transmission to the proximal two thirds of the urethra.

Table 5-4 Dynamic changes seen with urethral pressure profiles: dynamic function of the urethral sphincteric mechanism in normal women and in patients with genuine stress incontinence

	Closure Pressure Response	
	Normal Patient	Stress Incontinent Patient
Changes with urethral closure pressure profile in response to the following		
Cough	Increased	Minimal to none
Valsalva	Increased	Minimal to none
Holding urine	Increased	Minimal to none
Contraction of perineal muscles	Increased	Minimal to none
Bladder distension*		
Empty	—	—
Partially full	Increase	Minimal to none
Full distenstion	Further increase	Minimal to none
Position*		
Supine	—	—
Sitting	Increase	Minimal to none
Standing	Further increase	Minimal to none

From Tanagho EA, Stoller ML: Urodynamics: cystometry and urethral closure pressure profile. In Ostergard DR, Bent AE, editors: *Urogynecology and urodynamics theory and practice,* Baltimore, 1991, Williams & Wilkins.

*Response in pressure, length, or both.

(4) Dynamic: shows variation in sphincteric closure pressure under various physiologic events, various stresses, and various commands (Table 5-4). It uses the membrane catheter or microtransducer technique.

f. Fig. 5-3 shows a normal perfusion urethral pressure profile.

10. Cystometrogram (Fig. 5-4)

a. Measures changes in bladder pressure with increases in bladder volume; evaluates the bladder's ability to fill uniformly and store urine, by assessing detrusor activity, sensation, capacity, and compliance

b. Definitions[12]

(1) Intravesical pressure: the pressure within the bladder

(2) Abdominal pressure: the pressure surrounding the bladder

(3) Detrusor pressure: a measure of the passive and active forces within the bladder wall, obtained by subtracting abdominal pressure from intravesical pressure

(4) Bladder sensation: subjective; involves the following:

(a) First desire to void

(b) Normal desire to void: feeling that leads the patient to pass urine at the next convenient moment (can be delayed or postponed)

(c) Strong desire to void: persistent desire to void without fear of leakage or pain

(d) Urgency: the strong desire to void accompanied by fear of leakage and pain

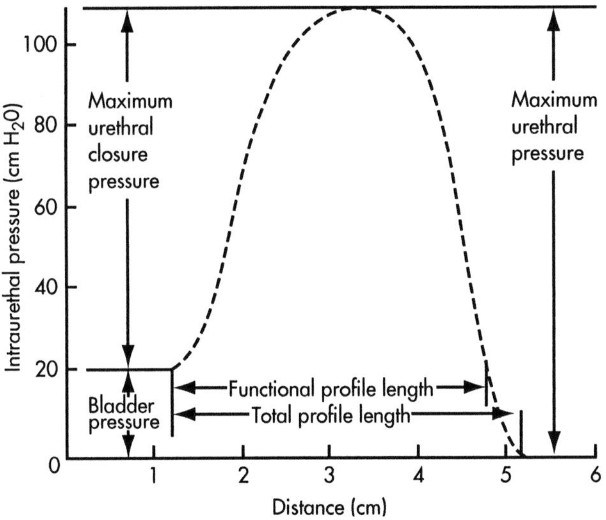

Figure 5-3
Normal perfusion urethral pressure profile.

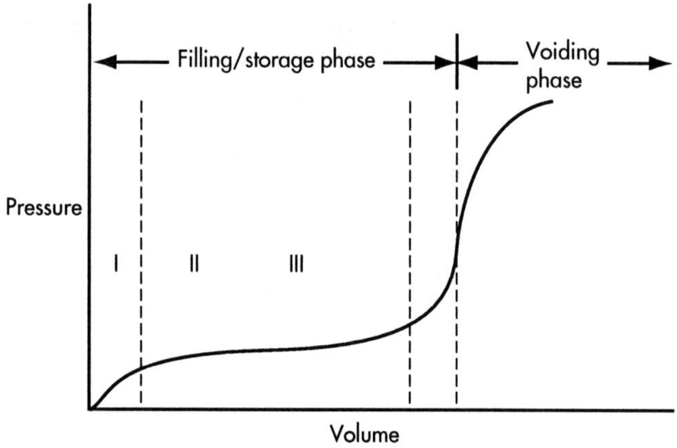

Figure 5-4
Normal adult cystometrogram. *I,* The compliance phase; *II,* the contraction phase; *III,* the voiding phase.

11. Three phases of bladder filling[6] (Fig. 5-5)
    a. The compliance phase is composed of the following:
        (1) An initial rise in pressure to achieve resting bladder pressure
        (2) A tonus limb that reflects the bladder's viscoelastic response to accommodating filling
            (a) Bladder compliance: the change in detrusor pressure that accompanies an increase in bladder volume during filling; not to exceed 15 cm of water. Compliance depends on the following:
                i. Rate of filling
                ii. The volume interval over which compliance is calculated
                iii. Bladder wall thickness
                iv. Mechanical bladder wall properties
                v. Shape of the bladder
                vi. Contractile and relaxant properties of the bladder wall
    b. The contraction phase characterizations
        (1) A rapid rise in intravesical pressure
        (2) Ability of patient to suppress voluntary voiding contractions
    c. The voiding phase
        (1) Requires an intact neural pathway to the brainstem micturition center
        (2) Coordination of the detrusor contraction with concomitant relaxation of the sphincter results in voiding
    d. Gas cystometry[15]
        (1) Clean and efficient
        (2) Allows rapid filling of the bladder

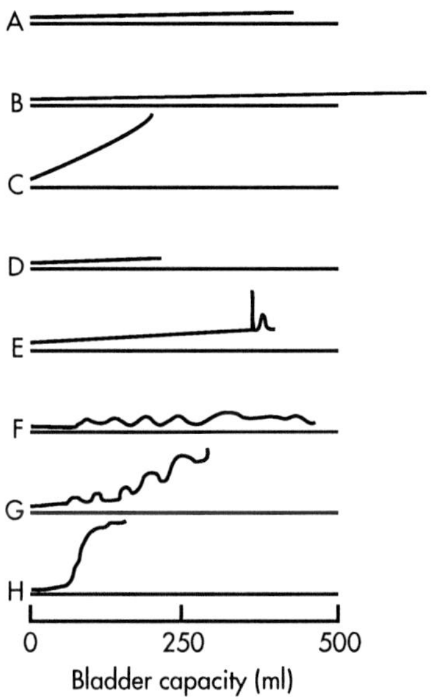

Figure 5-5
Various representative adult cystometrograms. **(A)** Normal filling curve in a patient with a bladder capacity of 450 ml, normal compliance, and no involuntary bladder contractions. Nothing can be said about bladder activity during the emptying phase of micturition from this tracing. **(B)** Large-capacity bladder with increased compliance at medium fill rate. This type of curve is characteristic of an individual with decreased sensation and bladder decompensation. Although most individuals will in fact have no or poor detrusor contraction, that conclusion cannot be made on the basis of this curve. **(C)** Decreased compliance. **(D)** Small-capacity bladder secondary to hypersensitivity without decreased compliance or involuntary bladder contraction. **(E)** Bladder contraction provoked by cough. This particular tracing represents total bladder pressure. To make this diagnosis from just this tracing would require either a very astute examiner or separate recordings of intravesical pressure and intra-abdominal pressure (intrarectal pressure). **(F)** Low-amplitude detrusor contractions. This is a subtracted bladder pressure, and this type of recording may be seen most characteristically in a patient with suprasacral neurologic disease or idiopathic detrusor instability. **(G)** Decreased compliance and involuntary bladder contractions. **(H)** High-amplitude early involuntary bladder contraction. (Redrawn from Wein AJ, English NS, Whitmore KE: *Urol Clin North Am* 15:609, 1988.)

(3) Impairs accommodation, producing a low-volume total capacity
(4) Irritating to the urothelium, producing discomfort and dysuria
(5) Gas compressibility may mask low-amplitude phasic contractions and blunt high-pressure contractions
(6) Gas can leak

e. Other terminology
   (1) Involuntary detrusor contraction: a phasic rise, uninhibited, in bladder pressure, generally provoked by a stimulus, which signifies a lack of accommodation on the part of the bladder during filling; pressures exceed 15 cm of water
   (2) Two phases of voluntary control
      (a) The ability to initiate a bladder contraction
      (b) The ability to inhibit the bladder contraction
   (3) Maximum functional capacity: the largest amount voided at any one time over a 24-hour observation period
   (4) Maximal cystometric capacity: the volume at which the patient feels micturition can no longer be delayed

12. Electromyography (EMG) (Fig. 5-6): defined as the study of electrical potentials generated by depolarization of muscle[12]
   a. Motor unit: functional unit in EMG
   b. Motor unit: described as a single motor neuron and the muscle fibers it innervates; comprises a single motor neuron and the muscle fibers it innervates
   c. Motor unit action potential: the recorded depolarization of muscle fibers that results from activation of a single anterior horn cell; muscle action potentials are detected by the following:
      (1) Surface electrode
         (a) Noninvasive
         (b) Comfortable
         (c) Determines gross motor activity
         (d) Cannot detect individual EMG potentials
         (e) Represents a total net record of anal or urethral sphincteric activity
      (2) Needle electrode
         (a) Monopolar/concentric
         (b) Invasive and uncomfortable
         (c) Produces an "injury potential"
         (d) Must be placed directly into the striated sphincter
         (e) Simultaneously records urethral, bladder, and rectal pressure changes and flow
   d. In a normal EMG tracing, with the bladder empty and at rest, there is a flat "quiet" baseline of activity with few random potentials.
   e. As bladder volume increases to 150 to 350 ml, more muscles depolarize and contract to maintain continence.
   f. As the bladder capacity is reached, maximal activation of perineal floor muscles occurs, producing a full interference pattern. With voiding there is silence.
   g. The progression from minimal activity to maximal activity with bladder filling is called the *guarding reflex.*
   h. Abnormal findings can be subdivided into the following categories[3]:
      (1) Upper motor neuron lesions
         (a) Loss of ability to contract or relax the sphincter voluntarily
         (b) Example: detrusor sphincter dyssynergia

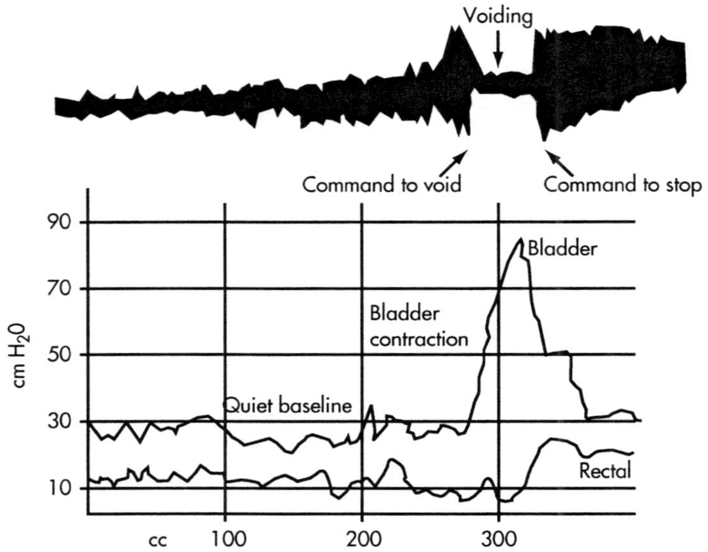

Figure 5-6
Normal pressure EMG tracing. (From Wein AJ, English WJ, Whitmore KE: *Urol Clin North Am* 15:609, 1988.)

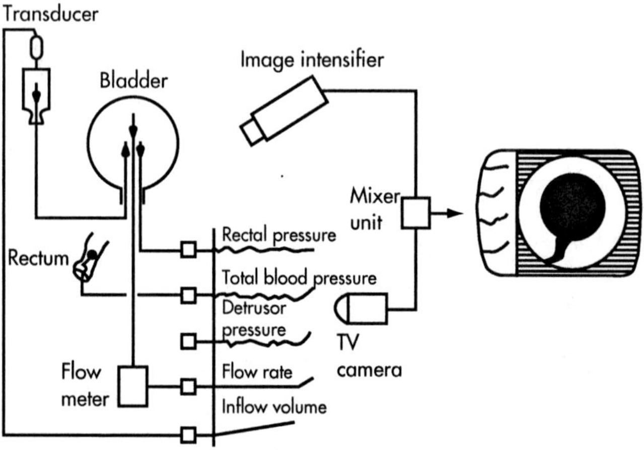

Figure 5-7
Typical videourodynamic system.

(2) Lower motor neuron lesions
   (a) Complete lesion: lesions of the spinal cord or cauda equina; total denervation of the striated sphincter
   (b) Incomplete lesion: partial denervation of the striated sphincter with consequent sphincteric contractions of poor magnitude
(3) Mixed neuron lesions
   (a) Demonstrate features of both upper and lower motor neuron lesions
   (b) Examples: myelodysplasia and multiple sclerosis

13. Videourodynamics (Fig. 5-7): Combines measurement of intravesical intraabdominal and striated urethral sphincter pressures with bladder filling, bladder emptying, and flow rate, all done simultaneously with fluoroscopy
14. Sacral evoked responses[17]
    a. This test quantitates the integrity of the innervation of the striated pelvic floor and perineal muscles along with the supraspinal pathways involved in lower urologic tract function.
    b. The nerve conduction time (latency) and the stimulation threshold are the two parameters most commonly measured.
    c. Bulbocavernosus reflex latency is clinically measured. Normal is 30 to 40 msec.
    d. Any neurologic process that interferes with the integrity of the reflex arc will result in a prolonged latency.
    e. The following are common disorders associated with prolonged latency:

(1) Diabetes mellitus
(2) Alcoholic neuropathy
(3) Disc disease

15. Abdominal-Valsalva Leak Point Pressures[9,16]
   a. This measures the amount of abdominal pressure required to induce urinary leakage.
      (1) A normal patient should remain continent regardless of the amount of abdominal pressure exerted on the lower urinary tract.
   b. This is used to document type III incontinence, associated with an incompetent sphincter.
      (1) These patients leak at low to moderate abdominal pressures.
      (2) Patients with types I and II incontinence require higher abdominal pressures to leak.
   c. The Abdominal-Valsalva Leak Point Pressure is the change in intravesical pressure documented before the valsalva maneuver to the pressure at which incontinence occurs.
   d. Abdominal-Valsalva Leak Point Pressures
      (1) >120 cm H_2O: Type I incontinence is characterized by the bladder neck gradually opening with heavy exercise or exertion. There is support for the pelvic floor and no movement of the bladder neck. Treatment: medication.
      (2) 60 to 100 cm H_2O: Type II incontinence is characterized by bladder neck hypermobility with herniation through the pelvic floor with straining, disrupting the ability of the bladder to remain closed. Treatment: bladder neck suspension.
      (3) <60 cm H_2O: Type III, or intrinsic sphincter deficiency is characterized by a dysfunctional bladder neck and proximal urethra. Treatment: pubovaginal sling, an injectable agent, or an artificial sphincter.
16. Detrusor Leak Point Pressure[9,16]
   a. This is the pressure obtained by filling the bladder until intravesical pressure overcomes urethral resistance and incontinence occurs. Detrusor pressure can force the sphincter open, whereas the abdominal pressure cannot.
   b. It is an indirect measure of bladder storage.
   c. It is an assessment of intravesical pressure, useful in the patient with a neuropathic bladder to determine if urine is being stored at pressures that will not cause upper urinary tract deterioration.
   d. Normal detrusor leak point pressure is below 40 cm H_2O. Pressures above this can over time cause upper tract damage.
17. Specialized Testing
   a. Rapid fill cystometry[19]
      (1) Used to rule out detrusor areflexia
      (2) Rapid filling of the bladder at rates of flow up to 300 cc/min
   b. Bethanechol supersensitivity test[10]
      (1) Bethanechol chloride
         (a) Parasympathomimetic
         (b) Selective for bladder and gut

(c) Cholinesterase resistant
(d) Causes bladder muscle to contract (spares ganglia and cardiovascular)
(e) Minimal effects on the normal bladder
  i. Decreases capacity slightly
  ii. Increases detrusor tone
  iii. Increases voluntary micturition pressure
  iv. Does not cause detrusor instability

(2) Basis for test: Cannon's law of denervation; when an organ is deprived of its nerve supply, it will develop hypersensitivity to its own neurotransmitter substance.[5]

(3) Method: Subcutaneous injection of 2.5 mg of bethanechol chloride followed in 15 to 30 minutes by repeat cystometrogram study.
(a) A rise of at least 15 cm of water after 100-cc infusion at a medium rate of between 100 and 200 cc/min in excess of the pretreated cystometrogram pressure is indicative of parasympathetic dysfunction (denervation). It is seen with lower motor neuron lesions (also called decentralized bladder).
(b) This test is contraindicated in patients with cardiac disease, asthma, hyperthyroidism, peptic ulcer disease, enteritis bowel obstruction, and bladder outlet obstruction.
(c) Blaivas reported a false-negative rate of 24%, attributing such testing factors as repeated overdistension of the bladder, bethanechol absorption, emotional stress, time, and bladder volume to the high false-negative rate.[4]
(d) False-positive test results occur in the presence of active urinary tract infections, azotemia, emotional stress, and detrusor hypertrophy.[17]
(e) Studies by Mattiason[8] and Malkowicz[7] suggest that end organ supersensitivity is not an end organ response to denervation but may measure supersensitivity at the pelvic reflex arc or demonstrates another aspect of vesical pressure generation such as detrusor muscle hypertrophy.

c. Phentolamine testing[1,7]

(1) Premise: Inappropriate smooth muscle or striated muscle activity with bladder outlet obstruction has been associated with the neurologically impaired bladder. Smooth muscle components are under the control of the autonomic nervous system. The striated muscle is under peripheral nervous system control. When symptoms are caused by the smooth muscle component, the pharmacologic manipulation of the sympathetic nervous system has been shown to be of benefit.

(2) The phentolamine test is used to select patients most likely to benefit from the use of adrenergic blocking agents. See relaxation of the urethral smooth muscle component of bladder neck.

(3) This test compares the urethral closure pressure profile before and after injection of phentolamine.
(4) An IV bolus of phentolamine mesylate, 0.1 mg/kg, is given, after which blood pressure and pulse are recorded every minute until a tachycardia of at least 10 beats per minute occurs. The urethral pressure profile is then repeated and the patient is observed for 30 minutes for any untoward effects from the drug.
(5) A positive test: A decrease of 30% or more occurs in the maximum urethral closure pressure after injection of phentolamine.

d. These patients can be offered a trial of alpha-1 blockers.
Glycopyrrolate test[17,18] (formerly pro-banthine stimulation test)
(1) Glycopyrrolate is an anticholinergic test.
(2) IV glycopyrrolate, 0.4 mg, is given.
(3) A cystometrogram is done before and 10 to 25 minutes after injection.
(4) The disappearance or decrease in the amplitude or the frequency of uninhibited contractions indicates that the patient may respond to outpatient therapy.
(5) Note: This test is almost never performed in clinical practice. The efficacy of newer anticholinergic medications, their rapid absorption (sublingual forms), and their different concentrations makes it far easier to use them than to expose a patient to intravenous glycopyrrolate.
(6) Glaucoma and obstructive gastrointestinal disease are contraindicated.

e. Urethral denervation sensitivity testing[15] (also listed as noradrenaline supersensitivity test of the urethra)
(1) The primary innervation of the urethra is through sympathetic alpha fibers.
(2) Baseline maximum urthral closure pressure is determined.
(3) Four mg IV ethylphenylephrine is given.
(4) Five minutes later, a repeat maximum closure pressure is obtained.
(5) Chronic urethral denervation is present when there is a rise of 15 cm of water or greater in the closure pressure from control.

f. Marshall-Marchetti-Bonney stress test[1] (also called the cough-stress test)
(1) The patient coughs with a full bladder while the examiner observes the urethra for urine loss.
(2) The examiner manipulates the urethrovesical angle either by placing Allis clamps on the anterior vaginal wall, lateral to the urethrovesical angle, or more commonly by inserting two fingers into the lateral fornices of the vagina, pushing the bladder base up and anteriorly without compressing the urethra closed. The patient coughs and bears down again. The practitioner observes for the following:
(a) Leak with cough but no leak with bladder base elevation: true stress urinary incontinence

(3) Controversy: This test presumes to simulate the results of the planned surgical procedure by elevation and stabilization of the urethra and vesical neck. Evidence by Bergman[1] has demonstrated that this test restores continence by occlusion of the urethra and vesical neck. Regardless, it remains a mainstay of tests in the evaluation of female incontinence.

g. Q-tip test
   (1) Using an orthopedic goniometer
      (a) Normal: with straining, 0° to 20° deflection
      (b) Urethral hypermobility (associated with genuine stress incontinence); greater than 25° deflection
   (2) NOTE: Recent evidence indicates that the Q-tip test is not specific for stress urinary incontinence because a positive result reflects anterior vaginal muscle relaxation rather than sphincteric incompetence. In addition, this test is thought to have a false-negative rate for the diagnosis of stress urinary incontinence of 30%, especially in elderly females.[6]

h. Pessary test[2]
   (1) Premise: The vaginal pessary may increase urethral closure and urethral functional length in women with a mild to moderate cystocele. The pessary restores continence by stabilization of the bladder base, allowing proper pressure transmission to the urethra, and by active enhancement of urethral resistance, by increasing urethral functional length and closure pressure.
      (a) Positive: surgical correction
      (b) Negative: urodynamic evaluation
   (2) NOTE: This test is thought to be unpredictable in the elderly.

References

1. Bergman A: Invalidity of the Marshall Marchetti and Bonney stress tests. In Ostergard DR, Bent AE, editors: *Urogynecology and urodynamics theory and practice,* Baltimore, 1991, Williams & Wilkins.
2. Bergman A: Nonsurgical treatment for stress urinary incontinence. In Ostergard DR, Bent AE, editors: *Urogynecology and urodynamics theory and practice,* Baltimore, 1991, Williams & Wilkins.
3. Bhatia NN: Neurourology and urodynamics: sphincter electromyography and electrophysiological testing. In Ostergard DR, Bent AE, editors: *Urogynecology and urodynamics theory and practice,* Baltimore, 1991, Williams & Wilkins.
4. Blaivas J et al: Failure of bethanechol denervation supersensitivity as a diagnostic aid, *J Urol* 123:199, 1980.
5. Cannon WB, Rosenbleuth A: *The supersensitivity of denervated structures,* New York, 1949, McMillan, pp. 96-105.
6. DuBeau CE, Resnick NM: Evaluation of the causes and severity of geriatric incontinence: a critical appraisal, *Urol Clin North Am* 18:243, 1991.
7. Malkowicz SB et al: The effect of parasympathetic decentralization on the feline urinary bladder, *J Urol* 133:521, 1985.
8. Mattiason A et al: Supersensitivity to carbachol in the parasympathetically decentralized feline urinary bladder, *J Urol* 131:562, 1984.
9. McGuire EJ et al: Clinical assessment of urethral sphincter function, *J Urol* 150:1452-1454, 1993.

10. Montella JM, Ostergard DR: Specialized testing procedures. In Ostergard DR, Bent AE, editors: *Urogynecology and urodynamics theory and practice,* Baltimore, 1991, Williams & Wilkins.
11. Olsson CA, Siroky MB, Krane RJ: The phentolamine test in neurogenic bladder dysfunction, *J Urol* 117:481, 1977.
12. Ostergard DR, Bent AE, editors: *Appendix I: the standardisation of terminology of lower urinary tract function,* Baltimore, 1991, Williams & Wilkins.
13. Robertson JR: Dynamic urethroscopy. In Ostergard DR, Bent AE, editors: *Urogynecology and urodynamics theory and practice,* Baltimore, 1991, Williams & Wilkins.
14. Siroky MB, Olsson CA, Krane RJ: The flow rate nomogram I: development, *J Urol* 122:665-668, 1979.
15. Snyder JA, editor: Urologic perspectives: urinary incontinence. Special Supplement to *Urology Grand Rounds,* Number 27, Chicago, McCann Healthcare Advertising.
16. Wan J et al: Stress leak point pressure: a diagnostic tool for incontinet children, *J Urol* 150:700-702, 1993.
17. Wein AJ: *Voiding dysfunction: neurogenic or non neurogenic?* AUA Update Series, vol VII, Lesson 23, Houston, 1988, American Urological Association, Inc, Office of Education.
18. Wein AJ, Barrett DM, editors: *Voiding function and dysfunction: a logical and practical approach,* Chicago, 1988, Yearbook Medical Publishers.
19. Wein AJ, English WS, Whitmore KE: Office urodynamics, *Urol Clin North Am* 15:609, 1988.

6 Contraception

Maria A. Corigliano, M.D.

Contraception is an integral and very important aspect of a general obstetric and gynecologic practice. Not only should the effectiveness of a method be considered but also what is best for each individual patient in regard to probable compliance with the method, medical history, and desire or lack of desire for future fertility. Emotional and social issues at the time of decision should also be discussed and evaluated.

Each patient should be informed of all options that are appropriate for her. Many times misconceptions about safety, fertility after use, and positive benefits of the different forms of contraception are very freely volunteered by the patient during a consultation. Many patients are pleasantly surprised by the fact that they are candidates for certain contraceptive methods that they never thought they would be eligible for because of misinformation given to them by friends. The clinician's job is not only to inform patients of their options and the risks of certain methods but also to stress the benefits of using them. The reason a particular method is not recommended for an individual patient may also be discussed at this time.

A full history and physical examination should be completed before a method is prescribed. History should include the usual data as follows:

1. Medical history
2. Surgical history
3. Obstetric history: establish whether patient could be already pregnant; desire for future fertility
4. Gynecologic history
5. History of sexually transmitted diseases
6. Numbers of partners
7. Previous difficulties with contraception use
8. Frequency of intercourse
9. Family history: include family members with history of vascular events or female cancers
10. A full physical examination: Papanicolaou smear and cultures of the cervix should be obtained

6.1 ORAL CONTRACEPTIVES

1. Oral contraceptive types
   a. Monophasic: Contain a constant dose of estrogen and progesterone in each of the 21 contraceptively active pills.

   b. Triphasic: Contain a varying dose of progestin. In some types the estrogen dose in the 21 contraceptively active pills is varied. The purpose of this manipulation is to keep the patient on the lowest dose possible throughout the cycle, while preventing pregnancy at the same rate.
   c. Progestin-only pill: Contains even lower doses of progestin in 28 contraceptively active pills.
2. The most commonly used estrogen is ethinyl estradiol in a dose containing less than 35 μg of estrogen.
3. Mestranol is the estrogen used in the higher dosed pills. Pills with estrogen levels greater than 50 μg are no longer available.
4. Most commonly used progestins are norethindrone, levonorgestrel, norgestrel, norethindrone acetate, or ethynodiol diacetate.
5. Less androgenic progestins are norgestimate and destogestrel. Gestodene is another new progestin.
6. Mechanism of action: Suppression of pituitary follicle stimulating hormone (FSH) and luteinizing hormone (LH) secretion, which suppresses ovulation. The progestin portion of the pill causes changes in cervical mucus and endometrium, which afford birth control because ovulation may occur on oral contraceptives.
7. Effectiveness rate: If taken correctly, *only* 1 in 1000 women is expected to get pregnant within the first year on combined oral contraceptives. The typical failure rate of combined oral contraceptives is about 3%. Progestin-only pills have about the same effectiveness rate as the combined pills.
8. Administration of combination oral contraceptives
   a. A daily ritual should be associated with oral contraceptive use. Many women are more likely to remember to take the pills at night before bedtime. This may prevent nausea because the patient will be sleeping. A woman should begin taking oral contraceptives either on the Sunday following the first day of her period or on the first day of her period.
   b. It should be stressed that taking the pills daily at the same time is necessary for optimum effectiveness.
   c. If one or two pills are missed, have the patient double up on the pills until she catches up.
   d. If two or more pills are missed, backup birth control should be used and the pack should be completed.
9. Antibiotic use and the Pill: The only antibiotic proven to decrease the effectiveness rate of the Pill is rifampin. The dermatologic literature has produced a guideline to follow regarding contraceptive pill and antibiotic mixing (see the box on p. 96).
10. Benefits of the Pill
   a. Menstruation becomes more regular; there is less dysmenorrhea (63% reduction of dysmenorrhea, and a 29% reduction of premenstrual syndrome [PMS]).
   b. There is decrease in the amount and duration of menstrual flow.
   c. The Pill corrects iron-deficiency anemia.

Categories of Antibiotics

CATEGORY A: ANTIBIOTIC THAT LIKELY REDUCES BIRTH CONTROL PILL EFFECTIVENESS

Rifampicin

CATEGORY B: ANTIBIOTICS ASSOCIATED WITH ORAL CONTRACEPTIVE FAILURE IN THREE OR MORE CASE REPORTS

Ampicillin
Amoxicillin
Metronidazole
Tetracycline

CATEGORY C: ANTIBIOTICS ASSOCIATED WITH ORAL CONTRACEPTIVE FAILURE IN AT LEAST ONE CASE REPORT

Cephalexin
Clindamycin
Dapsone
Erythromycin
Griseofulvin
Isoniazid
Phenoxymethylpenicillin
Telampicillin
Trimethoprim

From Miller DM et al: *J Am Acad Derm* 30:1009, 1994.

11. Preventions
    a. Benign breast disease: An Oxford study showed a 30% reduction in fibrocystic breast disease (FCBD) and 60% fewer fibroadenomas. An American study showed a 30% reduction with 13 to 24 months use, and a 65% reduction when used for 25 months or more.
    b. Hospitalization: The chance of hospitalization resulting from pelvic inflammatory disease (PID) is decreased secondary to thicker impenetrable cervical mucus. Menstrual blood flow is reduced by 50% to 60%. Smaller cervical openings, which do not prevent cervical *Chlamydia,* do decrease upper tract disease.
    c. Epithelial ovarian cancer: There is 40% to 50% reduction in occurrence if oral contraceptives are used for 5 years; an 80% to 90% reduction in occurrence if used for 10 years. Protection from cancer lasts up to 15 years after discontinuation. There is also a decrease in endometrial cancer (50% reduction, lasts for 15 years).
    d. Ectopic pregnancy: A 10-fold decrease in ectopic pregnancy is seen, compared with nonusers.

e. Acne: Decreasing serum testosterone improves acne.
f. Estrogen deficiency: Symptoms are improved.
g. Fear of pregnancy: The fear of pregnancy decreases, therefore sexual enjoyment is heightened.
h. Fibroid size: An Oxford study showed a 30% reduction in size over 10 years.

12. Possible benefits
    a. Prevention of rheumatoid arthritis: The onset may be postponed, but estrogen dose does not decrease the pain of rheumatoid arthritis.
    b. Prevention of ovarian cysts: The rate of recurrent hemorrhagic cysts is decreased.
    c. Increased bone density: The final word is not in.
    d. Decreased endometriosis and atherosclerosis with low-dose oral contraceptives.
13. Disadvantages or side effects that prompt discontinuation
    a. Nausea: usually disappears after first month
    b. Breast tenderness
    c. Breakthrough bleeding (initial months)
    d. Amenorrhea (prolonged use): may add estrogen or change pills
    e. Depression
    f. Decreased libido: may result from decreased free testosterone circulation
    g. Expense (pharmacy dependent)
    h. Headaches
        (1) Only classical migraine types should prompt stopping the Pill. Progestin-only pills may be tried in this case.
        (2) Often the headaches are experienced during the pill-free interval. This may be remedied through the use of continuous oral contraceptives (eliminate pill-free interval).
    i. *Chlamydia* infection
        (1) *Chlamydia* cervicitis (not PID) is more common in contraceptive pill users secondary to the increased ectropion caused by the pill than in nonusers (see the box on p. 98).
14. Major risks to health (see the box on p. 100 and Tables 6-1 and 6-2)
    a. Cardiovascular disease
        (1) Cardiovascular disease includes thrombophlebitis, pulmonary embolus, and stroke. All of these may occur in women who are at risk for these events (i.e., women who are smokers, sedentary, overweight, over 50 years old, and who have increased low-density lipoprotein/high-density lipoprotein [LDL/HDL] cholesterol ratio). History of hypertension, history of diabetes, a family history of cardiovascular events, and diabetes in a premenopausal women also indicate a higher risk level.
        (2) Estrogen and progesterone doses have decreased by 4-fold and 10-fold, respectively, from the original birth control pills, which were studied in the 1960s and 1970s. The use of low-dose oral contraceptives markedly decreases the risk of

Relation of Side Effects to Hormone Content

REPRODUCTIVE SYSTEM

Estrogen excess
- Breast cystic changes
- Cervical extrophy
- Dysmenorrhea
- Hypermenorrhea, menorrhagia, and clotting
  - Increase in breast size
  - Mucorrhea
  - Uterine enlargement
  - Uterine fibroid growth

Estrogen deficiency
- Absence of withdrawal bleeding
- Bleeding and spotting during pill days 1 to 9
- Continuous bleeding and spotting
- Flow decrease, hypomenorrhea
- Pelvic relaxation symptoms
- Vaginitis atrophic

Progestin excess
- Cervicitis
- Flow length decrease
- Moniliasis

Progestin deficiency
- Breakthrough bleeding and spotting during pill days 10 to 21
- Delayed withdrawal bleeding
- Dysmenorrhea (also estrogen excess)
- Heavy flow and clots (also estrogen excess), hypermenorrhea, menorrhagia

PREMENSTRUAL SYNDROME

Estrogen excess or progesterone deficiency
- Bloating
- Dizziness, syncope
- Edema
- Headache (cyclic)
- Irritability
- Leg cramps
- Nausea, vomiting
- Visual changes (cyclic)
- Weight gain (cyclic)

Relation of Side Effects to Hormone Content—cont'd

GENERAL

Estrogen excess
- Chloasma
- Chronic nasal pharyngitis
- Gastric influenza and varicella
- Hay fever and allergic rhinitis
- Urinary tract infection

Estrogen deficiency
- Nervousness
- Vasomotor symptoms

Progestin excess
- Appetite increase
- Depression
- Fatigue
- Hypoglycemia symptoms
- Libido decrease
- Neurodermatitis
- Weight gain (noncyclic)

Androgen excess
- Acne
- Cholestatic jaundice
- Hirsutism
- Libido increase
- Oily skin and scalp
- Rash and pruritus
- Edema

CARDIOVASCULAR SYSTEM

Progestin excess
- Hypertension
- Leg vein dilation

Estrogen excess
- Capillary fragility
- Cerebrovascular accident
- Deep vein thrombosis hemiparesis (unilateral weakness and numbness)
- Telangiectasias
- Thromboembolic disease

From Dickey R: *Managing Contraceptive Pill Patient,* ed 8, Durant, OK, 1994, Essential Medical Information Systems.

Contraindications to Using Oral Contraceptives

Present or past history of thrombophlebitis
Stroke
Coronary artery disease (CAD)
Breast cancer
Estrogen-dependent neoplasia
Hepatic disease, benign or malignant
Smokers over 35 years old
Women who smoke more than 15 cigarettes per day
Migraine headaches that started after oral contraception use
Hypertension
Pregnancy
Major surgery that involves immobilization
Lactation
Sickle cell disease (theoretical increase risk for thrombosis)
Active gall bladder disease
Undiagnosed vaginal bleeding
Gilbert's disease (congenital hyperbilirubinemia)
Women over 50 years old
Immediate postpartum period (up to 14 days still in hypercoagulable state)
Cardiac and renal disease (severe)
Mental illness, substance abusers (less likely to take pills correctly)
Family history of hyperlipidemia
Family history of female sibling or parents who died from myocardial infarction before menopause

cardiovascular side effects. For select outpatients that are at increased risk for cardiovascular events, it is wise to suggest alternate forms of birth control.

(3) Smokers: Smoking increases dangerous cardiovascular side effects. Smoking fewer than 15 cigarettes per day increases the risk of myocardial infarction (MI) 3-fold. Smoking more than 15 cigarettes a day increases the risk of MI to 21-fold. After age 35, smokers should not use the Pill.

b. Cancer: a major concern of women and the most common reason for women to decline use of oral contraceptives
   (1) Breast cancer: The final word on the Pill's influence on breast cancer is not in. There is no convincing evidence in the literature that birth control pill use increases the rate of breast cancer.
   (2) A recent study done in Canada shows a 50% reduction in breast cancer risk for women who used combination oral contraceptives for 5 years.
   (3) Cervical cancer: Five out of 13 studies have shown a significant increase in cervical cancer in women who use oral con-

Table 6-1 Symptoms of a serious or potentially serious nature

Symptom	Possible Cause
Serious: Pills should be stopped immediately.	
Loss of vision, proptosis, diplopia, papilledema	Retinal artery thrombosis
Unilateral numbness, weakness, or tingling	Hemorrhagic or thrombotic stroke
Severe pains in chest, left arm, or neck	Myocardial infarction
Hemoptysis	Pulmonary embolism
Severe pains, tenderness or swelling, warmth, or palpable cord in legs	Thrombophlebitis
Slurring of speech	Hemorrhagic or thrombotic stroke
Hepatic mass or tenderness	Liver neoplasm
Potentially serious: Pills may be continued with caution while patient is being evaluated.	
Absence of menses	Pregnancy
Spotting or breakthrough bleeding	Cervical, endometrial, or vaginal cancer
Breast mass, pain, or swelling	Breast cancer
Right upper quadrant pain	Cholecystitis, cholelithiasis, or liver neoplasm
Midepigastric pain	Thrombosis of abdominal artery or vein, myocardial infarction, or pulmonary embolism
Migraine (vascular or throbbing) headache	Vascular spasm, which may precede thrombosis
Severe nonvascular headache	Hypertension, vascular spasm
Galactorrhea	Pituitary adenoma
Jaundice, pruritus	Cholestatic jaundice
Depression	B_6 deficiency
Uterine size increase	Leiomyomata, adenomyosis, pregnancy

From Dickey R: *Managing contraceptive pill patients,* ed 8, Durant, OK, 1984, Essential Medical Information Systems.

traceptives. Seven studies showed no significant increase. One study showed a relationship between the Pill and dysplasia and carcinomas of the cervix, especially in women who were on oral contraceptives for prolonged periods of time. However this may be because pill users generally have multiple sexual partners and are screened more frequently by Papanicolaou smears than non–Pill users. Human papillomavirus (HPV) plays a large role in cervical cancer, and oral contraception users are less likely to use barrier methods than non–Pill users.

Table 6-2 Choosing oral contraceptives (OCs)

Step 1	Step 2	Step 3	Step 4
Can this individual be prescribed a pill with estrogen? →	YES, she can use an estrogen. →	Therefore, you may choose between any of the following OCs based on: • Number of micrograms of ethinyl estradiol • Availability of pill • Ease of remaining on schedule because of pills • Price of pills to clinic* • Price of pills to client* • Prior experience of this individual woman or the clinician caring for this woman with a special pill **Pills are listed from the lowest to the highest number of micrograms of ethinyl estradiol:** (see table below)	Other clinical considerations that may help in OC choice: A. To minimize the risk potential for *thrombosis* caused by estrogen in a woman 40 to 50 years of age or a woman at increased risk for thrombosis from another cause (e.g., diabetic or heavy smoker), prescribe: • Loestrin 1/20 B. To minimize *nausea, breast tenderness, vascular headaches,* and estrogen-mediated side effects, prescribe: • Loestrin 1/20 Or a 30 μg pill, such as: • Desogen • Levlen • Loestrin 1.5-30 • Lo-Ovral • Nordette • Ortho-Cept C. To minimize *spotting and/or breakthrough bleeding,* prescribe: • Lo-Ovral, Nordette, or Levlen
Definitely refrain from prescribing a pill with estrogen to women with a history of a cerebrovascular accident, ischemic heart diesease, uncontrolled hypertension, insulin-dependent diabetes with vascular disease, classic migraine with neurologic impairment that has increased with estrogen, breast cancer, estrogen-dependent neoplasia, active hepatic disease with impaired liver function at the present time, benign or malignant liver tumor, or deep vein thrombosis. Some clinicians would make an exception and provide combined OCs to women following postpartum pelvic vein →	NO, it would be best if she did not use an estrogen. Therefore, you can consider: • Progestin-only pills, such as: • Micronor (0.35 mg norethindrone daily) • NOR QD (0.35 mg nonrethindrone daily) • Ovrette (0.075 mg nogestrel daily) • Norplant (5-year levonorgestrel implants) • Depo-Provera (150 mg medroxyprogesterone acetate injection every 3 months) • Intrauterine device • Copper T 380-A • Progestasert System • Condoms (male or female) • Diaphragm, cervical cap • Foam, vaginal contraceptive film, suppository • Sponge		

Combined Pill	Estrogen (μg)	Availability/ Cost in Your Clinic	Company
Loestrin 1/20	20	______	Parke-Davis
Loestrin 1.5/30	30	______	Parke-Davis
Desogen	30	______	Organon
Lo-Ovral	30	______	Wyeth
Nordette	30	______	Wyeth
Levlen	30	______	Berlex
Ortho-Cept	30	______	Ortho
Tri-Levlen	30/40/30	______	Berlex
Triphasil	30/40/30	______	Wyeth
Ovcon 35	35	______	Mead Johnson

thrombosis or women whose thrombophlebitis has resulted from trauma or IV. Also, in most instances refrain from providing combined pills to women over 35 who smoke. Breast-feeding women, in general, should avoid estrogen.	Demulen 1/35	35	______	Searle	• A new progestin pill: Desogen, Ortho-Cept, Ortho-Cyclen, or Ortho Tri-Cyclen D. To minimize androgen effects such as *acne, hirsutism, oily skin, sebaceous cysts, pilonidal cysts, or weight gain,* prescribe: • Desogen, Ortho-Cept • Ortho Tri-Cyclen • Ortho Cyclen • Ovcon-35, Brevicon, or Modicon (of norethindrone pills) • Demulen-35 (of ethnodiol diacetate pills) E. To produce the most *favorable lipid profile,* prescribe: • Ortho Cyclen or Ortho Tri-Cyclen • Desogen or Ortho-Cept • Ovcon-35, Brevicon, or Modicon (of norethindrone pills)
	Ortho-Cyclen	35	______	Ortho	
	Ortho Tri-Cyclen	35	______	Ortho	
	Ortho Novum 777	35	______	Ortho	
	Ortho-Novum 1/35	35	______	Ortho	
	Modicon	35	______	Ortho	
	Brevicon	35	______	Syntex	
	Norninyl 1/35	35	______	Syntex	
	Tri-Norinyl	35	______	Syntex	
	Norcept-E 1/35†	35	______	Syntex	
	Nelova 0.5/35†	35	______	GynoPharma	
	Nelova 1/35†	35	______	Warner-Chilcott	
	NEE 0.5/35	35	______	Lexis	
	NEE 1/35	35	______	Lexis	
	Genora 0.5/35†	35	______	Rugby	
	Genora 1/35	35	______	Rugby	
	Jenest	35	______	Organon	
	NEE 10/11	35	______	Lexes	
	Norethin 1/35E	35	______	Schiaparelli-Searle	

From Hatcher RH et al: *Contraceptive technology,* ed 16, New York, 1994, Irvington Publishers.

*On December 11, 1992, *The Medical Letter* published the cost to pharmacists for a 1-month cycle of OCs based on "Average Wholesale Price Listing in Drug Topics Red Book 1992" and its November Update.

†The four pills costing pharmacists less than $10.00 per cycle were Norcept E ($5.72); Nelova 0.5/35; Nelova 1/35 ($6.25); and Genora 0.5/35 ($8.23). The cost of most pills to pharmacists was $17.00 to $22.33 per cycle. In some clinics, pills may be purchased at prices as low as $0.50 to $1.00 per cycle. These low prices are usually reflected in the prices clinics charge women.

(4) Ovarian and endometrial cancer: Many studies show a decreased risk of ovarian epithelial cancers and endometrial cancers for women on oral contraceptives. The longer the use, the more long term the protection.

(5) Hepatocellular carcinomas: Benign hepatic adenomas occur with oral contraceptive use. However, increased risk of hepatocellular cancer has not been proved in women using oral contraceptives.

(6) Adolescents: The Pill is not contraindicated; however, compliance and sexually transmitted disease (non–condom users) become issues.

6.2 PROGESTIN-ONLY CONTRACEPTION

1. Hormonal implants (Norplant) has the most use experience and clinical trials.
   a. Composition and mode of action: The implant consists of six soft plastic implants, each filled with 36 mg of levonorgestrel. It releases 85 μg daily and by the fifth year of use releases 30 μg daily. Levonorgestrel suppresses the LH surge responsible for ovulation. The LH peak is abolished. Ovulation occurs in about two thirds of all cycles with Norplant. Levonorgestrel thickens and decreases the amount of cervical mucus and blocks sperm penetration. It suppresses estrogenic maturation of the endometrial lining.
   b. Insertion: Six plastic capsules are inserted through a small anesthetized incision in the upper inner arm. They are removed after 5 years, or when the patient desires, through a 3 to 5 mm incision. Insertion should occur during the menses week to ensure that the patient is not pregnant.
   c. Effectiveness rate
      (1) About 1% of women are pregnant within the first 5 years of using Norplant. The rate goes up to 2% in the sixth year. Therefore removal and reinsertion is advised after 5 years.
      (2) Overweight women are more likely to get pregnant using the denser capsuled Norplant because they have lower serum levels. Using a less dense type of implant in these women will increase its effectiveness rate (Tables 6-3 and 6-4).

Table 6-3 Norplant capsules: gross cumulative pregnancy rates at 5 years of use by weight and type of tubing

Weight at insertion (kg)	*N*	Total	Pliable Tubing	Rigid Tubing
<50	532	0.2	0.0	0.3
50-59	1041	3.5	2.0	4.3
60-69	585	3.5	1.5	4.5
>70	309	7.6	2.4	9.3
Total	2469	3.5	1.6	4.9

From Darney PD: *Am J Obstet Gynecol* 170:1536-1543, 1994; data from Sivin IL: *Stud Fam Plann* 19:86, 1988.

(3) If fertilization does occur, it is more likely to be an ectopic pregnancy. Table 6-4 shows ectopic pregnancy rates per 1000 women-years with different types of birth control. The failure rate is increased by carbamazepine, phenytoin, phenobarbital, primidone, phenylbutazone, and rifampin.

d. Side effects most commonly occur in the first few months and can include irregular menses, headaches, weight change, breast tenderness, acne, hirsutism, depression, mood swings, galactorrhea, amenorrhea, and hair loss. Menstrual irregularities are the most common reason for discontinuation.

e. Fertility returns quickly after discontinuation. Plasma levels of levonogestrel are subcontraceptive level within 24 hours of removal.

f. Indications

(1) Women who breast-feed: The implant may be inserted in noncompliant patients while in hospital. However, most studies do not start the method before 4 weeks postpartum.

(2) Older women and women who cannot use estrogen.

g. Future implant systems

(1) Systems using fewer implants (Norplant 2 and Implanon) will make insertion and removal easier.

(2) Biodegradable systems, such as capronor and norethindrone pellets, will eliminate removal. Undesirable side effects will be eliminated by the use of less androgenic progestins such as desogestrel, gestodene, norgestimate, or ST 14356.

2. Depo-Provera

a. Depo-medroxy progesterone acetate (Depo-Provera) is the most commonly used injectable progestin in the world. It was finally approved for use in the United States in 1992. It is excellent for use in women who breast-feed or for short term use where estrogen is contraindicated.

b. Composition and mode of action

(1) Depo-medroxy progesterone acetate is given by deep intramuscular injections. A dosage of 150 mg must be given every 3 months.

Table 6-4 Rates of ectopic pregnancy per 1000 women-years by contraceptive method and for all U.S. women

Method	Rate
Norplant	0.28*
TCu380A	0.20†
Noncontraceptors	3.00‡
All U.S. women	1.50§

From Darney PD: *Am J Obstet Gynecol* 170:1536-1543; 1994.
*Sivin I. *Stud Fam Plann* 19:81, 1988.
†Sivin I. *Contraception* 19:151, 1979.
‡Franks AL et al: *Am J Obstet Gynecol* 163:1120, 1990.
§Centers for Disease Control and Prevention: *MMWR* 38:1, 1989.

(2) Its action is to shut down the LH surge and suppress LH and FSH levels. It also causes an atrophic endometrium and thick impenetrable cervical mucus. Depo-Provera is so effective that long-time users may be as much as 2 weeks late for their next injections.

c. Efficacy: Only 0.3% of women will experience accidental pregnancy within the first year of use. Giving 400 mg of Depo-Provera in the more concentrated form every 6 months decreases the effectiveness rate throughout the 6-month period.

d. Indications: Women who may not use estrogen, women who breast-feed, older women, women that need short-term but effective contraception may use Depo-Provera.

e. Advantages

(1) Risk of endometrial and ovarian cancer and PID is decreased.

(2) There is less menstrual blood loss, and therefore anemia is decreased.

(3) A decrease in dysmenorrhea and mittelschmerz is seen.

(4) Depo-Provera is a reversible form of birth control, even though the return of fertility is slower than it is for other types of hormonal contraception.

(5) Risk of ectopic pregnancies decreases to 1.3/1000 women-years as compared with 6.5/1000 women-years in women who use no contraception.

(6) Amenorrhea is of advantage in certain women because as many as 80% of women are amenorrheic after 3 years of use.

(7) Use with antibiotics is safe. The only drug known to decrease the effectiveness of Depo-Provera is cytodren. Because it is given parenterally, it is not dependent on the gastrointestinal (GI) tract. Improvement of seizure disorder results from the sedating effects of progestins.

f. Side effects

(1) The menstrual cycle changes (increased days of light bleeding but not increased blood loss).

(2) Amenorrhea develops with time.

(3) Weight gain: The patient may gain up to 14 pounds with 4 years of use.

(4) Breast tenderness may occur.

(5) Depression may occur.

(6) Bone density decreases, which is reversible after discontinuation.

(7) The return of fertility is delayed for 6 months to 1 year after discontinuing use.

3. Minipill

The progestin-only pill has many of the advantages of the Norplant and Depo-Provera injection. It is used very infrequently. It is known to be less effective than combination oral contraceptives, Norplant, and Depo-Provera. However, it is a viable alternative in women who breast-feed and are unable to use estrogen. It has the advantage of being stopped easily. Its effectiveness rate is intensified if it causes anovulation, menstrual irregularities, and amenorrhea.

a. Efficacy: The failure rate of the Minipill in the first year of typical use is 1.1% to 13.2%. If used perfectly, only 5 in 1000 women become pregnant in the first year. It is nearly 100% effective in lactating women and does not affect milk production.
b. Indications
    (1) Women for whom estrogen is contraindicated
    (2) Decreases blood loss during menses, therefore decreasing anemia, dysmenorrhea, and mittelschmerz
    (3) Decrease in endometrial and ovarian cancer and PID
    (4) Immediate reversibility
    (5) Indicated for women who develop headache and hypertension on combination oral contraceptives
c. Side effects
    (1) There are changes in menstrual cycles (more spotting and irregularity). These changes are sometimes unacceptable to women.
    (2) Interaction with anticonvulsants makes the Minipill less effective.
    (3) The risk of pregnancy is greater unless the cycles are disturbed.
    (4) The Pill must be taken with exact regularity.
    (5) The Minipill is less available.
    (6) Practitioners have less experience with the Minipill.
    (7) Ovarian cysts (functional) are increased with use of the Minipill.
    (8) Ectopic pregnancy is more common with failures.
d. Delivery systems (Table 6-5)

6.3 POSTCOITAL CONTRACEPTION

Postcoital contraception is used when condoms break, when combination oral contraceptives have been forgotten, or in cases of rape or misuse of present contraceptive method.

1. Types
    a. IUD insertion postcoitus: Insertion of a copper intrauterine device (IUD) within 7 days of coitus is very effective in preventing pregnancy. However, use in women who are at high risk for PID is discouraged. Also it is not to be used in rape situations or nulliparous women.
    b. Contraceptive pills: The so-called morning after pill is highly effective in preventing pregnancy if it is used within 12 to 24 hours after coitus. The most commonly used regimen is 100 μg ethinyl estradiol and 1 mg of norgestrel or 0.5 mg levonorgestrel given immediately and then repeated 12 hours later. Antiemetics are sometimes needed with this regimen. For example, Ovral, two double doses are given 12 hours apart totaling four; Loovral/Nordette/Levelen/Triphasil, four tablets are given every 12 hours, totaling eight pills; or Danazol, 400 mg given every 12 hours, two to three times, totalling 800 to 1200 mg are effective alternatives for women who are not able to use estrogen.

Table 6-5 Delivery systems for progestin-only contraceptives and combined pills

	Injectable	Implant	Oral	
	Depo-Provera	Norplant	Progestin-Only Pill	Combined OC
Administration				
Frequency	Every 3 months	5 years	Daily	Daily
Progestin dose	High	Ultra low	Ultra low	Low
Blood levels	Initial peak, then decline	Constant	Rapidly fluctuating	
First pass through liver	No	No	Yes	Yes
Major Mechanisms of Action				
Ovary: decreases ovulation*	+++	++	+	+++
Cervical mucus: decreases sperm penetrability	Yes	Yes	Yes	Yes
Endometrium: decreases receptivity to blastocyst	Yes	Yes	Yes	Yes
First-year failure rate (perfect use)	0.3	0.09	0.5	0.1
Menstrual pattern	Very irregular	Very irregular	Often irregular	Regular
Amenorrhea during use	Very common	Common	Occasional	Rare
Reversibility				
Immediate termination possible	No	Yes	Yes	Yes
By woman herself at any time	No	No	Yes	Yes
Median time to conception from first omitted dose, removal	6 months	About 1 month	<3 months	3 months

From Hatcher R: *Contraceptive technology*, ed 16, New York, 1994, Irvington Publishers.

*By several mechanisms—LH and FSH surges suppressed; preovulatory follicles suppressed.

c. IUD: An IUD is an excellent option for properly selected patients such as multiparous women who do not desire surgery for birth control. The IUD is indicated in monogamous women who have tested their fertility.

(1) Fewer than 2% of the women in the United States are IUD users. In the 1970s, before many of them were taken off the market, about 10% of American women were IUD users. There are presently two IUDs available. The Progestasert (the Alza corporation) is an IUD option for women who want short-term IUD use and who require decreased menstrual blood flow and dysmenorrhea. It must be removed and reinserted yearly. The copper 380A (Paragard) is a desirable IUD option because it has been recently approved for 10 years of use. It is produced by Gynopharma. It is the most commonly used IUD.

(2) Composition and mode of action

(a) The progesterone T (progestasert) consists of an ethylene vinyl acetate copolymer T. The vertical stem contains 38 mg of progesterone and barium sulfate in a silicone base. The base of the T attaches to a blue or black double string. This IUD releases 65 μg of progesterone daily.

(b) The CU T 380A (Paragard) also is shaped like a T. The polyethylene T is wrapped with a fine copper wire on all three arms of the T. A single-filament white string projects from the base of the T.

(c) The levonorgestrel IUD (LNG-20), the Nova T IUD, and the MLCU 375 devices are not available presently in the United States. The efficacy of the LNG-20 IUD may surpass that of the CU T 380A.

(d) The mechanism of action of the IUD includes sperm immobilization and increased speed of ovum transport through the fallopian tubes. It was once thought that IUDs caused abortion of the fertilized egg by preventing implantation. However, it is now known that the device prohibits the sperm from meeting the egg in the fallopian tube.

(3) Considerations before insertion of the IUD

(a) A detailed history must be completed and a thorough physical must be done. Cervical cultures for *Chlamydia* and gonorrhea must be negative. All abnormal Papanicolaou smears should be diagnosed and treated first.

(b) Discussion of risks and benefits for this form of birth control should be thorough. Patients with the following history should not be considered candidates for IUD insertion:

Known or possible pregnancy
History of recent PID
Recent postpartum endometritis
Postabortion infection

(c) The IUD should be used with caution in the following patient populations:
   i. Those at risk for sexually transmitted diseases and PID
   ii. Those with impaired immune response: HIV positive, diabetics, or patients on steroids
   iii. Patients with menorrhagia, undiagnosed irregular vaginal bleeding
   iv. Those who have had previous complications associated with IUDs such as pregnancies, expulsion, or perforation
   v. Women with anatomic uterine abnormalities that make insertion difficult (i.e., leiomyoma, cervical stenosis)
   vi. Those with valvular heart disease (Women with cardiac lesions are more susceptible to subacute bacterial endocarditis.)
   vii. History of a previous ectopic pregnancy is no longer a contraindication because IUDs actually decrease the risk of ectopic pregnancies.
   viii. Mitral valve prolapse is not a contraindication to IUD use.

(4) IUD insertion
(a) an IUD may be inserted any time in a menstrual cycle as long as pregnancy has been ruled out.
(b) The patient should be educated thoroughly before insertion. Gynopharma provides a very complete patient education pamphlet that reviews everything from composition to side effects, effectiveness rate, and how to check the IUD postinsertion. The patient should read this material carefully before the device is inserted. The more informed the patient is, the better selected the patient will be.
(c) Steps: The clinician should talk to the patient and let her know what is being done at all times during insertion to decrease fearfulness.
   i. A pelvic examination is performed to determine the size, shape, and position of uterus.
   ii. The speculum is inserted; adequate visualization of cervix is a must.
   iii. The cervix is cleaned with betadine or hibiclens (betadine allergy).
   iv. A tenaculum or long Allis clamp should be placed on the anterior lip of the cervix.
   v. Sounding the uterine cavity is essential.
   vi. The IUD is loaded into the barrel with its arms down. If sterile gloves are not available, sterility may be obtained by folding the arms of the IUD in a partially opened package on a flat surface.
   vii. The moveable flange on the insertion tube is adjusted to the depth of the patient's uterus. The plunger must be placed at the end of the insertion tube next to the IUD string.

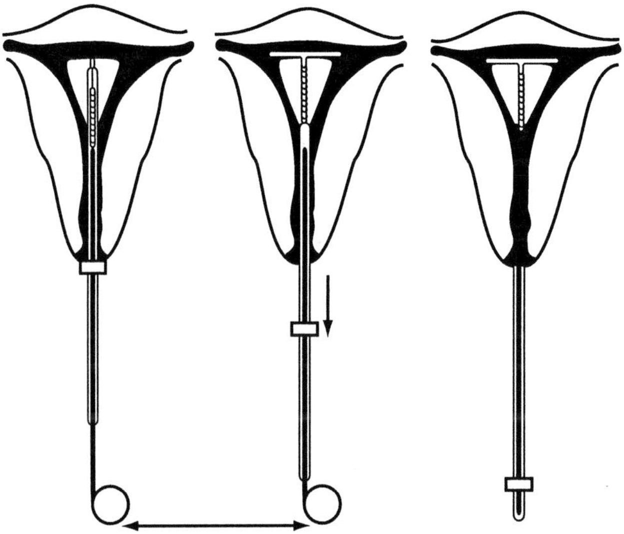

Figure 6-1
Withdrawal technique for an intrauterine device.

viii. The tube is gently inserted (loaded with IUD) through the cervix to the depth of the flange.

ix. Withdrawal technique: The IUD is inserted gently into the uterine cavity by withdrawing the insertion tube over the plunger.

x. The insertion tube is withdrawn ½ in. while the plunger is held still; this releases the IUD into the uterine cavity.

xi. The solid rod is withdrawn, leaving the insertion tube stationary; then the insertion tube is withdrawn.

xii. The IUD string is clipped to the length of 1 in. (2.5 cm) so the patient can feel for the string (Fig. 6-1).

(d) Prophylactic antibiotics: Two published studies differ on whether the use of antibiotics is necessary at the time of insertion. The author prefers to use them.

i. Giving 200 mg of doxycycline at the time of insertion and 100 mg 12 hours after insertion is appropriate in women who are not breast-feeding.

ii. In women who are breast-feeding erythromycin 500 mg PO 1 hour before insertion and 500 mg 6 hours after is appropriate.

(e) IUD removal: Paragard CU T 380A is now approved for 10 years of use. Removal should be done gently with ring forceps or any type of long grasping forceps.

i. Difficult removals may require cervical dilation with dilators or laminaria.

ii. An IUD hook or Novak's curette may be used to grasp an IUD in which strings are not visible.

(f) Pregnancy with an IUD

i. Ectopic pregnancy must be ruled out.

ii. The patient must be informed of signs and symptoms of infection and perforation if IUD strings are not seen.

iii. If IUD strings are seen, remove IUD gently.

(g) Perforation

i. There is 1/1000 incidence.

ii. The most common sites include fundus, body of the uterus, and cervical wall.

iii. If IUD partially perforates it can be removed as a simple IUD removal.

iv. If total perforation is diagnosed by ultrasound and x-ray film, PID or bowel obstruction may occur. In this case antibiotics and removal by laparoscopy is suggested. If no PID or obstruction occurs then patient has option of leaving the IUD and watching for signs or symptoms of PID or obstruction.

(h) If PID develops, treatment should be instituted, the IUD removed, and hospitalization with intravenous antibiotics started.

i. A simple mnemonic device* to remind patients of symptoms that indicate a problem with the IUD.

P Period late (pregnancy), abnormal bleeding
A Abdominal pain
I Infection exposure, abnormal discharges
N Not feeling well, fever, chills
S String missing, shorter, or longer

6.4 FEMALE BARRIERS

1. Diaphragms and cervical cap: These have about the same rate of effectiveness.
   a. Composition and use of diaphragm
      (1) The diaphragm is a dome-shaped rubber cup with a flexible rim.
      (2) It fits in the vagina between the symphysis pubis and the posterior fornix of the vagina, covering the cervix.
      (3) It must be used with contraceptive gel.
      (4) It is effective for 6 hours.
      (5) The diaphragm is not to be worn more than 24 hours (risk of toxic shock syndrome).
      (6) The size is 50 to 95 mm.
      (7) Disposable diaphragms packaged with spermicide are being developed for single use.

*Taken from *Contraceptional Tech,* p. 375.

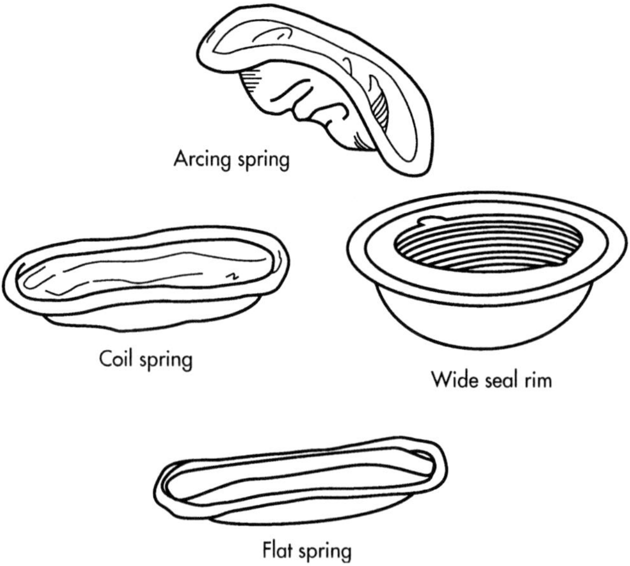

Figure 6-2
Types of diaphragms.

(8) Types (Fig. 6-2)
  (a) Flat spring rim: good for women with good vaginal muscle tone
  (b) Coil spring: good for women with average muscle tone and average pubic arch depth
  (c) Arcing spring: good for poor vaginal muscle tone
  (d) Wide seal: arcing or coil spring

b. Cervical cap (Fig. 6-3)
  (1) A deep rubber cup, smaller than the diaphragm and fits snugly over the cervix only (Prentif cavity rim cervical cap)
  (2) Must be one-third filled with contraceptive gel, effective continuously for 48 hours
  (3) May repeat intercourse without additional spermicide
  (4) Not to be left in more than 48 hours, may cause toxic shock syndrome
  (5) Fem cap and leahs shield—rubber caps now being tested

c. Fitting a diaphragm
  (1) Domed and fitting rings are available.
  (2) The average size is 70 to 75 mm.
  (3) Vaginal depth is estimated by inserting the middle and index finger into the posterior fornix of the vagina; the thumb will mark the pubic bone.

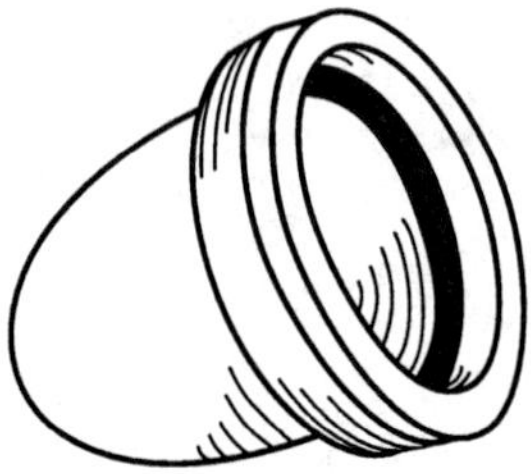

Figure 6-3
Cervical cap.

(4) Several rings or dome sizes should be used to get the best fit, which is the tighter but comfortable fit.

d. Fitting a cervical cap
   (1) The available sizes are 22, 25, 28, and 31 mm.
   (2) Six percent to 10% of patients are unable to be fitted.
   (3) When the cap is fitted, it should be the exact diameter (within a few millimeters only) of the base of the cervix.
   (4) The dome should not be tight to the cervix.
   (5) If the cap is too tight, it will cause cervical trauma.
   (6) The rim of the cap forms a suction around the cervix.

e. Efficacy of female barriers
   (1) All types of barriers have a failure rate of 5% to 9% in nulliparous and 5% to 26% in multiparous users in the first year of use.
   (2) Failures are also more likely to occur in women who have intercourse ≥3 times weekly or are less than 25 years old.
   (3) Increased failures result from use with oil-based lubricants such as mineral oil, baby oil, suntan oil, butter, vaginal medications, yeast preparations, estrogen creams, and Vagisil. Latex will break down.

f. Indications
   (1) No systemic side effects
   (2) Efficacy equal to condoms
   (3) Good for women who are much less sexually active
   (4) Protection against sexually transmitted diseases such as gonorrhea, *Chlamydia,* cervical intraepithelial neoplasia (CIN)

g. Side effects and contraindications
   (1) Allergy to spermicide, rubber, latex, or polyurethane
   (2) Abnormalities in anatomy (may affect the fit)
   (3) Patient insertion error
   (4) May cause recurrent urinary tract infections (UTIs)
   (5) History of toxic shock syndrome
   (6) Lack of experience in fitting cap/diaphragm
   (7) Vaginal bleeding
   (8) Should not be used before 6 weeks postpartum
   (9) Known malignancy (cervix, uterus)

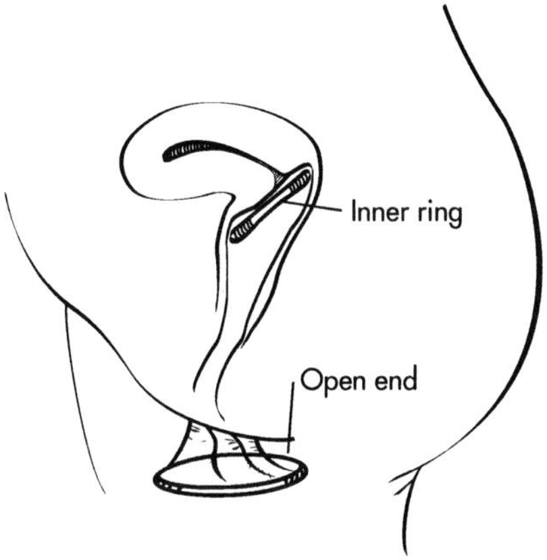

Figure 6-4
Position of female condom.

(10) Unresolved Papanicolaou smears or infections of the genital tract

2. Female condoms
   a. Female condoms look like a combination of a diaphragm and a condom.
   b. The condoms are composed of soft polyurethane, with one end closed, one end open.
   c. They come with extra lubricant.
   d. Insertion: The closed ring is inserted into the vagina and covers the cervix. The open end covers the labia and base of penis (Fig 6-4).
   e. Removal: The open end is twisted to contain semen and the condom is discarded; it should never be reused.
   f. Efficacy: There is a 5.1% pregnancy failure rate with perfect use; failure is 12.4% with average use. The FDA labeling states a 25% failure rate.
   g. Advantages
      (1) Highly effective protection against HIV (94% protection) and all other sexually transmitted diseases
      (2) May be used if male partner refuses to use a condom
3. Male condom
   a. Composition
      (1) Ninety-five percent are latex (rubber) condoms.
      (2) Five percent are skin or natural membrane.
      (3) Most condoms are 7 in. long (170 mm) and 2 in. (50 mm) wide.
      (4) Most condoms are 0.001 to 0.004 in. (0.03 to 0.10 mm) thick.
   b. Proper use of male condom (Fig. 6-5)
      (1) The condom should be placed on the erect penis before genital contact.
      (2) The condom is unrolled to the base of the penis; the rolled portion should remain on the outside of the condom.

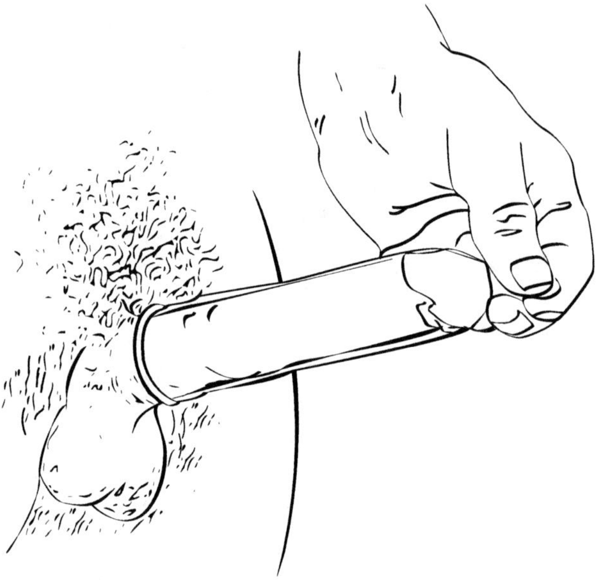

Figure 6-5
Placement of male condom.

(3) One-half inch of empty space is left at the tip of the condom.
(4) The condom must be lubricated; if it is dry it may tear.
(5) Oil-based lubricants should not be used.
(6) To prevent spillage, the condom is held to the base of penis while withdrawing.

c. Efficacy
  (1) Perfect use has a 3% failure rate. Typical use has a 12% failure rate.
  (2) Breakage rate is one or two per 100 condoms used.

d. Advantages
  (1) Accessibility
  (2) Hygienic
  (3) Erection enhancement
  (4) Prevention of sperm allergies
  (5) Prevention of sexually transmitted diseases: effective barrier against HIV, HPV, gonorrhea, herpes simplex, *Chlamydia*

e. Disadvantages
  (1) Interruption of foreplay
  (2) Decreased sexual pleasure for the female
  (3) Latex allergies (1% to 3% of the U.S. population)
  (4) Breakage of condoms

(5) Sheep skin condoms: do not act as a barrier to viruses

4. Spermicides
   a. Chemical methods of contraception are used alone or with other barriers.
   b. Types: Nonoxynol and octoxynol forms: Jellies, creams, foams, suppositories, tablets, and soluble films kill sperm.
   c. Effectiveness depends on correct use. Perfect use has a 3% failure rate, typical use a 36% failure rate.
   d. Use
      (1) Films and suppositories should be inserted into the vagina about 15 minutes before intercourse so they may dissolve.
      (2) They should be inserted deeply into the vagina.
      (3) Spermicide should be reapplied for each episode of intercourse.
      (4) Spermicide should be left in place for 6 to 8 hours after intercourse.
      (5) Users should not douche after intercourse.
      (6) Spermicides should be stored in a cool, dry place.
   e. Advantages
      (1) Sold over the counter
      (2) Inexpensive
      (3) Easy to use
      (4) Can also be used as a lubricant with other barriers
      (5) May help prevent sexually transmitted diseases
   f. Disadvantages
      (1) Irritation in either partner
      (2) May not prevent HIV transmission because of irritation
      (3) Needs to be used after every act of intercourse
      (4) Messy

6.5 LACTATION AMENORRHEA METHOD

The lactation amenorrhea method can provide contraception in the early postpartum months.

1. Mechanism of action
   a. There are decreased progesterone and estrogen levels after delivery.
   b. Ovulation suppression lasts 70 to 100 days after delivery.
   c. Nipple stimulation sends nerve impulses to the hypothalamus that cause release of beta-endorphin, which decreases gonadotropin-releasing hormone (GNRH) secretion; there is no follicle development.
   d. Increased levels of prolactin make ovaries unresponsive to LH, suppressing positive feedback effects of estrogen on the midcycle rise of GNRH or directly interfering with ovarian steroid production.
   e. The sucking mechanism is crucial for effectiveness. A woman who is fully or nearly fully breast-feeding and remains amenorrheic for 6 months postpartum is protected against pregnancy.
   f. Breast-feeding is effective as birth control for 6 months if 15 or more feedings lasting 10 minutes are accomplished daily.

g. This method depends on the intensity of breast-feeding and rate of menses return.
h. Most of the women in the United States do not practice full, on-demand breast-feeding, which is the basis of the lactation amenorrhea method; they need to use complementary contraceptive methods.

6.6 ABSTINENCE

Abstinence is defined as refraining from intercourse.

1. Abstainers outnumber people choosing to have intercourse in the United States until age 17.
2. Late 1980s surveys show that 12.4% of unmarried men and 13.2% of unmarried women 25 to 34 years old had no sexual partners in the past year.
3. In all, 13% of women 30 to 34 years old have never had sex.
4. The goal of abstinence is to avoid sexually transmitted diseases.
5. Abstinence should be seriously discussed with adolescents.
6. Adolescents should plan on how to say "No" to intercourse.
7. High-pressure sexual situations should be avoided.
8. "No" should be said clearly.

6.7 WITHDRAWAL

1. Mechanism: withdrawal of the penis from the vagina before ejaculation
2. Effectiveness: 4% failure rate for perfect use; a 19% failure in typical use
3. Advantages
   a. There are no costs, devices, or chemicals.
   b. This is a backup method that is always available.
   c. Only 2% of women use this method.
4. Disadvantages
   a. The excitement is interrupted.
   b. The method relies on self-control.
   c. The partners are not protected from transmission of sexually transmitted diseases before ejaculation.

6.8 RHYTHM METHOD—NATURAL FAMILY PLANNING

1. Mechanism of action
   a. This method depends on the awareness of the physiology of the male and female reproductive tracts.
   b. Sperm and ovum lifespans are as follows:
      (1) Sperm viability averages 3 days; however, the range is 2 to 7 days.
      (2) Ovum life span is about 24 hours.
   c. The unsafe period is considered to be up to 7 days before ovulation and 3 days after ovulation.
   d. Avoid intercourse at these unsafe times or use other methods such as barriers for backup.

2. Effectiveness rate
   a. There is a 20% failure rate for typical use in the first year.
   b. Perfect use has a failure rate of 1% to 9%.
   c. The most effective version is the postovulation method.
   d. If used perfectly, the symptothermal and ovulation method is very effective.
   e. The calendar method is the least effective.
3. Types include the postovulation method, the symptothermal method, the ovulation method, and the calendar method.
   a. Symptothermal
      (1) Cervical mucus basal body temperature (thermal) is measured.
      (2) Lower abdominal pain with ovulation is experienced (symptom).
      (3) Perfect use: Intercourse can be resumed only on the fourth day peak mucus and the third day after thermal rise.
   b. Ovulation method (Billings method)
      (1) Mucus is checked from the vagina before urination.
      (2) Mucus is checked for lubrication, elasticity, wetness, and tackiness (it ferns midcycle).
      (3) Ovulation occurs 1 day before, after, or during the last day of the most slippery and abundant mucus.
      (4) The fertile period is any time mucus is noted before ovulation.
      (5) NOTE: Some women have very insignificant mucus discharges at ovulation time.
   c. Basal body temperature (BBT) charting (temperature method)
      (1) Body temperature is taken every morning.
      (2) The temperature is charted on a BBT chart.
      (3) Look for a biphasic temperature chart (Fig. 6-6).
      (4) However, 6 out of 30 women ovulate but do not have biphasic changes on a temperature chart.
4. Advantages
   a. There are no side effects.
   b. Some couples like to be totally involved in fertility prevention.
5. Disadvantages
   a. There is no protection against sexually transmitted diseases.
   b. The male partner sometimes objects to participating.
   c. It is not as reliable a method of contraception with women who have irregular cycles, recent menarche, approaching menopause, or who are unable to keep records.

6.9 STERILIZATION

1. Male vasectomy
   a. Vasectomy interrupts the vas deferentia. This prevents the passage of sperm into the seminal ejaculate. It is about half as common as female sterilization in the United States.
   b. The failure rate of this method is about 0.1% in the first year. This does not include pregnancies that occur secondary to a couple's failure to wait for sperm to be cleared from the distal vas deferentia.

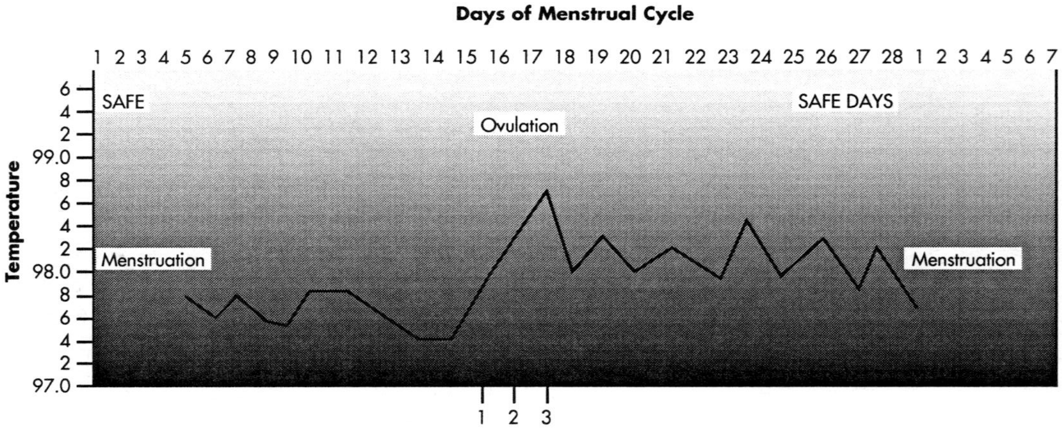

Figure 6-6
Basal body temperature variations during a model menstrual cycle.

c. Techniques: Sterilization is done under aseptic conditions with 1% lidocaine injection.
   (1) Scalpel technique
      (a) The vas deferentia are divided through an open skin incision (Fig. 6-7).
      (b) The divided ends are either fulgurated (more effective) or tied. A portion of the vas may be removed (not necessary).
      (c) The fascia may be sutured over one end of the divided vas; this may increase the effectiveness.
   (2) No-scalpel technique
      (a) The vas is grasped through the closed skin of the scrotum by a ring forceps (Fig. 6-8).
      (b) A sharp tipped forceps punctures the skin.
      (c) The vas is drawn out.
      (d) The same occlusion technique is used as for the scalpel technique.
      (e) The no-scalpel technique avoids skin incisions, decreases the rate of hematoma formation, affords bloodless surgery,

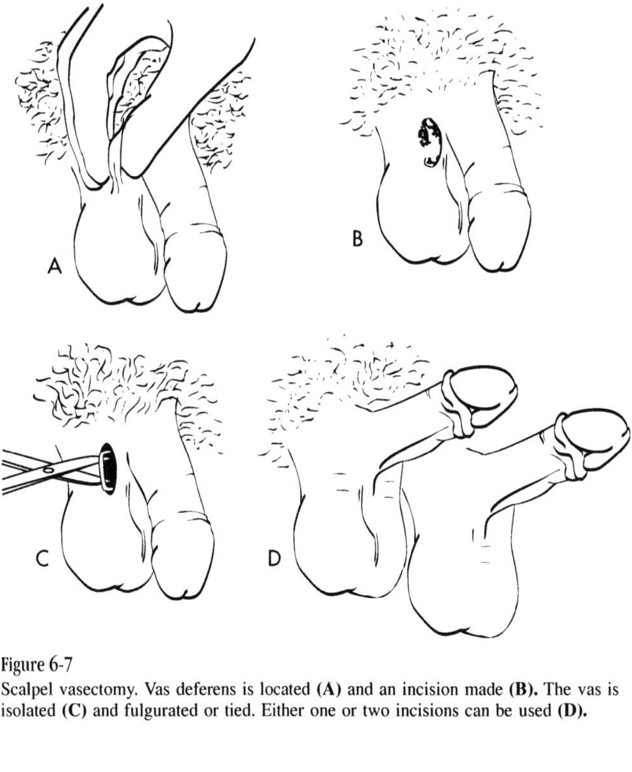

Figure 6-7
Scalpel vasectomy. Vas deferens is located **(A)** and an incision made **(B).** The vas is isolated **(C)** and fulgurated or tied. Either one or two incisions can be used **(D).**

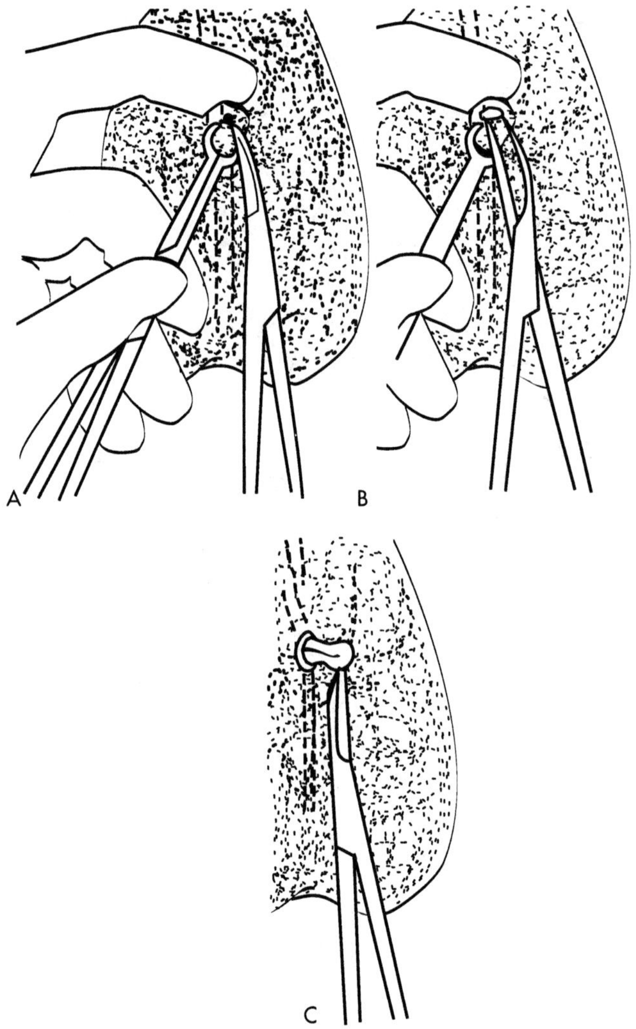

Figure 6-8
No-scalpel vasectomy. The vas (dotted line) is grasped by special ring forceps and the skin and the vas sheath are pierced by sharp-tipped dissecting forceps **(A).** The forceps stretch the opening **(B)** and the vas is lifted out **(C).**

and may be more acceptable in societies where skin scrotum incisions are not acceptable.

(3) Advantages: vasectomy vs. female sterilization
  (a) Safer procedure than female sterilization
  (b) More easily performed
  (c) Less expensive than female sterilization
  (d) Does not require general anesthesia

(1) Disadvantages
  (a) There is no protection against sexually transmitted diseases.
  (b) The procedure is permanent. Reversal cannot always be accomplished.
  (c) This is a "male only" form of birth control.
  (d) Five percent to 10% of men regret having the procedure.
  (e) One third to two thirds of men develop sperm antibodies postvasectomy.

(1) Safety of vasectomy: continually studied
  (a) Fears of increased risk of cardiovascular disease have been allayed by the Sichuan study, 1983-1986.
  (b) Also, studies have shown that there is no increased risk of developing prostate cancer postvasectomy.

2. Female sterilization
   a. Female sterilization is the leading popular method of fertility control in the United States, especially in women over 30 years old.
   b. Fifty percent are done at the time of delivery; 50% are done outside of pregnancy (interval).
   c. Women should be carefully counseled before they make such a permanent decision.
   d. All possible future situations should be discussed (i.e., divorce, remarriage, death of a spouse or child, future improvement of economic situation).
   e. Women younger than 30 years old have a greater tendency to regret the decision and seek reversal. Between 5% and 15% regret it. Only 1% to 2% seek reversal.
   f. Only the partner who has made the decision to end the possibility for child bearing should have the permanent procedure done.
   g. All other birth control options should be reviewed with the patient because she may not realize the benefits connected with other birth control options and the importance of keeping the option to have children in the future open.
   h. Also, it must be made very clear to the patient that this procedure should be viewed as permanent even though it has a failure rate.
   i. Types
      (1) Sterilization at the time of cesarean section
         (a) Pomeroy technique
            i. The technique was published in 1930; "the gold standard."
            ii. A loop of fallopian tube is grasped with a babcock clamp. An absorbable, plain, catgut suture is tied

around the loop; the loop is excised and is sent to pathology.

(b) Irving technique
  i. Described in 1924.
  ii. Destroys no tube, is highly effective, and is highly reversible.
  iii. The tube is divided at the isthmus. The proximal end is buried in the myometrium, and the distal end is buried in the broad ligament.
  iv. There is no known failure rate.
  v. The morbidity is higher than for other tubal ligation methods.

(2) Fimbriectomy
  (a) The procedure is not reversible; it is permanent.
  (b) Fimbria is totally excised, including the fimbria ovarica (portion of the tube connected to the ovary).

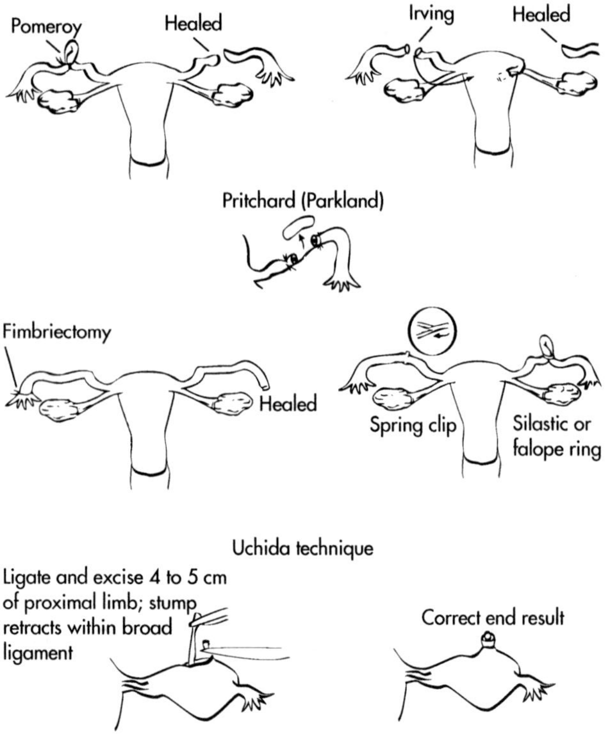

Figure 6-9
Techniques for tubal sterilization.

(c) Failures are secondary to not excising the fimbria ovarica.

(3) Postpartum tubal

(a) It is done 1 day postpartum.

(b) The incision is a small infraumbilical incision and may be done transversely very close to the umbilicus. Often the incision is hidden within the umbilicus and is no larger than a laparoscopic incision.

j. Techniques

(1) Pomeroy [see i.(1)(a)]

(2) Uchida technique

(a) A saline epinephrine solution is injected into tubal musculature to separate the serosa from the inner circular muscle of the tube.

(b) The edematous tube is incised on its antimesenteric side.

(c) The inner circular muscle of the tube is excised.

(d) The proximal stump is buried beneath the edematous serosa and the distal stump outside the serosa.

(e) The excised portions are sent to pathology.

(3) Clip application technique (Fig. 6-9)

(a) Spring loaded clips are used (same as for laparoscopy).

(b) The isthmus of the tube is stretched between two babcock clamps.

(c) The clip is put on by hand by holding the jaws of the clip between the thumb and the third finger. The index finger pushes the spring into locked position.

Table 6-6 Technical difficulties

Author	Electro-coagulation	Ring	Hulka Clip	Filshie Clip
Bhiwandiwal	3.03%	4.03%	6.06%	—
Khandwal	—	4.24%	8.50%	—
Parikh	—	—	—	10.72%

From Khandwala S: *J Reprod Med* 5:465, 1988.

Table 6-7 Technical failures

Author	Bipolar Coagulation	Endo-coagulation	Ring	Hulka Clip	Filshie Clip
Hirsch	0.08%	—	—	—	—
Kleppinger	0%	—	—	—	—
Riedel	—	0.1%	—	—	—
Bhiwandiwala	—	—	0.93%	0.74%	—
Khandwala	—	—	0.17%	0.3%	—
Chi	—	—	3.8%	—	—
Hulka	—	—	—	0.4%	—
Parika	—	—	—	—	0%

From Khandwala S: *J Reprod Med* 5:465, 1988.

Table 6-8 Effectiveness and mortality of contraceptive methods

	Pregnancies per 100 Women/ Years All Ages	
Method	Lowest Expected	Typical
No Contraception	85	85
Surgical Sterilization		
Tubal ligation	0.2	0.4
Combination Oral Contraceptives		
Nonsmokers	0.1	3
Smokers	0.1	3
Progestin-Only Oral Contraceptives	0.5	3
Progestin Injections		
Medroxyprogesterone acetate (MPA)	0.3	0.3
Norethindrone enanthanate (NET)	0.4	0.4
Progestin Implants		
Levonorgestrel (LNG)	0.3	0.3
Intrauterine Devices		
Progestasert	2.0	3
Copper T 380A	0.8	3
Barrier Methods*		
Diaphragm, cap	6	18
Condoms	2	12
Aerosol foam, jelly, cream, tablets	3	21
Sponge		
Parous women	9	28
Nulliparous women	6	18
Periodic Abstinence (rhythm)	1-9	20

From Dickey R: *Managing contraceptive pill patient,* Durant, OK, ed 8, 1994, Essential Medical Information Systems.

*In a comparative study of 1437 women using the sponge vs. diaphragm and a study of 1394 women using the cervical cap vs. diaphragm the 12 months failure rate was diaphragm, 5.2 and 6.9%; cervical cap 11.4%; sponge 11.7%. Failure rates increased to 26.4% for the cap and 20% for the sponge among parous users. The failure rate for condoms was estimated at 2.7%. J. Trussel, Office of Population Research, Princeton University, 1993.

3. Interval sterilization
   a. The procedure is done outside of pregnancy.
   b. Original unipolar technique was described by Steptoe.
   c. The introduction of laparoscopy made it a popular procedure not associated with pregnancy.

Estimated Annual Deaths Resulting from Contraceptive Method and/or Pregnancy per 100,000 Women/Years by Age

15-19	20-24	25-29	30-34	35-39	40-44
6	5	7	14	19	22
4	4	4	4	4	4
1	1	1	2	4	3
2	2	2	11	13	59
1	1	1	1	1	1
1	1	1	1	1	1
1	1	1	1	1	1
1	1	1	1	1	1
1	1	1	1	2	1
1	1	1	1	1	1
1-2	1-2	1-2	1-4	1-6	1-7
1-3	1-3	1-4	1-7	1-11	1-12
1-3	1-3	1-4	1-7	1-11	1-12
1-2	1-2	1-3	1-6	1-8	1-10
1-2	1-2	1-2	1-4	1-6	1-7
1-2	1-2	1-2	1-4	1-16	1-16

d. Vaginal sterilization by fimbriectomy was the only interval form of tubal ligation before laparoscopy.

e. Types (all done through the laparoscopy)
   (1) Unipolar coagulation
      (a) The tube was grasped and burned until blanching.
      (b) Scissors were used to excise the blanched portion, which was sent to pathology.
      (c) A current ran through patient's body. Morbidity is secondary to bowel and skin burn.
      (d) No longer used because morbidity, secondary to extensive tissue destruction is too high.

(2) Bipolar technique: developed independently in the 1970s by Kleppinger (United States), Rioux (Canada), and Hirsh (Germany)
    (a) This is the most common laparoscopic tubal ligation.
    (b) This technique is the easiest to perform.
    (c) The bipolar technique works by concentrating the electricity between two paddles; therefore, the patient does not carry the current.
    (d) Kleppinger recommends that the tube be burned in three places so there is at least a 3-cm gap between healthy portions of tube.
    (e) It is recommended that the cauterization begin 2 to 3 cm from the cornual angles, preventing uteroperitoneal fistulization and ectopic pregnancy formation.
(3) Falope Ring (silastic band)
    (a) The Falope Ring is safer than cautery.
    (b) It was developed in the 1970s.
    (c) The fallopian tube is grasped into a metal cylinder with grasping prongs.
    (d) The silastic ring occludes the base of a 3-cm portion of tube, which necroses.
    (e) It is associated with a 2.5% incidence of hemorrhage secondary to stretching of vessels beneath the tube or tearing of the tube.
    (f) The patient has pain from 48 to 96 hours from tubal hypoxia.
(4) Spring clip
    (a) Of the laparoscopic methods, it is the most difficult technically.
    (b) The clip must go across the whole tube.
    (c) The spring clip is applied across the isthmus of the tube.
    (d) Most procedures are reversible; destroys only 5 mm of the tube.
    (e) This is the best method for women under 30 years.
(5) Minilaparotomy tubal
    (a) Minilaparotomy tubal may be used if there is a contraindication to laparoscopy.
    (b) It is described as a technique using local anesthesia and intravenous sedation. General anesthesia also may be used.
    (c) A 2- to 5-cm suprapubic incision is made. The Pomeroy technique, clips, or silastic rings may be used on the tubes.
    (d) A dilator is placed in the uterus before the technique is done for manipulation and uterine elevation.

f. Failure rates of sterilization: All laparoscopic tubal ligations have a failure rate of between 2 and 10 pregnancies per 1000 operations (Tables 6-6 and 6-7).
g. Posttubal syndrome: an irregular cycle and dysmenorrhea post–tubual ligation

(1) Studies have been done, but none have been conclusive.
(2) Menstrual irregularities and dysmenorrhea are probably not caused by tubal ligation.
(3) It is more likely that the woman's own cycles are surfacing.
(4) Complication rate (Table 6-8)
    (a) Defined as those requiring laparotomy for repair
    (b) Has stayed below 2 in 1000 for the past decade
    (c) Mortality has not been reported since 1982
    (d) Major vessel laceration from trocar needle insertion in 1/1000 to 1/10,000 cases
    (e) Thermal bowel injury in 1/1000 cases

Suggested reading

ACOG Technical Bulletin, "Hormonal Contraception," 198:1994.
Burkman RT Jr: Non-contraceptive effects of hormonal contraceptive: review, *Am J Obstet Gynecol* 170:1569-1575, 1994.
Connell EB: The female condom: a new contraceptive option, *Contemp OB/GYN,* October 15, 1994.
Goldzieher JW: Are low dose oral contraceptives safer and better? (review), *Am J Obstet Gynecol* 171(3):587-590, 1994.
Grimes DA, editor: *The contraception report,* vol IV, no. 4, September, 1993.
Grimes DA, editor: *The contraception report,* vol IV, no. 5, November, 1993.
Grimes DA, editor: *The contraception report,* vol V, no. 4, September, 1994.
Grimes DA, editor: *The contraception report,* "Spermicides," vol V, no. 5, 1994, Patient Update 5.
Grimes DA, editor: *The contraception report,* vol V, no. 5, November, 1994.
Grimes DA, editor: *The contraception report,* "The Female Condom," vol V, no. 6, Patient Update 6, January, 1995.
Grimes DA, editor: *The contraception report,* vol V, no. 6, January, 1995.
Gynopharma Inc: Patient package insert, Paragard T 380A, May, 1994.
Hatcher RA et al: *Contraceptive technology,* ed 16 rev., New York, 1994, Irvington Publishers.
Khandwala, SD: Laparoscopic Sterilization, *J Reprod Med* 33(5):465-467, 1988.
Miller DM et al: A practical approach to antibiotic treatment in women taking oral contraceptives, *J Am Acad Dermatol* 30(6):1008-1011, 1994.
Mishell DR Jr, editor: *Dialogues in contraception,* Summer, 1992.
Mishell DR Jr, editor: *Dialogues in contraception II,* vol 4, no. 2, Winter, 1994.
Nichols DH, editor: *Gynecologic and obstetric surgery,* St Louis, 1993, Mosby.
Stratton P, Alexander NJ: Prevention of sexually transmitted infection, physical and chemical barrier methods, *Infect Dis Clin North* Am 7(4):841-859, 1993.
Waites GM: Male fertility regulation, *Br Med Bull* 49(1):56-63, 1994.
Wang IY et al: Reproductive function and contraception in the postpartum period, *Obstet Gynecol Surv* 49(1):56-63, 1994.

7 Infertility Evaluation

7.1 **FEMALE INFERTILITY**

Carolyn M. Doherty, M.D.

History and evaluation

1. Definition: Infertility is generally defined as the inability to achieve a conception after 1 year of unprotected intercourse.
2. Prevalence
   a. Infertility affects 13% to 15% of married couples in the United States.
   b. An episode of infertility will be experienced by 25% of women during their reproductive years.
3. Evaluation of the infertile female
   a. History: A detailed patient history is important.
      (1) Age of patient: fertility decreases with increasing age
      (2) Exposure to chemicals, toxins, or radiation in the work environment
      (3) Smokers: three to four times more likely to experience longer than a 1-year delay to conception when compared with nonsmokers; a relative risk of 3.1 for an ectopic pregnancy when compared with control pregnant patients
      (4) Caffeine: may be associated with an increased risk of miscarriage
      (5) Alcohol use
      (6) Current drugs or medications
         (a) Antihistamines: can decrease mucus production and also diminish vaginal lubrication
         (b) Nonsteroidal antiinflammatory drugs: can inhibit the luteinizing hormone (LH) surge
         (c) Barbiturates: can decrease or inhibit gonadotropin-releasing hormone (GNRH) release
      (7) Excessive physical activity: can lead to anovulatory cycles
      (8) Marital history
         (a) Number of years
         (b) Contraception used

(9) Sexual intercourse
  (a) Frequency: times per month
  (b) Adequate penetration
  (c) Ejaculation: retrograde, normal
  (d) Difficulties: impotence
  (e) Coital positions
  (f) Use of lubricants: type
  (g) Pain or discomfort: either partner
  (h) Orgasm
  (i) Masturbation: frequency, especially by the male partner
(10) Pregnancy history
  (a) All pregnancies: term, preterm, abortions
  (b) Dates
  (c) Outcome
  (d) Weight
  (e) Sex
  (f) Complications
  (g) Abortions: date, length of pregnancy, complications
  (h) Number of natural children
(11) Previous marriages: both partners
  (a) Number of years
  (b) Contraception use: number of years, type
  (c) Children
  (d) Miscarriages
(12) Past workup
  (a) Tests performed: repeating same tests should be avoided
  (b) Dates, results, physician's name
(13) Menstrual history
  (a) Age at onset of menses
  (b) Age of sexual development
  (c) Present menstrual cycle
    i. Length: start to start
    ii. Duration of flow
    iii. Date of last menstrual period
  (d) Dysmenorrhea
    i. What was the age of onset?
    ii. Does it occur with each cycle?
  (e) Vaginal discharge
    i. Color: Green or bright yellow is abnormal.
    ii. Odor: If odor present, it should be cultured.
    iii. Irritation: Wet mount and culture are probably required.
(14) Medical history
  (a) Allergies
  (b) Surgeries
  (c) Medications
  (d) Blood transfusion
  (e) Pelvic infection: syphilis, gonorrhea, *Chlamydia*
  (f) Thyroid disease
  (g) Other chronic medical problems

b. Physical examination
   (1) Head, ears, eyes, nose, and throat (HEENT)
      (a) Clinicians should be alert for exophthalmos (Graves disease).
      (b) The thyroid should be palpated for enlargement or nodules.
   (2) Breast
      (a) A complete breast examination is necessary.
      (b) Clinicians should be alert for galactorrhea; if present, prolactin and thyroid-stimulating hormone (TSH) should be checked.
      (c) Of patients with polycystic ovaries (PCO), 25% will have hyperprolactinemia.
   (3) Abdomen
      (a) Clinicians should palpate for masses.
      (b) Often, myomas can be palpated abdominally.
   (4) External genitalia
      (a) The size of the clitoris should be carefully examined. Enlargement is a sign of excessive androgens.
   (5) Cervix
      (a) A yearly Papanicolaou smear should be performed.
      (b) Clinicians should observe for scarring secondary to cones, cryotherapy, and LEEP.
      (c) Observe the canal for signs of stenosis.
   (6) Uterus, ovaries
      (a) Size
      (b) Position
      (c) Fixed vs. mobile
      (d) Contour: smooth vs. nodular
      (e) Pain

Common causes of infertility

1. Endometriosis
   a. Endometriosis is a condition characterized by ectopic endometrial glands and stroma.
   b. The etiology of endometriosis is unknown. Possible etiologies are as follows:
      (1) Retrograde menstruation
      (2) Vascular or lymphatic transport
      (3) Transformation of coelomic epithelium into endometrial type glands (coelomic metaplasia)
      (4) Immunologic alteration leading to a decreased cellular immunity to endometrial tissue
   c. Symptoms
      (1) Dysmenorrhea
      (2) Dyspareunia, especially with deep penetration
      (3) Low back pain
      (4) Infertility
   d. Examination: Certain findings should raise a physician's index of suspicion.
      (1) Retroverted uterus
      (2) Enlarged ovaries

(3) Fixed uterus or ovaries
(4) Tender, nodular uterosacral ligaments

e. Diagnosis
(1) Laparoscopy should be performed.
(2) Suspicious lesions on the cervix should be biopsied.

f. Treatment
(1) Surgical
(a) Operative laparoscopy to ablate all visible lesions and debulk ovarian endometriomas
(b) Laparotomy: debulking procedure
(2) Medical
(a) GNRH agonist (Depo-Lupron, Zoladex)
(b) Oral contraceptives: decidualize endometrial tissue
(c) Danazol: should be used only in cases of persistent pain
(d) Progestational agents (Depo-Provera, Provera)

2. Cervical factor
(1) Scarring
(a) Previous cone, LEEP, or cryotherapy
(2) Diethylstilbesterol (DES) exposure
(3) Clomiphene citrate
(a) Antiestrogenic mechanism of action leads to thick cervical mucus.

3. Uterine factor
(1) Müllerian anomalies
(2) Antatomic abnormalities
(a) Myomas
(b) Ashermans
(c) Adenomyosis: presence of endometriosis within the myometrium; these patients have chronic pelvic pain
(3) Diagnosis
(a) HSG: needed by all infertility patients
(b) Ultrasound
(c) Magnetic resonance imaging (MRI): especially for Müllerian anomalies and myomas
(4) Treatment
(a) Surgical: See Surgical Therapy for Infertility, p. 140.
(b) Medical: See Medical Management of Infertility, p. 137.

4. Male factor infertility
a. Semen analysis: Physicians should never make a diagnosis based on a single semen analysis (see also Section 7.2).
(1) Normal semen parameters[1]*
(a) Volume: 2.0 ml or greater
(b) pH: 7.2 to 8.0
(c) Concentration: 20×10^6 spermatozoa/ml or greater
(d) Motility: 50% or greater
(e) Morphology: 30% or greater normal forms
(f) White blood cells: 1×10^6/ml or fewer

*_WHO Laboratory Manual,_ ed 3.

5. Male factor infertility
   a. Specimen collection rules
      (1) Three days of abstinence is optimal.
      (2) Specimens should be produced via masturbation.
      (3) No lubricants may be used.
      (4) Specimens should be collected in a sterile specimen container.
      (5) Extremes of temperature should be avoided while transporting to the laboratory.
   b. See Section 7.2 for further information on male factor infertility.
6. Hormonal dysfunction
   a. Disorders of ovulation
      (1) Polycystic ovarian syndrome: LH/FSH (follicle-stimulating hormone) ratio of 3:1 or greater
      (2) Hypothyroidism: high TSH
      (3) Oligo-ovulation: etiology unknown
   b. Luteal phase defect: Defined as a lag of more than 2 days in the histologic development of the endometrium as compared with the actual day of the cycle. It is diagnosed by an appropriately timed endometrial biopsy. It is best to time the biopsy by the LH surge rather than the start of the menses. Luteal phase defects have one of the following etiologies:
      (1) Lack of adequate progesterone production
      (2) Inability of the endometrium to respond to the progesterone that is present
7. Pelvic adhesions
   a. Diagnosis
      (1) Hysterosalpingography (HSG): look for tubal occlusion or contrast loculation
      (2) Laparoscopy: direct evaluation of pelvic anatomy
   b. Therapy
      (1) Surgical lysis
      (2) Assisted reproductive technology (ART)
8. Ovarian failure
   a. Diagnosis
      (1) Serum FSH
         (a) <15: There is a good chance for successful ART.
         (b) >15 to <25: There is a diminished chance for success. Oocyte donation should be discussed with the patient.
         (c) >25: Estrogen replacement should be started and oocyte donation discussed.
9. Unexplained infertility
   a. This is a diagnosis of exclusion. A complete workup should be done before this diagnosis is made.

Diagnostic studies

1. Complete history and physical examination
   a. As previously outlined
2. HSG
   a. An HSG is a fluoroscopic examination used to demonstrate uterotubal disease.

b. An HSG should be performed early in the workup of the infertile female. Laparoscopy and HSG are complementary procedures. Chromotubation at the time of laparoscopy does not replace the HSG. Valuable information about the uterine cavity, such as intrauterine filling defects and the status of the fallopian tubes (i.e., the location of tubal occlusion), can be delineated by HSG.
c. HSG should be done before laparoscopy to verify and treat (if possible) at the time of surgery.
d. The timing of HSG should be just after the patient finishes her menses and well before the time of ovulation.
e. Indications for HSG
    (1) Infertility
    (2) Abnormal uterine bleeding
    (3) Repetitive pregnancy loss
    (4) Confirmation of uterine myomas
f. Contraindications
    (1) Current or suspected pelvic infection: HSG can lead to salpingitis or endometritis if performed during an active infection. Patients with a history of pelvic inflammatory disease (PID) have a 1% to 3% risk of recurrent infection after an HSG and therefore should be treated with antibiotics (doxcycline 100 mg, bid) beginning 24 hours before the examination.
    (2) Active bleeding: Active bleeding at the time of HSG can lead to contrast extravasation; passage of blood into the peritoneal cavity, possibly leading to endometriosis; and an inaccurate diagnosis of an intrauterine filling defect because of the presence of blood clots in the cavity.
    (3) Pregnancy: When HSG is inadvertently done during an early pregnancy, it is usually an "all-or-none phenomenon." If the fetus survives (which is usually the case), it will not be affected by the exposure.
g. Procedure technique
    (1) The physician inquires as to allergies to shellfish or iodine.
    (2) The physician inserts speculum and cleans cervix with betadine.
    (3) The physician places a single-tooth tenaculum on the anterior lip of the cervix and introduces the Kahn cannula into the os.
    (4) The speculum is removed slowly to avoid disrupting the cannula.
    (5) Contrast is injected slowly while always visualizing the uterine cavity for filling defects and the tubes for abnormal contour.
    (6) The physician should attempt to demonstrate tubal patency. However, the patient should not be tortured in the attempt.

3. Semen analysis
4. Hormonal development
    a. The menstrual cycle consists of three distinct phases.
        (1) Follicular phase (time during which the follicle develops): This phase is characterized by a rising estradiol.
            (a) The estradiol should peak at the time of ovulation at approximately 300 pg/ml.

(b) Progesterone in the follicular phase is always less than 1.
(c) It should be remembered that actual ovulation occurs 36 hours after the onset of the LH surge.
(d) An easy way to determine the day of ovulation is to subtract 14 days from the total cycle length to give the day of ovulation.

(2) Luteal phase (begins after ovulation, which is brought about by the LH surge)
(a) Any time the LH level rises two to four times above the baseline level, it is considered to be the ovulatory surge.
(b) This phase is characterized by rising progesterone levels (>2 ng/ml) and also by a secondary peak of the estradiol level on day 21.
(c) If a pregnancy occurs, then the hormone levels remain elevated.
(d) If no pregnancy occurs, then the hormone levels drop and menses begin.
(e) The basal body temperature (BBT) will rise 0.3° to 0.5° during the luteal phase and is associated with progesterone levels greater than 4 ng/ml.
(f) Care must be taken because BBT charts can be misleading.

(3) Menstrual phase: A drop in hormones leads the onset of menses.

5. Follicular development
   a. The follicle is a fluid-filled sac that contains the oocyte. It should be 18 to 25 mm at the time of ovulation.
   b. The development of the follicle can easily be followed by transvaginal ultrasound.
   c. An easy way to determine whether follicles of the correct size are being produced is to scan the patient 15 days before her expected menses. This should be just before ovulation.
6. Cervical mucus or postcoital testing
   a. Cervical mucus is estrogen dependent. There should be an increase in production at the time of ovulation.
   b. Mucus is evaluated for the following:
      (1) Consistency: should be thin, clear
      (2) Spinnbarkeit: thready stretchability
      (3) Ferning: product of estrogen influence
      (4) Cellularity
      (5) Volume: should be abundant
      (6) pH: 6.4 to 8.0
   c. A postcoital test (PCT) should be done 6 to 10 hours after intercourse. The endocervical specimen should contain 25 sperm per high-power field (HPF). Ten or more sperm with progressive motility should be considered an adequate PCT.
7. Endometrial biopsy
   a. The endometrial biopsy is used to diagnose a luteal phase defect (LFD). LFD is defined in one of the two following ways:

(1) An inadequate amount of progesterone being secreted by the corpus luteum
(2) The inability of the endometrium to respond to adequate progesterone concentrations

b. The diagnosis of LFD is made by two endometrial biopsies greater than 2 days out of phase.
c. Endometrial biopsy should be done 12 days after the LH surge.
d. Samples should be removed via a small pipette (Pipelle) from the anterior uterine wall to avoid possibly disrupting an early implantation, because the posterior surface is the most common site of implantation.
e. Pretreatment of patients with acetaminophen or Naprosyn is advised.

8. Laparoscopy/hysteroscopy
   a. Surgery should be the last step in the workup.
   b. Laparoscopy
      (1) Laparoscopy can be both diagnostic and therapeutic.
      (2) Visualization of the pelvis must be done to make the diagnosis of endometriosis or pelvic adhesions.
      (3) Laparoscopy can be done in the follicular or the luteal phase of the cycle. If chromotubation is planned, it should not be done during the menstrual cycle.
   c. Hysteroscopy
      (1) Hysteroscopy should be done when there is a suspected or known intrauterine defect. This is why hysterosalpingography is so important.
      (2) Tubal cannulation of proximal obstruction of the fallopian tubes can be accomplished hysteroscopically.
      (3) Intraoperative HSG can be done to assess the uterine cavity during an operative hysteroscopic procedure.

Medical management of infertility

The approach in this section is to take the most common causes of infertility as outlined in History and Evaluation and discuss medical management options.

1. Endometriosis: Endometriosis lesions have estrogen, androgen, and progesterone receptors. The concentration of these receptors is lower than that of eutopic endometrium. However, estradiol is the critical hormone regulating growth and development of endometriosis. Androgens and progestins produce atrophy in endometriosis lesions.
   a. Treatment options
      (1) Danazol
         (a) Derivative of 17-ethinyltestosterone
         (b) Produces a high-androgen, low-estrogen environment
         (c) Should *no longer be used* as first-line treatment for endometriosis
         (d) Dose > 100 mg/day leads to pain relief in most patients
         (e) Doses of 100 to 800 mg/day are most effective for treatment purposes

(2) GNRH analogs
   (a) The mechanism of action is effectively to shut down GNRH stimulation of FSH and LH, leading to a hypoestrogenic state.
   (b) The first 8 to 10 days after administration, the effects are stimulatory until downregulation occurs. Therefore, Depo-Lupron should be administered 8 to 10 days before expected menses (day 20) and then every 28 days after this for 6 months.
   (c) Most patients can be started on 3.75 mg of Depo-Lupron. Two weeks after the second shot, a serum estradiol level should be checked to make sure the patient is suppressed (E2 < 20 pg/ml). If the level is greater than 20 pg/ml, the next injection should be 7.5 mg.
   (d) Most patients require 6 months of therapy.

(3) Progestins
   (a) These agents produce a hypoestrogenic state by suppressing FSH and LH.
   (b) Good choices are Provera (10 to 30 mg day) and Depo-Provera 150 mg every 3 months.

(4) Oral contraceptives
   (a) There is a dual mechanism of action (i.e., suppression of LH and FSH as well as decidualization of the endometrium).
   (b) The most effective regime is a continuous regimen, but cyclic administration can also provide relief.
   (c) This is not a "treatment" for endometriosis; it is suppressive therapy.
   (d) Lo-Ovral is a good choice for this therapy.

2. Cervical factor
   a. The medical treatment of choice for cervical factor infertility is intrauterine insemination.
   b. The oral administration of estrogen does not improve cervical mucus or enhance pregnancy rates and should not be done.
3. Uterine factor
   a. Myomas
      (1) Indications for medical therapy of myomas
         (a) Bleeding
         (b) Pain
         (c) Preoperative therapy: to improve hemoglobin and decrease the risk of blood transfusion
      (2) GNRH agonists
         (a) They are the only real medical therapy.
         (b) They must suppress estradiol levels to less than 45 pg/ml.
         (c) Optimal therapeutic benefit comes after 3 months of therapy (Depo-Lupron, 3.75 mg, every 28 days).
         (d) Myomas will undergo rapid regrowth upon cessation of therapy.

b. Adenomyosis
    (1) Adenomyosis is a condition in which endometriosis is found within the myometrium.
    (2) It is characterized by chronic pelvic pain.
    (3) It is found in approximately one of every six patients at the time of hysterectomy (most are multiparous).
    (4) Its effect on fertility is unknown.
    (5) Medical therapy is the same as that for pelvic endometriosis.

4. Male factor (See Section 7.2.)
5. Hormonal dysfunction
    a. Disorders of ovulation. Usually require ovulation induction.
        (1) Clomid
            (a) Clomid works by blocking estrogen receptor binding or replenishment at hypothalamic or pituitary level, thus blocking estrogen feedback, leading to increased serum gonadotropins.
            (b) It is administered orally day 3 to day 7 or day 5 to day 9.
            (c) Dosage can be increased if ovulation does not occur. Recommended doses are 50 to 150 mg.
            (d) Human chorionic gonadotropin (HCG) (Profasi) can be added to increase ovulation rates. Administer IM 5000 or 10,000 IU when follicles are greater than 20 mm.
        (2) Humegon/Pergonal
            (a) These are injectable gonadotropins consisting of 75 IU of FSH and 75 IU of LH or HCG.
            (b) They act by directly stimulating the ovaries to produce follicles. Ovulation is accomplished by using HCG (Profasi).
            (c) Monitoring is by serum estradiol and LH. There should be a serum E2 level of approximately 250 pg/ml for each follicle.
            (d) Patients are also monitored by ultrasound.
            (e) Each follicle should be 18 to 20 mm at the time of ovulation.
        (3) Metrodin: partially purified FSH. It is the drug of choice in the treatment of patients with PCO.
        (4) GNRH pump (Factrel or Lutrepulse)
            (a) It is administered via an automatic portable infusion pump with a pulsatile mechanism.
            (b) It is a good choice for hypothalamic amenorrhea.
    b. LPD
        (1) The correction of a LPD is usually directed at enhancing the follicular phase, thus leading to an improved luteal phase with Clomid or Pergonal/Humegon.
        (2) Progesterone supplementation can benefit those patients with a LPD who produce inadequate amounts of progesterone.
6. Pelvic adhesions: The treatment of pelvic adhesions is surgical.
7. Ovarian failure: The current therapy for infertility associated with ovarian failure is egg donation.

8. Unexplained infertility
   a. Unexplained infertility is a diagnosis of exclusion.
   b. Therapy is usually ovulation induction with intrauterine insemination or an assisted reproductive procedure.

Surgical therapy for infertility

1. Endometriosis
   a. Basic tenets
      (1) The definitive diagnosis of endometriosis is by direct visualization and biopsy via laparoscopy.
      (2) Lesions can have a variety of appearances, including the following:
         (a) Clear: most likely early lesions
         (b) Red: histologically active
         (c) White: scarring
         (d) Brown-black: inactive endometrial glands and stroma
      (3) All patients found to have endometriosis should be surgically staged via the American Fertility Society Classification.
   b. Indications for surgery
      (1) Pain is present in 50% of patients with endometriosis.
      (2) Adnexal masses are unexplained ovarian enlargements that necessitate ultrasound and surgery.
      (3) Infertility: Endometriosis can lead to adhesions, ovarian dysfunction, tubal abnormalities, LPDs, and decreased fertilization.
   c. Surgical procedures
      (1) Conservative surgery by laparoscopy, the goal of which is to ablate and resect lesions and lyse adhesions with minimal disruption to normal surrounding tissue.
         (a) Electrosurgery
            i. This procedure is most commonly used.
            ii. Electrosurgery may be unipolar or bipolar.
            iii. A variety of instruments are available to operate with. A point coagulator is especially useful for small, individual lesions.
         (b) Thermocoagulator: causes tissue desiccation by increasing the temperature to 100° to 120° F and not by electric current
         (c) Laser
            i. This procedure offers precise tissue destruction.
            ii. CO_2 laser is best for vaporization.
            iii. Nd:YAG is best for coagulation.
      (2) Conservative surgery by laparotomy: The goal of this surgery is also to ablate and resect lesions and to lyse adhesions with minimal disruption to normal surrounding tissue.
         (a) Microsurgical technique: Tissues must be handled carefully to avoid trauma.
         (b) Ablation and resection of lesions: Uses the previously mentioned modalities to achieve the best results.
         (c) Preoperative suppression: Successful surgery can be more easily accomplished in certain cases with preoperation suppression with GNRH agonist. Some argue that this

makes the lesions more difficult to resect, but in most cases this is not the case.

(d) Laparoscopy vs. laparotomy

i. Laparoscopy is probably most dependent on the surgeon's skills.

ii. Current data supports the less costly, probably more effective laparoscopic approach.

(3) Definitive surgical therapy

(a) Hysterectomy with bilateral salpingoophorectomy is the definitive surgical therapy.

(b) Estrogen replacement should be instituted after surgery is completed with little risk of disease recurrence.

2. Cervical factor
   a. Stenosis: The surgical therapy for cervical stenosis is dilation.
   b. Myomas: Removal is via hysteroscope resectoscope.
   c. Polyps: Removal is via hysteroscope resectoscope.
3. Uterine factor
   a. Leiomyomata: They should only be removed if they impinge on the cavity or are thought to be causing repeated losses.

      (1) Hysteroscopic resection

      (2) Abdominal myomectomy

      (a) Abdominal myomectomy causes adhesions.

      (b) A second look laparoscopy 7 days after the myomectomy should be considered to lyse early adhesions.
   b. Polyps should be removed hysteroscopically.
   c. Intrauterine adhesions

      (1) Hysteroscopic resection with scissors

      (a) An intraoperative HSG should be performed to confirm complete lysis of the adhesions.

      (b) An 8-French, 3-cc pediatric Foley catheter should be placed in the endometrial cavity at the end of the procedure to prevent reformation of adhesions. The Foley should be left in place for 5 to 7 days, during which time the patient is on antibiotics and estrogen (Premarin, 2.5 mg, bid or Estrace, 4 mg, bid). The estrogen is continued for 25 days with 10 mg of Provera administered on days 16 to 25. Menses should occur 48 to 72 hours after the estrogen and Provera are discontinued.
   d. Congenital uterine anomalies

      (1) Unicornuate: No surgery is necessary unless a rudimentary horn is present and requires removal.

      (2) Bicornuate vs. septate uterus: This diagnosis can be made only by laparoscopy. A septum can be resected hysteroscopically. A bicornuate uterus requires a metroplasty if it is associated with repeated losses.

      (3) Uterine didelphys: Surgery is not generally required.
4. Male factor (See Section 7.2.)
5. Hormonal dysfunction
   a. This is usually corrected via contolled ovarian hyperstimulation, with or without insemination or assisted reproductive technology (see 6.b.).

6. Pelvic adhesions
   a. Surgical lysis of adhesions
      (1) Laparoscopy
      (2) Laparotomy
   b. Assisted reproduction
      (1) *In vitro* fertilization (IVF)
         (a) Indications
            i. Poor prognosis tubal factor
            ii. Endometriosis
            iii. Male factor
            iv. Immunologic infertility
            v. Diethylstilbesterol (DES) exposure
            vi. Unexplained infertility
         (b) Process
            i. Ovarian hyperstimulation
            ii. Oocyte retrieval
            iii. Oocyte insemination fertilization
            iv. Transcervical embryo transfer
         (c) Outcome
            i. Approximately 20% ongoing pregnancy rate
            ii. Multiple pregnancy rate of 30%
            iii. May need embryo manipulation, such as assisted hatching, to facilitate implantation
      (2) Gamete intrafallopian transfer (GIFT)
         (a) Indications
            i. Cervical factor
            ii. Mild to moderate male factor infertility
            iii. Pelvic adhesions: need one healthy tube
            iv. Unexplained primary or secondary infertility
            v. Ovarian failure: using donor oocytes
         (b) Process
            i. Ovarian hyperstimulation
            ii. Oocyte retrieval: usually transvaginal
            iii. Laparoscopy with tubal transfer of sperm and oocytes (usually four)
         (c) Outcome
            i. Approximately 30% ongoing pregnancy rate
            ii. Approximately 4% ectopic pregnancy rate
   c. Zygote intrafallopian transfer (ZIFT) and tubal embryo transfer (TET)
      (1) Indications
         (a) Severe male factor: allows fertilization to occur before laparoscopy
         (b) Immunologic infertility
         (c) Endometriosis
         (d) Oocyte donation
         (e) Unexplained infertility
      (2) Process
         (a) Ovarian hyperstimulation
         (b) Oocyte retrieval

(c) Oocyte insemination fertilization
(d) Laparoscopic zygote embryo transfer (24 to 56 hours after retrieval)
(3) Outcome
(a) A 30% to 35% ongoing pregnancy rate
d. Oocyte donation
(1) Indications
(a) Ovarian failure
(b) Genetic abnormalities
(c) Gonadal dysgenesis
(d) Poor oocyte quality
(2) Process
(a) Ovarian hyperstimulation of the donor
(b) Uterine preparation of the recipient
(c) Fertilization of the oocytes
(d) Transcervical embryo transfer (GIFT, ZIFT)
(3) Outcome
(a) Pregnancy rates approach 50%.
7. Ovarian failure: surgical therapy
a. Oocyte donation (See previous section.)
8. Unexplained infertility: surgical therapy
a. Assisted reproductive technologies
(1) IVF
(2) GIFT
(3) ZIFT/TET

7.2 MALE FERTILITY

Philip J. Aliotta, M.D., M.S.H.A., F.A.C.S.

Of patients presenting for fertility evaluation for their first pregnancy, 15% will fail. Over 50% of all cases can be ascribed to male factor involvement. The breakdown is as follows:

Male factor only	33%
Combined male and female factors	20%

The appropriate evaluation of the male partner is therefore very important.

Evaluation

The evaluation of the male partner should include the following:
1. Historical review (see the box on p. 144)
a. Childhood illnesses
b. Existing medical disease review
c. Prior surgeries
d. Family history
e. Sexual development
f. Exposure to toxins
(1) Alcohol
(2) Heat
(3) Radiation

Factors in Male Infertility History

History of infertility

Duration
Prior pregnancies
  Present partner
  Another partner
Previous treatments
Evaluation and treatment of wife

Sexual history

Potency
Lubricants
Timing of intercourse
Frequency of intercourse
Frequency of masturbation

Childhood and development

Undescended testicles, orchiopexy
Herniorrhaphy
Y-V plasty of bladder
Testicular torsion
Testicular trauma
Onset of puberty

Medical history

Systemic illness (i.e., diabetes mellitus, multiple sclerosis)
Previous or current therapy

Surgical history

Orchiectomy (testis cancer, torsion)
Retroperitoneal surgery
Pelvic injury
Pelvic, inguinal or scrotal surgery
Herniorrhaphy
Y-V plasty, transurethral prostate resection

Infections

Viral, febrile
Mumps orchitis
Venereal
Tuberculosis, smallpox (rare)

Factors in Male Infertility History–cont'd

Gonadotoxins

Chemicals (pesticides)
Drugs (chemotherapeutic, cimetidine, sulfasalazine, nitrofurantoin, alcohol, marijuana, androgenic steroids)
Thermal exposure
Radiation
Smoking

Family history

Cystic fibrosis
Androgen receptor deficiency

Review of systems

Respiratory infections
Anosmia
Galactorrhea
Impaired visual fields

From Sigman M, Lipshultz LI, Howards SS: The evaluation of the subfertile male. In Lipshultz LI, Howards SS, editors: *Infertility in the male,* ed 2, St Louis, 1991, Mosby.

(4) Toxic fumes
(5) Tobacco use
(6) Drug and recreational drug use (marijuana, cocaine, hallucinogens, etc.)

2. Physical examination: A "fertility focused" examination should seek to identify physical characteristics within organ systems that may contribute to or identify the male factor in a couple's infertility (see Table 7-1).
3. Tests
   a. Urinalysis and postejaculate urine: rule out urinary tract infections (UTI), retrograde ejaculation, and medical renal diseases
   b. *Chlamydia* and gonorrhea cultures (optional and where indicated)
   c. Endocrine evaluation: Knowledge of the hypothalamic–pituitary– gonadal (H–P–G) axis is important in the evaluation of the subfertile and infertile male. The H–P–G axis is a negative- feedback loop; the entire system is directed by pulsatile release from the hypothalamus of GNRH, which causes pituitary release of FSH and LH. The FSH acts on the Sertoli component of the testis with the release of inhibin, whereas the LH stimulates the Leydig cell component to release testosterone. The combination of high intratesticular levels of testosterone plus the effect of FSH on Sertoli cells is responsible for spermatogenesis. Both enter into the systemic circulation and, through negative feedback, inhibit the release of GNRH. The

Table 7-1 Focal points of the male physical examination

Examine	Look For	Suspect
1. Habitus	Eunuchoid proportions	Klinefelter's syndrome
2. Vital signs	Orthostatic hypotension	Autonomic insufficiency
3. Head, eyes, and nose	Diminished beard	Androgen deficiency
	Bitemporal hemianopsia	Pituitary tumor
	Retinopathy	Diabetes mellitus
	Anosmia	Kallmann's syndrome
4. Neck	Thyromegaly	Hypothyroidism or hyperthyroidism
5. Lungs	Wheezes, rhonchi, rales	Cystic fibrosis
		Young's syndrome
		Kartagener's syndrome
6. Breasts	Gynecomastia	Hyperprolactinemia
		Alcoholism
		Klinefelter's syndrome
		Reifenstein's syndrome
		Estrogen excess
7. Abdomen	Hepatomegaly	Alcoholism
	Inguinal hernia	Prior cryptorchidism
8. Genitalia		
a. Penis	Decreased length*	Hypospadias
Meatus	Ventral	Urethral distortion
	Occluded	Partial urethral obstruction
Foreskin	Phimosis	Local infection
		Dyspareunia
Shaft	Lateral deviation*	Peyronie's disease

b. Testes		
Volume	Bilateral decrease	Primary or secondary hypogonadism
		Selective germinal cell aplasia
	Unilateral decrease	Prior cryptorchidism or torsion
	Bilateral increase	Congenital adrenal hyperplasia
Scrotum	Varicocele	Varicocele
Epididymus	Pain	Acute epididymitis
	Painless mass	Chronic epididymitis
Vas deferens	Asymmetry	Bilateral absence of vas deferens
9. Prostate	Boggy, tender, enlarged	Prostatitis

From Spark RF: *The infantile male: the clinician's guide to diagnosis and treatment*, New York, 1988, Plenum, p. 186.
*Not evident in flaccid penis. Apparent only during spontaneous or pharmacologically induced erection.

endocrine evaluation allows for the categorization of male patients as follows[1]:

(1) Eugonadotropic
   (a) Normal FSH
   (b) Normal LH
   (c) Normal testosterone
(2) Hypogonadotropic (hypogonadotropic hypogonadism)
   (a) Low FSH
   (b) Low LH
   (c) Low testosterone
(3) Hypergonadotropic (hypergonadotropic hypogonadism)
   (a) Elevated LH → Leydig cell dysfunction → gonadal failure
   (b) Decreased testosterone → Leydig cell dysfunction → gonadal failure
   (c) Elevated FSH → spermatogenic dysfunction → gonadal failure
(4) Only in conditions associated with obstructive azoospermia or retrograde ejaculation are all hormonal levels within normal limits.

d. Semen analysis: Normal semen, as defined by the World Health Organization, is an admixture of spermatozoa suspended in secretions from the testes and epididymes, which are mixed at the time of ejaculation with secretions from the prostate, seminal vesicles, and bulbourethral glands. The final composition is a viscous fluid that comprises the ejaculate.[9]

(1) Requirements are as follows:
   (a) 48 to 72 hours of abstinence
   (b) Multiple analyses (I recommend a minimum of three) separated by 2 to 4 week intervals
   (c) A specimen: generally obtained through masturbation and delivered to the laboratory within 2 hours in a wide-mouth container (usually silicone); should be kept as close to body temperature as is possible
   (d) Postejaculate urine: tested to rule out retrograde ejaculation and possible retention of semen in the urethra secondary to obstruction[2]
   (e) Collecting jar: cap or top must not have a rubber lining because this will kill whatever spermatozoa are present
   (f) Collection, avoid the following:
      i. Ordinary condoms: interfere with sperm viability
      ii. Coitus interruptus: high potential loss of first part of the ejaculate, a possibility of cellular and bacterial contamination, and acid vaginal pH affects sperm motility
   (g) Safe handling: semen may contain harmful agents (e.g., HIV hepatitis viruses, herpes simplex viruses, *Chlamydia,* gonorrhea) and must be handled with care
(2) Table 7-2 shows the differential diagnosis based on sperm count.

(3) Macroscopic examination
  (a) pH of semen
    i. The pH of normal semen should be measured at a uniform time, usually within 1 hour of ejaculation, and should be in the range of 7.2 to 8.0.
    ii. If the pH is less than 7.0 in a sample with azoospermia, dysgenesis of the vas deferens, seminal vesicles, or epididymis may be present.
  (b) Color
    i. Opaque to opalescent = normal
    ii. Clear or translucent = oligospermia
    iii. Rust or red = hematospermia
    iv. Yellow, creamy, or milky = pyospermia
    v. In jaundice, the semen is bright yellow
(4) Liquefaction: In humans, semen forms a gellike clot after ejaculation, but within 15 to 20 minutes liquefaction of this clot has occurred. Coagulation of the human semen depends on the presence of a fibrinogen-like substance, manufactured by the seminal vesicles, that is acted on by the enzyme vesiculase produced by the prostate. Breaking down of the clot and the associated fibrin takes place as a result of the activities of a series of proteolytic enzymes secreted by the prostate. These include proteases, pepsinogen, and amylase, and even hyaluronidase. Concomitant release of transaminase enzymes can cause further peptide breakdown. Therefore, both clotting and liquefaction are induced by prostate secretions. Liquefaction of semen usually occurs within 10 to 20 minutes after ejaculation.[4]
  (a) Liquefaction is usually assessed visually.
    Grade 1: Semen that fails to liquefy forms a gellike coagulum.
    Grade 2: Partially liquefied semen will contain many small gellike clots.
    Grade 3: Fully liquefied semen has no gellike clots and the semen is completely fluid.
  (b) Treatment of liquefaction defects includes the following:
    i. Alpha-amylase
    ii. Alpha-chymotrypsin
    iii. Lysozyme
    iv. Hyaluronidase
(5) Viscosity
  (a) Viscosity is defined as the quality of semen that allows it to be poured drop by drop out of a container.
    i. The viscosity of the seminal fluid can vary from sample to sample.
    ii. Increased viscosity may be associated with infertility.[4]
  (b) Treatment of hyperviscous semen includes the following:

Table 7-2 Differential diagnosis based on sperm count in the infertile male

1. Azoospermia—severe oligospermia
   a. Central
      (1) Hypogonadotropic hypogonadism
      (2) Hyperprolactinemia
      (3) Hemochromatosis
      (4) Panhypopituitarism
      (5) Hypothalamic and pituitary sarcoidosis
   b. Genetic
      (1) Klinefelter's syndrome and variants
      (2) Noonan's syndrome (XX male)
      (3) Ring Y chromosome mosaicism
   c. Testicular
      (1) Anorchia
      (2) Cryptorchidism
      (3) Primary hypogonadism secondary to orchitis
      (4) Other causes
         (a) Germ cell dysfunction
         (b) Androgen resistance syndromes
         (c) Germ cell aplasia
         (d) Radiotherapy
         (e) Sertoli cell–only syndrome
         (f) Chemotherapy
   d. Obstruction or aplasia of the ductal system
      (1) Congenital
         (a) Aplasia of vas deferens
         (b) Aplasia of the epididymis
      (2) Acquired
         (a) Preepididymal
         (b) Epididymal
         (c) Postepididymal
      (3) Vas deferens occlusion
         (a) Vasectomy
         (b) Young's syndrome
   e. Retrograde ejaculation
      (1) Autonomic insufficiency
      (2) Ganglionic blockers
2. Oligospermia
   a. Central
      (1) Hypogonadotropic hypogonadism
      (2) Hypothalamic and pituitary sarcoidosis
      (3) Hemochromatosis
      (4) Panhypopituitarism
      (5) Hyperprolactinemia

From Spark RF: *The infantile male: the clinician's guide to diagnosis and treatment*, New York, 1988, Plenum, p. 195.

Table 7-2 Differential diagnosis based on sperm count in the infertile male—cont'd

- b. Other causes
  - (1) Selective germ cell dysfunction
  - (2) Chemotherapy
  - (3) Androgen resistance syndromes
  - (4) Germ cell aplasia
  - (5) Radiotherapy
  - (6) Sertoli cell–only syndrome
- c. Varicocele
- d. Idiopathic

3. Normospermia
   - a. Immunoinfertility
   - b. Varicocele
   - c. Unrecognized female factors
   - d. "Normal but infertile"

---

i. Passage through a wide-bore needle

ii. Mixing viscous semen with sperm free seminal fluid from another patient

(6) Count

(a) There is a large variance in the normal sperm count.

(b) Often cited are 20 million/ml to 200 million/ml.

(c) The World Health Organization established a count of 20 million/ml as the line between "normal" and "abnormal or infertile."

(d) The sperm concentration takes no account of total number of sperm in the overall ejaculate, because volumes can and do vary.

(e) It is known, too, that in a single individual, counts per milliliter can vary from some number less than 20 million/ml or exceed 200 million/ml.

(f) For that reason, I recommend at least three analyses, done at least 1 week or more apart, with 2 days of abstinence.

(g) Sperm counts can vary with the type of counting chamber used (Table 7-3). With respect to accuracy and using 35 million beads per milliliter as a standard, the following chambers were tested for their accuracy:

Cell VU	Mean count:	35.1 ± 2.5
Microcell	Mean count:	36.2 ± 9.3
Neubauer hemacytometer	Mean count:	51.4 ± 12.8
Makler	Mean count:	51.2 ± 7.4

Nomenclature for Semen Variables

Normozoospermia	Normal ejaculate
Oligozoospermia	Sperm concentration less than 20 million/ml
Azoospermia	No spermatozoa in the ejaculate
OligoAstheno-Teratozoospermia	Disturbance of all three variables: count, motility, and morphology
Teratozoospermia	Fewer than 30% spermatozoa with normal morphology
Asthenozoospermia	Fewer than 50% spermatozoa with forward progression of +3 or +4
Aspermia	No ejaculate
Polyzoospermia	Sperm concentration in excess of 250 million/ml
Necrospermia	Dead sperm

(7) Motility
  (a) Sperm must be able to move in such a manner as to demonstrate forward progression. This type of movement is necessary for a sperm to enter and pass through the female genital tract and also for it to achieve fertilization.
  (b) Sperm movement is evaluated both quantitatively and qualitatively.[7]
  (c) Quantitation motility (viability) is defined as the average percentage of sperm moving in 10 random high-power microscopic fields.
  (d) Qualitative assessment of sperm movement is based on the pattern displayed by the majority of motile spermatozoa.

Qualitative Assessment of Motility

0 = none	No forward progression
1 = poor	Sluggish forward progression
2 = moderate	Definite forward progression
3 = good	Good forward movement with progression
4 = excellent	Vigorous rapid forward progression

  (e) If motility is under 50%, a viability stain is done using eosin Y with nigrosin as counterstain. Greater than 50% of sperm should be viable. Abnormalities in motility and quality of movement can be seen with the following[8]:
    Infection
    Antisperm antibodies
    Partial ejaculatory duct obstruction
    Gonadotoxin exposure
    Varicoceles

Table 7-3 Comparison of chambers for counting sperm

	Cell VU	Hemacytometer	Makler	Microcell
Cells counted	Body fluids/sperm	Body fluids/sperm	Sperm	Body fluids/sperm
Disposal	Disposable	Nondisposable	Nondisposable	Disposable
Chamber depth	20 µm	100 µm	10 µm	12 and 20 µm
Grid	100 squares each 0.1 × 0.1 mm	Ruled Neubauer	100 squares each 0.1 × 0.1 mm	None (microscope reticle required)

From Seaman E, Bar-Chama N, Fisch H: Semen analysis in the clinical evaluation of infertility. In Carson CC III, Cooner WH, editors: *Mediguide to urology,* New York, 1994, Lawrence DellaCorte.

Protein–carboxyl methylase deficiency (induced by radiation exposure or environmental toxin)
Immotile cilia—Kartagener's syndrome

(8) Morphology
(a) According to the World Health Organization, a morphologically normal semen sample contains 50% normal forms, defined as sperm with oval heads and no neck or tail abnormalities (Figs. 7-1 and 7-2).
(b) The advanced technology of *in vitro* fertilization has made it necessary to redefine sperm morphologic criteria that may correlate with fertilization outcomes.
i. According to "strict criteria" established by Kruger et al., a normal spermatozoon has an oval configuration with a smooth contour; an acrosome comprising 40% to 70% of the distal part of the head; no abnormalities of the neck, midpiece, or tail; and no cytoplasmic droplets of more than half of the sperm head.
ii. Borderline forms are abnormal.[5,7]
(c) Kruger et al. grouped together the normal and borderline forms to obtain the "morphology index"; they proposed that more than 4% morphologically normal sperm and a morphology index greater than 30% predict a good fertilization outcome. Fertility rates per oocyte with a strict criteria score of under 4% was 7.6% compared to a fertility rate per oocyte of 64% with strict criteria score of greater than 4%.[5,7]

(9) Agglutination
(a) Simply put, motile spermatozoa stick to each other. These agglutinates can be as follows:
i. Head to head
ii. Tail to tail
iii. Midpiece to midpiece
iv. Mixed
(b) The adherence of immotile sperm to each other or of motile sperm to mucus threads, cells other than spermatozoa, or debris is considered to be "nonspecific aggregation" rather than agglutination.
(c) The presence of agglutination is suggestive of, but not sufficient evidence for, an immunologic cause of infertility.
(d) Sperm tend to agglutinate spontaneously with fairly high frequency. This phenomenon is observed in sperm of both fertile and infertile men.
(e) Agglutination can occur with exposure of sperm to the following:
i. Infection
ii. Fungi
iii. Antibodies

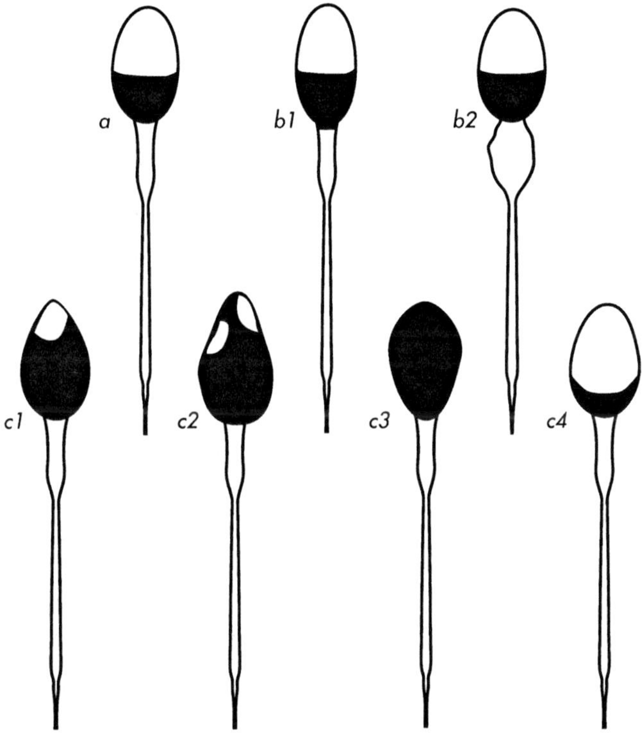

Figure 7-1
Diagrammatic representation of Diff-quick stained spermatozoa. *(a)* Normal form. *(b)* Slightly amorphous forms: *(1)* Head slightly elongated, loss of oval shape: *(2)* Thick neck but normal-shaped head. *(c)* Severely amorphous forms: (*1* and *2*) Abnormally small acrosome. *(3)* No acrosome. *(4)* Acrosome >70% of head. Adapted with permission, Kruger et al., 1988. Reproduced with permission of the publisher. The American Fertility Society. (From Seaman E, Bar-Chama N, Fisch H: Semen analysis in the clinical evaluation of infertility. In Carson CC III, Cooner WH, editors: *Mediguide to urology,* New York, 1994, Lawrence DellaCorte Publications.)

iv. Steroids:
Testosterone → tail to tail agglutination
Progesterone → head to head agglutination

(f) The severity of agglutination can be approximated as follows:

+ Fewer than 33% of sperm agglutinated
++ 33% to 66% of sperm agglutinated
+++ Greater than 66% of sperm agglutinated

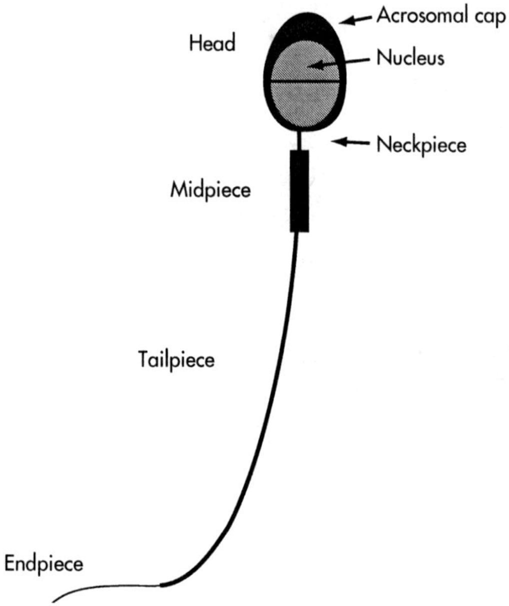

Figure 7-2
Basic components and morphologic characteristics of the normal spermatozoa. Note the following normal characteristics: oval shaped head with regular outline; acrosomal cap covering >⅓ of head surface; head length between 3 and 5 μm; head width between 2 and 3 μm; width must be between ½ and ⅔ of length; midiece <⅓ width of head, 7 to 8 μm long; and tail is uncoiled and at least 45 μm in length. (From Gilbert BR, Cooper GW, Goldstein M: Semen analysis in the evaluation of male factor subfertility. In *AUA Update 1992,* vol 11 no. 32, pp. 250-255, Houston, 1992, American Urological Association.)

(g) Furthermore, clinicians should endeavor to describe the nature of the agglutination (i.e., head to head, etc.).

(10) Antibody-agglutination testing (see the box on p. 157) should be done for the following[2]:

(a) Agglutination of spermatozoa
(b) Agglutination of motile dimers
(c) Idiopathic infertility
(d) Abnormal postcoital tests
(e) Historical factors that increase the risk of antibody formation

Vasectomy	Testicular biopsy
Infection	Trauma
Obstruction	Torsion
Cryptorchidism	Cancer
Varicocele	Genetic predisposition

(11) Cellular components of semen

(a) White blood cells (WBCs) and pyospermia

i. White blood cells are present in small numbers in normal semen. As a general guide, the normal ejaculate should not contain more than 5 to 10 WBCs per HPF.

ii. An abnormal number of WBCs in the semen is called *pyospermia*. The presence of WBCs lying together in aggregates is diagnostic of infection. Any sample demonstrating these findings must be cultured.

iii. Increased numbers of WBCs in the semen may also be the result of prostatic abnormalities.

iv. The four main sites for infection in the male genital tract are as follows:
Epididymis
Seminal vesicles
Prostate
Urethra and periurethral glands
By doing split ejaculate analysis and culture, the site of infection can be localized using the physiology of the emission and ejaculation process[4]:

Emission:	derived from the accessory or periurethral glands
Ejaculation:	The first part of the ejaculate derives from the testicular component, followed by secretions from the prostate; the last part derives from the seminal vesicles.

Tests for Agglutination and Antisperm Antibody[4,8,9]

1. Gel agglutination test (Kibrick): detects IgG or IgM
2. Sperm microagglutination test (Franklin-Dukes): detects clumping of motile sperm (>10% is considered positive for sperm antibodies): IgG, IgM, IgA
3. Sperm immobilization test (Isojima/SIT): detects those antibodies that interact with the surface of sperm, are complement dependent, and cause sperm immobilization: IgM and IgG; IgA: does not activate complement
4. Mixed agglutination reaction (MAR test): detects IgA and IgG
5. Immunobead test: detects IgG and IgA
6. Indirect immunofluorescence: detects IgG and IgA
7. Sperm–cervical mucus contact test (SCMC or Kremer): IgA and occasionally IgG within cervical mucus
8. Spermocytotoxicity tests: detect IgM and IgG
9. Enzyme-linked assay (ELISA)

v. Another method for detecting infection in the prostate is prostatic massage for expressed prostatic secretions (EPS). The sample can be examined under the microscope as well as sent for culture. A microscopic count of $\pm \geq 10$ WBCs per HPF is indicative of prostatitis.[4]

vi. Infection alters semen quality in the following ways:
Ductal damage with resultant obstruction
Interference with accessory gland secretion
Impaired motility of spermatozoa

vii. The most common organisms associated with pyospermia are as follows[4]:

Escherichia coli	*Mycobacterium tuberculosis*
Enterococci	*Chlamydia trachomatis*
Staphylococci	*Trichomonas vaginalis*
Neisseria gonorrheae	*Candida albicans*
Mycoplasmas	Viruses

(b) Epithelial cells
(c) Red blood cells
  i. Hematospermia
  ii. Can be a manifestation of infection and malignant disease or can be idiopathic
(d) Germ Cells
  i. Germ cells are generally considered normal in the semen.
  ii. The exact number of these immature cells felt to be abnormal has yet to be defined.
(e) Lymphocytes.
(f) Particulate Matter
  i. Spermine crystals
  ii. Prostatic calculi

e. Tests of sperm function[2]: Of the many tests of sperm function available, none unequivocally identify functional spermatozoa. These tests are not performed as a matter of routine examination of the subfertile male. They are highly selective.

(1) Sperm penetration assay (SPA): This test uses the golden hamster egg, which is unusual in that removal of its zona pellucida results in loss of all species specificity to egg penetration. It is used to yield information relative to sperm fertilization potential.
  (a) The SPA measures are as follows:
    i. Capacitation
    ii. The acrosome reaction
    iii. Sperm oolemma fusion
    iv. Sperm incorporation into the ooplasm
    v. Decondensation of chromatin

- (b) The SPA *does not* test for the following:
  - *i.* Penetration of the zona pellucida
  - *ii.* Normal embryonic development
- (c) The *positive* SPA test cannot therefore do the following:
  - *i.* Guarantee fertilization of intact human eggs
  - *ii.* Guarantee embryonic development of fertilized human eggs
- (d) The *negative* SPA test has not been found to correlate with poor fertilization in human IVF.

(2) The acrosin assay: This test measures acrosin, which is thought to be responsible for penetration of the zona pellucida and for triggering the acrosome reaction.

(3) The hemizona assay
- (a) This test measures the binding of sperm to the zona pellucida of human eggs.
- (b) In the human hemizona assay, unfertilized oocytes obtained through donation are bisected and the number of sperm tightly bound to the outer surface is counted.
- (c) The major advantages are as follows:
  - *i.* Using the two halves of the hemizona allows for controlled comparisons of binding.
  - *ii.* The limited number of human oocytes is amplified.
- (d) The results of this test show good correlation with Kruger "strict" morphology criteria and IVF fertilization rates.

(4) The hypoosmotic swelling test
- (a) This test measures the membrane integrity of sperm, important for metabolism but also for the successful union of male and female gametes.
- (b) When viable sperm are exposed to hypo-osmotic conditions, water enters the sperm, resulting in swelling. This places the tail fibers under tension, causing curling of the tails.

(5) Cervical mucus penetration
- (a) This test quantitates the sperm mucus interaction and yields information regarding the motility of the spermatozoa.
- (b) The postcoital test (PCT) is done at midcycle when the cervical mucus is less of a barrier to sperm. A good PCT done within 12 hours after coitus is defined as greater than 10 motile sperm per HPF.
- (c) Female factors affecting the PCT are as follows:
  - *i.* Inadequate estrogen priming
  - *ii.* Deficient endocervical tissue
  - *iii.* Previous surgery to the cervix
- (d) Male factors affecting the PCT are as follows:
  - *i.* Anatomical abnormality (i.e., hypospadias, resulting in inadequate delivery of sperm
  - *ii.* Oligozoospermia
  - *iii.* Asthenozoospermia
  - *iv.* Antibodies

References

1. Gangi GR, Nagler HM: Clinical evaluation of the subfertile man, *Infertil Reprod Med Clin North Am* 3:299, 1992
2. Gilbert BR, Cooper GW, Goldstein M: Semen analysis in the evaluation of male factor subfertility. In *AUA Update 1992,* vol 11 no.(32); pp. 250-255, Houston, 1992, American Urological Association.
3. Gilbert BR, Schlegel PN, Goldstein M: Office evaluation of the subfertile male, *AUA Update 1994,* vol 13 no. 9, pp. 70-75. Houston, 1994 American Urologic Association.
4. Jequier A, Crich J: *Semen analysis: A practical guide,* St Louis, 1986, Blackwell Mosby Book Company.
5. Kruger TF et al: Predictive value of abnormal sperm morphology in in vitro fertilization, *Fertil Steril* 49:112, 1988.
6. Lipshultz LI, Corriere JN Jr: Progressive testicular atrophy in the varicocele patient, *J Urol* 117:175, 1977.
7. Seaman E, Bar-Chama N, Fisch H: Semen analysis in the clinical evaluation of infertility. In Carson CC III, Cooner WH, editors: *Mediguide to urology.* New York, 1994, Lawrence DellaCorte Publications.
8. Spark RF: *The infertile male, the clinician's guide to diagnosis and treatment,* New York, 1988, Plenum.
9. World Health Organization: *WHO Laboratory Manual for the Examination of Human Semen and Sperm-Cervical Mucus Interaction,* Cambridge, England, 1992, Cambridge University Press.

Amenorrhea

8

Ivan D'Souza, M.D.

Amenorrhea is defined as the absence of menses for 6 consecutive months. Primary amenorrhea refers to a female who has never menstruated. Secondary amenorrhea is the cessation of menses after previous normal (6 months) menses.

8.1 CLASSIFICATION

The classification of amenorrhea is given in the box on p. 162.

1. Physiologic amenorrhea
   a. Physiologic amenorrhea can occur shortly after menarche, during pregnancy and lactation, and after menopause.
   b. All states except pregnancy are associated with a hypoestrogenic state with all the attendant clinical ramifications.
   c. Confirmation is with pregnancy test and pelvic examination.
2. Primary amenorrhea
   a. Absence of menses after age 16 indicates primary amenorrhea.
   b. Absence of pubertal development before age 14 may also indicate gonadal function.
   c. Gonadal abnormalities
      (1) Of patients with primary amenorrhea 60% have gonadal abnormalities:
         (a) Failure of gonadal differentiation
         (b) Inappropriate gonadal function during fetal and neonatal life; usually results in abnormal external genitalia
      (2) Up to one third of primary amenorrhea patients may be genetic males.
      (3) If a Y chromosome is present in dysgenic gonads, the gonads need to be removed for prophylaxis against malignant degeneration. Karyotyping is therefore an important part of the workup.
      (4) Gonadal dysgenesis (Turner's syndrome)
         (a) 1:2700 of newborn phenotypic females
         (b) Karyotypes: 45X, 45X/46XX, 45X/46XY
         (c) Clinical features are as follows:
            i. Short stature (<150 cm)
            ii. Webbed neck

The Classification of Amenorrhea

Physiologic

Pathologic

- Primary
  - Gonadal abnormalities
    - Gonadal dysgenesis (Turner's syndrome)
    - Pure gonadal dysgenesis
    - XY gonadal dysgenesis (Swyer's syndrome)
    - Mixed gonadal dysgenesis
    - Ovarian insensitivity syndrome (Savage syndrome)
    - 17-OH deficiency
  - Extragonadal abnormalities
    - Congenital anatomic defect of genital tract
    - Male pseudohermaphroditism
    - Female pseudohermaphroditism
    - Abnormal hypothalamic–pituitary function
- Secondary with the following
  - Normal ovarian function
  - Increased gonadotrophins
  - Normal or decreased gonadotrophins
    - Psychogenic
    - Weight related
    - Exercise induced
    - Pseudocyesis
    - Postpill
    - CNS lesions
    - Endocrinopathies
    - Drug induced
    - Acute or chronic illness
    - Estrogen-producing tumors
  - Androgen excess

iii. Shield chest
iv. High arched palate
v. Neck hairline low
vi. Cubitus vulgus
vii. CVS and renal abnormalities
viii. Gonads replaced by streaks of fibrous tissue in stroma without germ cells
ix. May have transient ovarian function if mosaic with 46XX; therefore variable sexual maturation

(5) Pure gonadal dysgenesis (all sexually immature)
(a) Height >150 cm
(b) Karyotype 46XX or 46XY
(c) Streak gonads

(d) Increased incidence in siblings
(e) Higher incidence of Y chromosome presence than in Turner's syndrome

(6) XY gonadal dysgenesis (Swyer's syndrome)
(a) Phenotypic females; normal female external and internal genitalia
(b) Karyotype XY
(c) Streak gonads; high incidence of malignant degeneration

(7) Mixed gonadal genesis (rare)
(a) Germ cell tumor or testis on one side and streak or no gonad on the other
(b) Abnormal external genitalia with pubertal virilization
(c) Y gonad: should be removed immediately

(8) Ovarian insensitivity syndrome (Savage syndrome)
(a) Phenotypic females, normal external and internal genitalia, and normal appearing ovaries
(b) Functional ovarian failure resulting from possible receptor defect that makes them unresponsive to gonadotrophins

(9) 17-OH deficiency: unable to synthesize androgens, estrogens, and some adrenal steroids
(a) Infantile external genitalia
(b) Hypertension, hypokalemic alkalosis
(c) Increased desoxycorticosterone, follicle stimulating hormone (FSH), luteinizing hormone (LH), and progesterone
(d) Ovarian function: cannot be restored

d. Extragonadal anomalies account for 40% of primary amenorrhea. There is normal ovarian functional capacity.

(1) Congenital anatomic defect of the genital tract
(a) Failure of normal Müllerian or urogenital sinus differentiation may lead to outlet obstruction or uterine agenesis.
(b) Phenotypic and genotypic females with normal external genitalia.
(c) Congenital absence of uterus and upper vagina is the most common defect (Mayer-Rokitansky-Kuster-Hauser syndrome). Incidence is 1:4000 female births. There is an association with renal abnormalities.
(d) Imperforate hymen or agenesis or stenosis of the proximal vagina, distal vagina, or cervix and transverse septa of the vagina are also contributing causes.
(e) Outlet obstruction results in retained menses with subsequent cyclic pain, hematocolpos, hematometra, and endometriosis.
(f) Physical examination and ultrasound will often make the diagnosis. Intravenous pyelogram (IVP) should be ordered.
(g) Surgical correction of the lower tract is often possible and should be done as soon as possible.

(2) Male pseudohermaphroditism
  (a) Male pseudohermaphroditism results from inadequate androgenic influence on the development of external genitalia in a genetic male.
  (b) Androgen insensitivity syndrome or testicular feminization (absence of testosterone receptors) is the most common cause. Clinical features include the following:
    i. Normal external genitalia
    ii. Blind vagina
    iii. Absent uterus
    iv. Scant pubic or axillary hair
    v. Normal breasts with immature, pale areolae
    vi. Often inguinal testis
    Testosterone levels are in the normal male range with normal gonadotrophins
  (c) Incomplete forms result from the presence of some functional androgen.
    i. Chromosomal abnormalities are often found. The spectrum varies from almost normal males with minor abnormalities of the external genitalia to almost normal females with Turner syndrome manifestations.
    ii. Causes include chromosomal mosaicism (45X and a cell line with a Y chromosome).
    iii. Enzymatic anomalies if steroid production with androgen overproduction, incomplete androgen insensitivity syndrome, hypospadias, multiple malformation syndromes, Müllerian derivative persistence, agonadia, and Leydig cell agenesis.
    iv. Breast development must always raise the suspicion of an estrogen-producing tumor.
(3) Female pseudohermaphroditism
  (a) Female pseudohermaphroditism results from anomalous production of androgen in genetic females.
  (b) Congenital adrenal hyperplasia is the most common cause, usually secondary to 21-hydroxylase or 11-beta-hydroxylase deficiency. Incomplete forms may manifest as amenorrhea in virilized females. Adequate treatment results in normal menses.
  (c) Androgen-producing tumors of the adrenals and ovaries can also result in virilization of external genitalia and amenorrhea.
(4) Hypothalamic–pituitary dysfunction
  (a) Destruction or abnormal development of the hypothalamus or anterior pituitary would result in hypogonadotrophic hypogonadism.
  (b) Craniopharyngiomas are the most common destructive lesion in this area, but primary and metastatic lesions need to be ruled out if this diagnosis is being considered. These are uncommon causes of primary amenorrhea.
  (c) Kallmann's syndrome: isolated gonadotrophin deficiency with anosmia.

8.2 CLINICAL ASSESSMENT

1. History
   a. Intrauterine environment to rule out teratogen
   b. Chronologic pubertal development, including growth spurt, pubarche, and thelarche
   c. Dietary habits or preferences, body weight perception and changes, psychosocial stress
   d. Family history: pubertal delay, menstrual patterns
   e. Social skills, school achievement
2. Physical examination
   a. External genitalia maturity, virilization, pubic hair distribution
   b. Internal genitalia, inguinal hernial sites
   c. Pubertal features: degree of pubic hair and breast development, galactorrhea
   d. Skin: consistency, acne, hair distribution, bruising and pigmentation
   e. Growth: height and weight
   f. Thyroid
3. Diagnostic procedures (Fig. 8-1)
   a. Ultrasound may be used to assess internal genitalia when office examination is difficult. It will also rule out flow-tract abnormalities and assess adnexal status.
   b. Progesterone withdrawal: Provera 10 mg, PO, for 5 days (or 100 mg progesterone in oil); bleeding within 1 week indicates significant endogenous estrogen and normal outflow tract and a likely diagnosis of anovulation.
   c. Karyotyping (or buccal smear chromatin) should be ordered, and if necessary human Y antigen assay (occasionally leukocyte karyotyping does not detect all forms of mosaicism).
   d. FSH + LH (high levels = ovarian failure), thyroid stimulating hormone (TSH), and prolactin are frequently also needed and can be used to assess pituitary status.
   e. Ambiguous genitalia
      (1) With Y chromosome presence a gonadal biopsy is needed (dd male pseudohermaphrodite, mixed gonadal dysgenesis, or true hermaphrodite).
      (2) Without Y chromosome consider virilizing tumors or 17-hydroxylase deficiency (late onset may require ACTH stimulation test.
   f. Elevated prolactin (>50 ng/ml) warrants an MRI or a CAT scan.
4. Treatment
   a. The cause should be treated if possible (i.e., dexamethasone for 17-OH deficiency).
   b. Phenotypic status should be attained with plastic surgery (i.e., clitoral recession for clitoromegaly and neovagina for blind nonfunctional vaginal pouches).
   c. Fertility should be achieved when possible and desired (i.e., parlodel for pituitary microadenomas, gonadotrophins for Kallmann's syndrome, *in vitro* fertilization for vaginal agenesis, donor eggs for gonadal dysgenesis, etc.).

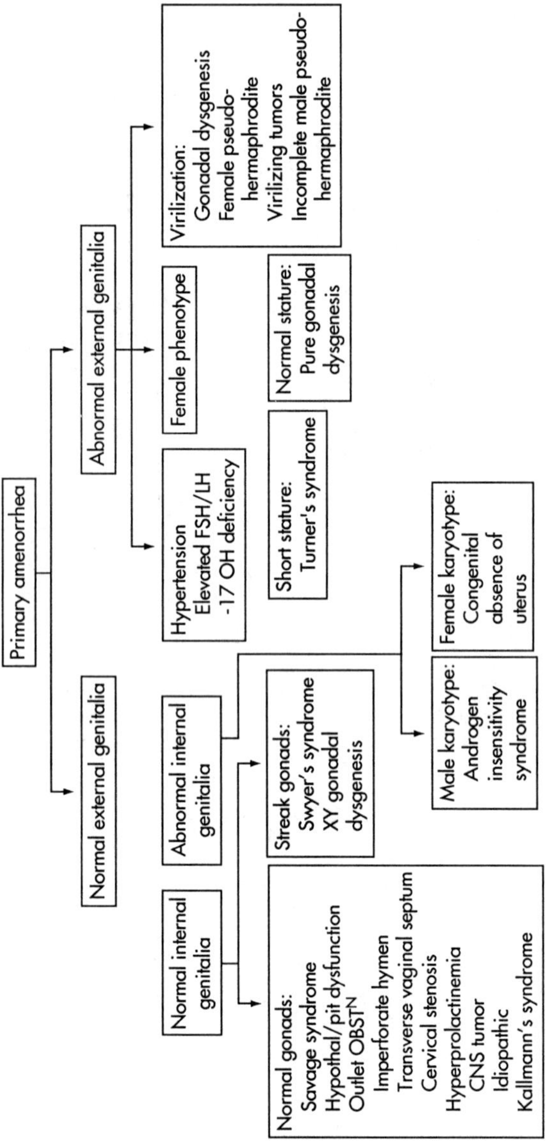

Figure 8-1
Steps in the assessment of primary amenorrhea.

The Classification of Secondary Amenorrheas

Functional ovaries
- Asherman's syndrome
- Endometrial destruction
  - Infectious
  - Iatrogenic

Hypergonadotrophic
- Premature ovarian failure
- Iatrogenic ovarian failure

Eugonadotrophic
- Hypothalamic–pituitary dysfunction
  - Psychogenic
  - Nutritional
    - Eating disorders
    - Starvation
  - Exercise induced
  - Pseudocyesis
  - CNS lesions
  - Nongonadal endocrinopathy
  - Pharmacologic
  - Acute and chronic disease
  - Idiopathic
- Central nervous system disease
- Feminizing ovarian tumors

Androgen excess
- Polycystic ovarian disease
- Masculinizing ovarian tumors

d. Excision of gonads in Y chromosome–positive individuals should be performed because of the increased risk of germ cell tumors. In testicular feminization, surgeons should wait until after puberty to allow normal long bone development. In others, surgery should occur before puberty to minimize risk of malignancy and virilization.
e. Estrogen replacement therapy can be used for hypoestrogenic states.

8.3 SECONDARY AMENORRHEA

Secondary amenorrhea is defined as the absence of menses for 6 months in a female who has had normal menstrual function for 12 months.

Classification

The classification of secondary amenorrheas appears in the box on p. 167.

1. Functional ovaries.
   a. Asherman's syndrome
      (1) Asherman's syndrome is the result of intrauterine synechiae, usually after curettage in association with endometritis (incomplete abortion or postpartum hemorrhage), but may occur with any operative procedure involving the uterine canal (myomectomy, septum resection etc.).
      (2) Diagnosis is made by hysteroscopy or, less reliably, by hysterosalpingogram.
      (3) Asherman's syndrome is divided into grades (grade 1, mucosal adhesions, to grade 4, uterine cavity obliteration), which reflect on surgical correctability and subsequent pregnancy rate.
      (4) Degree of menstrual flow or Provera withdrawal bleeding depends on amount of functional endometrium.
      (5) Treatment consists of hysteroscopically directed lysis of adhesions with 90% probability of menstrual return and 35% to 50% pregnancy rate.
   b. Endometrial destruction
      (1) By radiation or by infectious organisms (tuberculosis and schistosomiasis).
      (2) Uterine cavity may be maintained but is replaced by nonfunctional epithelium.
2. Hypergonadotrophic amenorrhea
   a. FSH and LH are increased and estrogen levels are low.
   b. Ten percent of secondary amenorrheas are caused by premature ovarian failure (menopause before age 40).
   c. It is associated with autoimmune disease, especially hypothyroidism.
   d. Antiovarian antibodies are present in 30% to 50%.
   e. Other causes include radiotherapy, chemotherapy (especially alkylating agents), chromosomal abnormalities, galactosemia, and postadnexal surgery.
   f. Reports of spontaneous remission and pregnancy are found in the literature, but the condition is usually irreversible.
   g. *In vitro* pregnancy with donor eggs or zygotes is an option for those requesting pregnancy.
3. Eugonadotrophic amenorrhea
   a. The majority of patients with secondary amenorrhea have eugonadotrophic amenorrhea.
   b. Hypothalamic–pituitary dysfunction is the most common cause but is a diagnosis of exclusion.
   c. Mechanism is likely a slowing of the hypothalamic gonadotropin-releasing hormone (GNRH) pulse generator with increased CRF (corticotropin), growth hormone, and nocturnal melatonin.
   d. There is a blunted response to GNRH stimulation.
   e. Prognosis is usually good if the underlying cause is treatable.

(1) Psychogenic amenorrhea
  (a) Increased CRF leads to decreased GNRH and therefore decreased LH.
  (b) The cause may be acute or chronic stress.
  (c) Treatment includes the following:
    i. Stress management
    ii. Antidepressants
    iii. Psychopharmaceutical
    iv. Estrogen replacement
    v. If necessary, ovulation induction
(2) Weight loss–induced amenorrhea
  (a) A minimum of 17% body fat is required for menarche.
  (b) Menstrual maintenance requires 22% body fat, but body fat is not the only determinant.
  (c) Anorexia nervosa is an extreme example and is associated with increased conversion of estradiol to catecholestrogens, which suppresses the hypothalamus.
  (d) Treatment includes the following:
    i. Dietary counseling
    ii. Behavior modification
    iii. Estrogen replacement
    iv. Ovulation induction (should be carried out only after careful consideration of underlying pathology)
(3) Exercise-induced amenorrhea
  (a) A combination of stress, weight loss, loss of body fat, and dietary control cause this.
  (b) Individuals' responses of CRF axis exercise intensity are important variables.
  (c) No consistent relationship to endogenous opiates exists.
  (d) Bone loss has been documented in amenorrheic athletes.
  (e) Treatment includes the following:
    i. Decreasing exercise
    ii. Increasing body fat
    iii. Estrogen replacement
  (f) Pregnancy counseling (should be carried out before ovulation induction)
(4) Pseudocyesis
  (a) All the symptoms and many of the signs of pregnancy are present.
  (b) Increased pulses of LH and prolactin with normal FSH are seen.
  (c) The LH/FSH ratio is high (>2).
  (d) Treatment includes counseling and ovulation induction.
(5) Postpill amenorrhea
  (a) Hypothalamic oversuppression syndrome.
  (b) Postpill amenorrhea occurs in <1% of women on the birth control pill (BCP).
  (c) There is no relationship to dose or duration of BCP use.
  (d) Spontaneous recovery may take years.
  (e) Treatment includes ovulation induction or sequential cyclic hormonal replacement.

(6) CNS lesions
  (a) These are most often pituitary or parapituitary lesions.
  (b) Amenorrhea with galactorrhea is a common presentation, but hyperprolactinemia can occur without galactorrhea.
  (c) Hyperprolactinemia requires a search for a pituitary microadenoma, especially with amenorrhea.
  (d) Pituitary gummas, nonfunctional pituitary tumors, postpartum ischemia (Sheehan's syndrome), and internal carotid aneurysms can cause pituitary insufficiency and present as amenorrhea.
  (e) Destructive lesions of the hypothalamus usually have neurologic symptoms preceding the amenorrhea.
  (f) Treatment requires an accurate diagnosis.
    i. Parlodel is the treatment of choice for prolactin-producing pituitary microadenomas.
    ii. Radiation or surgery is used for macroadenomas or other microadenomas.
    iii. Parlodel use has been shown to shrink the size of pituitary adenomas.

(7) Amenorrhea with other endocrinopathies
  (a) Thyroid dysfunction (usually hyperthyroidism) often presents with amenorrhea.
  (b) Juvenile diabetes mellitus and adrenocortical dysfunction may also cause amenorrhea.

(8) Drug-induced amenorrhea
  (a) Dopamine antagonists (phenothiazines, metoclopramide, etc.) can cause amenorrhea by elevation of prolactin.
  (b) Cytotoxic agents, especially alkylating agents, can cause ovarian follicular destruction that is often irreversible. Increased duration of therapy and patient age worsen prognosis.
  (c) Depo-Provera has been associated with prolonged amenorrhea.
  (d) Drug addiction has also been associated with amenorrhea.

(9) Chronic and acute disease
  (a) Often caused by nutritional or stress factors, but a variety of metabolic pathways may also be involved. Correction of the underlying disease often results in return of menses.

(10) Estrogen-producing tumors
  (a) These tumors are rare but should be considered if endometrial hyperplasia is noted.

4. Amenorrhea with androgenic excess: The source of androgen may be ovarian or adrenal.
   a. Polycystic ovarian disease
      (1) This is the main cause of ovarian hyperandrogenic state.
      (2) Results from altered feedback at hypothalamic level resulting in excessive suppression of FSH. Higher LH levels result in

increased androgen production by theca cell layer in developing follicles.
    (3) Oligomenorrhea, obesity, hirsutism, and infertility are often present.
    (4) Ovaries often have the characteristic smooth, thick, white capsule with multiple small developing follicles. This appearance can also be detected by ultrasound.
    (5) Increased LH/FSH ratio (>2), increased androstenedione, and free testosterone are present.
    (6) Treatment involves the following:
        (a) Cyclic progesterone (protection against endometrial hyperplasia)
        (b) Birth control pills (endometrial protection, suppression of ovarian androgenic production, and increased sex hormone binding globulin)
        (c) Ovulation induction
  b. Late-onset congenital hyperplasia
    (1) It presents with hirsutism and dysfunctional uterine bleeding.
    (2) Increased frequency is seen in Eastern European Jews, Hispanics, and Yugoslavians.
    (3) Diagnosis is made by adrenocorticotropic hormone (ACTH) stimulation test.
    (4) Treatment requires replacement therapy with prednisone or dexamethasone.
  c. Masculinizing ovarian tumors usually have high androgen levels.

Diagnostic workup

1. Ovulation
    a. If present, indicates unresponsive endometrium.
    b. Suggested by the presence of cyclic events (e.g., mittelschmertz, premenstrual complaints).
    c. Diagnosed by basal body temperature charts, progesterone level, or endometrial biopsy.
2. Estrogenic Status
    a. Hypoestrogenic states are associated with osteoporosis regardless of cause.
    b. Suggested by hot flushes and vaginal dryness.
    c. Lack of Provera withdrawal suggests hypoestrogenic state but 10% to 15% of hypoestrogenic females will have some bleeding.
    d. Estradiol is useful only when the estradiol level is high (estrogen tumor).
    e. Vaginal cytology is helpful.
3. Androgen excess
    a. Suggested by oily skin or hair, hirsutism, clitoromegaly, and defeminization
    b. Testosterone (50% ovarian, 50% adrenal), androstenedione (50% ovarian, 50% adrenal), dehydroepiandrosterone (DHEAS) (90% adrenal)
    c. 17-hydroxyprogesterone levels as necessary

4. Pituitary status
   a. Suggested by galactorrhea, visual field defects
   b. FSH, LH, TSH, and prolactin: necessary for evaluation
   c. Most patients require blood for FSH, LH, TSH, and prolactin.
      (1) A progesterone withdrawal confirms outflow tract integrity and suggests normal endogenous estrogen.
      (2) Absence of bleeding to even sequential estrogen and progesterone necessitates a hysteroscopy or hysterosalpingogram.
   d. Testosterone and DHEAS levels are useful when androgenic features are present.
   e. GNRH stimulation test will be diagnostic for pituitary failure.
   f. CAT scans and MRI are necessary with hyperprolactinemia.
   g. Counseling is imperative with eating or weight disorders.

Treatment modalities

1. Cyclic progesterone (Provera, 10 mg, for a minimum of 10 days for a minimum of every 2 months) helps protect against the development of endometrial hyperplasia and endometrial carcinoma.
2. BCP
   a. BCPs are useful when contraception is necessary but also protect against endometrial hyperplasia.
   b. BCPs improve hirsutism (reducing ovarian androgen production and increasing sex hormone binding globulin that does reduce free androgen).
   c. This is a useful and convenient method of estrogen replacement therapy.
   d. Certain BCPs are not acceptable by athletic organizations because of androgenic activity.
3. Ovulation induction
   a. Clomiphene citrate: There are increased incidence of symptomatic functional cysts, of multiple pregnancies, and a marginally increased risk of ovarian cancer.
   b. Pulsatile GNRH agonist therapy most closely mimics normal follicular development but is expensive and cumbersome.
   c. Gonadotrophin therapy is involved and expensive, with a higher risk of hyperstimulation, multiple pregnancy, and possibly ovarian carcinoma.
4. Hysteroscopic surgery often allows resumption of menses. Pregnancy rates depend on severity of the adhesions.
5. Prolactin antagonists are treatment of choice in pituitary microadenomas, idiopathic hyperprolactinemia, and pretherapy for macroadenomas (which usually require surgery or targeted radiation).
6. Estrogen therapy should be considered in all cases of hypoestrogenic states.
   a. Tamoxifen can be used in patients with breast cancer.
   b. Small doses of testosterone may improve quality of life and bone status.
7. Egg and zygote donation can be considered if pregnancy is desired in the presence of nonfunctional ovaries.

Abnormal Uterine Bleeding

9

George T. Danakas, M.D.

Abnormal uterine bleeding is defined as any bleeding that significantly deviates from the usual menstrual pattern. Normal menstruation varies among women in the amount and duration of blood flow and by the intervals between menstrual cycles. The average range of intervals between cycles is 21 and 35 days; the duration of normal menses is 3 to 7 days; blood lost during a normal cycle varies from 25 to 80 ml.

9.1 ETIOLOGY

1. Abnormal uterine bleeding can be divided into two major categories: organic and dysfunctional.
2. Dysfunctional uterine bleeding is abnormal bleeding from the uterine endometrium that is unrelated to anatomic lesions of the uterus.
   a. Of these cases, 80% are caused by anovulation.
   b. Twenty percent are caused by dysfunction of the corpus luteum or atrophic endometrium.
3. Organic causes can be subdivided into systemic disease and reproductive tract disease.

9.2 DEFINITIONS OF ABNORMAL BLEEDING

Amenorrhea	Absence or abnormal cessation of the menses
Hypermenorrhea	Menorrhagia; prolonged or profuse menses
Hypomenorrhea	A diminution of the flow or a shortening of the duration of menstruation
Menorrhagia	Excessively profuse or prolonged menstruation
Metrorrhea	Irregular, acyclic bleeding from the uterus, particularly between periods
Menometrorrhagia	Irregular or excessive bleeding during menstruation and between menstrual periods
Oligomenorrhea	Scanty menstruation; menses occurring at intervals greater than 35 days
Polymenorrhea	The occurrence of menstrual cycles of greater than usual frequency—usually at intervals less than 21 days

Systemic Diseases That Can Cause Abnormal Bleeding

I Blood Dyscrasia

Thrombocytopenia purpura
von Willebrand's disease
Leukemia
Increased fibrinolysin (endometrium)

II Hepatic Disease

Impaired synthesis of coagulation factors
Impaired metabolism of sex steroids (i.e., estrogen)
Impaired synthesis of sex hormone–binding globulin

III Renal Disease

Impaired excretion of estrogens
Obesity

IV Iatrogenic Causes

Anticoagulants, digitalis, oral contraceptives (breakthrough bleeding), aspirin, intrauterine device (IUD)

V Endocrine

Hypothyroidism or hyperthyroidism
Diabetes mellitus

Adapted from Copeland LJ: *Textbook of gynecology*, Philadelphia, 1993, Saunders.

9.3 DIAGNOSIS

History

1. Frequency, duration, and amount of bleeding
2. Current pregnancy
3. Contraceptive history
4. Systemic diseases (see the box above)
5. List of medications
6. Any recent surgical or gynecologic surgery

Physical examination

A complete physical examination, including a careful pelvic examination, should be performed. There are many anatomic causes of nonuterine bleeding (see the box on p. 175) and anatomic uterine abnormalities (see the box on p. 176).

Examination should include the following:

1. Thyroid
2. Breasts
3. Liver
4. Presence or absence of ecchymotic lesions on the skin
5. Obesity
6. Hirsutism

Anatomic Causes of Nonuterine Bleeding

Cervix
- Neoplasia (polyps or carcinoma)
- Cervicitis
- Ectropion and eversion
- Ulceration
- Condylomatous lesions
- Endometriosis

Vagina
- Neoplasia (carcinoma, sarcoma)
- Adenosis
- Trauma
- Foreign body
- Atrophic vaginitis
- Infection (vaginitis)
- Condylomas

Vulva
- Trauma
- Infections or inflammations
- Neoplasia
- Condylomas
- Dystrophy
- Varices

Urinary Tract
- Urethral caruncle
- Urethral diverticulum
- Hematuria

Gastrointestinal Tract
- Hemorrhoids
- Anal fissure
- Colorectal lesions

From Copeland LJ: *Textbook of gynecology*, Philadelphia, 1993, Saunders.

7. Inspection of vulva and vagina
8. Inspection and palpation of cervix and uterus
9. Determination of the size and shape of uterus
10. Palpation of adnexa for mass and to check for ovarian pathology

Diagnostic studies

Hemoglobin and hematocrit
Serum iron level and serum ferritin level
Chemistry profile including liver function tests

Anatomic Uterine Abnormalities

1. Endometrial hyperplasia
2. Endometrial or cervical carcinoma
3. Leiomyomas
4. Polyps: endometrial and endocervical
5. Infections: endometritis, cervicitis, vaginitis
6. Foreign bodies (IUD, tampon)
7. Pregnancy abnormalities
8. Estrogen-producing ovarian tumors
9. Medications: hormone replacement therapy, oral contraceptives (OCs)

Serum human chorionic gonadotropin (HCG)
Thyroid profile
Coagulation profile
Luteal phase progesterone
Prolactin, follicle stimulating hormone (FSH), luteinizing hormone (LH)
Serum androgens
Stool for occult blood
Urinalysis for hematuria
Papanicolaou smear
Pelvic ultrasound; include measurement of endometrial thickness
Hysterogram or hysteroscopy
Endometrial sampling

9.4 MANAGEMENT

In most patients abnormal uterine bleeding is a recurrent problem and long-term management depends on correct diagnosis for treatment (see the box above and the box on p. 177).

Systemic and anatomic causes should be managed with their specific treatments.

Medical therapy

1. Progestational agents
   a. Progesterone in oil, 100 to 200 mg (only in acute cases)
   b. Depo-Provera, 150 mg (acutely), followed by 150 mg q3mo for chronic management
   c. Medroxyprogesterone acetate
      (1) Acute: 20 to 40 mg/day × 15 days
      (2) Chronic: 10 mg/day × 12 days
      (3) Cyclically to induce monthly withdrawal bleeding
   d. Megestrol acetate, 40 to 120 mg/day (acute cases)
   e. Norethindrone
      (1) Acute: 1 to 5 mg/day (usually 2.5 mg, qd) × 15 days
      (2) Chronic: 1 mg/day × 12 days

Abnormal Uterine Bleeding

Pregnancy

- Threatened abortion
- Incomplete abortion
- Complete abortion
- Molar pregnancy
- Ectopic pregnancy
- Retained products of conception

Ovulatory

- Vulva: infection, laceration, tumor
- Vagina: infection, laceration, tumor, foreign body
- Cervix: polyps, cervical erosion, cervicitis, carcinoma
- Uterus: fibroids (submucous fibroids most likely to cause abnormal bleeding), polyps, adenomyosis, endometritis, IUD, atrophic endometrium
- Pregnancy complications: ectopic pregnancy; threatened, incomplete, complete abortion; retained products of conception
- Abnormality of clotting system
- Midcycle bleeding
- Halban's disease (persistent corpus luteum)
- Menorraghia
- Pelvic inflammatory disease

Anovulatory

- Physiologic causes
  - Puberty
  - Perimenopausal
- Pathologic causes
  - Ovarian failure (FSH over 40 IU/ml)
  - Hyperandrogenism
  - Hyperprolactinemia
  - Obesity
  - Hypothalamic dysfunction (polycystic ovaries); LH/FSH ratio greater than 2:1
  - Hyperplasia
  - Endometrial carcinoma
  - Estrogen-producing tumors
  - Hypothyroidism

f. Oral contraceptives
  (1) Acute: 1 to 4 tablets per day
  (2) Chronic: 1 tablet per day
g. For the management of acute, prolonged bleeding the author uses four tablets per day × 3 days followed by three tablets per day × 3 days. The patient will get a heavy withdrawal bleed; then the physician should follow with cyclic Provera or continue on oral contraceptives, one tablet daily.

2. Estrogen
   a. Conjugated estrogen (Premarin), 25 mg, IV, q4h until bleeding is under control in cases of prolonged heavy bleeding that is considered severe or life threatening (maximum: three doses).
   b. For prolonged bleeding that is not life threatening, Premarin, 1.25 mg (or Estrace 2 mg), q4h × 24 hours. This is followed by Provera to bring on a withdrawal bleed. After acute management, a sequential regimen of estrogen and Progestin (Premarin, 1.25 mg, qd × 24 days; Provera, 10 mg × 10 days) or OCs can be used.
3. Clomiphene citrate: Use in patients whose abnormal bleeding has been anovulatory and who wish to get pregnant.
4. Other
   a. Antiprostaglandins
   b. Danazol
   c. Gonadotropic-releasing hormone (GNRH) analogs
   d. Human menopausal gonadotropin (HMG)

Surgical therapy

1. Dilation and curettage
2. Endometrial ablation
3. Hysterectomy

Suggested reading

1. American College of Obstetricians and Gynecologists: *Dysfunctional uterine bleeding*, ACOG Technical Bulletin No. 134, Washington, DC, 1989, ACOG.
2. Boyd ME: Dysfunctional uterine bleeding, *Can J Surg* 29:305, 1986.
3. Devore GR, Owens O, Kase N: Use of intravenous Premarin in the treatment of dysfunctional uterine bleeding—a double-blind randomized controlled study, *Obstet Gynecol* 59:285, 1982.
4. Kim M: Dysfunctional uterine bleeding. In Copeland LJ: *Textbook of gynecology*, Philadelphia, 1993, WB Saunders, pp. 391-397.
5. Speroff L, Glass RH, Kase NG: *Dysfunctional uterine bleeding in clinical gynecologic endocrinology and infertility*, ed 5, Baltimore, 1994, Williams & Wilkins, pp. 531-546.

Endometriosis

10

Ronald E. Batt, M.D., and Germaine M. Buck, Ph.D.

Endometriosis is an extraordinarily complex, enigmatic chronic disease, although some investigators believe that some endometriotic lesions may be physiologic. Clinicians and scientists are unable to predict in which patients the endometriosis will progress to moderate, severe, or extensive disease. While the etiology, pathophysiology, and natural history of endometriosis are being studied, therapeutic trials with a "no-treatment" control arm are essential to discern treatment efficacy.

10.1 DEFINITION

Sampson defined endometriosis as "the presence of ectopic tissue which possesses the histologic structure and function of the uterine mucosa. It also includes the abnormal conditions which may result, not only from the invasion of organs and other structures by this tissue, but from its reaction to menstruation."[15] In light of new immunologic, biochemical, and physiologic findings, this pathologic definition of endometriosis is no longer adequate. A functional definition is needed to reflect prognostic and therapeutic issues.

10.2 EPIDEMIOLOGY

Traditionally, women with endometriosis were reported to be largely white, career-minded women of upper socioeconomic status who voluntarily delayed childbearing. This profile was based largely on convenient samples of women seeking treatment for infertility or pelvic pain associated with endometriosis. These early clinical studies did not fully adjust for biases arising from the selection of cases and other issues pertaining to medical care–seeking behaviors of affected women. More recent evidence suggests that endometriosis affects approximately 10% of women of reproductive age regardless of race, socioeconomic status, or childbearing intentions. Although limited in scope, findings from recent studies suggest that various factors may be associated with an increased or decreased risk of endometriosis, and these are summarized as follows.

Purported risk factors

1. Reproductive age
   a. Mean age at diagnosis is 25 to 29 years.[14]
   b. Adolescents are more likely to have Müllerian duct anomalies or cervical or vaginal obstruction.[10]
   c. Postmenopausal women are more likely to be on estrogen replacement therapy.[7]
2. Socioeconomic status: suggestion of greater risk for upper socioeconomic status (difference possibly from health care–seeking behaviors)[9]
3. Family history: primarily, first degree relatives (mother, sister, first cousin), although no clear inheritance pattern[12]
4. Menstrual characteristics: shorter cycles (< 27 days), longer flow (> 7 days), and greater menstrual pain[4,6]
5. Somatotype
   a. Weight: peripheral predominance of body fat among affected women under 30 years of age (i.e., risk inversely related to waist-to-hip and waist-to-thigh ratios)[13]
   b. Height: greater risk for tall women (> 166 cm)[8]
6. Reproductive history: history of infertility and impaired fecundity (e.g., spontaneous abortion)[5]

Factors decreasing risk

1. Strenuous exercise: physical exercise, especially if begun early and practiced regularly[4,8]
2. Cigarette smoking: early and regular use (Careful interpretation of these preliminary findings is warranted, especially in light of health hazards associated with smoking.)[4,8]

10.3 THEORIES OF HISTOGENESIS

1. General theories include the following:
   a. Coelomic metaplasia
   b. Transplantation of shed endometrium
   c. Direct extension, hematologic, and lymphatic spread
   d. Impaired immune system
2. Special theory of histogenesis to explain endometriosis in peritoneal pockets.
   a. Embryologic rudimentary duplication Müllerian ducts[1]

10.4 CLINICAL MANIFESTATIONS[3]

Endometriosis-associated pain

1. Acquired dysmenorrhea: possibly as early as third menstrual cycle in adolescents
2. Three or more emergency visits for unexplained pelvic pain
3. Low central backache and lower abdominal pain
4. Midcycle pain: mittelschmerz
5. Deep dyspareunia resulting from endometriosis of uterosacral ligaments and rectovaginal pouch of Douglas

6. Deep dyspareunia, worse before menses
7. Pain with bowel movements before and during menses

Endometriosis-associated infertility

1. Primary infertility: never pregnant
   a. Affects roughly 41% of women with endometriosis
   b. Monthly fecundity reduced
2. Secondary infertility: previously pregnant
   a. Roughly 35% of women with endometriosis state difficulty conceiving and carrying pregnancy to term.
3. Outcome of first pregnancy *before* diagnosis of endometriosis
   a. Decreased live births
   b. Increased spontaneous abortions
   c. Increased elective abortions
   d. Infrequent ectopic pregnancies

Endometriosis-associated health problems

1. Profuse, unremitting menorrhagia
   a. Risk of multiple blood transfusions
   b. Risk of pituitary ischemia
   c. Risk of multiorgan hormonal replacement
2. Intractable pelvic pain associated with frozen pelvis
3. Bowel pain or obstruction
4. Ureteral obstruction
   a. Risk of hydroureter and hydronephrosis
   b. Risk of hypertension
   c. Risk of autonephrectomy
   d. Risk of renal failure if obstruction is bilateral
5. Osteoporosis
   a. Risk increased by endometriosis
   b. Risk increased by gonadotropic-releasing hormone (GNRH) ovarian suppression
   c. Risk increased by early bilateral oophorectomy
   d. Risk increased by withholding estrogen replacement
6. Pneumothorax and hemothorax
7. Malignant transformation endometriosis posterior fornix
   a. Risk increased by unopposed estrogen replacement
   b. Risk removed by excising endometriosis

10.5 PHYSICAL EXAMINATION[3]

1. Inspection by examiner sitting at eye level of cervix
   a. Cervix displaced 1 cm or more lateral to midline
   b. Outflow obstruction favoring retrograde menstruation
      (1) Cervical stenosis
      (2) Imperforate hymen
      (3) Transverse vaginal septum
      (4) Uterine anomaly with blind uterine horn
   c. Tender, fixed angulation of rectum at sigmoidoscopy

2. Palpation: bimanual pelvic, rectovaginal, rectal examination
   a. Tenderness on stretching shortened cardinal ligament
   b. Tender rectovaginal pouch of Douglas
   c. Tender uterosacral ligaments
   d. Tender nodules in uterosacral ligaments
   e. Fixed retroverted uterus

10.6 TOOLS FOR ASSESSMENT[3]

1. Existing medical records (e.g., office, operative, pathology)
2. History and physical examination
3. Female anatomic grid map to localize pain graphically
4. Color duplex Doppler ultrasound of ovarian cysts
5. *Chlamydia* and *Neisseria* antibody titers
6. Hysterosalpingogram and hysteroscopy (selective)
7. Diagnostic laparoscopy
   a. Systematic inspection of abdomen and pelvis and palpation of suspicious lesions
   b. Photo documentation
   c. Biopsy confirmation
8. American Fertility Society Revised Classification of Endometriosis for pelvic pain and infertility
9. Dictation of operative report immediately after each surgery
10. Intravenous pyelogram (IVP) for ureteral involvement, left-frozen-pelvis, frozen pelvis
11. Sigmoidoscopy for bowel involvement
12. Original staging: benchmark from which to measure the regression, stability, or progression of the disease (as in cancer)
13. Staging: essential to establish early the clinical course of the disease in each patient

10.7 FINDINGS AT LAPAROSCOPY[3]

Organs at risk

1. Common organ involvement corresponds to those organs bathed in pelvic peritoneal fluid.
   a. Bladder
   b. Round ligaments
   c. Uterus
   d. Uterosacral ligaments
   e. Broad ligaments
   f. Ovaries
   g. Tubes
   h. Lateral pelvic peritoneum
   i. Rectovaginal pouch
   j. Rectum
   k. Sigmoid colon
   l. Cecum
   m. Appendix
   n. Distal ileum

2. Uncommon organ involvement
   a. Episiotomy
   b. Transverse colon
   c. Sciatic nerve
   d. Trigone of bladder
   e. Lung
3. Rare organ involvement
   a. Pancreas
   b. Liver
   c. Brain
   d. Skin

Asymmetry

1. Anteroposterior asymmetry: Endometriosis is common in the vesicouterine pouch when the uterus is sharply anteverted, and in the rectovaginal pouch when the uterus is retroverted.
2. Lateral asymmetry: Endometriosis tends to be more severe on one side of the pelvis, with sparing or relative sparing of the other side.

Invasion

1. Endometriosis elicits a foreign body reaction, fibrosis, to encapsulate and contain the disease.
2. Deep nodules form in the rectovaginal pouch and uterosacral ligaments.
3. Endometriotic cysts form in the ovaries.

Acute and chronic endometriosis

1. Acute endometriosis: exhibits red, angry, inflammatory host response to ruptured ovarian endometrioma, or aggressively active disease
2. Chronic endometriosis: exhibits firm, enveloping fibrosis in a quiescent pelvis

Peritoneal pockets with endometriosis

1. Located in broad ligaments and rectovaginal pouch of Douglas
2. Associated medial displacement of ureter(s) in some cases
3. Endometriosis presents as tan brim nodules and spider lesions

10.8 HOST RESPONSES TO ENDOMETRIOSIS [3]

Hypertrophy and relaxation

1. Uterine and ovarian hypertrophy, leiomyomas
2. Relaxation of round, uterosacral, utero-ovarian ligaments
3. Allow uterus and ovaries to adhere to rectovaginal pouch

Sclerosis of solid organs

1. Uterine sclerosis
2. Ovarian sclerosis: cartilaginous consistency

Stenosis to occlusion of hollow organs

1. Cervical stenosis
2. Cornual angle fallopian tube obstruction
3. Perifimbrial tubal stenosis
4. Fimbrial tubal phimosis
5. Ureteral stricture, obstruction
6. Bowel stricture, obstruction

Inflammation

1. Retrograde menstruation
2. Ruptured endometriomas
3. Autoimmune changes

Adhesions

1. Endometriotic adhesions
2. Surgical adhesions
3. Adhesions from sexually transmitted diseases
4. Adhesions from malignancy

10.9 DISEASE PATTERNS[3]

1. Simple disease pattern: corresponds to stages I and II disease
   a. Normal pelvic architecture serves as a platform for subtle and conspicuous endometriotic lesions.
   b. In our referral center, 75% of cases are simple.
      (1) Subtle forms of endometriosis
         (a) Peritoneal pockets with endometriosis (Müllerianosis)
         (b) Nonpigmented peritoneal and ovarian endometriosis
         (c) Slightly enlarged "normal ovary" with deep endometrioma
         (d) Ovarian endometriosis hidden by surface adhesions
         (e) Early bowel endometriosis
      (2) Conspicuous form of endometriosis
         (a) Deeply pigmented peritoneal and ovarian lesions
         (b) Ovarian endometriomas
         (c) Constricting endometriotic lesions of ileum and colon
2. Complex disease patterns: corresponds to stages III and IV
   a. Distorted pelvic architecture: There are thresholds of increased complexity until irreversible damage occurs. The surgeon must understand the evolution and development of complex disease patterns to resolve them successfully by surgery.
   b. In our referral center, 25% of cases are complex.
      (1) Centrifugal pattern: obliterated rectovaginal pouch with rectum and ovaries attached to retroverted uterus
      (2) Left-frozen-pelvis: sigmoid colonic adhesions obliterate the left adnexa, which is also densely adherent to left pelvic wall
      (3) Obliterated rectovaginal pouch of Douglas: rectum densely adherent to posterior uterus
      (4) Centripetal pattern: ovaries adherent laterally with or without an obliterated rectovaginal pouch of Douglas
      (5) Complete frozen pelvis

10.10 COMPLICATIONS OF TREATMENT OF COMPLEX DISEASE PATTERNS

Despite meticulous dissection by skilled surgeons, the following complications may occur when operating and reoperating severe and extensive pelvic endometriosis:

1. Premature menopause
2. Ovarian remnant syndrome
3. Ligation or severance of a ureter(s)
4. Ureterovaginal fistula
5. Vesicovaginal fistula
6. Rectovaginal fistula
7. Coloperitoneal fistula with abscess
8. Bowel obstruction
9. Sciatic nerve injury
10. Major arterial or venous injury

The risk of such complications may be minimized by the following:

1. Meticulous preoperative preparation
2. Mechanical and antibiotic bowel preparation
3. An experienced operative team
4. Good surgical exposure
5. Meticulous operative technique using dissection of retroperitoneal spaces
6. Ureteral catheters selectively

10.11 OPTIONS FOR TREATMENT

Endometriosis-associated pain[2,3,11,16]

The objective is to excise all visible endometriosis and treat with postoperative danocrine or GNRH for 3 months, then maintain the patient with combination oral contraceptive pills such as Orthonovum, 1:35-21, cyclically.

1. Stages I and II
   a. Danazol or GNRH in selected cases
   b. Laparoscopic surgery with postoperative danazol or GNRH
   c. Conservative surgery by laparotomy with preoperative danazol
2. Stage III: moderate disease
   a. Laparoscopic surgery with postoperative danazol or GNRH
   b. Conservative surgery by laparotomy with preoperative danazol
3. Stage IV: severe and extensive disease
   a. Conservative surgery by laparotomy with preoperative danazol
   b. Laparoscopic surgery with postoperative medical suppression

Endometriosis-associated infertility[2,3,11,16]

When surgery is indicated, the objective is to excise all visible endometriosis, and then allow the patient to conceive, using assisted reproductive technologies as indicated. Older patients and couples with prolonged infertility should be offered assisted reproductive therapies early.

1. Stages I and II
   a. Expectant treatment selectively
   b. Laparoscopic surgery with excision of endometriosis

   c. Menopausal gonadotropin or human chorionic gonadotropin (HCG) and intrauterine insemination
   d. Gamete intrafallopian transfer (GIFT), *in vitro* fertilization (IVF), and endotracheal tube (ET)
2. Stage III: moderate disease
   a. Laparoscopic surgery with excision of endometriosis
   b. Conservative surgery by laparotomy with preoperative danazol
   c. Menopausal gonadotropin or HCG and intrauterine insemination
   d. GIFT, IVF, and ET
3. Stage IV: severe and extensive disease
   a. Conservative surgery by laparotomy with preoperative danazol
   b. Laparoscopic surgery selectively
   c. GIFT, IVF, and ET

Endometriosis-associated health problems[2,3,11,16]

The objective of treatment is to control symptoms promptly and, where surgery is indicated, to excise all visible endometriosis.

1. Stages I and II
   a. Laparoscopic surgery with postoperative danazol or GNRH
   b. Conservative surgery by laparotomy with preoperative danazol or GNRH
   c. Excision of all endometriosis, hysterectomy –/+ bilateral salpingo-oophorectomy (SO)
2. Stage III: moderate disease
   a. Laparoscopic surgery with postoperative danazol or GNRH
   b. Conservative surgery with preoperative danazol or GNRH
   c. Excision of all endometriosis, hysterectomy –/+ bilateral
   d. Salpingo-oophorectomy with preoperative danazol or GNRH
3. Stage IV: severe and extensive disease
   a. Conservative surgery with preoperative danazol or GNRH
   b. Excision of all endometriosis, hysterectomy, bilateral salpingo-oophorectomy with postoperative estrogen or estrogen and progesterone hormone replacement (postoperative danazol or GNRH selectively)

Symptomatic bowel endometriosis[2]

In all cases, sigmoidoscopic examination for tender, fixed angulation of bowel is followed by double contrast barium enema. Selective colonoscopy. Mechanical and antibiotic bowel preparation in all cases. Estrogen hormone replacement therapy in patients without ovaries.

1. Conservative surgery for endometriosis and extraluminal, wedge, or segmental bowel resection
2. Excision of all pelvic endometriosis and hysterectomy with ovarian conservation and extraluminal, wedge, or segmental bowel resection
3. Excision of all pelvic endometriosis and hysterectomy, bilateral salpingo-oophorectomy, and extraluminal, wedge, or segmental bowel resection
4. Partial bowel obstruction
   a. Frozen section to rule out malignancy
   b. Wedge or segmental bowel resection
   c. Primary anastomosis if possible, colostomy if necessary

5. Complete bowel obstruction
   a. Frozen section to rule out malignancy
   b. Colostomy to relieve bowel obstruction
   c. Secondary bowel resection and closure of colostomy

Symptomatic ureteral endometriosis[2,3,11,16]

Intravenous pyelogram (IVP), sonogram of kidneys, and renal function studies selectively.

1. Ureterolysis or ureterovesical implantation and excision of all pelvic endometriosis
2. Ureterolysis or ureterovesical implantation and excision of all pelvic endometriosis with hysterectomy and ovarian conservation
3. Ureterolysis or ureterovesical implantation and excision of all pelvic endometriosis with hysterectomy, bilateral salpingo-oophorectomy, and hormone replacement therapy
4. Nephrectomy selectively, and appropriate pelvic surgery, dialysis, and kidney transplant selectively

Malignant endometriosis

Malignant ovarian endometriosis and malignant endometrosis of the posterior vaginal fornix should be treated by a gynecologic oncologist or by appropriate surgery and chemotherapy in consultation with a gynecologic oncologist.

Osteoporosis

Women with endometriosis are prone to osteoporosis. The object of treatment is removal of all endometriosis followed by estrogen or combined estrogen and progesterone hormone replacement therapy. The importance of excising all endometriosis at surgery cannot be overemphasized, so that patients can receive the benefits of hormonal replacement therapy.

10.12 PHYSICIAN–PATIENT FOLLOW-UP FROM DIAGNOSIS UNTIL POSTMENOPAUSE

1. Examine periodically.
2. Educate patient.
3. Maintain good physician records.
4. Ensure patient maintains good records also.
5. Minimize retrograde menstruation.
   a. Combination birth control pills cyclically
   b. Danazol selectively
   c. GNRH selectively
   d. Pregnancy when appropriate
   e. Lactation when desired
   f. Tubal ligation selectively
6. Repeat laparoscopic conservative surgery selectively.
7. Apply new research insights to patient care.

10.13 OVERVIEW OF MANAGEMENT

1. Patient education to encourage active informed cooperation is a must.
2. The diagnosis should be made early and accurately.

3. The disease should be staged by most up-to-date classification system.
4. Immediate and long-term treatment options should be discussed with patient.
5. Patient priorities should be respected: pain relief, fertility, health.
6. An appropriate treatment plan should be agreed on.
7. Copy of operative report and pathology reports should go to patient.
8. Endometriosis Association membership should be encouraged.

References

1. Batt RE et al: A case-series study of peritoneal pockets and endometriosis: Rudimentary duplications of the Müllerian system, *Adoles Pediatr Gynecol* 2:47-56, 1989.
2. Batt RE, Udagawa SM, Wheeler JM: Endometriosis: microconservative surgery. In Hunt RB, editor: *Atlas of female infertility surgery,* ed 2, St Louis, 1992, Mosby–Year Book, pp. 454-481.
3. Batt RE, Wheeler JM: Endometriosis: Advanced diagnostic laparoscopy. In Hunt RB, editor: *Atlas of female infertility* surgery, ed 2, St Louis, 1992, Mosby–Year Book.
4. Cramer DW et al: The relation of endometriosis to menstrual characteristics, smoking and exercise, *JAMA* 255:1904-1908, 1986.
5. Darrow SL et al: Sexual activity, contraception, and reproductive factors in predicting Endometriosis, *Am J Epidemiol* 140:500-509, 1994.
6. Darrow SL et al: Menstrual cycle characteristics and risk of endometriosis, *Epidemiology* 4:135-142, 1993.
7. Djursing H, Petersen K, Weberg E: Symptomatic postmenopausal endometriosis, *Acta Obstet Gynecol Scand* 60:529-530, 1981.
8. Goldman MB, Cramer DW: The epidemiology of endometriosis. In Chadra DR, Buttram VC Jr, editors: *Current concepts in endometriosis,* New York, 1990, Alan R. Liss.
9. Houston DE: Evidence for the risk of pelvic endometriosis by age, race and socioeconomic status, *Epidemiol Rev* 6:167-191, 1984.
10. Huffman JW: Endometriosis in young teenage girls, *Pediatr Ann* 10:44-49, 1981.
11. Hulka JF, Reich H: *Textbook of laparoscopy,* ed 2, Philadelphia, 1994, WB Saunders.
12. Malinak LR, Wheeler JM: Endometriosis. In Aiman J, editor: *Infertility: diagnosis and management,* New York, 1984, Springer-Verlag, pp. 255-275.
13. McCann SE et al: Endometriosis and body fat distribution, *Obstet Gynecol* 83:545-549, 1983.
14. Olive DL, Haney AF: Endometriosis. In DeCherney AH, editor: *Reproductive failure,* New York, 1986, Churchill Livingstone, pp. 153-203.
15. Sampson JA: The development of the implantation theory for the origin of peritoneal endometriosis, *Am J Obstet Gynecol* 40:549, 1940.
16. Soderstom RM: *Operative laparoscopy: the masters' techniques,* New York, 1993, Raven Press.

11 Gynecologic Infections

Lawrence J. Gugino, M.D.

11.1 GONORRHEA

Etiology

Neisseria gonorrhoeae, a gram-negative diplococcus is the causative agent for this disease.

1. Incidence
   a. Has been decreasing since 1975; fewer than 225 cases/100,000 in 1993
   b. Most commonly reported communicable disease in United States; one million reported cases plus an estimated 1.0 to 1.3 million additional cases in 1990
   c. Varies among populations and geographic areas, adolescents, minorities, and persons in southeastern United States
2. Prevalence
   a. Urban sexually transmitted disease (STD) clinics, 10% to 30% of cases
   b. Female family planning clinics, 0.5% to 5% of cases
   c. Female private MD office, 0% to 2% of cases
   d. Of all female infections, 75% occur in age group 15 to 24 years
3. Transmission
   a. By sexual contact
   b. Most efficiently by vaginal or anal intercourse
   c. Risk
      (1) Male to female: 80% to 90%
      (2) Female to male: 20% to 25%
4. Risk markers
   a. Homosexual male: 10× greater incidence
   b. Unmarried
   c. Urban residence
   d. Lower socioeconomic status
   e. Illicit drug use
   f. Prostitution
   g. Previous gonorrhea (GC)

h. No contraception or use of nonbarrier methods
i. Nonwhite race
5. Incubation period
a. Short
b. Urethritis, 2 to 5 days
c. Cervicitis, 5 to 10 days

Signs and symptoms

1. Ten percent of males and 20% to 40% of females are asymptomatic.
2. Uncomplicated anogenital female: Endocervix, urethra, Skenes's gland, Bartholin gland, and anus sites may be infected.
3. Common symptoms
a. Urethral or vaginal discharge
b. Dysuria, abnormal bleeding
c. Mucopurulent endocervical exudate
d. Nongenital symptoms may result from direct or contiguous spread and bloodstream dissemination.
(1) Pelvic inflammatory disease (PID) occurs in 15% to 20% of women with uncomplicated anogenital gonorrhea.
(2) Anorectal infection: 30% to 40% of patients with positive endocervical GC will have positive anorectal cultures.
(3) Perihepatitis (Fitz-Hugh-Curtis syndrome) may occur.
(4) Conjunctivitis may occur as well.
(5) Pharyngitis occurs in 10% to 20% of women with genital tract gonorrhea; it is most often asymptomatic.
e. Disseminated gonorrhea occurs when an infection of the genital tract, pharynx, or rectum invades the bloodstream.
(1) Prevalence: 0.1% to 0.3% of total gonorrhea
(2) The disease's two stages are as follows:
(a) Bacteremia
i. Chills
ii. Fever 38° to 39° C
iii. Skin lesions: erythematous macules 1 to 5 mm in diameter located on extremities secondary to gonococcal emboli
iv. Positive blood cultures in 50%
v. Endocarditis or meningitis: may ensue
(b) Septic arthritis
i. Purulent synovial effusion
ii. Knees, ankles, and wrists: erythema, edema, and pain
iii. Negative blood cultures

Gonococcal infection in pregnancy

1. Perinatal implications
a. Postabortal endometritis and salpingitis
b. Acute salpingitis in pregnancy
(1) Very rare and difficult to diagnose
(2) Occurs in first trimester

c. Perinatal complications
   (1) Increased incidence of premature rupture of membranes
   (2) Preterm delivery
   (3) Chorioamniotis
   (4) Neonatal sepsis
   (5) Postpartum sepsis
   (6) Neonatal conjunctivitis in 30% to 40%
2. All pregnant patients should be screened for *N. gonorrhoeae* at initial prenatal visit. The test should be repeated early in the third trimester.

Laboratory diagnosis

1. Gram-stain exudate
   a. Polymorphonuclear leukocytes (PMNs) intracellular gram-negative diplococci
   b. Diagnostic 90% male, 60% female
   c. Not useful for pharyngeal infection
2. Culture
   a. Isolation of organism in selective media (Thayer-Martin) is the gold standard.
   b. Culture detects 80% to 90% cervical, rectal, pharyngeal infections.
   c. Culture all symptomatic sites: Recovery of *N. gonorrhoeae* is improved by two consecutive endocervical specimens or combination endocervical and anal specimens.
3. Other tests: antigen detection (gonozyme)
   a. Less sensitive and specific
   b. Unable to measure antimicrobial susceptibility
   c. Use only when cultures are unavailable

Treatment of uncomplicated anogenital gonorrohea

1. Of gonococcal strains in the United States, 15% to 50% have a relative or absolute resistance to penicillin (PCN) or tetracycline (TCN).
2. 1993 Centers for Disease Control and Prevention (CDC) guidelines
   a. Ceftriaxone, 125 mg IM, single dose
   b. Cefixime, 400 mg orally, single dose
   c. Ciprofloxacin, 500 mg orally, single dose
   d. Ofloxacin, 400 mg orally, single dose, a regimen effective against coinfection with *C. trachomatis*

Treatment of disseminated gonorrhea

1. 1993 CDC guildelines
   a. Ceftriaxone, 1 g IM or IV, q24h
2. Alternative initial regimens
   a. Cefotaxime, 1 g IV, q8h, or
   b. Ceftizoxime, 1 g IV, q8h
3. β-Lactam allergic persons
   a. Spectinomycin, 2 g IM, q12h. Continue all regimens for 24 to 48 hours after improvement, then switch to one of the following regimens to complete a full week of therapy:
      (1) Cefixime, 400 mg orally, two times a day, or
      (2) Ciprofloxacin, 500 mg orally, two times a day

1993 CDC Screening Criteria for *Chlamydia*

Mucopurulent cervicitis
Sexually active <20 years
20 to 24 years age (one criterion)
>24 years age (both criteria)
  Inconsistent barrier contraception
  New or >1 partner in last 3 months

11.2 CHLAMYDIA

Etiology

Chlamydia is caused by *Chlamydia trachomatis,* an obligate intracellular parasite with 15 different serotypes.

1. The chlamydial organism has two forms.
   a. Elementary body (infectious)
      (1) Serotypes
         (a) L1, L2, L3: lymphogranuloma venereum
         (b) A, B, Ba, C: endemic blinding trachoma
         (c) D, E, F, G, H, I, J, K: oculogenital and STD strains
   b. Reticulate body (multiplies to form inclusions)
2. Epidemiology (see the box above)
   a. Emerging as most common STD
   b. 4 million cases per year
   c. Prevalence three to four times greater than GC
   d. Overall prevalence 3% to 5% (low risk), but greater than 20% of cases in STD clinics
   e. Transmission exclusively by sexual contact or perinatal contact
   f. Incubation period 6 to 14 days
3. Risk factors for acquiring *C. trachomatis*
   a. Unmarried and sexually active
   b. Multiple sexual partners
   c. Use of oral contraceptives
   d. Use of intrauterine device
   e. History of previous sexually transmitted disease
   f. Known exposure with partner having an STD
   g. Presence of concomitant STD especially *N. gonorrhoeae*
   h. Spotting after intercourse
   i. Intramenstrual spotting
   j. Vague complaints of lower abdominal pain

Lower genital tract infection

1. May often be asymptomatic and progress to upper genital tract disease
2. Bartholinitis: 33% of chlamydial infections
3. Endocervicitis: most common

a. Mucopurulent cervicitis
b. Specific for most nonciliated columnar or cuboidal epithelia (i.e., conjunctiva, urethra, endocervix, endometrium, fallopian tube mucosa)

4. Diagnosis suggested by the following:
    a. Positive swab test: a Q-Tip inserted into the endocervix stains yellowish-green
    b. Greater than 10 PMNS/oil immersion field gram stain
    c. Friable cervix
5. Acute urethral syndrome
    a. Indicated by dysuria and urinary frequency.
    b. Develops from 25% of cases of *C. trachomatis.*
    c. Sterile pyuria is found on urinalysis, or pyuria is found but with less than 10^5 organisms/ml.
    d. Culture cervix and urethra for diagnosis.
    e. *Chlamydia trachomatis* will not be recovered from urine.

Upper genital tract infection

1. Nonpuerperal endometritis
    a. Clinical signs of salpingitis are present.
    b. Patient has positive endometrial cultures or negative endocervical cultures.
    c. Infection is an intermediate step between endocervicitis and salpingitis.
2. Pelvic inflammatory disease
    a. The majority of serious acute illness and morbidity resulting from *Chlamydia* infections in women are caused by PID.
    b. Eight percent of females with *Chlamydia* have overt salpingitis.
    c. *Chlamydia* is found isolated or with other microorganisms in 5% to 50% of women with symptoms of PID.

Diagnosis

1. Cell cultures are the gold standard as specificity approaches 100%. This is essential for medical–legal situations.
2. Nonculture tests can detect *Chlamydia* antigens with 97% to 99% specificity.
    a. Direct fluorescent antibody (Micro Trak)
    b. Enzyme immunoassay (Chlamydiazyme)
    c. Nucleic acid hydridization (DNA probes)
    d. Polymerase chain reaction (PCR)
        (1) Gold standard of the future
        (2) Sensitivity >85%, specificity near 100%
            (a) Male urine
            (b) Female endocervix
            (c) Swabs: 90% to 100% sensitivity, specificity approaches 100%
            (d) Urine: 95% sensitivity
3. Disadvantages of cell culture
    a. Expensive
    b. Technically difficult

c. Requires 3 to 7 days to obtain result
d. Special transport media and storage temperatures required
4. Serology is rarely useful in clinical settings for genital tract infections.

Chlamydia treatment regimen, 1993 CDC guidelines

1. Recommended
   a. Doxycycline, 100 mg PO, bid × 7 days
   b. Azithromycin, 1 g PO, single dose
2. Alternative
   a. Ofloxacin, 300 mg PO, bid × 7 days
   b. Erythromycin base, 500 mg PO, qid × 7 days
   c. Erythromycin ethylsuccinate, 800 mg, qid × 7 days
   d. Sulfisoxazole, 500 mg PO, qid × 10 days
3. Pregnancy
   a. Erythromycin base
   b. Erythromycin ethylsuccinate
   c. Amoxicillin, 500 mg PO, tid 7 to 10 days

Follow-up

1. Test of cure culture is not necessary unless symptoms persist or reinfection is suspected.
2. Test of cure culture is recommended for pregnancy.
3. Reculture >3 weeks after initial treatment.

11.3 LYMPHOGRANULOMA VENEREUM (LGV)

Etiology

1. LGV is a sexually transmitted systemic disease.
2. *Chlamydia trachomatis* is the causative agent.
3. There are three serotypes: L1, L2, and L3.
4. LGV is rare in the United States (285 cases reported in 1993).
5. LGV is endemic in Africa, India, parts of Southeast Asia, South America, and the Caribbean.
6. Primary stage
   a. Primary lesion is caused by multiplication of organism at site of infection.
   b. Papule, shallow ulcer
   c. Herpetiform lesion at site of inoculation (most common)
   d. Incubation period is 3 to 21 days.
   e. Most common site of lesion in women is the posterior wall, fourchette, or vulva.
   f. Healing is spontaneous without scar.
7. Second stage
   a. Inguinal syndrome: Inguinal adenopathy is characteristic.
      (1) Begins 1 to 4 weeks after primary lesion.
      (2) Syndrome is the most frequent clinical sign of the disease.
      (3) Inguinal adenopathy is unilateral in 70% of cases.
      (4) Symptoms include painful, extensive adenitis (bubo) and suppuration may occur with numerous sinus tracts.

(5) "Groove sign" signals femoral and inguinal node involvement (20%); most often seen in men.
(6) Involvement of deep iliac and retroperitoneal lymph nodes in women may present as a pelvic mass.

8. Third stage (anogenital syndrome)
   a. Subacute: proctocolitis
   b. Late: tissue destruction or scarring sinuses, abscesses, fistulas, strictures of perineum, elephantiasis

Diagnosis

1. Positive Frei test
   a. Intradermal chlamydial antigen
   b. Nonspecific for all *Chlamydia*
   c. No longer available (historical significance only)
2. Complement fixation test
   a. Titer >1:64 in active infection
   b. Convalescent titers no difference
3. Cell culture of *Chlamydia*
   a. Aspiration of fluctuant node yields highest rates of recovery.

Treatment

1. Doxycycline, 100 mg PO, bid × 21 days (treatment of choice)
2. Erythromycin base, 500 mg PO, qid × 21 days
3. Sulfisoxazole, 500 mg PO, qid × 21 days
4. Surgical
   a. Aspirate fluctuant nodes
   b. Incise and drain abcesses

11.4 SYPHILIS

Etiology

1. Syphilis is a chronic sexually transmitted infection.
2. *Treponema pallidum* is the causative agent and is corkscrew shaped, microaerophilic; nonculturable, 10 to 14 μm length, 0.15 μm diameter, and very fragile.
3. Episodes of active clinical disease interrupted by periods of latency are characteristic of syphilis.
4. Transmission
   a. Direct contact with infectious lesion is required for infection. Organism does not survive outside the body.
   b. Incubation period is 9 to 90 days (2 to 6 weeks average).
5. Primary stage characteristics
   a. Painless, indurated chancre (genital, anal, oral)
   b. Firm, nontender, regional adenopathy
   c. Lasts 1 to 5 weeks
   d. Heals spontaneously if untreated
6. Secondary syphilis characteristics
   a. Systemic infection: all major organ systems
   b. Headache, fever, malaise: may precede rash

c. Generalized rash: macular (10%), papular (34%), pustular (6%), or maculopapular (51%); may be confused with other dermatoses
d. Generalized lymphadenopathy (86%)
e. Mucous patches (10%)
f. Condylomata lata (10%)
g. Persisting or unhealing chancre (15%)
h. Alopecia; liver or kidney involvement
i. Lasts 2 to 6 weeks; resolves spontaneously
j. Recurrent secondary symptoms possible within 1 year for 25% of cases

7. Latent syphilis characteristics
   a. Clinical manifestations will be absent.
   b. Positive serologic tests for syphilis are the mainstay of diagnosis.
      (1) Less than 1 year duration: early latent
      (2) More than 1 year duration: late latent
   c. Two thirds of patients with untreated syphilis remain in the latent phase for life.
8. Tertiary syphilis
   a. If untreated, 33% of patients will progress to the tertiary stage.
      (1) Late benign (gumma) (15%): Complete resolution is possible with treatment; bone skin, cartilage, and internal organs are involved.
      (2) Cardiovascular (10%): Ascending aorta is involved and results include the following:
         (a) Aortitis
         (b) Aortic insufficiency
         (c) Aneurysm
      (3) Neurosyphilis (symptomatic) occurs in 8% of patients.
9. Congenital syphilis
   a. Caused by transplacental transmission
      (1) Can occur at any time during gestation
      (2) Can occur at any stage of syphilis
         (a) Early active: 75% to 90% transmission
         (b) Late latent: 30% transmission
   b. Can result in the following:
      (1) Spontaneous abortion (second trimester)
      (2) Stillbirth
      (3) Infant with active or latent syphilis

Diagnosis

There is no gold standard and no culture technique is available. Diagnosis must rely on the following:

1. Clinical manifestations
2. Identification of *T. pallidum* from lesions using darkfield microscopy
3. Serology
   a. Nontreponemal
      (1) It measures IgM and IgG antibody directed against cardiolipin–lecithin–cholesterol antigen.

(2) It is nonspecific for *T. pallidum.*
(3) It is used to determine antibody titer and monitor therapy. Rising titer indicates an active infection that may be any one of the following:
(a) New infection
(b) Reinfection
(c) Reactivation of the latent disease
(4) Types of tests include the following
(a) Venereal Disease Research Laboratory (VDRL)
(b) Rapid plasma reagin (RPR)

b. Treponemal
(1) Measures IgM and IgG antibody against *T. Pallidum*-specific antigens
(2) Types are as follows:
(a) Fluorescent treponemal antibody test (FTA-ABS)
(b) *T. pallidum*–hemoglutinating antibody tests (MHA-TP, TPHA)

c. Specific treponemal antibody tests may remain active after adequate therapy.

Treatment

1. Early syphilis therapy 1993 CDC guidelines
   a. Benzathine penicillin G, 2.4 million units IM, single dose
   b. Penicillin allergy
      (1) Doxycycline, 100 mg, bid × 2 weeks, or
      (2) Tetracycline, 500 mg orally, qid × 2 weeks
2. Late syphilis therapy 1993 CDC guidelines
   a. Benzathine penicillin G, 2.4 million units IM, three doses at 1-week intervals
   b. Penicillin allergy
      (1) Doxycycline, 100 mg PO, bid × 4 weeks, or
      (2) Tetracycline, 500 mg PO, qid × 4 weeks
   c. Alternate drugs: should only be used after cerebrospinal fluid (CSF) examination to rule out neurosyphilis
3. Neurosyphilis therapy 1993 CDC guidelines
   a. Aqueous crystalline penicillin G, 12 to 24 million units IV daily for 10 to 14 days
   b. Aqueous procaine penicillin G, 2.4 million units IM daily, plus Probenicid, 500 mg, qid for 10 to 14 days
   c. Penicillin allergy: desensitize and treat with penicillin
4. Syphilis therapy in pregnancy
   a. Penicillin is the drug of choice. Therapy should be appropriate for the woman's stage of syphilis.
5. Penicillin allergy in pregnancy
   a. There are no alternatives to penicillin.
   b. The patient should be desensitized and treated with penicillin.
   c. Tetracycline and doxycycline are contraindicated during pregnancy.
   d. Erythromycin does not effectively cross the placenta and cannot be relied on to cure an infected infant.

11.5 CHANCROID

Etiology

1. *Haemophilus ducreyi,* a pleomorphic gram-negative facultative anaerobic bacillus, is the causative agent.
2. The disease is common in tropical countries.
3. It is now common in the United States.
   a. 900 cases per year 1980 through 1984
   b. 4000 to 5000 cases per year 1987 through 1990
   c. 2200 cases per year 1991 through 1993
4. Disease is a cofactor for HIV transmission: 10% coinfection rate.
5. Sexual contact is the only known method of transmission.

Signs and symptoms

1. Incubation period is 2 to 10 days; with a median of 4 to 7 days.
2. "Soft chancre" is the primary clinical sign.
   a. Shallow, tender, nonindurated ulcer with purulent base
   b. Multiple ulcers in women: lesions on fourchette, labia, vestibule, and clitoris
3. Unilateral or bilateral inguinal adenopathy (bubo) present in 50% of cases.
   a. Unilateral, 70%
   b. Spontaneous rupture if untreated
4. In HIV patients ulcers are larger, persist longer, and have less extensive lymphadenopathy.

Laboratory diagnosis

1. *H. ducreyi* should be isolated from lesion or node aspirate.
2. Gram stain is insensitive and nonspecific, revealing a pleomorphic gram negative "school of fish" pattern.
3. Cultures require special media, are 60% to 80% sensitive, and difficult to grow.
4. Rule out herpes simplex virus (HSV), syphilis, and lymphogranuloma venereum (LGV).
5. Diagnostic criteria
   a. Isolation of *H. ducreyi* is definitive.
   b. Otherwise, clinical diagnosis should include the following:
      (1) One or more painful genital ulcers
      (2) Negative darkfield examination, negative rapid plasma reagin (RPR)
      (3) Negative HSV, negative LGV
   c. Painful ulcer along with tender inguinal adenopathy is suggestive of chancroid.

Treatment

1. Azithromycin, 1 g PO, single dose
2. Ceftriaxone, 250 mg IM, single dose
3. Erythromycin base, 500 mg, qid × 7 days
4. Alternate:
   a. Amoxicillin, 500 mg, plus clavulanic acid, 125 mg PO × 7 days
   b. Ciprofloxacin, 500 mg PO, bid × 3 days

11.6 DONOVANOSIS (GRANULOMA INGUINALE)

Etiology

1. The infectious agent is *Calymmatobacterium granulomatis,* a gram negative bacillus that reproduces within PMNs, plasma cells, and histiocytes causing the infected cells to rupture 20 to 30 organisms.
2. Epidemiology
   a. Rare in the United States (<50 cases reported annually) and other developed countries
   b. Endemic in Australia, India, Caribbean, and Africa
3. Pathogenesis
   a. Indurated nodule is the primary lesion.
   b. Lesion erodes to granulomatous heaped ulcer, progresses slowly.
   c. Pathogenic features are as follows:
      (1) Large infected mononuclear cell containing many Donovan bodies
      (2) Intracytoplasmic location

Signs and symptoms

1. Incubation period is 8 to 80 days.
2. Lesions bleed easily.
3. Lesions are sharply defined and painless.
4. Secondary infection may ensue.
5. Inguinal involvement causes pseudobuboes; true lymph node involvement is unusual.

Diagnosis

1. Check for clinical manifestation.
2. Obtain stained crushed prep from lesion.
   a. Wright stain: Donovan bodies; organisms in vacuoles within macrophages.
3. Screen for other STDs.
4. Exclude other causes of lesions.
5. Differential diagnosis
   a. Carcinoma
   b. Secondary syphilis: condylomata lata
   c. Amebiasis: necrotic ulceration
   d. Concurrent infections

Treatment

1. Tetracycline, 500 mg, qid × 3 weeks
2. Chloramphenicol, 500 mg, q8h × 3 weeks
3. Gentamicin, 1 mg/kg, bid × 3 weeks
4. Streptomycin, 1.0 g IM, bid × 3 weeks
5. Ampicillin, 500 gm, qid × 12 weeks

Suggested reading

American College of Obststricians and Gynecologists: *Gonorrhea and Chlamydial Infections,* ACOG Technical Bulletin 190, Washington, DC, 1994, ACOG.

Cates W: Epidemiology and control of sexually transmitted diseases: strategic evaluation, *Infect Dis Clin North Am* 1:1-23, 1987.

Centers for Disease Control: 1993 Sexually transmitted diseases treatment guidelines, *MMWR* 42(RR-14), 1993.

Centers for Disease Control: Summary of notifiable diseases, United States 1993, *MMWR* 42(53), 1994.

Faro S: Lymphogranuloma venereum, chancroid, and granuloma inguinale, *Obstet Gynecol Clin North Am* 16:517, 1989.

Handsfield HH: Bacterial sexually transmitted diseases. In Handsfiels HH, editor: *Color atlas and synopsis of sexually transmitted diseases,* New York, 1992, McGraw-Hill, pp. 9-66.

Klein EJ et al: Anorectal gonococcal infection, *Ann Intern Med* 86:340-346, 1977.

Morales MJ: Gonococcal infections in pregnancy. In Mead PB, Hager DW, editors: *Infection protocols for obstetrics and gynecology,* 1992, Medical Economics Publishing, pp. 42-46.

Ronald AR, Albritten W: Chancroid and *Haemophilus ducreyi.* In Holmes KK, Mardh PA, Sparling PF, editors: *Sexually transmitted diseases,* ed 2, New York, 1990, McGraw-Hill, pp. 263-271.

Stamm WE, Holmes KK: Chlamydial infections in the adult. In Holmes KK, Mardh PA, Sparling PF, editors: *Sexually transmitted diseases,* ed 2, New York, 1990, McGraw-Hill, pp. 181-193.

Sweet RL, Gibbs RS: Sexually transmitted diseases. In Sweet RL, Gibbs RS, editors: *Infectious diseases of the female genital tract,* ed 2, Baltimore, 1990, Williams & Wilkins, pp. 109-143.

Sweet RL, Gibbs RS: Sexually transmitted diseases. In Sweet RL, Gibbs RS, editors: *Infectious diseases of the female genital tract,* ed 2, Baltimore, 1990, Williams & Wilkins, pp. 45-74.

Thin RN: Early syphilis in the adult. In Holmes KK, Mardh PA, Sparling PF, editors: *Sexually transmitted diseases,* ed 2, New York, 1990, McGraw-Hill, pp. 221-230.

Wager G: Lymphogranuloma venereum. In Mead PB, Hager DW, editors: *Infection protocols for obstetrics and gynecology,* 1992, Medical Economics Publishing, pp. 184-188.

11.7 GENITAL HERPES SIMPLEX VIRUS

Herpes simplex virus infection in the nonpregnant woman

1. Biology and epidemiology
   a. HSV is an exclusively sexually transmitted disease.
   b. It is a double-stranded DNA virus.
   c. Its two types are as follows:
      (1) HSV-1
         (a) Gingivostomatitis is the major clinical presentation but HSV-1 also causes 15% of primary genital herpes cases.
      (2) HSV-2
         (a) HSV-2 primarily affects the genital area.
   d. HSV is endemic in the United States with 500,000 new cases per year.
   e. Incidence is approximately 1% to 2% of the population.
   f. Genital HSV is prevalent: 20 million cases currently in the United States.
   g. About 50% to 80% of adults have antibodies to HSV-1 or HSV-2.
   h. The highest frequency of HSV occurs in the 15- to 29-year-old age group.

i. HSV is often associated with other STDs.
j. HSV may present as a primary, latent, or recurrent disease.

2. Signs and symptoms
   a. There are three distinct syndromes associated with HSV.
      (1) First episode primary genital herpes refers to the initial genital HSV infection and includes the following:
         (a) No evidence of HSV-1 or HSV-2 antibodies.
         (b) Severe local symptoms
         (c) Multiple painful lesions, vesicles, ulcers, inguinal adenopathy
         (d) Systemic symptoms such as fever, malaise, nausea, myalgia
         (e) First episode primary herpes is defined as three or more of the following:
            i. At least two extragenital symptoms
            ii. Multiple *bilateral* genital lesions
            iii. Persistence of genital lesions >16 days
            iv. Distal HSV lesions on the fingers, buttocks, or oropharynx
      (2) First episode nonprimary genital herpes is defined by the following:
         (a) Initial clinical episode
         (b) Antibodies to HSV-1 and HSV-2 present
         (c) Less severe clinical course
         (d) Symptoms similar to recurrent genital herpes
      (3) Recurrent herpes simplex infection involves the following:
         (a) Milder and shorter duration
         (b) Caused by reactivation of latent virus, not reinfection
         (c) Usual unilateral distribution of recurrent lesions
         (d) Typical lesion outbreak (preceded by prodromal symptoms such as paresthesias, itching, or pain)
         (e) Recurrent infection finished in 5 to 10 days
         (f) Systemic manifestations absent with few lesions
3. Clinical diagnosis
   a. Classical appearance of genital lesions is painful vesicles and ulcers in various stages of progression.
   b. History of prodrome and recurrences supports diagnosis.
4. Laboratory tests
   a. Viral culture is the gold standard for diagnosis; most positive cultures are identifiable in 48 to 72 hours.
      (1) More likely positive in first episode than recurrence
      (2) Positive culture more likely in early vesical lesions than later ulcerative crusted lesions.
   b. Tzanck smear is a cytologic test.
      (1) Presence of intranuclear inclusions and giant cells
      (2) Low sensitivity
   c. A negative Tzanck smear or negative culture does not exclude HSV.
   d. Indirect and direct immunoperoxidase stains are more sensitive than a Tzanck smear.
   e. The monoclonal antibody test can also be used.

(1) Positive predictive value: 93%
(2) Negative predictive value: 92%

f. Enzyme linked immunosorbent assay (ELISA) is also a testing option.

5. Treatment
   a. Acyclovir (Zovirax) was the first effect chemotherapeutic agent for genital herpes. The drug interferes selectively with viral thymidine kinase and ultimately inhibits viral DNA synthesis.
   b. 1993 CDC treatment guidelines
      (1) First clinical episode of genital herpes
         (a) Administer Acyclovir, 200 mg PO, five times a day × 7 to 10 days or until clinical resolution.
      (2) Recurrent episodes
         (a) Treatment instituted during prodrome or first 2 days of onset of lesions may provide limited benefit from therapy.
         (b) Recommended regimen is as follows:
            i. Acyclovir, 200 mg PO, five times a day × 5 days
            ii. Acyclovir, 400 mg PO, three times a day × 5 days
            iii. Acyclovir, 800 mg PO, two times a day × 5 days
      (3) Daily suppressive therapy
         (a) This therapy indicated in patients with frequent (≥6) recurrences per year.
         (b) Therapy may reduce frequency of HSV recurrence at least 75%.
         (c) Rate of recurrence should be reevaluated after 1 year of suppressive therapy.
         (d) Recommended regimen is acyclovir, 200 mg PO, three to five times a day.
         (e) Alternate regimen is acyclovir, 400 mg PO, two times a day.
      (4) Severe disease
         (a) Patients can be treated with intravenous therapy if indicated for complications of HSV such as encephalitis, pneumonitis or hepatitis.
         (b) Recommended regimen is acyclovir, 5 to 10 mg/kg body weight IV, q8h × 5 to 7 days or until clinical resolution.
      (5) Other management
         (a) Infected patients should abstain from sex during periods of active genital lesions.
         (b) Use of condoms during all sexual exposures should be encouraged.
         (c) Patients should be informed about the risks of neonatal infection.

Herpes simplex virus in pregnancy

1. Epidemiology
   a. HSV shedding occurs in 0.1% to 0.4% of deliveries.
   b. Frequency of neonatal infection is 0.01% to 0.04% of deliveries.
   c. Transmission rate of primary maternal infection to exposed neonate is estimated at 50%.

d. Transmission rate with recurrent maternal infection is estimated at 0% to 4%.
e. The risk of asymptomatic lower genital tract HSV infection on day of delivery is 1.4% in women with a confirmed history of recurrent herpes.
f. Nosocomial infection may also cause neonatal infection, most often HSV-1, at a rate of approximately 10%. Parents, family members, and health care workers may transmit the disease.

2. Neonatal infection
   a. Infection may result from HSV-1 or HSV-2.
   b. Neonatal complication is severe with third trimester maternal infection.
   c. Seventy percent of neonates with severe HSV infection are delivered from *asymptomatic* mothers.
   d. The risk of neonatal herpes from an asymptomatic mother with a history of recurrent genital herpes infection is estimated at <1 in 1000.
3. Neonatal complications of perinatal HSV
   a. Active HSV infection leads to a 50% chance of complications in primary episode HSV infection.
   b. Neonatal death may occur in 60% of cases.
   c. Fifty percent of surviving neonates have significant sequelae including the following:
      (1) Microcephaly
      (2) Mental retardation
      (3) Seizures
      (4) Microophthalmia
      (5) Retinal dysplasia
      (6) Chorioretinitis
      (7) Meningitis
      (8) Encephalitis
   d. Onset of neonatal herpes is often insidious. Delay in diagnosis without lesions approximates 72 hours.
4. Management: The American College of Obstetricians and Gynecologists has endorsed the following recommendations for pregnant women with HSV infections or a history of HSV infections:
   a. Antepartum
      (1) Cultures should be done when a women has active HSV lesions during pregnancy to confirm the diagnosis. If there are no visible lesions at the onset of labor, vaginal delivery is acceptable.
      (2) Weekly surveillance cultures of pregnant women with a history of HSV infection, but no visible lesions, are not necessary and vaginal delivery is acceptable.
      (3) Amniocentesis in an attempt to rule out intrauterine infection is not recommended for mothers with HSV at any stage of gestation.
   b. Intrapartum
      (1) Cesarean section in women with active infection will significantly decrease but not eliminate the risk and incidence of neonatal HSV infection.

(2) The American College of Obstetricians and Gynecologists recommends that term patients who have visible lesions and are in labor, or who have ruptured membranes, should undergo cesarean delivery.
(3) Cultures for HSV obtained at delivery in women with a history of HSV may aid in identifying potentially exposed neonates.

c. Medical therapy
(1) The safety of systemic acyclovir therapy among pregnant women has not been established.
(2) Acyclovir is indicated for life-threatening and disseminated HSV infection (i.e., encephalitis, pneumonitis, hepatitis).

References

1. American College of Obstetricians and Gynecologists: *Gynecologic herpes simplex virus infections,* ACOG Technical Bulletin 119, Washington, DC, 1988, ACOG.
2. American College of Obstetricians and Gynecologists: *Perinatal herpes simplex virus infections,* ACOG Technical Bulletin 122, Washington, DC, 1988, ACOG.
3. Andrews EB et al: Acyclovir in pregnancy register: six years experience, *Obstet Gynecol* 79:7-13, 1992.
4. Centers for Disease Control: 1993 sexually transmitted diseases treatment guidelines, *MMWR* 42(RR-14), 1993.
5. Gibbs RS, Amstey MS, Lezotte DC: Role of cesarean delivery in preventing neonatal herpes virus infection (editorial), *JAMA* 270:94-95, 1993.
6. Gibbs RS et al: Management of genital herpes infection in pregnancy, *Obstet Gynecol* 71:779-780, 1988.
7. Martens MG: Herpes simplex in pregnancy. In Gilstrap L, Faro S, editors: *Infections in pregnancy,* New York, 1990, Alan R. Liss, pp. 143-150.
8. Randolph GA, Washington AE, Prober CG: Cesarean delivery for women presenting with genital herpes lesions, *JAMA* 1993; 270:77-82.
9. Sweet RL, Gibbs RS: Herpes simplex virus infection. In Sweet RL, Gibbs RS, editors: *Infectious diseases of the female genital tract,* ed 2, Baltimore, 1990, Williams & Wilkins, pp. 144-157.

11.8 PELVIC INFLAMMATORY DISEASE

Definition

Pelvic inflammatory disease (PID) is a spectrum of inflammatory disorders of the upper genital tract including a combination of any of the following:

1. Endometritis, salpingitis, tuboovarian abscess, or pelvic peritonitis.
2. It results from an ascending lower genital tract infection.
3. It is not related to obstetric or surgical intervention.

Epidemiology

1. Incidence or prevalence
   a. There are an estimated 600,000 to 1 million cases annually in the United States.
   b. Disease is diagnosed in 2% to 5% of women seen in STD clinics.
   c. PID is the most common cause of female infertility and ectopic pregnancy.

d. Indirect and direct costs attributed to PID were estimated to be in excess of $4 billion in 1990.

2. Risk factors
   a. Adolescent sexually active females under age 20 (1:8 risk)
   b. Nonwhite race
   c. Previous episode of gonococcal PID
   d. Multiple sexual partners (more than two partners within 30 days)
   e. Vaginal douching (associated with 2× increased risk of PID)
   f. Use of intrauterine device (Users have a threefold to fivefold increased risk of developing acute PID.)
3. Risk reduction
   a. Other contraceptives *reduce* risk of PID.
      (1) Oral contraceptives
      (2) Condoms
      (3) Diaphragms with spermicide

Microbial etiology

1. *Neisseria gonorrhoeae*
   a. This bacteria causes many cases of PID in populations with high incidence rates of gonorrhea (i.e., inner city).
   b. Acute PID is developed in 10% to 20% of women with endocervical gonorrhea.
2. *Chlamydia trachomatis*
   a. This organism is an important cause of PID.
   b. It is the predominent etiologic agent among patients of middle and upper socioeconomic status with PID in the United States.
   c. More than 50% of PID cases are caused by *N. gonorrhoeae, C. trachomatis,* or both.
3. Polymicrobial infection
   a. Other microorganisms exist as causative agents for the disease, including facultative and anaerobic bacteria such as the following:
      (1) *Escherichia coli*
      (2) *Gardnerella vaginalis*
      (3) *Bacteroides* species
      (4) *Hemophilus influenza*
      (5) *Mycoplasma hominis*
4. *Mycobacterium tuberculosis* is an important cause of chronic PID in developing countries.

Signs and symptoms

1. Lower abdominal pain: usually bilateral, most common presenting symptom
2. Abnormal vaginal discharge
3. Abnormal uterine bleeding
4. Dysuria: 20% of patients
5. Dyspareunia: common
6. Nausea and vomiting: may suggest peritonitis
7. Fever
8. Right upper quadrant tenderness (perihepatitis): 5% of PID cases

Laboratory findings

1. Leukocytosis
2. Elevated acute phase reactants: ESR, C-reactive protein
3. Gram stain of endocervical exudate: >30 PMNs per high-power field (HPF) correlates with chlamydial or gonococcal infection
4. Endocervical cultures for *N. gonorrohoeae* and *C. trachomatis*
5. Fallopian tube aspirate or peritoneal exudate culture if laparoscopy performed

Diagnosis

1. Differential diagnosis
   a. Ectopic pregnancy
   b. Appendicitis
   c. Urinary tract infection (cystitis or pyelonephritis)
   d. Renal calculus
   e. Adnexal torsion
   f. Proctocolitis
2. Additional diagnostic procedures
   a. Human chorionic gonadotropin (β-HCG): to rule out ectopic pregnancy
   b. Endometrial biopsy: abnormal histology in 90% of patients with laparoscopic evidence of salpingitis
   c. Endocervical ultrasonography
      (1) Detects tuboovarian abscesses
      (2) May detect early salpingitis if tubal dilation, intratubal fluid, and tubal wall thickening found
   d. Laparoscopy
      (1) Gold standard for diagnosis of acute salpingitis
      (2) Should be considered when the diagnosis of PID is unsure
3. Diagnostic considerations
   a. Clinical diagnosis of PID is difficult and imprecise.
   b. Clinical diagnosis of symptomatic PID has a positive predictive value of 65% to 90% when compared with laparoscopy as the standard.
   c. No single historical, physical, or laboratory finding is both sensitive and specific for the diagnosis of PID.
4. 1993 CDC diagnostic criteria for PID
   a. Empiric treatment of PID should be initiated based on the presence of all of the following minimum criteria:
      (1) Lower abdominal pain
      (2) Adnexal tenderness
      (3) Cervical motion tenderness
   b. The following additional routine criteria may be used to increase the specificity of the diagnosis of PID in women with severe clinical signs:
      (1) Oral temperature >38.3° C
      (2) Abnormal cervical or vaginal discharge
      (3) Elevated ESR

(4) Elevated C-reactive protein
(5) Laboratory documentation of cervical infection with *N. gonorrhoeae* or *C. trachomatis*

c. Elaborate criteria for diagnosing PID are as follows:
(1) Laparoscopic abnormalitites consistent with PID
(2) Histopathologic evidence of endometritis on endocervical biopsy
(3) Tuboovarian abscess on sonography

Management of PID

1. Most patients are treated as outpatients.
2. Few studies exist comparing outpatient versus inpatient management.
3. Criteria for hospitalization (1993 CDC) (Table 11-1) are as follows:
   a. The diagnosis is uncertain.
   b. Pelvic abscess is suspected.
   c. Patient is pregnant.
   d. Patient is an adolescent.
   e. Patient is HIV positive.
   f. Severe illness, nausea, or vomiting precludes outpatient management.
   g. Patient cannot tolerate outpatient regimens.
   h. Patient has failed to respond clinically to outpatient therapy.

Table 11-1 Regimens for treatment of pelvic inflammatory disease recommended by the CDC 1993

Inpatient Treatment	Comment
Regimen A	
Defoxitin, 2 g IV, q6h, *or* Cefotetan, 2 g IV, q12h, *plus* Doxycycline, 100 mg IV or PO, q12h	Regimen should be continued for at least 48 hours after substantial clinical improvement, after which doxycycline, 100 mg PO, two times a day should be continued for a total of 14 days.
Regimen B	
Clindamycin, 900 mg IV, q8h, *plus* gentamycin, loading dose IV or IM (2 mg/kg of body weight), followed by a maintenance dose (1.5 mg/kg) q8h	Regimen should be continued for at least 48 hours after substantial clinical improvement, after which doxycycline, 100 mg PO, two times a day, or clindamycin, 450 mg PO, four times a day, to complete a total of 14 days of therapy.

i. Clinical follow-up within 72 hours of initiating antibiotic treatment cannot be arranged.

4. Outpatient treatment
   a. Regimen A
      (1) Cefoxitin, 2 g IM, plus probenicid, 1 g PO, or
      (2) Ceftriaxone, 250 mg IM, or
      (3) Equivalent cephalosporin (ceftizoxime or cefotaxime) plus doxycycline, 100 mg PO, bid × 10 to 14 days
   b. Regimen B
      (1) Ofloxacin, 400 mg PO, bid × 14 days, plus either clindamycin, 450 mg PO, qid, or metronidazole, 500 mg PO, bid × 14 days

Follow-up

1. Hospitalized patients receiving IV therapy should show significant clinical improvement characterized by defervescence, decreased abdominal tenderness, and decreased uterine, adnexal, and cervical motion tenderness within 3 to 5 days.
2. If no clinical improvement occurs, further diagnostic workup is necessary, including possible surgical intervention.
3. Clinical improvement for outpatient therapy should be observed within 72 hours.
4. Evaluation and treatment of male sex partners is essential.
5. Long-term sequelae of PID are as follows:
   a. Recurrent PID
   b. Chronic pelvic pain
   c. Ectopic pregnancy
   d. Infertility
6. The risk of tubal infertility related to episodes of PID is as follows:
   a. First episode: 8%
   b. Second episode: 20%
   c. Third episode: 40%

Suggested reading

1. Centers for Disease Control: 1993 sexually transmitted diseases treatment guidelines, *MMWR* 42(RR-15), 1993.
2. Hager WD et al: Criteria for the diagnosis and grading of salpingitis, *Obstet Gynecol* 61:113-114, 1983.
3. Handsfield HH: Pelvic inflammatory disease. In Handsfield HH, editor: *Color atlas and synopsis of sexually transmitted diseases,* New York, 1992, McGraw-Hill.
4. Holmes KK: Lower genital tract infections in women: cystitis, urethritis, vulvovaginitis, and cervicitis. In Holmes KK, Mardh PA, Sparling PF, editors: *Sexually transmitted diseases,* ed 2, New York, 1990, McGraw-Hill.
5. McCormack W: Current concepts = Pelvic inflammatory disease, *N Engl J Med* 330(4):115-118, 1994.
6. Soper D: Diagnosis and laparoscopic grading of acute salpingitis, *Am J Obstet Gynecol* 164:1370-1376, 1991.
7. Sweet RL: Acute salpingitis: diagnosis and management, *J Reprod Med* 19:21-30, 1977.
8. Westrom L et al: Pelvic inflammatory disease and fertility: a cohort study of 1844 women with laparoscopically verified disease and 657 control women with normal laparoscopic results, *Sex Transm Dis* 19:185-192, 1992.

9. Westrum L, Mardh PA: Acute pelvic inflammatory disease. In Holmes KK, Mardh PA, Sparling PF, editors: *Sexually transmitted diseases,* ed 2, New York, 1990, McGraw-Hill.

11.9 BACTERIAL VAGINOSIS (TABLE 11-2)

Etiology

1. Polymicrobial clinical syndrome
2. Disturbance of vaginal ecology
3. *Lactobacillus* replaced by anaerobes
4. Altered vaginal pH
5. Abnormal vaginal secretions
6. Most common vaginal disorder (35% to 45%)
7. Majority of cases: sexually active patients ages 15 to 44 years
8. Prevalence: general population (20% to 25%)
9. Normal vaginal ecosystem
   a. *Lactobacillus* predominant
   b. Usually fewer than 10^7 organisms/g
   c. Ratio of anaerobes to aerobes: 2:1 to 5:1
   d. *Gardnerella vaginalis:* 5% to 60%
   e. *Mobiluncus* spp.: 0% to 5%
   f. *Mycoplasma hominis:* 15% to 30% of sexually active women
10. Vaginal ecosystem in bacterial vaginosis
    a. Few hydrogen peroxide-producing lactobacilli
    b. 10^{11} organisms/g
    c. Ratio of anaerobes to aerobes: 100:1 to 1000:1
    d. *Gardnerella vaginalis:* 95%
    e. *Mobiluncus* spp. 50% to 70%
    f. *Mycoplasma hominis:* 60% to 75%
11. Possible causes
    a. Intercourse
    b. Spermicides
    c. Hormones
    d. Douches
    e. IUDs
    f. Other infections

Signs and Symptoms

1. Vaginal discharge evident at introitus (main symptom)
2. Foul vaginal odor
3. Vulvovaginal irritation less severe than other forms of vaginitis

Diagnosis

1. No single marker
2. Amsel's criteria
   a. pH >4.5
   b. Clue cells present
   c. Milky discharge
   d. Positive "whiff" test
   e. No diagnostic value of demonstrating *Gardnerella vaginalis* on culture

Table 11-2 Diagnostic features of vaginitis

	Normal	Yeast Vulvovaginitis	Trichomonal Vaginitis	Bacterial Vaginosis
Symptoms	None	Vulvar pruritis, discharge	Purulent discharge, vulvar pruritis	Malodor, discharge
Discharge				
Amount	Variable to scant	Scant to moderate	Profuse	Scant to moderate
Color	Clear or white	White or yellow	Yellow	White
Consistency	Floccular, nonhomogeneous	Clumped or adherent plaques	Homogeneous, frothy	Homogeneous, smooth or coats vaginal mucosa
Inflammation vulva/vagina	None	Erythema vagina, introitus, vulva	Erythema vagina, vulva or petechiae, ectocervix	None
pH vaginal fluid	<4.5	<4.5	>5.0	>4.7
Amino odor (KOH)	None	None	Present	Present
Microscopy	Normal epithelial cells, lactobacilli	Leukocytes, yeast pseudomycelia	Leukocytes, motile trichomonads	Clue cells, mixed flora, few lactobacilli

3. Do not treat based solely on *Gardnerella vaginalis* culture (40% to 60% of women's natural vaginal flora).

Bacterial vaginosis–associated diseases

1. Gynecologic
   a. Abnormal vaginal discharge
   b. Mucopurulent cervicitis
   c. Urinary tract infections
   d. Postoperative infections
   e. Cervical dysplasia
   f. Nonpuerperal endometritis
   g. PID
2. Obstetric
   a. Chorioamnionitis
   b. Premature labor
   c. Premature rupture of membranes
   d. Postpartum endometritis

Treatment

1. Metronidazole, 500 mg PO, bid × 7 days
2. Metronidazole, 2.0 g PO, single dose
3. Clindamycin cream, 2%, 5 g intravaginal, qhs × 7 days
4. Metronidazole gel, 0.75%, 5 g intravaginal, bid × 5 days
5. Clindamycin, 300 mg PO, bid × 7 days
6. Bacterial vaginosis in pregnancy
   a. Metronidazole is contraindicated first trimester.
   b. Clindamycin cream is preferred first trimester.
   c. Metronidazole orally, clindamycin cream, or metronidazole gel is preferred second and third trimester.
   d. Treatment may reduce risk of adverse pregnancy outcomes.

11.10 VULVOVAGINAL CANDIDIASIS (VVC) (SEE TABLE 11-2)

Etiology

1. This disease is the second most common cause of vaginitis in the United States.
2. *Candida* spp. can be isolated in 5% to 55% of asymptomatic women of childbearing age.
3. Hormonal dependence of infection: This is rare in premenarchal and in postmenopausal women.
4. There are three subpopulations of women with VVC.
   a. Those who never develop symptomatic VVC
   b. Those who suffer infrequent isolated episodes
   c. Those who have repeated, recurrent, often chronic infection (more than three episodes of symptomatic VVC annually)
      (1) Vulvovaginal candidiasis will be experienced by 75% of all women at least once.
      (2) Two or more episodes will be experienced by 40% to 50% of these women.

(3) Fewer than 5% of women experience recurrent vulvovaginal candidiasis.

5. Microbiology
   a. *Candida albicans* causes 85% to 90% of cases.
   b. Other *Candida* spp. (*C. glabrata, C. tropicalis*) can also cause the disease.
   c. Nonalbicans species of *Candida* are more resistant to conventional therapy.
   d. Uniquely virulent strains of *Candida* have not been identified.
6. Dimorphism of *Candida*
   a. Blastospores
      (1) Transmission or spread
      (2) Asymptomatic colonization
   b. Mycelia
      (1) Germination
      (2) Tissue invasive form
      (3) Symptomatic disease
7. *Candida* virulence factors
   a. *C. albicans* adhere to vaginal epithelial cells in very high numbers.
   b. Germination enhances colonization and tissue invasion.
8. Pathogenesis
   a. *C. albicans* may be a commensal or a pathogen in the vagina.
   b. Changes in the vaginal environment are necessary before disease is induced.
9. Predisposing factors
   a. Pregnancy
   b. Oral contraceptives
   c. Diabetes mellitus
   d. Antibiotics
   e. Hygiene
   f. Immunosuppression
10. Source of infection
    a. Intestinal reservoir: major source of vaginal colonization
    b. Sexual transmission: probable limited contribution; treatment of male partners rare
    c. Vaginal relapse: incomplete eradication of vaginal colonization after treatment
11. Natural vaginal defense mechanisms
    a. Humoral immunity: IgM, IgG, IgA
    b. Phagocytic system: PMNs and monocytes absent from vaginal fluid
    c. Cell-mediated immunity: reduced T-lymphocyte reactivity to *Candida* antigen
    d. Vaginal flora: most important defense

Signs and symptoms

1. Acute pruritus
2. Erythematous vulva and vagina
3. White vaginal discharge, white or yellow raised vaginal plaques
4. Dyspareunia

5. Dysuria
6. Minimal odor

Diagnosis

1. Signs and symptoms with low specificity
2. Pruritus without discharge (38% positive predictive value [PPV])
3. Microscopic examination: saline, 10% KOH, wet preparation, confirmed by observing mycelia or pseudohyphae (2.3% false-positive and 6.2% false-negative results)
4. Vaginal pH
5. Cultures: only if KOH negative and patient symptomatic (to exclude yeast)
6. Do not treat solely on presence of *Candida* on culture (10% to 20% normal vaginal flora)

Treatment

1. Topical
   a. Nystatin: 70% to 80% cure rate
   b. Imidazoles: 80% to 90% cure rate
2. Oral
   a. Ketoconazole
   b. Fluconazole (FDA approved for treatment of VVC, 1994)
3. Uncomplicated: short course
4. Severe: >1 week regimen
5. Recommended regimens (1993 CDC guidelines): All azole preparations: both oral and vaginal, have the same efficacy of cure: 90%.
   a. Intravaginal preparation:
      (1) Butoconazole* 2% cream, 5 g intravaginally, × 3 days
      (2) Clotrimazole* 1% cream, 5 g intravaginally, × 7 to 14 days
      (3) Clotrimazole,* 100 mg vaginal tablet, × 7 days
      (4) Clotrimazole, 100 mg vaginal tablet, two tablets × 3 days
      (5) Clotrimazole, 500 mg vaginal tablet, one tablet, single application
      (6) Miconazole 2% cream, 5 g intravaginally, × 7 days
      (7) Miconazole, 200 mg vaginal suppository, one suppository × 3 days
      (8) Miconazole, 100 mg vaginal suppository, one suppository × 7 days
      (9) Tiocinazole 6.5% ointment, 5 mg intravaginally, a single application
      (10) Terconazole 0.4% cream, 5 g intravaginally, × 7 days
      (11) Terconazole 0.8% cream 5 g intravaginally, × 3 days
      (12) Terconazole, 80 mg suppository, one suppository × 3 days
   b. Oral preparation
      (1) Fluconazole, 150 mg, one single oral dose: the only FDA approved oral agent for vulvovaginal candidiasis

*These preparations are available over the counter. Self-medication should be advised only for women who have been previously diagnosed with vulvovaginal candidiasis and have experienced a recurrence of the same symptoms.

c. Side effects
   (1) Vaginal preparations
      (a) Local burning or irritation
      (b) Usually free from systemic effects
   (2) Oral agents
      (a) Nausea
      (b) Abdominal pain
      (c) Headache
d. Alternative agents
   (1) Boric acid, 600 mg, qid × 2 weeks
   (2) 1% Gentian violet, two times a week × 2 weeks

6. Treatment of recurrent vulvovaginal candidiasis (RVVC)
   a. Optimal treatment has not been established.
   b. All cases should be confirmed by culture before therapy.
   c. All cases should be evaluated for predisposing conditions (i.e., diabetes mellitus, immunosuppression).
   d. Clinical trials have involved continuing therapy between episodes.
      (1) Ketoconazole, 100 mg PO, qd for up to 6 months
      (2) Clotrimazole, intravaginally, weekly

11.11 TRICHOMONIASIS

Etiology

1. *Trichomonas vaginalis* is the etiologic agent.
2. It is an anaerobic flagellated protozoan.
3. Humans are its only known hosts.
4. Epidemiology
   a. Trichomoniasis is responsible for 25% of all cases of clinically evident vaginitis.
   b. Incidence or prevalence is as follows:
      (1) 5% family planning clinics
      (2) 25% gynecology clinics
      (3) 75% prostitutes
   c. The disease is transmitted sexually.
   d. It often coexists with other STDs.
   e. Pathogenesis is uncertain for the disease.
   f. The disease is associated with preterm labor and premature rupture of membranes.

Signs and symptoms

1. Incubation period variable
2. Female: vagina, urethra, endocervix, or bladder infected
3. Male: most often asymptomatic, primary vector for transmission
4. Symptoms: profuse, malodorous vaginal discharge, postcoital bleeding
5. Signs: cervical "strawberry patches"; vaginal mucosal erythema; labial erythema

Diagnosis

1. Clinical manifestations
2. Laboratory diagnosis
   a. pH ≥5

b. Wet mount: motile trichomonads, PMNs; diagnostic 80%
c. Culture for *T. vaginalis* in rare circumstances of treatment failures
3. Differential diagnosis
a. Bacterial vaginosis
b. Vulvovaginal candidiasis
c. Mucopurulent cervicitis
d. Chemical vaginitis

Management

1. Metronidazole, 2.0 g PO, single dose
2. Metronidazole, 500 mg, bid × 7 days
3. Metronidazole gel: *not effective*
4. Concurrent treatment of sex partner
5. Screen for other STDs
6. Alcohol with metronidazole: avoid (disulfuram-like reaction may ensue)

Follow-up

1. Not necessary if patient becomes asymptomatic.
2. If treatment fails, retreat with metronidazole, 500 mg, bid × 7 days.
3. If treatment fails repeatedly, do the following:
   a. Treat with metronidazole, 2 g PO, daily × 3 to 5 days.
   b. Consider culture for possible resistant strain of *T. vaginalis.*
   c. Evaluate the patient's sex partner.
4. Special considerations
   a. Allergy: There is no effective alternative. Clotrimazole may inhibit growth of *T. vaginalis* but does not eradicate it.
   b. Pregnancy: Metronidazole is contraindicated in first trimester. Use cautiously in second and third for truly symptomatic cases.
   c. HIV positive: Treat with same regimen as HIV negative patients.

Suggested reading

1. Centers for Disease Control: 1993 sexually transmitted diseases treatment guidelines, *MMWR* 42(RR-14), 1993.
2. Faro S: Review of vaginitis, *Infect Dis Obstet Gynecol* 1:158-161, 1993.
3. Handsfield HH: Vaginal infections. In Handsfield HH, editor: *Color atlas and synopsis of sexually transmitted diseases,* New York, 1992, McGraw-Hill.
4. McGregor JA, French JI, Seo K: Premature rupture of membranes and bacterial vaginosis, *Am J Obstet Gynecol* 169:463-466, 1993.
5. Rein MF, Muller M: *Trichomonas vaginalis* and trichomoniasis. In Holmes KK, Mardh PA, Sparling PF, editors: *Sexually transmitted diseases,* ed 2, New York, 1990, McGraw-Hill.
6. Sobel JD: Candidial vulvovaginitis, *Clin Obstet Gynecol* 36(1):153-165, 1993.
7. Soper DE: Bacterial vaginosis and postoperative infections, *Am J Obstet Gynecol* 169:467-469, 1993.
8. Sweet RL, Gibbs RS: Infectious vulvovaginitis. In Sweet RL, Gibbs RS, editors: *Infectious diseases of the female genital tract,* ed 2, Baltimore, 1990, Williams & Wilkins.
9. Thomason JL, Gelbart SM: *Bacterial vaginosis: current concepts,* Kalamazoo, Michigan, 1990, The Upjohn Company.
10. Thomason JL, Gelbart SM, Scaglione NJ: Bacterial vaginosis: current review with indications for asymptomatic therapy, *Am J Obstet Gynecol* 165:1210-1217, 1991.

12 HIV Infection in Women

Lawrence J. Gugino, M.D.

12.1 BACKGROUND

1. The rate of human immunodeficiency virus (HIV) infection continues to increase dramatically among women.
2. Current estimates are that 1 to 1.5 million individuals in the United States are infected with HIV.
3. The rate of new infection in women has been more rapid than in any other risk group.
4. Obstetrician-gynecologists provide reproductive care to HIV-positive women and those at risk for HIV infection.

12.2 EPIDEMIOLOGY

1. There were more than 50,000 cumulative AIDS cases in women as of 1994.
2. Women represented 18% of all AIDS cases reported in 1994.
3. HIV/AIDS ranked as the fourth leading cause of death in women between ages of 25 and 44 years in 1994.
4. AIDS was the leading cause of death in approximately 20 large metropolitan areas on the eastern coast of the United States in 1994.
5. The national seroprevalence rate in childbearing women between the ages of 15 and 44 years was 1.6/1000 live births in 1993.
6. Among incarcerated women, mandatory HIV testing reveals HIV seroprevalence rates of 2.5% to 14.7%.
7. Approximately 7000 infants are born to HIV-positive mothers in the United States each year.
8. In 1994, 84% of women infected with HIV were in the childbearing ages of 15 to 44 years.
9. The highest incidence of HIV infection occurs in the age group of 30 to 39 years.
10. African-American and Hispanic women are disproportionately affected, accounting for greater than 70% of AIDS cases for women, although they collectively represent only 20% of the population of U.S. women.

Table 12-1 Changing patterns of HIV transmission to women: 1985-1992

Risk Categroy	1985 (%)	1990 (%)	1992 (%)
Injection drug use	56	48	45
Heterosexual sex	19	32	39
Transfusion	11	8	4

12.3 MAJOR ROUTES OF TRANSMISSION OF HIV-1

1. Blood and body fluids
2. Sexual contact
3. Perinatal transmission

Primary transmission categories in women

1. Injection drug use
2. Heterosexual contact
3. Transfusion recipient
4. Unknown

Modes of transmission (Table 12-1)

1. As of 1992, 45% women with AIDS acquired it by injection drug use.
2. As of 1992, 39% women with AIDS acquired it by heterosexual sex (21% with an injection drug user).
3. Preliminary 1994 data suggest that heterosexual transmission is now the most common mode of transmission.

12.4 PATHOPHYSIOLOGY

1. HIV is a retrovirus (RNA virus) converted to DNA copy by enzyme reverse transcriptase.
2. It preferentially infects cells with CD4+ receptor antigen, especially helper lymphocytes, but also cells of the placenta.
3. HIV infection results in progressive debilitation of the immune system.
4. Acute HIV infection may result in acute mononucleosis-like syndrome.
5. HIV antibodies may be detected in most individuals by 12 weeks after exposure (latent "window period").
6. The mean time from HIV infection to development of AIDS is greater than 10 years.

12.5 HIV TESTING AND COUNSELING IN WOMEN

Tests for HIV

1. Antibody (enzyme-linked immunosorbent assay, ELISA)
   a. Detects antibodies, not virus
   b. Screening test only
   c. Highly sensitive and specific test

   d. Needs confirmation by specific test: Western blot or indirect immunofluorescence assay (IFA)
   e. Negative result: infection unlikely
2. Antigen tests (p24)
3. Viral culture
4. Polymerase chain reaction (PCR)

"Window period"

1. Three months after infection with HIV, 80% of individuals seroconvert.
2. Six months after infection with HIV, 99% of individuals seroconvert.
3. A negative HIV test done today is indicative of the absence of HIV infection 6 months previously.
4. Twelve months after infection with HIV, there is a 1/5000 false-negative rate.

Why test for HIV infection?

1. Allows early HIV medical intervention
2. Assists in diagnosis
3. Assists in pregnancy decisions
4. Reinforces high-risk behavior change
5. Relieves anxiety of *not* knowing personal HIV status
6. *Decreases* pediatric HIV infection
7. Prevents HIV transmission to others

Who should be tested for HIV?

1. Women with current or past injection drug use
2. The current or past sexual partner of an injection drug user, a bisexual, or a person known to be HIV positive
3. Women with a history of blood or blood product transfusions between 1978 and 1985
4. Women with a history of multiple sexual partners
5. Women with a history of sexually transmitted disease

A widespread approach to HIV counseling and testing

1. A targeted approach to testing may fail to identify 50% to 70% of infected women.
2. Women may be unaware of their risk status.
3. Women may refuse testing to avoid the stigma of high-risk behaviors.
4. A universal approach to HIV counseling and testing is indicated for all women, regardless of the geographic prevalence of HIV.

12.6 CLINICAL MANIFESTATIONS AND DIAGNOSIS

Initial clinical manifestations

1. Symptoms are nonspecific in most women.
2. Constitutional symptoms such as night sweats, low-grade fevers, anorexia, and weight loss are common.
3. Recurrent, chronic, refractory vaginal candidiasis may be a sentinel indicator of HIV infection.

Table 12-2 1993 Revised classification system for HIV infection and expanded AIDS surveillance case definition for adolescents and adults

	Clinical Categories*		
CD4+ T-cell Categories	(A) Asymptomatic, Acute HIV or PGL	(B) Symptomatic, Not (A) or (C)	(C) AIDS Indicator Conditions
(1) ≥500/μl	A1	B1	C1
(2) 200 to 499/μl	A2	B2	C2
(3) <200/μl AIDS indicator T-cell count	A3	B3	C2

*Shaded areas illustrate the expanded AIDS surveillance case definition.

Centers for Disease Control and Prevention (CDC)-defined AIDS diagnosis

1. 1993 revised classification system for HIV infection
   a. CD4+ T-lymphocyte categories
      (1) Category 1: ≥500 cells/μl
      (2) Category 2: 200 to 499 cells/μl
      (3) Category 3: <200 cells/μl
   b. Clinical categories
      (1) Category A
         (a) Asymptomatic HIV infection
         (b) Persistent generalized lymphadenopathy
         (c) Acute HIV infection
      (2) Category B
         (a) Symptomatic HIV conditions
      (3) Examples
         (a) Oropharyngeal candidiasis
         (b) Vulvovaginal candidiasis
         (c) Cervical dysplasia (moderate or severe)
         (d) Cervical carcinoma-in-situ
         (e) Oral hairy leukoplakia
         (f) Pelvic inflammatory disease
      (4) Category C
         (a) All clinical conditions listed in AIDS surveillance case definition included
2. 1993 expanded CDC surveillance case definition for AIDS (Table 12-2)
   a. CD4+ T-lymphocyte count <200/μl or CD4+ percentage <14
   b. Also includes the following, in addition to previous 23 clinical conditions:
      (1) Pulmonary tuberculosis
      (2) Recurrent bacterial pneumonia
      (3) Invasive cervical cancer
3. Conditions included in the 1993 AIDS surveillance case definition
   a. Candidiasis of bronchi, trachea, or lungs
   b. Candidiasis, esophageal

c. Cervical cancer, invasive*
d. Coccidioidomycosis, disseminated or extrapulmonary
e. Cryptococcosis, extrapulmonary
f. Cryptococcosis, chronic intestinal (>1 month's duration)
g. Cytomegalovirus disease (other than liver, spleen, or nodes)
h. Cytomegalovirus retinitis (with loss of vision)
i. Encephalopathy, HIV related
j. Herpes simplex: chronic ulcer(s) (>1 month's duration); or bronchitis, pneumonia, or esophagitis
k. Histoplasmosis, disseminated or extrapulmonary
l. Isoplasmosis, chronic intestinal (>1 month's duration)
m. Kaposi's sarcoma
n. Lymphoma, Burkitt's (or equivalent term)
o. Lymphoma, immunoblastic (or equivalent term)
p. Lymphoma, primary, of brain
q. *Mycobacterium avium* complex or *M. kansasii,* disseminated or extrapulmonary
r. *Mycobacterium tuberculosis,* any site (pulmonary* or extrapulmonary)
s. *Mycobacterium,* other species or unidentified species, disseminated or extrapulmonary
t. *Pneumocystis carinii* pneumonia
u. Pneumonia, recurrent
v. Progressive multifocal leukoencephalopathy
w. *Salmonella* septicemia, recurrent
x. Toxoplasmosis of brain
y. Wasting syndrome resulting from HIV

Gynecologic manifestations

1. Menstrual disorders
   a. Amenorrhea, oligomenorrhea, metrorrhagia are anecdotally reported as common.
   b. Irregular bleeding may cause difficulty in predicting early pregnancy.
   c. Increased risk of transmission of HIV from menstrual blood.
2. *Candida* vaginitis
   a. Most common gynecologic infection in HIV-positive women
   b. Often presents as chronic and refractory to treatment
   c. May be a sentinel marker for HIV positivity
   d. Occurs with highest frequency with CD4 counts <100
   e. Treatment
      (1) Uncomplicated
         (a) Topical antifungal agent for 7 days
   f. Recurrent or unresponsive candidiasis
      (1) Oral imidazole agents
         (a) Ketoconazole, 400 mg, qd or fluconazole, 200 mg, qd for 14 days
   g. Chronic recurrence

*Added in 1993 expansion of AIDS surveillance case definition.

(1) Consider maintenance therapy
(a) Ketoconazole, 100 mg, qd
(b) Ketoconazole, 100 to 200 mg, 5 days each month at menses
(c) Fluconazole, 200 mg, qod

3. Herpes simplex
a. Herpes simplex (HSV) type 2 is the most clinically significant.
b. Outbreaks may be more severe and persistent.
c. Recurrence may be frequent and more severe.
d. Patients should be cultured for HSV and a serologic test for syphilis obtained before treatment.
e. Acyclovir therapy for acute episodes may require higher doses (400 mg, five times per day).
f. If recurrences are frequent, suppressive acyclovir therapy (400 mg bid) should be considered.
g. If lesions do not resolve, the possibility of acyclovir-resistant HSV should be considered.

4. Syphilis and other genital ulcers
a. Genital ulcers facilitate HIV transmission and acquisition secondary to interruption of epithelial barrier and presence of inflammatory cells in ulcer.
b. Syphilis
(1) Serologic titers may be higher than expected for the stage of disease.
(2) False-negative serologic tests or delayed seroreactive tests have been reported.
(3) Both treponemal and nontreponemal serologic tests for syphilis are accurate for the majority of patients with syphilis and HIV coinfection.
(4) Alternative tests such as lesion biopsy and darkfield examination may be helpful to confirm diagnosis if clinical suspicion suggests syphilis but serology is nonconfirmatory.
(5) Neurosyphilis should be considered in the differential diagnosis of neurologic disease in the HIV-positive female.
c. Treatment
(1) HIV-infected women with early syphilis may have increased neurologic complications and higher treatment failures.
(2) Careful follow-up after treatment for all stages of syphilis is essential.
(3) Treatment of primary and secondary syphilis is the same as for non–HIV-infected individuals.
(4) Patients with latent syphilis and HIV infection should undergo cerebrospinal fluid (CSF) examination before treatment.
(5) Latent syphilis, HIV infection, and a normal CSF examination should be treated with benzathine penicillin G, three weekly doses of 2.4 million units each.
d. Chancroid
(1) Patients coinfected with HIV should be closely monitored.
(2) Healing may be slower, and treatment failures occur.

(3) Longer courses of therapy may be required than standard CDC regimens.
(4) Azithromycin or ceftriaxone should be used only if follow-up is ensured.
(5) Some authorities recommend erythromycin base, 500 mg PO, four times daily for 7 days.

5. Pelvic inflammatory disease (PID)
 a. HIV seropositive rate is high in patients presenting with PID (6.7% to 13.6% in communities endemic for HIV).
 b. HIV infection does not predispose to PID.
 c. Clinical presentation may be altered in the following ways:
  (1) Lower abdominal tenderness scores
  (2) Lower admission white blood cells (WBC) (<10,000)
  (3) More likely to require surgical intervention
 d. Management should be based on the same diagnostic criteria and management protocols as for HIV-negative women.
 e. Patients should receive inpatient treatment for PID when HIV positive.
6. Condylomata accuminata
 a. Human papillomavirus (HPV) is the causative agent.
 b. Exophytic anogenital warts are most often caused by types 6 or 11.
 c. Disease is sexually transmitted.
 d. Disease can cause anogenital condylomata (warts) and anogenital dysplasia.
 e. The clinical course of anogenital condylomata may be accelerated.
 f. There is a high frequency of recurrence or persistence of infection.
 g. Disease may be confused with condylomata lata of secondary syphilis.
 h. These lesions may resist conventional treatment. If so, biopsy is indicated before therapy.
 i. Management
  (1) Goal of treatment is removal of exophytic warts and amelioration of signs and symptoms.
  (2) Current treatment modalities are 22% to 94% effective, with high recurrence rates with all modalities.
 j. Regimens
  (1) Cryotherapy with liquid nitrogen or cryoprobe.
  (2) Trichloroacetic acid (TCA), 80% to 90% should be applied only to warts. Repeat weekly if necessary. If warts persist after 6 weeks, reevaluate therapy.
  (3) Podophyllin, 10% to 25% in tincture of benzoin should be applied only to warts. Wash off in 1 to 4 hours. Systemic toxicity if absorbed. If warts persist after 6 weekly applications, reevaluate therapy. Podophyllin is *contraindicated during pregnancy.*
  (4) Podofilox, 0.5% solution, is used for self-treatment (genital warts) only. Apply to warts two times per day for 3 days followed by 4 days of no therapy. May be repeated for a total of four cycles. Podofilox is *contraindicated during pregnancy.*

(5) Surgical excision or CO_2 laser vaporization is useful in the management of extensive anogenital warts or for those patients who have not responded to other regimens.

7. Cervical neoplasia
   a. Women with impaired cellular immunity from other causes (i.e., renal transplant) have been shown to be more susceptible to HPV infection and cervical neoplasia.
   b. HPV infection is more common among HIV-infected women.
   c. HPV types 16, 18, 31, 33, and 35 are associated more often with cervical intraepithelial neoplasia.
   d. There is a 31% to 63% incidence of abnormal cervical cytology in HIV-positive women.
   e. Cervical intraepithelial neoplasia (CIN) is increased in HIV-infected women by 8 to 49 times compared with HIV-negative women.
   f. CIN may be more severe and extensive and may present with a higher grade (i.e., CIN II, CIN III, carcinoma *in situ* [CIS]) as compared with HIV-negative women.
   g. The natural history of CIN may be more aggressive with decreased time to progression of high-grade CIN or malignancy.
   h. Management
      (1) A Papanicolaou smear is an integral component of the HIV-positive woman's initial comprehensive medical evaluation.
      (2) If initial Papanicolaou smear results are within normal limits, repeat in approximately 6 months.
      (3) Repeat Papanicolaou smear annually when the initial two Papanicolaou smears are normal and reliability of follow-up is reasonably certain.
      (4) Papanicolaou smear should be repeated every 6 months when there is a history of the following:
         (a) HPV infection
         (b) Previous Papanicolaou smear showing squamous intraepithelial lesion (SIL) or other cellular abnormalities
         (c) Symptomatic HIV infection
      (5) If inflammation is noted, the patient should be evaluated and treated, and a repeat Papanicolaou smear should be collected within 3 months.
      (6) If Papanicolaou smear sampling is inadequate, repeat immediately.
      (7) If any Papanicolaou smear shows SIL or atypical squamous cells of undetermined significance (ASCUS), refer for colposcopic examination of the lower genital tract.
      (8) Treatment of CIN should be by standard modalities. Cryotherapy has been reported to have a higher failure rate.
      (9) There is a high likelihood of recurrence of CIN (40%) after standard therapy.

12.7 HIV INFECTION IN PREGNANCY

1. Perinatal transmission accounts for the majority of pediatric AIDS cases (~95% in 1995).

2. There are an estimated 7000 infants born to HIV-infected mothers yearly.
3. The estimated vertical transmission rate of HIV is 14% to 32% in developed countries.
4. Thus, 1000 to 2000 infants are born HIV infected each year.
5. Prevention of HIV infection of the fetus or infant is the most important current strategy.

Vertical transmission of HIV

1. Antepartum (transplacental): estimated at 30% to 50% of all cases
2. Intrapartum: exposure to maternal blood and cervical or vaginal secretions, estimated 50% to 70% of all cases
3. Postpartum: breast-feeding may increase risk of vertical transmission by 2% to 14%

Factors associated with an increased risk of mother-to-child transmission of HIV

1. Advanced maternal HIV stage
2. Increased maternal viral load
3. Decreased CD4+ lymphocytes
4. Presence of immune complex dissociated (ICD) p24 antigen
5. Preterm labor
6. Premature rupture of membranes
7. Chorioamnionitis

HIV counseling and testing of pregnant women

1. Recommend HIV testing to all prenatal patients.
2. Perform HIV risk assessment.
3. Women at high risk for HIV infection include those who have the following:
   a. Current or past history of injection drug use
   b. Sexual partners who are injection drug users
   c. HIV-positive partners
   d. Bisexual partners
   e. Current or past history of STDs
   f. Multiple sexual partners
   g. Past history of receiving blood products before 1985
4. Provide risk reduction counseling if HIV negative.

Counseling of HIV-positive pregnant women

1. Pregnancy concerns
   a. Perinatal transmission rate of HIV is 14% to 32%.
   b. Effect of HIV disease on pregnancy outcome: The same prevalence of intrauterine growth restriction (IUGR), prematurity, and early neonatal disease exists as for seronegative injection drug users.
   c. Effect of pregnancy on the course of HIV disease: Studies have not demonstrated a significant influence on the course of HIV disease.
   d. Information regarding measures to prevent perinatal transmission, including information on use of Zidovudine should be provided (see Obstetric Management, p. 225).

e. No evidence exists that HIV is teratogenic.
f. Informed choice about continuing pregnancy should be respected by caregivers.
g. Referrals for pregnancy termination should be made when the option is chosen by the patient.
h. Referral for HIV follow-up and prenatal care should be provided when appropriate.

Obstetric management

1. Antepartum
   a. The standard approach to the care of the asymptomatic and symptomatic HIV-positive woman, including laboratory tests, skin tests, vaccinations, and treatments should not be altered because of pregnancy.
   b. Screen for other STDs, including gonorrhea, *Chlamydia,* syphilis, and hepatitis B (present and past exposure).
   c. Pneumovax and hepatitis B vaccine are recommended.
   d. Rubella vaccine is contraindicated.
   e. Intradermal skin test for tuberculosis should be applied with two or more antigen controls (*Candida,* mumps, tetanus toxoid).
   f. Monitor CD4 counts once per trimester and more frequently if clinically indicated.
   g. At 14 weeks gestation, offer patients the option of Zidovudine (ZDV) to prevent perinatal transmission. Patients should be advised that ZDV has not been studied in patients who begin therapy after 34 weeks gestation, those who previously have received ZDV, and those whose CD4 count is less than $200/mm^3$.
      (1) Dose
         (a) Antepartum: 100 mg PO, five times daily until labor
         (b) Intrapartum: loading 2 mgk/kg over 1 hour, then 1 mg/kg/hr maintenance until delivery
         (c) Postpartum: neonate to receive oral ZDV syrup, 2 mg/kg, four times daily, for 6 weeks as per pediatrician
      (2) Maternal monitoring
         (a) Complete blood count, liver function tests, and serum creatinine monthly
      (3) Discontinue ZDV therapy if the following occur:
         (a) Hemoglobin <8 mg/dl
         (b) Platelet count $<100,000/mm^3$
         (c) Absolute neutrophil count $<750/mm^3$
         (d) Serum glutamic oxaloacetic transaminase (SGOT) or serum glutamic pyruvate transaminase (SGPT) >5 times normal
         (e) Serious cardiac, respiratory, neurologic, or gastrointestinal sequelae
      (4) Physicians should consider initiating ZDV for maternal indications when CD4 count is between 200 and 500 and patient is symptomatic or when CD4 count <200.
      (5) Didanosine (ddI) and Zalcitabine (ddC) are second-line therapies to supplement ZDV. Their efficacies in preventing vertical transmission of HIV have not been determined.

(6) If CD4 count <200/mm^3 or percentage CD4 <20%, begin *Pneumocystis carinii* pneumonia prophylaxis:
   (a) Double-strength trimethoprim sulfamethoxazole qd or 3 days each week. This drug remains the first-line agent.
      i. Sulfonamides pose a theoretical risk of kernicterus to fetus.
      ii. Benefits of therapy outweigh its possible risks.
   (b) Dapsone
      i. Risk of hemolytic anemia in glucose-6-phosphodiesterase (G6PD)-deficient individuals
      ii. G6PD level measured before initiating therapy
   (c) Aerosolized pentamidine, 300 mg, once per month
(7) Treatment of opportunistic infections
   (a) Recognize the possibility of opportunistic infections and obtain rapid consultation, diagnosis, and management.
   (b) These infections generally occur with increasing immunosuppression and decreasing CD4 counts <200/mm^3.
   (c) Aggressive therapy rarely needs to be altered because of pregnancy.
   (d) Provider and patient must weigh the benefits and possible fetal risks of each therapy.

2. Intrapartum
   a. Mode of delivery should be for obstetric indication only.
   b. Fetal scalp sampling or electrode placement is to be avoided if possible.
   c. Prolonged rupture of membranes may increase the chance for vertical transmission of HIV.
   d. Universal blood and body fluid precautions should be practiced:
      (1) Needles should not be resheathed.
      (2) Water barrier gowns should be worn.
      (3) Double gloving should be used in the operating room.
      (4) Goggles should be used.
      (5) Mouth operated suction traps should not be used.
   e. ZDV prophylaxis should be considered immediately if occupational exposure occurs.
3. Postpartum
   a. Continue universal blood and body fluid precautions.
   b. Counseling is against breast-feeding in the United States.
   c. Pediatric HIV follow-up should be arranged.
   d. Maternal HIV and gynecology referrals should be given.
4. Contraceptive counseling
   a. Contraceptive options should be discussed with *all* patients.
   b. Education about safer sexual practices should be provided.
   c. Barrier contraception (condoms and spermicide) should be recommended for vaginal, anal, and oral intercourse to reduce transmission of HIV.
   d. Hormonal contraception is not contraindicated in HIV-positive women. Barrier techniques should accompany hormonal methods.
   e. Intrauterine devices (IUD) may be contraindicated in women with HIV infection. There is an increased susceptibility to PID, a greater

risk of transmission because of increased blood flow, and the possibility of microabrasions on the head of the sexual partner's penis caused by the tail of the IUD.

f. The option of surgical sterilization should be discussed with full informed consent. It should neither be denied nor encouraged.

Suggested reading

1. American College of Obstetricians and Gynecologists: *Human immunodeficiency virus infections,* ACOG Technical Bulletin 169, Washington, DC, 1992, ACOG.
2. Carpenter CC et al: Human immunodeficiency virus infection in North American women: experience with 200 cases and a review of the literature, *Medicine* (Baltimore) 70:307-325, 1991.
3. Centers for Disease Control: *MMWR* 39(47), 1990.
4. Centers for Disease Control: Update: acquired immunodeficiency syndrome—United States, 1992, *MMWR* 42(28), 1993.
5. Centers for Disease Control: 1993 Sexually transmitted disease guidelines, *MMWR* 42(RR-14), 1993.
6. Centers for Disease Control: Update: mortality attributable to HIV infection/AIDS among persons aged 25-44 years—United States, 1990 and 1991, *MMWR* 42(25), 1993.
7. Centers for Disease Control: Update: barrier protection against HIV infection and other sexually transmitted diseases, *MMWR* 42(30), 1993.
8. Centers for Disease Control: Update: mortality attributable to HIV infection among persons aged 25-44 years—United States, 1991 and 1992, *MMWR* 42(45), 1993.
9. Centers for Disease Control: Recommendations for HIV testing services for inpatients and outpatients in acute care hospital settings and technical guidance on HIV counseling, *MMWR* 42(RR-2), 1993.
10. Centers for Disease Control: 1993 revised classification system for HIV infection and expanded surveillance case definition for AIDS among adolescents and adults, *MMWR* 41(RR-17), 1993.
11. Centers for Disease Control: Recommendations of the U.S. Public Health Service Task Force on the Use of Zidovudine to reduce perinatal transmission of human immunodeficiency virus, *MMWR* 43(RR-11), 1994.
12. Centers for Disease Control: Update: AIDS among women—United States, 1994, *MMWR* 44, 1995
13. Centers for Disease Control: USPHS/IDSA guidelines for the prevention of opportunistic infection in persons infected with human immunodeficiency virus: a summary, *MMWR* 44(RR-8), 1995.
14. Chin S, Wortley P: Epidemiology of HIV/AIDS in women. In Minkoff H, Dehovitz JA, Duerr A, editors: *HIV infection in women,* New York, 1995, Raven Press.
15. Dehovitz JA: Natural history of HIV infection in women. In Minkoff H, Dehovitz JA, Duerr A, editors: *HIV infection in women*, New York, 1995, Raven Press.
16. European Collaborative Study: Risk factors for mother-to-child transmission of HIV-1, *Lancet* 339:1007, 1992.
17. Gwinn M et al: Prevalence of HIV infection in childbearing women in the United States, *JAMA* 265:1704-1708, 1991.
18. Hoegsberg B et al: Sexually transmitted diseases and human immunodeficiency virus among women with pelvic inflammatory disease, *Am J Obstet Gynecol* 163:1175-1179, 1990.
19. Hook III EW: HIV/sexually transmitted disease interactions in women. In Minkoff H, Dehovitz JA, Duerr A, editors: *HIV infection in women,* New York, 1995, Raven Press.

20. Maiman M et al: Human immunodeficiency virus infection and cervical neoplasia, *Gynecol Oncol* 38:377-382, 1990.
21. Maiman M et al: Colposcopic evaluation of human immunodeficiency virus-seropositive women, *Obstet Gynecol* 70:84-88, 1991.
22. Mandelblatt JS et al: Association between HIV infection and cervical neoplasia: implications for clinical care of women at risk for both conditions, *AIDS* 6:173-178, 1992.
23. Minkoff H: Exposing offspring to HIV infection, *Contemporary Ob/Gyn* 40(4):60-66, 1995.
24. New York State Department of Health, AIDS Institute, Medical Care Criteria Committee, Women's HIV Care Subcommittee, Health Care Services for Women with HIV Infection (July 1995).
25. Safrin S et al: Seroprevalence and epidemiologic correlates of human immunodeficiency virus infection in women with acute pelvic inflammatory disease, *Am J Obstet Gynecol* 163, 1993.
26. Villari P et al: Cesarean section to reduce perinatal transmission of human immunodeficiency virus: potential benefits and costs, *T Online J Curr Clin Rev* 1993; Document 74.
27. Worth LA: HIV infection in women. In Cohen PT, Sande MA, Volberding PA, editors: *The AIDS knowledge base,* ed 2, Boston, 1994, Little, Brown.

13 Evaluation of Lower Abdominal and Pelvic Pain

Avi Sklar, M.D.

Lower abdominal and pelvic pain are the most common symptoms encountered in gynecologic practice and are clinically challenging despite recent technologic advances in pregnancy testing, diagnostic imaging, and endoscopy. A detailed and thorough history—physical examination, selective use of diagnostic tests, and a well-considered differential diagnosis—usually leads to an accurate diagnosis and appropriate therapy.

The initial classification scheme in the diagnosis of pelvic pain differentiates acute pain from chronic pelvic pain (CPP) that has been present for 6 months or more. CPP is further classified as episodic (e.g., dysmenorrhea) or continuous that waxes and wanes but is rarely or never completely absent. In each category, causes are further subdivided by gynecologic or nongynecologic origin. Some conditions (e.g., endometriosis) may be acute, episodic, or chronic. In the reproductive age, pregnancy-related events must always be considered.

13.1 ANATOMY AND PHYSIOLOGY

1. Stimuli that produce pain from lesions within the pelvic and lower abdomen arise from the following:
   a. Distension and subsequent high-amplitude contractions of a hollow viscus (e.g., bowel obstruction)
   b. Rapid stretching of an organ capsule (e.g., hematosalpinx)
   c. Chemical irritation of the parietal peritoneum (e.g., ruptured ovarian cyst)
   d. Tissue ischemia (e.g., degenerating fibroids)
   e. Neuritis secondary to inflammatory, neoplastic, or fibrotic processes in adjacent organs
2. Lesions involving the lower uterine segment, cervix, bladder trigone, or rectum tend to incite pain localized to the lower sacral area or the buttocks, with occasional radiation down the leg (sacral nerve roots 2 through 4).
3. Stimuli from the uterine fundus, adnexa, bladder dome, distal ileum, cecum, and appendix produce pain localized in the lower abdomen (hypogastric plexus).

4. Sensations from somatic structures (e.g., external genitalia and vagina) can be distinctly localized by the cerebral cortex, whereas those from visceral structures are poorly localized.
   a. Pain originating in any organ is felt in a skin area supplied by the corresponding spinal nerve (dermatome) rather than in the specific organ site.
   b. This lack of correlation between perceived site and organ of origin contributes to the difficulties encountered in the diagnosis of pelvic pain.

13.2 ASSESSMENT

1. History
   a. Onset: Pain of sudden onset usually indicates an acute intraperitoneal event that exposes the pelvic peritoneum to blood, pus, bowel contents, ovarian cyst contents, or ischemic infarction. Events include hemorrhage, torsion or rupture of an adnexal mass, bowel perforation, acute inflammation, ureteric calculi, and bowel obstruction. Pain of gradual onset suggests a more chronic process such as endometriosis or neoplasm.
   b. Character: Pain may be intermittent or constant, sharp, or dull.
      (1) Intermittent pain of a colicky nature suggests obstruction of a hollow viscus such as bowel, ureter, uterus, or fallopian tube.
      (2) An intraperitoneal catastrophe is associated with acute sharp pain.
      (3) Dull pain is usually associated with inflammation.
      (4) Constant pain is more likely caused by intraperitoneal hemorrhage, ischemia of a pelvic or abdominal organ, or ovarian cyst rupture.
   c. Degree: Severe pain usually denotes peritoneal irritation, tissue infarction, and colic of the uterus, ureter, and intestine.
   d. Duration
      (1) An acute incident (e.g., rupture, viscus perforation) causes the woman to present shortly after the onset.
      (2) Inflammatory conditions (e.g., pelvic inflammatory disease [PID], acute appendicitis) usually have a more indolent onset.
      (3) The duration of CPP is variable and often present for years.
   e. Relationship to menstrual cycle
      (1) In the reproductive age group, any pain following a short period of amenorrhea must be assumed to be a complication of pregnancy until disproved.
      (2) Cyclic pelvic pain is often functional in nature, related to ovulation, premenstrual tension, or dysmenorrhea.
   f. Radiation: Pain radiation is often indicative of the degree of parietal peritoneal involvement.
   g. Associated symptoms
      (1) Gastrointestinal symptoms
         (a) Anorexia
         (b) Nausea
         (c) Vomiting

(d) Diarrhea
(e) Tenesmus
(f) Dyschezia
(g) Bloody stools
(2) Urinary symptoms
(a) Frequency
(b) Urgency
(c) Dysuria
(d) Hesitancy
(e) Hematuria
(f) Flank pain
(3) Shoulder tip pain: secondary to diaphragmatic irritation from blood or pus
(4) Syncope: not uncommon with intraperitoneal bleeding, even in small amount
(5) Modifiers of the pain, including relieving and aggravating factors (e.g., medications)
(6) Fever and chills often indicate an infectious disorder (e.g., salpingitis, pyelonephritis, appendicitis)
(7) Dyspareunia
(8) Vaginal bleeding

2. Past medical, surgical, menstrual, sexual, and contraceptive history must be noted.
3. Review records from previous hospitalizations, surgeries, and radiologic investigations (especially for the patient with CPP)
4. Physical examination
   a. General appearance and vital signs
   b. Heart and lung examination
      (1) Abdominal pain may be referred from pulmonary and cardiac disease.
   c. Abdominal examination
      (1) Inspection for distension, contour, color changes (e.g., Cullen's sign), scars, area of greatest pain (patient should indicate where)
      (2) Auscultation for absent, hypoactive, or hyperactive bowel signs
      (3) Palpation for mass, tenderness, peritoneal signs (focal or diffuse), guarding, rebound tenderness, reflex rigidity, costovertebral angle tenderness (site of maximum pain should be evaluated last)
      (4) Percussion for ascites, shifting dullness
   d. Pelvic examination
      (1) Inspection of external genitalia and cervix for evidence of trauma, infection, hemorrhage, or asymmetry
      (2) Palpation of the vaginal wall for tenderness and palpation of the cervix for cervical motion tenderness
      (3) Bimanual examination starting with the side of least tenderness and noting the size, shape, location, tenderness, mobility, and consistency of any mass and position and mobility of the uterus
      (4) Rectovaginal examination including stool for occult blood and assessment of the uterosacral ligaments and rectovaginal septum

(5) Presence of a pelvic or abdominal tumor: should not necessarily lead to the conclusion that the pain is secondary to the lesion (e.g., a patient with a multinodular fibroid uterus is subject to a variety of acute pelvic processes unrelated to the myomas)
(6) Absence of palpable pathology: does not rule out the presence of organic disease (e.g., endometriosis)

5. Investigations: If a firm diagnosis cannot be made, a differential diagnosis should facilitate selection of the appropriate investigations among the following list (Table 13-1).
   a. Complete blood count (CBC) with differential
      (1) An increased white blood cell (WBC) count, especially with a left shift, may indicate systemic infection.
      (2) Decreased hemoglobin levels may indicate blood loss.
   b. Urinalysis: Presence of bacteria, WBC, or red blood cells (RBC) suggests urinary involvement.
   c. Blood type and antibody screen
      (1) Blood should be typed and screened for any surgical case.
      (2) Rhogam should be administered to unsensitized Rh negative patients with miscarriages or ectopic pregnancies.
   d. Pregnancy test: Urine human chorionic gonadotropin (HCG) immunoassay is quick and sensitive to 50 mIU/ml. Serum β-HCG can be quantitated and followed serially.
   e. Cervical cultures for gonorrhea and *Chlamydia* testing (enzyme immunoassays or antigen detection systems) are indicated when pelvic infection is suspected.
   f. Culdocentesis may be helpful in evaluating the peritoneal cavity for the following:
      (1) Blood (ectopic pregnancy, ruptured hemorrhagic ovarian cyst, ruptured spleen)
      (2) Free fluid (ruptured functional cyst)
      (3) Pus (PID, appendicitis)
      (4) Fixed mass in the cul-de-sac: contraindication
   g. Erythrocyte sedimentation rate is a nonspecific acute-phase reactive protein that indicates an inflammatory reaction when elevated.
   h. Ultrasound (U/S)
      (1) Transvaginal U/S avoids the thick abdominal wall and urine-filled bladder and generally has better resolution as the probe moves closer to the pelvic contents unobstructed by layers of fat and muscle.
      (2) A large pelvic–abdominal mass may be missed unless an abdominal U/S is performed.
      (3) U/S is helpful in the workup of early intrauterine pregnancy, ectopic pregnancy, adnexal mass, and in patients who cannot be examined otherwise because of pain, obesity, vaginal stenosis, or other conditions.
   i. Laparoscopy
      (1) Laparoscopy is a valuable tool to diagnosis and initiate therapy especially with ectopic pregnancy, salpingitis, appendicitis, adnexal accidents, endometriosis, and adhesions.
      (2) Contraindications include hypovolemic shock, bowel obstruction, and large pelvic–abdominal masses.

Table 13-1 Differential diagnosis of pelvic and lower abdominal pain

Acute

Early pregnancy complications
- Spontaneous abortion
- Septic abortion
- Ectopic pregnancy
- Hemorrhagic corpus luteum of pregnancy
- Gestational trophoblastic disease
- Uterine incarceration

Pelvic infections

Pain of adnexal origin
- Rupture
- Hemorrhage
- Torsion
- Ovarian hyperstimulation syndrome

Leiomyomas
- Degeneration
- Pedunculated myoma torsion
- Aborting submucous myoma

Intestinal sources of pain
- Appendicitis
- Inflammatory bowel disease
- Intestinal obstruction
- Gastroenteritis
- Diverticulitis
- Meckel's diverticulitis
- Colon tumors
- Torsion of appendices epiploicae

Urinary sources of pain
- Overdistended bladder
- Acute cystitis
- Ureteral calculi
- Pelvic kidney
- Urethral syndrome
- Interstitial cystitis

Vascular sources of pain
- Pelvic thrombophlebitis
- Mesenteric occlusion

Systemic causes of pain
- Sickle cell disease
- Diabetes mellitus
- Drug withdrawal
- Acute intermittent porphyria
- Connective tissue diseases
  - Familial Mediterranean fever
  - Henoch-Schlönlein purpura
  - Systemic lupus erythematous (SLE)
  - Hereditary angioneurotic edema
  - Periarteritis nodosa

Endocrine disorders
- Hyperthyroidism
- Addisonian crisis
- Hyperparathyroidism

Infections
- Syphilis
- Tubercular peritonitis
- Herpes zoster virus

Chronic
- Dysmenorrhea
- Endometriosis
- Adenomyosis
- Adhesions
- Mittelschmerz
- Ovarian remnant syndrome
- Pelvic congestion syndrome
- "Trigger point" abdominal wall pain

Functional bowel disorders
- Irritable bowel syndrome
- Chronic constipation

Chronic pelvic pain syndrome

13.3 EARLY PREGNANCY COMPLICATIONS

Pregnancy-related complications should be highly suspected in any women of reproductive age with acute or subacute pelvic and lower abdominal pain.

1. Abortions are characterized by vaginal bleeding and suprapubic crampy lower abdominal pain of variable intensity.
   a. Spontaneous abortions
      (1) Threatened abortion: vaginal bleeding or spotting and a closed cervical os
      (2) Inevitable abortion: prolonged, profuse bleeding with an open cervical os
      (3) Incomplete abortion: partial passage of tissue through an open cervical os
      (4) Complete abortion: complete passage of tissue, usually resulting in resolution of symptoms
   b. Induced abortions: Subsequent to an induced abortion, pelvic pain can occur secondary to the following:
      (1) Incomplete evacuation
      (2) Septic abortion
         (a) Septic abortion is associated with fever and sepsis secondary to infection of the uterine contents.
         (b) Treatment consists of obtaining appropriate cultures, broad-spectrum antiobiotics, resuscitative measures, and evacuation of the uterine contents.
2. Ectopic pregnancy

13.4 ECTOPIC PREGNANCY

Definition

An ectopic pregnancy (EP) is one in which a fertilized ovum implants outside the endometrial lining of the uterus; 97% are tubal, 78% ampullary, 12% isthmic, 5% fimbrial, 2% to 3% interstitial, 1% ovarian, 1% to 2% abdominal, 0.5% cervical.

Epidemiology

1. 1% to 2% of pregnancies
2. 13% of maternal deaths
3. Increasing number of EP in the United States: 17,800 reported cases in 1970 and 108,000 in 1992
4. Decreasing case fatality rate because of advances in diagnosis and therapy: 35.5/10,000 EP in 1970; 3.4/10,000 EP in 1987

Etiology

1. Anatomic obstruction to zygote passage
2. Abnormalities in tubal motility
3. Transperitoneal migration of the zygote

Risk factors

1. Salpingitis (laparoscopic proven)
   a. One episode: 5.3%
   b. Multiple episodes: 19%

2. Previous EP: 10% to 20%
3. Previous tubal sterilization: 16%
4. Previous tuboplasty: 17% to 20%
5. IUD: 3% to 16%
6. Progestin-only pill: 2% to 3%
7. Assisted reproductive techniques: 5% to 17%

Presenting symptoms

1. Abdominal pain: 87% to 99%
2. Abnormal bleeding: 48% to 64%
3. Amennorhea: 61% to 79%
4. Pregnancy symptoms: 23%
5. Syncope: 6% to 37%
6. Shoulder pain: 5% to 22%
7. Tissue passage: 6% to 7%

Presenting signs

1. Abdominal tenderness: 97% to 99%
2. Adnexal tenderness: 87% to 99%
3. Peritoneal signs: 71% to 76%
4. Adnexal mass: 33% to 53%
5. Enlarged uterus: 6% to 30%
6. Shock: 2% to 17%

Differential diagnosis

1. Corpus luteum cyst
2. Rupture or torsion of ovarian cyst
3. Threatened or incomplete abortion
4. PID
5. Appendicitis
6. Gastroenteritis
7. Dysfunctional uterine bleeding
8. Degenerating uterine fibroids

Diagnostic modalities (Fig. 13-1)

1. Pregnancy test
   a. Monoclonal urine HCG (ELISA)
   b. Serum QHCG
      (1) Of normal intrauterine pregnancies, 85% have a doubling time of 2 days.
      (2) Abnormal gestations show <66% increase of QHCG within 2 days.
      (3) Of EP, 13% may have a normal doubling time.
2. Progesterone
   a. Decreased production in EP
   b. Single determination
   c. Progesterone < 5 ng/ml: strongly predictive of abnormal pregnancy
   d. Progesterone > 25 ng/ml: strongly predictive of normal intrauterine pregnancy

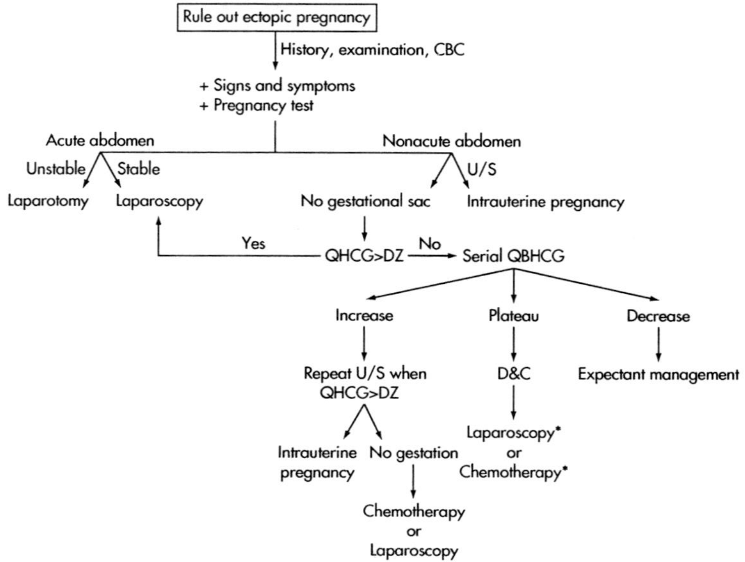

Figure 13-1
Steps in the diagnosis and treatment of lower abdominal or pelvic pain. (*DZ* , Discriminatory zone; *D&C*, dilation and curettage; *CBC*, complete blood count.)
*If clinically indicated.

3. Ultrasound
   a. Presence of an intrauterine pregnancy rules out EP. (Heterotopic pregnancy is rare in the nonreproductive assisted pregnancy.)
   b. Normal intrauterine gestation seen when QHCG > discriminatory zone (DZ):
      (1) DZ for abdominal U/S, 6000 mIU/(ml) (international reference preparation [IRP])
      (2) DZ for transvaginal U/S, 1500 mIU/ml (IRP)
   c. U/S findings in EP include the following:
      (1) Empty uterus
      (2) Increased decidual response
      (3) Adnexal mass or ring
      (4) Free peritoneal fluid
      (5) Fetal sac or pole in the tube
      (6) Active fetal heart in adnexa
4. Culdocentesis
   a. It is clinically useful when other diagnostic modalities not readily available.
   b. Positive tap means nonclotting blood with hematocrit (HCT) >12%. Positive tap in up to 70% of EP of which 65% are unruptured.
   c. Negative tap means clear or blood-tinged fluid.
   d. Nondiagnostic tap means clotted blood or no fluid.
5. Dilation and curretage (D&C)
   a. D&C may be useful with low progesterone or abnormal serial QHCG levels.
   b. Products of conception on pathology rules out EP.
6. Diagnostic laparoscopy
   a. Can diagnose and treat EP in the hemodynamically stable patient
   b. If performed too early, can miss the EP

Therapeutic options

1. Expectant management
   a. May consider in the compliant, stable patient with low falling HCG titers, mass <4 cm, and no U/S signs of rupture or bleeding
2. Medical management
   a. IM, IV, or PO methotrexate
      (1) Most common regimen is methotrexate 50 mg/m^2 body surface area
   b. Selection criteria
      (1) Compliant stable patient
      (2) No contraindication to methotrexate (hepatic or renal disease, thrombocytopenia, leukopenia, significant anemia)
      (3) < 4 cm mass
      (4) QHCG < 30,000 mIU/ml (IRP)
      (5) No evidence of hemoperitoneum on transvaginal sonogram
   c. A 95% success rate with minimal side effects (stomatitis, elevated hepatic transaminases, leukopenia, dermatitis)
   d. Require second dose or surgical intervention if QHCG increases or plateaus after 7 days
   e. Tubal mass: may take up to 3 months to resolve

3. Salpingiocentesis
   a. Direct injection of chemotherapy (e.g., methotrexate, 25 mg) into EP via laparoscopy, transvaginal U/S, or hysteroscopy
4. Conservative surgery (laparoscopy or laparotomy)
   a. Laparoscopy has the advantage of decreased recuperation time and shorter hospitalization.
   b. Salpingostomy or segmental resection depends on tubal location and size of EP.
      (1) In ampullary ectopics the trophoblast has invaded the mucosa and propagated in the extraluminal, subserosal space.
      (2) In contrast, isthmic pregnancies tend to propagate within and disrupt the lumen.
   c. Isthmic EP: Segmental resection is followed by delayed microsurgical anastomosis.
   d. Ampullary and fimbrial EP: Linear salpingostomy should be performed.
   e. Interstitial EP: Pregnancy should be resected with tubal preservation followed by delayed microsurgical anastomosis.
5. Salpingectomy
   a. Tubal rupture
   b. Fertility not desired
   c. Recurrent EP in the same tube
   d. Uncontrolled hemorrhage
6. Persistent ectopic pregnancy
   a. Persistent EP results from residual trophoblastic tissue or secondary implantation after conservative surgery.
   b. With conservative treatment, there is a 5% incidence of persistent EP.
   c. Follow QHCG every week until < 15 mIU/ml.
   d. Expect QHCG < 20% preoperative level within 72 hours.
   e. If QHCG increases or plateaus, medical or surgical intervention is required.

13.5 HEMORRHAGIC CORPUS LUTEUM OF PREGNANCY

1. Rupture or hemorrhage of the corpus luteum occurs occasionally in the first trimester.
2. It is associated with acute onset of unilateral lower abdominal pain, with or without an adnexal mass.
3. When an intrauterine gestation is not seen on U/S, this condition may be confused with an EP.

13.6 GESTATIONAL TROPHOBLASTIC DISEASE

1. Molar pregnancy generally becomes symptomatic late in the first trimester or early in the second.
2. It often presents with abnormal bleeding and cramps, suggesting a threatened abortion, and may be associated with uterine enlargement beyond that appropriate for dates.

3. U/S is often diagnostic.
4. Bilateral ovarian enlargements caused by massive luteinization of both ovaries may be present and may become symptomatic by torsion and necrosis.

13.7 PREGNANT UTERINE INCARCERATION

1. This rare complication results from the continued growth of a retroflexed pregnant uterus trapped in the concavity of the sacrum between the twelfth and sixteenth week of pregnancy.
2. Symptoms and signs of threatened abortion ensue.
3. They are generally relieved with repositioning of the uterus, which may require general anesthesia.
4. The condition is recognizable by the displacement of the cervix upward to a position directly behind the pubic symphysis, where it is found on pelvic examination to be firmly wedged.

13.8 PELVIC INFECTIONS

1. Pelvic infections include acute salpingitis and its complications of tuboovarian abscess, pyosalpingitis, and perihepatitis. Microorganisms produce an intitial cervicitis that subsequently spreads to cause an endometritis, salpingitis, and potentially peritonitis. Intraabdominal suppuration may continue, producing a pelvic abscess. Most upper tract infections are presumed to be polymicrobial and should be treated as such.
2. Classic presentation of acute PID includes a history of fairly acute lower abdominal pain, pyrexia, tachycardia, and sometimes gastrointestinal symptoms. The pain is usually poorly localized in the lower abdomen. There may be urinary frequency, dysuria, and often a vaginal discharge that may or may not be associated with vaginal bleeding.
3. On physical examination, the patient may appear flushed and distressed. The lower abdomen is very tender with guarding, but the epigastrium is usually soft. Pelvic examination is usually unsatisfactory because of the degree of bilateral adnexal tenderness and abdominal guarding. Cervical motion tenderness is present.
4. Early aggressive treatment may minimize the risks of sequelae such as infertility, CPP, adhesions, and ectopic pregnancy. Therefore, the clinician should have a lower threshold to hospitalize for parenteral antibiotic therapy and interventional laparoscopic treatment.
5. It is important to note that many cases of salpingitis have attenuated or even an absence of symptoms and clinical findings.
6. It is often difficult to distinguish between PID and other causes of pelvic pain such as endometriosis, ovarian cyst rupture, and appendicitis. Frequently, these patients are treated with antibiotics without establishment of the correct diagnosis and mislabeled as PID. (Full discussion of PID occurs in Chapter 11.)

13.9 PAIN OF ADNEXAL ORIGIN

The ovary is relatively insensitive to pain (e.g., an endometrioma may asymptomatically grow up to 15 cm in diameter because of the gradual nature of fluid accumulation). Pain in an adnexal mass is usually a result of rupture, intratumor hemorrhage, or torsion. Acute distension of the fallopian tube (e.g., EP, pyosalpynx) can cause intense colicky pain. An associated history of intercourse, intense physical activity, or abdominal trauma is commonly noted. U/S is often helpful in outlining an adnexal mass or fluid in the cul-de-sac because physical examination may be limited secondary to pain and abdominal guarding.

1. Ovarian cyst rupture
   a. Pain depends on the nature of the cyst's contents and the presence or absence of bleeding.
   b. Rupture or leakage of a benign cystic teratoma releases highly irritating material in the peritoneal cavity with potential development of the following:
      (1) Chemical peritonitis
      (2) Persistent spreading pelvic pain
      (3) Fever
      (4) Ileus
      (5) Abdominal distension
   c. Rupture of a folliular cyst is often painless or may cause only a temporary acute reaction that rapidly resolves.
   d. Corpus luteum cyst rupture is often associated with some degree of intraperitoneal bleeding and is frequently painful.
      (1) This condition should be suspected in patients on anticoagulant therapy who have repeated bouts of abdominal pain during the luteal phase.
   e. The escape of old blood from endometriomas may produce repetitive acute attacks of pain.
      (1) Occurring with menses, they may be associated with fever up to 101° F and may be mistaken for flare-ups of PID.
      (2) Because these attacks are self-limited, usually 7 to 10 days, mistakenly instituted antibiotic therapy appears to be repeatedly effective.
2. Internal hemorrhage can cause sudden distension of a cystic or solid ovarian tumor.
   a. Can cause sudden distension of a cystic or solid ovarian tumor producing a boring, throbbing pain of increasing severity.
   b. The mass usually has a tense consistency and is exquisitely tender.
   c. Delayed surgical intervention may result in infarction, tissue necrosis, and systemic toxity.
3. Torsion of an ovarian or tubal mass
   a. Torsion may be intermittent, producing characteristic recurrent attacks of colicky pain, nausea, vomiting, and low-grade fever.
   b. It may also be persistent proceeding to thrombosis of the infundibulopelvic vessels beyond the twist site and tissue necrosis.
   c. Occasionally, torsion with necrosis of the tumor can be sufficiently walled off by the bowel and omentum so that the process becomes low grade and chronic.

13.10 OVARIAN HYPERSTIMULATION SYNDROME

1. Ovarian hyperstimulation syndrome is an iatrogenic cause of multiple follicular cysts in infertility patients as a consequence of ovulation induction, generally with gonadotropins and rarely with clomiphene.
2. The syndrome, which is self-limiting, is worsened and prolonged with conception because of the continued stimulation by HCG.
3. Signs and symptoms include the following:
   a. Abdominal pain
   b. Abdominal distension
   c. Massive ovarian enlargement
   d. Ascites
   e. Pleural effusions
   f. Dyspnea
   g. Weight gain
   h. Electrolyte imbalance
   i. Hemoconcentration
   j. Oliguria
   k. Hypercoagulability
4. Patients usually respond to conservative management with particular attention to fluid status, correction of electrolyte imbalance, bed rest, and avoidance of any activity including coitus.
5. Mannitol may be used if renal failure is imminent and an ion-exchanged resin can reverse hyperkalemia.
6. Surgical intervention is rarely necessary except in cases of torsion or rupture.

13.11 LEIOMYOMAS

Uncomplicated uterine leiomyomas generally are asymptomatic. When acute pain is the presenting symptom, it is important to establish that no other coexisting pathology is responsible. Complications of myoma that commonly cause acute pain include the following:

1. Carneous degeneration that occurs in pregnancy and is associated with acute crampy moderate to severe pain.
   a. There are signs of adjacent peritoneal irritation ("point tenderness") and often ileus, fever, and leukocytosis.
   b. Management is conservative, with hydration and analgesics.
   c. Excision of these tumors from the hypervascularized myometrium of pregnancy may be accompanied by massive, uncontrollable hemorrhage.
2. Torsion of a pedunculated myoma with venous obstruction rapidly leading to edema and infarction produces acute colicky pain.
   a. These myomas require extirpation either by myomectomy or hysterectomy, depending on the age and reproductive desires of the patient.
3. Aborting submucous myoma is associated with laborlike crampy pain and prolonged menstrual bleeding.

a. With each succeeding menstrual cycle, the pain is of increasing severity, associated with gradual cervical dilation and protrusion of the aborting myoma.
b. Treatment is surgical with the myoma sent for frozen section to rule out a mixed Müllerian malignancy.

13.12 INTESTINAL SOURCES OF PAIN

1. Appendicitis
   a. The pain of appendicitis usually starts as a vague, dull, lower epigastric or periumbilical discomfort.
   b. After several hours, if the appendix is not retroperitoneal, the pain shifts to the RLQ, with the point of maximum tenderness at McBurney's point once the overlying parietal peritoneum becomes locally involved in the inflammatory process.
   c. Associated symptoms include the following:
      (1) Anorexia
      (2) Nausea
      (3) Vomiting
   d. Abdominal distension is unusual and bowel sounds are usually normal or slightly hypoactive.
   e. Guarding, rebound tenderness, and Rovsing's sign (pain felt in the RLQ resulting from palpation in the LLQ) are suggestive of the diagnosis.
   f. The presence of adductor pain (that produced by passive internal rotation of the flexed thigh) or the psoas sign (an increase in pain from passive extension of the right hip joint that stretches the iliopsoas muscle) may suggest both the anatomic location of the appendix and the progression of the inflammatory process.
   g. It is often a difficult diagnosis because of the variable position of the appendix and the spectrum of conditions with a similar form of presentation.
   h. When the differential diagnosis cannot be effectively established, laparoscopy or exploratory laparotomy is indicated, because the risk of morbidity and mortality of appendiceal rupture is significant.
2. Inflammatory bowel disease
   a. Ulcerative colitis involves the mucosa and submucosa of the gut and principally presents with lower abdominal cramping and diarrhea, often accompanied by rectal bleeding, tenesmus, and rectal urgency. The pain is usually LLQ and the initial course may be intermittent, with exacerbations or remissions lasting for up to a few months.
   b. Crohn's disease (ileitis) involves all tissue layers of the bowel.
      (1) The common symptoms include the following:
         (a) Diarrhea
         (b) Fever
         (c) RLQ pain
         (d) Sometimes associated with anorexia, nausea, vomiting, and perianal abscesses or fistulae

(2) Although the disease is chronic, the initial symptoms are usually significant enough that the patient is evaluated for acute abdominal pain, often confused with appendicitis.

3. Intestinal obstruction
   a. Pain is the primary complaint in all forms of small and large bowel obstruction arising from the following:
      (1) Adhesive bands
      (2) Tumors
      (3) Intussusception
      (4) Volvulus
      (5) Internal hernias
   b. The pain of obstruction is intermittent, colicky, and usually accompanied by nausea, vomiting, and progressive abdominal distension.
   c. Bowel sounds are characteristically hyperactive and high pitched.
   d. In distal small bowel or large bowel obstructions, the pain is less colicky and vomiting occurs late and often is feculent and foul smelling.
   e. The diagnosis can be established by flat plate and upright films of the abdomen.
4. Gastroenteritis: This is a complex clinical syndrome characterized by colicky abdominal pain, vomiting, and diarrhea.
   a. Causal agents include enteric viral pathogens, *Salmonella,* and certain bacterial exotoxins.
   b. The pain is diffuse throughout the abdomen and may occur in various quadrants at different times.
   c. On physical examination, bowel sounds are found to be hyperactive but not as high pitched as in bowel obstruction.
   d. The patient is often dehydrated.
   e. Stool studies for leukocytes, culture, ova, and parasites are indicated unless symptoms subside within 48 hours.
5. Diverticulitis
   a. Acquired diverticula are saclike profusions of the intestinal mucosa through the muscularis, which are covered only by the serosa.
   b. Most commonly located in the sigmoid, their frequency decreases as one ascends the intestinal tract.
   c. Their frequency increases with age, reaching 20% to 50% in persons over 50 years of age.
   d. This is in contradistinction to appendicitis and ileitis, which occur most frequently during the second and third decades.
   e. Diverticulitis results when diverticulae become infected or perforate, which may lead to the formation of a pericolonic abscess.
   f. The principal symptom is LLQ abdominal pain, but if the sigmoid mesentery is elongated, the pain and tenderness may be in the RLQ.
   g. The patient may report prolonged periods of constipation, with intermitent episodes of lower abdominal pain sometimes relieved by defecation.
   h. On physical examination, the patient may appear clinically ill, with a fever of 101° to 102° F and dehydrated.

i. Leukocytosis with a left shift is present.
j. There is marked tenderness in the lower abdomen, frequently associated with a palpable mass.
k. Flat and upright abdominal films do not reveal signs of pneumoperitoneum unless a sigmoid diverticulum has ruptured freely into the abdominal cavity.
l. In the absence of signs of peritonitis, abscess formation, or obstruction, treatment is conservative by "resting the bowel" with a nasogastric tube for gastrointestinal tract decompression, intravenous antibiotics, intravenous fluid therapy, and possibly hyperalimentation.
m. As soon as the acute inflammatory signs have subsided, the possibility of colon cancer should be excluded by either endoscopic or radiologic means.

6. Meckel's diverticulitis
   a. Meckel's diverticulum is an embryologic remnant of the omphaloenteric duct.
   b. It is typically located on the antimesenteric border of the terminal ileum approximately 2 ft from the ileocecal valve.
   c. The diverticulum may be lined by gastric mucosa or by exocrine pancreatic tissue and may produce painless gastrointestinal bleeding of obscure cause.
   d. If ulceration occurs, the diverticulum can become inflamed, producing lower abdominal pain with a midline or right of midline location.
   e. Seen infrequently, this condition is hard to differentiate from acute appendicitis, and the diagnosis of Meckel's diverticulitis is most often retrospective.
7. Colon tumors
   a. Tumors of the colon (adenomatous polyps, villous tumors, adenocarcinomas, carcinoids, lymphomas, melanomas, and leiomyosarcomas) usually do not cause pain until they have progressed to the point of obstruction or invasion of pelvic organs.
   b. The most frequent and early symptoms of bowel carcinomas are change in bowel habits and abdominal pain.
   c. There may also be tenesmus, melena, and weight loss.
   d. When a mass is present, it is often located at the pelvic brim and may be difficult to distinguish from the normal pelvic organs by palpation, but most rectal tumors can be palpated on rectal examination.
8. Torsion of appendices epiploicae
   a. Rarely, the appendices epiploicae may twist and undergo necrosis. The resultant peritoneal irritation produces pain deep in the pelvis.
   b. This pain often has a rectal reference and is at times associated with tenesmus.
   c. The diagnosis is seldom made preoperatively.
9. Functional bowel disorder: See under CPP.

13.13 URINARY TRACT SOURCES OF PAIN

Urinalysis (U/A) is essential to determine the presence of pyuria or hematuria. Other considerations include urine culture, urethral culture, and cystoscopy.

1. Overdistended bladder
   a. Pain may simulate that produced by distension of a genital organ.
   b. On palpation, the tense bladder resembles a large ovarian cyst or pregnant uterus.
   c. This may occur in association with other conditions (e.g., acute urethritis, postoperative period).
2. Acute cystitis
   a. Pain is suprapubic, related to micturition, and accompanied by a burning sensation at the external urethral meatus.
   b. Patients may initially present with lower abdominal pressure and soreness, urinary frequency, urgency, dysuria, and possibly hematuria.
   c. U/A reveals pyuria, and urine culture is subsequently positive.
   d. Symptoms usually respond to adequate hydration and antibiotics.
3. Ureteral calculi
   a. Pain begins as an aching sensation that rapidly becomes severe, colicky, and radiates from the flank around the abdomen and down into the groin and labia majora, depending on the position of the stone in the upper urinary tract.
   b. Agitation and a constant search for a comfortable position with episodes of pain so severe as to interfere with respirations are common.
   c. Unless obstruction is complete, hematuria is the rule with or without pyuria.
   d. KUB, intravenous pyelogram (IVP), or U/S will generally demonstrate the stone, particularly if it is radiopaque.
4. Pelvic kidney: A congenitally misplaced kidney located in the retroperitoneal area in front of the sacrum has an increased incidence of infectious complications because of stasis and retrograde reflux from the bladder.
5. Urethral syndrome
   a. Symptoms of suprapubic pain, dysuria, urgency, frequency, dyspareunia, and absence of nocturia are prominent and the diagnosis is one of exclusion.
   b. A negative urine and urethral culture, STD, and vulvovaginitis evaluation should raise the suspicion of this syndrome.
   c. Urethrocystoscopic evaluation should be performed and urethral diverticulae, interstitial cystitis, and cancer of the bladder, urethra, vulva, cervix, or vagina should be ruled out.
   d. Treatment consists of a trial of antibiotics and, if without success, consideration for urethral dilation in the reproductive aged women and vaginal estrogen for perimenopausal and postmenopausal women.
6. Interstitial cystitis (IC)
   a. IC is a chronic aseptic inflammation of the bladder of unknown etiology.

b. Typical presentation is urinary frequency (day and nighttime), urgency, and pelvic or suprapubic pain often relieved by voiding.
c. Dysuria is uncommon.
d. IC is often a diagnosis of exclusion and by cystoscopy with hydrodistension looking for Hunner's ulcers and glomerulations.

13.14 VASCULAR SOURCES OF PAIN

1. Pelvic thrombophlebitis
   a. Pelvic thrombophlebitis may occur in the postoperative period or after obstetric complications of pelvic infection.
   b. Disease may be septic or primarily thrombotic, and pain may accompany severe disease.
   c. The presence of spiking temperatures, chills, tachycardia, an aching type of pelvic pain, and lack of response to antibiotics are suggestive of the diagnosis.
   d. The absence of a pelvic mass associated with pelvic wall tenderness tends to confirm the diagnosis, which may be imaged by venography or computed tomography.
   e. Treatment involves effective anticoagulation with heparin.
2. Small bowel mesenteric occlusion
   a. The pain produced by small bowel mesenteric occlusion (arterial, venous, or embolic) leading to bowel ischemia and necrosis is initially colicky, periumbilical, and associated with hyperactive bowel sounds.
   b. If unrecognized, ischemia will progress to infarction with the development of an ileus, loss of bowel sounds, generalized peritonitis, sepsis, hemoconcentration, and shock.
   c. Patients often have a history of atrial fibrillation, extensive atherosclerosis, or poor tissue perfusion.
   d. Abdominal examination is notable for the presence of minimal tenderness, mild diffuse rebound, and the patient often appears sicker than the abdominal signs would suggest in the initial phase.
   e. Plain and erect abdominal films most often show evidence of an ileus and thickening of the bowel wall caused by mucosal edema or hemorrhage ("thumbprinting").
   f. Management requires immediate surgical intervention.

13.15 SYSTEMIC CAUSES OF ABDOMINAL PAIN

Numerous medical conditions may be associated with recurrent lower abdominal pain, but this is rarely an isolated or presenting symptom.

1. Sickle cell disease
2. Diabetes mellitus
3. Drug withdrawal
4. Acute intermittent porphyria
5. Connective tissue disease
   a. Familial Mediterranean fever
   b. Henoch-Schönlein purpura
   c. Systemic lupus erythematosus

   d. Hereditary angioneurotic edema
   e. Periarteritis nodosa
6. Endocrine disorders
   a. Untreated hyperthyroidism, Addisonian crisis, and hyperparathyroidism may be associated with vague and poorly localized lower abdominal pain.
7. Infections
   a. Syphilis
   b. Tubercular peritonitis
   c. Herpes zoster virus

13.16 DYSMENORRHEA

Painful menstruation, or dysmenorrhea, is defined as primary when there is no associated organic pathology and secondary when there is demonstrable organic pathology.

1. Primary dysmenorrhea
   a. Primary dysmenorrhea is caused by prostaglandin-induced uterine contractions and ischemia.
   b. Primary dysmenorrhea tends to occur with the onset of ovulatory cycles following menarche and usually improves with time; coincides with the onset of menstrual bleeding; and frequently is associated with other prostaglandin mediated symptoms (e.g., nausea, vomiting, diarrhea, headache, and dizziness).
   c. Pain is sharp, crampy, midline without a lower quadrant or adnexal component, but may have radiation to the lower back and upper thighs. Pelvic examination in a nonmenstruating patient is unremarkable.
   d. Treatment is with nonsteroidal antiinflammatory drugs (NSAIDs) or oral contraceptives. Laparoscopy is indicated for failed medical management (rule out endometriosis).
2. Secondary dysmenorrhea
   a. Secondary dysmenorrhea is usually caused by endometriosis, adenomyosis, leiomyomas, and, less commonly, chronic salpingitis, an IUD, or congenital or acquired outflow tract obstruction, including cervical stenosis.
   b. Secondary dysmenorrhea most commonly begins in women who are in their 20s and progressively worsens; it may improve temporarily after childbirth.
   c. Pain is midline, may include one or both lower quadrants, and may begin long before menses and continue during or after it. Dyspareunia is common.
   d. Bimanual pelvic–abdominal examination may demonstrate uterine or adnexal tenderness, fixed uterine retroflexion, uterosacral nodularity, a pelvic mass, or an enlarged irregular uterus.
   e. Treatment is aimed at evaluation and management of the underlying condition. U/S, laparoscopy, and hysteroscopy may be necessary to establish the diagnosis.

13.17 ENDOMETRIOSIS

1. There is a wide spectrum of presentation and clinical course, but the presentation is classically a gradual increase in the duration of dysmenorrhea, appearance of premenstrual pain, and cyclic dyspareunia that gradually becomes continuous but remains worst perimenstrually.
2. Symptoms may be acute (e.g., ruptured endometrioma with an acute abdomen), but they are typically of a gradually increasing and chronic nature.
3. Physical examination may reveal a tender, relatively immobile uterus and adnexa, adnexal mass (endometrioma), fixed uterine retroflexion, or thickening and nodularity of the uterosacral ligament.
4. The severity of pain does not correlate with the amount of endometriosis.
5. Therapy is medical and surgical, depending on the severity of disease and the patient's reproductive plans. (Management is discussed in Chapter 10.)

13.18 ADENOMYOSIS

1. Adenomyosis is a benign uterine disease characterized by the growth of endometrial glands and stroma in the uterine myometrium at a depth of at least 2.5 mm from the basalis endometrium layer.
2. The typical patient is multiparous in her late 30s or early 40s, with classic symptoms of progressive dysmenorrhea or menorrhagia.
3. During the premenstrual period, symptomatic patients describe pelvic heaviness, pressure, or an aching sensation.
4. With the onset of menses, the pain becomes more acute and crampy.
5. Pelvic examination is significant for a mildly enlarged, boggy, tender uterus, especially during menses.
6. It is important to note that adenomyosis is a common histologic finding in asymptomatic patients.
7. There is no long-term, satisfactory medical treatment.
8. Success is variable with cyclic oral contraceptives and NSAIDs.
9. GNRH agonists may suppress adenomyosis growth, but any benefits last only as long as the drug is continued.
10. Unlike myomata uteri, there is no conservative surgery for adenomyosis.
11. If a patient is perimenopausal with anticipated cessation of ovarian function, medical therapy with GNRHa may obviate the need for hysterectomy.
12. If appropriate for the women's age, parity, and future reproductive plans, hysterectomy remains the definitive treatment.

13.19 ADHESIONS

1. The role of adhesions in abdominal and pelvic pain is controversial.
2. Recent studies demonstrate no difference in prevalence of pelvic adhesions in patients with CPP as compared with pain-free infertile

controls and no correlation between location or severity of pain with the location or severity of adhesions.

a. These studies suggest that surgical adhesiolysis is of questionable benefit.
b. However, other studies of laparoscopic adhesiolysis suggest that pain relief may be obtained in up to 75% of patients.

3. The pain may start within weeks of the physical insult responsible (e.g., pelvic infections, surgery).
4. In most instances, pain duration varies from moments to an hour or so, and may be related to physical activity.
5. Over time, pain originating with adhesions may spread, as intestinal, muscular, and chronic pain syndrome factors come into play.
6. Depression and chronicity of pain, with a resultant lower pain threshold, serve to make the physical findings less distinct and treatment more complex.
7. The inability to diagnosis adhesions accurately by U/S or other imaging techniques makes laparoscopy essential to the diagnosis and treatment.
8. Preoperative evaluation should include studies to exclude more acute causes of pain.
9. Bowel studies (endoscopy or barium enema) should be limited to those women exhibiting signs (e.g., hematachezia, mucus) as opposed to only symptoms of bowel disease.
10. Laparotomy for pain attributed to adhesions should be reserved for cases of intestinal obstruction refractory to medical management.

13.20 OVULATORY PAIN (MITTELSCHMERZ)

1. Midcycle pelvic pain is usually a manifestation of peritoneal irritation caused by the release of blood or follicular fluid from the ovary at the time of ovulation.
2. Pain is generally unilateral, sharp, and dissipates within a few hours but may be intense and prolonged.
3. There may or may not be associated vaginal spotting.
4. When the pain is localized to the RLQ, the differential diagnosis of appendicitis can be challenging.
5. Less commonly, endometriosis or other organic conditions may be associated with isolated midcycle pain or midcycle exacerbation of continuous CPP.
6. Treatment is often expectant; otherwise NSAIDs, or ovarian suppression with oral contraceptives.

13.21 OVARIAN REMNANT SYNDROME

1. Results from residual ovarian cortical tissue that is left *in situ* after a difficult oophorectomy (severe endometriosis or PID).
2. Often the patient has had multiple pelvic operations with the uterus and adnexa removed sequentially.
3. Patient usually complains of cyclic pelvic pain that may be accompanied by peritoneal signs and usually arise 2 to 5 years after surgery.

4. Pelvic examination may reveal a tender mass in the lateral region of the pelvis and U/S usually confirms a mass with sonographic characteristics of ovarian tissue.
5. Estradiol and FSH assays reveal a premenopausal picture, although on occasion the remaining ovarian tissue may not be active enough to suppress FSH levels.
6. Medical treatment with danazol, progestins, or oral contraceptives has mixed results and GNRHa therapy is impractical for long-term therapy.
7. Definitive therapy is usually with surgical extirpation.

13.22 PELVIC CONGESTION SYNDROME

1. Pelvic congestion syndrome is an ill-defined syndrome marked by the presence of continuous lower abdominal pain, premenstrual or menstrual accentuation of pain, postcoital aching, dyspareunia, low back pain, increased intensity while standing or jumping, and often associated with premenstrual syndrome.
2. Pelvic examination is usually unremarkable except uterine retroversion is common, and often there is tenderness in the posterior fornix.
3. Laparoscopy may show a normal pelvis or prominent, enlarged, broad ligament veins, the significance of which in the pathophysiology in this condition is uncertain.
4. Treatment is as with the CPP syndrome.

13.23 "TRIGGER POINT" ABDOMINAL WALL PAIN

1. Trigger point pain is usually pinpoint, well localized, and of unknown etiology.
2. Diagnosis is confirmed if the patient's pain can be reproduced by pinching of the subcutaneous tissue directly beneath the point of maximal tenderness and by eliciting increased, rather than decreased, tenderness with palpation during voluntary guarding (rectus flexion).
3. Several treatment modalities have shown to be effective, including the following:
   a. Transcutaneous electric nerve stimulation (TENS)
   b. Accupuncture
   c. Massage
   d. Infiltration with a variety of agents (steroids and local anesthetics)
4. A common regimen is 5 to 10 cc of a long-acting topical anesthetic (e.g., bupivicaine, 0.25% to 0.5%) injected directly into the hyperpathic trigger points after it is first localized with the tip of a 25G 1½-inch needle.
5. Injections are repeated on a biweekly to monthly basis initially, followed by longer intervals, until a long-term or permanent response is achieved.
6. The overall response rate is approximately 75% to 90%, with most patients requiring three to five injections.

13.24 FUNCTIONAL BOWEL DISORDERS

1. Irritable bowel syndrome (IBS) and chronic constipation are symptomatic manifestations of altered bowel motility and are the most common medical diagnosis in women with CPP.
2. IBS is a common cause of lower abdominal pain that is usually intermittent, crampy, predominantly LLQ in location, but occasionally the pain is constant and often improved after defecation.
3. The pain may last for only a few minutes, but at least 50% of patients have pain for hours to days and 20% of patients may complain of pain for weeks or longer.
4. Associated symptoms include the following:
   a. Excessive flatulence
   b. Alternating diarrhea and constipation
   c. Passage of mucus
   d. Altered stool form
   e. Abdominal distension or bloating
5. Symptoms are usually worse during periods of stress, tension, anxiety, depression, and with the premenstrual and menstrual phases of the cycle.
6. The diagnosis is usually made by history and the exclusion of other disorders and therefore sigmoidoscopy and barium enema are often necessary.
7. IBS is a waxing and waning disorder and treatment consists of reassurance, dietary management, psychotherapy (stress reduction), and medical adjuncts, including anticholinergic agents.
8. *Psyllium* hydrophilic mucilloid, one tablespoon (or two wafers), once or twice daily with 8 oz of water or juice is a very effective regimen and often obviates the need for medical regimens.
9. To improve compliance, patients should be apprised of other advantages of a high-fiber diet, including reduced colon cancer and diverticular disease, and up to 15% mean reduction in serum cholesterol level.
10. Simethicone, 80 to 120 mg PO (chewable), pc, and qhs is a useful adjunct for abdominal distension and bloating.
11. Care must be exercised to avoid exacerbation of symptoms or substitution of one problem (diarrhea) for another (constipation).
12. Two medical adjuncts useful for treatment of unresponsive or severe hypermotile symptoms (diarrhea, distension, and gaseousness) are diphenoxylate/atropine (2.5 mg PO, qid, may be doubled to 5 mg PO qid, as indicated) and loperamide (two capsules initially, followed by one capsule after each unformed stool, not to exceed eight capsules or 16 mg/day).

13.25 CHRONIC PELVIC PAIN

1. Etiology and evaluation
   a. The interplay of psychosocial and sexual factors, coupled with the frequent involvement of nongynecologic organ systems into a

symptom complex, makes the approach to CPP clinically challenging.

b. The patient with CPP must be evaluated thoroughly and empathetically in a nonhurried fashion.
c. Many patients with CPP will develop the chronic pelvic pain syndrome in which the pain is accompanied by impaired function in daily activities.
d. These patients are often distraught, angry, and demanding and have a history of prolonged disability, loss of employment, sexual dysfunction, marital discord, divorce, and signs of depression (especially sleep disturbances).

2. Prevalence and occurrence
   a. CPP accounts for an estimated 10% to 20% of outpatient gynecologic visits, 30% of laparoscopies, and 12% to 16% of hysterectomies performed in the United States each year.
   b. CPP spans all age groups with an average age of 27 to 29 years and mean duration of pain greater than 2.5 years.
   c. Compared with pain-free age-matched controls, there is no significant difference with regard to mean gravidity, parity, rates of elective abortion, race, and educational level.
   d. However, CPP patients have undergone five times more previous surgeries, have sought treatment four times as many times for somatic complaints unrelated to CPP, and some studies show they are three to seven times more likely to have experienced major sexual or physical abuse.
3. Treatment
   a. Specific medical treatment of functional bowel disorders or abdominal trigger points, optimization of nonnarcotic analgesics, and empiric low-dose TCA therapy are the initial therapeutic modalities for CPP.
   b. In addition, cognitive behavioral pain management treatment to promote self-management of pain and to reduce associated affective symptomatology should be initiated simultaneously with a multidisciplinary team approach.
   c. Treatment includes reducing disability by progressive activities, pain behavior modification, reemployment, and substance abuse counseling.
   d. Cognitive distraction techniques, including relaxation and imagery, are taught to reduce attentional focusing on pain signals.
   e. Stress management and pain coping techniques are also dealt with.
   f. A comprehensive wellness program, focused on nutrition, sleep, hygiene, and increasing physical and constructive activity, is also critical.
   g. Additional interventions such as psychotherapy for depression, marital and family counseling, and sex therapy should be initiated as needed.
4. The goals of CPP therapy include the following:
   a. To rule out serious life-threatening pathology (e.g., cancer, or major depression with suicidal ideation)

b. To relieve suffering by treating identifiable symptoms and concurrent psychologic pathology
c. To restore normal function by managing symptoms and minimizing disability

5. Drug therapy plays an important role in CPP management.
   a. Analgesics
      (1) "As needed" (prn) dosing is discouraged because analgesics are more effective if taken before symptoms are severe.
      (2) Prn dosing can actually increase pain by encouraging the patient to focus on symptoms while monitoring pain severity.
      (3) Begin with less expensive NSAIDs (e.g., ibuprofen, 400 to 800 mg q6h to q8h) on a scheduled basis.
      (4) There is a wide variation in individual response to different agents; therefore, at least three different NSAIDs should be tried before therapy is declared ineffective (e.g., naproxen, 250 to 500 mg, q6h to q8h; naproxen sodium, 275 to 500 mg, q6h to q8h; mefenamic acid, 250 to 500 mg, q6h to q8h).
      (5) The most frequent side effects limiting NSAIDs are gastrointestinal upset and risk of peptic ulceration, which can be mitigated by the use of misoprostol (200 mg, qid for the duration of analgesic therapy) for those high-risk patients.
   b. Narcotics should be avoided because they are associated with tolerance, habituation, and an increase in baseline pain levels that may be caused by an endorphin-depleting effect.
      (1) These agents also relax smooth muscle and may complicate concurrent functional bowel disorder, especially constipation.
      (2) Narcotics may also cause sedation and altered cognition, which impairs restoration of normal function—the primary goal of CPP rehabilitation.
   c. Tricyclic antidepressants (TCAs)
      (1) TCAs have been shown to be effective in many chronic pain syndromes (e.g., arthritis, cancer, headache, backache, neuralgia).
      (2) The mechanism of action is unclear but believed to be caused by repletion of serum beta-endorphins, endogenous morphine-like peptides that can modulate systemic pain responses.
      (3) Higher doses are used to treat depression, which may complicate up to 60% of chronic pain of any organ.
      (4) Lower doses are used for CPP as well as sleep disorders.
      (5) CPP is commonly complicated by sleep disturbances that can further potentiate pain perception and impair pain tolerance and function.
      (6) TCA therapy for patients without significant mood disturbance is usually initiated with imipramine, amitriptyline, or doxepin, 10 to 25 mg qhs.
      (7) This is titrated to 50 or 75 mg as needed.
      (8) Full antidepressant dosages (up to 300 mg/day) are reserved for patients with documented major mood disturbances.
      (9) It is important to stress to patients that low doses of TCAs are used to treat pain and sleep disturbances and high doses are reserved for depression.

(10) Prozac, 20 mg PO, qm, is an effective and safe alternative for patients with moderate to severe depression or for patients with moderate mood disturbances failing appropriate titrated TCA therapy.

d. Functional Bowel disorder medications (Refer to Section 13.21.)
e. Local anesthetics (Refer to Section 13.20.)
f. Ovarian cycle suppressants
   (1) Functional cyclic pain is usually amenable to antiprostaglandin therapy and to cycle suppression.
   (2) For patients who fail at least three cycles of NSAIDs prescribed on a scheduled (usually tid) basis in appropriately titrated dosages, the choice of cycle suppressive therapy should be based on supply, cost, and patient acceptance.
   (3) Oral contraceptives (OBCP) and progestins are favored as primary therapy, although GNRHa may have a limited (primarily diagnostic) role in refractory cases.
   (4) Combination OBCP containing a sufficient dosage of estrogen to suppress folliculogenesis should be used such as monophasic ethinyl estradiol, 35 μg.
   (5) Synthetic progestin regimes are medroxyprogesterone acetate (MPA), 20 to 40 mg PO, qd, or 150 to 300 mg, IM, q3mo.
   (6) Duration of therapy may extend from months to years, depending on the rapidity of response, tolerance of the regimen, and family planning considerations.
   (7) Synthetic progestin therapy is frequently accompanied by breakthrough bleeding or spotting that may necessitate the addition of supplemental estrogen (ethinylestradiol, 20 μg/dl, or conjugated equine estrogen, 0.625 mg PO, qd, prn) to stabilize the endometrium.

6. Unfortunately, many patients who report relief of CPP after treatment may later present with other chronic disabling symptoms (e.g., headache, chronic fatigue) and, therefore, the ultimate goal of therapy is long-term freedom from disabling somatic symptoms and normalization of a health-related quality of life.

Suggested reading

ACOG Technical Bulletin: *Chronic pelvic pain*, #129, June 1989.
Howard F: The role of laparoscopy in chronic pelvic pain: promise and pitfalls, *Obstet Gyn Surv* 46:357-386, 1993.
Peters AAW et al: A randomized clinical trial to compare two different approaches in women with chronic pelvic pain, *Obstet Gynecol* 77:740, 1991.
Rapkin AJ, Reading AE: Chronic pelvic pain: current problems in obstetrics, *Gynecol Fertil* 14:99-137, 1991.
Silen W: *Cope's early diagnosis of the acute abdomen*, 1991, Oxford University Press.
Stovall T, Ling F: *Extrauterine pregnancy: denical diagnosis and management*, New York, 1993, McGraw-Hill.

14 Differential Diagnosis of Benign Gynecologic Conditions

Dennis M. Weppner, M.D.

14.1 ABNORMAL GENITAL TRACT BLEEDING

Premenarcheal

1. Trauma
2. Genital tract neoplasm
   a. Cervical
   b. Vaginal
   c. Uterine
3. Foreign body
4. Exogenous estrogen
5. Sporadic gonadotropin surge
6. Precocious puberty
7. Pseudopuberty
8. Neoplasm, hormone secreting
   a. Estrogen-granulosa cell tumor
   b. Human chorionic gonadotropin (HCG)-embryonal carcinoma
   c. Choriocarcinoma
9. Adrenal tumors
10. Craniopharyngioma
11. Albright's syndrome
12. von Recklinghausen's disease
13. Adrenal hyperplasia
14. Hypothyroidism
15. Idiopathic, gastiointestinal bleeding
16. Urinary tract bleeding

Reproductive age

1. Menorrhagia
2. Hypermenorrhea
3. Metrorrhagia
4. Oligomenorrhea
5. Polymenorrhea
6. Hypomenorrhea

Pregnancy

1. Intrauterine pregnancy with bleeding
   a. Placenta previa
   b. Vasa previa
   c. Abruptio placentae
   d. Spontaneous abortion
2. Ectopic pregnancy

Neoplasia

1. Genital tract
   a. Cervical
   b. Endometrial
   c. Gestational trophoblastic disease (GTD)
   d. Ovary: hormone producing
   e. Vaginal
   f. Vulvar
   g. Fallopian tube
2. Metastatic or contiguous involvement
3. Other
   a. Central nervous system (CNS)
   b. Adrenal
   c. Thyroid

Polyp

1. Cervical, endometrial
2. Leiomyoma: submucosal
3. Adenomyosis
4. Ectropion

Infection

Cervicitis: *Chlamydia trachomatis*

Endocrine dysfunction

1. Hypothalamic or pituitary
2. Polycystic ovaries (PCO)
3. Adrenal
4. Hypothyroidism or hyperthryoidism

Iatrogenic

1. Intrauterine device (IUD)
2. Drug use
   a. Estrogens
   b. Progestins
   c. Androgens
3. Nonhormonal drugs
   a. Phenothiazines
   b. Tricyclic antidepressants
   c. Reserpine
   d. Alpha-methyldopa

Blood dyscrasias

1. von Willebrand's
2. Thrombocytopenia
3. Disseminated intravascular coagulation (DIC)
4. Chronic anticoagulation
   a. Heparin
   b. Coumadin

Dysfunctional uterine bleeding

1. Ovulatory
   a. Midcycle: inadequate proliferative estrogen
   b. Late cycle: inadequate progesterone production
2. Altered prostaglandin metabolism: increased PGI
3. Anovulatory
   a. Disturbance
      (1) Hypothalmic
      (2) Pitituary
      (3) Ovarian axis
   b. Emotional stress
   c. Anorexia
   d. Strenuous exercise
   e. Weight gain

Postmenopausal Bleeding

1. Neoplasm
   a. Endometrial hyperplasia
   b. Endometrial cancer
   c. Other tumors of uterus (See Section 14.12.)
2. Other pelvic neoplasm
   a. Direct extension or metastatic
      (1) Vulva
      (2) Vagina
      (3) Cervix
      (4) Fallopian tube
      (5) Ovary
   b. Endometrial or cervical polyp
   c. Unopposed estrogen
      (1) Exogenous
      (2) Endogenous
         (a) Peripheral conversion
         (b) Tumor production
            i. Granulosa cell tumor
            ii. Thecoma
3. Trauma: vaginal
4. Infection
   a. Vaginitis
   b. Endometritis
   c. Vulvar dystrophy
   d. Vaginal atrophy

e. Idiopathic
f. Urinary tract bleeding
   (1) Urinary tract infection (UTI)
   (2) Cystitis
   (3) Bladder tumor
g. Gastrointestinal (GI) tract bleeding

14.2 AMENORRHEA

Primary amenorrhea (limited or no secondary sexual development)

1. Gonadal defects
   a. Gonadal dysgenesis
      (1) Turner's syndrome
      (2) Turner's mosaic
      (3) Swyer's syndrome
   b. "Pure" gonadal dysgenesis
   c. Resistant ovary (Savage) syndrome
   d. Ovarian
      (1) Trauma
      (2) Postinfection
      (3) Radiation
   e. 17-Alpha-hydroxylase deficiency
   f. Androgen insensitivity syndrome
      (1) Testicular feminization
      (2) Alpha-reductase deficiency
2. Hypothalmic
   a. Pituitary dysfunction: pituitary dwarfs
      (1) Craniopharyngioma
      (2) Tuberculosis (TB)
      (3) Trauma
      (4) Sarcoidosis
   b. Systemic illness
   c. Anorexia nervosa
   d. Isolated gonadotropin deficiency
      (1) Kallmann's syndrome
   e. Hypothyroidism

Primary or secondary amenorrhea (normal secondary sexual development)

1. Hypothalamic
   a. Stress induced
      (1) Psychogenic
      (2) Nutritional
   b. Environmental stress
   c. Anorexia nervosa
   d. Weight loss
   e. Exercise related
   f. Bulimia

2. Tumors
   a. Craniopharyngioma
   b. Glioma
   c. Endodermal sinus tumor
3. Psychotropic drug therapy, pseudocyesis
4. Pituitary abnormalities
   a. Postpartum infarction
      (1) Sheehan's syndrome
   b. Simmond's syndrome
   c. Pituitary stalk section
   d. Tumor
      (1) Prolactinoma
      (2) Craniopharyngioma
      (3) Radiation
      (4) Surgery or trauma
5. Thyroid abnormalities
   a. Hypothyroidism
   b. Hyperthyroidism
6. Adrenal abnormalities
   a. Congenital adrenal hyperplasia
   b. 21-Hydroxylase deficiency
   c. 3β-01-Dehydrogenase deficiency
   d. 11β-hydroxylase deficiency
   e. Cushing's syndrome
   f. Cushing's disease
   g. PCO
   h. Hyperthecosis
   i. Thecoma
   j. Adrenal tumor: hormone secreting
7. Ovarian abnormalities
   a. Ovarian failure
      (1) Constitutional
      (2) Chromosomally related
      (3) Postviral oophoritis
      (4) Postradiation
      (5) Postchemotherapy
   b. Polycystic ovary syndrome
   c. Premature ovarian failure
8. Neoplasm: hormone secreting
   a. Sertoli cell tumor
   b. Leydig cell tumor: androgen
   c. Granulosa cell tumor: estrogen
9. Endometrium and outflow tract: uterine synechiae (Asherman's syndrome)
10. Endometrial fibrosis
    a. TB
    b. Schistosomiasis
11. Endometrial atrophy
    a. Radiation
    b. Postmenopause

12. Congenital abnormality, uterus or outflow tract
    a. Imperforate hymen
    b. Transverse vaginal septum
    c. Atresia of vagina
    d. Absence of uterus and vagina
        (1) Complete agenesis
        (2) Müllerian aplasia
        (3) Rokitansky-Kuster-Hauser syndrome

14.3 ASCITES

1. Congestive heart failure
2. Portal vein obstruction
    a. Portal cirrhosis
    b. Hepatic amyloidosis
    c. Hilar lymphadenopathy, hepatic
3. Hepatic endothrombophlebitis
4. Budd-Chiari syndrome
5. Inferior vena cava thrombosis
6. Acute or chronic peritonitis
7. Neoplastic implant
8. Tuberculosis
9. Hydatid disease
10. Hypoproteinemia
    a. Nephrosis
    b. Anemia
11. Thoracic duct obstruction
    a. Injury thorax
    b. Abdomen
    c. Tuberculosis
    d. Filariasis
    e. Myxedema
    f. Primary amyloidosis
    g. Thiamine deficiency
    h. Wet beriberi
    i. Pancreatic ascites
    j. Pyogenic peritonitis
    k. Tuberculous peritonitis
    l. Neoplasm
        (1) Pelvic carcinomatosis
            (a) Ovarian
            (b) Peritoneal
    m. Ovarian hyperstimulation syndrome
12. Meigs syndrome
13. Constrictive pericarditis, myxedema

14.4 BREAST INFLAMMATORY LESION

1. Acute mastitis
   a. Infectous agent
      (1) *Staphylocccus aureus*
      (2) Streptocci
      (3) Foreign body
   b. Trauma
2. Chronic mastitis
3. Granuloma
   a. TB
   b. Actinomycosis
   c. Blastomycosis
   d. Cryptococosis
4. Foreign body mastitis
   a. Suture
   b. Silicone mammoplasty
5. Plasma cell mastitis
   a. Duct ectasia
6. Fat necrosis
   a. Postbiopsy
   b. Trauma
   c. Injection
   d. Mammoplasty
7. Necrosis or infarction
   a. Anticoagulant therapy
   b. Pregnancy
   c. Lactation
   d. Atherosclerosis in elderly
8. Breast malignancy (see Section 14.5)

14.5 BREAST MASS

Benign

1. Stromal fibrosis
2. Adenosis
3. Intraductal hyperplasia
4. Atypical epithelial hyperplasia
5. Sclerosing adenosis
6. Lobular hyperplasia
7. Juvenile hypertrophy
8. Galactocele
9. Duct papilloma
10. Fibroadenoma
11. Cystosarcoma phyllodes
12. Tubular adenoma
13. Lactating adenoma
14. Granular cell myoblastoma
15. Hemangioma
16. Fibroma

17. Schwannoma
18. Lipoma

Malignant

1. Ductal adenocarcinoma
   a. In situ
   b. Infiltrating
2. Lobular adenocarcinoma
3. Variants of carcinoma
   a. Carcinoid
   b. Squamous cell
   c. Spindle cell
   d. Other
4. Sarcoma, carcinosarcoma

14.6 ENDOCRINOPATHIES

Hirsutism

1. Regular menstruation
   a. Elevated alpha-reductase activity
   b. Genetic
      (1) Racial
      (2) Familial
   c. Physiologic
      (1) Premature pubarche
      (2) Precocious puberty
      (3) Puberty
      (4) Pregnancy
      (5) Menopause
   d. Idiopathic
   e. Local trauma
   f. Chronic skin irritation
   g. Drug related
      (1) Phenytoin
      (2) Diazoxide
      (3) Hexachlorobenzene
      (4) Adrenocorticotropic hormone (ACTH)
      (5) Corticosteroids
      (6) Progestogens
      (7) Anabolic agents
      (8) Androgen
   h. Hamartoma or nevi
      (1) Pigmented nevi with hair
      (2) Nevus pilosus
      (3) Pigmented hairy epidermal nevus
2. Irregular menstruation
   a. Adrenal origin
      (1) Congenital or adult-onset adrenal hyperplasia
      (2) Androgen-producing tumors

b. Ovarian origin
   (1) PCO
   (2) Androgen producing tumors
      (a) Arrhenoblastoma
      (b) Granulosa-theca cell tumor
      (c) Luteoma of pregnancy
   (3) Hyperthecosis
   (4) Chronic anovulation
      (a) Hypothalmic amenorrhea
      (b) Psychologic or emotional disorders
      (c) Hyperthyroidism
      (d) Hypothyroidism
c. Pituitary origin
   (1) Cushing's syndrome
   (2) Acromegaly
   (3) Sheehan's syndrome
   (4) Simmond's syndrome
d. Genetic
   (1) Male pseudohermaphroditism
   (2) Incomplete testicular feminization
   (3) Y-containing mosaics
   (4) Turner's syndrome

Hyperprolactinemia

1. Physiologic causes
   a. Sleep
   b. Nursing
   c. Breast stimulation
   d. Stress
   e. Vigorous exercise
   f. Coitus
   g. Pregnancy
2. Pharmacologic causes
   a. Phenothiazines
   b. Butyrophenones
   c. Thyrotrophin-releasing hormone (TRH)
   d. Opiates
   e. Endorphins
   f. Reserpine
   g. Metoclopramide
   h. a-Methyldopa
   i. Estrogens
3. Pathologic
   a. Hypothyroidism
   b. Idiopathic
   c. Pituitary adenoma
   d. Pituitary stalk section
   e. Chronic renal failure

Precocious puberty

1. True precocious puberty
   a. Constitutional
      (1) Increased gonadotropins
   b. Idiopathic
   c. Cerebral lesion
      (1) Rickets
      (2) Skull fracture
      (3) Craniopharyngioma
      (4) Optic glioma
      (5) Astrocytoma
      (6) Suprasellar teratoma
      (7) Hypothalamic tumor
      (8) Pineal tumor
      (9) Hypothalamic trauma or surgery
   d. Postinflammatory reaction
      (1) Toxoplasmosis
      (2) Congenital syphilis
      (3) TB
      (4) Encephalitis
      (5) Meningitis
      (6) Hydrocephalus
   e. Hypothyroidism
   f. von Recklinghausen's disease
   g. McCune-Albright syndrome
   h. Polyostotic fibrous dysplasia
   i. Hypothalamic hamartoma
   j. Tuberous sclerosis
   k. Cushing's disease
2. Precocious pseudopuberty: ectopic gonadotropin production
   a. Adrenal
      (1) Congenital adrenal hyperplasia
      (2) Steroid producing adrenal tumor
   b. Ovarian
      (1) Dysgerminoma
      (2) Teratoma
      (3) Choriocarcinoma
   c. Exogenous
      (1) Ingestion of estrogen
      (2) Birth control pills (BCP)
      (3) Estrogen-containing tonics, lotions, creams
   d. Chorioepithelioma
   e. Hepatoblastoma

Delayed puberty

1. Hypergonadotropic hypogonadism: gonadal dysgenesis
   a. Turner's syndrome or Turner's mosaic
2. 17-Alpha-hydroxylase deficiency

3. Ovarian damage
   a. Torsion
   b. Inflammation
4. Hypogonadotropic hypogonadism
   a. Physiologic
   b. Weight loss
   c. Anorexia nervosa
   d. Hypothyroidism
   e. Congenital adrenal hyperplasma (CAH)
   f. Cushing's syndrome
   g. Prolactinoma
   h. GNRH deficiency
   i. Hypopituitarism
   j. Congenital CNS defects
   k. Pituitary adenoma
   l. Craniopharyngioma
   m. Postsurgical hypopituitarism
5. Eugonadism
   a. Müllerian agenesis
   b. Vaginal septum
   c. Imperforate hymen
   d. Androgen insensitivity syndrome

14.7 FEMALE REPRODUCTIVE TRACT ABNORMALITIES

Congenital structural defects

1. Vaginal septum
   a. Longitudinal
   b. Transverse
2. Imperforate hymen
3. Upper vaginal atresia
4. Rokitansky-Kuster-Hauser syndrome
5. Pelvic kidney
6. Testicular feminization
7. Mesonephric duct remnants
   a. Appendix vesiculosa
   b. Epoophoron
   c. Paroophoron
   d. Gartner's duct cyst
8. Paramesonephric duct remnant
   a. Hydatid of Morgagni
9. Vaginal adenosis
10. Müllerian fusion defects
    a. Hypoplasia
    b. Agenesis
    c. Unicornuate
    d. Bicornuate
    e. Didelphus
    f. Arcuate

g. Septate
h. Diethylstilbesterol (DES) related

Acquired structural defect

1. Trauma perineal
2. Vaginal
3. Cervical
   a. Obstetric
      (1) Episiotomy: first, second, third degree tear
      (2) Sulcus tear
   b. Coitus
   c. Sexual assault
   d. Fall
   e. Motor vehicle accident (MVA)
4. Loss of pelvic support
   a. Hypoestrogenism
   b. Multiparity
   c. Congenital laxity of connective tissue
   d. Idiopathic
   e. Urethrocoele
   f. Cystocoele
   g. Rectocoele
   h. Enterocoele
   i. Uterine prolapse: first, second, third degree
   j. Vaginal vault prolapse

Genital tract fistulae

1. Vesicocolic
2. Ureterocolic
3. Vesicouterine
4. Vesicocervical
5. Vesicovaginal
6. Ureterovaginal
7. Rectovaginal
8. Urethrovaginal
9. Vaginoperianal

14.8 GENITAL DISCHARGE

1. Physiologic discharge
   a. Cervical mucus
   b. Vaginal transudation
   c. Bacteria
   d. Squamous epithelial cells
2. Individual variation
3. Pregnancy
4. Sexual response
5. Menstrual cycle variation
6. Infection (See Section 14.10.)

7. Foreign body
    a. Tampon
    b. Cervical cap
    c. Other
8. Neoplasm (See Section 14.12.)
9. Fistula
10. IUD
11. Cervical ectropion
12. Spermacide
13. Nongenital causes
    a. Urinary incontinence
    b. Urinary tract fistula
    c. Crohn's disease
    d. Rectovaginal fistula

14.9 INFERTILITY

Male factor

1. Abnormal semen
    a. History of testicular injury
    b. Surgery
    c. Mumps
    d. Heat
        (1) Sauna
        (2) Jockey shorts
    e. Allergy
    f. Radiation
    g. Industrial or environmental toxins
    h. Marijuana, cigarette smoking
    i. Cimetidine
    j. Spironolactone
    k. Furadantin
    l. Sulfasalazine
    m. Chemotherapy
    n. Ulcerative colitis
        (1) Sulfasalazine
    o. Coital timing
    p. DES
    q. Immunologic
    r. Incompatible cervical mucus
    s. Abnormal sperm production
2. Anatomic
    a. Hypospadias
    b. Retrograde ejaculation
    c. Prostatectomy
    d. Obstruction or absence of vas deferens
    e. Congenitally absent fructose
    f. Hyalinization of seminiferous tubules
    g. Mumps orchitis
    h. Cryptorchidism

i. Klinefelter's syndrome
j. Infection
(1) *Mycoplasma*
(2) *Chlamydia*
k. Varicocele
l. Vasectomy
3. Endocrine
a. Germ cell aplasia: increased follicle-stimulating hormone (FSH)
b. Hypogonadotropic hypogonadism: decreased testosterone
c. Hyperprolactinemia
d. Hypothyroidism or hyperthyroidism
e. Isolated gonadotropin deficiency

Female factor

1. Age
2. Delayed childbearing
3. Marriage postponement
4. Contraception
5. Abortion
6. Ovulatory disorders
a. Intracranial tumor
b. Stress
c. Obesity
d. Anorexia
e. Systemic disease
f. Physiologic
g. Noncyclic production
(1) FSH
(2) Luteinizing hormone (LH)
(3) Estrogen
h. Abnormal ovarian or adnexal steroid production
i. Luteal phase defect
7. Tubal peritoneal factors
a. Tubal obstruction
(1) Cornu
(2) Isthmus
(3) Fimbrial
(4) Peritube or adhesions
b. Pelvic adhesions
c. Inflammatory bowel disease (IBD)
d. Endometriosis
e. Appendicitis
f. Ovarian cyst rupture
(1) Dermoid
(2) Other
g. Previous abdominal surgery
h. Foreign body reaction
8. Cervical factors
a. Cervical canal stenosis
b. Abnormal or hostile mucus
c. Endocervical polyp

d. Endometriosis
e. TB
f. Surgical: cone or cautery
g. Synechiae
h. Preovulatory estrogen deficiency
i. Endocervicitis
   (1) *Chlamydia*
   (2) Other

9. Uterine factors
   a. Polyp
   b. Myoma
   c. Synechiae
   d. Asherman's anomaly
   e. Müllerian anomaly
      (1) Didelphys
      (2) Unicornuate
      (3) Septate
   f. Arcuate
   g. Bicornuate
   h. Hypoplasia or agenesis
   i. DES related
   j. Infection
      (1) *Mycoplasma*
      (2) *Toxoplasma gondii*
   k. Unexplained
   l. Idiopathic
   m. Immunologic
      (1) Sperm allergy
      (2) Antisperm antibody
   n. Hypothyroidism or hyperthyroidism
   o. Diabetes mellitus
   p. Collagen vascular disease (SLE)
   q. Disorders of ovulation
   r. Pituitary adenoma (See hyperprolactinemia, endocrinopathy, p. 263.)

14.10 LOWER REPRODUCTIVE TRACT INFECTION

Bacterial

1. *Neisseria gonorrhoeae*
   a. Bartholin
   b. Skene
   c. Periurethral
2. *Chlamydia trachomatis*
   a. Cervicitis
   b. Lymphogranuloma venereum
3. *Treponema pallidum*
   a. Primary, secondary, tertiary, and congenital syphylis
4. *Gardnerella vaginalis*
   a. *Bacteroides vivus*
   b. Mobiluncus

5. *Hemophilus ducreyi*
   a. Chancroid
6. *Calymmatobacterium granulomatis*
   a. Granuloma inguinale
7. Donovanosis
8. *Corynebacterium minutissimum*
   a. Erythrasma
9. Lower genital tract abscess
   a. Bartholin gland or duct
   b. Skene's gland
   c. Follicular abscess
   d. Hydradenitis suppurativa
   e. Surgical or obstetric site infection

Viral

1. Human papillomavirus: high-risk or low-risk subtype
2. Herpes simplex virus (HSV): HSV-1, HSV-2
   a. Primary
   b. Recurrent
3. Mulloscum contagiosum
4. Human immunodeficiency virus (HIV)

Fungal

1. *Candida albicans*
2. *C. tropicalis*
3. *C. stellatoidea*
4. *C. krusei*
5. *C. (Torulopsis) glabrata*
6. *Trichophyton rubium:* tinea cruris
7. *Pityrosporum orbiculare:* pityriasis versicolor

Protozoal

1. *Trichomonas vaginalis*

Parasitic

1. *Sarcoptes scabiei:* scabies
2. *Pthirus pubis:* pediculosis pubis

14.11 OVARIAN FAILURE

1. Menopause: climacteric
   a. Physiologic
      (1) Age
      (2) Heredity
      (3) Racial variation
      (4) Cigarette smoking
      (5) Nutritional status
2. Premature
   a. Genetic
   b. Turner's mosaic

   c. Iatrogenic
      (1) Surgical oophorectomy
      (2) Chemotherapy
      (3) Ionizing radiation
   d. Autoimmune endocrinopathy
   e. Idiopathic
3. Hypoestrogenemia
   a. Vasomoter instability
   b. Urogenital atrophy
   c. Psychosomatic complaints
   d. Osteoporosis
   e. Arteriosclerotic vascular disease
   f. Amenorrhea

14.12 PELVIC MASS—GYNECOLOGIC CAUSES

Vagina

1. Benign tumors
   a. Imperforate hymen: hematocolpos
   b. Transverse septum
   c. Longitudinal septum
   d. Vaginal duplication
   e. Gartner's duct cyst
   f. Inclusion cyst
   g. Uterine prolapse
   h. Cystocoele
   i. Rectocoele
   j. Enterocele
   k. Prolapsed fallopian tube
   l. Polyp
   m. Leiomyoma
   n. Fibroma
   o. Rhabdomyoma
   p. Mixed tumor
   q. Granular cell tumor
   r. Endometriosis
2. Malignant tumor
   a. Squamous carcinoma
   b. Verrucous carcinoma
   c. Basal cell carcinoma
   d. Adenocarcinoma
   e. Sarcoma
   f. Leiomyosarcoma
   g. Embryonal rhabdomyosarcoma
   h. Mixed Müllerian tumor
   i. Endodermal sinus tumor
   j. Melanoma
   k. Metastatic tumor
   l. Clear cell adenocarcinoma

Cervix

1. Benign
   a. Polyp
   b. Inclusion cyst
   c. Leiomyoma
   d. Hemangioma
   e. Adenofibroma
   f. Adenomyoma
   g. Fibroadenoma
   h. Papilloma
   i. Endometriosis
   j. Mesonephric remnant cyst
   k. Glioma
   l. Condyloma
   m. Cervical stenosis: hematometra
2. Malignant
   a. Squamous cell carcinoma
   b. Verrucous carcinoma
   c. Adenocarcinoma
      (1) Adenoma malignum
      (2) Adenoid cystic carcinoma
      (3) Mesonephric carcinoma
   d. Mixed epithelial
      (1) Adenosquamous carcinoma
      (2) Glassy cell carcinoma
      (3) Mucoepidermoid
      (4) Dual primary
   e. Neuroendocrine
      (1) Carcinoid
      (2) Small cell
   f. Metastatic tumors
   g. Rare tumors
      (1) Melanoma
      (2) Choriocarcinoma

Uterus

1. Pregnancy
   a. Congenital Müllerian defects
      (1) Didelphys
      (2) Bicornuate
      (3) Rudimentary horn
      (4) Cervix atresia
2. Tumor
   a. Polyp
   b. Atypical polyploid adenoma
   c. Teratoma
   d. Brenner tumor
   e. Heterologous tumor
   f. Glioma

- g. Endometrial carcinoma
  - (1) Papillary
  - (2) Secretory
  - (3) Ciliated cell
  - (4) Adenocanthoma
  - (5) Adenosquamous carcinoma
- h. Mucinous carcinoma
- i. Serous carcinoma
- j. Clear cell
- k. Squamous papillary serous
- l. Undifferentiated
- m. Mixed
- n. Glassy cell
- o. Metastatic
- p. GTD

3. Sarcoma
   - a. Homologous
     - (1) Leiomyosarcoma
     - (2) Stromal sarcoma
     - (3) Angiosarcoma
   - b. Heterologous
     - (1) Rhabdomyosarcoma
     - (2) Choridiosarcoma
     - (3) Osteosarcoma
   - c. Mixed
   - d. Mixed Müllerian
   - e. Malignant lymphoma
   - f. Unclassified sarcoma leiomyoma variants
     - (1) Myxoid
     - (2) Vascular
     - (3) Lipoid
     - (4) With tubules
     - (5) Intravenous
   - g. Benign metastasizing leiomyoma
   - h. Disseminated peritoneal leiomyomatosis
   - i. Adeonmyosis
   - j. Adenomyoma
   - k. Adenomatoid mesothelioma
   - l. Hemangioma
   - m. Angiosarcoma
   - n. Hemanogiopericytoma
   - o. Pseudotumor

Fallopian tube

1. Torsion
2. Pyosalpinx
3. Hydrosalpinx
4. Granulomatous salpingitis
5. Actinomycosis
6. Parasite salpingitis

   a. Enterbius vermicularis
   b. Schistosomiasis
   c. *Echinococcus granulosus*
7. Sarcoid
8. Crohn's disease
9. Foreign body
10. Ectopic pregnancy
11. Malignant
   a. Adenocarcinoma
      (1) Alveolar
      (2) Papillary
      (3) Medullary
   b. Squamous
   c. Transitional cell
   d. Clear cell carcinoma
   e. Sarcoma
      (1) Carcinosarcoma
      (2) Mixed mesodermal
   f. Metastatic
   g. Lymphoma
   h. GTD

Ovary

1. Benign
   a. Supernumerary ovary
   b. Adrenal rest
   c. Splenic gonadal fusion
   d. Actinomycosis
   e. Granulomas
   f. Parasitic infection
   g. Inclusion cyst
   h. Follicular cyst
   i. Corpus luteum cyst
      (1) Ruptured or unruptured: hemorrhagic
   j. Lutein cyst of pregnancy
   k. Ovarian hyperstimulation
   l. Hyperreaction luteinalis
   m. PCO
   n. Hyperthecosis
   o. HAIR-AN syndrome
   p. Fibromatosis
   q. Luteoma
   r. Torsion
   s. Endometrioma
   t. Retroperitoneal mucinous tumor
   u. Walthard rests
   v. Leiomyoma
   w. Mesothelioma

x. Oophoritis
y. Ovarian abscess
2. Serous tumor
   a. Benign and borderline
      (1) Cystadenoma
      (2) Papillary cystadenoma
      (3) Papilloma
      (4) Adenofibroma
      (5) Cystadenofibroma
   b. Malignant
      (1) Adenocarcinoma
      (2) Papillary adenocarcinoma
      (3) Papillary cystadenocarcinoma
      (4) Papillary carcinoma
      (5) Malignant adenofibroma
      (6) Cystadenofibroma
3. Mucinous tumor
   a. Benign and borderline
      (1) Cystadenoma
      (2) Adenofibroma
      (3) Cystadenofibroma
   b. Malignant
      (1) Adenocarcinoma
      (2) Cystadenocarcinoma
      (3) Malignant adenofibroma and cystadenofibroma
4. Endometrial tumors
   a. Benign and borderline
      (1) Adenoma
      (2) Cystadenoma
      (3) Adenofibroma
      (4) Cystadenofibroma
   b. Malignant
      (1) Adenocarcinoma
      (2) Adenocanthoma
      (3) Malignant adenofibroma
      (4) Cystadenofibroma
      (5) Endometrial stomal sarcoma
      (6) Mixed Müllerian tumor
      (1) Homologous
      (2) Heterologous
5. Clear cell tumor
   a. Benign
      (1) Adenofibroma
   b. Borderline and malignant
      (1) Carcinoma
      (2) Adenocarcinoma
6. Brenner's tumor
   a. Benign
   b. Borderline
   c. Malignant

7. Mixed epithelial tumor
   a. Undifferentiated
   b. Unclassified
8. Granulosa stromal cell tumor: adult, juvenile
   a. Thecoma
      (1) Typical
      (2) Luteinized
   b. Fibroma, fibrosarcoma
      (1) Fibroma
      (2) Cellular fibroma
9. Sertoli stromal cell tumors: Sertoli cell, Leydig cell, mixed
   a. Gynadroblastoma
   b. Sex cord tumor with annular tubules
   c. Unclassified
   d. Hilus cell tumor
   e. Steroid cell tumor
   f. Carcinoid
   g. Zollinger-Ellison syndrome
   h. Small-cell carcinoma
10. Dysgerminoma
   a. Endodermal sinus tumor
   b. Embryonal carcinoma
   c. Polyembryoma
   d. Choriocarcinoma
   e. Teratoma
      (1) Immature
      (2) Mature-solid
      (3) Cystic-dermoid
      (4) Dermoid with malignant transformation
      (5) Struma ovarii
      (6) Carcinoid
      (7) Strumal carcinoid
      (8) Other
   f. Mixed forms
11. Fibroma
   a. Fibrosarcoma
   b. Leiomyoma
   c. Leiomyosarcoma
   d. Rhabdomyoma
   e. Rhabdomyosarcoma
   f. Hemangioma
   g. Lymphangioma
   h. Chordoma
   i. Osteoma
   j. Osteosarcoma
   k. Giant-cell tumor
   l. Neural tissue tumors
   m. Mesothelial tumors
   n. Lymphoma
   o. Burkitt's lymphoma

12. Metastatic tumors
    a. Uterus
    b. Vulva
    c. Vagina
    d. Fallopian tube
    e. Breast
    f. Intestinal
    g. Krukenberg
    h. Appendix
    i. Carcinoid
    j. Pancreas
    k. Gall bladder
    l. Liver
    m. Esophagus
    n. Renal
    o. Bladder
    p. Ureter
    q. Urethra
    r. Adrenal gland
    s. Melanoma
    t. Lung
    u. Mediastinum
13. Obstetric
    a. Pregnancy
    b. Multiple pregnancy
    c. Ectopic pregnancy
    d. Abdominal pregnancy
    e. Hydatiform mole
        (1) Complete
        (2) Partial
    f. Invasive mole
    g. Choriocarcinoma
    h. Placenta site trophoblastic tumor
    i. Placenta percreta
    j. Fetus papyraceus
    k. Retained placenta

14.13 PELVIC MASS—NONGYNECOLOGIC CAUSES

1. GI tract
    a. Tuberculous granuloma
    b. Pericecal abscess
    c. Crohn's disease
    d. Carcinoma
    e. Constipation
    f. Obstipation
    g. Fecal impaction
    h. Polyp
    i. Bezoar
        (1) Tricho
        (2) Phyto

j. Volvulus
k. Intussusception
l. Diverticular abscess
m. Hemangioma
n. Carcinoid
o. Inguinal hernia
p. Femoral hernia

2. Genitourinary (GU) tract
   a. Distended bladder
   b. Ectopic kidney
   c. Supernumerary kidney
   d. Horseshoe kidney
   e. Polycystic kidney
   f. Benign neoplasm
   g. Wilm's tumor
   h. Carcinosarcoma
   i. Pelvic carcinoma
3. Other
   a. Hematoma rectus abdominis
   b. Retained sponge or instrument after surgery
   c. Ectopic spleen
   d. Inguinal endometriosis
   e. Mistaken normal structure
   f. Pseudomyxoma peritonei
   g. Lymphoma
   h. Burkitt's lymphoma
   i. Aneurysm
   j. Retroperitoneal hematoma
      (1) Postoperative
      (2) Postlaparoscopy
   k. Procedentia
   l. Incisional or epigastric hernia
   m. Obturator or spigelian hernia
   n. Metastatic tumor

14.14 PELVIC PAIN

Acute

1. Genital tract
   a. Pregnancy related
      (1) Abortion
         (a) Threatened
         (b) Inevitable
         (c) Complete
         (d) Induced
         (e) Septic
      (2) Ectopic pregnancy
         (a) Fallopian tube
         (b) Abdominal
         (c) Cervical
         (d) Ovarian

- b. Ovary
  - (1) Ruptured cyst
  - (2) Torsion of cyst
  - (3) Hemorrhagic corpus luteum
    - (a) Ruptured
    - (b) Unruptured
  - (4) Mittelschmerz
  - (5) Ovarian hyperstimulation syndrome
    - (a) Clomiphene
    - (b) Human menopausal gonadotropin (HMG)
- c. Fallopian tube
  - (1) Torsion
  - (2) Paratubal cyst
  - (3) Torsion of stump after sterilization
- d. Uterus
  - (1) Fibroid degeneration
  - (2) Fibroid torsion
  - (3) Pyometria
  - (4) Retrograde menstruation
- e. Acute pelvic inflammatory disease
  - (1) Endometriosis
  - (2) Salpingo-oophoritis
  - (3) Tuboovarian abscess

2. Nongenital tract
   - a. GI tract
     - (1) Appendicitis
     - (2) Meckel's diverticulitis
     - (3) Inflammatory bowel disease
       - (a) Crohn's disease
       - (b) Ulcerative colitis
     - (4) Mesenteric adenitis
     - (5) Bowel perforation
     - (6) Bowel obstruction
     - (7) Toxic megacolon
     - (8) Diverticulitis
   - b. Urinary tract
     - (1) Cystitis
     - (2) Pyelonephritis
     - (3) Renal calculus or colic
   - c. Other
     - (1) Abdominal wall hematoma: rectus
     - (2) Herpes zoster
     - (3) Acute intermittent porphyria
     - (4) Sickle cell crisis
     - (5) Idiopathic

Chronic

1. Cycle
   - a. Mittelschmerz
   - b. Primary dysmenorrhea

c. Secondary dysmenorrhea
   (1) Endometriosis
   (2) Endosalpingiosis
   (3) Adhesive disease
      (a) Chronic pelvic inflammatory disease (PID)
      (b) Endometriosis
      (c) Postsurgical
d. Uterine pathology
   (1) Adenomyosis
   (2) Leiomyoma
e. Congenital anomaly
   (1) Hematometria
   (2) Hematocolpos
f. Imperforate hymen
g. Transverse septum
h. Noncommunicating uterine horn
i. Acquired cervical stenosis
j. Congenital cervical absence
k. Other
   (1) Pedunculated myoma
   (2) Endometrial polyp
   (3) Intrauterine adhesions
   (4) Complete Asherman's
   (5) IUD use
   (6) Chronic PID

2. Acyclic
   a. Genital tract
      (1) Endometriosis
      (2) Pelvic adhesions
      (3) Pelvic congestion syndrome
      (4) Pelvic varicosities
      (5) Ovarian tumors
      (6) Leiomyoma
   b. Nongenital tract
      (1) Cystitis
      (2) Renal colic: renal calculi
      (3) Diverticulitis
      (4) Colitis
      (5) Spina bifida
      (6) Scoliosis
      (7) Osteoarthritis
      (8) Fibromyositis
      (9) Herniated intervertebral disc
3. No organic cause
   a. Sexual abuse
   b. Incest
   c. Spousal abuse
      (1) Physical
      (2) Mental
   d. Psychogenic etiologies

(1) Borderline personality
(2) Hypochondriasis
(3) Depression
(4) Hysteria
(5) Münchhaussen syndrome

14.15 PREMENSTRUAL SYNDROME

1. Normal physiology, psychologic factors, physiologic factors
   a. Estrogen excess
   b. Estrogen deficiency
   c. Progesterone deficiency
   d. Vitamin deficiency
   e. Disorder of renin–angiotensin–aldosterone
   f. Disorder of melanocyte-stimulating hormone (MSH), β-endorphins
2. Abnormality of psychosocial adjustment

14.16 SEXUAL DYSFUNCTION

Dyspareunia

1. Introital
   a. Vaginismus
   b. Intact or rigid hymen
   c. Clitoral problems
   d. Vulvovaginitis
   e. Vaginal atrophy: hypoestrogen
   f. Vulvar dystrophy
   g. Bartholin or Skene gland infection
   h. Inadequate lubrication
   i. Operative scarring
2. Midvaginal
   a. Urethritis
   b. Trigonitis
   c. Cystitis
   d. Short vagina
   e. Operative scarring
   f. Inadequate lubrication
3. Deep
   a. Endometriosis
   b. Pelvic infection
   c. Uterine retroversion
   d. Ovarian pathology
   e. Gastrointestinal
   f. Orthopedic
   g. Abnormal penile size or shape

Orgasm dysfunction

1. Anorgasmia: inadequate stimulation or learning
2. Spinal cord lesion or injury

3. Multiple sclerosis
4. Alcoholic neuropathy
5. Amyotrophic lateral sclerosis
6. Spinal cord accident
7. Spinal cord trauma
8. Peripheral nerve damage
9. Radical pelvic surgery
10. Herniated lumbar disc
11. Hypothyroidism
12. Addison's disease
13. Cushing's disease
14. Acromegaly
15. Hypopituitarism
16. Pharmacologic agents

Sexuality disorders

1. Primary or secondary sexual trauma
2. Incest
3. Abuse
4. Depression
5. Pharmacologic agents
   a. Anticholinergics
   b. Antiandrogens
   c. Alpha-blockers and beta-blockers
   d. Narcotics
   e. Sedatives
   f. Antidepressants
   g. Antihistamines
6. Malignancy
7. Hepatic renal disease
8. Chronic illness
9. Disfigurement
   a. Mastectomy
   b. Radical neck
   c. Burns
   d. Trauma
10. Multiple sclerosis
11. Cord injury
12. Diabetic nephropathy
13. Hypoadrenalism
14. Panhypopituitarism
15. Ovarian failure
16. Premenstrual syndrome

14.17 UPPER GENITAL TRACT INFECTION

1. PID
   a. Salpingitis
   b. Pyosalpinx
   c. Tuboovarian abscess

   - d. Endomyometritis
   - e. Parametritis
   - f. Pelvic peritonitis
   - g. Pelvic abscess
   - h. Generalized peritonitis
   - i. Fitz-Hugh-Curtis syndrome: perihepatitis
2. Ascending lower genital tract infection (See Section 14.10.)
3. IUD: Dalkon shield
4. Postpartum endomyometritis
5. Postsurgical manipulation
   - a. Hysteroscopy
   - b. Endometrial biopsy (EMB)
   - c. Dilation and curettage (D&C)
   - d. Hysterosalpingiogram (HSG)
6. Postsurgical procedure
7. Gynecologic procedure
   - a. Hysterectomy
   - b. Myomectomy
8. General surgical procedure
   - a. Appendectomy
   - b. Bowel resection
9. Adjacent ruptured viscus
   - a. Appendicitis
   - b. Diverticulitis
10. Hematogenous: pelvic tuberculosis
11. Chronic PID

14.18 URINARY INCONTINENCE

Intermittent

1. Genuine stress incontinence
2. Urethral sphincter incontinence
3. Detrusor instability
   - a. Inflammatory
   - b. Neurologic
   - c. Idiopathic
4. Diabetes
5. Surgery
6. Drugs
7. Spinal cord lesion
8. Spina bifida
9. Multiple sclerosis
10. Overflow incontinence
11. Detrusor or sphincter dyssynergia
12. Psychogenic
13. Mixed

Geniune stress incontinence (GSI)

1. Trauma
   - a. Childbirth
   - b. Pelvic surgery
   - c. Injury

2. Pelvic relaxation
   a. Congenital
   b. Childbirth
   c. Other
3. Drugs: alpha-blockers (i.e., Minipress)
4. Menopause: hypoestrogenism

Detrussor Instability

1. Inflammatory
   a. Chronic UTI
   b. Interstitial cystitis
   c. Bladder stone
   d. Neoplasm
   e. Suture
2. Neurologic
   a. Cerebrovascular accident (CVA)
   b. Multiple sclerosis
   c. Spinal cord tumor
   d. Cerebral degeneration
3. Miscellaneous
   a. Urethral diverticulum
   b. Psychogenic
      (1) Depression
      (2) Anxiety
      (3) Emotional conflict regarding process of urination
   c. Neglect
   d. Inability to ambulate

Continuous

1. Fistula
   a. Congenital
      (1) Ectopic ureter
   b. Acquired
      (1) Pelvic surgery
         (a) Hysterectomy
         (b) Radical hysterectomy
         (c) Pelvic irradiation
         (d) Crohn's disease

14.19 VULVAR LESIONS

Red lesion

Infection

1. Fungal infection
   a. Candida
   b. Tinea cruris
   c. Intertrigo
   d. Pityriasis versicolor

2. Sarcoptes scabiei
3. Erythrasma: *Corynebacterium minutissimum*
4. Granuloma inguinale: *Calymmatobacterium granulomatis*
5. Folliculitis: *Staphylococcus aureus*
6. Hidradenitis suppurativa
7. Behçet's syndrome

Inflammation

1. Reactive vulvitis
2. Chemical irritation
   a. Detergent
   b. Dyes
   c. Perfume
   d. Spermacide
   e. Lubricants
   f. Hygiene sprays
   g. Podophyllun
   h. Topical 5-FU
   i. Saliva
   j. Gentian violet
   k. Semen
3. Mechanical trauma: scratching
4. Vestibular adenitis
5. Essential vulvodynia
6. Psoriasis
7. Seborrheic dermatitis

Neoplasm

1. Vulvar intraepithelial neoplasia (VIN)
   a. Mild dysplasia
   b. Moderate dysplasia
   c. Severe dysplasia
   d. Carcinoma-in-situ
2. Vulvar dystrophy
3. Bowen's disease
4. Invasive cancer
   a. Squamous cell carcinoma
   b. Malignant melanoma
   c. Sarcoma
   d. Basal cell carcinoma
   e. Adenocarcinoma
   f. Paget's disease
   g. Undifferentiated

White lesion

1. Vulvar dystrophy
   a. Lichen sclerosis
   b. Vulvar dystrophy
   c. Vulvar hyperplasia
   d. Mixed dystrophy

2. VIN
3. Vitiligo
4. Partial albinism
5. Intertrigo
6. Radiation treatment

Dark lesion

1. Lentigo
2. Nevi (mole)
3. Neoplasm (see Neoplasm, Vulvar, below)
4. Reactive hyperpigmentation
5. Seborrheic keratosis
6. Pubic lice

Ulcerative lesion

1. Infection
   a. Herpes simplex
   b. Vaccinia
   c. *Treponema pallidum*
   d. Granuloma inguinale
   e. Pyoderma
   f. Tuberculosis
2. Noninfection
   a. Behçet's disease
   b. Crohn's disease
   c. Pemphigus
   d. Pemphigoid
   e. Hidradenitis suppurativa (see Neoplasm, Vulvar, below)

Neoplasm

1. Basal cell carcinoma
2. Squamous cell carcinoma
3. Vulvar tumor <1 cm
   a. Condyloma acuminata
   b. Mulluscum contagiosum
   c. Epidermal inclusion
   d. Vestibular cyst
   e. Mesenephric duct
   f. VIN
   g. Hemangioma
   h. Hidradenoma
   i. Neurofibroma
   j. Syringoma
   k. Accessory breast tissue
   l. Acrocordon
   m. Endometriosis
   n. Fox-Fordyce disease
   o. Pilonidal sinus
4. Vulvar tumor >1 cm
   a. Bartholin cyst or abscess
   b. Lymphogranuloma venereum

c. Fibroma
d. Lipoma
e. Verrucous carcinoma
f. Squamous cell carcinoma
g. Hernia
h. Edema
i. Hematoma
j. Acrocordon
k. Epidermal cysts
l. Neurofibromatosis
m. Accessory breast tissue

15

Gynecologic Oncology

Shashikant Lele, M.D., and Susan J. Littler, M.D., Ph.D.

15.1 CERVICAL CARCINOMA

Invasive cervical cancer is the third most frequent lower genital tract malignancy in the United States and is the second most common cause of gynecologic related deaths. The median age of onset for cervical cancer is 54 years, whereas the average age of intraepithelial neoplasia (CIN) is the early 30s. The predominant cell type is squamous carcinoma (85% to 90%), with adenocarcinoma being the second most frequent type (10% to 15%).

Etiology

1. The etiology is largely unknown; however certain behaviors are known to increase the risk of developing cervical cancer.
2. These behaviors are multiple sexual partners, early age of sexual intercourse, prostitution, and smoking.
3. Sexually transmitted agents, particularly the human papillomavirus (HPV) types 16, 18, 31, 33, 39, and 42, are strongly associated with the development of cervical cancer.
4. Patients with a history of cervical dysplasias (CIN) are at risk of progressing on to frank cervical cancer.
5. Patients who were exposed to diethylstilbestrol (DES) *in utero* are also at risk for developing abnormal cervical changes.

Signs and symptoms

1. Abnormal vaginal bleeding and brown discharge are the more common symptoms during the perimenopausal or menopausal period.
2. Patients may demonstrate prolonged, excessive menstrual bleeding or postcoital bleeding.
3. Advanced cases may present with pelvic pain, sciatic pain, difficulty voiding, or leg edema.

Diagnosis, screening

1. The Papanicolaou smear is currently the best screening technique available.

2. If an asymptomatic patient has an abnormal Papanicolaou smear, colposcopy with biopsy of all abnormal areas with endocervical curettage (ECC) is required.
3. If the results of the ECC are positive or the colposcopic examination differs with the Papanicolaou smear results, or if CIN II or CIN III changes are seen, further procedures are required.
   a. These procedures may vary from laser cone, LEEP, or cold knife conization.
4. If invasive carcinoma is found, clinical staging is done to determine the best treatment options.
5. The use of tissue markers such as carcinoembryonic antigen (CEA) or TA-4 (SCC) antigen is currently being studied for cervical cancer screening.
   a. CEA and SCC titers correlate with tumor volume and a persistent or rising titer after therapy may signal a recurrence.

Staging

1. Staging for cervical cancer is a clinical staging.
2. A thorough physical examination is done of the cervix, vaginal, rectovaginal, abdomen, and supraclavicular lymph nodes.
3. The workup should also include a chest x-ray examination, intravenous pyelogram (IVP), cystoscopy, and possible sigmoidoscopy.
   a. The FIGO system is found in Table 15-1.

Prognosis

1. Prognosis depends on the stage, age of the patient, and nodal involvement.
2. The 5-year survival depends on the stage and nodal involvement.
   a. Stage IA: 98% to 100%
   b. Stage IB: 90%
   c. Stage II: 65%
   d. Stage III: 35%
   e. Stage IV: 15%

Treatment

1. Treatment strategies depend on stage and health of the patient.
   a. Stage IA, IB (early IB) treatment would be radical hysterectomy with lymphadenectomy.
   b. Patients with IB >3 cm and stages II-IV are treated with radiation therapy.
   c. Radiation therapy may include the following:
      (1) Teletherapy: external beam
      (2) Brachytherapy: local implants
2. Pelvic exenteration procedures are reserved for local recurrences following radiation therapy.

15.2 UTERINE CANCER

Endometrial adenocarcinoma

1. The most common type of uterine cancer is endometrial adenocarcinoma (>90%)

Table 15-1 FIGO staging of cervial carcinoma

Stage	Criteria
I	Carcinoma strictly confined to cervix.
IA	Preclinical microscopic carcinoma of the cervix.
IAi	Minimal microscopically evident stromal invasion.
IAii	Microscopic lesions that can be measured. The upper limit of the measurement should not show a depth of invasion of >5 mm taken from base of epithelium, either surface or glandular; and a second dimension, the horizontal spread, must not exceed 7 mm. Larger lesions should be staged as IB.
IB	Lesion of greater dimensions than IA2 regardless of whether seen clinically. Preformed space involvement should not alter the staging but should be recorded for possible treatment decisions.
IIA	Extends to the upper two thirds of the vagina.
IIB	Extends to the paracervical tissue.
IIIA	Extends to the lower one third of the vagina.
IIIB	Pelvic sidewall extension or ureteral obstruction on IVP.
IVA	Bladder or rectal mucosal involvement.
IVB	Distant metastasis.

   a. Endometrial adenocarcinomas are the most common malignancy of the lower female genital tract but are one of the least common causes of cancer death.
   b. The median age of diagnosis is 60 (range 55 to 65) years old; therefore a disease primarily of postmenopausal women.
2. Uterine sarcomas comprise only 3% to 5% of all uterine tumors.

Etiology

1. Unopposed estrogen is thought to have the biggest influence on cancerous changes in the endometrium
2. Unopposed estrogen is seen with the following:
   a. Nulliparity
   b. Infertility
   c. Polycystic ovary syndrome
   d. Late menopause
   e. Obesity
   f. Use of exogenous estrogen without a progesterone agent
   g. Impaired liver function
   h. Estrogen-producing tumors
3. A history of atypical endometrial hyperplasia may also predispose to developing endometrial carcinoma.

Signs and symptoms

Abnormal uterine bleeding in the menopausal and perimenopausal phase is the most common symptom.

Diagnosis

1. The diagnosis of endometrial cancer is established by sampling the endometrium and performing histologic examination of the sample.
2. Routine Papanicolaou smear will detect only 35% of endometrial carcinomas.
3. Endometrial sampling may be done using a pipelle or by a dilation and curettage (D&C).
4. Transvaginal ultrasound may also be used to detect abnormalities in the uterus and assess endometrial stripe thickness.
5. An endometrial stripe thickness of <5 mm is considered to be normal.

Histology and grading (See the box on p. 292 and Table 15-2.)

Management, prognosis

1. Prognosis depends on the following:
   a. Surgical staging
   b. Age
   c. Histologic type
   d. Grade
   e. Depth of myometrial invasion
   f. Microscopic invasion of vascular spaces
   g. Lymph node metastases
   h. Peritoneal cytology (Table 15-3)

Histology of Endometrial Adenocarcinomas

1. Endometroid
   a. Adenoacanthoma (squamous metaplasia)
   b. Adenosquamous
   c. Papillary
   d. Ciliated
   e. Secretory
2. Squamous carcinoma
3. Papillary serous
4. Mucinous
5. Clear cell
6. Mixed

Table 15-2 FIGO surgical staging for carcinoma corpus uteri

Stage I	
Stage Ia G123	Tumor limited to endometrium
Stage Ib G123	Invasion to less than one half the myometrium
Stage Ic G123	Invasion to more than one half the myometrium
Stage II	
Stage IIa G123	Endocervical glandular involvement only
Stage IIb G123	Cervical stromal invasion
Stage III	
Stage IIIa G123	Tumor invades serosa and/or adnexa, and/or positive peritoneal cytology
Stage IIIb G123	Vaginal metastases
Stage IIIc G123	Metastases to pelvic and or para-aortic lymph nodes
Stage IV	
Stage IVa G123	Tumor invasion of bladder and or bowel mucosa
Stage IVb G123	Distant metastases including intraabdominal and/or inguinal nodes

Table 15-3 Five-year survival in endometrial cancer

Stage	% 5 Year Survival	Proportion (%) of Cases
I	72	75
II	56	11
III	32	11
IV	11	3

2. The best prognoses are with the histologic types contained in the endometroid group (80%), and poorer prognoses are seen with papillary serous, clear cell, and adenosquamous.
3. Stage I, no matter which histologic group, has the best prognosis.
4. Younger patients do better than older patients.
5. Before surgery, perform the following:
   a. Chest x-ray film
   b. IVP
   c. Barium enema
   d. Liver function tests
   e. Possibly abdominal pelvic CT scan
6. Tumor markers such as CA-125 are nonspecific and, if elevated, are thought to correlate with extrauterine disease. A pretreatment CA-125 is recommended.
7. Treatment for stage I, grade I lesions is total abdominal hysterectomy (TAH) and bilateral salpingo-oophorectomy (BSO) alone.
8. Lymph node dissection (pelvic and periaortic) is added for grade 2 and 3 diseases.
9. Stages II, III, and IV should undergo TAH/BSO and pelvic and periaortic lymph node dissection.
10. If extensive disease is present in the uterus or if metastases are present, radiation, progestins, and chemotherapy are given.
11. Most authors agree that postoperative external radiation should be used when the patient has periaortic and pelvic lymph node metastases.

Uterine sarcomas

1. Uterine sarcomas comprise only 3% to 5% of uterine tumors but account for 15% of uterine malignancy deaths.
2. The incidence is 1.7/100,000 women older than age 20.
3. The peak age depends on the tumor type.
   a. Leiomyosarcomas occur more in younger populations than other subtypes with peak age in the mid 50s.
   b. The incidence of mixed mesodermal sarcoma is low in middle age; then it sharply increases in the mid 60s.
4. Both tumor subtypes are more common in African-American women.

Classification

1. These neoplasms arise from mesenchymal tissue, and classification is based on the resemblance of sarcomatous elements to the mesenchymal tissue normally found in the uterus.
2. These tumors arise primarily from three tissues:
   a. Endometrial sarcoma from endometrial glands and stroma
   b. Leiomyosarcoma from uterine muscle
   c. Angiosarcomas, fibrosarcomas, etc. (arise in supporting structures)
3. Tumors are classified as cell type and tissue of origin.
   a. The term *pure* means the tumor contains one cell type, and the term *mixed* that the tumor contains more than one cell type.

Ober Classification of Uterine Sarcomas

Homologous	Heterologous
Pure	Pure
Stromal sarcoma (endolymphatic stromal myosis)	Rhabdomyosarcoma
Leiomyosarcoma	Chondrosarcoma
Angiosarcoma	Osteosarcoma
Fibrosarcoma	Liposarcoma
Mixed	Mixed
Carcinosarcoma	Mixed Müllerian tumors (mixed mesodermal tumor)

Classification of Uterine Tumors Endorsed by the Gynecologic Oncology Group

Leiomyosarcomas
Endometrial stromal sarcomas
Mixed homologous Müllerian sarcomas (carcinosarcoma)
Mixed heterologous Müllerian sarcomas (mixed mesodermal sarcoma)
Other uterine sarcomas

b. *Homologous* tumors contain tissue elements endogenous to the uterus, whereas *heterologous* tumors contain tissue foreign to the uterus (see the boxes above).

Signs and symptoms

1. Irregular vaginal bleeding
2. Vaginal discharge
3. Abdominal mass that is rapidly enlarging
4. Abdominal pain
5. Menorrhagia in younger patients
6. Friable polypoid mass extending through the cervix

Etiology

1. The etiology is largely unknown.
2. A prior history of pelvic irradiation is noted in 5% to 10% of women who develop uterine sarcoma.
3. Malignant transformation of a leiomyoma is rare (<1%).
4. Obesity may also be a predisposing factor.

Criteria for Differentiating Uterine Leiomyoma and Leiomyosarcoma

Leiomyosarcoma
- >10 mitoses per 10 high-power fields (HPF)
- 5 to 10 mitoses per HPF and cytologic atypia

Lesions of uncertain malignant potential
- 5 to 9 mitoses per HPF if well differentiated
- 2 to 4 mitoses per HPF with cytologic atypia

Leiomyoma
- 0 to 4 mitoses per HPF well differentiated

Diagnosis

1. Papanicolaou smears do not help in the diagnosis.
2. Biopsy of protruding mass from cervix and biopsy of endometrial lining by either fractional D&C or uterine sampling is important.
3. There are currently no tumor markers available.

Staging

Staging currently follows the same criteria as uterine adenocarcinoma (see Table 15-2).

Prognosis and management

The prognosis and management varies with the type of uterine sarcoma. Each type is briefly discussed here.

1. Leiomyosarcoma (LMS)
    a. LMS comprises approximately 35% of uterine sarcomas (second most common type).
    b. LMS is differentiated from the benign leiomyoma by the number of mitoses and presence of cellular atypia (see the box above).
    c. Premenopausal women have a better prognosis (Table 15-4).
    d. Development from a leiomyoma is rare.
    e. A rapidly enlarging uterus in the perimenopausal, menopausal period is suspicious for sarcoma.
    f. Treatment consists of removal of all tumor (TAH/BSO).
    g. An increased mitotic rate is associated with a poorer prognosis.
    h. Survival depends on stage (see Table 15-4).
    i. Essentially, neither radiation nor chemotherapy have proved effective in advanced disease.
2. Mixed Müllerian sarcoma (MMS)
    a. The malignant mixed Müllerian tumors are the most common type of uterine sarcomas (>45%).
    b. They contain both sarcomatous and a carcinomatous elements.
    c. These are often aggressive tumors with early spread to regional lymph nodes and adjacent tissue.

Table 15-4 Uterine sarcomas: 5-year survival rate in terms of stage, treatment, and pathology

Stage	Cell Type	S (%)	S + R (%)	R (%)
I	MMS	52	48	29
	LMS	58	75	33
	ESS	47	88	50
II-IV	MMS	5	16	0
	LMS	0	13	0
	ESS	0	33	0

S, Survival; *R*, remission.

d. Most recommend TAH/BSO for stage I and II and removal of all extrauterine tumor and postoperative radiation therapy.
e. Extent of tumor and depth of myometrial invasion are important to long-term outcome.

3. Endometrial stromal sarcoma (ESS)
   a. These tumors often present with tumor protruding from the cervical os (30% to 50%) and with irregular vaginal bleeding.
   b. These tumors are divided into two main groups:
      (1) Endolymphatic stromal myosis: low grade
      (2) Endometrial stromal sarcoma: high grade (>10 mitoses/HPF).
   c. The ESS are more aggressive and have a poorer prognosis.
   d. Treatment is the same as for MMS.
4. Adjuvant therapy
   a. Because prognosis is poor in uterine sarcoma, especially with extrauterine spread, chemotherapy regimes have been explored.
      (1) Doxorubicin is thought to be the single best agent.
      (2) Some authors use combinations of doxorubicin, cyclophosphamide, vincristine, and dimethyltriazenoimidazole carboxamide (DTIC).

15.3 VAGINAL CANCER

1. Vaginal cancers are rare and account for only 1.5% to 2% of all gynecologic malignancies.
2. FIGO uses strict criteria to define whether the vaginal lesion is primary to the vagina or metastatic.
   a. A vaginal growth that extends to the portio of the cervix is considered to be of cervical origin.
   b. A vaginal growth that has extended to the vulva should be classified as carcinoma of the vulva.
3. The majority of vaginal malignancies are metastatic from the cervix, endometrium, or vulva.
4. Less common metastases are from the ovary, rectosigmoid, or malignant trophoblastic disease.

Table 15-5 Vaginal tumor histology with clinical correlations

Tumor Type	Age (years)	Clinical Correlations
Squamous cell carcinoma	>50	Most common primary vaginal carcinoma
Endodermal sinus tumor	<2	Rare, alpha-fetoprotein secretion
Sarcoma botryoides	<8	Aggressive
Clear cell adenocarcinoma	>14	Associated with intrauterine DES exposure
Melanoma	>50	Rare, poor survival

Histology

Greater than 90% of primary vaginal cancers are squamous (Table 15-5).

Embryology

1. The vagina has two embryonic origins, which is important when considering lymphatic drainage.
   a. The upper two thirds of the vagina is formed fused Müllerian endoderm.
   b. The lower one third is derived from invagination of overlaying squamous epithelium, called the urogenital sinus.
2. The upper vagina drains with the cervix to the pelvic lymph nodes (i.e., obturator, iliacs)
3. The lower one third of the vagina has the same lymphatic drainage as the vulva to the inguinal and femoral nodes.

Etiology

1. The etiology is largely unknown and depends on the histologic type.
2. In general, exposure to HPV, prior radiation, immunosuppression, and chemotherapy may predispose a patient to vaginal cancer.
3. For clear cell carcinoma, exposure *in utero* (before 20 weeks gestation) to DES may predispose a patient to develop adenocarcinoma of the vagina.
4. Chronic exposure to pooled irritating substances, especially in the area of posterior fornix and upper vagina.

Diagnosis

1. Vaginal smear of multiple areas with Papanicolaou stain.
2. If suspicious lesions are seen or if positive smears, than colposcopy of the vagina should be done with biopsy of all areas in question.

Signs and symptoms

1. Vaginal bleeding (irregular, postmenopausal) is common.
2. Vaginal discharge may be seen.
3. Urinary symptoms such as frequency may be seen early with anterior wall tumors.

Table 15-6 FIGO staging for vaginal cancers

0	Carcinoma-in-situ, intraepithelial carcinoma
I	Carcinoma is limited to the vaginal wall mucosa
II	Spread to paravaginal tissue but not to the pelvic wall
III	Extension to one or both pelvic walls
IV	Carcinoma has extended beyond the true pelvis or has involved the mucosa of the bladder or rectum; bullous edema or tumor bulge into the bladder or rectum is not acceptable evidence of invasion
IVa	Spread of the growth to adjacent organs and/or direct extension beyond the true pelvis
IVb	Spread to distant organs

4. Constipation (tenesmus) may be seen with posterior wall tumors in advanced cases.
5. Pain is usually seen in advanced cases.

Staging

1. A thorough history and physical should be done because FIGO staging is a clinical, not a surgical staging.
2. All patients should have a chest x-ray examination, IVP, cystoscopy, and proctosigmoidoscopy.
3. See Table 15-6 for staging.

Treatment and survival

1. Squamous cell carcinoma is the most common type of primary vaginal cancer.
   a. It is often found in the upper half of the vagina; 50% are found in the upper one-third posterior wall; 30%, one-third anterior wall; and 19% are found in the middle.
   b. These tumors are often multicentric and may be fungating ulcerated masses producing a foul smell and discharge caused by secondary infection.
   c. Treatment depends on size, stage, location, age, and desire for sexual functioning.
      (1) Therapy is limited by the closeness of the rectum and bladder.
      (2) Location in vagina will determine areas of lymphatic spread.
      (3) If the uterus is present, external radiation is used, followed by local radiation.
      (4) If there is no uterus, local radiation is used.
   d. Patients with recurrences after radiation treatment may be treated with pelvic exenteration.
   e. Five-year survival depends on the stage.
      (1) Stage I: 71%
      (2) Stage II: 47%
      (3) Stage III: 25%
      (4) Stage IV: 8%

2. Clear cell adenocarcinoma is related to DES exposure in the first trimester of pregnancy and is seen in younger age groups.
   a. This disease is associated with adenosis of the vagina.
   b. This cancer is treated like squamous cell carcinoma.
   c. The best candidates for survival are low stage, tumor <2 cm and older age group, depth of invasion <3 cm.
3. Malignant melanoma is a rare vaginal tumor (<0.5%).
   a. It is seen in patients >60 years and primarily located in the lower one-third of the anterior vaginal wall.
   b. Treatment is based on surgical removal, and the type of surgery depends on location of the lesion.
   c. Radiation and chemotherapy treatments are not effective.
   d. Local recurrences and metastases to lung are common.
4. Endodermal sinus tumors and sarcoma botryoides are vaginal tumors of infants and children.
   a. Vaginal discharge, bleeding, and a mass protruding from the vagina are common symptoms.
   b. Sarcoma botryoides resembles a cluster of grapes, and strap cells (rhabdomyoblasts) are seen in histologic section.
   c. Treatment includes a combination of surgery and chemotherapy such as vincristine, cyclophosphamide, actinomycin D (VAC).
   d. Both have a poor prognosis.

15.4 OVARIAN CANCER

1. Ovarian cancer is found in about 20% of all ovarian masses investigated.
2. Ovarian neoplasms are solid, cystic, or mixed, and malignancy can only be diagnosed by histologic examination.
3. Ovarian masses that are irregular, solid, or semisolid; are fixed; and have surface excrescences; internal papillations and areas of necrosis are worrisome.
4. Ovarian cancer is the most common cause of death from female genital tract cancers (52% of gynecologic cancer deaths).
5. It is the second most common malignancy of the lower genital tract.
6. Ovarian cancer is the fifth leading cause of overall cancer-related deaths in women.
7. Approximately 12 out of every 1000 women in the United States over the age 40 will develop ovarian cancer.
8. Most patients with epithelial ovarian carcinoma display few symptoms and most are diagnosed at stage III or stage IV.
9. The incidence of ovarian cancer increases with age, becoming most prominent at ages greater than 50 and then decreases after age 80.
   a. Peak ages are between 55 and 79 years.
   b. Elderly women are more likely to be diagnosed with higher stage disease than younger women, and their 5-year survival rate is one half that of younger women (<65).

Etiology

1. The causes of ovarian cancer are unknown.
2. Ninety-five percent of new cases are sporadic with no family history.
3. The highest rates are in highly industrialized countries, which suggests an environmental factor.
4. Nulliparity with incessant ovulation may promote carcinogenic transformation of the epithelium, whereas prevention of ovulation, such as by use of the birth control pill, may decrease the risk of developing ovarian cancer.
5. The use of talc, carcinogens from the lower genital tract, and a high-fat diet are being studied.
6. There are family clusterings of ovarian cancer.
   a. There are thought to be at least three syndromes, all autosomal dominant pattern of inheritance.
   b. A 50% risk can be predicted in all offspring and siblings of affected individuals.
      (1) The first type of inherited ovarian cancer is thought to be site specific, wherein women are only at risk for developing ovarian cancer.
      (2) The second type is a breast–ovarian syndrome, wherein women have an increased risk of breast and ovarian cancer.
      (3) The third type (Lynch type) shows an association with colon, breast, endometrial, and ovarian cancers.
7. Prophylactic oophorectomy after childbearing may not be protective for these women because the ovarian carcinomas arise from the coelomic epithelium, from which the peritoneum also arises, and therefore the peritoneum is also a potential site of tumor formation.

Signs and symptoms

1. Signs and symptoms are nonspecific. Common signs and symptoms include the following:
   a. Vague abdominal discomfort
   b. Indigestion
   c. Pain
   d. Bloating
   e. Increasing abdominal girth
   f. Abnormal vaginal bleeding
2. Ascites is a late finding.
3. Because there are no early warning signs, greater than 70% of the cases are diagnosed at stages III and IV.
4. A finding of a 5-cm mass on one or both ovaries in a women 50 to 60 years old warrants an immediate workup.

Diagnoses

1. There are no specific screening techniques for ovarian cancer.
2. The primary tumor marker used is CA-125.
   a. CA-125 is a cell surface antigenic determinant on a high molecular weight glycoprotein that is recognized by the monoclonal antibody OC-125.

b. Approximately 80% of nonmucinous epithelial ovarian malignancies, including serous, endometroid, clear cell, and undifferentiated, express this antigen.
c. CA-125 is expressed by coelomic epithelium and amnion during fetal development and is not expressed by normal ovaries.
d. Fifty percent of stage I disease and 80% of stages III and IV express this antigen.
e. Normal reference range is 35 U/ml, whereas 99% of healthy people will have less than 35 U/ml and 99.7% will have less than 65 U/ml.
f. Unfortunately CA-125 is not specific for ovarian cancer.
   (1) Ca-125 may be elevated in other gynecologic cancers such as fallopian tube and endometrial.
   (2) CA-125 is also elevated in pancreatic, colon, lung, and breast carcinoma.
   (3) It is also elevated in nonmalignant conditions such as endometriosis, pelvic inflammatory disease (PID), pancreatitis, peritonitis, renal failure, and liver cirrhosis.
g. A normal CA-125 after chemotherapy and cytoreductive surgery is associated with a negative second look, whereas a persistently elevated or rising CA-125 is predictive of persistent disease.
h. Other tumor markers such as CA-15-3, NB/70K, TAG-72, M-CSF, and OVX1 are currently being studied to increase specificity and sensitivity.

3. Transvaginal ultrasound has shown to be a promising addition to CA-125 screening to improve sensitivity.
4. Measurements of ovarian volume, morphology index, and color flow Doppler (pulsatility index and neovascularity) are being studied.

Workup for ovarian cancer

1. Thorough history (including family back several generations)
2. Physical examination
3. Pelvic examination with Papanicolaou smear
4. CBC, SMA 18, CA-125
5. Chest x-ray examination
6. IVP
7. Pelvic ultrasound or abdominal, pelvic computerized tomography (CT) with contrast barium enema
8. Indications for surgical exploration of adnexal masses are as follows:
   a. Ovary >7 cm in diameter
   b. Enlargement of an "at-rest" ovary, meaning 1 year after menopause or 1 year preceding menarche
   c. After hormonal suppression (e.g., oral contraception or GNRH suppression)
   d. In second or third trimester of pregnancy
   e. Hormonally active ovarian neoplasm
   f. Bilateral ovarian neoplasm (excluding theca-lutein cysts)
   g. Solid ovarian neoplasms
   h. Signs or symptoms suggesting torsion or rupture of an ovarian cyst
   i. Unexplained malignant ascites

Histologic Classification of Malignant Ovarian Tumors

Common Epithelial Tumors

- Serous adenocarcinoma
- Mucinous adenocarcinoma
- Clear cell adenocarcinoma
- Endometrioid adenocarcinoma
- Undifferentiated carcinoma
- Small-cell carcinoma
- Borderline serous carcinoma
- Borderline mucinous carcinoma
- Borderline clear cell
- Borderline endometrioid carcinoma
- Brenner tumor

Germ Cell Tumors

- Dysgerminoma
- Endodermal sinus tumor
- Embryonal carcinoma
- Immature teratoma
- Choriocarcinoma
- Carcinoid struma ovarii
- Gonadoblastoma
- Mixed germ cell tumors

Sex Cord–Stromal Tumors

- Granulosa cell tumor
- Juvenile granulosa cell tumor
- Cellular fibroma
- Fibrosarcoma
- Thecoma
- Sertoli–Leydig cell tumor
- Sertoli–Leydig cell tumor with retiform pattern
- Sertoli cell tumor
- Stromal–Leydig cell tumor
- Lipid cell tumor
- Hilus tumor
- Gynandroblastoma

Histology

1. Ovarian neoplasms are classified into three main categories based on cells of origin:
   a. Epithelial tumors
   b. Germ cell tumors
   c. Gonadal (sex cord) stromal tumors (see the box above)
2. Metastatic neoplasms to the ovary also occur from the gastrointestinal (GI) tract (Krukenberg), breast, endometrium, and lymphoma.

3. Ninety percent of the ovarian cancers are epithelial in origin, with serous carcinomas being the most common (40% to 45%).
4. Mucinous tumors comprise about 10%; endometriod, 15%; and undifferentiated, 17%.
5. Staging for ovarian carcinoma is primarily a surgical staging technique (Table 15-7); suggestions for comprehensive surgical staging are in Table 15-7.
6. Accurate staging is very important in determining the prognosis and method of treatment.
7. The primary treatment for ovarian epithelial carcinomas is cytoreductive surgery (see the box on p. 305).
8. The decision to use adjuvant chemotherapy is individualized and based on adequate initial staging, clinicopathologic prognostic factors, medical condition of the patient, and desire to retain reproductive capacity.
9. Prognosis is related to age, clinical stage, amount of residual cancer, and histologic grade.
   a. Poorly differentiated have a poorer prognosis.

15.5 BORDERLINE TUMORS

There is a group of tumors that histologically are borderline between cystadenomas and invasive cystadenocarcinomas. They usually do not invade the stroma and are often called tumors of low malignant potential. These tumors are seen in younger population, ages 20 to 40. Survival for stage one is 100%. Unilateral salpingo-oophorectomies are performed.

Epithelial ovarian cancer

1. As mentioned, this is the most common type of ovarian cancer (90%).
2. The first procedure done is listed in the box on p. 305, the staging laparotomy and tumor debulking.
3. Stage I disease patients' treatment varies between institutions.
   a. In stage IA, IB, no further treatment may be done.
   b. In stage IC adjuvant therapy will be done with several possible chemotherapy regimes such as cisplatin and paclitaxel combinations or alkylating agents such as melphalan or cisplatin, adriamycin, cyclophosphamide (PAC). Intraperitoneal P_{32} is also found to be effective.
4. In higher stages other chemotherapy regimes may be used.
5. Second look laparotomies are usually limited to patients who have no clinical or radiographic evidence of persistent cancer after chemotherapy.
6. Prognosis depends on stage, age, grade, and amount of residual tumor.
7. Five-year survival stage IA and IB is about 65% to 90%; stage IC, 50% to 85%; stage IIA, 50%; stage IIB and C, 45%; stage III, 13%; and stage IV 4%.

Ovarian germ cell tumors

1. These tumors constitute only 15% to 20% of all primary ovarian neoplasms and 95% are benign.

Table 15-7 FIGO staging for ovarian cancer

Stage	Criteria
I	Growth limited to the ovaries.
IA	Growth limited to one ovary; no ascites. No tumor on the external surface; capsule intact.
IB	Growth limited to both ovaries; no ascites. No tumor on the external surfaces; capsule intact.
IC	Tumor either stage IA or IB but with tumor on the surface of one or both ovaries, or with capsule ruptured, or with ascites present containing malignant cells, or with positive peritoneal washings.
II	Growth involving one or both ovaries with pelvic extension.
IIA	Extension or metastases (or both) to the uterus or tubes (or both).
IIB	Extension to other pelvic tissues
IIC	Tumor either stage IIA or IIB but with tumor on the surface of one or both ovaries, or with capsule(s) ruptured, or with ascites present containing malignant cells, or with positive peritoneal washings.
III	Tumor involving one or both ovaries with peritoneal implants outside the pelvis or positive retroperitoneal implants outside the pelvis or positive retroperitoneal or inguinal nodes (or both). Superficial liver metastases indicates stage III. Tumor limited to the true pelvis but with histologically verified malignant extension to small bowel or omentum.
IIIA	Tumor grossly limited to the true pelvis with negative nodes but with histologically confirmed microscopic seeding of abdominal peritoneal surfaces.
IIIB	Tumor of one or both ovaries with histologically confirmed implants of abdominal peritoneal surfaces, none exceeding 2 cm in diameter. Nodes negative.
IIIC	Abdominal implants >2 cm in diameter or positive retroperitoneal or inguinal nodes (or both).
IV	Growth involving one or both ovaries with distant metastasis. If pleural effusion is present there must be positive cytologic test results to allot a case to stage IV. Parenchymal liver metastasis indicates stage IV

Comprehensive Staging Laparotomy for Early Epithelial Ovarian Carcinoma

Midline abdominal incision
Washings for cytology
- Ascites
- Pelvis
- Pericolic gutters
- Diaphragm

Total abdominal hysterectomy with bilateral salpingo-oophorectomy
Omentectomy
Meticulous peritoneal exploration
Biopsies of adhesions or suspicious lesions
Random peritoneal biopsies
- Anterior and posterior cul-de-sac
- Pelvic sidewalls
- Pericolic gutters
- Small bowel serosa or mesentery
- Diaphragm

Bilateral selective pelvic and periaortic lymphadenectomy

2. The dysgerminoma is the most common type of germ cell tumor.
   a. These are tumors of younger women.
   b. A young women with suspected malignant germ cell tumor should have tumor markers drawn besides the routine laboratory tests and chest x-ray films.
   c. These markers should include the following:
      (1) Human chorionic gonadotropin (HCG)
      (2) Alpha-fetoprotein (AFP)
      (3) Lactic dehydrogenase (LDH)
   d. The malignant germ cell tumors may produce these tumor markers and can be used to follow the success of therapy.
   e. In dysgerminomas LDH and HCG may be elevated.
3. Endodermal sinus tumors are the second most common malignant germ cell tumor and may be characterized by an elevated AFP.
   a. AFP is a nonspecific marker that may be elevated in other tumors such as liver, colon pancreatic, and bronchogenic.
   b. Karyotyping should be considered in young women with a suspected malignant germ cell tumor because XY females with gonadal dysgenesis run a 25% risk of malignancy.
   c. Treatment depends on the desire to preserve fertility and stage.
      (1) Tumor debulking is always the first step
      (2) TAH/BSO with radiation follows if fertility is not an issue.
   d. Dysgerminomas are particularly radiosensitive. Some combinations of chemotherapy such as vinblastin, etopside, bleomycin, and platinum are used successfully.

Sex cord–stromal tumors

1. Comprise 5% of ovarian tumors and have no specific markers associated with them.
2. May produce excessive estrogen, progesterone, testosterone, corticosteroids, and signs of overproduction of any of these hormones should prompt further investigation.
3. Usually benign or tumors of low malignant potential.
   a. Fifty percent of these tumors are fibromas and are benign.
   b. The rest of these tumors are predominantly granulosa cell tumors.
4. Granulosa cell tumors may be suspected when an adnexal mass is seen with signs of excess estrogen production, such as isosexual precocious puberty or postmenopausal bleeding.
5. Treatment includes tumor debulking, radiation, and chemotherapy combinations such as VAC.
6. Prognosis is good for stage I (85%); 55%, stage II; and 25%, stage III.

Suggested reading

1. Boente MP, Godwin AK, Hogan WM: Screening, imaging, and early diagnosis of ovarian cancer, *Clin Obstet Gynecol* 37(2):377-391, 1994.
2. Daunter B: Review: tumor markers in gynecology oncology, *Gynecol Oncol* 39:1-15, 1990.
3. Disaia PJ, Creasman WT: *Clinical gynecologic oncology,* ed 4, St Louis, 1993, Mosby–Year Book.
4. Herbst AL et al: *Comprhensive gynecology,* ed 2, St Louis, 1992, Mosby–Year Book.
5. Montag TW: Tumor markers in gynecologic oncology, *Obstet Gynecol Surv* 45(2):94-105, 1990.
6. Nagell JR et al: Ovarian cancer screening, *CANCER* Suppl. 71(4):1523-1528, 1993.
7. Piver SM: *Manual of gynecologic oncology and gynecology.* Boston, 1989, Little, Brown.
8. Rubin SC, Lewis JL: Tumor antigens in ovarian malignancy, *Clin Obstet Gynecol* 29(3):693-700, 1986.
9. Soper JT: Management of early-stage epithelial ovarian cancer, *Clin Obstet Gynecol* 37(2):423-438, 1994.
10. Sutton G: Chemotherapy of epithelial ovarian cancer: an overview, *Clin Obstet Gyncol* 37(2):461-474, 1994.
11. Wolfson AH et al: A multivariant analysis of clinicopathologic factors for predicting outcome in uterine sarcomas, *Gynecol Oncol* 52:56-62, 1994.

Abdominal Surgical Approaches

16

J. Kevin Fitzpatrick, M.D.

16.1 ANATOMY OF THE ANTERIOR ABDOMINAL WALL

Skin and subcutaneous tissue

1. The skin is composed of epidermis and dermis.
2. It is traversed by lines of cleavage called Langer's lines. First described by Langer in 1861, these lines represent parallel rows of collagen bundles present in the dermal tissue. When these lines are transected the skin edges are pulled apart.
3. Skin incisions following these lines generally heal with a thinner scar.
4. The Langer's lines on the abdomen run in a transverse fashion (Fig. 16-1).

Fascial layers (Fig. 16-2)

1. Camper's fascia
   a. Superficial fatty layer that can be several centimeters thick in an obese patient
2. Scarpa's fascia
   a. A membranous layer lying beneath Camper's fascia
   b. Continuous with Colle's fascia of the perineum and joins the deep fascia lata of the anterior thigh 2 cm inferior to the inguinal ligament
3. Rectus fascia
   a. The rectus fascia is a tough band of connective tissue that is composed of the aponeuroses of the external oblique, internal oblique, and transversus abdominis muscles and their point of insertion at the midline in the avascular linea alba.
   b. Superior to the arcuate line, a landmark found in the midline at the level of the anterior superior iliac spine, the aponeuroses form an anterior and posterior sheath to the rectus abdominis muscles.
      (1) The anterior rectus sheath consists of the aponeuroses of the external oblique and the split aponeurosis of the internal oblique.
      (2) The posterior rectus sheath consists of the remaining portion of the internal oblique coupled with the aponeurosis of the transversus abdominis muscle.

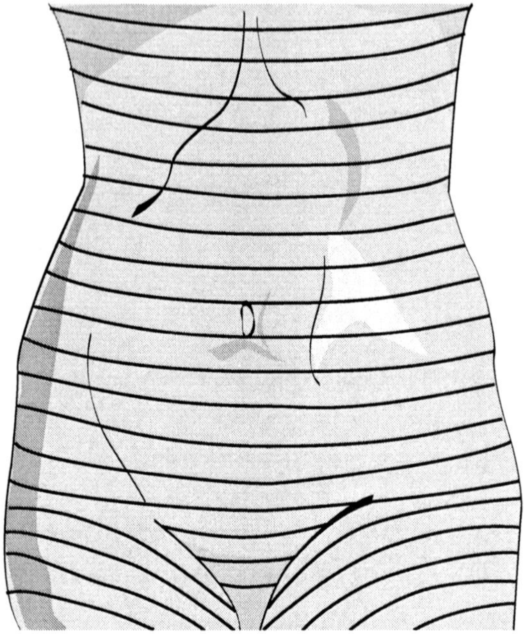

Figure 16-1
Langer's lines of the abdomen.

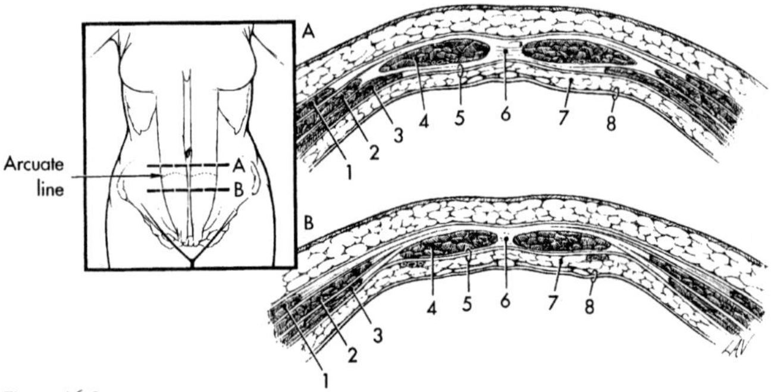

Figure 16-2
A, Transverse section of the anterior abdominal wall above the arcuate line. The posterior leaf of the aponeurosis of the internal oblique muscle and the aponeurosis of the transversus abdominis muscle unite to form the posterior wall of the rectus sheath. **B,** A transverse section through the anterior abdominal wall. Below the arcuate line, the posterior wall of the rectus sheath is formed only by the transversalis fascia. *1,* External oblique; *2,* internal oblique; *3,* transversus abdominis; *4,* rectus abdominis; *5A,* posterior rectus sheath; *5B,* transversales fascia; *6,* linea alba; *7,* perperitioneal fat; *8,* peritoneum. (From Nichols DH, editor: *Gynecologic and obstetric surgery,* St Louis, 1993, Mosby.)

c. Inferior to the arcuate line, the posterior rectus sheath disappears.
d. The transversus abdominus and the entire internal oblique aponeurosis is found anterior to the rectus abdominus muscle.
e. Therefore, below the arcuate line, the anterior rectus sheath consists of the aponeuroses of the external and the entire internal oblique and transversus abdominus.
f. In this region the anterior abdominal wall is weaker and there is an increased incidence of incisional hernias.

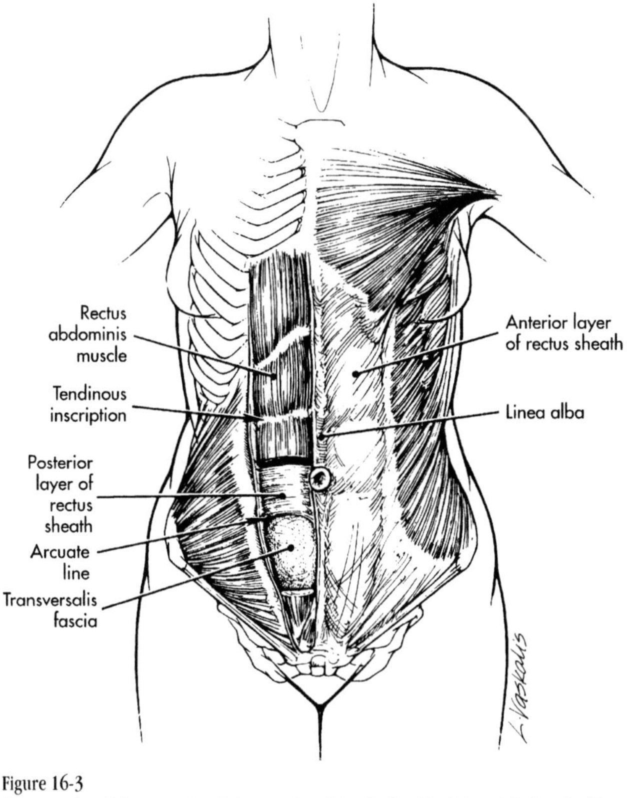

Figure 16-3
A composite of the muscles of the anterior abdominal wall of the adult female. The superficial muscles are shown in the left side of the drawing, and the rectus abdominis and external and internal oblique muscles have been removed in the right side of the drawing. (From Nichols DH, editor: *Gynecologic and obstetric surgery,* St Louis, 1993, Mosby.)

g. Tendinous insertions between the rectus abdominus muscles and the anterior rectus sheath exist in several horizontal bands along the course of the muscle.
4. Transversalis fascia: a membranous layer that lies deep to the rectus muscles and superficial to the peritoneum

Muscle layers (Fig. 16-3)

1. Rectus abdominis
   a. The rectus abdominis is a paired group of longitudinal muscles found in the midline.
   b. They are separated by the linea alba and held in the rectus sheath as described above.
   c. Their origin is on the symphysis pubis and the pubic crest and the rectus abdominis runs to the xiphoid process and lower costal cartilage.
   d. There are also tendinous insertions between the muscle and the anterior rectus sheath found mainly above the arcuate line.
      (1) These function to anchor the muscle to the anterior sheath.
   e. Function of the rectus abdominis is in locomotion and increasing intraabdominal pressure.
   f. The inferior epigastric artery supplies the lower portion of the muscle and enters the rectus sheath posteriorly at the arcuate line.
      (1) This vessel anastomoses with the superior epigastric artery, which supplies the upper portion of the muscle.
   g. Nerve supply to the rectus abdominis is derived from the intercostal and lumbar nerves, which enter the rectus sheath laterally.
2. External oblique muscle
   a. The most superficial of the lateral abdominal muscles.
   b. It runs from its origin on the lower eight ribs to its insertion on the pubic crest, pubic tubercle, linea alba, and xiphoid process.
   c. This muscle functions mainly to assist respirations and increasing abdominal pressure.
      (1) It has a minor role in locomotion.
   d. Its aponeurosis forms part of the anterior rectus sheath.
3. Internal oblique muscle
   a. This muscle is found deep to the external oblique.
   b. Its origin is on the lumbar fascia, iliac crest, and inguinal ligament.
   c. It inserts on the symphysis pubis, linea alba, lower ribs, and xiphoid process.
   d. The rectus sheath is partially formed by its aponeurosis, as mentioned previously.
   e. Its fibers run perpendicular to the external oblique's fibers.
   f. It, too, functions mainly in respiration, increasing abdominal pressure, and locomotion.
4. Transversus abdominis
   a. This muscle lies deep to the internal oblique.
   b. It arises from the lower costal cartilages, lumbar fascia, iliac crest, and inguinal ligament.

c. Its insertion is found on the symphysis pubis, linea alba, and xiphoid process.
d. Functions include respiration, increasing abdominal pressure, and locomotion.
e. Its aponeurosis is part of the anterior and posterior rectus sheath, as mentioned.

Blood supply (Fig. 16-4)

1. The blood supply for the anterior abdominal wall arises mainly from the inferior and superior epigastrics near the midline.
2. Laterally, the blood supply is derived from the intercostal, lumbar, and deep circumflex iliac arteries.

Nerve supply (Fig. 16-5)

1. The intercostal and lumbar nerves run between the internal oblique and transversus muscles.
2. These enter the rectus sheath at various points laterally and innervate the rectus abdominis.
3. The skin over the symphysis pubis and upper, lateral thigh is innervated by branches of the iliohypogastric and ilioinguinal nerves.
4. This is important in transverse incisions, in which numbness over the abdomen and upper thigh may result from transection of these branches.

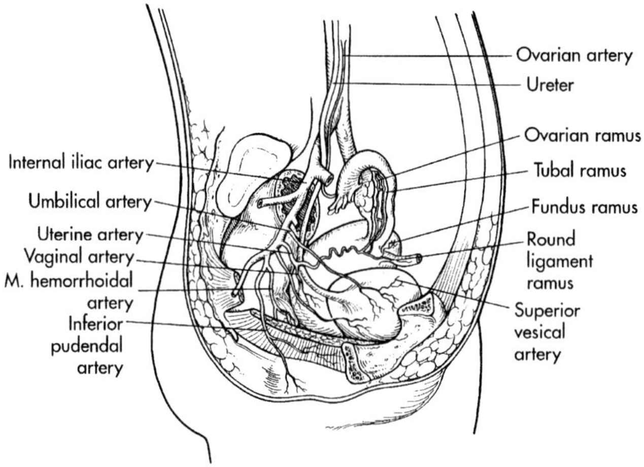

Figure 16-4
Arteries of the internal female genitalia. (From Nichols DH, editor: *Gynecologic and obstetric surgery,* St Louis, 1993, Mosby.)

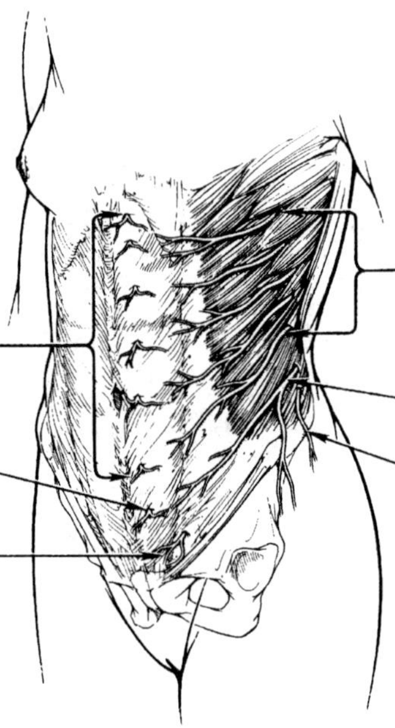

Figure 16-5
A, Superificial nerves of the anterior abdominal wall.

Continued.

16.2 ABDOMINAL INCISIONS

Selection of the appropriate incision (Fig. 16-6)

There are several considerations when selecting an abdominal approach. The main factor is exposure. It is absurd to select a limited incision that will not grant adequate exposure to perform the necessary surgery.

1. Midline incisions
   a. Midline incisions provide excellent exposure.
   b. They can be extended cranially without compromising the strength of the abdominal wall.
   c. These incisions, however, do not heal as well as the transverse incision and are less cosmetically appealing.
   d. The midline incision is generally reserved for cases in which a transverse incision would not allow for adequate exposure.
   e. Another factor is the speed of entry in an emergency situation. In this regard, the low midline incision is again generally considered the incision of choice.

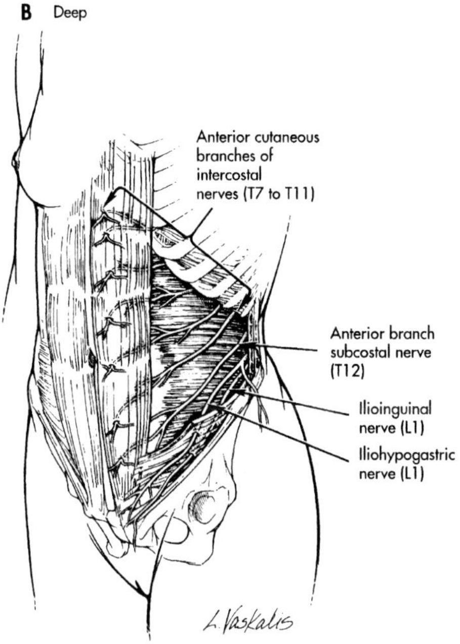

Figure 16-5, cont'd
B, Deep nerves of the anterior abdominal wall. (From Nichols DH, editor: *Gynecologic and obstetric surgery,* St Louis, 1993, Mosby.)

2. Transverse incisions
   a. The transverse incisions usually provide adequate exposure, are stronger, and are more cosmetically appealing than the midline incisions.
   b. The transverse incisions are the most common abdominal incisions in gynecologic and obstetric surgery.

Transverse incisions

There are several types of transverse incisions. As mentioned previously, these incisions are used preferentially, provided adequate exposure can be achieved. This is because they heal better, with less incidence of incisional hernias than the midline incision. Also, since they follow Langer's lines, they heal with a thinner scar. They do, however, have a higher incidence of skin numbness inferior to the incision and damage to the femoral nerve by crushing it to the psoas with the deep blades of retractors.

1. Pfannenstiel incision (Fig. 16-7)
   a. This is a transverse incision that is generally considered to have the best postoperative strength.

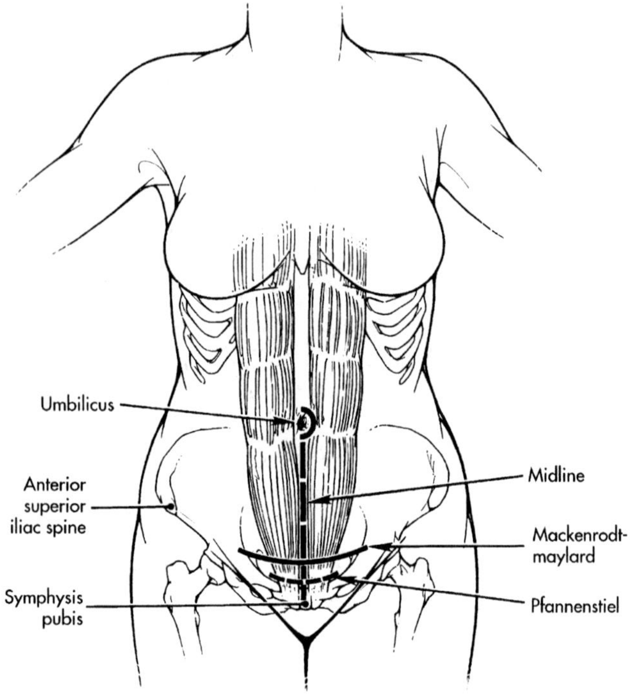

Figure 16-6
The frequent incisions of the anterior abdominal wall are shown in relation to the anterior superior iliac spines. (From Nichols DH, editor: *Gynecologic and obstetric surgery,* St Louis, 1993, Mosby.)

b. However, it offers probably the least exposure of any abdominal incision.
c. To perform this incision, the following is done:
   (1) The skin is incised approximately 2 cm above the symphysis pubis in a transverse fashion.
   (2) This incision is carried down through Camper's and Scarpa's fascia to the rectus fascia with either the scalpel or electrocautery.
   (3) The rectus fascia is then nicked in the midline, again in a transverse fashion.
   (4) This incision is then carried laterally through the rectus fascia with either Mayo scissors, scalpel, or cautery.
   (5) Often, the fascia can be elevated with a Rochester clamp to allow incision without extension into the deeper tissues.

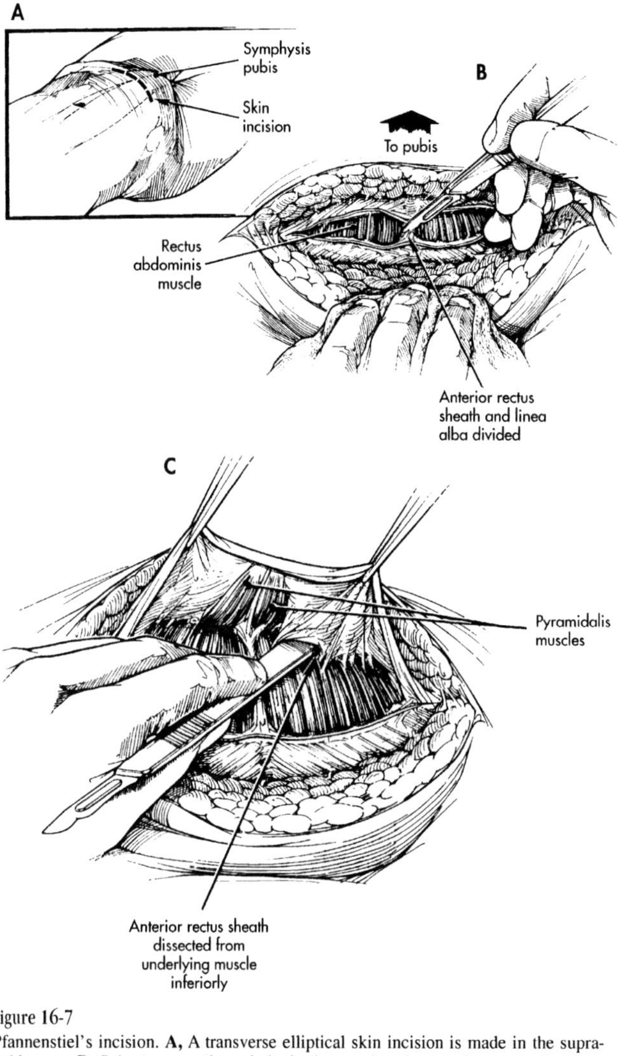

Figure 16-7

Pfannenstiel's incision. **A,** A transverse elliptical skin incision is made in the suprapubic area. **B,** Subcutaneous tissue is incised, exposing the anterior rectus sheath, which is incised to expose the underlying rectus abdominis muscle. The anterior sheath is separated from the muscle by sharp and blunt dissection (**C**), first in the caudal portion of the incision, and then beneath the cranial portion of the anterior rectus sheath (**D**).

Continued.

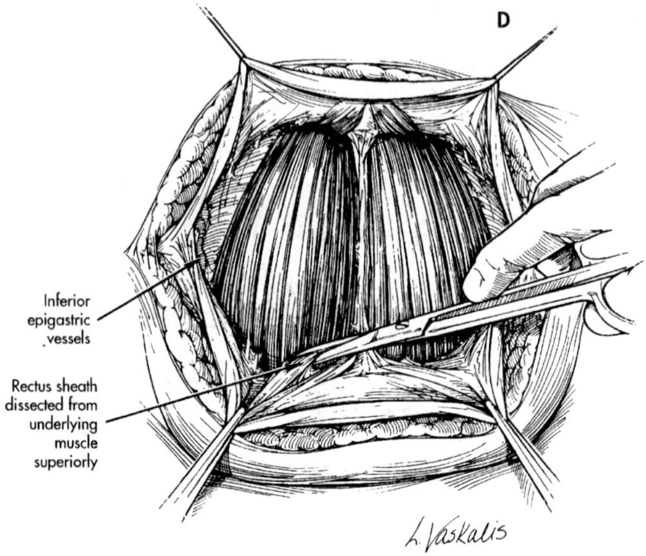

Figure 16-7, cont'd
For legend, see previous page.

(6) Once the rectus fascia has been incised, Kocher clamps are used to grasp the superior leaf of the fascia.
(7) This is then dissected off the rectus abdominis and pyramidalis muscles using either blunt or sharp dissection.
(8) While dissecting the fascia off the muscle, it is important to be aware of perforating vessels that come through the rectus muscle, mainly lateral to the midline, to give a blood supply to the anterior rectus sheath.
   (a) These can be controlled with either cautery or fine free ties.
(9) After dissection of the superior leaf of the fascia is complete, attention is given to the inferior leaf of the incised fascia.
   (a) This too is grasped with two Kocher clamps and dissected off the pyramidalis muscle using either blunt or sharp dissection.
   (b) The dissection should be carried down to the level of the pubic symphysis.
(10) Following this, the rectus muscles are separated in the midline and retracted laterally, exposing the transversalis fascia and peritoneum.

E

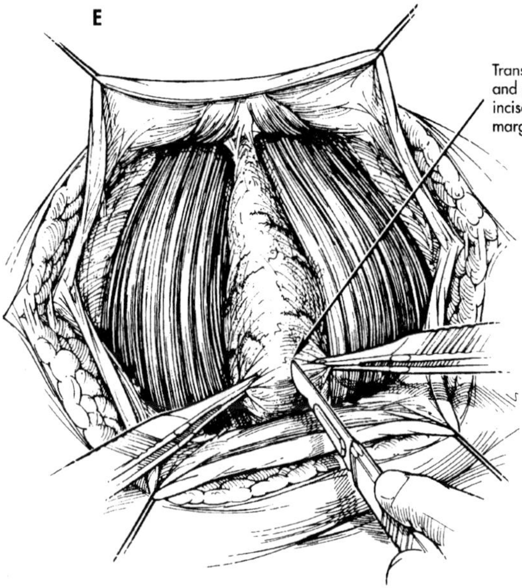

Figure 16-7, cont'd
The peritoneum is identified between the bellies of the rectus muscles, and the transversalis fascia and peritoneum are grasped with forceps and incised in the midline at the cranial margin of the exposure **(E)**.

Continued.

(11) This layer is then grasped with two clamps and elevated.
   (a) It is important at this point to make sure that the peritoneum is grasped sufficiently cranially to ensure the bladder is not included in the clamp.
   (b) The possibility of picking up adherent bowel or omentum in the clamp should also be considered, particularly in a patient with previous abdominal surgery, endometriosis, or intraabdominal infection.

(12) Once the presence of bowel or omentum in the clamp has been ruled out by palpation, Metzenbaum scissors can be used to sharply enter the peritoneum.

d. This incision can be extended cranially using the Metzenbaum scissors.

e. When extending the incision caudally, the transversalis fascia can be dissected sharply off the peritoneum and incised.
   (1) Care must be taken at this point not to enter the bladder.
   (2) Transillumination should be used while extending the peritoneal incision to ensure this does not occur.
   (3) It may also be necessary to split the pyramidalis muscle in the midline to provide adequate exposure.

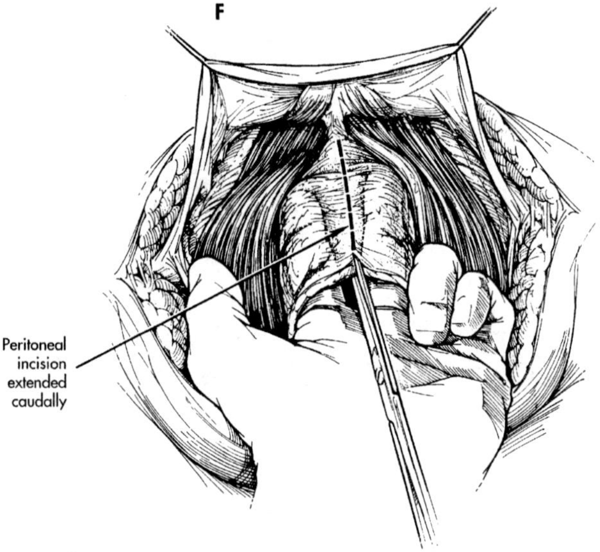

Figure 16-7, cont'd

F, The surgeon's fingertips are inserted caudally beneath the peritoneum, and the incision is extended downward between the surgeon's fingers, with care being taken to recognize and avoid the cranial margin of the apex of the bladder at the inferior pole of the incision. At the completion of surgery, it is optional whether the parietal peritoneum and transversalis fascia are closed. (From Nichols DH, editor: *Gynecologic and obstetric surgery,* St Louis, 1993, Mosby.)

f. This completes the steps necessary to enter the abdomen through a Pfannenstiel incision.

As mentioned previously, this incision is limited by the amount of exposure it provides. If a Pfannenstiel incision is done and exposure is suboptimal, it can be converted to a Cherney incision. It is important that this incision not be converted to a Maylard, because once the fascia has been dissected off the rectus muscles, as in the Pfannenstiel, transecting the rectus abdominis muscle corpus, as is done in the Maylard, may cause the rectus muscle to retract and, without its insertions to the anterior sheath, it may not heal well.

2. Maylard incision (Fig. 16-8)
    a. This incision allows for greater exposure than the Pfannenstiel as the rectus abdominis muscle is transected and retracted superiorly and inferiorly.
    b. Through this incision, pelvic and paraaortic node dissections can be done, as well as the removal of large pelvic tumors.
    c. When compared with the midline incision, the Maylard has less postoperative pain, stronger healing, and fewer adhesions, although accessibility to the upper abdomen through this incision is limited.

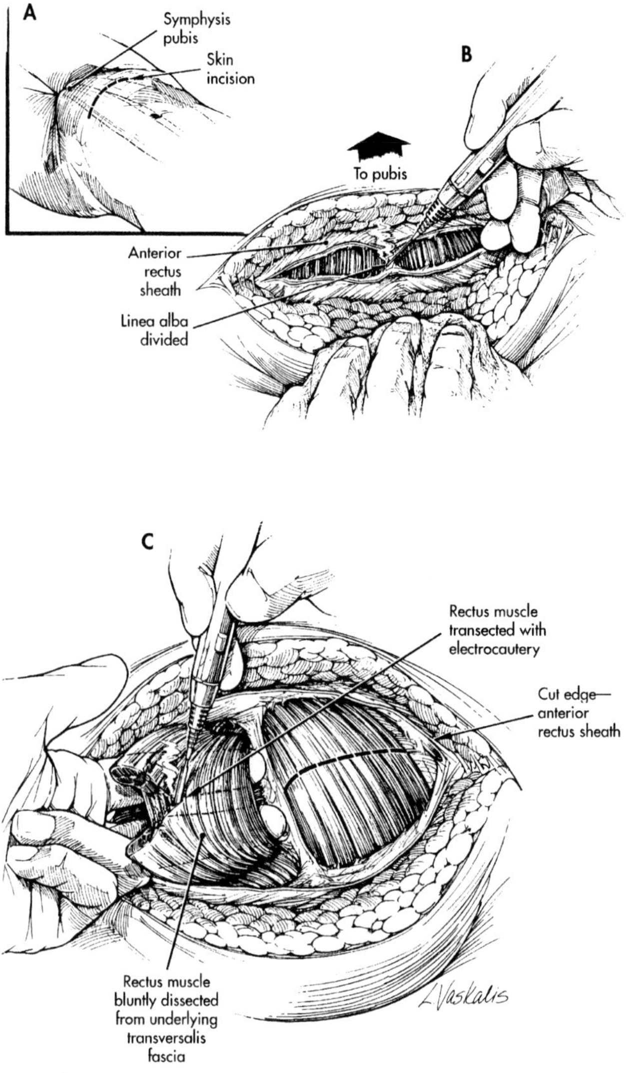

Figure 16-8

The Maylard incision. **A,** A transverse skin incision is made 5 cm above the superior border of the pubis. **B,** The anterior rectus sheath is incised in the same line, exposing the bellies of the rectus abdominis muscles. The muscle is bluntly dissected from the underlying transversalis fascia and incised transversely on each side, along the path of the broken side, using the electrosurgical scalpel (**C**). *Continued.*

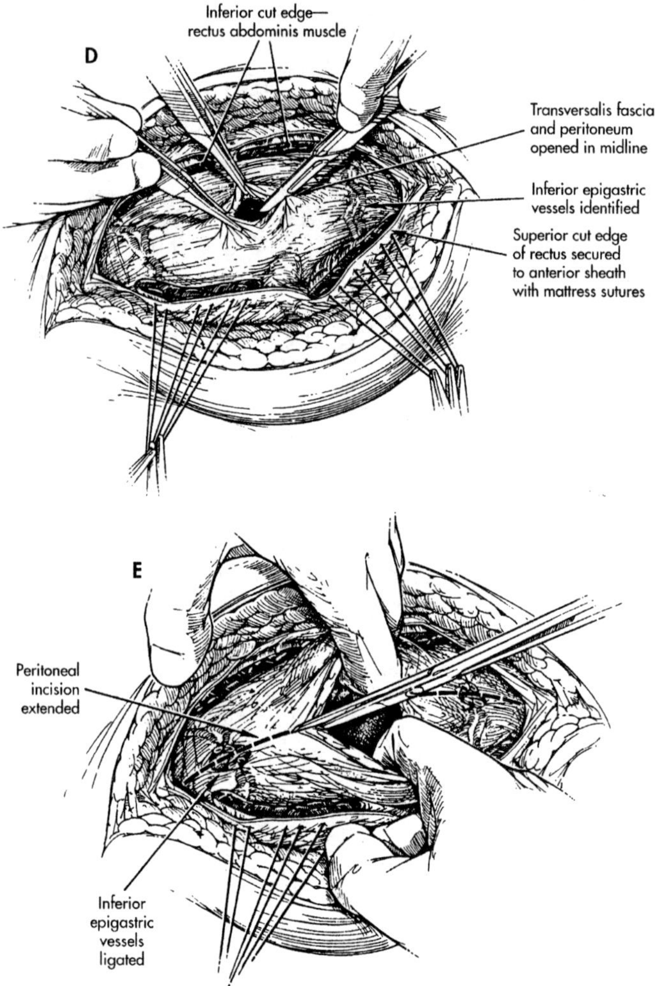

Figure 16-8, cont'd

D, The transversalis fascia and peritoneum are opened, and the superior cut edge of the rectus abdominis is secured to the anterior sheath with mattress sutures. **E,** The peritoneal incision is extended laterally, and the inferior epigastric vessels must usually be ligated and cut. (From Nichols DH, editor: *Gynecologic and obstetric surgery,* St Louis, 1993, Mosby.)

d. To perform the Maylard incision, the following is done:
   (1) An incision is made 2 to 3 cm above the pubic symphysis and carried down to the rectus fascia, as is done in the Pfannenstiel incision.
   (2) Once the rectus fascia has been identified, it is nicked using the scalpel and extended bilaterally using sharp dissection.
   (3) At this point, the incision differs from the Pfannenstiel in that the rectus fascia is not dissected off the rectus abdominis muscles. Instead, the inferior epigastric arteries are isolated in the connective tissue lying at the lateral border of the rectus muscles.
      (a) These can be identified by palpation and dissected out using blunt dissection with a clamp.
      (b) Once identified, they should be ligated by passing a free 2-0 Vicryl tie around the vessel on a right angle clamp.
      (c) They should be doubly ligated and incised in between the ligatures.
   (4) After the epigastrics are ligated, attention can be turned to the rectus abdominis muscles. These can be transected, about 3 to 5 cm above their origin on the pubic symphysis, using electrocautery, and proceeding across the muscle in a zigzagging motion to achieve adequate hemostasis.
   (5) Often, a Penrose drain can be passed beneath each rectus muscle, allowing elevation of the muscle while the incision is made.
   (6) This also serves to protect the underlying tissues from extending beyond the limits of the muscle with the electrocautery.
   (7) Once the rectus muscle has been transected, it can be retracted superiorly and inferiorly and the transversalis fascia and peritoneum can be entered using the technique mentioned previously, with the only difference being that the peritoneum is opened in a transverse fashion parallel to the skin incision.
   (8) When closing this incision, it is not necessary to reapproximate the rectus muscles because these will spontaneously heal provided their tendinous insertions to the anterior rectus sheath remain intact.

3. Cherney incision (Fig. 16-9)
   a. This incision differs from the Maylard in that the rectus muscle is not transected through its corpus; instead, it is cut across its tendinous origin on the pubic symphysis.
   b. The muscle is then retracted cranially.
   c. Following the surgery, the tendinous insertion is reattached to the pubic symphysis.
   d. This incision is strong and allows adequate exposure to the pelvis.
   e. Like the Maylard it is limited in its exposure of the upper abdomen.
      (1) A Cherney incision begins like the Maylard and Pfannenstiel in that the skin and superficial fascia are cut down to the level of the rectus fascia.
      (2) The rectus fascia is then nicked in the midline and the incision is extended transversely with sharp dissection as described.

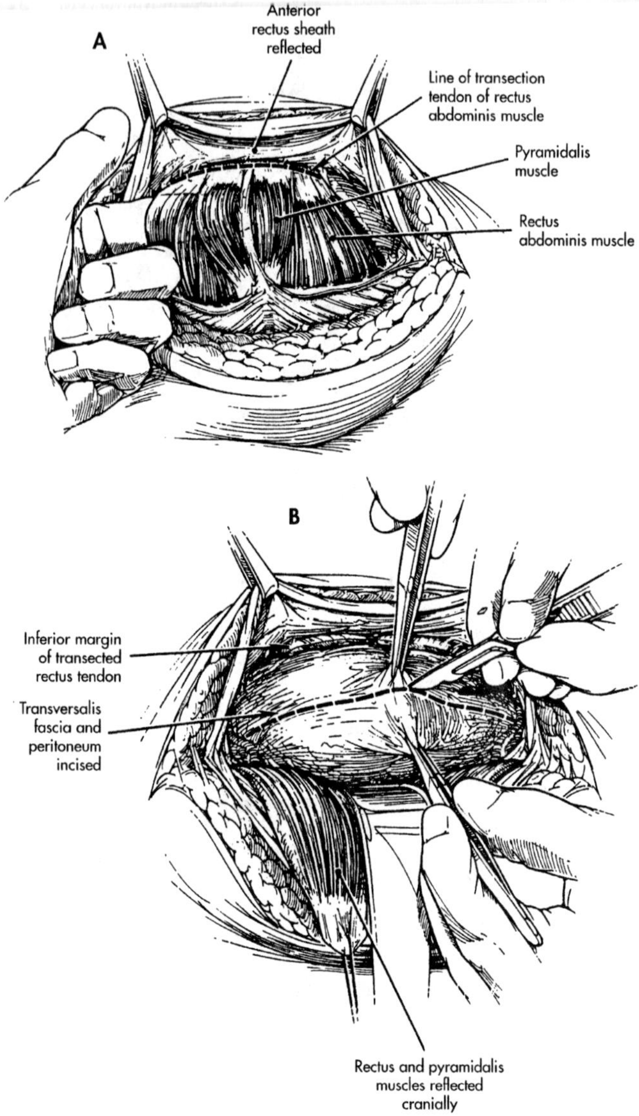

Figure 16-9

The Cherney incision. **A,** A transverse elliptical skin incision is made through the skin and subcutaneous tissue. The tendon of the rectus abdominis muscle and pyramidalis is transsected on each side as shown by the broken line. **B,** The muscles are reflected cranially, and the peritoneum and transversalis fascia are picked up between forceps and incised transversely. *Continued.*

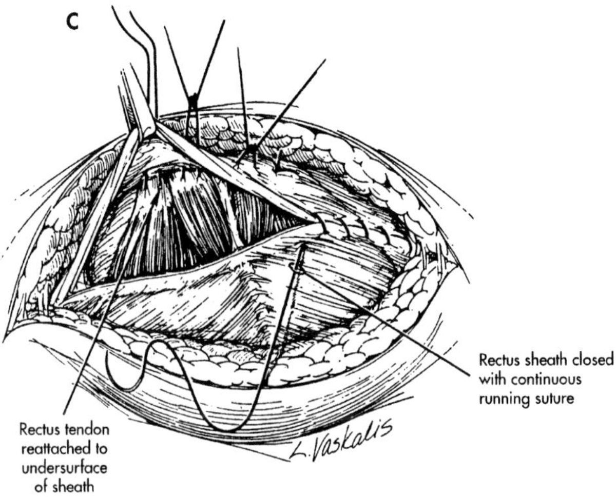

Figure 16-9, cont'd
C, At the conclusion of surgery, the tendon of the rectus muscle is attached to the undersurface of the rectus sheath by several interrupted stitches, and the original incision in the rectus aponeurosis is closed with a continuous running suture. The skin incision is closed with staples or a subcuticular closure. (From Nichols DH, editor: *Gynecologic and obstetric surgery,* St Louis, 1993, Mosby.)

(a) At this point, the Cherney differs from the Maylard in that the inferior leaf of the split fascia is grasped with two Kocher clamps, is elevated, and is dissected off the rectus abdominis and pyramidalis muscles using either sharp or blunt dissection.

(b) This dissection is carried down to the level of the pubic symphysis, where the aponeurosis of the rectus and pyramidalis muscles are identified.

(3) The tendon is then incised with Mayo scissors, releasing the muscles from their origin on the pubic symphysis.

(4) This allows the muscles to be retracted superiorly, and out of the operative field.

(5) Once retracted, the transversalis fascia and peritoneum can be entered as described.

(6) Following the operation, the tendon of the rectus and pyramidalis muscles should be reattached to the pubic symphysis using interrupted permanent suture.

(7) Because this incision reattaches the muscle to the pubic symphysis, the rectus muscle cannot retract cranially into the rectus sheath. Therefore, a Pfannenstiel incision, if found to be inadequate intraoperatively, can be converted to a Cherney without compromising the integrity of the midline musculature.

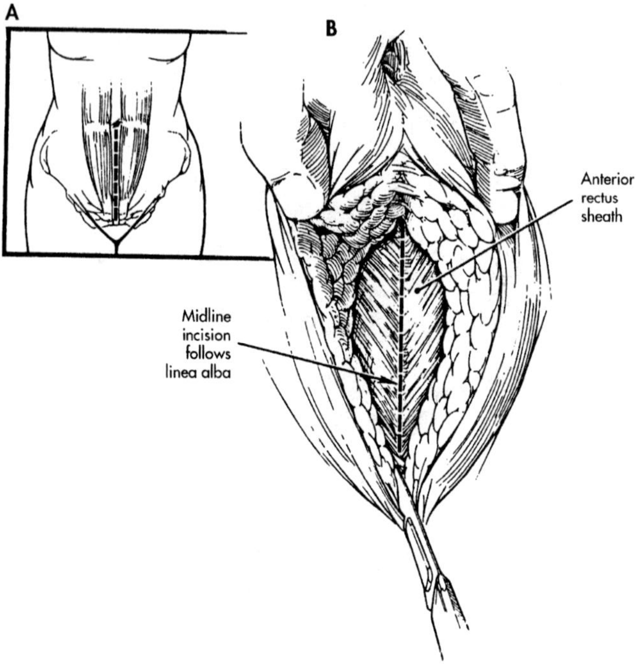

Figure 16-10
The technique of a midline incision in the lower abdomen. **A,** Site of the incision between the umbilicus and the pubis. **B,** The midline incision continues through the subcutaneous tissue to expose the linea alba of the anterior rectus sheath. *Continued.*

Vertical incisions

As mentioned, the vertical incisions allow for unparalleled exposure to both the pelvis and upper abdomen and can be extended from xiphoid to pubis if need be. They are, however, not as strong as the transverse incisions and, because Langer's lines are transected, heal with a larger, less cosmetically appealing scar.

1. Median incision (Fig. 16-10)
   a. In this procedure, the following is done:
      (1) An incision is made between the umbilicus and pubic symphysis.
      (2) This is carried down through the superficial fascia to the level of the rectus fascia, using either the scalpel or cautery.
      (3) The fascia is then nicked in a vertical direction and a Rochester clamp is placed beneath the fascia to elevate it and allow it to be incised without extension into the deeper tissues.

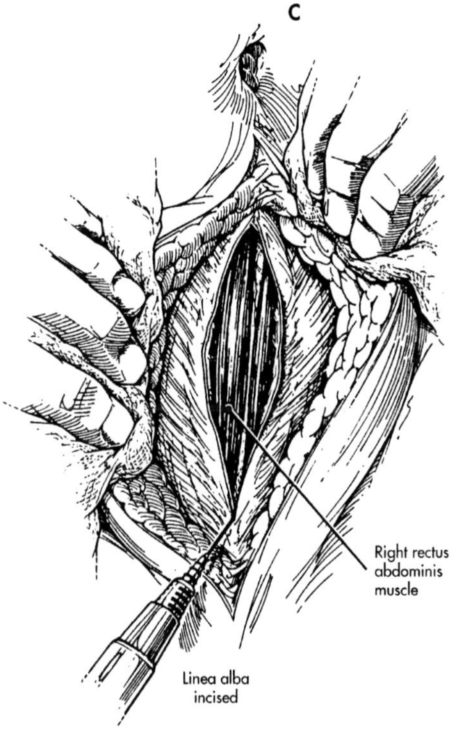

Figure 16-10, cont'd
C, This sheath is incised.

Continued.

(4) A scalpel or cautery can then be used to incise the fascia, opening it to the limits of the skin incision.
(5) The rectus muscles are then split in the midline along the linea alba and retracted laterally.
(6) Using clamps, the deeper tissues are then bluntly dissected and the transversalis fascia and peritoneum are identified and elevated between two clamps.
    (a) As described previously, the peritoneum is palpated to ensure no bowel or omentum is adherent to the posterior surface of the peritoneum.
(7) The peritoneum is then entered sharply using Metzenbaum scissors.
(8) This incision is then carried cranially using the Mayo scissors and transecting the posterior rectus sheath, transversalis fascia, and peritoneum in the midline.

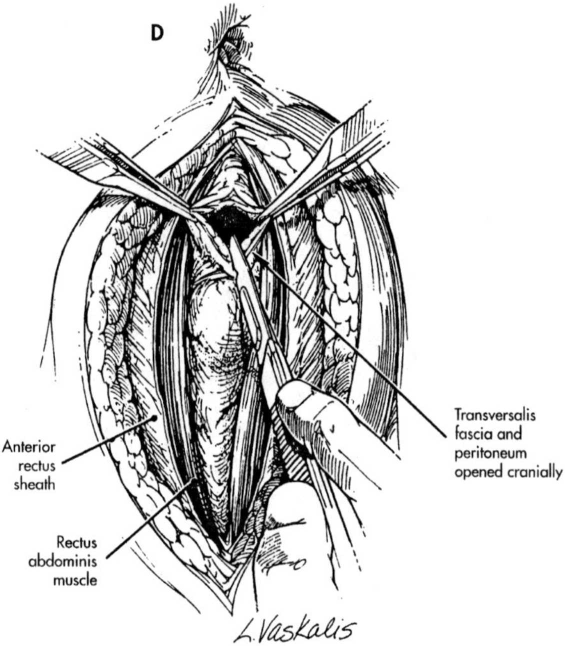

Figure 16-10, cont'd

D, The peritoneum and transversalis fascia are grasped between forceps and opened at the cranial end of the incision.

Continued.

(a) While making this portion of the incision, the posterior surface of the peritoneum should be explored intermittently to ensure that no bowel or omentum is adherent to the posterior surface.

(9) Once the incision has been extended to the length of the skin incision, the peritoneum can be incised in a caudal direction.
   (a) Again, the position of the bladder should be demonstrated by transillumination to avoid entering it with extension of the incision.
   (b) Once complete, this incision will allow adequate exposure for pelvic surgery and exploration of the upper abdomen and paraaortic lymphatics.
   (c) Should the need arise, the incision can be carried around the umbilicus and as far cranially as the xiphoid process, allowing exposure to the entire upper abdomen.

E

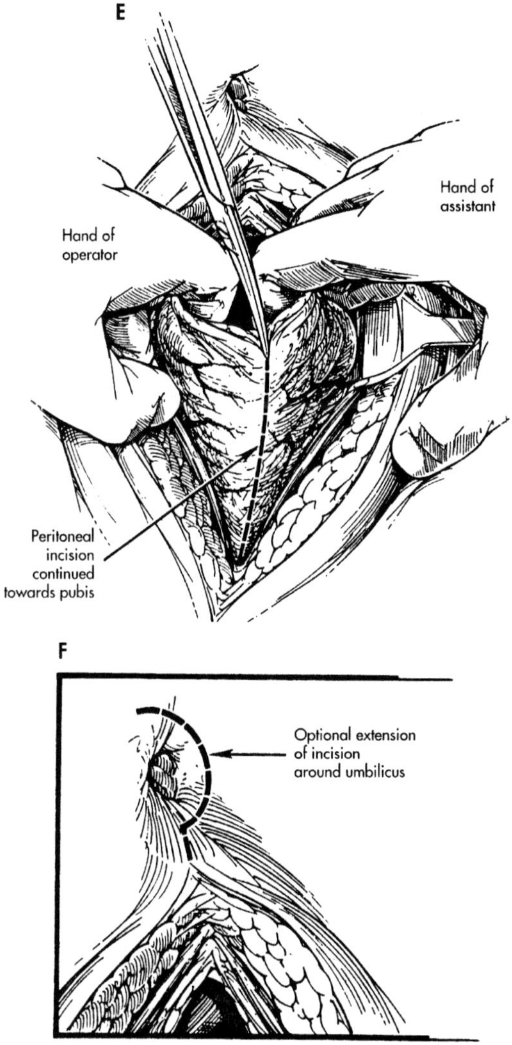

Figure 16-10, cont'd
Transillumination of this flap by looking through its peritoneal side discloses the outline of the apex of the bladder, marking the caudal limit of the pubic peritoneal dissection (**E**). When it is necessary to extend the midline incision cranially to obtain additional exposure, it should be performed around the left side of the umbilicus to avoid the ligamentus teres (**F**). (From Nichols DH, editor: *Gynecologic and obstetric surgery,* St Louis, 1993, Mosby.)

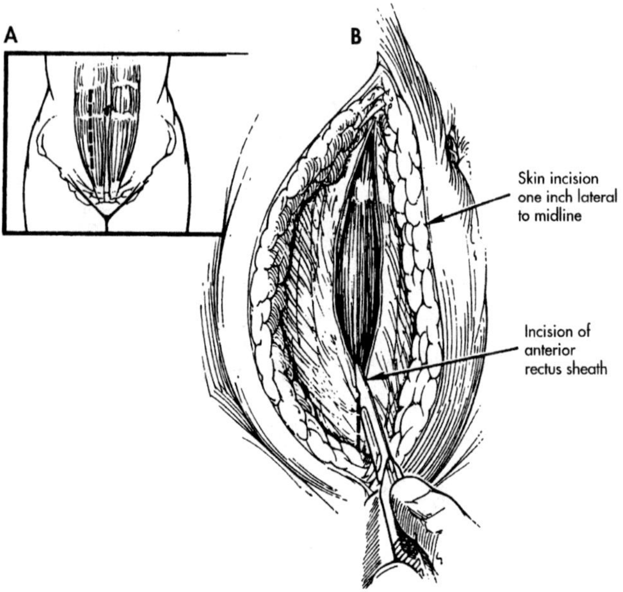

Figure 16-11
Paramedian incision. The skin incision is made on either the right or the left side of the abdomen along the path of the dashed line as shown in **A,** 1 inch lateral to the midline. The anterior rectus sheath is incised over the midportion of the underlying rectus muscle (**B**) and retracted laterally. *Continued.*

2. Paramedian Incision (Fig. 16-11)
   a. This incision is made to one side of the midline, usually on the side of the expected pathology.
      (1) Instead of entering the peritoneal cavity through the linea alba, the rectus muscle is split longitudinally and retracted laterally.
      (2) Or the abdomen is entered lateral to the rectus muscle following ligature of the inferior epigastric artery.
   b. This incision is reported to be stronger than the median incision, as the avascular linea alba is left intact.
   c. Denervation of the rectus muscle can occur if the incision is extended too far along the lateral border of the muscle. This can result in muscle atrophy.

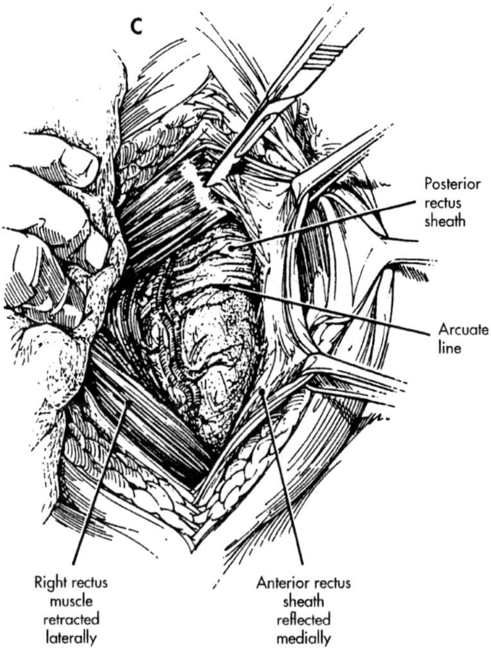

Figure 16-11, cont'd
The anterior rectus sheath is reflected immediately (**C**). *Continued.*

16.3 CLOSING THE ABDOMEN

Transverse incisions

1. Peritoneum
   a. It is currently controversial whether to close the peritoneum following laparotomy or leave it to heal spontaneously.
   b. Several recent studies have shown no benefit in closing the peritoneal membrane; however, surgeons are still concerned that failure to close this layer will result in pelvic and abdominal organs becoming adherent to the anterior abdominal wall.
   c. One exception is with the Maylard incision; in this case, the peritoneum should be closed to keep the split ends of the rectus muscles outside the peritoneal cavity.
   d. To close the peritoneum, the following is done:
      (1) The entire length of the defect can be grasped with clamps. This allows definition of the membrane and its elevation to aid in suturing.

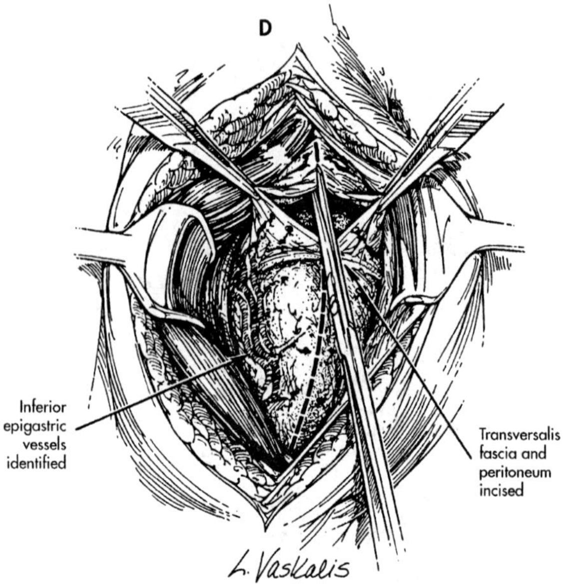

Figure 16-11, cont'd
The posterior rectus sheath, transversalis fascia, and peritoneum are incised in the bed temporarily vacated by the muscle (**D**). (From Nichols DH, editor: *Gynecologic and obstetric surgery,* St Louis, 1993, Mosby.)

(2) Using an absorbable or delayed absorbable suture, this layer can be closed in a running stitch, which generally begins at the cranial apex of the incision and extends to the inferior apex.
(3) When suturing near the caudal aspect of the incision, more superficial stitches should be used to avoid including the bladder.
(4) A malleable ribbon can be used to protect the bowel from inadvertent needle punctures.

e. Manipulation of this layer in patients under regional anesthesia, as at cesarean section, can result in discomfort, nausea, and vomiting.

2. Muscle
   a. Closing the muscle defect in the Maylard incision is not useful in providing extra strength for the incision because the rectus will be reapproximated when the rectus fascia is closed and will heal spontaneously.
   b. Reapproximation of the rectus muscles in the Pfannenstiel incision is also of little value.
   c. In the Cherney incision, it is necessary to reattach the aponeurosis of the rectus and pyramidalis muscles to their origin on the pubic symphysis using a permanent suture.

   (1) Should one choose to close the muscle layer in a Pfannenstiel incision, wide bites of a delayed absorbable or absorbable suture should be used and these should be loosely tied, just allowing for gentle reapproximation of the musculature.

3. Rectus fascia
   a. This layer should be closed using a delayed absorbable or permanent suture of sufficient strength.
      (1) The apex of the defect should be identified and the initial suture placed behind the apex, through both leaves of the fascia.
      (2) Care should be taken not to include the corpus of the oblique or transverse musculature because ligature of these could result in damage to the ilioinguinal and iliohypogastric nerves, causing numbness inferior to the incision and over the upper thigh.
      (3) The sutures should be placed at 1- to 2-cm intervals and at least 1.5 cm away from the cut edge.
         (a) This avoids strangulation of the fascia and weakening the incision.
      (4) Again, the fascia should be approximated with gentle pressure and not pulled taut.
         (a) This too avoids strangulation of the tissues and postoperative pain.
4. Superficial fascia
   a. Recent reports have shown that closure of the superficial fascia in patients with greater than 3 cm of tissue in this plane results in a decreased incidence of wound separation.
   b. When dealing with an obese patient, it is often prudent to leave this layer and the skin open to heal by secondary intention or by a delayed primary closure.
   c. Other cases in which leaving this layer open is desirable include infected or contaminated cases.
   d. Leaving the skin and superficial fascia open with aggressive wound care allows the area to remain clean and for good granulation tissue to accumulate before closure.
      (1) Closure of this layer can be achieved by using a fine absorbable or delayed absorbable suture that can be run from apex to apex of the incision.
      (2) Again, it is only necessary to approximate the edges of the tissue gently.
      (3) Apart from allowing fewer wound separations, this stitch serves to support the skin and allows better anatomical reapproximation at skin closure.
5. Skin
   a. There are multiple methods for closing the skin; these include the following:
      (1) Skin clips
      (2) A running subcuticular stitch
      (3) Mattress stitches
      (4) Interrupted through-and-through stitches
   b. An important consideration when closing the skin is potential compromise of the microvasculature.

c. This can be avoided with any of the above techniques provided that the tissue is not strangulated at closure.
d. An advantage to the skin clips is their ease of removal to allow opening and drainage of the wound should a hematoma, seroma, or wound infection develop.
e. Another consideration when closing the skin is whether it should be closed at all.
   (1) As mentioned previously, in certain cases (such as infected cases, contaminated cases, and in obese patients) leaving the skin open has certain advantages.
f. In these cases, permanent mattress sutures can be placed in the skin and subcuticular tissues and not tied.
   (1) These can be left loose until adequate granulation tissue has developed in the wound and then tied at the bedside giving a delayed primary wound closure.

Vertical incisions

1. A running mass closure is an excellent means of closing a midline incision.
2. With this technique, a permanent, thick suture is used to grasp the peritoneum, the posterior and anterior rectus sheath, and the superficial fascia.
3. This is carried in a running fashion from apex to apex, avoiding the inclusion of muscle in the suture.
4. Stitches should be taken at 1- to 2-cm intervals and at least 1.5 cm from the fascial edge.
5. This allows the microcirculation to remain intact and results in a decreased incidence of wound eviscerations.

Hirsutism

17

Marcia Soler, M.D.

17.1 DEFINITIONS

1. Hirsutism: androgen stimulated excess hair growth
2. Virilization: hirsutism accompanied by the following:
   a. Temporal hairline recession
   b. Deepening of the voice
   c. Loss of female body contour
   d. Enlargement of the clitoris

17.2 PHYSIOLOGY OF HAIR GROWTH

1. Definitions
   a. Vellus hairs: fine, short, nonpigmented hairs
   b. Terminal hairs: long, course, pigmented and responsive to hormones in certain parts of the body
2. Hair growth cycle
   a. Anagen: growing phase
   b. Catagen: rapid involution phase
   c. Telogen: resting phase
3. Hair growth is influenced by the following:
   a. Genetics: Certain ethnic groups have more hair follicles per surface area of skin.
   b. Androgens initiate growth and increase rate of matrix cell mitosis; estrogens have the opposite effect.
   c. Ratio of growth phase/resting phase: Length of hair is determined by duration of the growth phase (anagen); shorter hair is produced by a short anagen, long telogen.
   d. Degree of asynchrony: marked synchrony
      (1) All hair undergoes telogen at the same time, which leads to shedding, as seen in pregnancy.
      (2) Anagen at the same time to produce increased hair growth.
   e. Once the pattern of hair growth is established, it persists despite withdrawal of androgens.

17.3 ANDROGEN PRODUCTION

1. Testosterone
   a. Normal female: produces 0.2 to 0.3 mg/day
   b. Peripheral conversion: 50%
   c. Adrenal gland: 25%
   d. Ovary: 25%
   e. Bound to sex hormone–binding globulin (SHBG): 80%
   f. Bound to albumin: 19%
   g. Unbound: 1%, which is the active portion
2. Dehydroepiandrosterone sulfate (DHEAS)
   a. Produced exclusively by the adrenal gland

17.4 ETIOLOGY OF HIRSUTISM

Etiology can be divided into the following four categories.

Altered androgen metabolism

1. Exemplified by the idiopathic form of hirsutism
2. Caused by an increase in 5-α-reductase activity in the skin, which leads to an increased conversion of testosterone to dihydrotestosterone (DHT)
3. Diagnosed by measuring 3-androstanediol glucuronide, a metabolite of DHT, which correlates well with 5-α-reductase activity

Decrease in androgen binding

1. SHBG
   a. Produced in the liver
   b. Decreased by androgens
      (1) Therefore, men have a decreased binding capacity and increase level of free testosterone.
   c. Increased by estrogen and thyroid hormone
      (1) Therefore, binding capacity is increased in women, pregnancy, hyperthyroidism, and when taking estrogen-containing medications
      (2) Pathologic states with decreased binding capacity are as follows:
         (a) Hypothyroidism
         (b) Anorexia
         (c) Dermatomyositis
         (d) Porphyria

Exogenous androgen ingestion

1. Danazol: gonadotropin-releasing hormone (GNRH) agonist used to treat endometriosis
2. Anabolic steroids
3. Minoxidil: antihypertensive
4. Androgen-containing creams: used for vulvar dystrophies
5. Dilantin
6. Streptomycin
7. Penicillamine
8. Diazoxide

Increased androgen production

Increased androgen production arises from one of two sources: adrenal gland or ovary.

1. Adrenal gland
   a. Cushing's syndrome
      (1) Common reason for referral, but rare cause
      (2) Associated with cortisol hypersecretion
      (3) Related to malignant pituitary adrenocorticotropic hormone (ACTH)-producing tumor (Cushing's disease) or ectopic ACTH-producing tumor
      (4) Clinical signs and symptoms
         (a) Truncal obesity
         (b) Purple striae over abdomen
         (c) Buffalo hump
         (d) Hypertension
         (e) Easy bruisability
      (5) Diagnosis
         (a) Unlikely if clinical signs and symptoms are lacking
         (b) 24-hour urinary-free cortisol excretion; normal level: 20 to 90 μg
         (c) Single-dose overnight dexamethasone suppression test
            i. There is a very low incidence of false results.
            ii. Give 1 mg dexamethasone at 11 PM, and measure 8 AM serum cortisol, which should be less than 5 μg/dl.
   b. Congenital adrenal hyperplasia (CAH)
      (1) Most commonly caused by 21-hydroxylase deficiency
      (2) May also result from 11-hydroxylase deficiency
      (3) Diagnosis
         (a) Increased DHEAS
            i. Greater than 325 μg/dl considered elevated
            ii. Greater than 700 μg/dl suspicious for tumor
         (b) Increased 17-hydroxyprogesterone
            i. Greater than 200 μg/dl considered elevated
            ii. between 200 and 800 μg/dl suspicious for adult-onset CAH (perform ACTH stimulation test)
            iii. Greater than 800 μg/dl virtually diagnostic for adult-onset CAH
   c. Androgen-producing tumors: rare, but should be suspected if testosterone level greater than 200 μg/dl
      (1) Adenomas
         (a) Usually benign
         (b) More common in reproductive age
         (c) Characterized by acute onset of hirsutism
         (d) Produce testosterone or DHEAS
      (2) Carcinomas
         (a) Usually malignant
         (b) More likely to develop in postmenopausal women
         (c) Progressive onset of hirsutism
         (d) Rarely produce DHEAS, lack sulfotransferase enzyme

activity to convert dehydroepiandrosterone (DHEA) to DHEAS

2. Ovary
   a. Polycystic ovarian syndrome or hyperandrogenic chronic anovulation
      (1) Most common cause of excess androgen production
      (2) Characterized by menstrual irregularity, hirsutism, obesity, and acne
      (3) Increased risk for developing endometrial cancer at an early age
      (4) Definition: endocrinologic disorder beginning soon after menarche consisting of inappropriate luteinizing hormone (LH) and follicle stimulating hormone (FSH) secretion associated with increased GNRH pulse amplitude, which leads to chronically elevated LH and anovulation
      (5) Diagnosis
         (a) Increased levels of the following:
            i. Testosterone
            ii. DHEAS
            iii. LH
            iv. LH/FSH ratio >3
         (b) Decreased SHBG
      (6) HAIR-AN syndrome: subgroup of polyceptic ovaries (PCO) characterized by the following:
         (a) Hyperandrogenism
         (b) Insulin resistance
         (c) Acanthosis nigricans: velvety pigmented lesion found in the nape of the neck and intertriginous areas
   b. Ovarian neoplasms: Nearly every type of primary or metastatic tumor can have stromal cells that secrete excess amounts of androgens.
      (1) Krukenberg tumor: tumor metastatic to the ovary consisting of signet ring cells that usually originate from the gastrointestinal tract—stomach, colon
      (2) Brenner tumor: epithelial neoplasm that consists of cells resembling urothelium mixed with ovarian stroma
      (3) Germ cell tumors
         (a) Sertoli–Leydig cell tumors
            i. Rare; <1%
            ii. Most common in 20 to 40 year olds
            iii. Palpable ovarian mass in 85%
         (b) Hilus cell tumor
            i. Usually postmenopausal
            ii. Not always palpable
            iii. Diagnosis: testosterone level greater than two times normal with normal DHEAS
      (4) Lipoid cell tumors: increase in testosterone, DHEAS, or both
      (5) Granulosa-theca cell tumors: can occasionally produce increased testosterone in addition to increased estradiol

17.5 EVALUATION

1. Complete history and physical.
2. Document extent of hirsutism (i.e., Ferriman-Galloway score), age of onset, and rapidity of onset.
3. Perform laboratory studies (purpose is to rule out neoplasm).
   a. Testosterone level: >200 μg/dl = tumor
   b. DHEAS: adrenal is the only source; >700 μg/dl = tumor
   c. 17-Hydroxyprogesterone: marker of late-onset congenital adrenal hyperplasia
   d. Prolactin: to rule out pituitary tumor
4. Perform additional laboratory studies: because other metabolic problems are very common in hirsute women and because they have increased risk factors for heart disease
   a. Thyroid-stimulating hormone (TSH)
   b. Lipid profile and glucose tolerance test
5. Radiology
   a. Ultrasound
   b. CT
   c. Selective adrenal or ovarian vein catheterization

17.6 TREATMENT

Once androgen-producing tumors, Cushing's syndrome, and CAH have been ruled out, medical treatment is generally successful in limiting new hair growth but does not affect existing hair.

1. Oral contraceptive pills
   a. First-line therapy
   b. Very effective in the majority of cases
   c. Suppress ovarian function and decrease ovarian androgen secretion
   d. Takes at least 6 months to get results
   e. Mechanism of action
      (1) Estrogen component decreases LH, which decreases testosterone production and, in turn, decreases free testosterone.
      (2) Estrogen component also increases SHBG, which increases testosterone binding capacity and thus decreases free testosterone.
      (3) Progestin component decreases plasma ACTH, which decreases adrenal androgen secretion (DHEAS).
2. Depo-Provera can also be used.
3. Spironolactone
   a. Inhibits 5-α-reductase
   b. Competes at the androgen receptor level in the hair follicle
   c. Dose-dependent: 100 to 200 mg PO qd
   d. Side effects: initial diuresis, mastodynia, and irregular menses (when used without oral contraceptive pills (OCPs)
   e. May combine peripheral action of spironolactone with OCPs for a more dramatic result
   f. Acne: effectively treated with 2% to 5% spironolactone topical cream

4. Dexamethasone
   a. Treatment of choice for patients with CAH (i.e., deficiency in 21-hydroxylase, 11-β-hydroxylase, or 3-β-hydroxysteroid dehydrogenase-isomerase)
   b. Mechanism: ACTH suppression decreases testosterone derived from adrenal steriod precursors
   c. Androgens more sensitive than cortisol
   d. May be effective in inducing ovulation when added to clomiphene citrate (clomid)
5. Cimetidine
   a. Inhibits androgen receptor activity
6. GNRH agonist (synarel, lupron depot)
   a. May be required in addition to OCPs in severe cases
   b. Mechanism: Downregulation of GNRH receptors leads to LH/FSH suppression and thus ovarian androgen decrease

Premenstrual Syndrome

18

George T. Danakas, M.D., and JoAnne Arnold, M.D.

18.1 DEFINITION

Premenstrual syndrome (PMS) is a cyclic recurrence, during the luteal phase of the menstrual cycle, of somatic, affective, and behavioral disturbances that are of sufficient severity to affect interpersonal relationships adversely or interfere with normal activities.

18.2 EPIDEMIOLOGY

1. PMS is thought to be extremely prevalent, intermittently affecting approximately one third of all premenopausal women.
2. Approximately 2% to 10% of women with PMS are severely affected.
3. Most women who seek treatment for PMS are in their 30s or 40s.
4. The natural history of PMS has yet to be clearly elucidated.

18.3 DIAGNOSTIC CRITERIA[6]

1. Cyclic, recurrent physical, emotional, and behavioral symptoms are present in the luteal phase of the menstrual cycle and remit shortly after the onset of menstruation.
2. The luteal phase symptoms are present in the majority of menstrual cycles.
3. The luteal phase symptoms do not represent simply a worsening of a chronic physical or emotional disorder.
4. Luteal phase symptoms are severe enough to cause physical or emotional distress or deterioration in psychosocial functioning.
5. The recurrent, cyclic nature of the disorder can be confirmed by prospective daily monitoring by the woman and her significant other for at least two menstrual cycles.

18.4 ETIOLOGY

1. The etiology of PMS remains obscure.
2. Because of the multifactorial–multiorgan nature of PMS, a single etiologic cause is unlikely.

3. Current research regarding the pathophysiology and etiology of PMS is focusing on the interaction of cuing factors and context or vulnerability factors.[6]

18.5 SYMPTOMS[5]

1. The symptoms of PMS are diverse and potentially disabling.
2. There are more than 150 psychologic, physical, and behavioral symptoms associated with PMS (Table 18-1).
3. Treatment is most frequently sought because of emotional symptoms.
4. The most common emotional symptoms are as follows:
   a. Depression
   b. Irritability
   c. Anxiety
   d. Mood swings
5. The most common physical (somatic) complaints are the following:
   a. Headache
   b. Bloating
   c. Cramps
6. The most common behavioral symptom is food cravings.

18.6 DIAGNOSIS

1. PMS is a diagnosis of exclusion (Fig. 18-1).
2. Other medical or psychologic disorders must be ruled out.
3. No laboratory test is available that can specifically confirm the diagnosis of PMS.
4. Premenstrual dysphoric disorder (PDD) is a diagnostic category for PMS included in the *Diagnostic and Statistical Manual of Mental Disorders*[1] (DSM-IV) (see box on p. 342).

Text continued on p. 343

Table 18-1 Common premenstrual syndrome symptoms

Emotional	Physical	Behavioral
Anxiety	Headache	Food cravings
Irritability	Migraines	Increased appetite
Labile moods	Breast tenderness	Increased alcohol intake
Depression	Swelling of extremities	Decreased motivation
Anger	Bloatedness	Decreased efficiency
Sadness	Fatigue	Activities avoidance
Crying easily	Abdominal cramps	Staying home
Nervous tension	Aches and pains	Sleep changes
Overly sensitive	Weight gain	Libido changes
	Skin problems	Reduced cognitive function
	Hot flashes	Social isolation
	Gastrointestinal	Poor concentration
	Dizziness	Forgetfulness
	Palpitation	

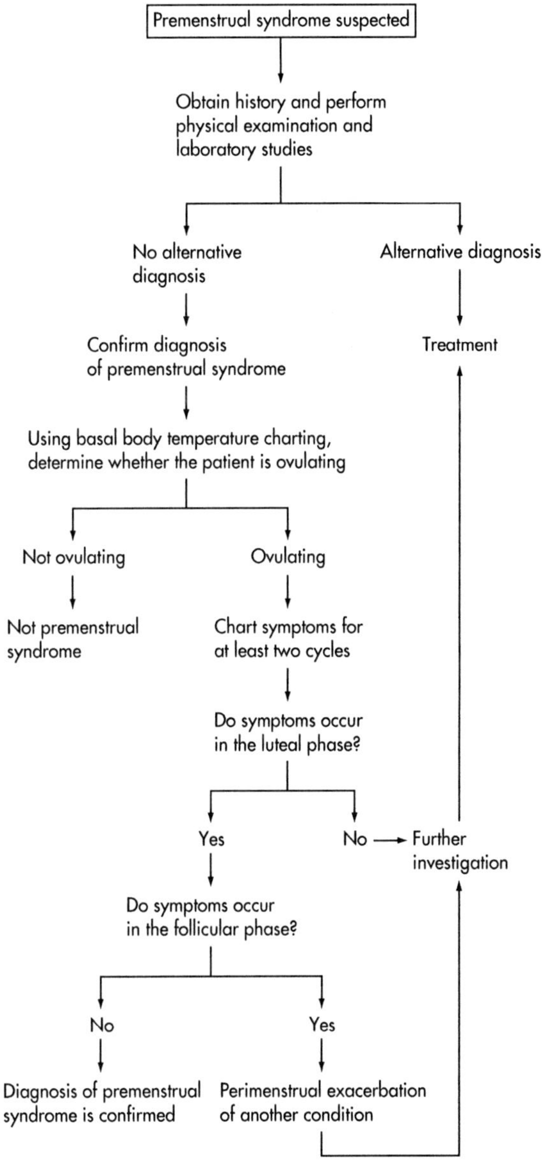

Figure 18-1
An approach to the diagnosis of premenstrual syndrome. (Adapted from Parker PD: Premenstrual syndrome, *Am Fam Physician* 50:1312, 1994.)

Research Criteria for Premenstrual Dysphoric Disorder

1. In most menstrual cycles during the past year, five (or more) of the following symptoms have been present for most of the time during the last week of the luteal phase, have begun to remit within a few days after the onset of the follicular phase, and have been absent in the week of postmenses, with at least one of the symptoms being either a, b, c, or d.
   a. Markedly depressed mood, feelings of hopelessness, or self-deprecating thoughts
   b. Marked anxiety, tension, feelings of being "keyed up" or "on edge"
   c. Marked affective lability (e.g., feeling suddenly sad or tearful or increased sensitivity to rejection)
   d. Persistent and marked anger or irritability or increased interpersonal conflicts
   e. Decreased interest in usual activities (e.g., work, school, friends, hobbies)
   f. Subjective sense of difficulty in concentrating
   g. Lethargy, easy fatigability, or marked lack of energy
   h. Marked change in appetite, overeating, or specific food cravings
   i. Hypersomnia or insomnia
   j. A subjective sense of being overwhelmed or out of control.
   k. Other physical symptoms, such as breast tenderness or swelling, headaches, joint or muscle pain, a sensation of "bloating," weight gain
2. The disturbance markedly interferes with work or school or with usual social activities and relationships with others (e.g., avoidance of social activities, decreased productivity and efficiency at work or school).
3. The disturbance is not merely an exacerbation of the symptoms of another disorder, such as major depressive disorder, panic disorder, dysthymic disorder, or a personality disorder (although it may be superimposed on any of these disorders).
4. Criteria 1, 2, and 3 must be confirmed by prospective daily ratings during at least two consecutive symptomatic cycles. (The diagnosis may be made provisionally before this confirmation.)

From American Psychiatric Association: *Diagnostic and statistical manual of mental disorders,* ed 4, Washington, DC, 1994, American Psychiatric Association.

5. PDD is a subset of PMS in which mood disturbance predominates.
6. A woman may have both a psychiatric or physical disorder and PMS.
7. Confirming PMS by symptom charting for 2 months (Fig. 18-2) is important to the diagnostic process.

18.7 MANAGEMENT[2,3,4,7]

1. The key to the management of PMS is early and correct diagnosis using prospective methods of documentation.
2. Initial management consists of education, support, and stress reduction.
3. Interventions should include psychosocial, nutritional, and pharmacologic approaches, with consideration for surgical intervention in severe cases.
   a. Psychosocial
      (1) Individualization of the treatment plan will maximize therapeutic response.
         (a) Education
         (b) Stress management
         (c) Environmental changes
         (d) Adequate rest and sleep
         (e) Regular exercise
   b. Nutritional
      (1) Whereas the effectiveness of dietary management of PMS has never been evaluated in a controlled scientific manner, widely accepted recommendations include the following:
         (a) Well-balanced meals should be eaten regularly.
         (b) Food should contain adequate amounts of protein, fiber, and complex carbohydrates and be low in fat.
         (c) Foods that are high in salt and simple sugars should be avoided because they may promote water retention, weight gain, and physical discomfort.
         (d) Caffeine-containing beverages should be avoided because the stimulant effects of caffeine may worsen tension, irritability, and insomnia.
         (e) Alcohol and illicit drugs should be avoided because their use may worsen emotional lability.
         (f) Calcium supplementation (1 g/day) reduces the physical and emotional symptoms of PMS.
         (g) Magnesium (360 mg/day) reduces water retention and the negative affect associated with PMS.
         (h) Pyridoxine (vitamin B_6) has been shown to improve depression, fatigue, and irritability. Neurotoxicity (paresthesia, hyperesthesia, muscle weakness, numbness, bone pain), however, has been observed at 50-mg doses.
   c. Pharmacologic
      (1) Intervention needs to be individualized and targeted to the symptoms.
      (2) Pharmacotherapy should be initiated only after a diagnosis is made (based on medical evaluation and confirmed by prospec-

Name:																																					
Day of cycle:		1	2	3	4	5	6	7	8	9	10	11	12	13	14	15	16	17	18	19	20	21	22	23	24	25	26	27	28	29	30	31	32	33	34	35	36
Date																																					
Menses																																					
Irritability																																					
Anxiety																																					
Nervous tension																																					
Mood swings																																					
Anger/Rage																																					
Violent behavior																																					
Depression																																					
Crying easily																																					
Despondency																																					
Overemotionality																																					
Fatigue																																					
Skin problems																																					
Swelling (legs, hands)																																					
Breast tenderness																																					
Abdominal bloating																																					
Headaches																																					
Migraine headaches																																					
Abdominal cramps																																					
General aches/pains																																					
Hot flushes																																					
Nausea																																					
Gastrointestinal																																					
Food cravings																																					
Insomnia																																					
Increased naps																																					

Clumsiness																																					
Confusion																																					
Inability to concentrate																																					
Forgetfulness																																					
Avoid activities																																					
Weight																																					
BBT																																					
Scale:																																					
No symptom	0																																				
Mild	1																																				
Moderate	2																																				
Severe	3																																				
Menstrual flow	M																																				
Therapy:																																					

Figure 18-2

Example of a daily symptom calendar. The patient records her symptoms on a 1 to 3 severity scale for mild, moderate, and severe, respectively. Boxes are left blank if symptom severity is zero. (From Smith S: Diagnosis of premenstrual syndrome. In Smith S, Schiff I, editors: *Modern management of premenstrual syndrome,* New York, 1993, WW Norton.)

tive daily symptom ratings) and after psychosocial and nutritional strategies have been attempted (Table 18-2).[4]

(a) No treatment has consistently withstood the test of double-blind placebo-controlled studies; therefore, no single treatment for PMS is universally accepted or recommended.

(b) Because of confusing and contradictory findings and the inability to predict which form of therapy will be most effective for a specific patient, therapy is to a large extent trial and error, the goal being to provide effective treatment with the safest and simplest therapy.

(3) Pharmacologic treatments include the following:

(a) Hormonal treatments that alter the menstrual cycle

i. Progesterone: Data indicate that little or no benefit can be expected; progesterone has not been established as a treatment for PMS.

ii. Estradiol: Overall, studies suggest that estradiol administration with cyclic progestin may be effective in treating PMS.

iii. Danazol: It may be useful in suppressing ovulation, leading to symptomatic relief, especially in patients with mastalgia; studies of safety and efficacy are needed.

iv. Oral contraceptives: Additional research is required before these are recommended as a therapeutic regimen.

v. Testosterone: The risks of birth defects and of possible irreversible masculinization seem to outweigh the potential benefits.

vi. GNRH agonists: Treatment should be limited to 6 months because of the risk of osteoporosis and cardiovascular disease.

(b) Drugs that alter fluid balance

i. Atenolol: Research data do not support its use as a treatment for PMS.

ii. Spironolactone: It probably should be avoided in the treatment of PMS.

(c) Prostaglandin-related treatments

i. Mefenamic acid: It does not appear to have an important role in the treatment of PMS.

ii. Prostaglandin precursors (evening primrose oil): It is not recommended as a treatment for PMS.

(d) Psychotropic drugs

i. Alprazolam: Women with primarily affective premenstrual symptoms may benefit from this; however, the risks (sedation, adverse effects, tolerance, and dependence) of its use must be considered.

ii. Buspirone: Additional research is indicated.

iii. Tricyclic antidepressants: Although good results have

Table 18-2 Pharmacologic therapy for premenstrual syndrome

Suppression of Ovulation	
Oral contraceptives	One pill per day
Progestin-only oral contraceptive	One pill per day
Oral micronized progesterone	100 mg every morning and 200 mg every evening on days 17 through 28 of menstrual cycle
Progestin suppository	200 to 400 mg, bid, on days 17 through 28 of menstrual cycle
Medroxyprogesterone (depot)	150 mg, IM, q3mo
Levonorgestrel implants	Surgical insertion q5yr
Transdermal estradiol	One or two 100 µg patches q3d
Danazol	100 to 200 mg/day (This dose will not suppress ovulation.)
Gonadotropin-releasing hormone (GNRH) agonists	Daily by intranasal spray or monthly by depot injection
Suppression of Physical Symptoms	
Spironolactone	25 to 50 mg, bid, on days 14 through 28 of menstrual cycle
Mefenamic acid	For fluid retention: 250 mg, tid, on days 24 through 28 of cycle For pain: 500 mg, tid, on days 19 through 28 of cycle
Bromocriptine	5 mg/day on days 10 through 26 of cycle
Danazol	200 mg/day on days 19 through 28 of cycle
Naproxen	Anaprox: 550 mg, bid, on days 17 through 28 of cycle Naprosyn: 500 mg, bid, on days 17 through 28 of cycle
Suppression of Psychologic Symptoms	
Nortripyline	50 to 125 mg/day
Fluoxetine	20 mg/day
Buspirone	10 mg, bid or tid, on days 16 through 28 of cycle, then taper drug
Alprazolam	25 mg, tid, on days 16 through 28 of cycle, then taper drug
Fenfluramine	15 mg, bid
Clonidine	0.1 mg, bid
Naltrexone	0.25 mg/day on days 9 through 18 of cycle
Atenolol	50 mg/day
Propranolol	20 to 40 mg, bid
Verapamil	100 to 320 mg qd
Pyridoxine	50 mg/day
Calcium	1 gm/day
Magnesium	360 mg/day

From Parker PD: Premenstrual syndrome, *Am Fam Physician* 50(6):1309, 1994.

been documented, additional controlled trials are warranted.

iv. Fluoxetine: It appears promising for women with PDD: additional studies are needed to test the efficacy of fluoxetine for women with less severe affective symptoms associated with PMS.

v. Fluvoxamine: Additional studies are indicated.

vi. Fenfluramine: It appears to have efficacy for treating affective and food-craving symptoms; however, a larger trial is indicated before its use can be generalized to women with PMS or PDD.

vii. Lithium: An overall beneficial effect on premenstrual symptoms has not been demonstrated.

viii. Clonidine: Although case reports indicate efficacy in treating anxiety, tension, irritability, and depression, additional research is necessary before generalization of these results can occur.

ix. Verapamil: There is possible efficacy in treating symptoms such as irritability, emotional lability, depression, and agitation; further study indicated.

x. Naltrexone: It is associated with fewer PMS symptoms than placebo; however, side effects are serious: Hepatotoxicity, insomnia, anxiety, nausea, and headache.

(e) Nonprescription preparations

i. Combinations of an analgesic (e.g., acetaminophen), an antihistamine (e.g., pyrilamine maleate), and a diuretic (e.g., pamabrom)

ii. No empirical testing of this combination of ingredients has appeared in the literature.

(f) Other

i. Bromocriptine: It is useful for treatment of mastalgia; its effectiveness for other symptoms of PMS is not clearly established.

d. Surgical

(1) Severe intractable PMS responds well to hysterectomy with bilateral ovariectomy.

(2) Before surgery, a trial of GNRH therapy or danazol is recommended.

(3) Estrogen replacement therapy is recommended postoperatively to reduce the risk of osteoporosis, heart disease, and genitourinary atrophy.

References

1. American Psychiatric Association: *Diagnostic and statistical manual of mental disorders,* ed 4, Washington, DC, 1994, American Psychiatric Association.
2. Goldstein S, Halbreich U: Psychotropic medications as treatment of dysphoric premenstrual syndrome. In Smith S, Schiff I, editors: *Modern management of premenstrual syndrome,* New York, 1993, WW Norton.

3. Moline M: Therapy reviews: pharmacologic strategies for managing premenstrual syndrome, *Clin Pharm* 12:181, 1993.
4. Parker PD: Premenstrual syndrome, *Am Fam Physician* 50(6):1309, 1994.
5. Smith S: Diagnosis of premenstrual syndrome. In Smith S, Schiff I, editors: *Modern management of premenstrual syndrome,* New York, 1993, WW Norton.
6. Smith S, Schiff I: Premenstrual syndrome: Controversy and consensus. In Smith S, Schiff I, editors: *Modern management of premenstrual syndrome,* New York, 1993, WW Norton.
7. Smith S, Schiff I: Practical approach to evaluation and management of premenstrual syndrome. In Smith S, Schiff I, editors: *Modern management of premenstrual syndrome,* New York, 1993, WW Norton.

19 Menopause

Maria Elena Soler, M.D., and George T. Danakas, M.D.

19.1 MENOPAUSE

Definitions

1. Menopause: no menstrual periods for 1 year after age 40 or permanent cessation of ovulation following lost ovarian activity
2. Climacteric: reproductive stage of life marked by waxing and waning estrogen levels followed by decreasing ovarian function
3. Premature ovarian failure: no menstrual periods, because of depletion of ovarian follicles, before age 40

Epidemiology

1. Average age of menopause in the United States is 51.
2. Age at which menopause occurs is genetically determined.
3. Smokers experience menopause an average of 1.5 years earlier than nonsmokers.
4. More than one third of a woman's life will be spent after the menopause.

Pathophysiology

1. Degenerating theca cells fail to react to endogenous gonadotropins.

   ↓

2. Less estrogen is produced.

   ↓

3. There is decreased negative feedback on the hypothalamic–pituitary axis.

   ↓

4. There is increased follicle stimulating hormone (FSH) (and luteinizing hormone [LH]) production.

   ↓

5. Stromal cells continue to produce androgens as a result of increased LH stimulation.

Menopausal symptoms

1. Hot flashes (flushes)
   a. Definition: A hot flash is a sudden, transient sensation ranging from warmth to intense heat that spreads over the body, particularly over the chest, face, and head, typically accompanied by flushing and perspiration and often followed by a chill.
   b. Menopause as the cause for hot flashes can be documented by elevated FSH level.
   c. Hot flashes are caused by a decrease in circulating estrogen.
   d. Seventy-five percent of women experience hot flashes; one third will require treatment of their symptoms.
   e. Hot flashes frequently occur at night and produce insomnia.
   f. Usually one hot flash a day is experienced; 20% of women experience more than one per day.
   g. Management of hot flashes includes the following:
      (1) Clinician should determine the level of impact for the woman and how she is coping with them.
      (2) Estrogen is the most effective treatment, but the full benefit may not be realized for several months. The most commonly used regimens are as follows:
         (a) Conjugated equine estrogen (Premarin) 0.625 to 1.25 mg/day
         (b) Transdermal estradiol (Estraderm) 0.05 to 0.1 mg, biw
         (c) Climera 0.05 to 0.1 mg qwk
      (3) Nonestrogenic treatments include the following:
         (a) Medroxyprogesterone 150 mg, IM, qmo
         (b) Clonidine, an α-adrenergic receptor agonist, 0.05 to 0.15 mg/solids day
         (c) Propranolol, a peripherally and centrally acting β-receptor antagonist, 60 mg/solids day
         (d) Bellargel-S
      (4) Nonpharmacologic treatments include the following:
         (a) Change in the ambient temperature (may ameliorate hot flashes and reduce night sweats)
         (b) Vitamin E
         (c) Paced respirations
         (d) Acupuncture
         (e) Exercise
         (f) Caffiene, alcohol, and spicy foods avoidance if they trigger hot flashes
2. Atrophic vaginitis
   a. Etiology: decreased maturation of the vaginal mucosal epithelium; vagina shortens and narrows, vaginal walls become thinner and less elastic, are pale in color, and lose rugations
   b. Symptoms are as follows:
      (1) Burning
      (2) Itching
      (3) Bleeding
      (4) Dyspareunia

c. Differential diagnosis: Physician should rule out other causes for vulvovaginitis such as the following:
   (1) Malignant and nonmalignant tumors
   (2) Infection
   (3) Trauma
   (4) Foreign body

d. Treatment: Systemic and local estrogens are both effective.
   (1) Start with a loading dose of 2 to 4 g (½ to 1 full applicator) of an estrogen-containing cream nightly for 1 to 2 weeks; when symptoms improve, 2 g once or twice weekly is adequate maintenance.
   (2) Lubricants such as KY jelly or Nivea cream may be useful for temporary relief of vaginal dryness with intercourse.
   (3) For hyperplastic dystrophy, corticosteroids (0.025% or 0.01% fluocinolone acetonide), applied two to three times daily, relieve pruritis; they should be stopped once the itching is under control (to prevent atrophy of the treated tissues with long-term use), and a steroid cream containing hydrocortisone should be used.
   (4) Lichen sclerosis is treated with 2% testosterone proprionate two to three times daily for 3 to 6 months; then gradually decreased over the next 1 to 2 years to a dose of one or two times weekly.

3. Incontinence
   a. Definition: the demonstrable involuntary loss of urine that is a social or hygienic problem
   b. Etiology
      (1) The bladder and urethra are embryologically derived from estrogen-dependent tissues.
      (2) Hypoestrogenism leads to atrophy of these tissues, producing dysuria, urinary frequency and urgency, incontinence, and increased frequency of urinary tract infections.
   c. Evaluation and treatment: Estrogen vaginal cream, with or without systemic estrogen, is helpful in alleviating the irritative and urgency symptoms; for a complete discussion refer to Chapter 5.

4. Psychologic dysfunction: Several researchers have found that women during the climacteric have an increased prevalence of affective and behavioral symptoms (depressed mood, difficulty falling asleep), often accompanied by somatic complaints (sexual problems and vasomotor symptoms). However, no increased incidence of major depression is found menopausally.
   a. Etiology
      (1) Psychosocial: Studies should emphasize the importance of losses at the time of menopause; has not been substantiated in controlled studies.
      (2) Biologic: Estrogen has been shown to affect the hypothalamus and the hippocampus and to impact neurotransmitter synthesis, receptor number, and sensitivity, especially for norepinephrine and dopamine.
   b. Treatment
      (1) Hormone replacement therapy (HRT) has been shown to elevate mood, improve sleep, and improve somatic symptoms.

c. Evaluation
   (1) Nature, duration, and severity of symptoms must be assessed.
   (2) Clinician should inquire about the quality of the patient's work life, interpersonal life, overall health, use of medications, substance abuse, sexual life, and any significant stresses.
   (3) Menopause should be documented by FSH determination.
   (4) Contraindications to HRT must be ruled out:
      (a) History of estrogen-dependent cancer
      (b) Undiagnosed vaginal bleeding
      (c) Active thromboembolic disease
      (d) Uncontrolled hypertension
      (e) Active liver disease
   (5) Reasons for a psychiatric referral include the following:
      (a) Suicidal ideas or behavior
      (b) Persistent symptoms that do not respond to treatment
      (c) New onset, depressed mood, or loss of interest or pleasure that has been present for at least 2 weeks, associated with at least three of the following:
         i. Significant weight loss or gain or change in appetite
         ii. Insomnia or hypersomnia
         iii. Observable restlessness or slowing
         iv. Fatigue
         v. Feelings of worthlessness or excessive guilt
         vi. Difficulty concentrating or indecision
         vii. Recurrent thoughts of death or suicide
      (d) Significant interpersonal difficulties
      (e) First manifestation of preexisting psychiatric condition

5. Sleep disturbance
   a. Definition: difficulty falling asleep and disrupted sleep, usually because of hot flashes (Lack of sleep can cause fatigue and lead to irritability, impaired memory, and disrupted concentration; sleep is less efficient and there is longer time to the onset of rapid eye movement [REM] sleep.)
   b. Etiology
      (1) Hypothalamic alterations may cause vasomotor instability and sleep disruption.
      (2) Estrogen affects serotonin and norepinephrine, the neurotransmitters involved in sleep.

6. Sexual changes
   a. Sexual responsiveness is diminished.
   b. Dyspareunia occurs, usually caused by vaginal dryness.
   c. Sexual activity is decreased.
   d. Sexual desire declines.
   e. Male partner becomes dysfunctional.
   f. Etiology: Although the sexual response cycle is a multidetermined process, estrogen affects it via its influence on the peripheral nervous system, the cardiovascular system, and neurotransmitters.
   g. Treatment: HRT has been shown to be effective in relieving many sexual complaints, especially vaginal dryness associated with dyspareunia, decreased desire, and arousal.

19.2 OSTEOPOROSIS

Definition

Loss of bone mass

Epidemiology

1. Osteoporosis affects at least 30% of white women over the age of 45.
2. In the United States, 1.2 million fractures a year result from osteoporosis.
3. Risk factors include the following:
   a. Northern European heritage
   b. Petite body frame
   c. Smoking
   d. Sedentary life style
   e. Family history
   f. Low calcium intake
   g. Early menopause or oophorectomy
4. Hip fractures represent one of the most devastating consequences of osteoporosis.
   a. In the United States, 250,000 hip fractures occur every year.
   b. Subsequent to the fracture, 50% of cases will not be able to ambulate independently; 20% will die within 6 months.

Pathophysiology

1. Estrogen promotes bone formation by doing the following:
   a. Stimulating osteoblastic activity
   b. Enhancing calcium absorption from the gut
   c. Increasing blood levels of the active vitamin D metabolite, 1,25-dihydroxyvitamin D_3
2. Loss of ovarian function is associated with increase rate of bone loss, especially in the first 3 to 4 years, by increasing bone resorption.
3. Early loss is primarily trabecular bone, leading to vertebral crush fractures, followed by long-term loss of both cortical and trabecular bone, leading to other fractures such as those of the wrist and hip.

Diagnosis

1. X-ray film: may pick up fractures occurring with no or low impact trauma
2. Radiogrammetry: measures the thickness of the cortex of the metacarpal or phalangeal bones on standard radiographs of the hand; no information about trabecular bone
3. Radiographic absorptiometry
   a. A standardized radiograph of the hand is made along with an aluminum reference wedge.
   b. Bone density is compared with that of the wedge using an optical densitometer or a videodensitometric technique after the radiograph is digitalized.
4. Single-photon absorptiometry
   a. A highly collimated photon beam from a radionuclide source is used

to measure the photon attenuation of the radius, which is converted to bone mineral content in grams using a known standard.
   b. A constant tissue path length, which is achieved by scanning the extemity in a water bath of known dimensions, is required.
   c. Trabecular and cortical bone cannot be differentiated.
5. Dual-photon absorptiometry
   a. This is used for bone mass measurements in the femur or spine or assessment of total body bone mineral content.
   b. A radionuclide source emitting photons at two effective energies is used, and the attenuation is measured at the site.
   c. Cortical and trabecular bone cannot be differentiated.
6. Dual x-ray absorptiometry: A dual energy spectrum is generated by rapid switching of the x-ray tube voltage supply or by K-edge filtering.
7. Quantitative computed tomography
   a. This is the only method that can separate trabecular and cortical bone.
   b. This is the only method that can give a true density estimate.

Differential diagnosis

1. Osteomalacia: This is a defect in collagen matrix mineralization caused by an abnormality in vitamin D metabolism. This may occur with renal failure, steatorrhea, vitamin D–resistant rickets, or severe hypophosphatemia (usually because of excess ingestion of phosphate-binding antacids).
2. Multiple myeloma: Plasma cells produce osteoclast activating factor or transforming growth factor, which induce bone resorption.
3. Hyperparathyroidism and hyperthyroidism: Excess hormone induces bone resorption.
4. Carcinoma: Squamous cell, renal, bladder, and ovarian carcinomas may secrete humoral factors that induce bone resorption.
5. Hypercortisolism: Glucocorticoid excess causes osteoporosis by inhibiting intestinal calcium absorption, leading to a compensatory bone resorption.
6. Idiopathic postmenopausal osteoporosis is the most common form.
7. Evaluation of osteoporosis should include the following:
   a. Serum calcium
   b. Phosphorus
   c. Alkaline phosphatase
   d. Complete blood count (CBC)
   e. Protein electrophoresis
   f. Thyroid function tests
   g. Parathyroid hormone
   h. Serum cortisol level
   i. 24-Hour urinary calcium excretion

Treatment

1. Estrogens as recommended on p. 360
2. Calcium
   a. 1500 mg PO per day is necessary to maintain zero calcium balance in postmenopausal women.

   b. 1000 mg PO per day when taking HRT.
   c. Epidemiologic studies suggest that a lifetime of adequate calcium intake reduces fracture risk.
3. Biphosphonates
   a. These compounds have a strong affinity for hydroxyapatite and at low concentrations inhibit bone resorption.
   b. Cyclical therapy with etidronate (Didronel) has been shown to increase bone density, decrease fracture rate, and reduce the loss of height that accompanies vertebral fractures.
   c. These drugs are not FDA approved for the treatment of osteoporosis.
4. Calcitonin
   a. Calcitonin is a potent inhibitor of osteoclastic bone resorption.
   b. Studies show that it increases bone mass by 20% per year in women with high turnover osteoporosis.
5. Vitamin D_3
   a. In elderly women, vitamin D_3 deficiency may contribute to bone loss.
   b. Treatment with vitamin D, 800 U, qd, and calcium has been shown to decrease hip fractures.

19.3 CARDIOVASCULAR DISEASE

Epidemiology

1. Heart disease is the leading cause of death in postmenopausal women.
   a. Of deaths in women, 46% are caused by cardiovascular disease.
   b. Four percent risk of death from breast cancer; 2.5% for osteoporotic fractures; 2% for genital tract cancers.
2. Women lag behind men in the incidence of coronary artery disease (CAD) by 10 years and have a 20 year advantage for myocardial infarction (MI) and sudden death.
3. HRT decreases the incidence and mortality of heart disease in postmenopausal women by approximately 50%.
4. Evidence seems to support the protective effect of HRT in cerebrovascular accidents, even though the number of studies is small.

Pathophysiology

1. The following changes contribute to improved vascular function and may be associated with reduced risk of heart disease:
   a. Lowers the level of low-density lipoprotein (LDL) cholesterol
   b. Raises high-density lipoproteins (HDL) cholesterol
   c. Decreases progression of atherosclerosis
   d. Directly affects the arterial wall and endothelium-mediated vascular responses
2. Effects of progestins
   a. Additions of progestins have been found to reduce the risk of endometrial cancer resulting from unopposed estrogen.
   b. The Postmenopausal Estrogen/Progestin Interventions (PEPI) Trial found that the combined regimens, as well as estrogen alone,

increased HDL levels, decreased LDL levels, lowered fibrinogen levels, and had little effect on insulin levels and blood pressure.

c. The PEPI study also confirmed the benefits of combination therapy in decreasing the rate of endometrial hyperplasia.

3. Risk factors and management strategies for preventing CAD are as follows:
   a. Cigarette smoking
      (1) Smoking is the leading preventable cause.
      (2) After smoking cessation the risk of CAD begins to decline within a few months and reaches the level of risk among nonsmokers within 3 to 5 years.
   b. Cholesterol: Increased level of HDL cholesterol is a strong predictor of decreased risk of CAD in women.
   c. Hypertension
      (1) Treatment of severe hypertension reduces the risk of CAD and stroke.
      (2) Treatment of mild to moderate hypertension has reduced the incidence of cardiovascular events and may decrease the incidence of CAD.
      (3) Treatment of isolated systolic hypertension has been shown to reduce the incidence of stroke and CAD.
   d. Obesity
      (1) There is a direct association between obesity and the risk of CAD.
      (2) Weight loss decreases blood pressure and LDL cholesterol.
      (3) There is up to a 60% lower risk of MI in women who maintain their ideal body weight.
   e. Diabetes mellitus
      (1) Diabetes mellitus is a strong risk factor for CAD.
      (2) The mechanism may involve impaired estrogen binding and thus decrease the protective effect of endogenous estrogens.
      (3) Gestational diabetes may be a marker for increased risk of CAD, because there is a 30% risk of subsequently developing non–insulin dependent diabetes mellitus (NIDDM).
   f. Exercise: The Healthy Women Study has shown an association between physical activity and reduced blood pressure, lower weight, and decreased cholesterol in perimenopausal women.
   g. Alcohol consumption: Although heavy alcohol use is associated with an increased risk of CAD, the Nurse's Health Study showed that women who consumed 10 to 15 g of alcohol daily (i.e., 12 ounces of beer, one glass of wine, or one drink of hard liquor) reduced their risk of heart disease by 40%.
   h. Low-dose aspirin: The benefits to women are currently unclear; this issue is being addressed in the ongoing Women's Health Study, a randomized, controlled trial of 40,000 healthy women greater than 45 years of age taking 100 mg of aspirin every other day.
   i. Antioxidant vitamins: Although some basic research has suggested that antioxidants such as beta carotene, vitamin E, and vitamin C inhibit the oxidation of LDL cholesterol or its uptake into the coronary artery endothelium, and some observational studies

support this, there have been no randomized trials of antioxidant-vitamin supplementation in women.

j. Oral contraceptives
   (1) The high-dose oral contraceptive pills (OCPs) raised LDL levels, lowered HDL levels, decreased glucose tolerance, elevated blood pressure, and promoted clotting and acted synergistically with cigarette smoking to increase the risk of MI.
   (2) Studies suggest that the newer OCPs carry less risk of CAD.
   (3) There is no increased risk among past users.

19.4 HORMONE REPLACEMENT THERAPY

Indications and contraindications of HRT

1. Indications are as follows:
   a. Vasomotor symptoms and atrophy of genitourinary tissues
   b. Osteoporosis prophylaxis and treatment
   c. Prevention of cardiovascular morbidity and mortality
   d. Gonadal dysgenesis
   e. Premature ovarian failure
   f. Some perimenopausal women
   g. Menopausal or postmenopausal women
2. Contraindications and risks are as follows:
   a. Liver function impairment
   b. Presence of acute vascular event, such as embolus or thrombosis
   c. Hypertension, fibroids, diabetes, or varicose veins are *not* contraindications.
   d. HRT may increase the risk of gallbladder disease.
   e. Endometrial cancer
      (1) Incidence in postmenopausal women is 1/1000 per year.
      (2) Unopposed estrogen increases risk 2 to 10 times.
      (3) Adding progestins decreases this risk (PEPI study).
      (4) Hysterectomized women should get combination therapy if they have had the following:
         (a) Stage I endometrial cancer
         (b) Previous treatment for endometrioid tumors of the ovary
         (c) A history of endometriosis (because adenocarcinoma has been reported in patients with pelvic endometriosis who are on unopposed estrogen)
      (5) HRT in women with endometrial cancer is a controversial topic.
         (a) In 1990, the American College of Obstetricians and Gynecologists (ACOG) published a committee opinion that concluded that the beneficial effects of estrogen might outweigh the risk of stimulating cancer growth.
         (b) However, the specifics of when to initiate therapy and the effect of adding progestins remain unknown.
         (c) The Gynecologic Oncology Group trial currently underway should help answer some of these questions.

f. Breast cancer
   (1) The relationship between breast cancer and HRT is still a controversial and widely debated topic.
      (a) Although some studies indicate that there may be an increased risk of breast cancer associated with the prolonged use of estrogen, they are not randomized controlled studies.
      (b) Clinicians must await the results of the Women's Health Initiative, which was developed to investigate the effects of hormone replacement therapy on cardiovascular disease, osteoporosis, and the incidence of breast and endometrial cancer.
      (c) In the meantime, clinicians must take into account the incidence of CAD, osteoporosis, and breast, endometrial, and ovarian cancer in the general population, as well as the individual patient's risk factors, in counseling her on the risks and benefits of HRT.
   (2) Treating the postmenopausal symptoms of women with a history of breast cancer also presents a difficult problem.
      (a) Again, there are no clear-cut answers in the literature.
      (b) In patients with intraductal carcinoma or minimally invasive intraductal carcinoma, which has an almost 100% cure rate, the addition of HRT probably carries the same risk and benefits as with any postmenopausal woman.
      (c) In patients with node-negative disease, the greatest risk of recurrence is within the first 5 years, and HRT should probably not be initiated during this time.
      (d) Clinicians must also take into account the estrogen receptor status of the tumor.
         i. In this group, it is interesting to note the positive estrogenic effects of tamoxifen.
         ii. Although tamoxifen is a nonsteroidal antiestrogen, which has been shown to inhibit estrogen receptor–positive tumor growth, it has beneficial effects on the lipid profile and bone metabolism in postmenopausal women.
      (e) In patients with positive nodes, the risk is probably greater.
   (3) The addition of progestins to HRT as it concerns breast cancer is poorly defined at this time. This should not overshadow the well-proven protective effect of progestins in preventing endometrial cancer.

g. Ovarian cancer
   (1) Because castration is the primary treatment for ovarian cancer, these women would benefit from HRT for symptom management and health benefits.
   (2) However, because of the theoretical impact on survival, estrogen use had been contraindicated in these patients.
   (3) More recently, some oncologists have begun to prescribe estrogen as concerns about quality of life and the beneficial medical effects of estrogen have become more routinely addressed.

3. In summary, the decision to begin HRT must be made on an individual basis, taking into account the risk of CAD, osteoporosis, severity of climacteric symptoms, and family history. Once the woman is presented with the risks and benefits, she can make an informed decision that will provide her with the best quality of life.

Methods of hormone replacement therapy

1. Oral preparations
   a. Conjugated equine estrogens (Premarin), 0.625 to 1.25 mg PO per day
   b. Conjugated estrogens, 0.625 mg, plus medroxyprogesterone, 2.5 mg, packaged together in a 4-week continuous combined dosage regimen (Prempro)
   c. Conjugated estrogens, 0.625 mg, a 28-day supply to be taken continuously, plus a 14-day supply of medroxyprogesterone, 5 mg, to be taken days 15 through 28 (Premphase)
   d. Estradiol, 1 mg/day (Estrace)
   e. Esterified estrogens (Estratab), 0.3 to 1.25 mg qd
      (1) The lowest dose that will control symptoms should be chosen.
      (2) Administration should be cyclic (i.e., 3 weeks on and 1 week off).
      (3) Attempts to decrease or discontinue medication should be made at 3- to 6-month intervals.
   f. Estropipate (Ogen), 0.625 to 1.25 mg, qd
2. Vaginal preparations
   a. Estradiol vaginal cream 0.01% (Estace), 2 to 4 g (marked on the applicator), daily for 1 or 2 weeks
      (1) Then gradually reduce to one-half the initial dose for a similar period.
      (2) Maintenance dose of 1 g may be used one to three times per week after the vaginal mucosa has been restored.
   b. Estropipate vaginal cream (Ogen), 2 to 4 g/day, as described in 2.a.
3. Dermal preparations
   a. Estradiol transdermal system (Estraderm), 0.05 to 0.1 mg, applied to the skin twice weekly
   b. Estradiol patch (Climera), 0.05 to 0.1 mg, used once a week.

Suggested reading

1. Lobo RA, editor: *Treatment of the postmenopausal woman,* New York, 1994, Raven Press.
2. Mishell DR Jr: In Herbst AL et al, editors: *Comprehensive gynecology: menopause,* St Louis, 1992, Mosby–Year Book.
3. Ravnikar VA, editor: Primary care of the mature woman, *Obstet Gynecol Clin North Am* 21:2, 1994, Philadelphia, 1994, W.B. Saunders.

Laboratory Values and Interpretation of Results

20

Dilara E. Samadi, M.D.

This chapter covers over 150 of the most common laboratory tests. Each test is approached with the following format:

1. Laboratory test
2. Normal range in adult patients
3. Common abnormalities, such as positive test, increased or decreased value
4. Causes of abnormal result

The normal ranges may differ slightly, depending on the laboratory. The reader should be aware of the "normal range" of the particular laboratory performing the test. Every attempt has been made to present current laboratory test data, with emphasis on practical considerations. Normal values are given using the present (traditional) reference interval, followed by the Systeme Internationale (SI) reference interval, the conversion factor (CF), and the suggested minimum increment (SMI). The following is an example:

Test	Present Reference Interval	SI Reference Interval	CF	SMI
Fasting glucose	70–110 mg/dl	3.6–6.1 mmol/L	0.05551	0.1 mmol/L

ACETONE (serum or plasma)
Normal:
Negative
Elevated in:
Diabetic ketoacidosis (DKA), starvation, isopropanol ingestion, hyperemesis gravidarum

ACE LEVEL; *see* ANGIOTENSIN-CONVERTING ENZYME

ACID PHOSPHATASE (serum)
Normal range:
0 to 5.5 U/L (0 to 90 nkat/L) (CF: 16.67, SMI: 2 nkat/L)

Elevated in:

Carcinoma of prostate, other neoplasms (breast, bone), Paget's disease, osteogenesis imperfecta, malignant invasion of bone, Gaucher's disease, multiple myeloma, myeloproliferative disorders, benign prostatic hypertrophy, prostatic palpation or surgery, hyperparathyroidism, liver disease, chronic renal failure

ACID SERUM TEST; *see* HAM TEST

ACTIVATED PARTIAL THROMBOPLASTIN TIME (APTT, aPTT); *see* PARTIAL THROMBOPLASTIN TIME

ALANINE AMINOTRANSFERASE (ALT, SGPT)

Normal range:

0 to 35 U/L (0.058 μkat/L) (CF: 0.02 μkat/L)

Elevated in:

Liver disease (hepatitis, cirrhosis, Reye's syndrome), hepatic congestion, infectious mononucleosis, myocardial infarction (MI), myocarditis, severe muscle trauma, dermatomyositis or polymyositis, muscular dystrophy, drugs (antibiotics, narcotics, antihypertensive agents, heparin, labetalol, lovastatin, nonsteroidal antiinflammatory drugs (NSAIDs), amiodarone, chlorpromazine, phenytoin), malignancy, renal and pulmonary infarction, convulsions, eclampsia, HELLP syndrome, shock liver

ALBUMIN (serum)

Normal range:

4 to 6 g/dl (40 to 60 g/L) (CF: 10, SMI: 1 g/L)

Elevated in:

Dehydration

Decreased in:

Liver disease, nephrotic syndrome, poor nutritional status, rapid IV hydration, protein-losing enteropathies (inflammatory bowel disease), severe burns, neoplasia, chronic inflammatory diseases, pregnancy, oral contraceptives, prolonged immobilization

ALDOLASE (serum)

Normal range:

0 to 6 U/L (0 to 100 nkat/L) (CF: 16.67, SMI: 20 nkat/L)

Elevated in:

Muscular dystrophy, rhabdomyolysis, dermatomyositis or polymyositis, trichinosis, acute hepatitis and other liver diseases, MI, prostatic carcinoma, hemorrhagic pancreatitis, gangrene, delirium tremens

Decreased in:

Loss of muscle mass, late stages of muscular dystrophy

ALKALINE PHOSPHATASE (serum)

Normal ranges:

30 to 120 U/L (0.5 to 2 μkat/L) (CF: 0.01667, SMI: 0.1 μkat/L)

Elevated in:

Biliary obstruction, cirrhosis (particularly primary biliary cirrhosis), liver disease (hepatitis, infiltrative liver diseases, fatty metamorphosis), Paget's disease of bone, osteitis deformans, rickets, osteomalacia, hypervitaminosis D, hyperparathyroidism, hyperthyroidism, ulcerative colitis, bowel perforation, bone metastases, healing fractures, bone neoplasms, acromegaly, infectious mononucleosis, cytomegalovirus

(CMV) infections, sepsis, pulmonary infarction, congestive heart failure (CHF), hypernephroma, leukemia, myelofibrosis, multiple myeloma, drugs (estrogens, albumin, erythromycin and other antibiotics, cholestasis-producing drugs [phenothiazines])

Decreased in:

Hypothyroidism, pernicious anemia, hypophosphatemia, hypervitaminosis D, malnutrition

ALPHA-1-FETOPROTEIN (serum); *see* α-1-FETOPROTEIN

ALT; *see* ALANINE AMINOTRANSFERASE

AMMONIA (serum)

Normal range:

10 to 80 μg/dl (5 to 50 μmol/L) (CF: 0.5872, SMI: 5 μmol/L)

Elevated in:

Hepatic failure, hepatic encephalopathy, Reye's syndrome, portacaval shunt, drugs (diuretics, polymyxin B, methicillin)

Decreased in:

Drugs (neomycin, lactulose, tetracycline), renal failure

AMYLASE (serum)

Normal range:

0 to 130 U/L (0 to 2.17 μkat/L) (CF: 0.01667, SMI: 0.01 μkat/L)

Elevated in:

Acute pancreatitis; pancreatic neoplasm; abscess; pseudocyst; ascites; macroamylasemia; perforated peptic ulcer; intestinal obstruction; intestinal infarction; acute cholecystitis; appendicitis; ruptured ectopic pregnancy; salivary gland inflammation; peritonitis; burns; DKA; renal insufficiency; drugs (morphine); carcinomatosis of lung, esophagus, ovary; acute ethanol ingestion

Decreased in:

Advanced chronic pancreatitis, hepatic necrosis

AMYLASE, URINE; *see* URINE AMYLASE

ANA; *see* ANTINUCLEAR ANTIBODY

ANGIOTENSIN-CONVERTING ENZYME (ACE level)

Normal range:

<40 nmol/ml/min (<670 nkat/L) (CF: 16.67, SMI: 10 nkat/L)

Elevated in:

Sarcoidosis, primary biliary cirrhosis, alcoholic liver disease, hyperthyroidism, hyperparathyroidism, diabetes mellitus, amyloidosis, multiple myeloma, lung disease (asbestosis, silicosis, berylliosis, allergic alveolitis, coccidioidomycosis), Gaucher's disease, leprosy

ANION GAP

Normal range:

8 to 16 mEq/L

Elevated in:

Lactic acidosis, ketoacidosis (DKA, alcoholic starvation), uremia (chronic renal failure), ingestion of toxins (paraldehyde, methanol, salicylates, ethylene glycol)

Decreased in:

Hypoalbuminemia, severe hypermagnesemia, IgG myeloma, lithium toxicity, laboratory error (falsely decreased sodium or overestimation of bicarbonate or chloride)

ANTICOAGULANT; *see* CIRCULATING ANTICOAGULANT

ANTI-DNA

Normal range:

Absent

Present in:

Systemic lupus erythematosus (SLE), chronic active hepatitis, infectious mononucleosis, biliary cirrhosis

ANTIGLOMERULAR BASEMENT ANTIBODY; *see* GLOMERULAR BASEMENT MEMBRANE ANTIBODY

ANTIMITOCHONDRIAL ANTIBODY

Normal range:

<1:20 titer

Elevated in:

Primary biliary cirrhosis (85% to 95%), chronic active hepatitis (25% to 30%), cryptogenic cirrhosis (25% to 30%)

ANTINUCLEAR ANTIBODY (ANA)

Normal range:

<1:20 titer

Positive test:

SLE (more significant if titer >1:160), drugs (phenytoin, ethosuximide, primidone, methyldopa, hydralazine, carbamazepine, penicillin, procainamide, chlorpromazine, griseofulvin, thiazides), chronic active hepatitis, age over 60 years (particularly age over 80), rheumatoid arthritis, scleroderma, mixed connective tissue disease, necrotizing vasculitis, Sjögren's syndrome (SS), tuberculosis, pulmonary interstitial fibrosis

ANTI-RNP ANTIBODY; *see* EXTRACTABLE NUCLEAR ANTIGEN

ANTI-Sm (anti-Smith) ANTIBODY; *see* EXTRACTABLE NUCLEAR ANTIGEN

ANTI-SMOOTH MUSCLE ANTIBODY; *see* SMOOTH MUSCLE ANTIBODY

ANTI-STREPTOLYSIN O TITER (STREPTOZYME, ASLO titer)

Normal range for adults:

<160 Todd units

Elevated in:

Streptococcal upper airway infection, acute rheumatic fever, acute glomerulonephritis, increased levels of β-lipoprotein

NOTE: A fourfold increase in titer between acute and convalescent specimens is diagnostic of streptococcal upper airway infection regardless of the initial titer.

ANTITHROMBIN III

Normal range:

81% to 120% of normal activity; 17 to 30 mg/dl

Decreased in:

Hereditary deficiency of antithrombin III, disseminated intravascular coagulation (DIC), pulmonary embolism, cirrhosis, thrombolytic therapy, chronic liver failure, postsurgery, third trimester of pregnancy, oral contraceptives, nephrotic syndrome, IV heparin >3 days, sepsis

Elevated in:
Warfarin drugs, post-MI
ARTERIAL BLOOD GASES
Normal range:
Po_2: 75 to 100 mm Hg
Pco_2: 35 to 45 mm Hg
HCO_3^-: 24 to 28 mEq/L
pH: 7.35 to 7.45
ASLO TITER; *see* ANTI-STREPTOLYSIN O TITER
ASPARTATE AMINOTRANSFERASE (AST, SGOT)
Normal range:
0 to 35 U/L (0 to 0.58 μkat/L) (CF: 0.01667, SMI: 0.01 μkat/L)
Elevated in:
Liver disease (hepatitis, cirrhosis, Reye's syndrome), hepatic congestion, infectious mononucleosis, MI, myocarditis, severe muscle trauma, dermatomyositis or polymyositis, muscular dystrophy, drugs (antibiotics, narcotics, antihypertensive agents, heparin, labetalol, lovastatin, NSAIDs, phenytoin, amiodarone, chlorpromazine), malignancy, renal and pulmonary infarction, convulsions, eclampsia
BASOPHIL COUNT
Normal range:
0.4 to 1% of total WBC; 40 to $100/mm^3$
Elevated in:
Leukemia, inflammatory processes, polycythemia vera, Hodgkin's lymphoma, hemolytic anemia, after splenectomy, myeloid metaplasia
Decreased in:
Stress, hypersensitivity reaction, steroids, pregnancy, hyperthyroidism
BILE, URINE; *see* URINE BILE
BILIRUBIN, DIRECT (conjugated bilirubin)
Normal range:
0 to 0.2 mg/dl (0 to 4 μmol/L) (CF: 17.10, SMI: 2 μmol/L)
Elevated in:
Hepatocellular disease, biliary obstruction, drug-induced cholestasis, hereditary disorders (Dubin-Johnson syndrome, Rotor's syndrome)
BILIRUBIN, INDIRECT (unconjugated bilirubin)
Normal range:
0 to 1 mg/dl (2 to 18 μmol/L) (CF: 17.10, SMI: 2 μmol/L)
Elevated in:
Hemolysis, liver disease (hepatitis, cirrhosis, neoplasm), hepatic congestion secondary to congestive heart failure, hereditary disorders (Gilbert's disease, Crigler-Najjar syndrome)
BILIRUBIN, TOTAL
Normal range:
0 to 1 mg/dl (2 to 18 μmol/L) (CF: 17.10, SMI: 2 μmol/L)
Elevated in:
Liver disease (hepatitis, cirrhosis, cholangitis, neoplasm, biliary obstruction, infectious mononucleosis), hereditary disorders (Gilbert's disease,

Dubin-Johnson syndrome), drugs (steroids, diphenylhydantoin, phenothiazines, penicillin, erythromycin, clindamycin, captopril, amphotericin B, sulfonamides, azathioprine, isoniazid, 5-aminosalicylic acid, allopurinol, methyldopa, indomethacin, halothane, oral contraceptives, procainamide, tolbutamide, labetalol), hemolysis, pulmonary embolism or infarct, hepatic congestion secondary to CHF

BILIRUBIN, URINE; *see* URINE BILE

BLEEDING TIME (modified Ivy method)

Normal range:

2 to 9½ min

Elevated in:

Thrombocytopenia, capillary wall abnormalities, platelet abnormalities (Bernard-Soulier, Glanzmann's), drugs (aspirin, warfarin, antiinflammatory medications, streptokinase, urokinase, dextran, β-lactam antibiotics, moxalactam), DIC, cirrhosis, uremia, myeloproliferative disorders, von Willebrand's disease

BUN; *see* UREA NITROGEN

C3; *see* COMPLEMENT C3

C4; *see* COMPLEMENT C4

CALCITONIN (serum)

Normal range:

<100 pg/ml (<100 ng/L) (CF: 1, SMI: 10 ng/L)

Elevated in:

Medullary carcinoma of the thyroid (particularly if level >1500 pg/ml), carcinoma of the breast, APUDomas, carcinoids, renal failure, thyroiditis

CALCIUM (serum)

Normal range:

8.8 to 10.3 mg/dl (2.2 to 2.58 mmol/L) (CF: 0.2495, SMI: 0.02 mmol/L)

CALCIUM, URINE; *see* URINE CALCIUM

CARBON MONOXIDE; *see* CARBOXYHEMOGLOBIN

CARBOXYHEMOGLOBIN

Normal range:

Saturation of hemoglobin <2%, smokers <9% (coma: 50%; death: 80%)

Elevated in:

Smoking, exposure to smoking, exposure to automobile exhaust fumes, malfunctioning gas-burning appliances

CARCINOEMBRYONIC ANTIGEN (CEA)

Normal range:

Nonsmokers: 0 to 2.5 ng/ml (0 to 2.5 μg/L) (CF: 1, SMI: 0.1 μg/L)

Smokers: 0 to 5 ng/ml (0 to 5 μg/L) (CF: 1, SMI: 0.1 μg/L)

Elevated in:

Colorectal carcinomas, pancreatic carcinomas, and metastatic disease usually produce higher elevations (>20 ng/ml).

Carcinomas of the esophagus, stomach, small intestine, liver, breast, ovary, lung, and thyroid usually produce lesser elevations.

Benign conditions (smoking, inflammatory bowel disease, hypothyroidism, cirrhosis, pancreatitis, infections) usually produce levels <10 ng/ml.

CAROTENE (serum)
Normal range:
50 to 250 μg/dl (0.9 to 4.6 μmol/L) (CF: 0.01863, SMI: 0.1 μmol/L)
Elevated in:
Carotenemia, chronic nephritis, diabetes mellitus, hypothyroidism, nephrotic syndrome
Decreased in:
Fat malabsorption, steatorrhea, pancreatic insufficiency, lack of carotenoids in diet
CATECHOLAMINES, URINE; *see* URINE CATECHOLAMINES
CBC; *see* COMPLETE BLOOD COUNT
CEA; *see* CARCINOEMBRYONIC ANTIGEN
CEREBROSPINAL FLUID (CSF)
Normal range:
Appearance: clear
Glucose: 40 to 70 mg/dl (2.2 to 3.9 mmol/L) (CF: 0.055, SMI: 0.1 mmol/L)
Protein: 20 to 45 mg/dl (0.20 to 0.45 g/L) (CF: 0.01, SMI: 0.1 g/L)
Chloride: 116 to 122 mEq/L (116 to 122 mmol/L) (CF: 1, SMI: 1 mmol/L)
Pressure: 100 to 200 mm H_2O
Cell count (cells/mm^3) and cell type: <6 lymphocytes, no polymorphonucleocytes
CERULOPLASMIN (serum)
Normal range:
20 to 35 mg/dl (200 to 350 mg/L) (CF: 10, SMI: 10 mg/L)
Elevated in:
Pregnancy, estrogens, oral contraceptives, neoplastic diseases (leukemias, Hodgkin's lymphoma, carcinomas), inflammatory states, SLE, primary biliary cirrhosis, rheumatoid arthritis
Decreased in:
Wilson's disease (values often <10 mg/dl), nephrotic syndrome, advanced liver disease, malabsorption, total parenteral nutrition, Menkes' syndrome
CHLORIDE (serum)
Normal range:
95 to 105 mEq/L (95 to 105 mmol/L) (CF: 1, SMI: 1 mmol/L)
Elevated in:
Dehydration, excessive infusion of normal saline; hyperparathyroidism, renal tubular disease, metabolic acidosis, prolonged diarrhea; drugs (ammonium chloride administration, acetazolamide, boric acid, triamterene)
Decreased in:
CHF, syndrome of inappropriate secretion of antidiuretic hormone (SIADH), Addison's disease, vomiting, gastric suction, salt-losing nephritis, continuous infusion of D_5W, thiazide diuretic administration, diaphoresis, diarrhea, burns
CHLORIDE, URINE; *see* URINE CHLORIDE
CHOLESTEROL, TOTAL
Normal range:
Varies with age
Generally <200 mg/dl (<5.20 mmol/L) (CF: 0.02586, SMI: 0.05 mmol/L)

Elevated in:

Primary hypercholesterolemia, biliary obstruction, diabetes mellitus, nephrotic syndrome, hypothyroidism, primary biliary cirrhosis, high-cholesterol diet, third trimester of pregnancy, MI, drugs (steroids, phenothiazines, oral contraceptives)

Decreased in:

Starvation, malabsorption, sideroblastic anemia, thalassemia, abetalipoproteinemia, hyperthyroidism, Cushing's syndrome, hepatic failure, multiple myeloma, polycythemia vera, chronic myelocytic leukemia, myeloid metaplasia, Waldenstrom's macroglobulinemia, myelofibrosis

CHOLESTEROL, LOW-DENSITY LIPOPROTEIN; *see* LOW-DENSITY LIPOPROTEIN CHOLESTEROL

CHOLESTEROL, HIGH-DENSITY LIPOPROTEIN; *see* HIGH-DENSITY LIPOPROTEIN CHOLESTEROL

CIRCULATING ANTICOAGULANT (lupus anticoagulant)

Normal:

Negative

Detected in:

SLE, drug-induced lupus, long-term phenothiazine therapy, multiple myeloma, ulcerative colitis, rheumatoid arthritis, postpartum, hemophilia, neoplasms, chronic inflammatory states

CK; *see* CREATINE KINASE

CO; *see* CARBOXYHEMOGLOBIN

COAGULATION FACTORS

Factor reference ranges:

V: >10%
VII: 50% to 170%
IX: 60% to 136%
X: >10%
XI: 50% to 150%
XII: >30%

COLD AGGLUTININS TITER

Normal range:

<1:32

Elevated in:

Primary atypical pneumonia (mycoplasma pneumonia), infectious mononucleosis, CMV infection

Other: hepatic cirrhosis, acquired hemolytic anemia, frostbite, multiple myeloma, lymphoma, malaria

COMPLEMENT (C3, C4)

Normal range:

C3 70 to 160 mg/dl (0.7 to 1.6 g/L) (CF: 0.01, SMI: 0.1 g/L)
C4 20 to 40 mg/dl (0.2 to 0.4 g/L) (CF: 0.01, SMI: 0.1 g/L)

Abnormal values:

Refer to Tables 20-1 and 20-2.

COMPLETE BLOOD COUNT

WBC 3200 to 9800/mm^3 (3.2 to 9.8 $\times 10^9$/L) (CF: 0.001, SMI: 0.1 $\times 10^9$/L)

RBC

Male: 4.3 to 5.9 $\times 10^6$/mm^3 (4.3 to 5.9 $\times 10^{12}$/L) (CF: 1, SMI: 0.1 $\times 10^{12}$/L)

Table 20-1 Summary of complement deficiencies in humans and their association with repeated infection and collagen disease

Deficient Component	Patients	Disease/Symptoms
Clr	4	SLE, renal disease, repeated infections
Cls	2	SLE
C4	3	SLE
C2	23	LE, vasculitis, membrane proliferative glomerulonephritis (MPGN), dermatomyositis
C3	4	Repeated infections, fever or rash or arthralgias Antiphospholipid syndrome
C5	3	SLE, gonococcal disease
C6	5	Relapsing meningococcal meningitis, gonococcal disease
C7	5	Raynaud's disease, chronic renal disease, gonococcal disease, SLE
C8	3	SLE, gonococcal disease

Adapted from Sonnenwirth AC, Jarrett L, (editors): *Gradwohl's clinical laboratory methods and diagnosis,* ed 8, St Louis, 1980, Mosby.

Female: 3.5 to $5 \times 10^6/mm^3$ (3.5 to $5 \times 10^{12}/L$) (CF: 1, SMI: $0.1 \times 10^{12}/L$)

Hemoglobin

Male: 13.6 to 17.7 g/dl (136 to 172 g/L) (CF: 10, SMI: 1 g/L)

Female: 12 to 15 g/dl (120 to 150 g/L) (CF: 10, SMI: 1 g/L)

Hematocrit

Male: 39% to 49% (0.39 to 0.49) (CF: 0.01, SMI: 0.01)

Female: 33% to 43% (0.33 to 0.43) (CF: 0.01, SMI: 0.01)

MCV: 76 to 100 μm^3 (76 to 100 fL) (CF: 1, SMI: 1 fL)

MCH: 27 to 33 pg (27 to 33 pg) (CF: 1, SMI: 1 pg)

MCHC: 33 to 37 g/dl (330 to 370 g/L) (CF: 10, SMI: 10 g/L)

RDW: 11.5% to 14.5%

Platelet count: 130 to $400 \times 10^3/mm^3$ (130 to $400 \times 10^9/L$) (CF: 1, SMI: $5 \times 10^9/L$)

Differential:

2 to 6 stabs (bands, early mature neutrophils)

60 to 70 segs (mature neutrophils)

1 to 4 eosinophils

0 to 1 basophils

2 to 8 monocytes

25 to 40 lymphocytes

CONJUGATED BILIRUBIN; *see* BILIRUBIN, DIRECT

COOMBS, DIRECT

Normal:

Negative

Table 20-2 General guide to the evaluation of C4 and C3 protein levels in the presence of decreased hemolytic complement activity

	Normal C4	Decreased C4
Normal C3	Alterations *in vitro* (e.g., improper specimen handling)	Immune complex disease
	Coagulation-associated complement consumption	Hypergammaglobulinemic states
	Inborn errors (other than C4 or C3)	Cryoglobulinemia
		Hereditary angioedema
		Inborn C4 deficiency
Decreased C3	Acute glomerulonephritis	Active SLE
	Membranoproliferative glomerulonephritis	Serum sickness
	Immune complex disease	Chronic active hepatitis
	Active SLE	Subacute bacterial endocarditis
	Inborn C3 deficiency	Immune complex disease

Adapted from Sonnenwirth AC, Jarrett L (editors): *Gradwohl's clinical laboratory methods and diagnosis*, ed 8, St Louis, 1980, Mosby.

Positive:
Autoimmune hemolytic anemia, erythroblastosis fetalis, transfusion reactions, drugs (α-methyldopa, penicillins, tetracycline, sulfonamides, levodopa, cephalosporins, quinidine, insulin)
False positive:
May be seen with cold agglutinins
COOMBS, INDIRECT
Normal:
Negative
Positive:
Acquired hemolytic anemia, incompatible cross-matched blood, anti-Rh antibodies, drugs (methyldopa, mefenamic acid, levodopa)
COPPER (serum)
Normal range:
70 to 140 μg/dl (11 to 22 μmol/L) (CF: 0.1574, SMI: 0.2 μmol/L)
Decreased in:
Wilson's disease, Menkes' syndrome, malabsorption, malnutrition, nephrosis, total parenteral nutrition (TPN)
COPPER, URINE; *see* URINE COPPER
CORTISOL (plasma)
Normal range:
Varies with time of collection (circadian variation):

8 AM: 4 to 19 μg/dl (110 to 520 nmol/L) (CF: 27.59, SMI: 10 nmol/L)
4 PM: 2 to 15 μg/dl (50 to 410 nmol/L) (CF: 27.59, SMI: 10 nmol/L)

Elevated in:

Ectopic adrenocorticotropic hormone (ACTH) production (i.e., oat cell carcinoma of lung), loss of normal diurnal variation, pregnancy, chronic renal failure, iatrogenic, stress, adrenal or pituitary hyperplasia or adenomas

Decreased in:

Primary adrenocortical insufficiency, anterior pituitary hypofunction, secondary adrenocortical insufficiency, adrenogenital syndromes

CPK; *see* CREATINE KINASE

C-REACTIVE PROTEIN

Normal range:

6.8 to 820 μg/dl (68 to 8200 μg/L) (CF: 10, SMI: 10 μg/L)

Elevated in:

Rheumatoid arthritis, rheumatic fever, inflammatory bowel disease, bacterial infections, MI, oral contraceptives, third trimester of pregnancy (acute phase reactant), inflammatory and neoplastic diseases

CREATINE KINASE (CK, CPK)

Normal range:

0 to 130 U/L (0 to 2.16 μkat/L) (CF 0.01667, SMI: 0.01 μkat/L)

Elevated in:

MI, myocarditis, rhabdomyolysis, myositis, crush injury or trauma, polymyositis, dermatomyositis, vigorous exercise, muscular dystrophy, myxedema, seizures, malignant hyperthermia syndrome, IM injections, cerebrovascular accident (CVA), pulmonary embolism and infarction, acute dissection of aorta

Decreased in:

Steroids, decreased muscle mass, connective tissue disorders, alcoholic liver disease, metastatic neoplasms

CREATINE KINASE ISOENZYMES

CK-MB

Elevated in: MI, myocarditis, pericarditis, muscular dystrophy, cardiac defibrillation, cardiac surgery, extensive rhabdomyolysis, strenuous exercise (marathon runners), mixed connective tissue disease, cardiomyopathy, hypothermia

CK-MM

Elevated in: crush injury, seizures, malignant hyperthermia syndrome, rhabdomyolysis, myositis, polymyositis, dermatomyositis, vigorous exercise, muscular dystrophy, IM injections, acute dissection of aorta

CK-BB

Elevated in: CVA, subarachnoid hemorrhage, neoplasms (prostate, GI tract, brain, ovary, breast, lung), severe shock, bowel infarction, hypothermia

CREATININE (serum)

Normal range:

0.6 to 1.2 mg/dl (50 to 110 μmol/L) (CF: 88.4, SMI: 10 μmol/L)

Elevated in:

Renal insufficiency (acute and chronic), decreased renal perfusion (hypotension, dehydration, CHF), urinary tract infection, rhabdomyolysis, ketonemia

Drugs (antibiotics [aminoglycosides, cephalosporins], hydantoin, diuretics, methyldopa)
Falsely elevated in:
DKA, administration of some cephalosporins (e.g., cefoxitin, cephalothin)
Decreased in:
Decreased muscle mass (including amputees and the elderly), pregnancy, prolonged debilitation

CREATININE CLEARANCE
Normal range:
75 to 124 ml/min (1.24 to 2.08 ml/sec) (CF: 0.01667, SMI: 0.02 ml/sec)
Elevated in:
Pregnancy, exercise
Decreased in:
Renal insufficiency, drugs (cimetidine, procainamide, antibiotics, quinidine)

CREATININE, URINE; *see* URINE CREATININE

CRYOGLOBULINS (serum)
Normal range:
Not detectable
Present in:
Collagen-vascular diseases, chronic lymphocytic leukemia (CLL), hemolytic anemias, multiple myeloma, Waldenström's macroglobulinemia, chronic active hepatitis, Hodgkin's disease

CSF; *see* CEREBROSPINAL FLUID

ELECTROLYTES, URINE; *see* URINE ELECTROLYTES

ELECTROPHORESIS, HEMOGLOBIN; *see* HEMOGLOBIN ELECTROPHORESIS

ELECTROPHORESIS, PROTEIN; *see* PROTEIN ELECTROPHORESIS

ENA-COMPLEX; *see* EXTRACTABLE NUCLEAR ANTIGEN

EOSINOPHIL COUNT
Normal range:
1% to 4% eosinophils (0 to 440/mm^3)
Elevated in:
Allergy, parasitic infestations (trichinosis, aspergillosis, hydatidosis), angioneurotic edema, drug reactions, warfarin sensitivity, collagen-vascular diseases, acute hypereosinophilic syndrome, eosinophilic nonallergic rhinitis, myeloproliferative disorders, Hodgkin's lymphoma, radiation therapy, non-Hodgkin's lymphoma (NHL), L-tryptophan ingestion

ERYTHROCYTE SEDIMENTATION RATE (Westergren)
Normal range:
Male: 0 to 15 mm/hr
Female: 0 to 20 mm/hr
Elevated in:
Collagen-vascular diseases, infections, MI, neoplasms, inflammatory states (acute-phase reactant)

EXTRACTABLE NUCLEAR ANTIGEN (ENA complex, anti-RNP antibody, anti-Sm, anti-Smith)
Normal:
Negative

Present in:
SLE, rheumatoid arthritis, Sjögren's syndrome, mixed connective tissue disease (MCTD)
FDP; *see* FIBRIN DEGRADATION PRODUCT
FECAL FAT, QUANTITATIVE (72-hour collection)
Normal range:
2 to 6 g/24 hour (7 to 21 mmol/dl) (CF: 3.515, SMI: 1 mmol/dl)
Elevated in:
Malabsorption syndrome
FERRITIN (serum)
Normal range:
18 to 300 ng/ml (18 to 300 μg/L) (CF: 1, SMI: 10 μg/L)
Elevated in:
Hyperthyroidism, inflammatory states, liver disease (ferritin elevated from necrotic hepatocytes), neoplasms (neuroblastomas, lymphomas, leukemia, breast carcinoma), iron replacement therapy, hemochromatosis
Decreased in:
Iron-deficiency anemia
α-1-FETOPROTEIN
Normal range:
0 to 20 ng/ml (0 to 20 μg/L) (CF: 1, SMI: 1 μg/L)
Elevated in:
Hepatocellular carcinoma (usually values >1000 ng/ml), germinal neoplasms (testis, ovary, mediastinum, retroperitoneum), liver disease (alcoholic cirrhosis, acute hepatitis, chronic active hepatitis), fetal anencephaly, multiple gestation, spina bifida, neural tube defects, and fetal GI anamolies
Decreased in:
Down's syndrome
FIBRIN DEGRADATION PRODUCT (FDP)
Normal range:
<10 μg/ml
Elevated in:
DIC, primary fibrinolysis, pulmonary embolism, severe liver disease
NOTE: The presence of rheumatoid factor may cause falsely elevated FDP.
FIBRINOGEN
Normal range:
200 to 400 mg/dl (2 to 4 g/L) (CF: 0.01, SMI: 0.1 g/L)
Elevated in:
Tissue inflammation or damage (acute-phase protein reactant), oral contraceptives, pregnancy, acute infection, MI
Decreased in:
DIC, hereditary afibrinogenemia, liver disease, primary or secondary fibrinolysis, cachexia
FLUORESCENT TREPONEMAL ANTIBODY; *see* FTA-ABS
FOLATE (FOLIC ACID)
Normal range:
Plasma: 2 to 10 ng/ml (4 to 22 nmol/L) (CF: 2.266, SMI: 2 nmol/L)
RBC: 140 to 960 ng/ml (550 to 2200 nmol/L) (CF: 2.266, SMI: 10 nmol/L)

Decreased in:
Folic acid deficiency (inadequate intake, malabsorption), alcoholism, drugs (methotrexate, trimethoprim, phenytoin, oral contraceptives, azulfadine), vitamin B_{12} deficiency (defective red cell folate absorption)

FREE T4; *see* T4, FREE

FREE THYROXINE INDEX

Normal range:
1.1 to 4.3

FTA-ABS (serum)

Normal:
Nonreactive

Reactive in:
Syphilis, other treponemal diseases (yaws, pinta, bejel)

GAMMA-GLUTAMYL TRANSFERASE (GGT); *see* γ-GLUTAMYL TRANSFERASE

GASTRIN (serum)

Normal range:
0 to 180 pg/ml (0 to 180 ng/L) (CF: 1, SMI: 10 ng/L)

Elevated in:
Zollinger-Ellison syndrome (gastrinoma), pernicious anemia, hyperparathyroidism, retained gastric antrum, chronic renal failure, gastric ulcer, chronic atrophic gastritis, pyloric obstruction, malignant neoplasms of the stomach, H2 blockers, omeprazole

GLOMERULAR BASEMENT MEMBRANE ANTIBODY

Normal:
Negative

Present in:
Goodpasture's syndrome

GLUCOSE, FASTING

Normal range:
70 to 110 mg/dl (3.9 to 6.1 mmol/L) (CF: 0.05551, SMI: 0.1 mmol/L)

Elevated in:
Diabetes mellitus, stress, infections, MI, CVA; Cushing's syndrome, accromegaly, acute pancreatitis, glucagonoma, hemochromatosis, drugs (glucocorticoids, diuretics [thiazides, loop diuretics]), glucose intolerance

Decreased in:
Fractitious hypoglycemia, insulinoma, non-islet cell neoplasmas, hormonal deficiency, liver disease, renal disease, and ethanol-induced hypoglycemia

GLUCOSE, POSTPRANDIAL

Normal range:
<140 mg/dl (<7.8 mmol/L) (CF: 0.0551, SMI: 0.1 mmol/L)

Elevated in:
Diabetes mellitus, glucose intolerance

Decreased in:
Postgastrointestinal resection, reactive hypoglycemia, hereditary fructose intolerance, galactosemia, leucine sensitivity

GLUCOSE TOLERANCE TEST

Normal values above fasting:
30 min: 30 to 60 mg/dl (1.65 to 3.3 mmol/L) (CF: 0.05551, SMI: 0.1 mmol/L)

60 min: 20 to 50 mg/dl (1.1 to 2.75 mmol/L) (CF: 0.05551, SMI: 0.1 mmol/L)
120 min: 5 to 15 mg/dl (0.28 to 0.83 mmol/L) (CF: 0.05551, SMI: 0.1 mmol/L)
180 min: fasting level or below

Elevated in:
Glucose intolerance, diabetes mellitus; Cushing's syndrome, acromegaly, pheochromocytoma

GLUCOSE-6-PHOSPHATE DEHYDROGENASE (G6PD) SCREEN (blood)

Normal:
G6PD enzyme activity is detected.

Abnormal:
If a deficiency is detected, quantitation of G6PD is necessary; a G6PD screen may be falsely interpreted as "normal" after an episode of hemolysis because most G6PD-deficient cells have been destroyed.

γ-GLUTAMYL TRANSFERASE (GGT)

Normal:
0 to 30 U/L (0.050 μkat/L) (CF: 0.01667, SMI: 0.01 μkat/L)

Elevated in:
Chronic alcoholic liver disease, neoplasms (hepatoma, metastatic disease to the liver, carcinoma of the pancreas), SLE, CHF, trauma, nephrotic syndrome, sepsis, cholestasis, drugs (phenytoin, barbiturates)

GLYCATED (GLYCOSYLATED) HEMOGLOBIN (HbA_{1c})

Normal range:
4.0% to 6.7%

Elevated in:
Uncontrolled diabetes mellitus (Glycated hemoglobin levels reflect the level of glucose control over the preceding 120 days.)

Decreased in:
Hemolytic anemias, decreased RBC survival, pregnancy, chronic blood loss, chronic renal failure, insulinoma

HAM TEST (acid serum test)

Normal:
Negative

Positive in:
Paroxysmal nocturnal hemoglobinuria (PNH)

False positive in:
Hereditary or acquired spherocytosi, recent transfusion with aged RBC, aplastic anemia, myeloproliferative syndromes, leukemia, hereditary dyserythropoietic anemia type II (HEMPAS)

HAPTOGLOBIN (serum)

Normal range:
50 to 220 mg/dl (0.50 to 2.2 g/L) (CF: 0.01, SMI: 0.01 g/L)

Elevated in:
Inflammation (acute-phase reactant), collagen-vascular diseases, infections (acute-phase reactant), drugs (androgens)

Decreased in:
Hemolysis (intravascular > extravascular), megaloblastic anemia, severe liver disease, large tissue hematomas, infectious mononucleosis, drugs (oral contraceptives)

HDL; *see* HIGH-DENSITY LIPOPROTEIN CHOLESTEROL

HEMATOCRIT

Normal range:

Male: 39% to 49% (0.39 to 0.49) (CF: 0.01, SMI: 0.01)

Female: 33% to 43% (0.33 to 0.43) (CF: 0.01, SMI: 0.01)

Elevated in:

Polycythemia vera, smoking, chronic obstructive pulmonary disease (COPD), high altitudes, dehydration, hypovolemia

Decreased in:

Blood loss (GI, genitourinary [GU]), anemia, pregnancy

HEMOGLOBIN

Normal range:

Male: 13.6 to 17.7 g/dl (136 to 172 g/L) (CF: 10, SMI: 1 g/L)

Female: 12 to 15 g/dl (120 to 150 g/L) (CF: 10, SMI: 1 g/L)

Elevated in:

Hemoconcentration, dehydration, polycythemia vera, COPD, high altitudes, false elevations (hyperlipemic plasma, WBC >50,000/mm^3), stress

Decreased in:

Hemorrhage (GI, GU), anemia

HEMOGLOBIN ELECTROPHORESIS

Normal range:

HbA1: 95% to 98%

HbA2: 1.5% to 3.5%

HbF: <2%

HbC: Absent

HbS: Absent

HEMOGLOBIN, GLYCATED; *see* GLYCATED HEMOGLOBIN

HEMOGLOBIN, GLYCOSYLATED; *see* GLYCATED HEMOGLOBIN

HEMOGLOBIN, URINE; *see* URINE HEMOGLOBIN

HEMOSIDERIN, URINE; *see* URINE HEMOSIDERIN

HEPATITIS A ANTIBODY

Normal:

Negative

Present in:

Viral hepatitis A; can be IgM or IgG (if IgM, acute hepatitis A; if IgG, previous infection with hepatitis A).

HEPATITIS B SURFACE ANTIGEN (HBsAg)

Normal:

Not detected

Detected in:

Acute viral hepatitis type B, chronic hepatitis B

HIGH-DENSITY LIPOPROTEIN (HDL) CHOLESTEROL

Normal range:

Male: 30 to 70 mg/dl (0.8 to 1.8 mmol/L) (CF: 0.02586, SMI: 0.05 mmol/L)

Female: 30 to 90 mg/dl (0.8 to 2.35 mmol/L) (CF: 0.02586, SMI: 0.05 mmol/L)

Increased:

Use of gemifibrozil, nicotinic acid, estrogens, regular aerobic exercise, small (1 ounce) daily alcohol intake

Table 20-3 HLA antigens associated with specific diseases

Antigen	Condition
HLA-B27	Ankylosing spondylitis Reiter's syndrome Psoriatic arthritis
HLA-A10, B18, Dw2	C2 deficiency
HLA-A2, B40, Cw3	C4 deficiency
HLA-B7, Dw2	Multiple sclerosis
HLA-A3	Hemochromatosis
HLA-B8, Dw3	Celiac disease
HLA-B8, Dw3	Dermatitis herpetiformis
HLA-B8	Myasthenia gravis
HLA-B8	Chronic active hepatitis in children
HLA-Drw4	Active chronic hepatitis in adults
HLA-B13, Bw17	Psoriasis

From Cerra FB: *Manual of critical care,* St Louis, 1987, Mosby.

Decreased:

Deficiency of apoproteins, liver disease, probucol ingestion, Tangler disease

NOTE: A cholesterol/HDL ratio >4.5 is associated with increased risk of coronary artery disease.

HLA ANTIGENS

Associated disorders:

See Table 20-3.

5-HYDROXYINDOLEACETIC ACID, URINE; *see* URINE 5-HYDROXYINDOLEACETIC ACID

IMMUNE COMPLEX ASSAY

Normal:

Negative

Detected in:

Collagen-vascular disorders, glomerulonephritis, neoplastic disease, malaria, primary biliary cirrhosis, chronic acute hepatitis, bacterial endocarditis, vasculitis

IMMUNOGLOBULINS

Normal range:

IgA: 50 to 350 mg/dl (0.5 to 3.5 g/L) (CF: 0.01, SMI: 0.01 g/L)

IgD: <6 mg/dl (<60 mg/L) (CF: 0.01, SMI: 0.01 g/L)

IgE: <25 μg/dl (<0.00025 g/L) (CF: 0.01, SMI: 0.01 g/L)

IgG: 800 to 1500 mg/dl (8 to 15 g/L) (CF: 0.01, SMI: 0.01 g/L)

IgM: 45 to 150 mg/dl (0.45 to 1.5 g/L) (CF: 0.01, SMI: 0.01 g/L)

Elevated in:

IgA: Lymphoproliferative disorders, Berger's nephropathy, chronic infections, autoimmune disorders, liver disease

IgE: Allergic disorders, parasitic infections, immunologic disorders, IgE myeloma

IgG: Chronic granulomatous infections, infectious diseases, inflammation, myeloma, liver disease

IgM: Primary biliary cirrhosis, infectious diseases (brucellosis, malaria), Waldenström's macroglobulinemia, liver disease

Decreased in:

IgA: Nephrotic syndrome, protein-losing enteropathy, congenital deficiency, lymphocytic leukemia, ataxia-telengiectasia, chronic sinopulmonary disease

IgE: Hypogammaglobulinemia, neoplasm (breast, bronchial, cervical), ataxia-telengiectasia

IgG: Congenital or acquired deficiency, lymphocytic leukemia, phenytoin, methylprednisolone, nephrotic syndrome, protein-losing enteropathy

IgM: Congenital deficiency, lymphocytic leukemia, nephrotic syndrome

IRON-BINDING CAPACITY (TIBC)

Normal range:

250 to 460 μg/dl (45 to 82 μmol/L) (CF: 0.1791, SMI: 1 μmol/L)

Elevated in:

Iron-deficiency anemia, pregnancy, polycythemia

Decreased in:

Anemia of chronic disease, hemochromatosis, chronic liver disease, hemolytic anemias, malnutrition (protein depletion)

LACTATE (blood)

Normal range:

0.5 to 2 mEq/L (0.5 to 2 mmol/L) (CF: 1, SMI; 0.1 mmol/L)

Elevated in:

Lactic acidosis

LACTATE DEHYDROGENASE (LDH)

Normal range:

50 to 150 U/L (0.82 to 2.66 μkat/L) (CF: 0.01667, SMI: 0.02 μkat/L)

Elevated in:

Infarction of myocardium, lung, kidney

Diseases of cardiopulmonary system, liver, collagen, central nervous system (CNS)

Hemolytic anemias, megaloblastic anemias, transfusions, seizures, muscle trauma, muscular dystrophy, acute pancreatitis, hypotension, shock, infectious mononucleosis, inflammation, neoplasia, intestinal obstruction, hypothyroidism, pregnancy

LACTATE DEHYDROGENASE (LDH) ISOENZYMES

Normal range:

LDH1: 22% to 36% (cardiac, RBC) (0.22 to 0.36) (CF: 0.01, SMI: 0.01)

LDH2: 35% to 46% (cardiac, RBC) (0.35 to 0.46)

LDH3: 13% to 26% (pulmonary) (0.15 to 0.26)

LDH4: 3% to 10% (striated muscle, liver) (0.03 to 0.1)

LDH5: 2% to 9% (striated muscle, liver) (0.02 to 0.09)

Normal ratios:

LDH1 < LDH2

LDH5 < LDH4

Abnormal values:

LDH1 > LDH2: MI (can also be seen with hemolytic anemias, pernicious anemia, folate deficiency, renal infarct)

LDH5 > LDH4: liver disease (cirrhosis, hepatitis, hepatic congestion)

LAP SCORE; *see* LEUKOCYTE ALKALINE PHOSPHATASE
LDH; *see* LACTATE DEHYDROGENASE
LDL; *see* LOW-DENSITIY LIPOPROTEIN CHOLESTEROL
LEGIONELLA TITER
Normal:
Negative
Positive in:
Legionnaire's disease (presumptive: ≥1:256 titer; definitive: fourfold titer increase to ≥1:128)
LEUKOCYTE ALKALINE PHOSPHATASE
Normal range:
13 to 100 (33 to 188 U)
Elevated in:
Leukemoid reactions, neutrophilia secondary to infections (except in sickle cell crisis—no significant increase in LAP score), Hodgkin's disease, polycythemia vera, hairy cell leukemia, aplastic anemia, Down's syndrome, myelofibrosis
Decreased in:
Acute and chronic granulocytic leukemia, thrombocytopenic purpura, PNH, hypophosphatemia, collagen disorders
LEUKOCYTE COUNT; *see* COMPLETE BLOOD COUNT
LIPASE
Normal range:
0 to 160 U/L (0 to 2.66 μkat/L) (CF: 0.01667, SMI: 0.02 μkat/L)
Elevated in:
Acute pancreatitis, perforated peptic ulcer, carcinoma of pancreas (early stage), pancreatic duct obstruction
LIPOPROTEIN CHOLESTEROL, LOW DENSITY; *see* LOW-DENSITY LIPOPROTEIN CHOLESTEROL
LIPOPROTEIN CHOLESTEROL, HIGH DENSITY; *see* HIGH-DENSITY LIPOPROTEIN CHOLESTEROL
LOW-DENSITY LIPOPROTEIN (LDL) CHOLESTEROL
Normal range:
50 to 190 mg/dl (1.30 to 4.90 mmol/L) (CF: 0.02586, SMI: 0.05 mmol/L)
Elevated in:
Primary hyperlipoproteinemia, diet high in saturated fats, acute MI, hypothyroidism, primary biliary cirrhosis, nephrosis, diabetes mellitus
Decreased in:
Abetalipoproteinemia, advanced liver disease, malabsorption, malnutrition
LUPUS ANTIOCOAGULANT; *see* CIRCULATING ANTICOAGULANT
LYMPHOCYTES
Normal range:
15% to 40%: total lymphocyte count 800 to 2600/mm^3
total T-lymphocytes 800 to 2200/mm^3
CD2 65% to 85% lymphocytes
helper-inducer T-lymphocytes (T4) >400/mm^3
CD4 45% to 75% of T-lymphocytes
suppressor-cytotoxicity T-lymphocytes 250 to 750/mm^3
T8 (CD8) 18% to 40% of T-lymphocytes
helper/suppressor ratio >0.9

Elevated in:
Chronic infections, infectious mononucleosis and other viral infections, CCL, Hodgkin's disease, ulcerative colitis, hypoadrenalism, idiopathic thrombocytopenic purpura (ITP)
Decreased in:
AIDS, AIDS-related complex (ARC), bone marrow suppression from chemotherapeutic agents or chemotherapy, aplastic anemia, neoplasms, steroids, adrenocortical hyperfunction, neurologic disorders (multiple sclerosis, myasthenia gravis, Guillain-Barré syndrome)

MAGNESIUM (serum)
Normal range:
1.8 to 3 mg/dl (0.80 to 1.20 mmol/L) (CF: 0.4114, SMI: 0.02 mmol/L)

MEAN CORPUSCULAR VOLUME (MCV)
Normal range:
76 to 100 μm^3 (76 to 100 fL) (CF: 1, SMI: 1 fL)
Elevated in:
Vitamin B_{12} deficiency, folic acid deficiency, liver disease, alcohol abuse, reticulocytosis, hypothyroidism, marrow aplasia, myelofibrosis
Decreased in:
Iron deficiency, thalassemia syndrome and other hemoglobinopathies, anemia of chronic disease, sideroblastic anemia, chronic renal failure, lead poisoning

METANEPHRINES, URINE; *see* URINE METANEPHRINES

MONOCYTE COUNT
Normal range:
2% to 8%
Elevated in:
Viral diseases, parasites, infections, neoplasms, inflammatory bowel disease, monocytic leukemia, lymphomas, myeloma, sarcoidosis
Decreased in:
Aplastic anemia, lymphocytic leukemia, glucocorticoid administration

MYOGLOBIN, URINE; *see* URINE MYOGLOBIN

NEUTROPHIL COUNT
Normal range:
50% to 70%
Subsets
Stabs (bands, early mature neutrophils): 2% to 6%
Segs (mature neutrophils): 60% to 70%
Elevated in:
Acute bacterial infections, acute MI, stress, neoplasms, myelocytic leukemia
Decreased in:
Viral infections, aplastic anemias, immunosuppressive drugs, radiation therapy to bone marrow, agranulocytosis, drugs (antibiotics, antithyroidals), lymphocytic and monocytic leukemias

5′-NUCLEOTIDASE
Normal range:
2 to 16 IU/L (3 to 27 $\times 10^{-8}$ kat/L) (CF: 1.67×10^{-8}, SMI: 1×10^{-8} kat/L)

Elevated in:

Biliary obstruction, metastatic neoplasms to liver, primary biliary cirrhosis

OSMOLALITY, SERUM

Normal range:

280 to 300 mOsm/kg (280 to 300 mmol/kg) (CF: 1, SMI: 1 mmol/kg)

It can also be estimated by the following formula:

$$2([Na]+[K])+\frac{\text{Glucose}}{18}+\frac{\text{BUN}}{2.8}$$

Elevated in:

Dehydration, hypernatremia, diabetes insipidus, uremia, hyperglycemia, mannitol therapy, ingestion of toxins (ethylmethyl + glycol, methanol, ethanol)

Decreased in:

SIADH, hyponatremia, overhydration

OSMOLALITY, URINE; *see* URINE OSMOLALITY

PARTIAL THROMBOPLASTIN TIME (PTT), ACTIVATED PARTIAL THROMBOPLASTIN TIME (APTT)

Normal range:

25 to 41 seconds

Elevated in:

Heparin therapy, coagulation factor deficiency (I, II, V, VIII, IX, X, XI, XII), liver disease, vitamin K deficiency, DIC, circulating anticoagulant, warfarin therapy, specific factor inhibition (penicillin [PCN] reaction, rheumatoid arthritis), thrombolytic therapy

NOTE: Useful to evaluate the intrinsic coagulation system.

pH, BLOOD

Normal values:

Arterial: 7.35 to 7.45

Venous: 7.32 to 7.42

pH, URINE; *see* URINE pH

PHOSPHATASE, ACID; *see* ACID PHOSPHATASE

PHOSPHATASE, ALKALINE; *see* ALKALINE PHOSPHATASE

PHOSPHORUS (serum)

Normal range:

2.5 to 5 mg/dl (0.8 to 1.6 mmol/L) (CF: 0.3229, SMI: 0.05 mmol/L)

Elevated in:

Renal failure, dehydration, Addison's disease, myelogenous leukemia, hypervitaminosis D, hypoparathyroidism, pseudohypoparathyroidism, bone metastases, sarcoidosis, mild-alkali syndrome, immobilization, magnesium deficiency, transfusions, hemolysis

Decreased in:

Starvation (e.g., alcoholics), DKA, TPN, continuous IV dextrose administration, vitamin D deficiency, hyperparathyroidism, pseudohyperparathyroidism, antacids containing aluminum hydroxide, insulin administration, nasogastric suctioning, vomiting, diuretics, steroids, gram negative septicemia

PLATELET COUNT

Normal range:

130 to $400 \times 10^3/mm^3$ (130 to $400 \times 10^9/L$) (CF: 1, SMI: $5 \times 10^9/L$)

Elevated in:

Neoplasms (GI tract), chronic myelogenous leukemia (CML), polycythemia vera, myelopibrosis with myeloid metaplasia, infections, after splenectomy, postpartum, after hemorrhage, hemophilia, iron deficiency, pancreatitis, cirrhosis

Decreased in:

HELLP syndrome, preeclampsia.

POTASSIUM (serum)

Normal range:

3.5 to 5 mEq/L (3.5 to 5 mmol/L) (CF: 1, SMI: 0.1 mmol/L)

POTASSIUM, URINE; *see* URINE POTASSIUM

PROLACTIN

Normal range:

<20 ng/ml (<20 μg/L) (CF: 1, SMI: 1 μg/L)

Elevated in:

Prolactinomas (level >200 highly suggestive), drugs (phenothiazines, cimetidine, tricyclic antidepressants, metoclopramide, estrogens, antihypertensives [methyldopa], verapamil, haloperidol), postpartum, stress, hypoglycemia, hypothyroidism

PROTEIN (serum)

Normal range:

6 to 8 g/dl (60 to 80 g/L) (CF: 10, SMI: 1 g/L)

Elevated in:

Dehydration, multiple myeloma, Waldenstrom's macroglobulinemia, sarcoidosis, collagen-vascular diseases

Decreased in:

Malnutrition, low-protein diet, overhydration, malabsorption, pregnancy, severe burns, neoplasms, chronic diseases, cirrhosis, nephrosis

PROTEIN ELECTROPHORESIS (serum)

Normal range:

Albumin: 60% to 75% (0.6 to 0.75) (CF: 0.01, SMI: 0.01)
- a-1: 1.7% to 5% (0.02 to 0.05)
- a-2: 6.7% to 12.5% (0.07 to 0.13)
- b: 8.3% to 16.3% (0.08 to 0.16)
- y: 10.7% to 20% (0.11 to 0.2)

Albumin: 3.6 to 5.2 g/dl (36 to 52 g/L) (CF: 0.01, SMI: 1 g/L)
- a-1: 0.1 to 0.4 g/dl (1 to 4 g/L)
- a-2: 0.4 to 1 g/dl (4 to 10 g/L)
- b: 0.5 to 1.2 g/dl (5 to 12 g/L)
- y: 0.6 to 1.6 g/dl (6 to 16 g/L)

Elevated:

Albumin: dehydration
- a-1: neoplastic diseases, inflammation
- a-2: neoplasms, inflammation, infection, nephrotic syndrome
- b: hypothyroidism, biliary cirrhosis, diabetes mellitus
- y: *see* IMMUNOGLOBULINS

Decreased:

Albumin: malnutrition, chronic liver disease, malabsorption, nephrotic syndrome, burns, SLE

a-1: emphysema (a-1 antitrypsin deficiency), nephrosis
a-2: hemolytic anemias (decreased haptoglobin), severe hepatocellular damage
b: hypocholesterolemia, nephrosis
y: *see* IMMUNOGLOBULINS

PROTHROMBIN TIME (PT)

Normal range:
10 to 12 seconds

Elevated in:
Liver disease, oral anticoagulants (warfarin), heparin, factor deficiency (I, II, V, VII, X), DIC, vitamin K deficiency, afibrinogenemia, dysfibrinogenemia, drugs (salicylate, chloral hydrate, diphenylhydantoin, estrogens, antacids, phenylbutazone, quinidine, antibiotics, allopurinol, anabolic steroids)

Decreased in:
Vitamin K supplementation, thrombophlebitis, drugs (gluthetimide, estrogens, griseofulvin, diphenhydramine)

PROTOPORPHYRIN (free erythrocyte)

Normal range:
16 to 36 μg/dl of RBC (0.28 to 0.64 μmol/L) (CF: 0.0177, SMI: 0.02 μmol/L)

Elevated in:
Iron deficiency, lead poisoning, sideroblastic anemias, anemia of chronic disease, hemolytic anemias, erythropoietic protoporphyria

PT; *see* PROTHROMBIN TIME

PTT; *see* PARTIAL THROMBOPLASTIN TIME

RDW; *see* RED BLOOD CELL DISTRIBUTION WIDTH

RED BLOOD CELL COUNT

Normal range:
Male: 4.4 to 5.9 $\times 10^6$/mm^3 (4.3 to 5.9 $\times 10^{12}$/L) (CF: 1, SMI 0.1 $\times 10^{12}$/L)
Female: 3.5 to 5 $\times 10^7$/mm^3 (3.5 to 5 $\times 10^{12}$/L) (CF: 1, SMI 0.1 $\times 10^{12}$/L)

Elevated in:
Polycythemia vera, smokers, high altitude, cardiovascular disease, renal cell carcinoma and other erythropoietin-producing neoplasms, stress, hemoconcentration or dehydration

Decreased in:
Anemias, hemolysis, chronic renal failure, hemorrhage, failure of marrow production

RED BLOOD CELL DISTRIBUTION WIDTH (RDW)

Measures variability of red cell size (anisocytosis)

Normal range:
11.5 to 14.5

Normal RDW and:
Elevated mean cell volume (MCV): aplastic anemia, preleukemia
Normal MCV: normal, anemia of chronic disease, acute blood loss or hemolysis, CLL, CML, nonanemic enzymopathy or hemoglobinopathy
Decreased MCV: anemia of chronic disease, heterozygous thalassemia

Elevated RDW and:

Elevated MCV: vitamin B_{12} deficiency, folate deficiency, immune hemolytic anemia, cold agglutinins, CLL with high count, liver disease

Normal MCV: early iron deficiency, early vitamin B_{12} deficiency, early folate deficiency, anemic globinopathy

Decreased MCV: iron deficiency, RBC fragmentation, HbH, thalassemia intermedia

RED BLOOD CELL FOLATE; *see* FOLATE, RBC

RED BLOOD CELL MASS (VOLUME)

Normal range:

Male: 20 to 36 ml/kg of body weight (BW) (1.15 to 1.21 L/m^2 body surface area [BSA])

Female: 19 to 31 ml/kg of BW (0.95 to 1.00 L/m^2 BSA)

Elevated in:

Polycythemia vera, hypoxia (smokers, high-altitude, cardiovascular disease), hemoglobinopathies with high O_2 affinity, erythropoietin-producing tumors (renal cell carcinoma)

Decreased in:

Hemorrhage, chronic disease, failure of marrow production, anemias, hemolysis

RETICULOCYTE COUNT

Normal range:

0.5% to 1.5%

Elevated in:

Hemolytic anemia (sickle cell crisis, thalassemia major, autoimmune hemolysis, hemorrhage, postanemia therapy (folic acid, ferrous sulfate, vitamin B_{12})

Decreased in:

Aplastic anemia, marrow suppression (sepsis, chemotherapeutic agents, radiation), hepatic cirrhosis, blood transfusion, anemias of disordered maturation (iron-deficiency anemia, megaloblastic anemia, sideroblastic anemia, anemia of chronic disease)

RHEUMATOID FACTOR

Normal:

Negative

Present in titer >1:20:

Rheumatoid arthritis, SLE, chronic inflammatory processes, old age, infections, liver disease

RNP; *see* EXTRACTABLE NUCLEAR ANTIGEN

SEDIMENTATION RATE; *see* ERYTHROCYTE SEDIMENTATION RATE

SGOT; *see* ASPARTATE AMINOTRANSFERASE

SGPT; *see* ALANINE AMINOTRANSFERASE

SHILLING TEST; see Fig. 24-1.

SMOOTH MUSCLE ANTIBODY

Normal:

Negative

Present in:

Chronic active hepatitis (≥1.80), primary biliary cirrhosis (≥1.80), infectious mononucleosis

SODIUM (serum)
Normal range:
135 to 147 mEq/L (135 to 147 mmol/L) (CF: 1, SMI: 1 mmol/L)
STREPTOZYME; *see* ANTI-STREPTOLYSIN O TITER
SUCROSE HEMOLYSIS TEST (sugar water test)
Normal:
Absence of hemolysis
Positive in:
Paroxysmal nocturnal hemoglobinuria (PNH)
False positive: Autoimmune hemolytic anemia, megaloblastic anemias
False negative: May occur with use of heparin or ethylenediamine tetraacetate (EDTA)
T3 (TRIIODOTHYRONINE)
Normal range:
75 to 220 ng/dl (1.2 to 3.4 nmol/L) (CF: 0.01536, SMI: 0.1 nmol/L)
T3 RESIN UPTAKE (T3RU)
Normal range:
25% to 35% (0.25 to 0.35) (CF: 0.01, SMI: 0.01)
T4, FREE (free thyroxine)
Normal range:
0.8 to 2.8 ng/dl (10 to 36 pmol/L) (CF: 12.87, SMI: 1 pmol/L)
THROMBIN TIME (TT)
Normal range:
11.3 to 18.5 seconds
Elevated in:
Thrombolytic and heparin therapy, DIC, hypofibrinogenemia, dysfibrinogenemia
THYROID-STIMULATING HORMONE (TSH)
Normal range:
2 to 11.0 μU/ml (2.11 mU/L) (CF: 1, SMI: 1 mU/L)
Elevated in:
Hypothyroidism, drugs (haloperidol, chlorpromazine, metoclopramide, droperidol), TSH antibodies, pituitary resistance to thyroid hormone
Decreased in:
Hyperthyroidism, acute medical illness, drugs (dopamine, corticosteroids, bromocriptine, levodopa, pyridoxine), hyponatremia, malnutrition
THYROXINE (T4)
Normal range:
4 to 11 μg/dl (51 to 142 nmol/L) (CF: 12.87, SMI: 1 nmol/L)
TIBC; *see* IRON BINDING CAPACITY
TRANSFERRIN
Normal range:
170 to 370 mg/dl (1.7 to 3.7 g/L) (CF: 0.01, SMI: 0.01 g/L)

Elevated in:
Iron-deficiency anemia, oral contraceptive administration, viral hepatitis
Decreased in:
Nephrotic syndrome, liver disease, hereditary deficiency, protein malnutrition, neoplasms, chronic inflammatory states, chronic illness, thalassemia

TRIGLYCERIDES
Normal range:
<160 mg/dl (<1.80 mmol/L) (CF: 0.01129, SMI: 0.02 mmol/L)
Elevated in:
Hyperlipoproteinemias (types I, IIb, III, IV, V), hypothyroidism, pregnancy, estrogens, acute MI, pancreatitis, alcohol intake, nephrotic syndrome, diabetes mellitus, glycogen storage disease
Decreased in:
Malnutrition, congential abetalipoproteinemias, drugs (e.g., gemfibrozil, nicotinic acid, clofibrate)

TRIIODOTHYRONINE; *see* T3

TSH; *see* THYROID STIMULATING HORMONE

TT; *see* THROMBIN TIME

UNCONJUGATED BILIRUBIN; *see* BILIRUBIN, INDIRECT

UREA NITROGEN
Normal range:
8 to 18 mg/dl (3 to 6.5 mmol/L) (CF: 0.357, SMI: 0.5 mmol/L)
Elevated in:
Drugs (aminoglycosides and other antibiotics, diuretics, lithium, corticosteroids), dehydration, gastrointestinal bleeding, decreased renal blood flow (shock, CHF, MI), renal disease (glomerulonephritis, pyelonephritis, diabetic nephropathy), urinary tract obstruction (prostatic hypertrophy)
Decreased in:
Liver disease, malnutrition, third trimester of pregnancy, overhydration

URIC ACID (serum)
Normal range:
2 to 7 mg/dl (120 to 420 μmol/L) (CF: 59.48, SMI: 10 μmol/L)
Elevated in:
Renal failure, gout, excessive cell lysis (chemotherapeutic agents, radiation therapy, leukemia, lymphoma, hemolytic anemia), hereditary enzyme deficiency (hypoxanthine-guanine-phosphoribosyl transferase), acidosis, myeloproliferative disorders, diet high in purines or protein, drugs (diuretics, low doses of aspirin [ASA], ethambutol, nicotinic acid), lead poisoning, hypothyroidism, Addison's disease, nephrogenic diabetes insipidus, active psoriasis, polycystic kidneys
Decreased in:
Drugs (allopurinol, high doses of ASA, probenecid, warfarin, corticosteroid), deficiency of xanthine oxidase, SIADH, renal tubular deficits (Fanconi's syndrome), alcoholism, liver disease, diet deficient in protein or purines, Wilson's disease, hemochromatosis

URINALYSIS
Normal range:
Color: Light straw
Appearance: Clear
pH: 4.5 to 8 (average, 6)
Specific gravity: 1.005 to 1.030
Protein: Absent
Ketones: Absent
Glucose: Absent
Occult blood: Absent
Microscopic examination:
RBC: 0 to 5 (high-power field)
WBC: 0 to 5 (high-power field)
Bacteria (spun specimen): Absent
Casts: 0 to 4 hyaline (low-power field)

URINE AMYLASE
Normal range:
35 to 260 U Somogyi/hr (6.5 to 48.1 U/hr) (CF: 0.185, SMI: 1 U/hr)
Elevated in:
Pancreatitis, carcinoma of the pancreas

URINE BILE
Normal:
Absent
Abnormal:
Urine bilirubin: hepatitis (viral, toxic, drug induced), biliary obstruction
Urine urobilinogen: hepatitis (viral, toxic, drug induced), hemolytic jaundice, liver cell dysfunction (cirrhosis, infection, metastases)

URINE CALCIUM
Normal range:
<250 mg/24 hr (<6.2 mmol/dl) (CF: 0.02495, SMI: 0.1 mmol/dl)
Elevated in:
Primary hyperparathyroidism, hypervitaminosis D, bone metastases, multiple myeloma, increased calcium intake, steroids, prolonged immobilization, sarcoidosis, Paget's disease, idiopathic hypercalciuria renal tubular acidosis
Decreased in:
Hypoparathyroidism, pseudohypoparathyroidism, vitamin D deficiency, vitamin D–resistant rickets, diet low in calcium, drugs (thiazide diuretics, oral contraceptives), familial hypocalciuric hypercalcemia, renal osteodystrophy

URINE CATECHOLAMINES
Normal range:
Norepinephrine: <100 μg/24 hr (<590 nmol/day) (CF: 5.911, SMI: 10 nmol/day)
Epinephrine: <10 μg/24 hr (<55 nmol/day) (CF: 5.458, SMI: 5 nmol/day)
Elevated in:
Pheochromocytoma, neuroblastoma, severe stress

URINE CHLORIDE
Normal range:
110 to 250 mEq/day (110 to 250 mmol/day) (CF: 1, SMI: 1 mmol/day)
Elevated in:
Corticosteroids, Bartter's syndrome

Decreased in:

Chloride depletion (vomiting, diuretics), colonic vilous adenoma

URINE COPPER

Normal range:

<40 μg/24 hr (<0.6 μmol/day) (CF: 0.01574, SMI: 0.2 μmol/day)

URINE CORTISOL, FREE

Normal range:

10 to 110 μg/24 hr (30 to 300 nmol/day) (CF: 2.759, SMI: 10 nmol/day)

Elevated:

Refer to CORTISOL (serum)

URINE CREATININE (24 hour)

Normal range:

Male: 0.8 to 1.8 g/day (7 to 16 mmol/day) (CF: 8.840, SMI: 0.1 mmol/day)

Female: 0.6 to 1.6 g/day (5.3 to 14 mmol/day)

NOTE: Useful test as an indicator of completeness of 24-hour urine collection

URINE GLUCOSE (qualitative)

Normal:

Absent

Present in:

Diabetes mellitus, renal glycosuria (decreased renal threshold for glucose), glucose intolerance

URINE HEMOGLOBIN, FREE

Normal:

Absent

Present in:

Hemolysis (with saturation of serum haptoglobin binding capacity and renal threshold for tubular absorption of hemoglobin)

URINE HEMOSIDERIN

Normal:

Absent

Present in:

PNH, chronic hemolytic anemia, hemochromatosis

URINE 5-HYDROXYINDOLEACETIC ACID (URINE 5-HIAA)

Normal range:

2 to 8 mg/24 hr (10 to 40 μmol/day) (CF: 5.23, SMI: 5 μmol/day)

Elevated in:

Carcinoid tumors, after ingestion of certain foods (bananas, plums, tomatoes, avocados, pineapples, eggplant, walnuts), drugs (monoamine oxidase [MAO] inhibitors, phenacetin, methyldopa, glycerol guaiacolate, acetaminophen, salicylates, phenothiazines, imipramine, methocarbamol, reserpine, metamphetamine)

URINE INDICAN

Normal:

Absent

Present in:

Malabsorption secondary to intestinal bacterial overgrowth

URINE KETONES (semiquantitative)

Normal:

Absent

Present in:
DKA, alcoholic ketoacidosis, starvation, isopropanol ingestion

URINE METANEPHRINES

Normal range:
0 to 2 mg/24 hr (0 to 11.0 μmol/day) (CF: 5.458, SMI: 0.5 μmol/day)

Elevated in:
Pheochromocytoma, neuroblastoma, drugs (caffeine, phenothiazines, MAO inhibitors), stress

URINE MYOGLOBIN

Normal:
Absent

Present in:
Severe trauma, hyperthermia, polymyositis or dermatomyositis, carbon monoxide poisoning

URINE NITRITE

Normal:
Absent

Present in:
Urinary tract infections

URINE OCCULT BLOOD

Normal:
Negative

Positive in:
Trauma to urinary tract, renal disease (glomerulonephritis, pyelonephritis), renal or ureteral calculi, bladder lesions (carcinoma, cystitis), prostatitis, prostatic carcinoma, menstrual contamination, hematopoietic disorders (hemophilia, thrombocytopenia), anticoagulants, ASA

URINE OSMOLALITY

Normal range:
50 to 1200 mOsm/kg (50 to 1200 mmol/kg) (CF: 1, SMI: 1 mmol/kg)

Elevated in:
SIADH, dehydration, glycosuria, adrenal insufficiency, high-protein diet

Decreased in:
Diabetes insipidus, excessive water intake, IV hydration with D_5W, acute renal insufficiency, glomerulonephritis

URINE pH

Normal range:
4.6 to 8 (average 6)

Elevated in:
Bacteriuria, vegetarian diet, renal failure with inability to form ammonia, drugs (antibiotics, sodium bicarbonate, acetazolamide)

Decreased in:
Acidosis (metabolic, respiratory), drugs (ammonium chloride, methenamine mandelate), diabetes mellitus, starvation, diarrhea

URINE POTASSIUM

Normal range:
25 to 100 mEq/24 hr (25 to 100 mmol/day) (CF:1, SMI: 1 mmol/day)

Elevated in:
Aldosteronism (primary, secondary), glucocorticoids, alkalosis, renal tubular acidosis, excessive dietary potassium intake

Decreased in:

Acute renal failure, potassium-sparing diuretics, diarrhea, hypokalemia

URINE PROTEIN (quantitative)

Normal range:

<150 mg/24 hr (<0.15 g/day) (CF: 0.001, SMI: 0.01 g/day)

Elevated in:

Renal disease (glomerular, tubular, interstitial), CHF, hypertension, neoplasms of renal pelvis and bladder, multiple myeloma, Waldenström's macroglobulinemia

URINE SODIUM (quantitative)

Normal range:

40 to 220 mEq/day (40 to 220 mmol/day) (CF: 1, SMI: 1 mmol/day)

Elevated in:

Diuretic administration, high sodium intake, salt-losing nephritis, acute tubular necrosis, vomiting, Addison's disease, SIADH, hypothyroidism, CHF, hepatic failure

URINE SPECIFIC GRAVITY

Normal range:

1.005 to 1.03

Elevated in:

Dehydration, excessive fluid losses (vomiting, diarrhea, fever), x-ray contrast media, diabetes mellitus, CHF, SIADH, adrenal insufficiency, decreased fluid intake

Decreased in:

Diabetes insipidus, renal disease (glomerulonephritis, pyelonephritis), excessive fluid intake or IV hydration

URINE VANILLYLMANDELIC ACID (VMA)

Normal range:

<6.8 mg/24 hr (<35 μmol/day) (CF: 5.046, SMI: 1 μmol/day)

Elevated in:

Pheochromocytoma; neuroblastoma; ganglioblastoma; drugs (isoproterenol, methocarbamol, levodopa, sulfonamides, chlorpromazine); severe stress; after ingestion of bananas, chocolate, vanilla, tea, or coffee

Decreased in:

Drugs (MAO inhibitors, reserpine, guanethidine, methyldopa)

VDRL (Venereal Disease Research Laboratories test for syphilis)

Normal range:

Negative

Positive test:

Syphilis, other treponemal diseases (yaws, pinta, bejel)

NOTE: A false-positive test may be seen in patients with SLE and other autoimmune diseases, infectious mononucleosis, atypical pneumonia, malaria, leprosy.

VISCOSITY

Normal range:

1.4 to 1.8 relative to water (1.10 to 1.22 centipoise)

Elevated in:

Monoclonal gammopathies (Waldenström's macroglobulinemia, multiple myeloma), hyperfibrinogenemia, SLE, rheumatoid arthritis, polycythemia, leukemia

WESTERGREN; *see* ERYTHROCYTE SEDIMENTATION RATE

D-XYLOSE ABSORPTION

Normal range:

21% to 31% excreted in 5 hours (0.21 to 0.31) (CF: 0.01, SMI: 0.01)

Decreased in:

Malabsorption syndrome

21 Labor and Delivery

Armando Fuentes, M.D.

21.1 NORMAL

Parturition is the process of giving birth. This process incorporates two major events, labor and delivery. Labor is defined as the progressive cervical dilation in response to repetitive uterine contractions. Delivery is the expulsion of the fetus as a result of uterine contractions and cervical dilation.

The initiation and maintenance of labor is complex. Prostaglandins, cytokines, and sex-steroid hormones appear to play pivotal roles in this process.

The gestational age is used to classify the type of delivery. Premature labor occurs before 37 weeks gestation. A delivery before 24 weeks of gestation is referred to as an abortion. Term labor is defined as labor occurring after 37 weeks gestation.

Essential factors

Before labor, several factors need to be considered to ensure good progress and to minimize risks to the fetus and mother. An abnormality of any one of these factors is often a contraindication to labor and results in dystocia.

1. Pelvic architecture

   The classic work of Caldwell and Moloy in the 1930s provided the framework for the evaluation of the female bony pelvis. The four basic types of bony pelvis are characterized in Fig. 21-1. Although most pelves are mixed, these four types provide us with a basic configuration.

   The clinical evaluation of the bony pelvis has replaced x-ray pelvimetry over the years. The focus of the evaluation of the pelvis is on the true rather than the false pelvis. The true pelvis includes the pelvic inlet, the midpelvis, and the outlet. Fig. 21-2 illustrates the pelvic landmarks.

   a. Pelvic inlet: The pelvic inlet is evaluated by measuring the diagonal conjugate diameter. The diagonal conjugate diameter is the distance between the lower edge of the symphysis and the sacral promontory. Subtracting 1.5 to 2 cm from the diagonal conjugate provides an estimate of the true conjugate diameter. The true conjugate should measure 11 cm or more. The critical distance is known as the

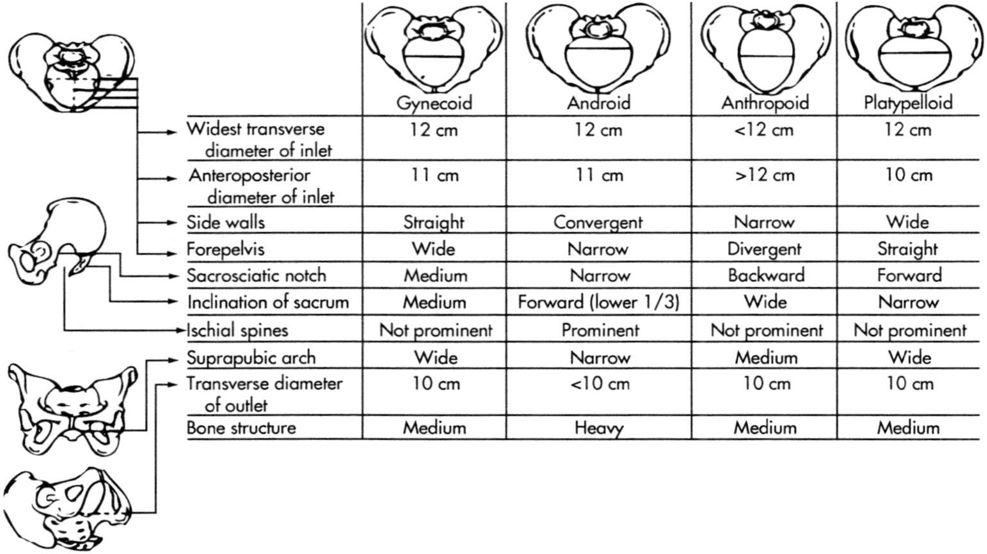

	Gynecoid	Android	Anthropoid	Platypelloid
Widest transverse diameter of inlet	12 cm	12 cm	<12 cm	12 cm
Anteroposterior diameter of inlet	11 cm	11 cm	>12 cm	10 cm
Side walls	Straight	Convergent	Narrow	Wide
Forepelvis	Wide	Narrow	Divergent	Straight
Sacrosciatic notch	Medium	Narrow	Backward	Forward
Inclination of sacrum	Medium	Forward (lower 1/3)	Wide	Narrow
Ischial spines	Not prominent	Prominent	Not prominent	Not prominent
Suprapubic arch	Wide	Narrow	Medium	Wide
Transverse diameter of outlet	10 cm	<10 cm	10 cm	10 cm
Bone structure	Medium	Heavy	Medium	Medium

Figure 21-1
Architecture and dimensions of the four basic pelvic types. (From Niswander KR: *Manual of obstetrics: diagnosis and therapy,* ed 3, Boston, 1987, Little, Brown.)

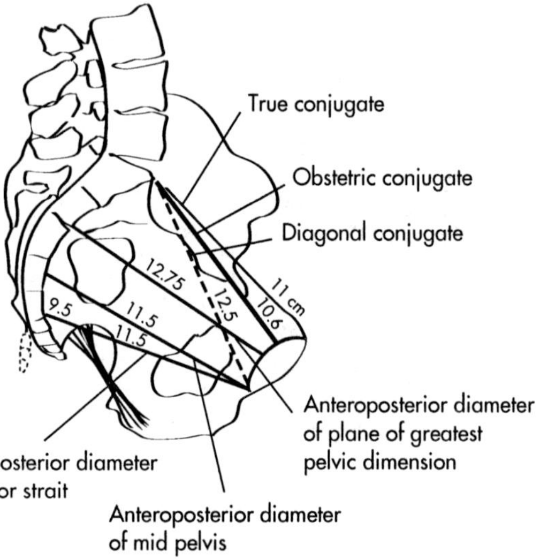

Figure 21-2
Obstetrical measurements of the bony pelvis. (From Niswander KR: *Manual of obstetrics: diagnosis and therapy,* ed 3, Boston, 1987, Little, Brown.)

obstetric conjugate diameter. This represents the shortest distance of the inlet and is measured just below the upper edge of the symphysis to the sacral promontory. A diagonal conjugate diameter greater than 12.5 cm has been shown to be a reliable estimate of the pelvic inlet.

b. Midpelvis: The midpelvis is the plane with the narrowest dimensions. The transverse diameter is measured between the ischial spines. The normal length is approximately 10 cm. Clinically, the evaluation has centered on the side walls. The side walls are determined by sweeping the digits laterally from the inlet to the intertuberous diameter during the pelvic examination. The side walls are normally straight. A converging side may limit descent of the fetal presenting part. Midpelvis contraction is also recognized if the distance between the spines is less than 9.5 cm. The sacral curvature should also be examined. A flat or prominent sacrum may result in either failure of the fetus to descend or inability to complete the rotation necessary.

c. Pelvic outlet: The pelvic outlet is evaluated by the angle of the pubic symphysis and the intertuberous diameter. The intertuberous diameter is the most critical and is normally 8 cm or greater. The angle of the symphysis should be equal to or greater than 90°. It should be noted that contractions of both the midpelvis and the outlet are usually concomitant.

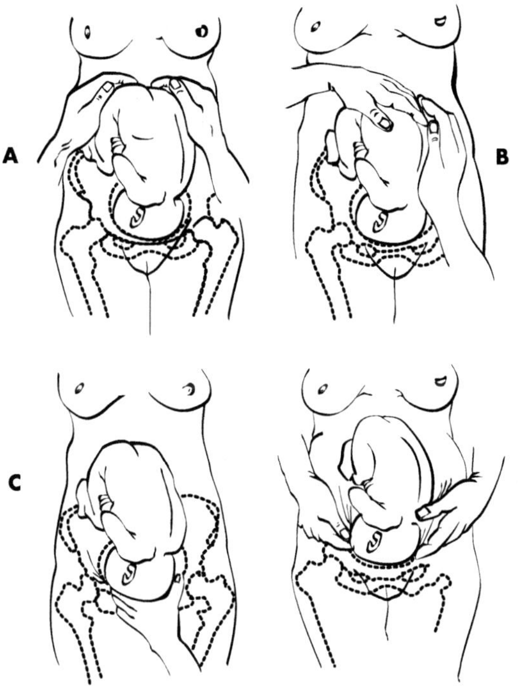

Figure 21-3
Leopold maneuvers, **A, B, C, D.** (From Niswander KR: *Manual of obstetrics: diagnosis and therapy,* ed 3, Boston, 1987, Little, Brown.)

2. Fetal presentation
   Fetal presentation refers to the part that lies over the pelvic inlet. At term, more than 95% of infants present as vertex. Breech presentation may occur in 3% to 5% of pregnancies at term. Fetal position is defined as the relationship of the lowest presenting part to one of the four quadrants of the bony pelvis. In most cases, the fetal occiput is the lowest part and the position is described as occiput anterior or posterior. The left or right designation is given if the occiput is rotated to the right or left of the pelvis. Dystocia may occur if any malposition or malpresentation occurs. Leopold maneuver and a pelvic examination in early labor is crucial to identify any malpresentations (Fig. 21-3). Leopold maneuvers assist in determining whether the presentation is vertex or breech. The pelvic examination confirms an abnormal presentation and identifies a face, brow, or compound presentation.

3. Fetal weight
   Fetal macrosomia is defined as a birth weight greater than 4000 g. The most common complications encountered are shoulder dystocia and postpartum hemorrhage. Clinical and sonographic techniques have been used to identify macrosomic infants. Clinical assessment has been shown to be very inaccurate. Sonography suffers from low sensitivity and high false-positive rates. Shoulder dystocia has been found to occur in over 8% of infants weighing more than 4500 g. Also, the risk of fetal injury increases fourfold in infants over 4000 g. Nevertheless, attempts should be made to estimate fetal weight using both techniques. Women carrying a fetus weighing over 4500 g should be given the option of a cesarean delivery.

Initial evaluation

The initial evaluation should determine whether the woman is in labor and identify any conditions that will impact the labor and delivery process. A complete history and physical examination is required. Laboratory tests are also indicated before admission.

1. History
   a. Proper evaluation of the laboring patient should begin with a complete history. The gravidity and the gestational age should be determined. The gestational age may be determined from the last menstrual period and confirmed by any sonograms obtained during the pregnancy.
   b. The onset of contractions and their frequency and duration should be determined next. This assists in determining true labor from false labor. False labor, or Braxton-Hicks contractions, is usually mild, is irregular, and generally does not result in any cervical change.
   c. Any history of leakage of fluid or bleeding should be sought. Spontaneous rupture of membranes may be very obvious, with copious amounts of watery discharge from the vagina, or it may be very subtle. A woman may complain of only a small amount of moisture on her underpants. A history of bleeding or spotting may simply be a result of a "bloody show," or it may be something more ominous such as a placenta previa.
   d. Information should also be obtained regarding the antepartum course. Any problems, such as infections, hospitalizations, and medications used, may become relevant during the labor process. A history of abnormal glucose tolerance test and any treatment should be noted.
   e. History from any past pregnancies and general medical history need to be obtained. The past pregnancy outcomes need to be elicited to assess any risks to this labor. Attention should be paid to any history of preeclampsia, placental abruptio, and postpartum hemorrhage. Any general medical problems that may impact the labor should be identified. Women with pulmonary, cardiac, hematologic, or autoimmunologic disorders may need very careful observation and prophylactic therapy during labor.

2. Physical examination
   a. The physical examination during labor is usually brief, but it should be as thorough as possible. The difficulty encountered is usually a result of the painful labor contractions, and examination is best performed at intervals between the contractions. Vital signs are also best taken between contractions to avoid any reactive elevation of maternal heart rate or blood pressure. The emphasis is on the abdominal and the pelvic examination.
   b. The abdominal examination should focus on the fundal height, the fetal presentation, and assessment of the fetal heart rate. The fundal height can be measured with a tape measure. Fundal height measurement in centimeters is from the pubic symphysis to the top of the uterine fundus. This method is a good approximation of gestational age between 16 and 38 weeks.
   c. The fetal presentation can be assessed from Leopold maneuvers. The four maneuvers are shown in Fig. 21-3. The first maneuver attempts to determine the fetal pole in the uterine fundus. The second step determines on which side of the maternal abdomen lies the fetal small parts or the fetal back. The third step is performed to determine the presenting part in the pelvis and whether engagement has occurred. The fourth maneuver confirms the presentation.
   d. The fetal heart rate can be determined by Doppler. The baseline heart rate and any decelerations or accelerations in relation to contractions should be noted. The pattern and frequency of contractions should also be determined to assist in the determination of an adequate labor pattern or an abnormal one.
3. Pelvic examination
   a. The pelvic examination begins by inspecting the perineum, vagina, and cervix. Close inspection is required to identify any herpetic lesions or other vaginal or cervical lesions. The diagnosis of ruptured membranes is often made by noting pooling of amniotic fluid in the posterior fornix; confirmation may be made by nitrazine test and ferning. Amniotic fluid air dried on a slide develops a "ferning" pattern under the microscope. The basic pH of amniotic fluid turns yellow nitrazine paper deep blue. A cotton swab is used to obtain the sample from the lateral and upper wall of the vaginal fornix. False-positive tests can be obtained from cervical mucus, blood, and urine. Any green discoloration to the amniotic fluid suggesting meconium should be noted.
   b. Digital examination of the cervix and vagina is carried out to determine the dilation and effacement. The dilation refers to the opening of the cervical os. The effacement describes the thinning of the cervix. This process has usually been described very subjectively in terms of percentage. The normal length of the cervix is usually approximately 3 to 4 cm long. When the cervix shortens to 1.5 to 2 cm long, it is usually described as 50% effaced. To add some consistency to the description, the length in centimeters is being used more frequently. The description in terms of percentage has been plagued with high interobserver variability, which often creates discrepancies during examination.

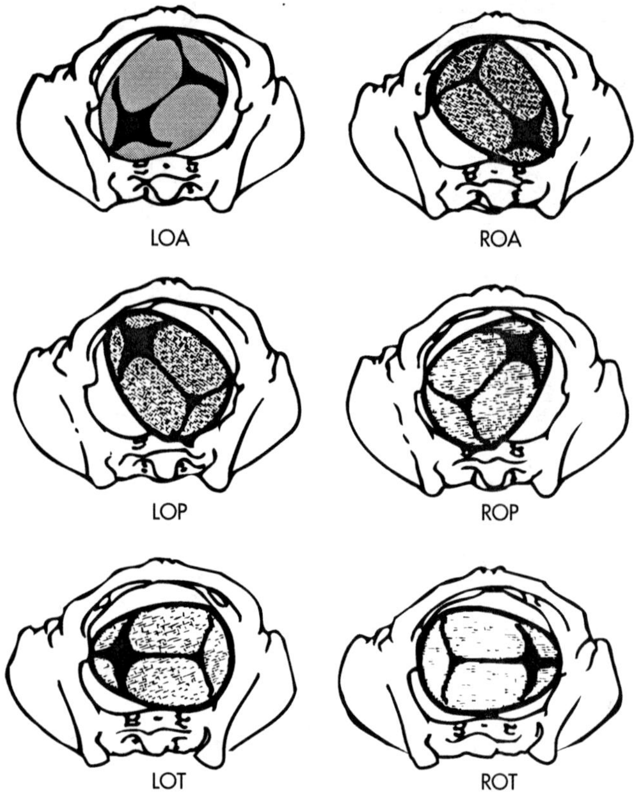

Figure 21-4
Fetal positions in the bony pelvis. (From Pernoll ML, Benson RC: *Current obstetrics and gynecologic diagnosis and treatment,* ed 6, Norwalk, CT, 1987, Appleton & Lange.)

c. The digital examination also assists in identifying the presenting part. The station should be noted. This refers to the relationship between the presenting part and the ischial spines. The level of the ischial spines is referred to as zero station. Each centimeter above the spines is termed minus and below the spines is termed plus. Therefore, a presenting part 2 cm below the spines is referred to as +2 station.

d. Every attempt to evaluate the position of the presenting part should also be made. The landmark in a vertex presentation is the occiput, which is identified by the junction of the lamboidal and sagittal sutures. The term used for the position is the relationship between the occiput and the pelvis (Fig. 21-4).

4. Laboratory tests
   a. Most of the routine tests may already be on a patient's prenatal form. In normal laboring patients, very few laboratory tests are required. A laboring woman requires an evaluation of the blood count and the blood type with an indirect Coombs test in the event of a blood transfusion.
   b. In the event any complication or concurrent medical disorders are identified, other laboratory tests are required. These may involve evaluation of platelet counts and liver function tests (aspartate aminotransferase [AST], alanine aminotransferase [ALT]) if a suspicion of preeclampsia is raised.

Labor

Labor has traditionally been divided into three stages. The first stage is recognized from the onset of labor until complete cervical dilation. The second stage is defined from complete dilation until the delivery of the infant. The interval from delivery of the infant until the delivery of the placenta is known as the third stage. Some have attempted to add a fourth stage, defined as the first hour following the delivery of the placenta, which carries an increased risk of hemorrhage (Fig. 21-5).

1. Mechanism of labor
   a. During labor, the fetus undergoes certain movements to maneuver through the pelvis. These movements are known as the seven cardinal movements of labor. They consist of engagement, flexion, descent, internal rotation, extension, external rotation, and expulsion. These movements apply to both vertex and breech presentations. These movements allow the fetus to pass through the pelvis with the least resistance.
   b. Engagement occurs early in labor or before labor. The presenting part reaches the level of the ischial spines. The most common position is occiput anterior. As engagement occurs, the head often rotates transversely. However, the position is usually dictated by the size of the pelvic inlet.
   c. Flexion allows the smallest diameter of the head to pass through the pelvis. Once again, this is dependent on the shape of the pelvis. A platypelloid pelvis may cause some deflexion in some cases and result in a brow or face presentation.
   d. Fetal descent progresses constantly. It is dependent on the uterine contractions and the size of the fetus. The position of the presenting part also plays a role.
   e. As descent takes place, the presenting part undergoes internal rotation. The fetal head rotates from a transverse position to an anterior or posterior position so as to maneuver through the ischial spines. The rotation is complete by the time the head reaches the perineum.
   f. At the level of the perineum, a combination of uterine contractions and maternal expulsive efforts assist in extension. The extension of the fetal head also allows it to maneuver under the pubic symphysis.
   g. The external rotation occurs after the head is delivered. The rotation restores the fetal head to the initial position it occupied when it became engaged.

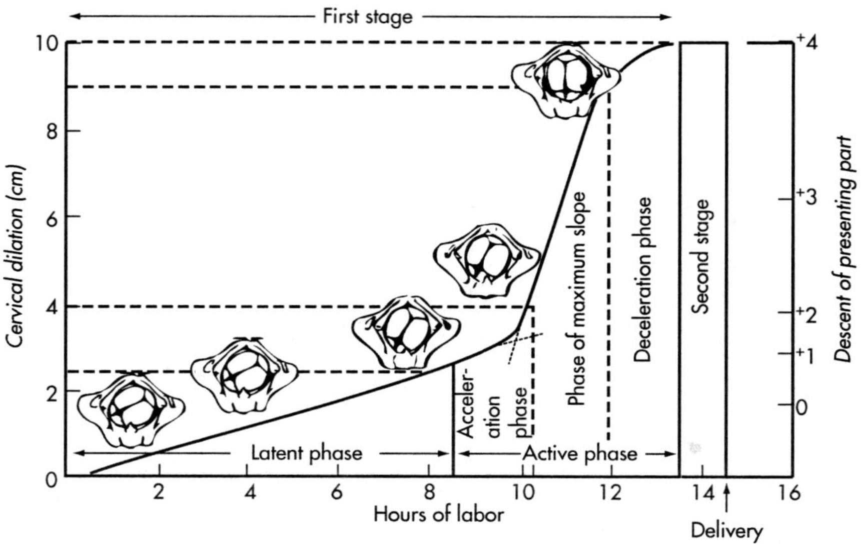

Figure 21-5
Normal labor curve and the fetal position. (From Niswander KR: *Manual of obstetrics: diagnosis and therapy,* ed 3, Boston, 1987, Little, Brown.)

h. The complete expulsion of the infant occurs with the delivery of the shoulders and the rest of the body.

2. First stage
   a. The first stage of labor is composed of two phases. The latent phase is the period of gradual cervical effacement and dilation. This period begins with the onset of labor and ends when cervical dilation is approximately 4 to 5 cm. The active phase begins at the conclusion of the latent phase and ends with complete cervical dilation. This period is recognized by rapid cervical dilation. Nulliparous women should dilate at least 1.2 cm/hr and multiparous women at least 1.5 cm/hr during the active phase. The average duration of the entire first stage in nulliparous women is 8 hours; in multiparous women it averages 5 hours (see Fig. 21-4).
   b. Analgesia is offered to a woman once labor has started and her level of pain has risen. The goal should be to allow her to participate as fully as possible in the labor process without compromising the fetus. Most women have been encouraged to take prenatal classes emphasizing the Lamaze method or another psychoprophylaxis method to alleviate stress and anxiety during labor.
   c. Other methods, such as narcotics and regional anesthetics, are available. Some of the most common narcotics used, such as butorphanol or meperidine, are parenterally administered and have little effect on the progress of labor in the active phase. They generally are best avoided in the latent phase because of their effect of prolonging it. The most common regional block used is an epidural anesthesia. Similar to narcotic analgesics, epidurals are best used in the active phase of labor. Prolongation of the second stage and an increase in operative deliveries have been reported with the use of epidural anesthetics.
3. Second stage
   a. The second stage is defined as the period between complete cervical dilation and delivery of the infant. Maternal expulsive efforts are usually spontaneous during this stage if no regional anesthetic is used. These expulsive efforts and the uterine contractions drive the presenting part to the pelvic floor. Delivery is anticipated as the perineum begins to distend.
   b. Delivery is generally performed with a woman in a lithotomy position, although in some European countries a left lateral position (Sims) is preferred for delivery. The goal is to control the delivery of the infant to avoid excessive force or a rapid release of pressure on the fetal head. A modified Ritgen maneuver is often used for control. A gloved hand covered with a towel is used to apply pressure on the fetal chin upwards, and the other hand is used to control the extension of the fetal head superiorly.
   c. An episiotomy is performed to avoid any lacerations of the perineum and to provide an adequate space to minimize any soft tissue dystocia.
   d. As the head is delivered, external rotation follows. The rotation is often assisted and gentle traction is exerted downward to aid the progress of the anterior shoulder under the symphysis. It is

imperative to avoid excessive traction on the head and neck to avoid a brachial plexus injury. The head is then lifted upward to deliver the posterior shoulder.

e. After the shoulders, the rest of the infant is delivered by gentle traction.

4. Third stage
   a. The period between the delivery of the infant and the delivery of the placenta is termed the third stage of labor. The placenta separates within 5 minutes following the delivery of the infant. This process is often assisted by administering oxytocin to the intravenous fluid. The separation of the placenta is believed to occur by the rapid reduction of the uterine size resulting in "buckling" of the placental surface area and forming a retroplacental bleed. This bleed eventually propagates and shears off the remaining surface of the placenta.
   b. Spontaneous separation of the placenta can be determined by certain signs. Three commonly noted signs are a change in the shape of the uterus, a flow of blood, and a relative lengthening of the umbilical cord. A fourth sign often noted is a release of the tension on the umbilical vessels when gently compressed.
   c. Caution should be applied when traction is applied to the umbilical cord to deliver the placenta. Brandt-Andrews is a technique used to minimize any risk of a uterine inversion. With one hand placed on the abdomen, the uterus is gently massaged near the fundus; the other hand applies gentle traction to the umbilical cord once separation has started. As the placenta is delivered, the abdominal hand is lowered to the suprapubic area to identify any signs of a uterine inversion. A Crede maneuver has been described that uses the abdominal hand to massage the uterus and uses the fundus as a piston to drive the placenta out of the uterine cavity. This maneuver carries great risk for uterine hemorrhage and inversion. There is no role for this maneuver in modern obstetrics.
   d. Manual removal of the placenta may be indicated if the placenta has not separated after 20 minutes or if there is excessive vaginal bleeding. After adequate anesthesia is given, one hand is introduced into the uterine cavity and the other hand is placed on the uterine fundus. The intrauterine hand cleaves off the placenta from the uterine wall in a circumferential pattern. The uterus is then aggressively massaged to minimize any excessive bleeding.
   e. The placenta should always be examined to determine whether the entire placenta has been delivered. Missing cotyledons may suggest retention in the uterine cavity. The inspection should also note any placental pathology. Three vessels of the umbilical cord should be confirmed. Any evidence of succenturiate lobes or of circumvallate or marginal insertion of the umbilical cord should be documented.
5. Fourth stage

   This stage has been recognized as the first hour following the delivery of the placenta. It appears to be a critical period for postpartum hemorrhage. The use of oxytocin and uterine massage will minimize any significant bleeding. The perineal region needs to be frequently noted for any signs of excessive bleeding.

Episiotomy/lacerations

Episiotomy is a surgical incision of the perineum performed during a delivery to provide sufficient area for the delivery of the infant and minimize or avoid lacerations of the perineum and rectum.

1. Types
   a. Lacerations of the perineum have been classified as first, second, third, and fourth degree.
      (1) A first-degree laceration involves a tear of the vaginal mucosa but spares any underlying muscle and tissue.
      (2) If the tear extends through the muscle and fascia, a second-degree laceration is noted.
      (3) A tear into the rectal sphincter is classified as a third-degree laceration.
      (4) A fourth-degree laceration encompasses the entire thickness of the perineal body and into the rectal mucosa.
   b. Episiotomies are classified as either midline or mediolateral.
      (1) Midline episiotomies are incisions directed downward from the middle of the fourchet, including the vaginal mucosa and the underlying fascia and muscle.
      (2) A mediolateral episiotomy begins at the same point but is directed laterally to avoid the rectum.
         (a) Mediolateral episiotomies have the advantage of rarely extending, and damage to the rectal mucosa is avoided.
         (b) The disadvantage is an increase in blood loss and greater postpartum pain.
2. Oxytocics
   The three commonly used oxytocics in modern obstetrics are oxytocin, methylergonovine maleate, and prostaglandin F2-alpha. They are used primarily in the third stage of labor to reduce blood loss and stimulate uterine contractions.
   a. Oxytocin
      (1) Oxytocin is an octapeptide commonly used to stimulate uterine contractions. It is often used for induction and augmentation of labor. Intravenously, its half-life is approximately 3 to 5 minutes.
      (2) Administration is usually carried out using controlled infusion pumps, and the dose is diluted to avoid any side effects.
      (3) The most common side effects are significant hypotension if given as a large intravenous bolus, or antidiuresis if given as a continuous infusion of greater than 20 mU/min.
   b. Methylergonovine
      (1) Methylergonovine is a synthetic alkaloid created from lysergic acid. It is a very potent uterotonic substance. Its use is primarily confined to the third stage of labor.
      (2) Caution should be used because of its ability to cause vasoconstriction, resulting in hypertension.

(3) Its administration is confined to intramuscular dosing. Intravenous administration is contraindicated.

c. Prostaglandin F2

(1) A 15-methyl derivative of prostaglandin F2 has been noted to be a potent oxytocic agent. Its use is limited for the control of postpartum hemorrhage.

(2) It is administered intramuscularly or directly into the myometrium.

(3) Some side effects reported have involved hypertension, diarrhea, vomiting, and fever.

21.2 ABNORMAL LABOR

Abnormalities of labor are generally described as dystocia. Since 1980, the incidence of cesarean births has increased significantly in the United States. One of the major indications for cesarean births has been dystocia. The exact incidence has been difficult to ascertain because the definition has been vague and generalized. Frequently, generic terms such as cephalopelvic disproportion or failure to progress have been used to describe various dystocias. Every effort should be made to characterize the dystocia encountered precisely so that the correct diagnosis is made.

Dystocias can be classified into three categories. The categories are a result of problems with uterine contractions, the size of the maternal pelvis, or the size of the fetus. These have been referred to as abnormalities of the power, the passenger, and the passage.

1. Power

a. Normal uterine contractions during labor complete their purpose by developing a rhythmic pattern beginning in the fundus near a cornual end. The average resting tone is approximately 10 to 15 mm Hg. During the active phase of labor, contractions reach 40 to 60 mm Hg. One of the most common quantitative measurements developed to assess uterine contractions has been the Montevideo unit. The Montevideo unit is calculated by multiplying the average intensity of contractions by the number of contractions in a 10-minute window. Adequate contractions are recognized as over 180 Montevideo units. Intrauterine pressure catheters are pivotal in evaluating the adequacy of uterine contractions.

b. Abnormalities of the power are usually classified into protraction disorders, arrest disorders, or a prolonged latent phase. Understanding the definition of each assists in the proper diagnosis.

(1) Prolonged latent phase

(a) A prolonged latent phase is defined as a latent phase exceeding 20 hours in nulliparous women and 14 hours in multiparous women. The most common etiology is heavy sedation or early analgesia. False labor can be another common etiology.

(b) Treatment is usually accomplished by sedating the patient with meperidine, butorphanol, or morphine. Oxytocin augmentation can be used to organize the frequency of the contraction pattern.

(2) Protraction disorders
    (a) Protraction disorders can be a protraction either of cervical dilation or of fetal descent. In nulliparous patients, cervical dilation in the active phase should be at least 1.2 cm/hr, 1.5 cm/hr in multiparous women. Fetal descent should also be 1 cm/hr for multiparous women and 2 cm/hr in multigravidas.
    (b) Common causes of protraction disorders are fetopelvic discrepancy from either size or fetal presentation abnormalities. Factors such as macrosomia, occiput transverse, brow presentation, or narrow inlet should be investigated. Heavy sedation or anesthesia may play a role in multigravidas.
    (c) Attempts should be made to determine the cause of the protraction. Macrosomic infants or fetal malpresentation may require a cesarean section. An intrauterine catheter should be inserted and the contractions quantified. Augmentation is attempted with oxytocin for hypotonic dysfunction.

(3) Arrest disorders
    (a) The most common arrest disorder recognized is an arrest of dilation. This is defined as failure to dilate in the active phase for 2 hours or more. It is found in approximately 5% of nulliparous labor. An arrest of descent is defined as failure to descend for 1 hour or more.
    (b) The most common causes of arrest disorders are fetopelvic discrepancy. Many are as a result of positional abnormalities such as occiput transverse or occiput posterior. Uterine dystocia also accounts for a large percentage of arrest disorders. Fetal macrosomia or pelvic contractions account for many of the abnormalities encountered with arrest of descent.
    (c) Intrauterine catheters should be placed in these cases to identify any evidence of uterine inertia. Oxytocin augmentation may be required. Careful pelvic examination may be required to assess the fetal position and sonography may be indicated to evaluate the estimated fetal weight.

2. Passenger

Dystocia from the fetus is usually caused by a large infant, malposition of the presenting part, or a malpresentation. Treatment for many of these disorders is often an operative delivery by a cesarean section or forceps.

a. Macrosomia

(1) Fetal macrosomia occurs in approximately 5% of infants and is defined as a fetal weight in excess of 4000 g. A fetal weight over 4500 g has been used by others for the definition. Several risk factors for macrosomia have been encountered. Women with previous macrosomic infants, diabetic women, obese women, women with postdate pregnancies, and those with a prolonged second stage are at increased risk. Unfortunately, clinical

estimates of fetal weight have been poor. Sonographic evaluation has not provided sufficient sensitivity.

(2) Macrosomic infants have a fivefold increased risk of perinatal mortality. Shoulder dystocia occurs in approximately 8% to 10% of infants weighing over 4500 g. A thorough review of the maneuvers performed in the event of a shoulder dystocia should be performed when a labor abnormality occurs.

b. Malpresentation

Approximately 5% of all labors at term are complicated by malpresentations. These are abnormalities related to the fetal position, or presentation. Malpresentations are the most common cause of fetal dystocia.

(1) Breech

(a) A breech is an abnormal fetal lie in which the head of the infant lies in the uterine fundus. Breeches are described as frank, complete, or footling based on the position of the fetal hips and knees (Fig. 21-6). A frank breech is a fetus who is lying with flexed hips and extended knees. If both the knees and the hips are flexed, it is referred to as a complete breech. When one or both hips are extended, a footling breech is identified. The infants may be designated as single or double footling breeches.

(b) The incidence of breech infants is dependent on the gestational age. Pregnancies less than 28 weeks have an incidence of approximately 25%. This decreases to 7% to 9% by 32 weeks. At term, the incidence of all breeches is 3% to 4%.

(c) Breech presentations have been associated with fetal and uterine anomalies. A careful sonographic evaluation is warranted in persistent breech infants to rule out any anomalies. The perinatal mortality rate of breech presentations varies from 9% to 25%. However, controversy exists because many breeches have anomalies and are premature. The corrected estimates of perinatal mortality at term may not be different from those of infants presenting as vertex.

(d) The mode of delivery remains controversial. A cesarean section should be considered for any breech between 800 and 1500 g. The optimal mode of delivery between 1500 and 2500 g has not clearly been established. A trial of labor may be considered with a breech presentation between 2500 and 3800 g. The box on p. 408 demonstrates prerequisites needed for the management of a trial of labor.

(2) Occiput posterior

(a) An occiput posterior occurs when the vertex fails to rotate once it has reached the pelvic floor. Dystocia occurs because of partial deflexion of the fetal head. It is often a result of a contracted pelvis, an anthropoid pelvis, or poor uterine contractions.

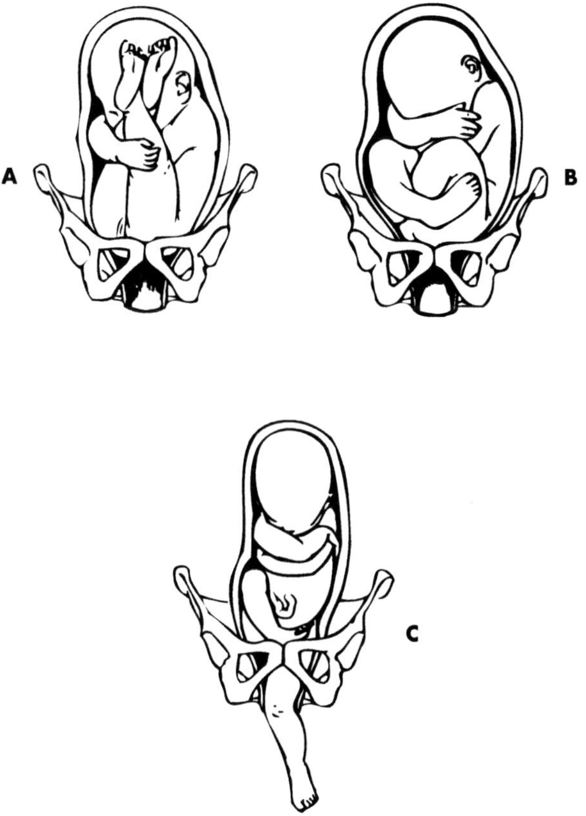

Figure 21-6
Breech presentations: **A,** Frank. **B,** Complete. **C,** Footling. (From Pernoll ML, Benson RC: *Current obstetrics and gynecologic diagnosis and treatment,* ed 6, Norwalk, CT, 1987, Appleton & Lange.)

(b) The diagnosis can be made on pelvic examination as the anterior fontanel is palpated on the anterior aspect of the pelvis. Confirmation may be made by palpating the orientation of the fetal ear.

(c) Management may involve oxytocin augmentation if the contractions are inadequate. A vaginal delivery of a posterior occiput may be considered if fetal descent progresses. In skilled hands and with no evidence of fetal macrosomia, midforceps rotation and extraction may be

Prerequisites of a Vaginal Delivery of a Breech

Estimated fetal weight between 2500 and 3800 g
Frank breech
Adequate x-ray pelvimetry
Flexed head
Continuous fetal monitoring
Normal progress of labor
Experienced clinician

considered. A cesarean section may be necessary if the vertex fails to descend and a rotation is not possible.

(3) Occiput transverse
  (a) The occiput transverse is considered to be a transient position. As labor progresses, the occiput rotates to either an anterior or a posterior position. The etiology may be a platypelloid pelvis or inadequate contractions. A deep transverse arrest occurs when the vertex has failed to negotiate the inlet.
  (b) The diagnosis is made on the pelvic examination. The axis of the sagittal suture is used for orientation.
  (c) A cesarean section is indicated in infants with deep transverse arrest. In other cases of a transverse arrest, evaluation of the contractions may be warranted and, if adequate, patience may be necessary.

(4) Brow presentation
  (a) Brow presentations are also recognized as transient positions. They occur in approximately 0.06% of deliveries. Pelvic contractures, prematurity, and grand multiparity are associated with this position.
  (b) The diagnosis is made on pelvic or speculum examination.
  (c) Management is usually expectant. Spontaneous rotation occurs in most of the cases. Inadequate uterine contractions may be encountered in cases with a contracted pelvis.

(5) Face presentation
  (a) Face presentations are noted in approximately 0.2% of deliveries. In this position, the fetal head is deflexed from its longitudinal axis. The most common causes are fetal anomalies, prematurity, grand multiparity, and a contracted pelvis.
  (b) The diagnosis is often made on pelvic examination. The palpation of the fetal mouth, orbit, or malar prominence can often shock an examiner. The diagnosis of either a breech or umbilical cord can sometimes be made.
  (c) Management depends on the location of the mentum. Mentum posterior presentations are unable to extend any further and require a cesarean section. Infants with mentum

anterior may be able to negotiate the pelvis; however, the presenting submentobregmatic diameter may be too large and dystocia may occur. No attempts should be made to flex the fetal head or manually rotate a mentum posterior.

(6) Shoulder dystocia

(a) A shoulder dystocia is defined as the when the anterior shoulder of the infant fails to maneuver the pubic symphysis after the head is delivered. The incidence is approximately 0.15%. The incidence rises to approximately 2% in infants over 4000 g.

(b) The most common cause of a shoulder dystocia is maternal obesity, diabetes, fetal macrosomia, and a previous history of a shoulder dystocia.

(c) Management should always be reviewed before any delivery, and the clinician should remain calm and proceed in a systematic fashion. Once the diagnosis is made, attention should be placed on the perineum, and a large episiotomy is made to ensure adequate space. An assistant and an anesthesiologist should be notified immediately. Suprapubic pressure is applied downward along with gentle traction downward on the fetal head. Fundal pressure should be avoided because this can wedge the shoulder under the symphysis and also the risk of a uterine rupture is increased.

(d) A McRoberts maneuver is next attempted if suprapubic pressure fails. The woman's legs are flexed extensively toward her abdomen and chest. This may rotate the symphysis cephalad and straighten the sacrum, allowing the anterior shoulder to be freed.

(e) A Wood's screw maneuver may be tried after the McRoberts maneuver. In this procedure, the clinician places two fingers on the anterior aspect of the posterior shoulder and rotates the shoulder anteriorly and in an oblique position. This allows the posterior shoulder to be delivered and the anterior shoulder, which is now in the posterior space of the pelvis, is delivered.

(f) Delivery of the posterior arm may also be performed by inserting a hand into the hollow of the sacrum and sweeping the posterior arm across the chest and out of the vagina. This often leads to clavicular or humeral fractures.

(g) Birth asphyxia, clavicular or humeral fractures, and Erbs palsy may occur in up to 50% of cases of shoulder dystocia.

3. Passage

a. Dystocia from the passage should be considered in every woman with protraction or arrest disorders in labor. X-ray pelvimetry was used extensively to examine for any evidence of pelvic contractures. However, clinical pelvimetry has replaced x-ray pelvimetry in modern obstetrics. There is still some limited use for x-ray pelvimetry, particularly in cases of breech presentations.

b. The contractions of the pelvis are defined by the location of the abnormality. They are described as either inlet, midpelvis, or outlet contractions.
   (1) Inlet dystocia
      (a) An inlet contraction is often suspected if the diagonal conjugate diameter is less than 12.5 cm. Other clinical indications may be a floating vertex failure of descent or deep transverse arrest.
      (b) Considerable molding is evident in these infants because of the prolonged use of oxytocin and the failure of fetal descent.
      (c) A caput succedaneum can often be misleading and the clinician may determine that descent is occurring.
      (d) Treatment is often a cesarean section.
   (2) Midpelvic–outlet dystocia
      (a) Contractions of the midpelvis and the outlet are very commonly indistinguishable. The diagnosis is often made on pelvic examination because the sidewalls are convergent, the ischial spines are prominent, and the pubic arch is 90° or less.
      (b) The diagnosis is often confirmed by a prolonged second stage, a persistent occiput posterior, or a deep transverse arrest. A caput is often found on the fetus.
      (c) As a result of the contracted pelvis, rotation and extension are often difficult. Careful applications of forceps may be attempted if the vertex has managed to descend to the pelvis floor. A cesarean section is often indicated in those infants who have failed to descend appropriately.

4. Operative delivery

An operative delivery is defined as any delivery requiring an active maneuver. The three most common methods are with forceps, by vacuum or by a cesarean section.

a. Forceps
   (1) The obstetric forcep is composed of two matched instruments. Each instrument consists of a blade, a shank, a lock, and a handle. The cephalic curve is the area of the blade that is applied to the infant's head. The area of the blade placed on the mother's pelvis is known as the pelvic curve. There is a left and a right blade on all forceps, which correspond to the left and right side of the mother's pelvis when placed.
   (2) There are a variety of classic and modern or special forceps available (Fig. 21-7). The clinician should become familiar with just a few of the forcep types and the unique conditions required for each.
   (3) The indications for forcep use are divided between maternal and fetal.
      (a) Maternal indications may include maternal exhaustion and concurrent medical problems requiring a shortened second stage.

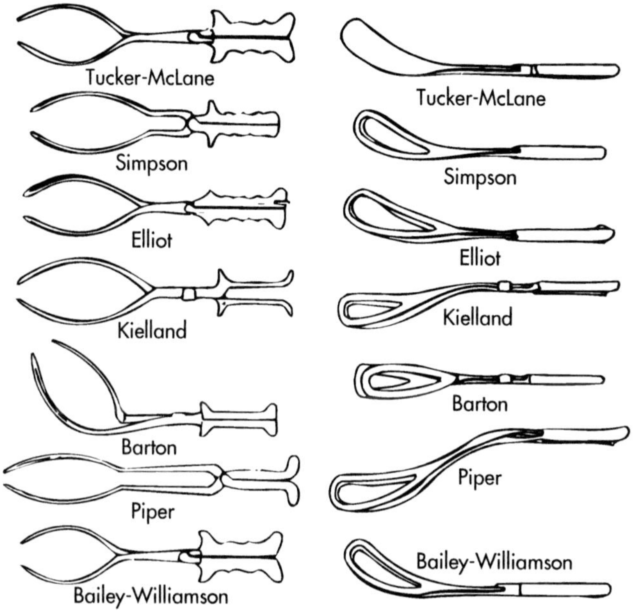

Figure 21-7
Types of forceps. (From Pernoll ML, Benson RC: *Current obstetrics and gynecologic diagnosis and treatment,* ed 6, Norwalk, CT, 1987, Appleton & Lange.)

(b) Fetal indications are usually limited to any evidence of fetal distress requiring immediate delivery.

(4) Several conditions need to be met before forceps are used. The box on p. 412 lists the six conditions required to minimize any trauma to the infant or mother.

(5) Forcep deliveries are classified as either mid, low, or outlet.

(a) Mid forceps deliveries occur when the fetal head is engaged, but above +2 station. If the vortex is rotated >45°, despite the station, it is also classified as a mid forcep.

(b) A low forceps delivery occurs when the head is beyond +2 station but has not reached the pelvic floor.

(c) Outlet forceps are recognized when the head has reached the pelvic floor, the scalp is visible at the introitus, and the rotation of the sagittal suture is <45°.

b. Vacuum

(1) The vacuum is composed of either a 65-mm soft, silastic cup or a more firm, disposable 60-mm cup. Its use has increased over the past several years secondary to data suggesting less perinatal morbidity.

Conditions for Forceps Delivery

Cervix is fully dilated.
Membranes are ruptured.
Head must be engaged.
Fetal head position is known.
There is no evidence of cephalopelvic disproportion.
The bladder is empty.

(2) The indications for application of the vacuum are similar to those of forceps. The classification of vacuum deliveries is similar as well.

(3) The prerequisites for vacuum extraction are similar to those of forceps; however, the identification of the sagittal suture may not be as critical.

c. Cesarean section

(1) Cesarean section is a surgical incision through the abdominal wall and the uterus, performed to deliver a fetus. Its use has increased significantly over the past several years, and numerous attempts are underway to reduce the cesarean births in the United States. Most hospitals report a 10% to 35% cesarean birth rate.

(2) Cesareans are classified as either classical or low cervical.

(a) Classical cesarean section refers to a delivery of an infant through a vertical incision on the corpus of the uterus. It is associated with increased blood loss and an increased risk of uterine rupture in a subsequent pregnancy.

(b) Low cervical cesarean sections apply to transverse incisions (Kerr incision) performed in the lower, noncontractile portion of the uterus.

(3) Major risk during cesarean sections are infection, anesthetic complications, and hemorrhage. The mortality rate for cesarean section is approximately 5.8 per 100,000 live births.

Suggested reading

1. Acker DB, Sachs BP, Friedman EA: Risk factors for shoulder dystocia, *Obstet Gynecol* 66:762-765, 1985.
2. ACOG Technical Bulletin: *Operative vaginal delivery* February 1991, p. 152.
3. ACOG Technical Bulletin: *Fetal macrosomia* September 1991, p. 159.
4. Bigrigg A, Chissell S, Read MD: Use of intra myometrial 15-methyl prostaglandin F2-alpha to control atonic postpartum haemorrhage following vaginal delivery and failure of conventional therapy, *Br J Obstet Gynaecol* 98:734-736, 1991.
5. Brandt ML: Mechanism and management of the third stage of labor, *Am J Obstet Gynecol* 25:662-663, 1933.
6. Caldwell WE, Moloy HC: Anatomical variations in the female pelvis and their effect in labor with a suggested classification, *Am J Obstet Gynecol* 26:479-483, 1933.

7. Caldwell WE, Moloy HC, D'Espo DA: Further studies on the pelvic architecture, *Am J Obstet Gynecol* 28:482-486, 1934.
8. Cunningham FG et al: *Williams obstetrics,* ed 19, Norwalk, CT, 1993, Appleton & Lange.
9. Friedman EA: *Labor: clinical evaluation and management,* ed 2, New York, 1978, Appleton-Century-Crofts.
10. Gabbe SG, Niebyl JR, Simpson JL: *Obstetrics: normal and problem pregnancies,* ed 2, New York, 1991, Churchill Livingstone.
11. Harris AP, Michitsch RU: Anesthesia and analgesia for labor, *Curr Op Obstet Gynecol* 4:813-817, 1992.
12. Keirse MJ: Therapeutic uses of prostaglandins, *Baillieres Clin Obstet Gynaecol* 6:787-808, 1992.
13. Okazaki T et al: Initiation of human parturition. XII. Biosynthesis and metabolism of prostaglandins in human fetal membranes and uterine decidua, *Am J Obstet Gynecol* 39:373-376, 1981.
14. Ott WJ: The diagnosis of altered fetal growth, *Obstet Gynecol Clin* 15:237-263, 1988.
15. Santos AC, Pedersen H: Current controversies in obstetric anesthesia, *Anesthesia Analgesia* 78:753-760, 1994.
16. Wittels B: Does epidural anesthesia affect the course of labor and delivery? *Sem Perinatol* 15:358-367, 1991.

22 Analgesia and Anesthetics in Obstetrics

22.1 ANALGESIA AND ANESTHETICS IN NORMAL PREGNANCY

Jeffery R. Graves, M.D.

Characteristics of labor pain

1. Severe, exceeded only by the following:
   a. Causalgia
   b. Traumatic amputation
   c. Terminal cancer pain
2. Labor pain is physiologic.
3. Variable in onset and severity. Not all parturients experience pain; however, 35% to 77% of parturients characterize their pain as severe or intolerable. Factors associated with increased severity are as follows:
   a. Nulliparity
   b. Occiput posterior position
   c. History of severe dysmenorrhea
   d. Young maternal age
   e. Increased maternal and/or fetal weight
   f. Absence of supportive companion
   g. Unrealistic expectations
   h. Maternal fear and anxiety
4. Predictive: Early onset and increased severity may indicate dysfunctional labor and malpresentation of the fetus, resulting in a higher likelihood of operative or instrumented delivery.
5. Retrospectively devalued: Postpartum recall will minimize the intensity of the pain experienced.
6. Labor pain is treatable.

Harmful physiologic effects of labor pain

The pain is generally well tolerated by most parturients; however, for parturients with compromised cardiopulmonary function, the provision of adequate laboring analgesia can be life saving.

1. Cardiovascular
   a. Increased heart rate
   b. Increased stroke volume

c. Increased systemic vascular resistance
d. Increased cardiac output
e. Increased myocardial workload and oxygen (O_2) requirements
2. Pulmonary (hyperventilation or hypoventilation syndrome)
a. Maternal hyperventilation during contractions
(1) Hypocarbia
(2) Alkalemia
(3) Deleterious leftward shift of the oxyhemoglobin dissociation curve
b. Maternal hypoventilation between contractions
(1) Maternal hypoxemia
(2) Less O_2 available to the uteroplacental circulation
3. Metabolic
a. Increased systemic O_2 consumption
b. Decreased O_2 available to the uteroplacental circulation
4. Increased levels of circulating catecholamines
a. Uterine artery vasoconstriction
b. Decreased uteroplacental blood flow
5. Decreased uterine activity and delayed progress of labor
6. Increased maternal anxiety and fear

Stages of labor and pain pathways

1. First stage of labor
a. Pain source
(1) Cervical distension
(2) Lower uterine distension
(3) Uterine contractions
b. Pain pathway
(1) Visceral sensory afferent nerves pass via:
(2) Frankenhauser's ganglion (paracervical region); to exit pelvis via:
(3) Inferior, middle, and superior hypogastric plexi, to pass via:
(4) Lumbar sympathetic chain at L2-L3, to terminate in the:
(5) Dorsal horn of the spinal cord at the T10-L1 segmental level.
2. Second stage of labor
a. Pain source
(1) Distension of pelvic floor
(2) Distension of vagina
(3) Distension of perineum
b. Pain pathway
(1) Perineal somatic sensory afferents travel via the:
(2) Pudendal nerve, which arises from the:
(3) Spinal cord at the S2-S4 segmental level.
3. Third stage of labor
a. Uncomplicated placental delivery is generally well tolerated.
b. Anesthesia is often required for the following:
(1) Manual extraction of a retained placenta
(2) Difficulties relating to placental invasion of uterine components

4. Transitional stage of labor
   a. Definition: the time frame occuring within the first stage of labor from onset of somatic (second stage pain) to the complete dilation of the cervix
   b. Experienced more often, at an earlier cervical dilation, and with greater severity by nulliparous women
   c. Pain sources: those of first and second stages of labor

Analgesic or anesthetic interventions (Table 22-1)

1. Psychoprophylactic or nonpharmacologic techniques
2. Systemic intravenous agents
   a. Intermittent bolus dosing
   b. Patient-controlled (demand) dosing
3. Inhalation analgesia
4. Neuraxial anesthesia
   a. Continuous techniques
      (1) Continuous lumbar epidural
      (2) Continuous subarachnoid catheter
      (3) Continuous caudal epidural
   b. Single-injection techniques
      (1) "Saddle" block
      (2) "Modified saddle" block
      (3) Spinal anesthesia
      (4) Intrathecal opioids
   c. Combined spinal and epidural
5. Paracervical block
6. Lumbar sympathetic block
7. Bilateral pudendal nerve blocks with or without local infiltration

Psychoprophylactic or nonpharmacologic techniques

1. Techniques are as follows:
   a. Lamaze and other childbirth preparatory classes
   b. Emotional support
   c. Massage or touch therapy
   d. Hydrotherapy
   e. Biofeedback and self-hypnosis
   f. Acupuncture
   g. Transcutaneous electrical nerve stimulation (TENS)
2. Purported advantages are hotly debated.
   a. Purported advantages not consistently demonstrated
      (1) Decreased use of systemic analgesics
      (2) Decreased use of regional anesthesia
      (3) Shorter labor
      (4) Decreased incidence of instrumented vaginal delivery
      (5) Decreased incidence of operative delivery
      (6) Decreased incidence of fetal distress
   b. Advantages
      (1) Increased maternal control or cooperation
      (2) Reduced maternal anxiety
      (3) Reduced perception of pain

Table 22-1 A comparison of analgesic techniques

Psychoprophylactic Nonpharmacologic Techniques	Systemic Intravenous Analgesia	Neuraxial Anesthesia (Epidural or Spinal)
May require specialized equipment, supportive partner, or attendance at prenatal classes	Technically easy to administer	Requires specialized equipment and personnel
Progressively ineffective, poor late first-stage efficacy, poor second-stage efficacy	Incomplete analgesia, improves tolerability of labor, poor second-stage efficacy	Superior laboring analgesia; offers excellent first-stage and second-stage analgesia
Maternal safety unquestioned	Maternal side effects	Procedural risks incurred
Avoids systemic medications, fetal or neonatal effects	Fetal or neonatal effects of systemically administered agents possible	Systemic absorption minimal; fetal or neonatal effects are rare
Has no effect on harmful physiologic effects of labor pain	Blunts the harmful physiologic changes of labor pain	Largely ablates the harmful physiologic changes of labor pain
Operative anesthesia absent	Operative anesthesia absent	Operative anesthesia capability readily inherent in continuous techniques

3. Risks and disadvantages are as follows:
   a. Attendance at prenatal classes may be required.
   b. Presence of supportive partner may be required.
   c. Instructor bias may lead women to believe they have "failed" if they require additional analgesic techniques.
4. No psychoprophylactic or nonpharmacologic technique consistently provides the quality of relief provided by neuraxial analgesia.

Placental transfer of maternally administered medications

1. Passive transport
   a. Diffusion of substance across a membrane is secondary to a concentration or electrochemical gradient.
   b. Passive transport does not expend energy and depends on the following factors:
      (1) Extent of concentration or electrochemical differences
      (2) Lipid solubility
      (3) Molecular weight
      (4) Degree of ionization
      (5) Membrane surface area
      (6) Membrane thickness
   c. Examples include almost all maternally administered pharmacologic agents.
2. Facilitated transport
   a. Carrier-mediated transport of relatively lipid-insoluble molecules down their concentration or electrochemical gradient.
   b. Facilitated transport does not expend energy and exhibits the following characteristics:
      (1) Saturation kinetics
      (2) Competitive inhibition
      (3) Noncompetitive inhibition
      (4) Sterospecificity
      (5) Temperature effect
   c. Examples include the transplacental transport of glucose.
3. Secondary active transport
   a. This is a type of facilitated transport in which a secondary molecule is transported across a membrane against its diffusion gradient because it is "coupled" with a "carrier" molecule being transported "down" its concentration or electrochemical gradient.
   b. Examples include transplacental transport of amino acids.
4. Active transport
   a. Active transport is the transport of any substance across a membrane that occurs in an energy-expending fashion.
   b. Although generally occurring against a substance's concentration or electrochemical gradient, any energy-requiring transport is considered active regardless of the substance's concentration or electrochemical gradient
5. Pinocytosis
   a. This is an invagination of membrane wall and energy-requiring transport across the membrane wall or to intracellular structures.
   b. Examples include large protein molecules.

Systemic intravenous analgesics

1. Opioids
   a. Opioids are equally effective at equianalgesic doses; choice is largely a matter of provider preference.
   b. Adverse maternal effects occur with equal frequency or severity at equianalgesic doses.
   c. Morphine's longer duration of action and the heightened sensitivity of the neonate to its respiratory depressent effect limit its use in labor.
   d. Fentanyl's short duration of action and accumulative effect (loss of short duration of action with repeated dosing) limits its use in labor.
2. Opioid agonist or antagonists
   a. Possess respiratory depressent "ceiling effect" (ceiling effect: Beyond a certain "ceiling" dose, increased effect no longer occurs)
   b. Possess analgesic ceiling effect
   c. Increased incidence of dysphoria relative to the opioids
3. Ketamine
   a. Amnesia, short duration of action limit use for first-stage analgesia.
   b. Intense analgesia useful for the following:
      (1) Painful vaginal delivery
      (2) Instrumented vaginal delivery in the absence of regional anesthesia
      (3) Adjunctive therapy when regional anesthesia is inadequate
   c. Neonatal depression, abnormal muscle tone, and low Apgar score occur at maternal doses >1.5 to 2 mg/kg.
4. Ketorolac: The efficacy and safety of ketorolac for laboring analgesia is unproven.
5. Dosing (Table 22-2)

Table 22-2 Systemic analgesics

Drug	Dose	Onset	Duration
Fentanyl	IV: 25-50 μg	2-3 min	30-60 min
	IM: 50-100 μg	7-10 min	1-2 hr
Meperidine	IV: 25-50 mg	5-10 min	2-3 hr
	IM: 50-100 mg	40-50 min	3-4 hr
Morphine	IV: 2-5 mg	5-10 min	3-4 hr
	IM: 5-10 mg	20-40 min	4-6 hr
Butorphanol	IV: 1-2 mg	5-10 min	3-4 hr
	IM: 1-2 mg	5-10 min	3-4 hr
Nalbuphine	IV: 10-20 mg	2-3 min	3-4 hr
	IM: 10-20 mg	10-15 min	4-6 hr
Pentazocine	IV: 10-20 mg	2-3 min	2-3 hr
	IM: 20-40 mg	10-20 min	3-4 hr
Ketamine	IV: 10-20 mg	30-60 sec	2-5 min

Risks and disadvantages of systemic analgesics

1. Maternal
   a. Do not provide complete analgesia (opioids, opioid agonists or antagonists)
   b. Respiratory depression (opioids, opioid agonists or antagonists)
   c. Sedation, drowsiness (opioids, opioid agonists or antagonists, ketamine)
   d. Nausea or vomiting (opioids, opioid agonists or antagonists)
   e. Delayed gastric emptying (opioids, opioid agonists or antagonists)
   f. Pruritis (opioids, opioid agonists or antagonists)
   g. Orthostatic hypotension (opioids, opioid agonists or antagonists)
   h. Dysphoria (opioids, opioid agonists or antagonists, ketamine)
   i. Decreased uterine activity (opioids, opioid agonists or antagonists, ketorolac)
   j. Slowed cervical dilation (opioids, opioid agonists or antagonists)
   k. Delayed progress of labor (opioids, opioid agonists or antagonists)
   l. Amnesia (ketamine)
   m. Short duration of action limits use during first stage (ketamine)
   n. Hallucinations (ketamine)
   o. Sympathetic nervous system activation (ketamine)
   p. Obstetric safety unproven (ketorolac)
   q. Platelet dysfunction (ketorolac)
   r. Readily enter fetal circulation (opioids, opioid agonists or antagonists, ketamine, ketorolac)
2. Fetal
   a. Decreased beat-to-beat variability (opioids, opioid agonists or antagonists)
   b. Premature closure of ductus arteriosus (ketorolac)
3. Neonatal
   a. Respiratory depression (opioids, opioid agonists or antagonists, ketamine)
   b. Neurobehavioral changes (opioids, opioid agonists or antagonists, ketamine)
   c. Premature closure of ductus arteriosus (ketorolac)

Intravenous analgesia, patient-controlled (demand) dosing (PCA)

1. To date none of the purported benefits (with the exception of higher patient satisfaction) have been consistently demonstrated in the obstetric population.
2. Purported benefits and advantages are as follows:
   a. Superior analgesia compared with intermittent dosing
   b. Decreased total drug requirements, resulting in decreased placental transfer and fetal or neonatal accumulation
   c. Decreased incidence of untoward side effects, particularly respiratory depression and nausea or vomiting
   d. Higher patient satisfaction
3. Risks and disadvantages are those of the agent chosen.

Systemic intravenous adjuvants

1. Commonly used adjuvant agents include the following:
   a. Antihistamines (diphenhydramine, hydroxyzine)
   b. Barbiturates (pentobarbital, secobarbital)
   c. Benzodiazepines (diazepam, lorazepam, midazolam)
   d. Narcotic antagonists (naloxone)
   e. Phenothiazine derivatives (promethazine, propriomazine)
2. Indications
   a. Treatment of untoward effects of systemic analgesics
      (1) Opioid overdose (naloxone)
      (2) Opioid-induced pruritis (diphenhydramine, naloxone, opioid agonist or antagonists)
      (3) Nausea or vomiting (promethazine, propriomazine)
      (4) Local anesthetic induced central nervous system (CNS) excitability (diazepam, lorazepam)
   b. Sedation anxiolysis (pentobarbital, secobarbital, diazepam, lorazepam, midazolam)
   c. Amnesia, generally an undesired effect (diazepam, lorazepam, midazolam)
   d. Analgesic adjuvant (hydroxyzine)
3. Dosing (Table 22-3)

Adverse effects of intravenous adjuvants

1. Maternal
   a. Sedation (pentobarbital, secobarbital, diazepam, lorazepam, midazolam, promethazine, diphenhydramine, hydroxyzine)
   b. Hypotension (pentobarbital, secobarbital)
   c. Reversal of opioid analgesic effect (naloxone)
   d. Elicitation of acute opioid withdrawal syndrome (naloxone)
   e. Painful injection (hydroxyzine)
2. Fetal and neonatal
   a. Elicitation of acute opioid withdrawal syndrome (naloxone)
   b. Respiratory depression (pentobarbital, secobarbital, diazepam, lorazepam, midazolam)
   c. Hypotonia, loss of thermoregulation (diazepam, lorazepam, midazolam)

Inhalation analgesia

1. Definition: Inhalational analgesia is the administration of subanesthetic doses of inhalational agents to provide analgesia.
2. This is largely impractical for first-stage analgesia because of the following:
   a. Episodic crescendo–decrescendo pattern of labor pain
   b. Need for specialized vaporizers
   c. Environmental pollution by agent
   d. Undesirable maternal amnesia
   e. Potential for maternal overdose
3. Indications
   a. Painful vaginal delivery
   b. Instrumented vaginal delivery in the absence of regional anesthesia
   c. Adjunctive therapy when regional anesthesia is inadequate

Table 22-3 Adjuvant agents

Drug	Dose	Drug	Dose
Diphenhydramine, antihistamine	IV: 12.5-25 ng IM: 25-50 mg	Midazolam, benzodiazepine	IV: 1-5 mg IM: 1-5 mg
Hydroxyzine, antihistamine	IM: 25-50 mg	Naloxone, opioid antagonist	IV bolus: 40-400 μg (in 40 μg increments) IV infusion: 5-10 μg/kg/min IM: 400 μg
Pentobarbital, barbiturate	PO: 100-200 mg IM: 100-200 mg		
Secobarbital, barbiturate	PO: 100 mg IM: 100 mg		
Diazepam, benzodiazepine	IV: 2.5-5 mg IM: 5-10 mg	Promethazine, phenothiazine	IV: 12.5-25 mg IM: 25-50 mg
Lorazepam, benzodiazepine	IV: 1-2 mg IM: 2-5 mg	Propriomazine, phenothiazine	IV: 10-20 mg IM: 20-40 mg

4. Many prefer low doses of ketamine (0.10 to 0.25 mg/kg) titrated to effect to the risks of inhalational analgesia.
5. *Major* risk of this technique is accidental maternal overdose with loss of protective airway reflexes and increased risk for maternal aspiration.
6. Pharmacology: See General anesthesia, Inhalational agents.

Neuraxial anesthesia

Anatomy (internal to external)

1. Spinal cord, terminating at L1 level (continues as the cauda equina)
2. Pia mater
3. Subarachnoid space containing the cerebrospinal fluid (CSF) and transversed by the spinal nerves as they exit or enter the spinal cord
4. Arachnoid membrane
5. Dura mater, a tough fibrous sheath tethered at the S2 level
6. Epidural space, transversed by the spinal nerves, and bounded by the following:
   a. Vertebral bodies and intervertebral discs anteriorly
   b. Vertebral pedicles laterally
   c. Vertebral laminae and spinous processes posteriorly
   d. Ligamentum flavum, connecting the anterior aspects of laminae and spinous processes, thus forming the posterior border of the epidural space in the interspinous space

Mechanism of action

1. Epidural
   a. Local anesthetic diffuses through the dural sheath to exert its influence on the nerve roots as they exit the central neuraxis.
   b. Opioids diffuse through the dural membrane to enter the CSF and exert antinociceptive actions via interaction with spinal cord and higher CNS opioid receptors.
2. Subarachnoid
   a. Local anesthetic is directly injected into CSF to exert influence on spinal cord neural transmission.
   b. Opioids are directly injected into the CSF to exert antinociceptive actions via interaction with spinal cord and higher central nervous system opioid receptors.

Absolute contraindications

1. Patient refusal
2. Localized infection at skin puncture site
3. Septicemia
4. Coagulopathy
5. Increased intracranial pressure

Epidural versus spinal (Table 22-4)

Continuous techniques

1. Continuous lumbar epidural (CLE)
   a. Analgesia
      (1) First stage: excellent

Table 22-4 A comparison of neuraxial techniques

Characteristic	Subarachnoid Administration (Single Injection)	Epidural Administration (Continuous)
Ease of administration	Technically easy	Technically more difficult than subarachnoid
Efficacy	Failure rate under 1%	Operative failure rate 2% to 4%
Onset	Rapid	Slower onset
Segmental level	Dependent on characteristics of technique	Segmental level titratable
Motor block	Dense	Dependent on local anesthetic concentration
Dose required	Less than epidural	Greater dosing requirement
Systemic absorption	Negligible to nonexistent	Does occur, but maternal, fetal, and neonatal effects are rare
Use as laboring analgesic	Dense motor block, limits use as laboring analgesic	Superior laboring analgesic
Operative anesthesic	Operative anesthesia available with initial or repeat injection	Operative anesthetic capability present throughout labor

(2) Second stage: variable; may require a "sitting" dose or a segmental level to T6 or greater to provide adequate sacral coverage or perineal anesthesia
(3) Operative: capability present throughout duration of catheterization

b. Technically easier to place than caudal epidural
c. Motor block: can be minimized by using dilute local anesthetic
d. Disadvantages: none, relative to other continuous techniques; surpassed only by combined spinal and epidural technique in its usefulness
e. Dosing
(1) Local anesthetic only (intermittent dosing or continuous infusion)
  (a) Advantage is relatively long history of safety and efficacy.
  (b) Disadvantages are as follows:
    i. Motor block usually present at effective doses
      • Decreases maternal satisfaction
      • May increase the likelihood of operative or instrumented delivery
    ii. Increased incidences of hypotension
    iii. Increased risk for local anesthetic toxicity
(2) Continuous infusion of local anesthetic and opioid combination
  (a) Advantages are as follows:
    i. Decreased concentration (i.e., 1⁄16% bupivicaine) of local anesthetic
    ii. Minimal motor block
    iii. May provide superior analgesia compared to infusion of local anesthetic only
    iv. May provide superior second-stage analgesia without increasing the incidence of malrotation or instrumented vaginal delivery
  (b) Disadvantages (introduces the risks of neuraxial opioids) include the following:
    i. Maternal respiratory depression (less than with systemic administration)
    ii. Increased incidence of opioid-induced pruritis
    iii. Neonatal respiratory depression (less than with systemic administration, but more than with spinal administration)
(3) Continuous infusion of opioid only
  (a) Advantages: avoids local anesthetic effects entirely
  (b) Disadvantages are as follows:
    i. Required analgesic doses can cause maternal and fetal or neonatal effects comparable to systemic opioids (epidural only; subarachnoid administration results in negligible maternal systemic uptake)
    ii. Poor second-stage analgesia
    iii. Not an operative anesthetic
  (c) Usually reserved for parturients with coexisting disease who would not tolerate even the minimal afterload reduction caused by a dilute local solution

2. Caudal epidural anesthesia
   a. Analgesia
      (1) First stage: excellent; requires significantly more infusate
      (2) Second stage: excellent; more effective sacral coverage than lumbar technique
      (3) Operative: capability present throughout duration of catheterization
   b. Advantages: particularly useful for parturients in whom lumbar techniques are technically difficult (e.g., parturients who have had prior back surgery)
   c. Disadvantages
      (1) Technically more difficult or painful to place than lumbar epidural
      (2) Motor block: generally greater than lumbar, particularly pelvic floor
      (3) Potential for direct fetal injury with the needle
   d. Dosing: as for lumbar epidural
3. Continuous subarachnoid catheter
   a. Possesses characteristics of epidural or spinal depending on the dosing or infusion agent chosen.
   b. Can be dosed as "spinal" for operative anesthesia.
   c. Risks and benefits profile dependent on dosing agent.
   d. Systemic absorption of agents negligible.
   e. Major disadvantages are as follows:
      (1) Potential for unexpected high block
      (2) Potential avenue for infection directly into CNS
   f. Rarely used, but ideally suited for the following:
      (1) Continuous intrathecal opioids in parturients with coexisting disease who would tolerate neither the pain of labor nor regional blockade from local anesthetic (e.g., parturients with stenotic valvular disorders)
      (2) Neuraxial anesthesia when epidural placement is technically difficult or impossible (e.g., status post [s/p] back surgery, morbidly obese parturients)

Single-injection techniques

1. Subarachnoid block (SAB, "spinal," "saddle block")
   a. True saddle block (dense motor and sensory block S1-S5)
      (1) Second-stage analgesia.
      (2) Perineal anesthesia.
      (3) Patient must be sitting for placement.
      (4) First stage analgesia is not provided.
      (5) Dense motor block may increase incidence of malrotation or instrumented vaginal delivery.
   b. Modified saddle block (dense motor and sensory block to T-10)
      (1) First and second stages of analgesia.
      (2) Perineal anesthesia.
      (3) Dense motor block (to T-10 level) limits use of this technique.
   c. Spinal (dense motor and sensory block to T-4 level)
      (1) Indicated for operative anesthesia.

2. Intrathecal opioids
   a. Opioids provide analgesia for the latent and early active phases of the first stage of labor.
   b. Opioids avoid local anesthetic (local anesthetic during early labor may increase the incidence of operative and instrumented delivery).
   c. Analgesia for the late first stage and second stage of labor are of doubtful effectiveness (intrathecal opioids appear ineffective past 6 to 8 cm of cervical dilation).
   d. Opioids do not provide surgical anesthesia.
   e. With the advent of the combined spinal and epidural technique, the use of intrathecal opioids as sole laboring analgesic is rarely, if ever, indicated.
   f. Dosing
      (1) Morphine: 0.1 to 0.3 mg, duration 4 to 6 hours
      (2) Fentanyl: 15 to 25 μg, duration 1 to 3 hours
      (3) Sufentanil: 10 to 15 μg, duration 1 to 3 hours
   g. Maternal systemic absorption and fetal or neonatal effects are negligible.

Combined spinal and epidural (CSE)

1. CSE possesses all the capabilities and benefits of the intrathecal single-injection techniques and continuous lumbar epidural techniques.
2. CSE is ideally suited for parturients who hurt early in labor. The combination of intrathecal narcotics for latent and early active laboring analgesia and epidural catheter placement for later laboring analgesia avoids local anesthetic or systemic analgesics in early labor and offers these patients their single best opportunity at an uncomplicated vaginal delivery while maintaining all the benefits of an epidural catheter.

Complications

1. Complications associated with placement
   a. Inadvertent dural puncture
      (1) Incidence: provider dependent, generally 1% to 4% at teaching institutions
      (2) Signs: frank CSF from epidural needle
      (3) Treatment
         (a) Catheter is placed and used as continuous intrathecal catheter.
         (b) Or, needle is removed and epidural catheter is placed in an adjacent interspace.
   b. Post–dural puncture headache (PDPH, spinal headache)
      (1) Incidence
         (a) 35% to 80% past puncture of dural membrane with epidural needle; overall incidence associated with epidural placement is 1% to 2%
         (b) 1% to 2% with small-gauge spinal needles
      (2) Signs
         (a) New onset of headache 12 to 72 hours after neuraxial anesthesia
         (b) Postural, worsened by upright position
         (c) Absence of other causes for headache

(3) Treatment
   (a) Other causes must be ruled out, although PDPH can be superimposed on other types of headaches
   (b) Increased PO fluid intake
   (c) Systemic analgesics (rarely effective)
   (d) Intravenous hydration
   (e) Intravenous caffeine (500 mg, q6h $\times$ 2)
   (f) Epidural blood patch (95% effective)

c. Inadvertent intrathecal catheter placement (unrecognized)
   (1) Incidence: extremely rare
   (2) Signs: unexpected high block if dosed as epidural catheter
   (3) Treatment: ventilatory and hemodynamic support

d. Recognized intrathecal catheter placement
   (1) Incidence: extremely rare
   (2) Signs
      (a) CSF aspirated from catheter
      (b) Epidural test dose positive for spinal anesthesia
   (3) Treatment
      (a) Used as continuous intrathecal catheter
      (b) Or, epidural catheter is removed and replaced in an adjacent interspace

e. Intravascular catheter placement (unrecognized)
   (1) Incidence: extremely rare
   (2) Signs
      (a) Inadequate or absent anesthesia
      (b) Signs of systemic toxicity
   (3) Treatment: Catheter removed and systemic toxicity is treated as needed.

f. Intravascular catheter placement (recognized)
   (1) Incidence: rare
   (2) Signs: blood aspirated from catheter
   (3) Treatment: catheter removed and replaced at adjacent interspace

g. Direct neurologic injury or paresthesia
   (1) Incidence: extremely rare
   (2) Signs: postpartum neurologic deficit, prolonged block
   (3) Treatment: immediate neurologic, neurosurgical consultation

h. Epidural hematoma
   (1) Incidence: extremely rare
   (2) Signs: neurologic deficits compatible with mass effect or spinal cord compression; often painful
   (3) Treatment: immediate neurosurgical consultation

i. Infection (epidural abcess)
   (1) Incidence: extremely rare
   (2) Signs:
      (a) Mass effect (spinal cord)
      (b) Systemic signs of infection
   (3) Treatment: immediate neurosurgical consultation

2. Complications associated with dosing
   a. Hypotension
      (1) Cause
         (a) Lower extremity and splanchnic sympathectomy (decreased venous return leading to decreased preload and subsequent decreased cardiac output resulting from decreased venous return)
         (b) Lower extremity and splanchnic vasodilation (play minor role)
      (2) Treatment
         (a) Best avoided by adequate prehydration, maintenance of left uterine displacement, and slow onset of block
         (b) Intravenous boluses of balanced salt solution
         (c) Vasopressors (Table 22-5)
   b. Unexpected high segmental level ("high spinal," "total spinal")
      (1) Cause: unexpectedly high sensory or motor block
      (2) Signs
         (a) Dyspnea
            i. Cause: loss of chest wall proprioception
            ii. Treatment: reassurance, ventilatory support as needed
         (b) Apnea
            i. Cause: brain stem hypotension; rarely caused by phrenic nerve blockade
            ii. Treatment: immediate ventilatory and hemodynamic support
         (c) Hypotension: The severity of hypotension is directly related to the rapidity of onset and segmental height of sympathetic blockade.
   c. Systemic local anesthetic toxicity
      (1) Cause
         (a) Inadvertent intravascular injection
         (b) Systemic absorption
      (2) Toxic doses of local anesthetics

	Dose (mg/kg) (without epinephrine)	Dose (mg/kg) (with epinephrine)
(a) Bupivicaine	2.5	3.0
(b) Chlorprocaine	11.0	14.0
(c) Etidocaine	3.0	5.0
(d) Lidocaine	4.0	7.0
(e) Mepivicaine	4.0	7.0
(f) Procaine	6.0	9.0
(g) Tetracaine	1.5	2.5

      (3) Signs
         (a) Tremulousness
         (b) Perioral tingling, numbness
         (c) Muscle twitching
         (d) Convulsions
         (e) Cardiovascular collapse

NOTE: Bupivicaine, the most commonly used local anesthetic in

Table 22-5 Vasoactive agents

Drug	Dose	Effects
Ephedrine, indirectly acting sympathomimetic	5-50 mg IV, IM titrated to desired effect	Minimal direct effect on uterine blood flow; initial vasopressor of choice to treat neuroaxial anesthesia-induced hypotension
Phenylephrine, directly acting vasoactive amine	50-100 μg IV titrated to desired effect	May cause uterine artery vasoconstriction; will improve uteroplacental perfusion when systemic hypotension is significant
Dopamine, directly acting vasoactive amine	2.5-20 μg/kg/min titrated to desired effect	May cause uterine artery vasoconstriction; will improve uteroplacental perfusion when systemic hypotension is significant
Dobutamine, directly acting vasoactive amine	2.5-20 μg/kg/min titrated to desired effect	Positive inotrope; will improve uteroplacental perfusion with improved cardiac output
Epinephrine, endogenous catecholamine	0.025 μg/kg/min titrated to desired effect	May cause uterine artery vasoconstriction; will improve uteroplacental perfusion when systemic hypotension is significant
Norepinephrine, endogenous catecholamine	0.025 μg/kg/min titrated to desired effect	May cause uterine artery vasoconstriction; will improve uteroplacental perfusion when systemic hypotension is significant
Isoproterenol, directly acting vasoactive amine	0.025 μg/kg/min titrated to desired effect	Positive inotrope; will improve uteroplacental perfusion with improved cardiac output

Nitroglycerin, vasodilator	0.25 μg/kg/min titrated to desired effect	Can be dosed in 50 μg increments for uterine myometrial and cervical relaxation in the event of retained placenta or difficult breech delivery
Nitroprusside, vasodilator	0.25 μg/kg/min titrated to desired effect	Rarely used because of concerns about fetal or neonatal cyanide toxicit
Esmolol, cardioselective beta-blocker	10-mg IV increments, 25 μg/kg/min, titrated to desired effect	May cause fetal or neonatal bradycardia; generally well tolerated
Labetolol, mixed alpha-blocker/beta-blocker	5-mg IV increments, 0.25 μg/kg/min titrated to desired effect	Very useful in obstetrics; may cause fetal or neonatal bradycardia; generally well tolerated
Lidocaine, local anesthetic	0.5-1 mg/kg IV load, 25 μg/kg/min titrated to desired effect	Useful as antiarrhythmic; beware systemic toxicity when neuraxial anesthesia is used concurrently
Trimethaphan, ganglionic blocker	25 μg/kg/min titrated to desired effect	Peripheral vasodilator; rarely used in obstetrics
Phentolamine, peripheral alpha-blocker	0.025 μg/kg/min titrated to desired effect	Peripheral vasodilator; rarely used in obstetrics

obstetric practice, may manifest cardiovascular toxicity before CNS toxicity.

(4) Treatment (see treatment of local anesthetic toxicity)
  (a) Provide 100% O_2.
  (b) Maintain airway.
  (c) Ensure adequate breathing, support ventilation as necessary.
  (d) Stop all local anesthetic infusion or infiltration.
  (e) Maintain hemodynamic parameters and treat circulatory collapse.
    i. Establish adequate cardiopulmonary resuscitation (CPR) (may require stat delivery of the fetus).
    ii. Treat arrhythmias with bretyllium.
  (f) Treat CNS manifestations.
    i. Convulsions do not require intubation if airway patency, breathing, and circulatory stability are maintained.
    ii. Convulsions generally respond to treatment with sodium thiopental and diazepam.
    iii. Signs of CNS excitability should be treated with sodium thiopental (50 to 100 mg) or diazepam (2.5 to 5 mg).

d. Urinary retention
  (1) Cause: exact mechanism unknown
  (2) Treatment: bladder catheterization until retention resolves

e. Pruritis
  (1) Activation of CNS opioid receptors
  (2) Treatment
    (a) Diphenhydramine
    (b) Naloxone
    (c) Opioid agonist or antagonist

f. Failed block
  (1) Treatment
    (a) Further attempts at neuraxial anesthesia
    (b) Alternative laboring analgesic techniques
    (c) Supplemental intravenous agents or inhalational analgesia

Technique

1. Continuous catheter technique
   a. Anesthesiologist should discuss risks and benefits with patient and obtain witnessed informed consent (preferably before the onset of active labor).
   b. Anesthesiologist should ensure proper rescuscitative personnel and equipment are present.
   c. Patient is prehydrated with 500 to 1000 ml of balanced salt solution.
   d. Patient is properly positioned (lateral decubitus/fetal or sitting).
   e. Anesthesiologist performs appropriate antiseptic measures.
   f. Local infiltration at L2-L3 or L3-L4 interspace is the appropriate approach to be used (midline or paramedian).
   g. The lumen of the hollow-bore needle is placed in the epidural space (identified by loss of resistance as the needle passes through the

ligamentum flavum) or subarachnoid space (identified by the tactile sensation of a "pop" as the needle penetrates the dura mater).

h. The catheter is placed to the appropriate depth into the space.
i. Needle is removed.
j. Catheter placement is tested.
   (1) Aspiration should be negative for blood and negative for CSF if epidural, positive for CSF if subarachnoid.
   (2) Test dose of local anesthetic is administered with or without epinephrine to rule out inadvertent intrathecal or intravascular placement if placing epidural catheter.
k. Catheter is dosed.

2. Single-injection technique
   a. Spinal needle is placed as in continuous catheter technique (a through g, on p. 432)
   b. Needle placement is tested as in (j), above).
   c. Dose is administered through the needle.
   d. Needle is removed.
3. Combined spinal and epidural technique
   a. Epidural needle is placed (as in continuous catheter technique a through g, above).
   b. Spinal needle is placed through epidural needle.
   c. Placement is confirmed by aspirating CSF.
   d. Dose is administered intrathecally.
   e. Spinal needle is removed.
   f. Epidural catheter is placed.
   g. Epidural needle is removed.
   h. Epidural catheter is tested.
   i. Epidural catheter is secured for later use.

Additional regional techniques

1. Paracervical block
   a. Technique: With the patient in a modified lithotomy position, local anesthetic is infiltrated into Frankenhauser's ganglion located near the left and right vaginal fornix.
   b. Characteristics
      (1) First-stage analgesia only; does not provide second-stage analgesia
      (2) Useful anesthetic for uterine procedures not involving a viable fetus
      (3) Largely abandoned because of harmful effects
   c. Complications
      (1) Fetal bradycardia
      (2) Direct fetal injury with the needle
      (3) Fetal toxicity from direct injection of local anesthetic
      (4) Increased uterine activity, hyperstimulation
      (5) Uterine artery vasoconstriction
      (6) Decreased uteroplacental blood flow
2. Lumbar sympathetic block
   a. Technique: With the patient in the sitting position a needle is introduced to the anterolateral aspect of the vertebral body of L2 and then repeated on the opposite side.

b. Characteristics
   (1) First-stage analgesia (for 2 to 3 hours) in parturients for whom neuraxial analgesia is not practical or technically impossible
   (2) Absent motor block
   (3) Technically more difficult to perform than neuraxial techniques
   (4) Pain caused by needle placement
   (5) Does not provide second-stage analgesia
   (6) Rarely used in current practice
c. Complications
   (1) Maternal hypotension (less than with neuraxial techniques)
   (2) Systemic toxic reactions
   (3) Unexpected high neuraxial block ("high spinal")
   (4) Retroperitoneal hematoma

3. Pudendal block or local perineal infiltration
   a. Technique: With the patient in the lithotomy position, local anesthetic is injected transvaginally, infiltrating the area where the pudendal nerve passes in close proximity to the ischial spines. Local infiltration is usually accomplished just before delivery or initiation of an episiotomy and involves the infiltration of local anesthetic into the posterior vaginal fourchette.
   b. Characteristics
      (1) Second-stage analgesia only
      (2) Failure rate inversely proportional to provider experience technique
   c. Complications
      (1) Maternal toxicity from local anesthetic (usually as a result of repeated injections, failed attempts)
      (2) Direct fetal injury with the needle
      (3) Fetal toxicity from direct injection of local anesthetic

General anesthesia

1. Indications
   a. Dire fetal distress in the absence of preexisting epidural anesthesia
   b. Acute maternal hypovolemia
   c. Any patient for whom regional anesthesia is contraindicated or refused
   d. Inadequate regional anesthesia
   e. Need for uterine relaxation (e.g., difficult breech delivery, retained placenta), failing to respond to IV nitroglycerin
2. Advantages
   a. Rapid induction: allows surgery to begin immediately
   b. Optimal control of airway
   c. Decreased incidence of hypotension in the hypovolemic patient
3. Complications
   a. Maternal death or hypoxic brain injury caused by airway complications
   b. Maternal aspiration
   c. Maternal awareness: rare
   d. Untoward effects of systemically administered agents

(1) Medication errors
(2) Untoward extension of physiologic effect
(3) Allergic reactions

e. Fetal or neonatal demise: rare
(1) Perioperative fetal or neonatal demise is generally a result of the underlying condition necessitating operative delivery.

f. Neonatal depression
(1) Preexisting uteroplacental insufficiencies
(2) Prolonged uterine incision to delivery time
(3) Systemically administered analgesics during labor
(4) Rarely caused by placental transfer of general anesthetics unless skin incision to delivery time is prolonged

Induction

1. Sodium thiopental (3 to 5 mg/kg)
   a. Long history of safety; relatively contraindicated in hypovolemic patients
   b. Rarely a source of neonatal depression because of rapid redistribution and dilution by the fetal circulation
2. Ketamine (1 to 2 mg/kg)
   a. Sympathetic nervous system stimulation makes ketamine ideal in cases of maternal hypovolemia or reactive airway disease.
   b. Ketamine is relatively contraindicated in cases of maternal hypertension and cocaine intoxication.
   c. Minimal neonatal depression occurs.
3. Etomidate (0.2 to 0.3 mg/kg)
   a. Useful for stable cardiovascular induction
   b. Suppression of maternal and neonatal cortisol secretion; clinical significance unknown
4. Propofol (1 to 2 mg/kg)
   a. Obstetric information lacking
   b. Unclear whether it offers any advantages over sodium thiopental
5. Neurolept anesthesia (droperidol or fentanyl)
   a. Rarely used; significant neonatal depression, high incidence of maternal dysphoria
6. Narcotic and benzodiazepine inductions
   a. Rarely used; significant neonatal depression
   b. Useful for parturients who require hemodynamically stable induction
7. "Combined" induction (sodium thiopental [1 to 2 mg/kg] and ketamine [0.5 to 0.7 mg/kg])
   a. May represent ideal induction agent in patients whose vital signs are stable but whose hemodynamic status is uncertain
   b. Combines the benefits of both induction agents while minimizing adverse effects

Neuromuscular relaxing agents

1. Depolarizing muscle relaxant (succinylcholine)
   a. Rapid onset (30 to 45 seconds); relaxant of choice in rapid sequence induction

   b. Highly polar; crosses placenta in clinically insignificant amounts
   c. Relative contraindications
      (1) Preexisting neuromuscular disease
      (2) History of spinal cord injuries
      (3) Burn patients
      (4) Hyperkalemia
2. Nondepolarizing muscle relaxants (rocuronium, mivacurium, vecuronium, atracurium)
   a. Less rapid onset and longer duration of action as compared with succinylcholine
   b. Inadequate reversal (may be cause of delayed emergence from general anesthesia)
   c. Highly polar; crosses placenta in clinically insignificant amounts
   d. Relatively similar risks and benefits profiles; choice of agent largely dependent on provider preference

Inhalational agents

1. Nitrous oxide
   a. Maternal effects
      (1) Analgesia at 50% inspired concentration
      (2) Does not interfere with uterine activity
   b. Fetal or neonatal effects
      (1) Neonatal depression: rare; treatment: ventilatory support with 100% O_2
2. Potent halogenated agents (halothane, isoflurane, enflurane, desflurane)
   a. Maternal effects
      (1) Dose-related smooth muscle, including uterine and relaxation
      (2) Decreases uterine activity but does not interfere with uterine response to oxytocics
      (3) Maternal sedation and amnesia (limit popularity of these agents)
   b. Fetal or neonatal effects
      (1) Neonatal depression: rare, usually only after prolonged exposure; treatment: ventilatory support with 100% O_2

Technique

1. Risks and benefits are discussed with patient and witnessed informed consent is obtained.
2. Aspiration prophylaxis
   a. 30 ml of nonparticulate antacid
   b. 10 mg metoclopramide, IV
   c. H2 blocker, IV
3. Appropriate monitors are placed in the operating room.
4. Preoxygenation (denitrogenation of the functional residual capacity)
   a. 3 to 5 minutes of 100% O_2 (tidal volume breathing)
   b. Four vital capacity breaths of 100% O_2
5. Surgical field is prepared and draped; surgeons prepared to operate.
6. Rapid sequence induction

   a. Cricoid pressure (maintained until endotracheal tube placement is confirmed)
   b. Intravenous induction
   c. Neuromuscular relaxation
7. Endotracheal intubation: In emergencies, the procedure may begin with induction; but, ideally, the procedure should not start until the airway is secured. In the event that the airway cannot be secured, but the surgery must proceed, mask inhalation anesthesia with the maintenance of cricoid pressure is the best option until the airway can be secured with additional interventions (e.g., fiberoptic bronchoscopy). An operative airway is indicated if mask ventilation cannot be established.
8. Maintenance anesthetic (predelivery)
   a. 50% nitrous oxide
   b. 0.3 to 0.5 maximal allowable concentration (MAC) of potent halogenated agent
9. Maintenance anesthetic (postdelivery)
   a. Increased nitrous oxide concentration
   b. Discontinuance of potent halogenated agent
   c. Intravenous amnestic or hypnotic agent as needed
   d. Additional muscle relaxant
   e. Opioid
10. Emergence or awake extubation

Anesthesia for operative delivery

1. General anesthesia
   a. Offers most rapid establishment of operating conditions
   b. Rarely contraindicated
2. Epidural anesthesia: establishment of dense motor and sensory block to T4 level
   a. Establishment of dense motor and sensory block to T4 segmental level using local anesthetic with or without opioids added.
   b. Extension with an *in situ* epidural catheter requires 5 to 10 minutes for operating conditions.
   c. *De novo* institution can require considerably longer than extension of preexisting epidural blockade.
   d. It is contraindicated in the following:
      (1) Acute maternal hypovolemia
      (2) Uterine rupture
      (3) Cord prolapse with fetal distress
      (4) Agonal fetal distress
3. Spinal anesthesia
   a. Establishment of dense motor and sensory block to T4 segmental level using local anesthetic with or without opioids added.
   b. Technically easy, rapid onset: Operating conditions can generally be established in 5 to 10 minutes.
   c. Technical ease, quicker onset allow *de novo* institution much more rapidly than epidural blockade.
   d. Contraindications are those of extension of preexisting epidural blockade.

4. Local infiltration
   a. Extremely rare
   b. Use 0.5% lidocaine
   c. Infiltrate
      (1) Intracutaneous (10 ml)
      (2) Subcutaneous (10 to 20 ml)
      (3) Intrarectus (40 to 50 ml)
      (4) Parietal peritoneum (5 to 10 ml)
      (5) Visceral peritoneum (10 ml)
      (6) Paracervical (5 to 10 ml, bilaterally)
   d. Disadvantages
      (1) Maternal distress
      (2) Potential for local anesthetic toxicity
      (3) Prolonged skin incision to delivery time
5. Anesthetic options
   a. Stat
      (1) Indications
         (a) Maternal hemorrhage
         (b) Ruptured uterus
         (c) Cord prolapse with fetal bradycardia
         (d) Agonal fetal distress, prolonged bradycardia, late decelerations without recovery of variability
      (2) Anesthesia (in order of preference)
         (a) General anesthesia
         (b) Local infiltration (only in instances where general anesthesia is unavailable)
   b. Urgent
      (1) Indications
         (a) Dystocia
         (b) Failed forceps
         (c) Active genital herpes with rupture of membranes
         (d) Previous classical cesarean section and active labor
         (e) Cord prolapse without fetal distress
         (f) Variable decelerations with prompt recovery
         (g) Abnormal fetal presentation with ruptured membranes (in active labor)
      (2) Anesthesia (in order of preference)
         (a) Extension of preexisting epidural blockade
         (b) Spinal (NOTE: Provider should not persist if initial attempts at locating the subarachnoid space are unsuccessful)
         (c) General anesthesia
   c. Emergent
      (1) Indications
         (a) Chronic uteroplacental insufficiency
         (b) Abnormal fetal presentation with ruptured membranes (not in active labor)
         (c) Deteriorating maternal illness
      (2) Anesthesia (in order of preference)
         (a) Spinal or epidural
         (b) General anesthesia

d. Elective
    (1) Anesthesia (in order of preference)
        (a) Spinal or epidural
        (b) General anesthesia

Controversies in obstetric anesthesia

1. Effect of the progress of labor
    a. Early onset of severe pain is associated with a higher incidence of operative and instrumented vaginal delivery and a higher likelihood of receiving neuraxial analgesia.
    b. Continuous epidural anesthesia is associated with an increased incidence of operative and instrumented vaginal delivery.
    c. Continuous epidural anesthesia has not been shown to cause an increased incidence of operative and instrumented vaginal delivery.
    d. Continuous epidural anesthesia is associated with prolonged first and second stages of labor.
    e. Local anesthetic may play a role in prolonging first and second stages of labor.
    f. Dense perineal motor block is associated with an increased incidence of fetal malrotation or instrumented delivery.
    g. Continuous epidural analgesia does not cause failure of maternal expulsive efforts unless dense motor block to T4 segmental level is achieved.
    h. Withholding analgesia because of concerns about its effect on labor is *never* warranted.
2. Effect on uteroplacental perfusion
    a. In the absence of systemic hypotension, neuraxial analgesia has no effect on uteroplacental perfusion and may offer improved flow through uterine artery vasodilation.
3. Back pain
    a. Incidence is 40% to 60%.
    b. Presence or absence of neuraxial anesthesia has no effect on the incidence or severity of postpartum back pain.
    c. Factors associated with postpartum back pain include the following:
        (1) History of pregestational or gestational back pain
        (2) Short stature
        (3) Maternal obesity
        (4) Difficult or prolonged labor
4. Neonatal effects
    a. In the absence of hypotension, neuraxial anesthesia has no effect on the neonate.
    b. General anesthesia can result in significant neonatal depression if skin incision to delivery time is prolonged.
    c. One-minute Apgar scores are highest with neuraxial anesthesia. Five-minute scores are similar for general and neuraxial anesthesia.
5. Neurologic injury
    a. Permanent neurologic injury from neuraxial anesthesia is rare.
    b. Sacral neuropraxia secondary to birth trauma is the leading cause of postpartum neurologic deficit.

Anesthesia for nonobstetric surgery during pregnancy

1. General principles
   a. The surgical disease and maternal perioperative complications pose the greatest risk to the fetus.
   b. Physiologic changes of pregnancy increase maternal risk for anesthetic complications, most notably airway complications.
   c. Surgery and anesthesia do not increase the risk of congenital abnormalities. No anesthetic is a proven teratogen (use of nitrous oxide is controversial because it has been shown to be teratogenic is some animals when given in excessive, nonclinical doses).
   d. No anesthetic or anesthetic technique has shown a difference relative to maternal and fetal or neonatal outcome.
   e. Surgical disease or operative treatment located in or near the uterus will have an associated increased incidence of preterm labor or spontaneous abortion.
2. Anesthetic goals
   a. Avoidance of hypoxemia, hypercarbia, hypocarbia, hypertension, hypotension, and other exremes of physiologic changes associated with surgery
   b. Prevention of preterm labor

Lactation and maternally administered drugs

1. General principles
   a. Almost all drugs can be detected in breast milk.
   b. Almost all drugs are detected in clinically insignificant amounts.
   c. Physiologic status (e.g., prematurity) may decrease the dose required for clinical effect.
2. Breast-feeding is contraindicated with the following:
   a. Lithium
   b. Ergotamine preparations (Use of ergotamine preparations in the treatment of uterine atony does not contraindicate breast-feeding.)
3. Breast-feeding is relatively contraindicated with the following:
   a. Psychotropic drugs
      (1) Anxiolytics
      (2) Antidepressants
      (3) Antipsychotics
   b. Metronidazole
4. Drugs compatible with breast-feeding are as follows:
   a. Opioids
   b. Sedatives
   c. Anticonvulsants
   d. Antihistamines
   e. Cimetidine
   f. Corticosteroids
   g. Antibiotics
   h. Phenothiazines
   i. Aminophylline
   j. Amphetamines
   k. Antihypertensives
   l. Digoxin
   m. Antibiotics
   n. Caffeine

Suggested reading

1. Chestnut DJ: *Obstetric anesthesia: principles and practice,* St Louis, 1994, Mosby.
2. Shnider SM: *Anesthesia for obstetrics,* ed 3, Baltimore, 1993, Williams & Wilkins.

3. Stoelting RK: *Pharmacology and Physiology in anesthetic practice,* ed 2, Philadelphia, 1991, JB Lippincott.

22.2 HIGH-RISK OBSTETRIC ANESTHESIA

Mushtaque Juneja, M.D.

Parturients are considered to be high risk to the anesthesiologist if they have a preexisting medical condition, obstetric complication, a problem that can potentially necessitate an emergent cesarean section, or a potential uncertainty regarding anesthetic management. It is important to understand the pathophysiology of anesthetic management which is outlined here.

1. Disorders related to pregnancy
   a. Preeclampsia
   b. Hemorrhage
      (1) Placenta previa
      (2) Placenta accreta
      (3) Abruptio placenta
2. Problems unrelated to pregnancy
   a. Diabetes mellitus
   b. Cardiac disorders
   c. Respiratory disorders
   d. Neurologic disorders
   e. Renal disorders
   f. Hematologic disorders
   g. Endocrinologic disorders
3. Fetal conditions
   a. Prematurity
   b. Fetal distress
4. Morbid obesity
5. Difficult airway

Preeclampsia and eclampsia

Anesthetic considerations in preeclampsia are related to drug interactions. Magnesium sulfate interacts with both depolarizing and nondepolarizing neuromuscular blocking drugs.

1. Analgesia for vaginal delivery
   a. Epidural analgesia is the preferred method if there is no coagulation abnormality.
   b. Epidural analgesia offers several advantages, including the following:
      (1) Helps with blood pressure management
      (2) Increases uteroplacental perfusion by decreasing endogenous catecholamines
      (3) Allows a rapid route for cesarean section, if necessary, without the use of general anesthesia
      (4) Maintains epidural block at T10 level for labor pain
      (5) Ensures left uterine displacement (LUD)
      (6) Treats hypotension: decrease in systolic blood pressure >25%, <100 mm Hg, or causing deleterious change in fetal heart rate

2. Anesthesia for cesarean section
   a. Epidural: If epidural is in place, the sensory block level should be gradually increased to T4.
   b. Points to consider
      (1) Epinephrine-containing local anesthetics should be avoided.
      (2) Central line should be considered before initiation of epidural if volume status is in question.
      (3) Ephedrine should be used in small incremental doses to treat hypotension.
   c. Subarachnoid block
      (1) May be used in less severe preeclamptics
      (2) 0.75% hyperberic bupivacaine (12 to 15 mg)
3. General anesthesia
   Indications
   a. Epidural contraindicated (coagulopathy, hypovolemia, septicemia, etc.)
   b. Maternal refusal of other means
   c. Very severe fetal distress
4. Problems of general anesthesia in preeclampsia
   a. Upper airway edema
      (1) Thorough evaluation is required before induction.
      (2) Small endotracheal tube is used.
      (3) Intubation is difficult and traumatic.
      (4) Nasal airways and suction must be avoided.
   b. The need to blunt the severe hypertensive response associated with laryngoscopy, intubation, and emergence
      (1) Techniques to modify response include the following:
         (a) Adequate induction dose of thiopentone, 4 mg/kg
         (b) Intravenous lidocaine, 1.5 mg/kg
5. Antihypertensives on induction and emergence
   a. Hydralazine
   b. Nitroprusside
   c. Labetalol
   d. Trimethaphan
   e. Nitroglycerin
6. Two thirds MAC potent inhalation drug throughout surgery
7. Other considerations with general anesthesia
   a. Need for LUD until delivery
   b. Need to avoid hyperventilation: monitor $ETCO_2$
   c. Pulmonary aspiration on induction and emergence
      (1) Use of clear antacids, metoclopramide and H2 blockers
      (2) Requires a rapid sequence induction and cricoid pressure

Antepartum hemorrhage

1. Placenta previa
   a. Actively bleeding or major blood loss: General endotracheal anesthesia
      (1) Get help, second IV placement.
      (2) Fluid administration (via rapid infusion device with warmer, if available)

(3) Rapid sequence induction: Consider ketamine, 1 mg/kg.

b. No active hemorrhage, hemodynamic stable

(1) If no hypovolemia, epidural or spinal anesthesia may be used.

2. Placenta accreta
   a. Placenta previa in a patient for a repeat cesarean section may be associated with placenta accreta; these patients should be treated as though major blood loss will occur.
   b. Two intravenous lines should be placed, blood should be available, and the patient should be made aware that a cesarean hysterectomy may become necessary and that general anesthesia may be used to provide appropriate operating conditions and to protect her airway in the event of massive hemorrhage and cesarean hysterectomy.
   c. In an elective repeat cesarean section in a patient with a placenta previa, regional anesthesia may be used and, if hemodynamics remain stable, may be continued even if a cesarean hysterectomy is performed.
3. Abruptio placenta
   a. Actively bleeding or major blood loss: general endotracheal anesthesia as in a placenta previa
   b. No active hemorrhage: Regional anesthesia can be initiated if the following occur:
      (1) There is no evidence of maternal hypovolemia.
      (2) Clotting studies are within normal limits.

Diabetes mellitus

Figs. 22-1 and 22-2 show the effects of diabetes mellitus.

Anesthetic considerations

1. For labor and vaginal delivery, small doses of narcotics will provide moderate pain relief.
2. Lumbar epidural block can provide excellent pain relief both for labor and delivery.
3. A separate intravenous line should be used for the rapid infusion of solutions not containing dextrose if necessary to treat hypotension without producing hyperglycemia.

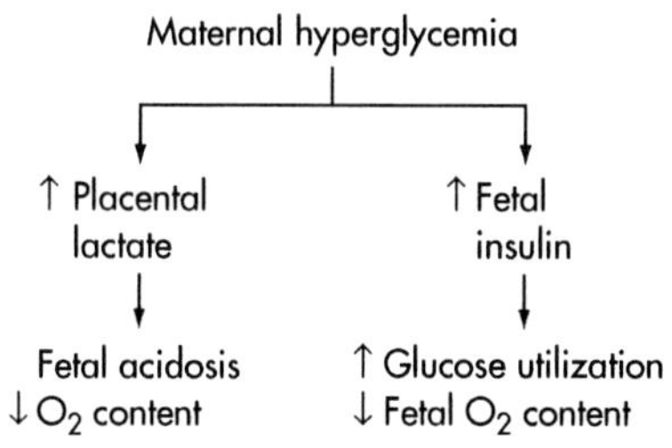

Figure 22-1

Maternal hyperglycemia contributes to fetal acidosis and reduced fetal oxygen (O_2) content.

Maternal hyperglycemia

↓

$\uparrow$ Fetal insulin
$\uparrow$ Fetal glucose

↓

Delivery

↓

Persistent $\uparrow$insulin in neonate
Loss of maternal glucose source

↓

Neonatal hypoglycemia

Figure 22-2
Maternal hyperglycemia results in neonatal hypoglycemia.

4. The following criteria should be considered in the use of anesthesia for cesarean delivery in diabetic parturients:
   a. Acute hydration by nondextrose solution before induction of anesthesia. A separate intravenous line should be used for this purpose.
   b. Routine LUD starting from induction of anesthesia until the delivery of the baby.
   c. Prompt treatment of hypotension with intravenous ephedrine (increments of 5 mg).
   d. Amide local anesthetics with long fetal or neonatal half-life (e.g., mepivacaine) should be avoided in these cases.
   e. Well-conducted general anesthesia can be used if necessary with good neonatal outcome.

Anesthetic considerations for patients with cardiac disease

The prevalence of heart disease during pregnancy ranges from 0.4% to 4.1%. A patient with severe valvular disease requires a team approach involving the anesthesiologist, the obstetrician, and nursing and cardiology personnel.

1. Maternal monitoring
   a. A parturient with heart disease warrants continuous monitoring during labor and delivery.
      (1) New York Heart Association class I or II may not require invasive monitoring.
      (2) Class III or IV may need invasive monitoring.
   b. Central venous pressure (CVP) may help on fluid management.
   c. Pulmonary artery catheter may be required in severe cases for better assessment of left ventricular (LV) filling pressure.
   d. Risk of thromboembolism is increased in the cardiac patient and the

use of elastic stockings or other mechanical device should be considered.

2. General considerations
   a. Regional anesthetic technique should be used unless contraindicated.
   b. All parturients must receive nonparticulate antacid.
   c. For general anesthesia (GA), preoxygenation, rapid sequence induction, cricoid pressure, and cuffed endotracheal (ET) tube must be used.
   d. Continuous monitoring of pulse oximetry and capnography are essential.
   e. Patients are positioned with LUD to optimize uterine blood flow and increase venous return.

Mitral valve prolapse (MVP)

1. MVP is a common finding in women.
   a. Sympathetic stimulation should be minimized.
   b. Regional anesthetic technique is preferable.
   c. Use of epinephrine-containing solutions should be avoided if history of palpitation.
   d. Antibiotic prophylaxis before procedure may prevent bacteremia.
   e. If GA, ketamine and pancuronium should be avoided.
   f. If vasopressors are needed and MVP is severe, phenylephrine, rather than ephedrine, should be used.
2. Mitral stenosis: anesthetic considerations
   a. Prevention of rapid ventricular rates
   b. Minimization of increases in central blood volume
   c. Avoidance of marked decreases in systemic vascular resistance
   d. Prevention of increases in pulmonary artery pressure
      (1) Digoxin may be required to control atrial fibrillation (AF).
      (2) Rapid AF dramatically reduces cardiac output and produces pulmonary edema.
      (3) Marked increases in central blood volume are poorly tolerated.
         (a) Overtransfusion, Trendelenburg position, or autotransfusion via uterine contraction can precipitate right ventricular failure, pulmonary hypertension, pulmonary edema, or AF.
         (b) Increases in CVP or pulmonary capillary wedge (PCW) pressure may be used to assess increases in central blood volume.
      (4) Marked decreases in systemic vascular resistance may not be tolerated.
         (a) With severe stenosis, decreases in systemic vascular resistance are compensated by increases in heart rate (stroke volume is fixed).
         (b) This response is limited, and marked increases in heart rate may lead to decompensation.
         (c) If necessary, systemic vascular resistance may be maintained with an intravenous infusion of metaraminol (10 mg in 250 ml of saline).
         (d) Because ephedrine may increase heart rate, it is not recommended.

(5) Exacerbation of pulmonary hypertension and right ventricular failure can be precipitated by multiple factors.
   (a) Any degree of hypercarbia, hypoxia, acidosis, lung hyperinflation, or increased lung water can elevate pulmonary vascular resistance.
   (b) Prostaglandins to treat uterine atony should be used with caution because they may have effects on the pulmonary vasculature.
(6) Segmental lumbar epidural is the preferred anesthetic.

3. Mitral insufficiency: anesthetic considerations
   a. Prevention of peripheral vasoconstriction
   b. Avoidance of myocardial depressants
   c. Immediate treatment of acute atrial fibrillation
   d. Maintenance of a normal or slightly elevated heart rate
   e. Monitoring of PCW pressure and intensity of murmur
   f. Labor and vaginal delivery: lumbar epidural analgesia recommended to prevent the peripheral vasoconstriction associated with the pain of labor and to increase the forward flow of blood
   g. Constant LUD and a 10° Trendelenburg position: used to maintain venous return (The positive inotropic and chronotropic effects of ephedrine are especially useful in preventing and treating hypotension.)
4. Aortic insufficiency: anesthetic considerations
   a. Avoidance of marked increases in systemic vascular resistance
   b. Maintenance of a normal or slightly elevated heart rate
   c. Avoidance of myocardial depressants
   d. Monitoring of arterial diastolic pressure, PCW pressure, and intensity of murmur
      (1) Continuous lumbar epidural analgesia prevents peripheral vasoconstriction and is recommended for vaginal delivery.
5. Aortic stenosis: anesthetic considerations
   a. Avoidance of decreases in systemic vascular resistance
   b. Avoidance of bradycardia
   c. Maintenance of venous return and left ventricular filling
   d. Sympathetic blockade: should be avoided when possible; if regional anesthesia is necessary, a gradually administered continuous epidural technique is indicated (Because hypotension is poorly tolerated, maternal blood pressure should be sustained with LUD, fluids, and metaraminol or ephedrine.)
6. Congenital heart lesions
   a. Hypotension will reverse the left to right shunt. For this reason, high spinal anesthesia should always be avoided.
   b. Epidural anesthesia using proper invasive cardiovascular monitoring can be used for labor and delivery. This will be beneficial for complete relief of pain and abolition of bearing down efforts, which might further increase the right atrial, right ventricular, and pulmonary pressures.
   c. Combination of systemic analgesics and tranquilizers during the early first stage, and bilateral pudendal block during delivery.
   d. Regional anesthesia is contraindicated if the patients receive anticoagulants for any reason.

e. A dilute oxytocin solution should be infused to prevent postpartum uterine relaxation and needless blood loss.
   (1) Bolus intravenous injection of oxytocin may cause serious hypotension, whereas intramuscular ergonovine preparations may produce severe peripheral vasoconstriction followed by hypertension.
   (2) Both these drugs should be used carefully during this situation.

Anesthesia for the pregnant patient with asthma

1. Drugs to avoid in pregnancy complicated by asthma

Aspirin	Tartrazine dyes
Iodine-containing preparations	Tetracycline
Hydroxyzine	Prostaglandin $F_{2\alpha}$
Brompheniramine maleate	β-Blockers

2. Anesthetic considerations
   a. Regional anesthesia is recommended for labor and delivery and a cesarean section if necessary.
   b. Ketamine is recommended over thiopental for induction of general anesthesia because of its beneficial effects on airway resistance if not contraindicated.
   c. The administration of 1 to 2 mg/kg of lidocaine, IV, before extubation of the trachea may prevent bronchospasm on extubation.
   d. The ET should not be removed until the patient has regained laryngeal and pharyngeal reflexes. A lidocaine infusion of 2 mg/kg/hr may be of benefit in attenuating airway stimulation until the patient can be extubated.
3. Causes of wheezing during general anesthesia
   a. Bronchial asthma
   b. Mechanical obstruction of the ET
   c. Inadequate anesthesia for the surgical stimulation, resulting in active expiratory efforts
   d. Inadequate neuromuscular blockade
   e. Endobronchial intubation
   f. Overinflation of the ET cuff
   g. Pulmonary edema
   h. Aspiration of gastric contents
   i. Anaphylactic or anaphylactoid reaction
   j. Amniotic fluid embolism
   k. Pneumothorax
4. Management of acute asthmatic attack during pregnancy
   a. Initial therapy
      (1) Supplemental oxygen
      (2) Inhaled bronchodilator (i.e., isoetharine, 0.5 ml in 2.5 ml saline, or metaproterenol, 0.3 ml in 2.5 ml saline) or subcutaneous injection of β-agonist (i.e., 0.3 ml of 1:1000 epinephrine or 0.25 mg terbutaline sulfate); repeat, if needed
      (3) Initial laboratory examinations (i.e., arterial blood gas [ABG], complete blood count, [CBC], spirometry as therapy is begun)
   b. If no improvement, add the following:
      (1) Intravenous hydration
      (2) Intravenous aminophylline

(a) Loading dose
i. No prior theophylline: 5.6 mg/kg lean body weight over 20 min (400 mg maximum)
ii. Previous inadequate theophylline: 2.5 mg/kg lean body weight over 20 min (400 mg maximum)
iii. Previous adequate theophylline: no loading dose
(b) Then, continuous infusion
i. 0.5 mg/kg/hr: normal
ii. 0.7 mg/kg/hr: smokers, teenagers
iii. 0.3 mg/kg/hr: coexisting heart disease, liver disease, or cimetidine therapy
(3) Intravenous corticosteroid therapy
(a) Cortisol sodium succinate (Solu-Cortef), 100 to 200 mg, q2h to q6h or
(b) Methyl prednisolone sodium succinate (Solu-Medrol), 40 mg, q2h to q6h

Neurologic problems

Uncommon during the childbearing age. Possible causes are as follows:

1. Infectious disease
   a. Regional anesthesia is absolutely contraindicated in the presence of an active inflammatory disease in the spinal canal: acute meningitis or superficial infection at the site of the lumbar puncture.
   b. However, regional anesthesia is not contraindicated in old inflammatory problems (i.e., parturient with history of poliomyelitis).
2. Paralysis
   a. With spinal cord lesions above T7, one must observe for autonomic hyperreflexia.
   b. Bradycardia, hypertension, and severe headaches may be observed.
   c. Contraction of a hollow viscus (i.e., uterus) can result in sympathetic nervous system stimulation.
   d. Lesions above T10 result in painless labor.
   e. Anesthetic considerations
      (1) Succinylcholine should be avoided if intubation is necessary.
      (2) A nondepolarizing muscle relaxant should be used for intubation.
      (3) Subarachnoid or epidural anesthesia may be used for cesarean section and vaginal delivery and may prevent autonomic hyperreflexia.
      (4) Treatment of autonomic hyperreflexia includes phentolamine, 2 to 5 mg IV (onset of 1 to 2 minutes with a duration of about 10 minutes) or sodium nitroprusside by intravenous infusion beginning at 0.1 mg/kg/min (immediate onset).
3. Cerebrovascular accidents
   a. Arterial or venous thrombosis is not common.
   b. Cerebral hemorrhage can be seen in association with severe eclampsia.
   c. Subarachnoid hemorrhage can occur during pregnancy because of a leaking aneurysm or arteriovenous malformation.

d. Cardiovascular stresses during pregnancy, labor, delivery, and the immediate postpartum period can precipitate subarachnoid hemorrhage.
e. Anesthetic management
   (1) For labor and delivery continuous epidural block is advisable.
   (2) The use of forceps is indicated to shorten the second stage.
   (3) In the immediate postpartum period, physicians should be prepared to treat hypertension aggressively if it occurs.
   (4) For cesarean delivery, epidural block is the choice of anesthesia; however, if there is fetal distress or if general anesthesia is indicated for some other reason, the anesthesiologist should be careful about the hypertensive response following endotracheal intubation, which can be blocked by intravenous lidocaine given before induction.

4. Multiple sclerosis
   a. Although the choice of anesthesia is controversial, epidural anesthesia can be used for vaginal delivery in such cases.
   b. Most experts do not recommend spinal block because of possible neurotoxicity from local anesthetic.
   c. If GA for cesarean section, use of succinylcholine should be avoided.
5. Space-occupying lesions (brain tumors)
   a. Spinal anesthesia may be relatively contraindicated because of reduction of CSF pressure, which, if it occurs rapidly, may produce cerebral herniation and sudden death.
   b. Some anesthesiologists may consider epidural or caudal anesthesia in such cases.
   c. However, the possibility of dural puncture and the sequelae secondary to the rapid decrease in CSF remains.
6. Epilepsy
   a. There is no evidence that epileptic patients are more susceptible to local anesthetics than the normal population.
   b. Spinal or epidural anesthesia are not contraindicated in such patients.
   c. For GA, drugs that have potential convulsive action should be avoided (i.e., enflurane, ketamine, etc.).
7. Myasthenia gravis
   a. Major problems
      (1) Chance of prolonged second stage because of muscle weakness
      (2) Postdelivery pulmonary complications because of respiratory muscle weakness
      (3) Possible complications during anesthesia
      (4) Possibility of neonatal myasthenia gravis
   b. Anesthesia management
      (1) For labor and delivery:
         (a) Segmental epidural block is used for pain relief.
         (b) If systemic narcotics used, the anesthesiologist should use a smaller dose.
         (c) The anesthesiologist should avoid ester-type local anesthetic in patients receiving anticholinesterase medications.

(d) The anesthesiologist should avoid aminoglycoside antibiotics and magnesium therapy.

(2) For cesarean section:

(a) Carefully titrated epidural anesthetic is better than high spinal.

(b) Epidural narcotics for postoperative pain relief.

(c) For GA, use succinylcholine for intubation and monitor neuromuscular block.

(d) May need postoperative ventilation.

Renal disorders

1. Major physiologic changes
   a. Effective renal plasma flow (RPF) and glomerular filtration rate (GFR) increase by 50% by 16 weeks gestation.
   b. The high RPF and GFR result in an increase in creatinine clearance.
   c. During normal pregnancy, the blood urea nitrogen (BUN) averages 8 to 9 mg/dl and creatinine 0.46 mg/dl. Therefore, during pregnancy, a "normal" nonpregnant BUN (10 to 20 mg/dl) and creatinine (0.51 to 2 mg/dl) may represent renal compromise.
   d. One of the most common disorders in pregnancy that involves kidney function is toxemia of pregnancy.
   e. Acute renal failure in pregnancy can occur in conjunction with hemorrhage, sepsis, or toxemia.
2. Anesthetic management
   a. Nephrotoxicity occasionally follows after using methoxyflurane and enflurane; therefore, these agents should be avoided in the presence of renal compromise.
   b. Spinal and epidural anesthesia do not sufficiently alter renal function unless there is significant hypotension.
   c. Ephedrine can maintain renal blood flow without affecting the uterine flow; it should be the vasopressor of choice if there is hypotension.

Sickle cell disease

Parturients with sickle cell trait usually have no problems during pregnancy; however women with sickle cell anemia (S/S) or sickle cell hemoglobin C (S/C) disease are poor obstetric risks. Their anemia becomes more severe during pregnancy and the incidence of toxemia is increased.

1. Anesthesia management: Hypoxia and hypotension must be prevented because of the increased chance of sickling.
2. For labor and delivery, if regional anesthesia is administered, it must be used cautiously. Oxygen should be administered throughout the procedure and aortocaval compression should be avoided.
3. Avoid the following:
   a. Hypoxia
   b. Cold
   c. Acidosis
   d. Dehydration
   e. Vasopressors

4. Adequate prehydration and slow onset of epidural block are essential.
5. Spinal should be avoided because it can cause hypotension and may need vasopressors. If vasopressor is essential, ephedrine should be used instead of phenylepheine.

Anesthetic considerations for the patient with thyroid disease

1. Hypothyroidism
   a. Patients with hypothyroidism may have a history of paresthesias and hoarseness. These patients can be sensitive to inhalational anesthetics, as well as narcotics and benzodiazepines.
2. Hyperthyroidism
   a. Tachycardia, elevated temperature, and increased blood pressure may occur under general anesthesia, making it difficult to assess anesthesia depth.
   b. Either epidural or spinal anesthesia is preferred for cesarean section.
   c. Ketamine should be avoided in the patient with hyperthyroid disease.
   d. If ephedrine must be used to treat hypotension following regional anesthesia, it should be given intravenously in 2.5-mg increments.

Prematurity

1. Prematurity is defined as birth occurring between 20 and 37 weeks of gestation. The incidence in the United States is approximately 7%, but it accounts for the majority of perinatal deaths.
2. Anesthetic implications
   a. Patients are often placed on tocolytic therapy, which may have profound maternal effects and interact with anesthetics.
      (1) Beta-adrenergic agents (Terbutaline, Ritodrine): tachycardia, hypotension, chest pain, myocardial ischemia, arrhythmias, pulmonary edema, anxiety, nausea or vomiting, hyperglycemia, hypokalemia
      (2) Magnesium sulfate: pulmonary edema, chest pain, nausea or vomiting, drowsiness, increased sensitivity to muscle relaxants
   b. Regional anesthesia may be used for labor analgesia in the patient who is delivering a premature infant.
      (1) It has the advantage of obviating the need for parenteral narcotics.
      (2) This is advantageous because the premature fetus may be more susceptible to the effects of these drugs.
      (3) It also decreases catecholamine levels, may improve uteroplacental blood flow, and gives a route for fast administration of a regional anesthetic should fetal distress occur and require a cesarean section.
      (4) By allowing the patient (and the obstetrician) more control, a labor epidural can prevent a precipitous delivery, which can have devastating effects on a premature infant.
      (5) Prior administration of a beta-sympathomimetic tocolytic agent is not a contraindication to a regional anesthetic.

c. Subarachnoid or epidural anesthesia may be used for cesarean section.
   (1) Administration of general anesthesia is the same as for the term parturient, except that the general anesthetics may depress the preterm infant more than the term infant.
   (2) Techniques, dosages, and choices or agents are the same as for the full-term parturient.
   (3) If general anesthesia is to be initiated shortly after discontinuation of a beta-sympathomimetic tocolytic, drugs that cause maternal tachycardia (atropine, glycopyrolate, pancuronium) should be avoided.

Fetal distress (nonreassuring fetal heart rate pattern)

The American College of Obstetricians and Gynecologists (ACOG) has issued a committee opinion entitled "Anesthesia for Emergency Deliveries." They suggest the following:

1. Failed intubation and pulmonary aspiration remain prominent causes of maternal morbidity and mortality from anesthesia.
2. The obstetric care team should be alert to the presence of risk factors that place the parturient at increased risk for complications from emergency general or regional anesthesia.
3. When risk factors are identified, the obstetrician should obtain an antepartum anesthesia consultation.
4. Strategies should be developed to help minimize the need for emergency induction of general anesthesia. Such strategies might include early placement of an epidural.
5. "Although there are some situations in which general anesthesia is preferable to regional anesthesia, the risk of general anesthesia must be weighed against the benefit for those patients who have a greater potential for complications."

Anesthetic considerations for the morbidly obese patient

1. Epidural analgesia decreases respiratory work and oxygen consumption.
2. Oxygen should be administered throughout labor because of increased oxygen consumption.
3. Technical difficulties may be encountered when performing regional anesthesia because of fat over the spinous processes. Special long needles may be necessary.
4. The sitting position may provide the anesthetist with the easiest identification of the midline.
5. The volume of anesthetic needed for spinal anesthesia may be less. It is controversial whether or not decreased volume is needed for epidural anesthesia.
6. Aortocaval compression must be avoided.
7. Histamine H2-receptor antagonists should be administered before surgery.
8. Metoclopramide (10 mg, IV) may be of benefit.

9. All patients should receive 30 ml of 0.3 *M* sodium citrate.
10. Obese patients can have laryngeal edema. Therefore, a smaller diameter (6.5 mm) ET should be prepared if GA is anticipated.
11. A short-handled laryngoscope blade may make intubation easier if GA is necessary.
12. Postoperative analgesia is helpful to encourage deep breathing as well as atelectasis. Epidural narcotics may be administered.
13. A massive panniculus can make intubation potentially difficult. The panniculus may be taped to the ether screen.

The difficult airway

1. Failed intubation remains a major problem facing the obstetric anesthesiologist.
2. Studies have shown that failed intubations occur more commonly in obstetric patients than in the nonpregnant patient.
3. Difficult intubation in obstetrics may be caused by the following:
   a. Increased weight
   b. Increased breast size
   c. Easy bleeding of oral cavity
   d. Pharyngeal or laryngeal edema
4. In addition, the use of cricoid pressure to minimize aspiration risk may make visualization more difficult.
5. To minimize difficult intubations in the obstetric patient, the following should be done:
   a. A preoperative airway examination should always be performed.
   b. The patient should be placed in the sniffing position. A wedge can be placed to achieve LUD.
   c. The patient should be preoxygenated to ensure appropriate denitrogenation.
   d. A trained assistant should administer cricoid pressure.
   e. A small ET tube with a stylet should be used even if the anesthesiologist does not think it is necessary. The first attempt is the best chance!
   f. Laryngoscopy should not be initiated until the patient is relaxed.
   g. ET tube position should be confirmed with $ETCO_2$ monitoring and auscultation before the surgeon begins.
   h. Algorithm and equipment should be readily available for failed intubation.
6. Management of the failed intubation in the pregnant patient includes the following steps:
   a. Call for help
   b. Maintenance of cricoid pressure
   c. Communication with obstetrician; determination whether surgery can be delayed (i.e., fetal distress or no fetal distress)
   d. Ventilation with 100% O_2
      (1) If surgery can be delayed the following is done:
         (a) The patient is ventilated with 100% O_2 until she awakens.
         (b) A regional anesthetic or an awake fiberoptic intubation is performed.

(2) If surgery cannot be delayed the following is done:
   (a) Cricoid pressure is maintained throughout.
   (b) Oxygen and a volatile agent are used to ventilate.
   (c) If any difficulty occurs with ventilation, laryngeal mask airway should be considered.
   (d) In the event of a lost airway and inability to use LMA or combitube, placement of an intravenous cannula through the cricothyroid membrane to administer transtracheal oxygenation and ventilation should be considered.

Suggested reading

Chestnut DJ: *Obstetric anesthesia: principles and practice,* St Louis, 1994, Mosby.
Shnider SM: *Anesthesia for obstetrics,* ed 3, Baltimore, 1993, Williams & Wilkins.
Stoelting RK: *Pharmacology and physiology in anesthetic practice,* ed 2, Philadelphia, 1991, JB Lippincott.

High-Risk Obstetrics

23

23.1 DIABETES IN PREGNANCY

Bruce D. Rodgers, M.D

Classification of diabetes mellitus

1. Type I
   a. Accounts for 10% of all cases of diabetes
   b. Inadequate pancreatic insulin secretion
   c. Autoimmune destruction of pancreatic beta cells
   d. Body habitus thin
   e. Usually diagnosed <30 years of age
   f. Patients usually symptomatic
   g. Strong predisposition to ketosis and ketoacidosis
   h. Some familial predisposition (common HLA haplotypes)
   i. Therapeutic principles
      (1) Diet
      (2) Insulin
2. Type II
   a. Accounts for 90% of all cases of diabetes
   b. Heterogenous causes (one or more of the following):
      (1) Subnormal beta-cell function
      (2) Insulin resistance in muscle and adipose tissue
      (3) Increased hepatic production of glucose
   c. Body habitus usually obese
   d. Usually presents >30 years of age
   e. Patients often asymptomatic and undiagnosed
   f. Little predisposition to ketosis
   g. Strong familial predisposition
   h. Often accompanied by hypertension and hyperlipidemia
   i. Therapeutic principles (one or combination of the following):
      (1) Diet
      (2) Weight loss
      (3) Oral antidiabetic drugs
      (4) Insulin
3. Other type of diabetes
   a. Associated with other conditions or syndromes
   b. Rare cause of diabetes

4. Impaired glucose intolerance
   a. Higher than normal plasma glucose levels
   b. Glucose levels not diagnostic of diabetes
5. Gestational diabetes
   a. Onset or discovery of glucose intolerance during pregnancy
   b. May include preconceptionally undiagnosed overt diabetes

Classification of diabetes during pregnancy

1. White classification of diabetes in pregnancy (Table 23-1)
   a. Basis of classification
      (1) Age of onset
      (2) Duration of diabetes
      (3) Presence of vascular disease
   b. Largely of historical interest
   c. Still used as a descriptive tool in clinical practice
2. A more clinically relevant classification scheme is as follows:
   a. Type I pregestational diabetes
   b. Type II pregestational diabetes
   c. Pregestational diabetes with vascular disease
      (1) Nephropathy
      (2) Retinopathy; background, proliferative
      (3) Arteriosclerotic heart disease
      (4) Renal transplant
      (5) Hypertension
   d. Gestational diabetes
      (1) Diet controlled
      (2) Insulin required

Gestational diabetes

1. Risk factors for glucose intolerance in pregnancy (see the box on p. 457)
   a. Risk of gestational diabetes is increased.
   b. Risk that pregestational glucose intolerance present is increased.
   c. Of patients with gestational diabetes, 50% have no risk factors.
   d. Universal screening should be undertaken on all pregnant women.
2. Screening (Fig. 23-1)
   a. All patients between 24 and 28 weeks
   b. Significant risk factors: First trimester, 24 to 28 weeks, 32 weeks
3. Diagnosis
   a. Based on 3-hour oral glucose tolerance test (OGTT) (Table 23-2)
   b. National Diabetes Data Group (NDDG) criteria
      (1) Criterion modified from original O'Sullivan criteria.
      (2) Modification based on plasma glucose measurements.
   c. Carpenter and Coustan criteria (modified)
      (1) Also adjusts for inaccuracy of older laboratory technique for measuring glucose
      (2) Cutoffs lower then NDDG criteria
      (3) More sensitive for diagnosis of gestational diabetes
   d. Positive test: two or more values ≥ cutoff values
   e. Borderline test: 1 value ≥ cutoff value
      (1) Retest in several weeks, *or*
      (2) Treat as gestational diabetes

Table 23-1 White classification of diabetes in pregnancy

Class	Description
A1	Gestational diabetes, diet controlled
A2	Gestational diabetes, requiring insulin
B	Age of onset ≤20 yr, *or* duration <10 yr
C	Age of onset 10-19 yr, *or* duration >10-19 yr
D	Age of onset <10 yr *or* duration ≥20 yr
F	Nephropathy
R	Proliferative retinopathy
H	Arteriosclerotic heart disease
T	Postrenal transplantation

Risk Factors for Gestational Diabetes

Obesity
Age >30 years
Family history; first-degree relative with type II diabetes
Previous baby >4000 g (8 lb, 10 oz)
Previous baby with congenital anomaly(ies)
Previous fetal or neonatal death
Hypertension
Excessive weight gain in index pregnancy
Fasting glycosuria in index pregnancy
Hydramnios in index pregnancy
Suspected macrosomia in index pregnancy
Somatic disproportion on ultrasound in index pregnancy
Previous pregnancy with gestational diabetes
History of pregestational impaired glucose tolerance

4. Goals of treatment
   a. Attenuation and prevention of fetal hyperinsulinemia
   b. Prevention of macrosomia
   c. Prevention of fetal or neonatal birth trauma
   d. Reduction of need for cesarean section
   e. Prevention of neonatal complications
   f. Prevention of long-term complications
      (1) Childhood obesity
      (2) Type II diabetes in offspring
   g. Prevention of stillbirth
5. Risk
   a. Most common
      (1) Macrosomia
      (2) Shoulder dystocia
      (3) Neonatal hypoglycemia

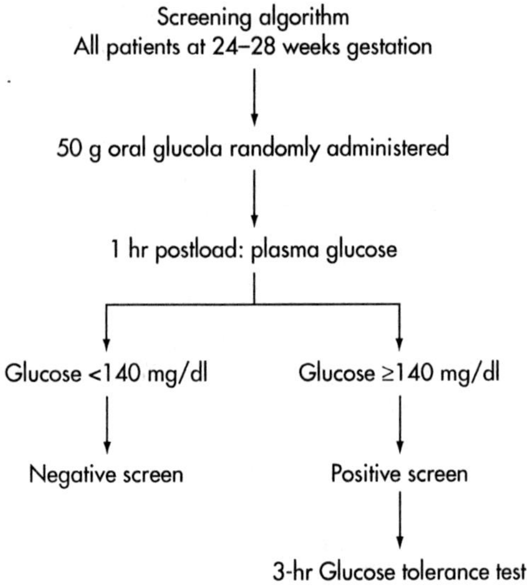

Figure 23-1
GCT: 50-g, 1-hour glucose challenge test.

Table 23-2 Three hour glucose tolerance test criteria (plasma glucose values; mg/dl)

Time	NDDG Criteria	Modified Criteria
Fasting	≥105	≥95
1 hour	≥190	≥180
2 hour	≥165	≥155
3 hour	≥145	≥140

b. Less common
  (1) Intrapartum hypoxia or acidosis
  (2) Intrauterine fetal death
c. High-risk gestational diabetes (see the box on p. 459)
  (1) Ten percent to 20% of gestational diabetes are high-risk.
  (2) High-risk gestational diabetes may include patients with undiagnosed pregestational diabetes.
  (3) Risk may be similar to pregestational diabetes in some cases.

6. Treatment
  a. Maternal glycemic control
    (1) Diet
    (2) Selective insulin therapy

High-Risk Gestational Diabetes
Maternal age >35 years
Hypertension
Previous intrauterine fetal death
Noncompliance
Poor glucose control
Macrosomia
Diabetic fetopathy
Hydramnios
Therapeutic insulin therapy
Insulin dose >100 U/day

b. Fetal surveillance
   (1) Optional in low-risk gestational diabetes
   (2) Mandatory in high-risk gestational diabetes
c. Elective delivery in select high-risk gestational diabetes
d. Selective delivery by primary cesarean section
e. Expert management of shoulder dystocia

Pregestational diabetes

1. Differs from gestational diabetes
   a. Complexity of medical management
   b. Maternal risk
      (1) Hypoglycemia
      (2) Diabetic ketoacidosis
      (3) Infection
      (4) Poor wound healing
   c. Diversity and level of perinatal risk
   d. Risk of congenital anomalies
2. May require team approach
   a. Maternal–fetal medicine specialist
   b. Diabetic teaching nurse
   c. Medical endocrinologist
   d. Nephrologist
   e. Ophthalmologist
3. Goals of management
   a. Preconception counseling and diabetes management
   b. Establishment of the extent of maternal disease
   c. Establishment of pregnancy viability and gestational age
   d. Detection of congenital anomalies
   e. Prevention and treatment of preterm labor
   f. Prevention and treatment of fetal growth aberrancy
   g. Establishment of euglycemia

h. Prevention of intrauterine fetal death (IUFD)
i. Prevention of intrapartum asphyxia
j. Prevention of fetal and maternal birth trauma
k. Prevention and treatment of neonatal complications

Preconception counseling and diabetes management

1. Establishment of extent of maternal disease and submission for treatment
   a. Presence of microvascular and macrovascular disease
      (1) Nephropathy
      (2) Retinopathy
      (3) Coronary artery disease
   b. Neuropathy
   c. Gastroenteropathy
   d. Hypertension
2. Contraceptive counseling
3. Establish periconception glucose control
   a. May reduce fetal anomaly risk
   b. May reduce first-trimester pregnancy loss
   c. Pregnancy standards of glucose control
      (1) Insulin therapy
      (2) American Diabetes Association (ADA) diet
      (3) Risk of first-trimester hypoglycemia

Establishment of the extent of maternal disease

1. Formal eye ground examination
   a. No retinopathy; examination repeated if clinically indicated.
   b. Background retinopathy; examination repeated each trimester.
   c. Proliferative retinopathy:
      (1) Referral for treatment
      (2) Frequent examinations
      (3) May progress during pregnancy
   d. Macular edema; referral for treatment.
2. 24-Hour urine collection
   a. Creatinine clearance
   b. Total protein excretion
      (1) >300 mg: suspect nephropathy
      (2) >500 mg: nephropathy present
3. Hypoglycemia unawareness
   a. Unawareness poses a significant risk for hypoglycemia and insulin coma.
   b. Hypoglycemia is common in long-standing type I insulin-dependent diabetes mellitus (IDDM).
   c. Patient should not live alone.
   d. Family members should be trained to do the following:
      (1) Recognize symptoms of hypoglycemia
      (2) Treat hypoglycemia
      (3) Administer glucagon
   e. Avoid excessively rigid glucose control.

4. Hypertension
   a. Medications
      (1) Angiotensin-converting enzyme (ACE) inhibitors should be discontinued.
      (2) Beta-blockers should be avoided.
      (3) Alpha-methyldopa, nifedipine, labetalol may be used.
   b. Consider preeclampsia prophylaxis
      (1) Calcium, 1500 mg/day
      (2) Aspirin, 80 mg/day
   c. Long-standing or severe hypertension
      (1) Electrocardiogram (EKG)
      (2) Echocardiogram
5. Symptoms of coronary insufficiency
   a. Exertional chest pain or dyspnea
   b. Referred pain
   c. Arrhythmia
   d. Heart failure
   e. Treatment
      (1) EKG
      (2) Echocardiogram
      (3) Referral to cardiologist
6. Gastroenteropathy
   a. Intermittent constipation and diarrhea
   b. Emesis
   c. Early satiety
   d. Problems include the following:
      (1) Dehydration and ketoacidosis
      (2) Erratic blood sugar control
      (3) Hypoglycemia
      (4) Poor maternal weight gain

Establishment of pregnancy viability and gestational age

1. Viability and gestational age
   a. Accurate dating imperative
      (1) Increased risk of later perinatal complications
      (2) Timing of delivery at term
   b. Increased risk of first-trimester pregnancy loss
      (1) Higher in pregestational diabetes
      (2) Early diagnosis important for diabetes management
      (3) Correlates with periconceptional hyperglycemia
2. Pregnancy dating
   a. Serum human chorionic gonadotropin (HCG)
   b. Vaginal probe ultrasound: 6 to 12 weeks
      (1) Date pregnancy accurately within ±4 days.
      (2) Establish intrauterine pregnancy.
      (3) Rule out missed abortion.
      (4) Rule out multiple gestation.
      (5) Diagnose gross fetal anomalies.

Detection of congenital anomalies

1. Overall risk is twofold to threefold over general population.
2. All major organ systems may be involved.
3. Risk related to poor first-trimester glucose control.
4. Detection
   a. First-trimester glycosylated hemoglobin
      (1) Elevated: increased risk of anomalies
      (2) Normal: risk approaches general population
   b. First trimester vaginal ultrasound
      (1) Ultrasound is performed at 10 to 12 weeks.
      (2) Detection of major anomalies is possible.
      (3) Sensitivity and specificity are not well defined.
   c. Maternal serum alpha-fetoprotein (AFP)
      (1) Performed at 14 to 16 weeks.
      (2) Level is lower in diabetic women.
      (3) Level is lower in obese women.
   d. Transabdominal ultrasound
      (1) Perform at 15 to 20 weeks
      (2) Fetal anomaly screen
      (3) Four-chambered cardiac view
   e. Fetal echocardiography
      (1) Echocardiography is performed at 22 to 24 weeks.
      (2) Fetal anomaly screen repeated.

Prevention and treatment of preterm labor

1. Risk increased in diabetic pregnancy
   a. Hydramnios increases risk.
   b. Poor glucose control increases risk.
   c. Vascular disease increases risk.
2. Frequent prenatal visits
3. Patient education and counseling
4. Screening and treatment for bacterial vaginosis
5. Treatment
   a. Avoid betasympathomimetic tocolytics
      (1) Cause hyperglycemia
      (2) May precipitate diabetic ketoacidosis
   b. Tocolytic agents
      (1) Magnesium sulfate; first choice
      (2) Nifedipine; second choice (may also be used for long-term oral prophylaxis)
      (3) Indomethacin; third choice
   c. Betamethasone
      (1) Betamethasone can be used for fetal lung maturation.
      (2) It may cause hyperglycemia.
      (3) It may precipitate diabetic ketoacidosis.
      (4) Careful monitoring of blood glucose is required.
      (5) Insulin drip may be necessary during acute phase of treatment.

Fetal growth aberrancy

1. Macrosomia
   a. Neonatal weight >90th percentile for gestational age
   b. Characterized by central obesity
   c. Associated with the following:
      (1) Poor maternal glucose control
      (2) Elevated third-trimester glycosylated hemoglobin
      (3) Excessive maternal weight gain
      (4) Maternal obesity
      (5) Diabetic classes A through C
      (6) Hydramnios
      (7) Previous macrosomic infant
   d. Increases risk of the following:
      (1) Neonatal metabolic complications
      (2) Neonatal physiologic complications
      (3) Intrauterine fetal death
      (4) Intrapartum hypoxia and acidosis
      (5) Fetal birth trauma and shoulder dystocia
      (6) Cephalopelvic disproportion and cesarean section
      (7) Maternal genital trauma
      (8) Uterine atony and postpartum hemorrhage
2. Intrauterine growth retardation (IUGR)
   a. Associated with the following:
      (1) Diabetic classes C, R, F, T, H
      (2) Hypertension
      (3) Vascular disease
      (4) Oligohydramnios
      (5) Preeclampsia
      (6) Chronic maternal hypoglycemia (mean daily glucose <95 mg/dl)
   b. Increased risk of the following:
      (1) Intrapartum and neonatal hypoxia or acidosis
      (2) Intrauterine fetal death
      (3) Long-term developmental impairment
      (4) Meconium aspiration syndrome

Establishment of glucose control (Table 23-3)

1. Establishment defines most perinatal risk.
   a. Fetal anomalies
   b. First-trimester pregnancy loss
   c. Preterm labor
   d. Intrauterine fetal death
   e. Intrapartum hypoxia
   f. Macrosomia
   g. Neonatal metabolic and physiologic complications (e.g., hypoglycemia)
2. Perinatal outcome correlates better with postprandial glucose levels.
3. Self-monitoring of blood glucose
   a. Glucometer should be used.

Table 23-3 Standards of glucose control in diabetic pregnancy

Time	Ideal Glucose Range (mg/dl)
Fasting	60-95
Premeal	60-105
1 hour postprandial	110-140
2 hour postprandial	80-120
2 AM-6 AM	60-120

   b. Glucometer should be used at least four times a day in pregestational diabetics.
   c. Standards are more stringent then in nonpregnant state.
   d. Recommended standards are estimates based on clinical consensus.
   e. Poor control: Mean daily blood glucose is >120 mg/dl.
4. Complications of glucose control
   a. Diabetic ketoacidosis: Associations are as follows:
      (1) Patient noncompliance
      (2) Use of betasympathomimetic drugs
      (3) Use of betamethasone
      (4) Emesis with dehydration
      (5) Maternal infection
      (6) Can occur more readily and at lower glucose levels in pregnancy
   b. Hypoglycemia
      (1) Hypoglycemia is more frequent in first trimester.
      (2) It is more frequent in type I IDDM.
      (3) It is associated with overzealous insulin administration.
      (4) Hypoglycemia is associated with maternal dietary noncompliance.
      (5) Insulin coma may result in face of hypoglycemia unawareness.
      (6) Chronic hypoglycemia may lead to IUGR (mean daily plasma glucose <95 mg/dl)

Prevention of IUFD

1. Risk is increased in *complicated* diabetes mellitus
   a. Poor third-trimester glucose control
   b. Maternal age >35 years or teenage pregnancy
   c. Insulin requirement >100 U/day
   d. Fetal macrosomia or diabetic fetopathy
   e. Maternal vascular disease
   f. Maternal hypertension
   g. Preeclampsia
   h. Previous IUFD
   i. IUGR
   j. Hydramnios or oligohydramnios
   k. Patient noncompliance
   l. Fetal anomalies

2. Fetal surveillance
   a. Uncomplicated diabetes; to begin at 30 to 32 weeks
   b. Complicated diabetes; to begin 28 to 30 weeks
   c. Ultrasound
      (1) Every 2 to 4 weeks after 20 weeks
      (2) Assessment of fetal growth and amniotic fluid volume
   d. Doppler ultrasound
      (1) Generally not predictive of fetal health in diabetic pregnancy
      (2) May be useful in presence of hypertension or vascular disease
      (3) Should be interpreted with caution
      (4) Should be interpreted in conjunction with other surveillance methods
3. Timed delivery
   a. No risk factors for IUFD, good glycemic control, compliant:
      (1) Vigilant expectancy until 40 weeks
      (2) Induction at 40 weeks if labor has not occurred
   b. Risk factors for IUFD, poor glycemic control, noncompliant:
      (1) Assess fetal lung maturity by amniocentesis.
      (2) Phosphatidyl glycerol is required for confirmation of lung maturity.
      (3) Amniocentesis is generally performed between 37 and 38 weeks.
      (4) Induction at confirmation of fetal lung maturity: 4s ≥2.0 and phosphatidyl glycerol is positive or 4s ≥3.0 and phosphatidyl glycerol is negative.

Prevention of intrapartum asphyxia

1. Continuous fetal monitoring
2. Adjunctive fetal scalp sampling
3. Amniotomy
   a. Internal monitor placement
   b. Detection of meconium
4. Amnioinfusion
   a. Recurrent severe variable decelerations
   b. Presence of thick meconium
5. Skilled pediatric personel in attendance at delivery

Prevention of birth trauma

1. Primary cesarean section should be considered for either of the following:
   a. Estimated fetal weight is >4000 g, head circumference to abdominal circumference ratio is <10th percentile.
   b. Estimated fetal weight is >4200 g.
2. Attention to dysfunction labors associated with cephalopelvic disproportion
   a. Protraction of descent or dilation
   b. Arrest of descent or dilation
   c. Failure of descent
3. Attention to pelvic findings associated with cephalopelvic disproportion.

a. Excessive fetal cranial molding
b. Fetal caput
c. Fetal cranium overriding maternal symphysis
4. Use of intrauterine pressure catheters for management of dysfunctional labor
5. Avoidance of unnecessary operative delivery with vacuum or forceps
a. Especially in face of dysfunctional labor
b. Especially if fetal macrosomia suspected
6. Anticipation and expert management of shoulder dystocia
a. Selective use of formal delivery room setting
(1) Large baby suspected clinically or by ultrasound
(2) Risk factors for macrosomia present
b. Rehearsed protocol for clinical management
c. Anesthesia on standby
d. Skilled pediatric personnel in attendance at delivery

Prevention and treatment of neonatal complications

1. Variables associated with complications
a. Poor glycemic control
b. IUGR
c. Macrosomia
d. Premature delivery
e. Preeclampsia
f. Maternal noncompliance
g. Congenital anomalies
h. Hyperglycemia during labor
i. Complicated diabetes mellitus
2. Categories of complications
a. Anatomic
(1) Occult fetal anomalies
(2) Birth trauma
b. Metabolic
(1) Hypoglycemia: most common and most immediate problem
(2) Hypocalcemia
(3) Hypomagnesemia
(4) Polycythemia and hyperviscosity syndrome
(5) Hyperbilirubinemia
c. Physiologic
(1) Respiratory distress
(2) Renal vein thrombosis
(3) Cardiomyopathy
(4) Asphyxia
3. Prevention
a. Glycemic control during pregnancy and labor
b. Ultrasound detection of growth aberrancy
c. Ultrasound detection of congenital anomalies
d. Selective delivery at tertiary centers
(1) Complicated diabetes
(2) Poor glycemic control or noncompliance
(3) Premature gestational age
(4) Suspected IUGR or oligohydramnios

(5) Preeclampsia
(6) Suspected fetal anomalies
(7) Suspected extreme macrosomia (>4500 g)
(8) Premature labor

e. Confirmation of fetal pulmonary maturity before onset of labor
(1) <40 weeks gestation
(2) Uncertain dating

General management principles

1. Applicable to both gestational and pregestational diabetes
   a. Standards of glycemic control
   b. Perinatal risk assessment
   c. Fetal surveillance strategies
   d. Timing of delivery
   e. Intrapartum surveillance
2. Diet
   a. ADA diet
   b. Must minimize hyperglycemia
   c. Must meet nutritional needs of pregnancy (Tables 23-4 and 23-5)
   d. Calories determined by maternal weight at time of diagnosis
      (1) 10% of calories at breakfast
      (2) 20% to 30% of calories at lunch
      (3) 30% to 40% of calories at dinner
      (4) 30% of calories as snacks
   e. Prevent excessive maternal weight gain (see Table 23-5)
3. Maternal glucose monitoring (see the box on p. 470)
   a. Fasting and postprandial blood sugar determinations
      (1) Gestational diabetes
         (a) Self-monitoring of blood glucose by reflectance meters; 2 to 3 days per week, *or*
         (b) Office monitoring of blood glucose
      (2) Pregestational diabetes; daily, at least four times a day
      (3) Office determination of maternal glucose every 2 to 4 weeks
   b. Glycosylated hemoglobin determinations
      (1) Indicator of chronic glycemic control over prior 4 to 6 weeks
      (2) Limited use in gestational diabetes
      (3) Insensitive indicator of subtle but perinatally significant maternal hyperglycemia usually seen in gestational diabetes
      (4) Measure every 6 to 12 weeks in pregestational diabetes
      (5) Not a substitute for frequent maternal glucose measurement
4. Insulin therapy; pregestational diabetes
   a. Split dose insulin used
      (1) Intermediate acting (neutral protamine Hagedorn [NPH] preferred)
      (2) Short acting
   b. Human insulin used
   c. First trimester: Dose = approximately 0.5 U/kg/day
   d. Second trimester: Dose = approximately 0.8 U/kg/day
   e. Third trimester: Dose = approximately 1 to 2 U/kg/day
5. Insulin therapy; gestational diabetes
   a. Therapeutic insulin treatment

Table 23-4 Ideal weight for height and percentage deviations from ideal

Height (ft/in.)	Ideal Weight (lb)	80% Ideal Weight	90% Ideal Weight	120% Ideal Weight	135% Ideal Weight	150% Ideal Weight
4/8	101	81	91	121	136	152
4/9	104	83	94	125	140	156
4/10	106	85	95	127	143	159
4/11	109	87	98	131	147	164
5/0	112	90	101	134	151	168
5/1	115	92	104	138	155	173
5/2	119	95	107	143	161	179
5/3	122	98	110	146	165	183
5/4	126	101	113	151	170	189
5/5	130	104	117	156	176	195
5/6	134	107	121	161	181	201
5/7	138	110	124	166	186	207
5/8	142	114	128	170	192	213
5/9	147	118	132	176	198	221
5/10	151	121	136	181	204	227

Table 23-5 Nutritional indices for pregestational and gestational diabetes

---

Pregestational Diabetes
Weight Before Pregnancy (Expressed as % of Ideal Weight)
<90
90-120
>120
Recommended Daily Caloric Intake (kcal/kg)
36-40
30
24

Gestational Diabetes
Weight at Time of Diagnosis (Expressed as % of Ideal Weight)
<80
80-120
120-150
>150
Recommended Daily Caloric Intake (kcal/kg)
35-40
30
24
12-15

Pregestational and Gestational Diabetes
Recommended Caloric Composition
40%-50% carbohydrate
20% protein
30%-40% fat
Recommended Caloric Distribution
10% of calories at breakfast
20%-30% of calories at lunch
30%-40% of calories at dinner
30% of calories as snacks

Pregestational and Gestational Diabetes
Prepregnancy Weight (Expressed as % of Ideal Weight)
<90
90-135
>135
Recommended Total Weight Gain (lb) (For Entire Pregnancy)
28-40
25-35
15-25

Recommendations for Maternal Glucose Monitoring in Diabetic Pregnancies

Gestational Diabetes

Self-monitoring of blood glucose: reflectance meter
- four times a day; fasting blood sugars and 1-hr or 2-hr postprandials, 2-3 times a week, *or*
- Office blood glucose determinations weekly; fasting blood sugar and 1-hr or 2-hr postprandial

Pregestational Diabetes

Self-monitoring of blood glucose: reflectance meter
- Minimum of four times a day; fasting blood sugar, and 1-hr or 2-hr postprandials daily
- Select patients: additional determinations, before meals, bedtime, 2 a.m.

Urine dipsticks for ketones
- During acute illness

Glycosylated hemoglobin determination
- At least once per trimester; more frequently in select patients

(1) Failure to achieve glycemic control by diet in gestational diabetes
(2) Human insulin used.
(3) Initial dose: 20 U intermediate, 10 U short-acting insulin before breakfast
(4) Further dose adjustments according to initial dose response

b. Prophylactic insulin
   (1) Prophylactic insulin is used in patients with glycemic control.
   (2) Dose: 20 U are given intermediate, 10 U short-acting insulin are given before breakfast.
   (3) Prophylactic insulin may reduce macrosomia in patients with glycemic control.
   (4) Obese patients appear to benefit the most.
   (5) Prophylactic insulin is presently not standard of practice.
   (6) Prophylactic insulin is presently not a method of patient selection.

6. Oral hypoglycemic agents
   a. Classes of drugs are as follows:
      (1) Sulfonylureas: potentiate pancreatic insulin secretion
      (2) Biguanides: reduce hepatic glucose production, reduce intestinal glucose absorption, and increase insulin sensitivity
      (3) α-Glucosidase inhibitors: reduce intestinal glucose absorption
   b. May potentiate fetal hyperinsulinemia
   c. May cause neonatal hypoglycemia

   d. Clinical data presently lacking
   e. None presently approved for use in pregnancy
   f. New generation agents: potentially beneficial in the future in the treatment of gestational diabetes
7. Ultrasound surveillance
   a. First-trimester vaginal sonography
      (1) Principally for pregestational diabetes
      (2) Detect early pregnancy loss
      (3) Accurate pregnancy dating
      (4) Detection of gross fetal anomalies
   b. Second-trimester sonography
      (1) Pregnancy dating
      (2) Detect fetal anomalies in pregestational diabetes (15 to 18 weeks)
   c. Third-trimester sonography
      (1) Applicable for both pregestational and gestational diabetes
      (2) Detection of diabetic fetopathy
      (3) Detection of fetal macrosomia and cardiomyopathy
   d. Fetal echocardiography: pregestational diabetes
      (1) Four-chambered view (15 to 18 weeks)
      (2) Formal study (22 to 24 weeks)
      (3) Detection of diabetic cardiomyopathy (third trimester)
8. Ultrasound predictors of growth aberrancy
   a. Macrosomia (*most predictive)
      (1) Third trimester fetal abdominal circumference growth >1.5 cm/week*
      (2) Head circumference to abdominal circumference ratio <10th percentile
      (3) Femur length to abdominal circumference ratio <20%
      (4) Estimated fetal weight >4200 g at term
      (5) Hydramnios
   b. IUGR: pregestational diabetes
      (1) Poor interval fetal abdominal circumference growth
      (2) Head circumference to abdominal circumference ratio >90th percentile
      (3) Femur length to abdominal circumference ratio >24%
      (4) Transcerebellar diameter to abdominal circumference ratio >15%
      (5) Elevated umbilical artery doppler systolic/diastolic (S/D) or pulsatility index
      (6) Decreased middle cerebral artery doppler S/D or pulsatility index
      (7) Elevated uterine artery doppler S/D ratio
      (8) Oligohydramnios
9. Congenital anomalies
   a. Anomalies are increased twofold to threefold in pregestational diabetes.
   b. This applies to all fetal organ systems.
   c. Most anomalies present by the seventh gestational week.
   d. There is no increased risk in gestational diabetes.

e. Risk correlates with first-trimester hyperglycemia.
   (1) Documented hyperglycemia by self-glucose monitoring
   (2) Elevated first-trimester glycosylated hemoglobin
f. Independent risk is possibly related to vascular disease.
g. Congenital abnormalities are the leading cause of perinatal mortality.
h. Incidence has remained constant in diabetic pregnancies.
i. Risk is not related to first-trimester hypoglycemia.
j. Small risk is possibly related to first-trimester oral hypoglycemic drugs.
k. Detection
   (1) First-trimester sonography: limited to gross anomalies
   (2) Second-trimester sonography
   (3) Fetal echocardiography
   (4) Second-trimester maternal alpha-fetoprotein screening
l. Prevention
   (1) Preconception counseling and glycemic control
   (2) Planned pregnancy
   (3) Cannot be effectively prevented postconception

10. Diabetic fetopathy: refers to ultrasound-detected fetal somatic disproportion, reflecting accelerated growth of insulin-senstive tissues (liver, adipose tissue, skeletal muscle) in response to fetal hyperinsulinemia
   a. Implies presence of fetal hyperinsulinemia
      (1) May suggest poor maternal glucose control
      (2) Increased risk of macrosomia
      (3) Increased risk of intrauterine fetal death
      (4) Increased risk of intrapartum hypoxia
      (5) Increased risk of neonatal morbidity
   b. Sonogram findings (one or more of the following):
      (1) Low head circumference to abdominal circumference (HC/AC)
      (2) Low femur to abdominal circumference (F/AC)
      (3) Accelerated third-trimester abdominal circumference growth (≥1.2 cm/wk)
      (4) Abdominal circumference ≥90th percentile for gestational age
      (5) Estimated fetal weight ≥90th percentile for gestational age
11. Hydramnios
   a. Frequent complication of pregestational and gestational diabetes
   b. Exact mechanism not well understood
   c. Sonographic findings
      (1) Amniotic fluid index ≥25 cm any time during gestation
      (2) Amniotic fluid index >2 standard deviations (S.D.) from mean for gestational age
   d. Correlates somewhat with poor maternal glycemic control.
   e. Correlates somewhat with fetal macrosomia.
   f. May indicate the presence of a fetal anomaly.
   g. Increases risk of the following:
      (1) Preterm labor, preterm rupture of membranes
      (2) Maternal preeclampsia
      (3) Intrauterine fetal death

(4) Fetal macrosomia
(5) Fetal malpresentation
(6) Cord prolapse
(7) Placenta separation
(8) Uterine atony

12. Surveillance of fetal well-being
    a. Timing and intensity depends on risk of fetal death
        (1) 32 to 24 weeks: all pregestational diabetics and high-risk gestational diabetics (see box on p. 459)
        (2) <32 weeks: selected pregestational diabetics
        (3) 35 weeks: low-risk gestational diabetics
    b. Fetal risk is increased by the following:
        (1) Pregestational diabetes in general
        (2) High-risk gestational diabetes
        (3) Diabetic fetopathy or fetal macrosomia
        (4) IUGR
        (5) Hydramnios or oligohydramnios
        (6) Poor maternal glucose control (especially third trimester)
        (7) Poor prior pregnancy history
        (8) Prior intrauterine fetal death
        (9) Maternal hypertension
        (10) Maternal vascular disease
        (11) Abnormal umbilical artery doppler indices
        (12) Patient noncompliance
        (13) Advanced maternal age (>35 years of age)
        (14) Large doses of maternal insulin (>100 U/day)
        (15) Maternal smoking
        (16) Maternal substance abuse
    c. Surveillance strategies
        (1) Daily maternal fetal movement counts
        (2) Formal fetal surveillance
    d. Surveillance techniques
        (1) No method has been definitively demonstrated superior
        (2) One of three modalities can be used for pregestational and high-risk gestational diabetics:
            (a) Weekly contraction stress testing (CST)
            (b) Twice weekly biophysical profile assessment (BPP)
            (c) Twice weekly nonstress testing (NST) with adjunctiive BPP
    e. Low-risk gestational diabetics: weekly NST

13. Umbilical artery doppler ultrasound
    a. Poor predictor of perinatal outcome in diabetic pregnancy
    b. Some efficacy in diabetics with hypertension or vascular disease
        (1) Initial assessment at 28 weeks
        (2) Repeat at intervals depending on 28-week findings

14. Timing of delivery
    a. Fetal lung maturity
        (1) Lung maturity may be delayed in diabetic fetuses.
        (2) Risk of delay is correlated to maternal glucose control.
        (3) Amiotic lecithin/sphyngomyelin (L/S) ratio may not be predictive of fetal lung maturity.

(4) Presence of amniotic fluid phosphatidyl glycerol may be more predictive of fetal lung maturity.
(5) Amniotic fluid lung maturity should be confirmed before elective delivery <40 weeks.

15. Timing of delivery
    a. Pregestational and high-risk gestational diabetes
        (1) Assessment of fetal lung maturity beginning at 37 to 38 weeks
        (2) Delivery at fetal lung maturity
    b. Gestational diabetes
        (1) Spontaneous labor should be allowed.
        (2) If undelivered at 40 to 41 weeks, labor should be induced.
    c. Low-risk pregestational diabetes
        (1) Allowing spontaneous labor should be considered.
        (2) Delivery should be considered in presence of fetal lung maturity and high cervical Bishop score.
        (3) If undelivered at 40 weeks, labor should be induced.
16. Mode of delivery
    a. Vaginal birth is the preferred mode of delivery.
    b. Cervical ripening agents should be used in the presence of low cervical Bishop score:
        (1) Prostaglandin gel
        (2) Mechanical cervical dilators
    c. Cesarean section is reserved for specific indications
        (1) Failed induction in high-risk pregestational diabetics
        (2) Selected cases of suspected fetal macrosomia
17. Prevention of birth trauma and shoulder dystocia
    a. Selective primary cesarean section
    b. Careful management of arrested and protracted labors
    c. Avoidance of operative vaginal delivery
        (1) In cases of suspected fetal macrosomia
        (2) In cases of dysfunctional labors
    d. Anticipation and expert management of shoulder dystocia
18. Prelabor and labor management
    a. General guidelines
        (1) Patient should take usual dose of intermediate and short-acting insulin the evening before delivery.
        (2) Patient should take dinner and evening snack the evening before delivery.
        (3) No food or subcutaneous insulin the day of delivery.
        (4) Fasting blood sugar should be measured the day of delivery.
        (5) Blood glucose and urine dipstick for ketones every 1 to 2 hours during labor.
        (6) Blood glucose should be maintained at 70 to 120, and urine maintained free of ketones.
        (7) Rapid glucose infusions for conduction anesthesia should be avoided.
    b. Suggested insulin regimen
        (1) Type I pregestational diabetes
            (a) Type I diabetics have a propensity toward ketosis and hypoglycemia, and labor may predispose toward both conditions.

(b) Therefore it is prudent in general to begin dextrose and insulin infusions from the onset.

(2) Five percent dextrose solution is instituted IV at 125 ml/hr.

(3) Insulin drip at 0.5 U/hr is instituted.

(4) Insulin and dextrose infusions are adjusted according to glucose and urinary ketone values.

c. Suggested insulin regimen

(1) Type II and gestational diabetes

(a) Many type II and gestational diabetics may not need any dextrose or insulin infusions during labor.

(b) Therefore a more conservative approach to these patients is permissible.

(2) Dextrose-free crystalloid is instituted.

(3) Dextrose solution is administered IV for persistent glucose <70 or for persistent ketonuria.

(4) Insulin drip is administered starting at 0.5 U/hr for glucose >120.

(5) Insulin and dextrose infusions are adjusted according to glucose and urinary ketone values.

19. Neonatal management

a. Delivery of select patients at tertiary facilities

(1) Diabetics with vascular disease or hypertension

(2) Diabetics with brittle glucose control

(3) Diabetes of long standing

(4) Fetuses suspected of IUGR

(5) Gestational age <37 weeks

(6) Poorly compliant patients

(7) Hydramnios

(8) Suspected or proven fetal anomalies

(9) Poor maternal glucose control

b. Anticipation and management of neonatal complications

(1) Unanticipated congenital anomalies

(2) Respiratory distress

(3) Hypoglycemia

(4) Hypocalcemia

(5) Birth trauma

(6) Birth asphyxia

(7) Polycythemia and hyperviscosity syndrome

(8) Jaundice

(9) Diabetic cardiomyopathy and cardiac failure

Suggested reading

American Diabetes Association: Clinical practice recommendations, *Diabetes Care* (Suppl 1), 1996.

American Diabetes Association: *Physicians guide to insulin-dependent (type I) diabetes; diagnosis and treatment,* VA, 1988, American Diabetes Association.

American Diabetes Association: *Physicians guide to insulin-dependent (type II) diabetes; diagnosis and treatment,* VA, 1989, American Diabetes Association.

American Diabetes Association: *Medical management of pregnancy complicated by diabetes,* VA, 1993, American Diabetes Association.

American Diabetes Association: Diabetes and pregnancy; part I, *Diabetes Reviews* 3:1995.
American Diabetes Association: Diabetes and pregnancy; part II. *Diabetes Reviews* 4:1996.
Reece EA, Coustan DR: *Diabetes mellitus in pregnancy,* ed 2, New York, 1995, Churchill Livingstone.
Rodgers BD, Rodgers DE: Clinical variables associated with diabetic ketoacidosis during pregnancy, *J Reprod Med* 36:797, 1991.

23.2 INSULIN TREATMENT IN PREGNANCY

Harold Bays, M.D., F.A.C.P., and Mary Self, M.D.

1. Scientifically, studies such as the Diabetes Control and Complication Trial (DCCT) have confirmed that "tight" blood sugar (BS) control can decrease progression of many of the chronic complications of diabetes mellitus (DM). Similarly, studies have demonstrated that normalization of BS control may normalize the risks associated with pregnancy complicated by gestational diabetes or pregestational DM.
2. Practically, the advancement in medical technology, along with the influences of managed health care systems, has increasingly diverted DM medical care toward an outpatient basis.
3. Health care providers recognize the scientific need to maximize BS control and the ability to incorporate technologies and outpatient care systems to implement maximal BS control in the outpatient setting.
   a. Use of new technologies (e.g., home glucose monitors, insulin pumps)
   b. Use of outpatient, health systems (e.g., hospital-based, insurance-based, or private educational facilities, or home health care or visiting nurse instruction)

Gestational diabetes mellitus (GDM)

Definitions, etiology, and diagnosis

1. GDM is glucose intolerance with onset during pregnancy.
2. The etiology of hyperglycemia during pregnancy is probably multifactorial and is thought to be significantly caused by placental production of human placental lactogen hormone (HPL), which results in insulin resistance.
3. Hyperglycemia in GDM is most accentuated after meals.
4. GDM accounts for about 90% of all pregnant women who have DM.
5. Diagnosis
   a. A 50-g oral glucose screening or challenge test is recommended for all women (regardless of risk factors) between 24 and 28 weeks gestation. If subsequent 1-hour BS level is greater than 140 mg/dl, then a glucose tolerance test (GTT) is indicated.
   b. The GTT includes at least an 8-hour fast, followed by a fasting BS. After 100 g of oral glucose, BS levels are obtained at 1, 2, and 3 hours. Interpretation of GTT is described in the box on p. 477.
      (1) It should be noted that some authors feel that these guidelines are not sensitive enough. Other, more rigid suggestions have been made.

Interpretation of 100 G Oral GTT

Gestational diabetes mellitus is diagnosed if two or more subsequent blood sugar values (after 100 g oral glucose) are above:

Fasting	105 mg/dl
1 hour	190 mg/dl
2 hours	165 mg/dl
3 hours	145 mg/dl

(2) Furthermore, other authors suggest that GDM is present if the fasting blood sugar is greater than 105 mg/dl, regardless of other values.

Risks

1. Before delivery, the most common potential fetal complication associated with GDM is macrosomia.
   a. Macrosomia can be defined as birth weight >90th percentile, adjusted for sex and gestational age.
   b. Development of macrosomia is related to increased nutrient transport across the placenta (such as "facilitated" glucose transport, and "active" amino acid transport), and subsequent fetal hyperinsulinemia.
2. At delivery, if macrosomia is present, potential fetal complications may include birth trauma such as the following:
   a. Brachial plexus injury
   b. Facial nerve injury
   c. Cephalohematoma
3. After delivery, potential fetal complications associated with GDM may include the following:
   a. Respiratory distress
   b. Hypoglycemia
   c. Electrolyte imbalances
   d. An increased risk of obesity
   e. Type II (adult-onset) DM later in the newborn's life.
4. The most common potential maternal complications associated with GDM include the following:
   a. Increased thirst
   b. Increased urination
   c. Increased fetal amniotic fluid
   d. An increased rate of urinary tract infections
   e. Increased rate of yeast infections
   f. Increased rate of spontaneous abortions
   g. Increased rate of hypertension
   h. Increased rate of toxemia

5. If fetal macrosomia occurs, potential maternal complications may include the following:
   a. Difficult delivery
   b. Prolonged labor
   c. Vaginal wall trauma
   d. Need for a cesarean section

Monitoring of gestational diabetes mellitus

1. Once the diagnosis of GDM is made, one monitoring strategy is to recommend that BS be obtained (by home glucose monitoring) fasting and 1 or 2 hours after each meal (four times a day).
2. Monitoring BS levels before meals is not sensitive enough in women with GDM and misses many women with GDM who may benefit from more aggressive treatment.
3. The goal is to maintain fasting BS less than 90 mg/dl, 1-hour postprandial BS less than 140 mg/dl, and 2-hour postprandial BS less than 120 mg/dl.
4. Unless the initial BS is found to be high enough to warrant immediate intervention, glucose monitoring is usually recommended for about a week while on appropriate diet before any decision is made concerning need for insulin therapy.
5. Urinary ketone determination measures starvation states and ketosis, both of which may be harmful to the fetus. Testing is usually recommended fasting, whenever meals are omitted, during periods of nausea or vomiting, or with medical stresses such as during infections.
   a. If the metabolic needs of mother and fetus exceed the carbohydrate consumption and stores of the mother, then a "starvation" state may occur wherein maternal body fat becomes a major source of calories. Fat metabolism may result in the formation of "ketone bodies."
   b. The kidneys are very efficient in clearing ketones so that even if urinary ketones are moderate, it is unlikely that ketone levels in the blood are significantly elevated. However, if urinary ketones become highly positive, this may mean that acidemia is present. Therefore, maintaining urinary ketones less than moderate is a reasonable treatment goal.
   c. Fasting (before breakfast) urinary ketosis can be treated by simple interventions such as an increase in the bedtime snack, or 3 AM glass of milk. Because, for most women, the risk for relative "starvation" is greatest after an overnight fast, a single fasting urinary ketone test each morning may be the most cost efficient way to detect women at risk for significant ketosis.
6. The total glycated hemoglobin (TGH), or hemoglobin A1C (Hgb A1C) determines the overall BS control for the previous 6 to 8 weeks.
   a. TGH/Hgb A1C may detect patients who had substantial elevations in BS before the glucose tolerance testing.
   b. If the initial blood testing indicates normal TGH/Hgb A1C, and if BS is found to be well controlled by home glucose monitoring, subsequent repeat TGH/Hgb A1C blood testing is usually not necessary.

c. If the patient develops significant hyperglycemia or requires intensive insulin therapy, or if doubts exist as to the accuracy of home glucose monitoring, then repeat TGH/Hgb A1C blood level testing may be appropriate.
7. Fructosamine and glycated albumin blood levels are of questionable additional clinical benefit in most women with GDM.
8. After diagnosis through glucose tolerance testing, and after obtaining a baseline TGH/Hgb A1C, the best method for determining BS control is home glucose monitoring.
   a. Many current home glucose monitoring meters are very "user friendly" and quite accurate.
   b. Some companies may provide "loaner" glucose meters to help reduce cost.

Dietary treatment

1. Many of the dietary recommendations for women with GDM are similar to the recommendations to any patient with DM. In general, women with GDM should be encouraged to adhere to healthy, low–concentrated sweet diets. If high blood pressure occurs, then reduction in dietary sodium is also important. Some recommendations unique to women with GDM include the following:
   a. To reduce the postprandial glycemic effects of carbohydrates, the recommended diet composition is 40% carbohydrate, 20% protein, and 40% fat.
   b. Women with GDM who are underweight should consume about 40 kcal/kg/day.
   c. Women with GDM at normal weight should consume about 30 kcal/kg/day.
   d. Women with GDM moderately overweight should consume about 25 kcal/kg/day.
   e. Women with GDM massively overweight should consume about 15 kcal/kg/day.
2. However, because the goals of DM control in GDM are often more rigid than for nonpregnant patients with type I or type II DM, dietary compliance and education about the glycemic response to foods is often essential.
   a. The glycemic response to mixed meals is most dependent on the amount (or percentage) of carbohydrates.
   b. The glycemic response to isolated foods may be anticipated by the "glycemic index" (see the box on p. 480).
   c. Perhaps the best method to educate patients of the glycemic properties of food is through intensive home glucose monitoring. Monitoring postprandial BS three times a day, 7 days a week, quickly educates women with GDM as to which foods result in postprandial hyperglycemia.
   d. If the woman with GDM declines to avoid foods with high glycemic potential, then it is recommended that such foods be incorporated into mixed meals. This may blunt glycemic excursions. For example, consumption of cornflakes, potatoes, or bread alone may cause unacceptable elevations in BS, suggesting the need of insulin

Glycemic Indexes of Some Foods*

80% to 90% Cornflakes, carrots, potatoes (instant or mashed), honey
70% to 79% Whole wheat or whole meal bread, white rice, potatoes
60% to 69% White bread, shredded wheat, brown rice, raisins, beets, bananas, Mars bar
50% to 59% Bran, many biscuits, white spaghetti, sweet corn, green peas, potato chips, sucrose, pastry
40% to 49% Oatmeal, whole meal spaghetti, sweet potatoes, navy beans, dry peas, grapes, oranges
30% to 39% Butter beans, chick and blackeye peas, ice cream, milk, yogurt, tomatoes, apples, pears
20% to 29% Sausage, kidney beans, lentils, fructose, peaches, grapefruit, plums, cherries
10% to 19% Soybeans, peanuts

The glycemic index (GI) is defined as the rise in BS after ingestion of a fixed amount of a certain food, as determined for an individual. For example, if 100 g of glucose ingestion caused a rise in BS by 50 mg/dl, then this is the standard by which other foods are compared. If ingestion of another food only caused a 25 mg/dl rise in BS, then the GI would be 50%. (Please note that sucrose—table sugar—has a GI of about 50%.)

treatment. However, if these foods are eaten with other foods, insulin treatment may not be needed.

3. To limit postprandial hyperglycemia and limit ketosis, it is often best to recommend spreading the daily caloric consumption to six small meals a day.

Insulin treatment

1. If initial fasting BS on GTT is >105 mg/dl, then insulin treatment is indicated, along with dietary counseling.
2. If initial fasting BS on GTT is <105 mg/dl, but the patient meets the criteria of GDM, then dietary treatment is attempted.
3. If, despite dietary treatment, the fasting BS exceeds 90 mg/dl, or if other goals of BS control are not achieved, then insulin therapy is indicated. In the past, it was commonplace that such women were admitted to the hospital for initiation of such therapy. However, because of the improvement in technology in home glucose monitoring, and the influence of health care systems, outpatient initiation of insulin therapy is becoming the rule.
4. Insulin does not cross the placenta and is not harmful to the fetus. However, insulin treatment of elevated BS in women with GDM has favorable effects on fetal and maternal outcome.
5. The choice of the initial dose of insulin should be based on BS readings. However, different providers may differ with regard to their preferences of insulin dosing, even given the same home glucose monitoring readings.

6. If a woman with GDM is initially found to have marked elevations in BS, and if access to appropriate diabetes education and instruction are not readily accessible, then hospitalization is indicated.
7. If a woman with GDM is initially found to have mild to moderately elevated BS despite diet and is able and willing to receive appropriate DM instruction, then beginning with small doses of insulin may be the safest and most prudent way to initiate insulin therapy. Further adjustments in dosing can be made every 2 to 3 days afterward, based on the patient's home glucose monitoring.

Follow-up during pregnancy

1. Many women who develop GDM are recommended to monitor fasting and 1-hour or 2-hour postprandial BS, as well as fasting urinary ketones, throughout the pregnancy.
2. It is often recommended that women who maintain acceptable BS control with dietary therapy alone reduce their home glucose monitoring and urinary ketone testing to three or four times a week. This recommendation reduces the cost and inconvenience to the patient, yet maintains an acceptable level of monitoring.

Management during labor and delivery

1. For most women with diet-controlled GDM who deliver within a few hours of labor, no special treatment or evaluation is usually necessary other than glucose monitoring.
2. If the labor is prolonged, it is the goal that BS readings be maintained between 60 and 100 mg/dl. Furthermore, it is probably best that urinary ketones be kept no higher than moderate.
3. A practical strategy might include glucose monitoring performed every 2 hours until delivery.
   a. If the BS goes below 60 mg/dl and this is not as the result of a hypoglycemic reaction from previously administered insulin, then simply changing the intravenous fluids to something containing dextrose is often sufficient to stabilize the BS.
   b. If the BS exceeds 100 mg/dl, then a low-dose insulin drip (1 to 5 U/hr), is often the safest and easiest way to prevent hyperglycemia.
4. BS should be maintained less than 100 mg/dl during and at delivery to avoid fetal hypoglycemia.
5. Also, the potential for ketosis can be monitored by requesting that urine ketone testing be performed at each void.
   a. If the urinary ketones are found to be greater than moderate, then the patient may be entering into a "starvation state." Intravenous fluids should be be changed to something that includes dextrose.
   b. If the BS level subsequently exceeds 100 mg/dl as result of the start of this intravenous dextrose, then an insulin drip should be initiated.
   c. It should be remembered that *both* glucose and insulin are necessary to prevent ketosis.

After delivery

1. Once the child has been delivered, insulin therapy is no longer needed for the majority of insulin-treated women with GDM.

2. Some women (particularly if treated with significant amounts of insulin during their pregnancy) may have underlying type I or type II DM. For these women, close follow-up of BS after delivery is indicated.
3. A GTT is recommended 6 weeks postpartum, or when breast-feeding is stopped. At the very least, women with history of GDM should have fasting BS within weeks after delivery. During this postdelivery visit, the likelihood of developing GDM during future pregnancies and the substantial risk of developing type II DM in the future should be emphasized in patient education.
   a. Women with history of GDM should be encouraged to adopt and maintain lifestyle habits such as appropriate diet, attaining ideal body weight, and regular physical exercise.
   b. BS monitoring, possibly including GTT, should be performed before any future pregnancy.
   c. Periodic BS monitoring should be recommended to detect potential type II DM later in the mother's lifetime.

Miscellaneous issues

1. The occasional high BS
   a. Particularly during initial dietary counseling, some women with GDM will experience an occasional high BS after meals as detected by home glucose monitoring.
   b. Little evidence supports that rare, mild, postprandial elevation in BS affords any significant adverse effect to the pregnancy.
   c. Therefore, although it is necessary to counsel women with GDM as to the need for strict BS control, it is also important to reassure them that, if the vast majority of BS levels are well within treatment goals, an occasional mild elevation in BS is unlikely to have any adverse effect to the unborn child.
2. Mixed versus premixed insulin
   a. Insulin administration ameliorates many of the metabolic abnormalities found in patients with DM. Numerous acceptable regimens have proven efficacy, as long as the goals of treatment are met.
   b. Some physicians make extensive use of the premixed insulins.
      (1) These include "70/30" preparations which contain 70% NPH (long acting), and 30% regular insulin (short acting).
      (2) There is a 50/50 premixed insulin preparation as well.
   c. Conversely, other physicians rarely use premixed insulin. They may feel that appropriate BS control can be achieved only through the greater flexibility of dosing achieved through the uncoupled, independent adjustment of moderately long-acting NPH or lente and short-acting regular insulin.
   d. In most cases, adequate achievement of glycemic controls can be achieved with either regimen. In either case, the goal is to reach a fasting BS of less than 90 mg/dl, and 1-hour postprandial BS of less than 140 mg/dl, or 2-hour postprandial BS less than 120 mg/dl.
3. Hypocaloric diets
   a. Pregnancy is not the time to enter into an aggressive, calorie-restricted dietary program for the sole purpose of losing weight.
   b. Most women gain about 25 pounds over the course of pregnancy.

c. However, some overweight pregnant mothers may not gain or, in fact, may lose weight during pregnancy while adhering to the recommended diet.
   (1) This is usually acceptable, as long as the weight loss is not excessive, is not the result of an underlying illness, is not caused by uncontrolled BS, and as is not associated with positive urinary ketones.
d. Severe hypocaloric diets (such as greater than 50% caloric restriction) may result in significant urinary ketosis.
e. Some studies suggest that less severe hypocaloric diets (such as a 33% caloric restriction) may prevent the need of insulin treatment and may result in minimal urinary ketosis.

4. Attitudes and realities of GDM and insulin administration
   a. Normalization of BS during pregnancy normalizes the risks of pregnancy complicated by DM.
   b. Most women with GDM are very willing and quite able to learn how to normalize BS with insulin.
   c. Some health care providers are reluctant to recommend insulin treatment to women with GDM for the purpose of normalizing BS.

Diabetes mellitus before pregnancy or pregestational diabetes mellitus (PGDM)

Concerns before conception

1. Just as among patients with DM in the general population, the range of BS control, the level of access to quality DM health care, the commitment to self-care and the severity of the complications of DM varies among women with PGDM.
2. Some women of childbearing potential may have BS well controlled with diet or oral DM drugs.
3. Some women in the childbearing years have "brittle" DM, with wide swings in BS and possibly, significant complications of DM, including recurrent diabetes ketoacidosis, hyperosmolar states, retinopathy, neuropathy, nephropathy, cardiomyopathy, and dermopathy.
4. In either event, the risk to the mother and fetus of PGDM is greater than that of GDM. For this reason, one of the most important measures to prevent the complications affiliated with DM and pregnancy is appropriate DM education and treatment before conception.
5. Women with DM treated with diet should be instructed to monitor fasting and 1-hour or 2-hour postprandial BS for months before potential conception.
   a. If the woman's fasting BS exceeds 90 mg/dl, or if postprandial BS consistently exceeds 120 mg/dl, then she may be a candidate for insulin treatment before conception.
6. Women treated with oral DM drugs should be instructed to discontinue these medications months before potential conception and to closely monitor fasting, and 1-hour or 2-hour postprandial BS for months before potential conception.
   a. If the woman's fasting BS exceeds 90 mg/dl, or if postprandial BS consistently exceeds 120 mg/dl, then she may be a candidate for insulin treatment before conception.

7. It has been suggested that oral DM drugs may cause congenital malformations in humans and in animals.
   a. Sulfonylureas such as glipizide and glyburide have shown no evidence of impaired fertility or harm to the fetus in rats and rabbits given 500 times the human dose.
   b. Biguanides such as phenformin have been shown to produce neural tube closure defects, craniofacial hypoplasia, and other congenital malformations in a dose-dependent manner in rats.
   c. Other biguanides, such as metformin, may not produce such effects.
   d. Prolonged, severe hypoglycemia may occur in newborns whose mothers are treated with oral DM drugs at delivery.
   e. Because no well-controlled clinical trials have demonstrated safety in humans with the use of oral DM drugs in pregnancy, such medications should be used only if the benefit is perceived to outweigh the potential risk.
8. For childbearing women with type I DM, "tight" BS control should be initiated before the potential for conception.
   a. In isolated cases, this may be achieved with diet and two shots of insulin per day.
   b. However, in most cases, women with type I DM who wish to become pregnant usually require intensive insulin regimens such as three or four shots of insulin per day, or the use of the insulin pump.

Risks

1. In general, the fetal and maternal risks associated with pregnancy in women with type I DM include those of women with GDM (see Gestational Diabetes Mellitus, Risks).
2. In addition, pregnancies complicated by type I DM have other, often more serious potential complications as well.
   a. Other fetal complications are as follows:
      (1) Fetal malformations or congenital anomalies (with or without spontaneous abortions) are the most common cause of perinatal death of the fetus in diabetic mothers.
      (2) The most common congenital defects include congenital heart disease and neural tube defects with caudal regression syndrome being the most common and most specific.
         (a) Because these complications will have occurred within the first several weeks of pregnancy, it is crucial that women with type I diabetes inform their doctors for diabetes counseling before considering pregnancy.
      (3) Other potential congenital malformations include anencephalus, anal or rectal atresias, and renal abnormalities.
      (4) Infants of women with DM before pregnancy are also at risk for polycythemia, hypocalcemia, hyperbilirubinemia, respiratory distress syndrome, and hypoglycemia.
      (5) If BS control is good at the time of conception, the risk of fetal malformations is very low—only about 3% to 5%.
      (6) If BS is under very poor control at time of conception, the risks of fetal malformations is about 20% to 25%.
      (7) The percentage risk to the fetus of congenital malformations is roughly equal to the TGH/Hgb A1C. For example, studies have

shown that women who conceive with glycated hemoglobin blood levels of 25% have approximately the same percentage risk of congenital malformations.

b. Other maternal complications
   (1) For women with type I DM without complications, pregnancy has not been shown to increase the risk or progression of diabetes complications later in life.
   (2) Type I DM kidney or vascular disease increases the risk of spontaneous abortion and low birth weight.
   (3) Type I DM complications such as diabetes retinopathy, neuropathy, and nephropathy may substantially worsen during pregnancy. The risks of worsening diabetes complications should be incorporated in any counseling of diabetic women before conception.

Monitoring of the woman with diabetes mellitus before pregnancy

1. If initial BS levels are under good control at conception (as documented by home glucose monitoring and TGH/Hgb A1C), then BS and urinary ketone measurements may be recommended similar to that of women with GDM (see Gestational Diabetes Mellitus). In some cases, BS may also need to be monitored before meals and at bedtime as well.
2. If initial BS levels are not under good control at conception or if the mother has difficulty in controlling BS ("brittle diabetes"), measurements may initially need to be performed before meals and at bedtime until better control is reached. Later during the pregnancy, after significant insulin resistance occurs (which may blunt wide glycemic excursions), BS may become easier to control. Insulin treatment decisions may then more safely be made on fasting, and 1 to 2 hours after meal BS.
3. Dietary treatment: Dietary therapy is essentially the same as for women with GDM (described in Gestational Diabetes Mellitus).

Insulin treatment

1. Hospitalization may be required if close outpatient follow-up and successful outpatient management of BS cannot be achieved.
2. "Tight" BS control is the goal for most pregnant mothers with type I DM. Women with type I DM should try to keep fasting (before breakfast) BS less than 90 mg/dl and 1-hour postprandial BS less than 140 mg/dl or 2-hour postprandial BS less than 120 mg/dl.
3. During the early months of pregnancy, optimal control of BS may not be safely obtainable, particularly among type I DM women with histories of widely unpredictable BS.
   a. If attempts at "tight control" are too aggressive, this may increase the risk of severe hypoglycemic reactions, possibly resulting in coma, seizures, car accidents, falls, etc.
   b. As the pregnancy progresses, and insulin resistance develops (blunting glycemic excursions), the ability to control BS may improve.

4. In some cases, women with type I DM can achieve adequate BS control with an insulin regimen of two daily injections. However, in most cases, adequate BS control requires intensive insulin treatment of four daily injections, preferably started months before conception.
5. Insulin pump treatment is indicated if intensive insulin treatment is inadequate in achieving adequate BS control. The use of insulin pumps may not only improve BS control but may also reduce the frequency of hypoglycemic reactions.

Follow-up during pregnancy

1. In addition to close monitoring of BS, urinary ketones, and TGH/Hgb A1C, women with PGDM should be monitored for hypertension, which not only is more frequent but may also increase the progression of many of the complications of DM.
2. In women with PGDM, progression of prior DM eye disease may occur. Therefore, it is essential that all women with PGDM have eye examinations before conception and regularly during the pregnancy.
3. In women with PGDM, progression of prior neuropathy may occur. For example, DM gastroparesis or delayed stomach emptying may worsen during pregnancy, requiring hospitalization if feeding is not tolerated.

Management during labor and delivery

1. During labor, it is the goal that BS readings be maintained between 60 and 100 mg/dl. Furthermore, it is probably best that urinary ketones should be kept no higher than moderate.
2. A practical strategy might include glucose monitoring performed every 2 hours until delivery.
   a. If the BS goes below 60 mg/dl and this is not as the result of a hypoglycemic reaction from previously administered insulin, then simply changing the intravenous fluids to something containing dextrose is often sufficient to stabilize the BS.
   b. If the BS exceeds 100 mg/dl, then a low-dose insulin drip (1 to 5 U/hr) is often the safest and easiest way to prevent hyperglycemia.
3. BS should be maintained less than 100 mg/dl during and at delivery to avoid fetal hypoglycemia.
4. Also, the potential for ketosis can be monitored by requesting that urine ketone testing be performed every 2 hours, or at least at each void.
   a. If the urinary ketones are found to be greater than moderate, then the patient may be entering into a "starvation state." Intravenous fluids should then be changed to something that includes dextrose.
   b. If the BS level subsequently exceeds 100 mg/dl as result of the start of this intravenous dextrose, then insulin drip should be initiated.
   c. It should be remembered that both glucose and insulin are necessary to prevent ketosis.

After delivery

1. During active labor, the need for insulin therapy is markedly decreased. In fact, many women with DM before pregnancy often require little or no insulin for several hours to days after the delivery.

2. Nevertheless, in women with type I DM before pregnancy, the need for insulin treatment will soon return, necessitating close follow-up blood sugar monitoring

Miscellaneous issues

1. Breast-feeding
   a. If BS levels remain high after delivery (glucose levels consistently >140 to 180 mg/dl), the glucose may "spill" into breast milk.
   b. Excess sugar in breast milk has been suggested to cause the newborn to be overweight or overactive. It may also cause the baby to prefer sweets in the future.
   c. BS should be well controlled before and during breast-feeding.
2. Need for other testing
   a. Thyroid disease is more common in patients with type I Diabetes.
      (1) Because thyroid disease often has few symptoms but can adversely affect the fetus, thyroid testing is recommended for pregnant women with type I Diabetes.
      (2) However, thyroid scans should never be obtained during pregnancy.
   b. Women with PGDM with the National Diabetes Data Criteria class A1 and A2-diet may not require antepartum fetal "stress" or "nonstress" testing, if their blood sugars remain under acceptable control.
   c. On an individual basis, women with PGDM with class A2-insulin or class B may benefit from weekly or biweekly NST or BPP around 32 to 34 weeks of pregnancy, especially if there is a suggestion of intrauterine growth restriction, hypertension, poorly controlled BS, or decreased or increased amniotic fluid volumes.
   d. In high-risk pregnant women with PGDM (class R or F), particularly if associated with a growth-retarded fetus, hypertension, poorly controlled BS, or increase or decrease in amniotic fluid, antepartum testing may start as early as 26 to 28 weeks and may be performed more frequently.
3. Drugs that affect BS
   a. Many drugs can increase BS in women with PGDM. For example, terbutaline and betamethasone may substantially increase BS in susceptible women.
   b. Although it has been suggested that some oral diabetes drugs may eventually prove beneficial in women with DM, these drugs have yet to be approved during pregnancy.
4. Glucosuria
   a. Glucosuria may result when BS exceeds 160 to 200 mg/dl.
   b. Because the timing of the onset of action of insulin delivered by subcutaneous insulin administration may not identically match the insulin secretion from a normal pancreas, glucosuria may result.
   c. Even in those patients with otherwise excellent BS control, some asynchrony of the timing of insulin action and insulin need is not uncommon. This may account for the occasional finding of significant glucosuria in a woman with type I DM who has excellent TGH/Hgb A1C, and excellent BS recorded by home glucose monitoring.

d. One method to improve the match of the hypoglycemic effects of insulin and the hyperglycemic effects of meals is to administer insulin ½ to 1 hour before meals.
e. Shorter acting insulin may soon be available that may improve the ability to better match the timing of insulin action and insulin need.

Practical examples (Tables 23-6 through 23-9)

Table 23-6 Illustrative blood sugar* level presentations of women with gestational diabetes treated with diet only

Example 1: Fasting Hyperglycemia

Fasting Urine Ketones†	Fasting Blood Sugar (mg/dl)	After-Breakfast Blood Sugar (mg/dl)	After-Lunch Blood Sugar (mg/dl)	After-Supper Blood Sugar (mg/dl)
Large	90-110	110-125	100-120	100-120

*"Blood sugar" represents a range of glucose blood levels as determined by home glucose monitoring for several days, after dietary counseling.
†"Fasting urine ketones" represents self–urine ketone testing by urine monitoring strips before breakfast

Comment and insulin recommendations: This woman with GDM (treated with diet alone) shows a common presentation of morning hyperglycemia with fasting urinary ketosis. A possible insulin regimen may include 6 U of NPH or lente at supper or bedtime. These long-acting insulins, given in the evening, would be expected to lower morning BS and resolve ketosis. Further adjustments or increases in insulin doses are made based upon future BS readings.

Example 2: After Supper Hyperglycemia

Fasting Urine Ketones†	Fasting Blood Sugar (mg/dl)	After-Breakfast Blood Sugar (mg/dl)	After-Lunch Blood Sugar (mg/dl)	After-Supper Blood Sugar (mg/dl)
Mild	80-100	100-120	100-120	120-160

Comment and insulin recommendations: This woman with GDM (treated with diet alone) shows a common presentation of after-supper hyperglycemia, accompanied by mild, occasional increases in morning BS. A possible insulin regimen may include 6 U of regular insulin at supper. This short-acting insulin would be expected to lower after-supper BS. And lowering the evening BS may have residual effect on the morning BS and urinary ketone levels. Alternatively, a combined regimen of 3 NPH or lente and 3 U regular, or 6 U of 50/50 insulin, may also have favorable effects on both the after-supper and before-breakfast BS, and fasting urinary ketone levels. Further adjustments or increases in insulin doses are made based upon future BS readings.

Table 23-7 Illustrative blood sugar level presentation of a women with pregestational diabetes mellitus before conception treated with a twice a day insulin regimen (before-breakfast and before-supper split dose NPH or Lente and regular insulin)

Example 1: Variable Blood Sugar After Supper

Fasting Urine Ketones	FBS (mg/dl)	PPBrkPS (mg/dl)	ACLunBS (mg/dl)	PPLunBS (mg/dl)	ACSupBS (mg/dl)	PPSupBS (mg/dl)	Bedtime BS (mg/dl)
Mild	60-180	80-120	60-100	80-120	60-100	100-180	60-180

FBS, Fasting blood sugar; *PPBrkBS*, postprandial breakfast blood sugar; *ACLunBS*, anteciba (before) lunch blood sugar; *PPLunBS*, postprandial lunch blood sugar; *ACSupBS*, before-supper blood sugar; *PPSupBS*, postprandial supper blood sugar.

Comment and insulin recommendations: This woman, with diabetes before pregnancy (treated with before-breakfast and before-supper insulin) presents with variable BS levels after supper and before breakfast. Because the BS levels are sometimes low at bedtime, increasing the before-supper regular insulin may increase the risk of bedtime hypoglycemia. Therefore, it may be recommended that supper meals be more consistent in composition, particularly with regard to amount and type of carbohydrates. However, another strategy may be to recommend three or four shots of insulin a day. Three shots of insulin a day would likely include (1) before-breakfast NPH or lente mixed with regular, (2) before-supper regular, and (3) bedtime NPH or lente. This would allow greater flexibility in insulin dosing, particularly before supper. Four shots of insulin a day may include before-meal regular, with nighttime NPH or lente. Before-breakfast NPH is also sometimes mixed with before-breakfast regular in patients treated with four shots of insulin a day. Afterwards, further adjustments or increases in insulin doses are made based upon future blood sugar readings.

Table 23-8 Illustrative blood sugar level presentations of women with type I diabetes mellitus, before conception, treated with a four times a day insulin regimen (premeal regular and nighttime NPH or lente)

Example 1: Gradually Increasing Blood Sugars

Fasting Urine Ketones	FBS (mg/dl)	PPBrkBS (mg/dl)	ACLunBS (mg/dl)	PPLunBS (mg/dl)	ACSupBS (mg/dl)	PPSupBS (mg/dl)	BedtimeBS (mg/dl)
Negative	60-90	80-120	90-110	90-130	100-140	100-140	80-120

FBS, Fasting blood sugar; *PPBrkBS,* postprandial breakfast blood sugar; *ACLunBS,* anteciba (before) lunch blood sugar; *PPL unBS,* postprandial lunch blood sugar; *ACSupBS,* before-supper blood sugar; *PPSupBS,* postprandial supper blood sugar.

Comment and insulin recommendations: This woman, with diabetes before pregnancy treated with intensive, four times a day insulin (premeal regular—before breakfast, before lunch, and before supper, and bedtime NPH or lente) presents with a gradual increase in before-meal blood sugars *and* a gradual increase in postprandial blood sugars throughout the day. One option would be to increase the before-lunch and before-supper regular insulin. Another option would be to add NPH or lente to before-breakfast regular insulin.

Example 2: Unpredictable Blood Sugars

Fasting Urine Ketones	FBS (mg/dl)	PPBrkBS (mg/dl)	ACLunBS (mg/dl)	PPLunBS (mg/dl)	ACSupBS (mg/dl)	PPSupBS (mg/dl)	BedtimeBS (mg/dl)
Negative	40-150	80-200	40-150	80-200	40-150	80-200	40-150

FBS, Fasting blood sugar; *PPBrkBS,* postprandial breakfast blood sugar; *ACLunBS,* anteciba (before) lunch blood sugar; *PPLunBS,* postprandial lunch blood sugar; *ACSupBS,* before-supper blood sugar; *PPSupBS,* postprandial supper blood sugar.

Comment and insulin recommendations: This woman, with diabetes before pregnancy treated with intensive, four times a day insulin treatment (premeal regular—before breakfast, before lunch, and before supper, and bedtime NPH or lente) presents with wide fluctuations in blood sugars. Any increase in before-meal insulin may result in hypoglycemia before the next meal or at bedtime. Therefore, recommendations would include improved dietary compliance and better adjustment of regular insulin dosing based on blood sugar, amount and type of carbohydrate consumption, anticipated level of physical activity, anticipated amount of physical or mental stress, etc. If these measures are not successful, then the use of an insulin pump should be considered.

Table 23-9 Illustrative blood sugar level presentation of a woman with type I diabetes mellitus before conception, treated with insulin pump

Example 1: Fasting Hyperglycemia								
Fasting Urine Ketones	FBS (mg/dl)	PPBrkBS (mg/dl)	ACLunBS (mg/dl)	PPLunBS (mg/dl)	ACSupBS (mg/dl)	PPSupBS (mg/dl)	BedtimeBS (mg/dl)	2 AM
Mild	90-120	80-120	60-110	80-120	60-110	80-120	60-110	60-110

Comment and insulin recommendations: This woman is treated with an insulin pump. She is receiving basal rate insulin and bolus insulin. Her basal insulin includes 2.0 U of regular insulin per hour between 7 AM and 10 PM, 1.0 U regular insulin per hour between 10 PM and 3 AM, and 2.5 U regular insulin per hour between 3 AM and 7 AM. She also receives bolus insulin based on her blood sugar, amount and composition of meals, anticipated exercise, and anticipated physical and mental stress. Her BS levels demonstrate fasting hyperglycemia with mild ketosis. This suggests a persistent effect of the "dawn phenomenon," despite the increased insulin basal rate of 3 AM to 7 AM. A reasonable approach would be to further increase the 3 AM to 7 AM basal rate.

Suggested reading

Bevier WC, Jovanovic-Peterson L, Peterson CM: Pancreatic disorders of pregnancy: diagnosis, management, and outcome of gestational diabetes, *Endo Metab Clin North Am* 24(1):103-138, 1995.

Burkart W, Hanker JP, Schneider HP: Complications and fetal outcome in diabetic pregnancy: intensified conventional versus insulin pump therapy, *Gynecol Obstet Invest* 26(2):104-112, 1988.

Healy K, Jovanovic-Peterson L, Peterson CM: Pancreatic disorders of pregnancy: pregestational diabetes, *Endo Metab Clin North Am* 24(1):73-102, 1995.

Hemachandra A et al: The influence of pregnancy on IDDM complications, *Diabetes Care* 18(7):950-954, 1995.

Knopp RH et al: Metabolic effects of hypocaloric diets in management of gestational diabetes, *Diabetes* 40(2):165-171, 1991.

Kuhl C: Insulin secretion and insulin resistance in pregnancy and GDM: implications during pregnancy, *Diabetes Care* 16(1):310-314, 1993.

23.3 INTRAUTERINE GROWTH RETARDATION

Mark Williams, M.D.

Significance

1. Low birth weight (LBW) is a worldwide problem.
   a. Usually defined as birthweight <2500 g, irrespective of gestational age
   b. Associated with increased perinatal morbidity and mortality
   c. Widely used as marker of increased neonatal risk
   d. Not an ideal marker of fetal growth and development
      (1) Combines both prematurity and varying degrees of growth retardation
2. Morbidity is associated with LBW and growth retardation.
   a. Twenty-one million LBW babies a year are born internationally, 90% in developing countries.
   b. Proportion of LBWs varies by type of society.
      (1) 3% to 12% rates of LBW in developed countries
         (a) 60% premature, 40% growth retarded
      (2) 12% to 40% rates of LBW in developing countries
         (a) 20% premature, 80% growth retarded
   c. There are high rates of perinatal morbidity in growth-retarded infants.
      (1) Perinatal depression is three times more likely.
      (2) Hypoglycemia is four to six times more likely.
      (3) Hypothermia is five times more likely.
      (4) Meconium aspiration is 13 times more likely.
      (5) Fetal distress in labor is six times more likely.
3. Components of LBW are as follows:
   a. Proportion of LBW varies by gestational age:
      (1) Of infants at 32 to 33 weeks gestation, 90% are LBW.
      (2) Of infants at 34 to 35 weeks gestation, 50% are LBW.
      (3) Of infants at 37 to 38 weeks gestation, 10% are LBW.
   b. Degree of growth retardation increases as gestational age increases.

4. It is important to distinguish between prematurity and degrees of growth retardation to better understand the etiology of perinatal morbidity and mortality.

Patterns of growth

1. General concepts
   a. Two overlapping periods of fetal cellular activity, cellular hyperplasia, and cellular hypertrophy, result in three phases of fetal growth and development.
      (1) First phase, occurring from 4 to 20 weeks gestation, is characterized by proportional increases in fetal weight, protein content, and DNA content (cellular hyperplasia).
      (2) Second phase, occurring from 20 to 28 weeks gestation, is characterized by increases in protein and weight and lesser increases in fetal DNA content (hyperplasia and concomitant hypertrophy).
      (3) Third phase, occurring from 28 weeks to term, is characterized by continued increases in fetal protein and weight but no increase in DNA content (hypertrophy).
   b. Population data
      (1) Numerous delivery populations have been described.
         (a) All populations show generally similar growth curves.
         (b) Infants from generally larger (sea level) populations weigh approximately 10% more than infants from smaller (altitude) populations in given racial, gender, gestational age, and birth weight for gestational age centile groups.
      (2) Fetal weight has a sigmoid growth pattern.
         (a) Linear growth occurs between 24 and 37 weeks gestation.
      (3) Fetuses tend to maintain a given centile range during pregnancy.
      (4) Increased variation in birth weights is noted in postterm infants.
      (5) Absolute birth weights drop in postterm infants.
   c. Timing of the insult to the fetus (predisposes to the type of growth retardation)
      (1) Early insults usually result in symmetric growth retardation.
         (a) Probably by restricting fetal cellular hyperplasia
      (2) Third-trimester insults restrict cellular hypertrophy.
         (a) Usually result in asymmetric growth retardation
            i. Uteroplacental insufficiency and other similar insults result in stresses on the fetus that cause the fetus to redistribute blood flow, maintaining perfusion of the head, heart, and adrenal glands.
            ii. Particularly severe insults to the fetus may cause asymmetric growth retardation to progress to symmetric growth retardation, as redistribution of blood flow fails to maintain growth of the head.
   d. Multiple gestation
      (1) Twins and higher order multiple gestation infants are at increased risk of growth retardation.
         (a) Increased rates of LBW for gestational age

(b) Increased rates of asymmetric growth restriction (abnormally lean body morphology)
(2) Twins have distinct patterns of growth.
(a) Growth patterns generally overlap singletons until 32 weeks gestation.
(b) Twins do not maintain singleton average birth weight growth in the last 6 to 8 weeks of pregnancy.
(c) The value of separate growth tables for twins is controversial.
(d) Discordance of more than 20% to 25% in birth weight relative to the larger twin is associated with IUGR and increased perinatal morbidity.

Definitions of growth retardation

1. Ideal criteria not well established
   a. Birthweight and length vary by many factors.
      (1) Gestational age (term > preterm)
      (2) Gender (male > female)
      (3) Ethnicity (white > black)
      (4) Multiple gestations (singletons > multiples)
      (5) Altitude (low altitude > high altitude)
      (6) Others (see later text)
   b. Some data are poorly documented.
      (1) Accuracy of gestational age assessment may vary.
      (2) Measures such as crown to heel length at term may be inaccurate.
      (3) Some measures of neonatal nutritional status are not always obtained.
         (a) Crown to heel length
         (b) Midarm circumference
         (c) Skin fold thickness
2. Gestational age assessment
   a. It is necessary to assign centile rankings of fetal weight properly by gestational age.
   b. Dubowitz scoring of infants often varies 1 or 2 weeks from menstrual dating.
      (1) Unavailable until after delivery of infant
   c. Obstetric dating is often inaccurate.
      (1) 15% of patients with proper dating criteria have sonographic dating findings that differ by more than 2 weeks from menstrual dating determinations.
3. Prenatal sonographic estimation of fetal weight
   a. Accuracy limited to ±15%
   b. Should be used with caution
   c. Accuracy less at extremes of estimated weight
   d. Decreased accuracy if fetal positioning precludes accurate measurements or if oligohydramnios is present
4. Types of markers of neonatal growth and development include the following:

a. Absolute measures
   (1) Example: LBW
   (2) Reproducible
   (3) Tend to "lump" prematurity and growth retardation into the same marker
b. Birth weight relative to gestational age, gender, ethnicity, etc.
   (1) Examples include the following:
      (a) Small for gestational age (LBW centile for gestational age)
      (b) Low fetal growth ratio (observed birth weight/adjusted birth weight)
   (2) Gestational age is not always accurately documented.
c. Body symmetry relative to gestational age
   (1) Examples include the following:
      (a) Ponderal index
      (b) Weight/length ratio
      (c) Body mass index (BMI)
      (d) Midarm circumference/head circumference ratio
   (2) Require gestational age and another body measure, such as length or midarm circumference.
      (a) Need for other measures increases possibility of erroneous values.
   (3) Identify abnormal growth patterns independent of absolute birth weight.
   (4) Identify groups of infants with otherwise normal birth weights who are at increased risk for perinatal mortality and morbidity.
      (a) Sixfold to 10-fold increases in rates of hypoglycemia, perinatal depression, meconium aspiration, and prolonged hospitalization.
   (5) Ponderal index may be better correlates of perinatal morbidity than birthweight for gestational age.

5. Correlation between markers and neonatal outcome
   a. Birth weight centile is the most commonly used marker of neonatal status.
   b. Some argue that markers incorporating weight for length, such as the weight/length ratio, may be better correlates of neonatal morbidity than LBW centile for gestational age.
6. Indices of growth retardation
   a. Small for gestational age (low percentile birth weight for gestational age)
      (1) Most commonly used method of neonatal and fetal assessment.
         (a) Birth weight <10% for gestational age usually used in the United States
         (b) Birth weight <2 S.D. (birth weight <2.5%) often used in Europe
      (2) Sensitivity and specificity can be adjusted by choice of centile range for population screening vs. more specific categorization of growth-retarded infants.
   b. Low birth weight (<2500 g)
      (1) Commonly used criterion to screen for neonatal risk
      (2) Robust, as error in weight determination is minimal

(3) Confounded by conflicting influences of prematurity and growth retardation
(4) Does not require accurate knowledge of gestational age

c. Fetal growth ratio (FGR)
(1) FGR = observed birth weight/adjusted mean birth weight.
(2) Reference mean values for gestational age are relatively easy to determine.
(3) Adjustments for gender and ethnicity are easy to determine.
(4) Correlates well with birth weight centiles.
(a) FGR <0.90 occurs in 18% of patients.
(b) FGR <0.85 occurs in 9.0% of patients.
(c) FGR <0.80 occurs in 4.3% of patients.
(d) FGR <0.75 occurs in 1.7% of patients.

d. Ponderal index
(1) Ponderal index = 100 (birth weight in g)/(length in cm)^3.
(2) Ponderal index requires length, as well as other standard data regarding birth weight, gestational age, and occasionally race and gender.
(3) Use of body length in ratios may decrease sensitivity of marker because of inaccuracy often associated with crown to heel measurements.
(a) Use of cubed length term may further decrease accuracy of this marker.
(4) Index varies by gestational age, and by gender and ethnicity to a much smaller degree.

Weeks	10%	3%
30 weeks	2.05	2.00
32 weeks	2.10	2.05
34 weeks	2.15	2.10
36 weeks	2.23	2.15
≥38 weeks	2.30	2.20

(5) Low ponderal index, a marker of asymmetric growth restriction, is associated with increased perinatal morbidity.

e. Weight/length ratio
(1) Weight/length = birth weight in g/length in cm.
(2) This requires length, as well as other standard data regarding birth weight, gestational age, and occasionally race and gender.
(3) Use of body length in ratios may decrease sensitivity of marker because of inaccuracy often associated with crown to heel measurements.
(4) Ratio varies by gestational age, and by gender and ethnicity to a much smaller degree.
(5) Weight/length ratio <5% or 10%, asymmetric growth restriction, is associated with increased perinatal morbidity.

f. BMI
(1) BMI = birth weight in g/(length in cm)^2.
(2) BMI requires length as well as other standard data regarding birth weight, gestational age, and occasionally race and gender.
(3) Use of body length in ratios may decrease sensitivity of marker because of inaccuracy often associated with crown to heel measurements.

(4) BMI varies by gestational age, and by gender and ethnicity to a much smaller degree.
(5) BMI has not been extensively evaluated as a marker of neonatal status.

g. Midarm circumference/head circumference (MAC/HC).
(1) HC/MAC = head circumference/midarm circumference
(2) Possibly a better marker of neonatal status than ratios of weight to length or birthweight for gestational age
(3) Varies by gestational age.

Weeks	MAC/HC (±1 S.D.)
30	0.23 (0.02)
32	0.24 (0.02)
34	0.26 (0.02)
36	0.27 (0.01)
38	0.28 (0.01)
40	0.29 (0.02)
42	0.30 (0.01)

7. Markers for abnormal fetal growth in multiple gestation
a. Discordance in estimated sonographic fetal weights of 20% to 25% using the larger twin as the index case
b. Intratwin pair differences in biparietal diameter: >5 mm
c. Intratwin pair differences in abdominal circumference: >20 mm
d. Intratwin pair differences in femur length: >4 mm

8. Sonographic (antenatal) markers of abnormal fetal growth
a. Estimated fetal weight
(1) Many formulas are available.
(2) Combinations of biparietal diameter, head circumference, and femur length with the abdominal circumference should be used.
(3) Estimated fetal weight is generally accurate to ± 15%.
(a) Larger margins of error at extremes of weight range and if oligohydramnios is present

b. Head circumference/abdominal circumference ratio
(1) This ratio is useful to detect asymmetric growth restriction caused by "head sparing effect" active in most cases of growth retardation late.
(2) Values vary by gestational age.

c. Femur length/abdomen circumference ratio
(1) Minimal variation is seen during pregnancy: 0.224 ± 0.015 (mean ± 1 S.D.).
(2) The ratio is altered if skeletal dysplasia is present.

9. Doppler sonography
a. Systolic/diastolic flow velocity ratios correlate with placental resistance.
(1) Decrease over the course of pregnancy.
(2) Increased values for gestational age indicate increased placental resistance.
(3) Absent or reversed end diastolic flow is often associated with imminent fetal compromise.
(a) Reversed flow has occasionally been noted to resolve.

(4) Fetuses with estimated fetal weights in the growth retarded range and normal Doppler flow indices are at increased risk of aneuploidy.

Causes of growth retardation

1. Incorrect dates
   a. Overestimation of gestational age causes centile birth weight to be lower than is actually the case.
   b. Underestimation of gestational age may mask the presence of growth retardation.
2. Aneuploidy
   a. Autosomal trisomies
      (1) Trisomy 13
      (2) Trisomy 18
      (3) Trisomy 21
   b. Triploidy
   c. Turner's syndrome
   d. Extra sex (X) chromosomes (47 XXY, etc.)
      (1) Average birth weight decreases by 300 g per each additional X chromosome.
   e. Autosomal deletion syndromes
      (1) 5p- (cri du chat)
      (2) 5q-
      (3) 4p-
      (4) 4q-
      (5) 18p-
      (6) 18q-
      (7) Others
3. Open neural tube disorders
4. Renal agenesis
5. Chondrodystrophies
6. Single umbilical artery
7. Maternal factors
   a. Medical conditions
      (1) Advanced stage diabetes (>White class B)
      (2) Collagen vascular disease
         (a) Polymyositis or dermatomyositis
         (b) Systemic lupus erythematosus
      (3) Cyanotic heart disease
      (4) Hypertension
      (5) Renal disease (chronic) without hypertension
      (6) Thyrotoxicosis
   b. Obstetric factors
      (1) Pregnancy-induced hypertension
      (2) Primigravidity
      (3) Prior miscarriage, stillborn, or growth-retarded infant
      (4) Multiple gestation
   c. Medications
      (1) Chemotherapeutic antimetabolites
      (2) Coumadin

   (3) Phenytoin
   (4) Systemic steroid usage
d. Socioeconomic factors
   (1) Poor nutritional status
      (a) Low prepregnancy weight
      (b) Low pregnancy weight gain
      (c) Dietary deficiencies (zinc, others?)
   (2) Substance abuse
      (a) Tobacco
      (b) Ethanol
      (c) Drugs
e. Ethnicity
f. Infection
   (1) Bacterial
      (a) *Listeria*
      (b) Malaria
      (c) Syphilis
      (d) Toxoplasmosis
      (e) Tuberculosis
   (2) Viral
      (a) Cytomegalovirus
      (b) Rubella

Detection of growth retardation

1. Firm obstetric dates should be established.
   a. Dates are established on the first obstetric visit.
   b. Dating should be modified later in gestation with caution and always with proper documentation.
   c. Menstrual and sonographic dating information must be coordinated.
      (1) Sonograms are generally accurate to within 10% of the composite gestational age.
      (2) Sonography before 22 to 24 weeks gestation is relatively reliable for the purposes of pregnancy dating.
         (a) If a reliable menstrual history of completely regular cycles for the prior 3 months, no hormonal interventions for at least 3 months, and certain dating of the last normal menses is obtained, menstrual dating is accepted if those dates place the gestational age within 10% of the ultrasonographic dates.
         (b) Even if all criteria in 1.c.(2).(a). are met, but the sonographic dating places the gestational age more than 10% earlier or later, the sonographic dating criteria are accepted.
         (c) In the first trimester, trisomy 18 causes significant growth retardation but is sufficiently rare that it does not cause significant problems with pregnancy dating in the first half of pregnancy.
      (3) Sonography after 22 to 24 weeks gestation to establish pregnancy dating can allow cases of early fetal growth disturbances to go undiagnosed.

(a) Caution should be used if sonographic dating after 22 to 24 weeks gestation is necessary.

(b) If significant disparity is present between sonographic fetal dating information and menstrual dating information, it may be necessary to perform interval fetal surveillance until serial growth measures allow distinctions between incorrect dating and growth retardation to be made.

i. Factors that should heighten concern for significant growth retardation include oligohydramnios, presence of fetal anomalies, and asymmetric growth indices (abnormally small abdominal circumference for gestation or abnormally elevated HC/AC or femur length [FL]/abdominal circumference [AC] ratios)

(c) Symmetric growth retardation will be categorized as having a gestational age less than the actual value if no other credible dating information is available, and symmetric growth retardation will escape detection in such circumstances.

(d) Early macrosomic fetal growth trends may cause an overestimate of the gestational age.

2. The risk of growth retardation in the pregnancy should be evaluated based on initial history, physical findings, and laboratory evaluations of the patient.
   a. Although commonly employed and inexpensive, fundal height assessment has an unacceptably low negative predictive value for growth retardation in high-risk populations, such as hypertensives, insulin-dependent diabetics, and patients with collagen vascular disorders.
   b. Serial sonographic evaluations during the pregnancy should be considered if a significant risk of growth retardation exists.
3. Methods of serial assessment include the following:
   a. Weight gain
      (1) Monitoring the patient's weight gain and ensuring minimum standards are achieved
   b. Symphisio fundal height measurements
      (1) The symphyseal to fundal height measurement (in cm) approximates the menstrual gestational age in weeks from 20 weeks to approximately 37 weeks.
         (a) Less reliable if the maternal body habitus is obese
         (b) Not useful in multiple gestations
      (2) Sonography is used to evaluate deviations of more than 3 cm in fundal height from expected values.
      (3) Sonography detects approximately 50% to 60% of cases of growth retardation.
         (a) Suitable for screening of low-risk populations
         (b) Not sufficiently reliable as the only screening modality in patients at high risk of growth retardation
   c. Serial sonographic estimated fetal weights
      (1) Gestational age should be established, preferably in the first trimester.

(2) Estimated fetal weight should be assessed after 24 weeks, at 3-week to 6-week intervals.
   (a) Intervals of less than 2 weeks may fail to detect ongoing growth.
(3) Various parameters are useful to assess fetal growth.
   (a) Estimated fetal weight for gestational age
   (b) Abdominal circumference
   (c) Ratios of head circumference or femur length to abdominal circumference

d. Doppler sonography
   (1) Normal Doppler waveforms indicate normal placental resistance.
      (a) Normal waveforms in growth retardation
         i. May indicate genetic predisposition to small fetal size
         ii. Indicate increased risk of aneuploidy
   (2) Doppler sonography is not useful for screening in low-risk populations.

Management of growth retardation

1. Accuracy of obstetric dating must be determined.
   a. Dating should be reassigned with care.
2. Possibility of aneuploidy should be considered.
   a. Symmetric growth retardation is often associated with aneuploidy.
   b. Normal umbilical Doppler flow or normal amniotic fluid volume in fetuses with apparent ultrasonographic growth retardation indicate increased risk for aneuploidy.
   c. Negative targeted sonograms decrease likelihood of syndromes associated with high rates of structural anomalies, such as trisomy 13 or 18.
   d. Negative targeted sonograms in syndromes with low rates of detectable sonographic anomalies, such as trisomy 21, do not appreciably lower the *a priori* risk of this in a given pregnancy.
   e. Karyotypic evaluation by amniocentesis, placental biopsy, umbilical arterial blood sampling, and occasionally karyotype from the fetal urinary bladder are possible if documentation of the fetal karyotype is judged necessary.
3. Clinical circumstances must be evaluated.
   a. Is the index of suspicion for severe growth retardation and imminent fetal death high?
   b. Do the potential benefits of ongoing fetal assessment and (hopefully) continued growth and development sufficiently balance the perceived risks of continuing the pregnancy?
      (1) Benefits of delaying delivery
         (a) Allows time to reassess interval growth and possibly identify cases of incorrect dating.
         (b) Allows time for further growth of the fetus and maturation of critical fetal organ systems
         (c) Decreases subsequent need for neonatal care
         (d) Increases likelihood of subsequent labor induction, if necessary

(2) Risks of delaying delivery
   (a) Ongoing disease processes may put fetus at risk of increased morbidity or mortality.
   (b) Temporization in fetuses near term or at term gestation may not yield any significant gain in growth, development, or maturation of fetal organ systems.
   (c) Cases of falsely diagnosed growth retardation (i.e., incorrectly dated pregnancies) may receive unnecessary interventions, including cesarean delivery after failed induction of labor.
   (d) Increases the need for emergency (cesarean) delivery if fetal status unexpectedly deteriorates.

c. Common clinical presentations
   (1) Size–dates discrepancy noted in the third trimester, no early sonogram.
      (a) Presentation
         i. A patient presents for care in the mid-second trimester and no significant disparity between menstrual dating and physical examination findings (16-cm fundal height at 18 weeks gestation) is noted.
         ii. Maternal serum alpha-feloprotein (MSAFP) testing shows a low normal value (0.6 multiple of median [MOM]).
         iii. Menstrual dates are accepted.
         iv. The pregnancy progresses and a fundal height discrepancy is noted at 32 weeks gestation by dates (28-cm fundal height).
         v. A sonogram is performed that shows biparietal diameter, head circumference, abdominal circumference, and femur length all approximate 28 weeks size, and amniotic fluid volume is normal.
         vi. Doppler flow indices show normal diastolic flow.
      (b) Differential diagnosis
         i. Symmetric growth retardation (rare)
         ii. Incorrect dates (very common)
      (c) Plan
         i. Patient is questioned regarding accuracy of menstrual dating.
         ii. If history remains consistent with reliable dates, fetal electronic assessment weekly, weekly amniotic fluid assessment, and a follow-up sonogram in 3 weeks to assess for interval growth are considered.
         iii. Amniocentesis for karyotype may also be a consideration, depending on maternal age and sonographic findings.
         iv. If normal interval growth for a 28 week gestation fetus occurs, the most likely diagnosis is incorrect dates.
         v. If inadequate growth occurs, growth retardation is more likely.

vi. If growth retardation appears likely, careful evaluation with serial fetal assessment and delivery when risks to the fetus appear to outweigh perceived benefit of waiting are done.

vii. Severe degrees of growth retardation may increase the clinical utility of karyotypic evaluation.

(2) Size–dates discrepancy, early sonographic dating

(a) Presentation

i. A patient presents for care in the mid-second trimester and no significant disparity between menstrual dating and physical examination findings (16-cm fundal height at 18 weeks gestation) is noted.

ii. MSAFP testing is low (0.4 MOM).

iii. Ultrasonography in preparation for genetic amniocentesis reveals biparietal diameter, head circumference, and femur length consistent with 15 weeks gestation at the time of MSAFP testing, when 18 weeks gestation had been assumed.

iv. The 3-week disparity is greater than 10% of the menstrual dating gestational age, and sonographic dates are accepted.

v. The MSAFP is recomputed based on new dating information, and a new MSAFP value of 0.7 MOM is determined.

vi. The pregnancy continues and fundal height discrepancy is noted at 32 weeks gestation by dates (28-cm fundal height).

vii. A sonogram is performed that shows biparietal diameter, head circumference, abdominal circumference, and femur length all approximate 28-weeks size, and amniotic fluid volume is normal.

viii. Doppler flow indices show normal diastolic flow.

(b) Diagnosis: symmetric growth retardation

(c) Comment: Because of the mid-second trimester sonography, the dating of the pregnancy is firmly established and, in rare cases, adjustment of the dates to a lower value may have temporarily masked the presence of early fetal growth retardation (sometimes associated with aneuploidies such as trisomy 18). The normal Doppler flow pattern indicates that placental (vascular) disease is not likely the cause and increases the risk of aneuploidy.

(d) Plan

i. Targeted sonography is performed; electronic fetal assessment, serial evaluation of amniotic fluid volume, and interval sonography for fetal growth are begun, in 2 to 3 weeks.

ii. Amniocentesis should be considered for karyotype.

iii. Given the presentation, it is unlikely that growth will normalize.

iv. The principle goal of surveillance is to allow adequate time to exclude the presence of semilethal aneuploidies such as trisomy 13, trisomy 18, and triploidy.
v. If such aneuploidies are detected, cesarean section for fetal distress is not recommended, after careful explanation of the rationale for avoiding such surgery, where it will provide minimal fetal benefit and much more potential for maternal harm.
vi. Delivery should be considered if fetal assessment yields information suggesting imminent fetal compromise before documenting the fetal karyotype.
vii. If a normal fetal karyotype is present, timing of delivery will depend on results of ongoing fetal assessment, cervical ripeness for induction, degree of growth retardation (i.e., perceived fetal risk), and gestational age.

(3) Size–dates discrepancy, late access to care
(a) Presentation
i. A patient presents for care in the third trimester and no significant disparity between menstrual dating and physical examination findings (26-cm fundal height at 28 weeks gestation) is noted, although the patient's recollection of her menstrual history is somewhat unclear.
ii. No sonographic assessment is performed.
iii. The pregnancy continues and, 4 weeks later, a fundal height discrepancy is noted at 32 weeks gestation by dates (28-cm fundal height).
iv. A sonogram is performed that shows biparietal diameter, head circumference, abdominal circumference, and femur length all approximate 28-weeks size, and the amniotic fluid volume is normal.
v. Doppler flow indices show normal diastolic flow.

(b) Differential diagnosis
i. Symmetric growth retardation (rare)
ii. Incorrect dates (very common)

(c) Comment:
i. Because of the lack of any proper dating criteria, accurate pregnancy dating is impossible.
ii. Because of the rarity of symmetric growth retardation and the high incidence of incorrect dating in such circumstances, the likelihood of significant fetal pathology is minimal.
iii. Because dating is at best uncertain, growth retardation cannot be strongly suspected in such circumstances, and further invasive clinical evaluation with amniocentesis is usually best deferred until the diagnosis is better established.

(d) Plan

i. Interval sonography for fetal growth is performed in 3 weeks, and serial electronic fetal assessment on a weekly basis until fetal growth has been reevaluated is considered.

ii. Repeat evaluation of the fetal size in such circumstances will usually show normal interval growth for a fetus of the indicated sonographic age.

iii. If normal growth is seen, pregnancy dates are changed to sonographic dates, the reasons for the change are documented in the chart, and the pregnancy is allowed to continue.

iv. In the rare event of inadequate growth, the plan of evaluation and management would be as noted in 3.c.(2).

Methods of fetal assessment

1. General principles
   a. The possibility of false-positive results (i.e., disease indicated when not present) should always be considered.
   b. A positive result in a high-risk patient population has a stronger positive predictive value than a similar result in a low-risk patient.
   c. The minimum interval for many tests is not well established.
      (1) The number of patients necessary to establish distinctions between weekly and twice weekly surveillance precludes the possibility of performing such a study at any individual center.
      (2) Anecdotal reports suggest twice weekly testing is somewhat more sensitive than weekly testing.
   d. Most assessments are valid after 31 weeks gestation.
      (1) In expert hands, may be applied in range of 24 to 31 weeks gestation
2. Fetal movement counts
   a. Counts are not proven useful by prospective studies.
   b. Retrospective reports often document decreased fetal movement within 24 to 48 hours before fetal demise.
   c. Time to achieve 10 perceived fetal movements from waking up is noted.
      (1) Lack of 10 movements by noon or 1 PM should be investigated by electronic fetal assessment.
      (2) Significantly increased time required to achieve 10 movements should be investigated by electronic fetal assessment (NST, contraction stress testing [CST], or biophysical profile [BPP]).
3. NST
   a. NSTs should be performed weekly or twice weekly, depending on index of suspicion of growth retardation and perceived degree of growth retardation.
   b. Depending on gestational age and cervical ripeness, abnormal testing (nonreactive test) should usually be reevaluated with contraction stress testing or biophysical profiling.

4. CST
   a. CSTs may be administered by controlled nipple stimulation or oxytocin infusion.
   b. Uterine hyperstimulation may occasionally occur.
   c. Once weekly testing is usually adequate.
   d. Depending on gestational age, delivery should be considered for abnormal (positive) test result.
5. BPP
   a. Uses 10-point system (usually)
      (1) Two points are awarded during 30-minute observation for each of the following five criteria:
         (a) Presence of at least one 2 cm × 2 cm amniotic fluid pocket
         (b) Reactive NST
         (c) Presence of 30 seconds of fetal breathing movements
         (d) Presence of one episode of active extension and return to flexion of the fetal limbs, spine, or trunk, or opening and closing of a hand
         (e) Presence of three discrete body or limb movements (Episodes of active continuous movements are considered one movement.)
   b. Biophysical score used to plan obstetric management
      (1) Scores of 8 or 10 indicate low risk for ongoing fetal hypoxia.
      (2) Score of 6 indicates mild suspicion of ongoing fetal hypoxia.
         (a) Testing with BPP repeated in 4 to 6 hours, or with CST.
         (b) If oligohydramnios and gestational age >35 weeks, delivery is considered.
      (3) Score of 4 indicates moderate suspicion of ongoing fetal hypoxia.
         (a) If >35 weeks gestation, delivery is considered.
         (b) if <35 weeks gestation, benefits of CST or repeated serial BPP are evaluated vs. delivery.
      (4) Score of 0 to 2 indicates high risk for ongoing fetal hypoxia.
         (a) If preterm, testing time is extended to up to 120 minutes.
         (b) Persistent scores of 0 or 2 indicate need for delivery.
         (c) If at term, delivery may be appropriate before completion of 120-minute extended evaluation.
   c. Modified BPP
      (1) Normal amniotic fluid volume in combination with either reactive NST or 30 seconds fetal breathing movements is strongly predictive of adequate fetal oxygenation.
      (2) If normal modified criteria are present, other components of biophysical profile are unnecessary.
6. Amniotic fluid volume
   a. Two common methods of assessment are as follows:
      (1) Single-pocket technique
         (a) Presence of at least one 2 cm × 2 cm (or one 1 cm × 1 cm) pocket of amniotic fluid indicates adequate amniotic fluid volume.
      (2) Amniotic fluid index
         (a) Deepest vertical amniotic fluid pocket in each of four uterine quadrants is measured.

(b) Need for pocket to be completely free of umbilical cord is controversial.
(c) Values vary with gestational age.
(d) Values less than 5 to 6 cm quadrants indicate oligohydramnios.
(e) Values in excess of 25 cm quadrants indicate polyhydramnios.
i. If present, evaluation of maternal and fetal correlates of polyhydramnios is indicated.

b. Weekly evaluations are done for patients at risk for oligohydramnios.
c. If oligohydramnios is present, the possibility of ruptured membranes should always be considered.
d. Consider delivery if oligohydramnios is present at term.

7. Sonographic assessment of fetal growth
   a. Many formulas are available to estimate fetal weight.
   b. Physician should use weight derived by the same formula to perform interval comparisons.
   c. An interval of 3 or more weeks is usually necessary for meaningful comparisons of serial growth.

Suggested reading

Divon M, editor: *Abnormal fetal growth,* New York, 1991, Elsevier Science Publishing.

Gross TL, Sokol RJ, editors: *Intrauterine growth retardation—a practical approach,* Chicago, 1989, Year Book Medical Publisher.

Kurjak A, Beazley JM, editors: *Fetal growth retardation: diagnosis and treatment,* Boca Raton, 1989, CRC Press.

23.4 GENETIC COUNSELING

Beth Buehler, M.S.

Guiding principles in genetic counseling

1. Philosophy
   a. Genetic counselors encourage their clients to make informed decisions that reflect the clients' own personal beliefs and values.
   b. Genetic counseling requires knowledge of the specific condition, including the following:
      (1) The clinical presentation
      (2) The natural prognosis
      (3) The diagnosis capabilities, including carrier and prenatal testing if available
   c. A genetic counselor must have communication skills, counseling skills, and time necessary to transmit complex medical information to the family and encourage decision making.
   d. Genetic counselors recognize their own biases but provide nondirective counseling.
   e. They support the informed decisions made by their clients.
2. Goals of genetic counseling in the prenatal setting
   a. Understanding of the medical information
      (1) The client is given the most current and accurate information concerning the pregnancy and the fetus requiring diagnosis,

appropriate therapies, management of the condition, and etiology of the condition.

b. Comprehending the recurrence risk
   (1) The mode of inheritance should be clearly explained (using the client's own pedigree to show inheritance) to the couple or family members
   (2) Recurrence risks may include empirical data (example: nonspecific mental retardation with cause unknown), calculated risks, or Mendelian genetics risks (25% recurrence risk for cystic fibrosis when a couple are known carriers).
   (3) Clients appreciate risks in many different ways.
      (a) Numerical risk (Risk for 35-year-old woman to have a child born with chromosomal abnormality is $1/192$ or 0.5%.)
      (b) Inverse numerical risk (Risk for 35-year-old woman to have a child without a chromosomal abnormality is $191/192$ or 99.5%.)
      (c) Concrete thinking (Either the event will occur or it will not.)
      (d) Comparison of losses and gains (The condition is analyzed comparing what is the benefit versus what is the risk, positive versus negative aspects of decision.)
   (4) Genetic counselors should encourage clients to evaluate risks in more than one way to understand their implications fully.

c. Realization of options:
   (1) When deciding whether or not to have prenatal testing clients understand advantages and disadvantages and may choose from a variety of options including no testing (example: chorionic villus sampling [CVS], early amniocentesis, ultrasound alone, or no testing).
   (2) Options are listed in no particular order to ensure nondirective counseling and examples of different options for different families are emphasized.

d. Empowering clients to make decisions
   (1) The couple is encouraged to choose the best course of action for themselves in light of the medical information, their values and beliefs, the psychological implications (e.g., anxiety over knowing the fetus has Tay-Sachs disease but knowing they would not choose to terminate for religious reasons), and the goals of the family.
   (2) Encouraging the couple to make their own decisions puts control of the pregnancy back in their hands.
      (a) Many families feel decisions are made around them or because their doctor told them to do something.
      (b) These are the clients more likely to blame the doctor if there is a problem or to have unresolved guilt concerning an unhealthy pregnancy.
   (3) If the client becomes a part of the team deciding what is best for the pregnancy she will more easily adjust to the outcome.

The prenatal genetic session

Individuals are referred for genetic counseling for expert information on specific genetic conditions, possible carrier and prenatal testing, risk evaluation, and guidance in decision making for the family or individual.

1. Indications for genetic counseling referral are as follows:
   a. Advanced maternal age (amniocentesis or CVS is offered to pregnant woman who will be age 35 years or older at time of delivery; see Table 23-10)
   b. Known or suspected hereditary condition in family
   c. Exposure to known or suspected teratogens
   d. A fetus or child with birth defects
   e. Previous multiple miscarriages (three or more) or stillbirth baby
   f. Mental retardation in client or family member
   g. Ethnic population with increased risk for genetic condition (Tay-Sachs in Ashkenazi Jewish population)
   h. Consanguinity
   i. Individual with known genetic condition or birth defect
2. Gathering information
   a. It is important to have all the medical information concerning a client before appropriate genetic counseling can be accomplished.
   b. Analysis of multiple pieces of information is routine in genetics before the most likely diagnosis and recurrence risk can be determined.
   c. Genetic disorders carry with them some stigma, and clients are reluctant to divulge information to individuals they do not trust.
   d. Establishing a good rapport and feelings of trust is imperative to obtaining accurate information from the client.

Table 23-10 Chromosome abnormalities in liveborn deliveries

Maternal Age	Risk for Down Syndrome	Any Chromosome Abnormality
35	1/378	1/192
36	1/289	1/156
37	1/224	1/127
38	1/173	1/102
39	1/136	1/83
40	1/106	1/66
41	1/82	1/53
42	1/63	1/42
43	1/44	1/33
44	1/38	1/26
45	1/30	1/21
46	1/23	1/16
47	1/18	1/13
48	1/14	1/10
49	1/11	1/8

e. The pedigree
  (1) This is the most important tool for establishing the mode of inheritance in a family.
  (2) How to construct a pedigree.
    (a) Specific questions should be asked. (How many pregnancies have you had with Mr. B? versus How many pregnancies have you had?)
    (b) Information should never be assumed. (Three pregnancies does not mean three living children.)
    (c) Clearly defined symbols should be used, with a key for interpretation.
    (d) The informant and the historian should be identified, and the interview dated. (This will make sure the pedigree can be understood and updated in the future by anyone who reviews it.)
    (e) Counselor should ask specifically about mental retardation, birth defects, multiple miscarriages, consanguinity, genetic conditions, reasons for death, and age at time of death.
  (3) Analysis of pedigree: Careful analysis of the pedigree can establish mode of inheritance (see Mode of Inheritance, on p. 512, for detail).

f. Reviewing past medical information
  (1) Autopsy findings
  (2) Photography of affected family member
  (3) Reports of surgical procedures
  (4) Laboratory reports (chromosomes, DNA studies, complete blood count [CBC])
  (5) Ultrasound reports

g. Clinical diagnosis
  (1) Visual assessment
    (a) Counselor should make eye contact with the client throughout genetic counseling session.
      i. Does the client understand the information?
      ii. Does he or she have any unusual physical characteristics, peculiar movements, or obvious medical problems not discussed (example: the client has a suspicious scar on lip and nasal speech but has not mentioned having a cleft lip or palate)?
  (2) Referral to clinical geneticist
    (a) The client or family member has one or more multiple congenital anomalies but no diagnosis.
      i. Counselor should refer client to clinical geneticist for diagnosis.
      ii. An incorrect diagnosis can change a client's recurrence risks, prenatal testing, and family planning options.
      iii. If after the medical literature is reviewed the diagnosis is suspected to be incorrect, client should be referred to a specialist to make the appropriate diagnosis.

3. Counseling parents
   a. Counselor should establish rapport.
      (1) The first 1 to 3 minutes of the session should be used to introduce oneself and find out a little about the client.
      (2) These 3 minutes will establish a foundation for trust from the client.
   b. Counselor should investigate the client's agenda.
      (1) The client may be concerned about issues different from those he or she was referred for.
      (2) Ascertaining what the client feels is important and alerts the counselor to additional issues for the session and lets the client know he or she is being heard and that his or her concerns will be addressed.
   c. Counselor should explain personal agenda.
      (1) Counselor should explain what he or she will do during the genetic counseling session and in what order.
      (2) Explaining the counseling agenda before starting helps to keep the genetic counseling session focused and the client aware of its goals.
   d. Counselor should repeat information.
      (1) Counselor should be prepared to repeat the medical information more than once and in more than one way. (It is desirable to use pictures, diagrams, and visual aids, as well as giving examples.)
      (2) A follow-up letter should be sent to review complex information.
   e. Counselor should invite questions.
      (1) Counselor should stop several times to invite questions on each subtopic before moving to the next agenda items.
      (2) Counselor should make sure the client understands the information without intimidating him or her. (Am *I* making myself clear? vs. Do *you* understand?)
4. Giving bad news
   a. In person
      (1) Counselor should insist that a client come to the office to get bad news.
      (2) The telephone should be used only as a means to get the client into the office. (Mrs. Jones, the chromosome analysis is finalized, and we would like you and your husband to come in to discuss the information as soon as possible.)
   b. Counselor should never call client at work.
      (1) Only when a client has specifically asked ahead of time to be called with bad news at work and he or she understands the awkwardness and shock this will cause, or when he or she cannot be reached otherwise, should the client be called at work.
      (2) It is devastating to receive bad news in the workplace.
   c. Counselor should give news humanely.
      (1) Counselor should always express sympathy for the diagnosis.
      (2) In retrospect, the simple act of saying "I'm sorry" helps the patient in the grieving process.

d. The actual news
   (1) The information discussed during the bad news session varies depending on what type of testing has been done, the accuracy of the testing, and the degree of severity of the problem.
   (2) A specific diagnosis necessitates that clients be given appropriate medical information, be able to review their options and recurrence risks for themselves and family members, and have support information.
   (3) Nonspecific problems without diagnosis necessitate explanation of follow-up medical procedures or tests and support.
      (a) The emotional impact of not having a diagnosis is many times far worse for families because they are left with many unanswered questions and unresolved anxiety.

e. Follow-up
   (1) A written letter is sent to the client with the information discussed, recurrence risk, natural prognosis of condition, and the decision to use as a permanent record and to review for the future, or as reference when explaining to the other family members what has happened.
      (a) A follow-up telephone call after a termination of pregnancy helps the client grieve.
      (b) Referral to specific specialist (example: a neurologist needs to talk with a client who chooses to continue a pregnancy with myelomeningocele).

Mode of inheritance

Autosomal dominant inheritance

One gene on an autosomal chromosome (chromosome 1 through 22) causes the condition.

1. Criteria
   a. Chromosome affects both male and female equally since the gene is contained on an autosomal chromosome.
   b. Trait appears in every generation.
      (1) The pedigree is vertical (example: III-A).
      (2) Exceptions to this rule include new mutations in a family and decreased expressivity.
   c. There is a 50% recurrence risk in any pregnancy of affected individuals.
   d. Unaffected family members do not transmit the trait to their children.
      (1) If an individual does not have the gene, the risk of having an affected child is no greater than the general population risk.
2. Genetic counseling
   a. Counselor should establish diagnosis.
      (1) Counselor should examine the client and question siblings and other possible relatives for characteristics of the disorder.
      (2) Counselor should rely on a medical geneticist to establish the diagnosis or should obtain medical records with stated diagnostic criteria.

b. Counselor should explain recurrence risk for individual.
c. Counselor should explain developmental pathology and how the condition originates from a single dominant gene.
d. Counselor should outline natural history and management.

3. Examples of autosomal dominant disorders are as follows:
   a. Neurofibromatosis type I
      (1) Characterized by café-au-lait spots, axillary freckling, external and internal tumors, and growth abnormalities.
      (2) Highly variable expressivity with 50% being new mutations with no family history.
      (3) The gene is located on chromosome 17.
   b. Achondroplasia
      (1) Eighty percent are new mutations.
      (2) Mating of two individuals with achondroplasia can cause lethal dwarfism in 25% of offspring.

Autosomal recessive inheritance

Condition is caused by two genes inherited from specific autosomal chromosome of each parent or of affected individual.

1. Criteria
   a. Males and females are equally likely to be affected since the gene is on an autosomal chromosome.
   b. Pedigree is typically horizontal, with siblings affected, not parents or offspring (III-B).
   c. There is a 25% recurrence risk when both parents are found to be carriers (having one gene each).
2. Genetic counseling
   a. Individuals with one gene are not affected (heterozygous).
   b. Condition is expressed only when a double dose of the gene is present (homozygous).
   c. Chance to have normal children is 75% when both parents are carriers.
   d. Counselor should explain the nature of the condition, carrier testing or prenatal testing and newborn screening if available, and management.
3. Examples are as follows:
   a. Cystic fibrosis (see Genetic Screening by Ethnic Background, Cystic Fibrosis, below.)
   b. Phenylketonuria (PKU)
      (1) PKU is a defect in enzyme phenylalanine hydroxylase.
      (2) Children are normal at birth but cannot digest phenylalanine.
      (3) If children are not put on a specific diet low in phenylalanine, they will become mentally retarded.
      (4) Women of childbearing age should also be on a restrictive diet to prevent having mentally retarded children because of the high maternal plasma phenylalanine.

X-Linked recessive

The gene is inherited on the X chromosome and expressed in males with one gene and only in homozygous females. Consequently, the condition is usually seen only in males and very rarely in females (Pedigree III-C).

1. Criteria
   a. The incidence is much higher in males than in females.
   b. The gene is passed from an affected male to all of his daughters, who in turn pass it to 50% of their sons.
   c. The gene is never passed from father to son.
   d. When the mother is a carrier, there is a 50% recurrence risk for affected males and a 50% chance for carrier daughters.
2. Counseling
   a. Counselor should obtain a pedigree to evaluate the origin of the gene or to determine whether it is a new mutation.
   b. Counselor should explain that the condition is caused by genes from both parents because the mother has given the X chromosome with the gene on it and the father has given the Y chromosome to make the individual male.
   c. Counselor should explain recurrence risk if the mother is carrier or possibility of gonadal dysgenesis.
3. Examples are as follows:
   a. Duchenne muscular dystrophy
      (1) Also known as pseudohypertrophic muscular dystrophy.
      (2) Males have progressive muscle weakness and are usually confined to a wheelchair by early teens.
      (3) Individuals have decreased IO ≤75.
      (4) Seventy percent of individuals affected will have a deletion or a duplication of the X chromosome.
      (5) Thirty percent are new mutations; 5% to 15% of cases that appear to be new mutations will actually be germline mosaicism.
      (6) Prenatal and carrier testing is available and should be offered to any women with an affected son.
   b. Hemophilia A
      (1) Blood fails to clot because of lack of factor VIII.
      (2) Internal hemorrhage into joints is the primary clinical characteristic.
      (3) Prenatal testing is available though linkage and direct mutation analysis in some families.
      (4) Fifty percent of severely affected males will have an inversion on the X chromosome.

Multifactorial inheritance

Multifactorial inheritance is said to occur when a condition is said to be caused by a combination of genetic and nongenetic (environmental) conditions (III-D).

1. Criteria
   a. Condition does not follow any particular single-gene pattern of inheritance but tends to be familial.
   b. Condition tends to occur more frequently in one sex than in the other but is seen in both. (Cleft lip with or without cleft palate is more common in boys. Spina bifida is more common in girls.)
   c. The recurrence risk is the same in all relatives who share the same proportion of genes. (Recurrence risk for all first-degree

relatives of an individual with a neural tube defect would be the same.)
    d. The recurrence risk drops off quickly as the relationship to an affected individual becomes more remote. (The possibility of the condition diminishes in individuals who share fewer genes.)
    e. In monozygotic twins the chance that the second twin is also affected is under 100% and usually under 50%.
    f. In dizygotic twins the concordinance is less than monozygotic twins and usually similar to the recurrence risk in ordinary twins.
2. Counseling
    a. Counselor should explain that parents have not done anything to cause this condition. It is a combination of multiple genetic and nongenetic factors that contribute to making the condition and therefore is unlikely to occur again.
    b. Counselor should explain the treatment, the severity of the condition, and current options.
    c. Counselor should explain future prenatal diagnosis and prevention. (Giving high doses of folic acid before conception and during the first trimester, 4 mg/day, reduces the risk of neural tube defects [NTD] in future pregnancies.)
3. Examples
    a. Pyloric stenosis
    b. Anencephaly

Mitochondrial inheritance

Mutations involving the mitochondrial DNA are known to cause a limited number of genetic conditions. It is important to remember that only the egg cell contains inheritable mitochondria. The sperm's mitochondria are contained in the tail, which is released during fertilization and therefore not of inheritable significance.

1. Criteria
    a. Pedigree should show both males and females affected; however, inheritance is never through the father.
    b. Specific tissues have different proportions of mitochondria. The more mitochondria, the more severely affected. High areas of mitochondria include cardiac muscles, central nervous system (CNS), and kidney.
    c. Mothers pass mitochondria on to all their offspring.
2. Counseling
    a. It is important that the individual understands that the variability of these conditions is directly caused by the concentration of mitochondria, and this is very difficult to predict.
    b. Currently there is no prenatal diagnosis.
    c. Sons will not transmit the condition to their children.
3. Examples of mitochondrial disorders
    a. Leber's optic neuropathy: optic atrophy, occasional movement disorders, electrocardiography abnormalities
    b. Kearns-Sayre syndrome: progressive external ophthalmoplegia, retinal pigment abnormalities, heart disease, and cerebellar ataxia; onset usually before age 20

Genetic screening by ethnic background

Tay-Sachs disease

Tay-Sachs disease affects 1/3600 conceptions and is caused by the lack of an enzyme, hexosaminidase A. Individuals with this condition usually die between the ages of 2 and 5 years from an accumulation of GM_2-ganglioside in the brain and nervous system. Individuals are symptomatic by age 6 to 10 months.

1. Population at risk includes the following:
   a. Ashkenazi Jewish descent (carrier incidence 1/25)
   b. French Canadian (carrier incidence 1/25)
   c. Cajun (carrier incidence 1/12)
2. Carrier testing: When at least one partner is from a population at risk, both partners should be tested to determine whether they are carriers.
3. Inheritance
   a. Tay-Sachs disease has an autosomal recessive inheritance pattern.
   b. Therefore if one parent is determined not to be a carrier, the pregnancy is not a risk.
   c. If both parents are carriers, there is a 75% chance for a healthy child and 25% chance of an affected child.
4. Prenatal diagnosis is available through CVS and amniocentesis by an assay to determine the level of hexosaminidose A activity.

Cystic fibrosis

Cystic fibrosis affects about 1/5000 infants in Northern European populations. Its clinical characteristics include chronic respiratory infection, malabsorption, failure to thrive, and thick secretions of the lung and gut when sodium chloride levels are high. Chronic pulmonary disease begins before 1 year of age and is the cause of death in 90% of individuals. Average life span is 35 years. Treatment includes digestive enzyme replacement therapy, chest physiotherapy, and antibiotics.

1. Population at risk includes the following:
   a. Individuals with a family history
   b. Gamete donors
   c. Individuals with an ultrasound indicative of fetal echogenic bowel, obstructive bowel, or meconium ileus
2. Inheritance is autosomal recessive.
   a. The gene is located on chromosome 7p; however, there are many mutations of the gene that cause it not to work properly.
   b. All of the mutations are not known; however, most labs will determine 85% of carriers by analysis of the most common mutations.
   c. Specific linkage analysis can be done for families with living affected members.
3. Prenatal diagnosis
   a. Analysis of six of the common mutations will identify 85% to 90% of carriers.
   b. Family linkage studies can be done for a specific family with a more rare mutation and a living affected family member.

c. Prenatal diagnosis is possible by CVS and amniocentesis when the mutation in question is known.
   (1) Tests have a 2% to 5% false-positive rate and a 2% to 10% false-negative rate.
   (2) Specific laboratories should be consulted concerning their accuracy.

Sickle cell anemia

Sickle cell anemia is a blood disorder involving a structural abnormality in one of the globin chains. Clinical manifestations appear in the first year of life, and repeat episodes may cause organ damage, musculoskeletal infarcts, delay in growth, delay in secondary sex characteristics, increased susceptibility to infections, seizures, ocular abnormalities, pulmonary infarcts, renal abnormalities, skin ulcers, and gall stones. Individuals may have severe pain associated with crisis but variability exists. The only cure is bone marrow transplant, which carries a 15% mortality rate.

1. Populations at risk include the following:
   a. African-Americans including Haitians, Jamaicans, and individuals from the Caribbean islands
   b. Hispanics from South America, the Caribbean, Puerto Rico, Cuba, and Southeast Asia
   c. Screening: best done by hemoglobin electrophoresis
2. Prenatal diagnosis is available by CVS or amniocentesis using direct site-specific recombinant DNA analysis.
   a. For prenatal diagnosis of a sickle-cell gene in combination with another hemoglobinopathy, family studies or DNA polymorphism by restriction enzyme analysis may be necessary.
   b. Evaluation for these studies should be done by a genetic counselor early in pregnancy.

Beta-thalassemia

Beta-thalassemia is a blood disorder affecting the globin chain synthesis, resulting in severe anemia with an onset at 2 to 3 months. The disorder is characterized by stunted growth, skull bossing (particularly in frontal and parietal areas), increased susceptibility to infection, bone deformities, fractures, delayed or absent sexual maturation, hepatomegaly, splenomegaly, and shortened life span (second or third decade). Treatment includes blood transfusions, iron chelation, therapy to prevent iron overload, and splenectomy.

1. Population at risk: India, Pakistan, South China, Southeast Asia (Laos, Cambodia, Thailand, Vietnam, Philippines, Malaysia), North Africa
2. Screening should be done by a CBC, mean corpuscular hemoglobin (MCH), or electrophoresis.
   a. Mean corpuscular volume (MCV) is <79.
   b. Mean corpuscular hemoglobin count (MCHC) is normal.
   c. HbA_2 is increased (1% to 6%).
   d. HbF is increased (2% to 5%).
3. Prenatal diagnosis: Direct DNA analysis by PCR can be done following CVS or amniocentesis or through fetal blood samples later in pregnancy.

Using genetic resources

1. Genetic counselors
   a. Genetic counselors are individuals with Masters degrees who have been formally trained in genetics.
   b. They are certified by the American Board of Genetic Counseling.
   c. Genetic counselors can be of enormous help to obstetricians.
      (1) They have the expertise and training to decide what type of genetic testing might be necessary for a patient.
      (2) They are usually compassionate individuals who can provide invaluable insight into helping families make decisions because they have extensive experience working with individuals with genetic conditions.
2. Medical geneticists
   a. Medical geneticists are medical specialists with additional training in genetics.
   b. The medical geneticist can establish a genetic diagnosis and review the medical prognosis of the disorder.
   c. Medical geneticists, like genetic counselors, have specific knowledge of genetic disease and how it affects families from first-hand experience.
3. Genetic laboratories
   a. It is important to build up a relationship with the genetic laboratory, whether it is academic or commercial.
   b. A good rapport with a laboratory will provide confidence in results and lead to referrals for research and support groups.
4. Support groups
   a. Counselors should get to know the support groups in their area and those available on a national level.
   b. Directing patients to these valuable organizations can put them in direct contact with others affected by the same condition.
   c. Many of these groups also have newsletters, links to research groups, and local chapters, and some even have yearly conventions.

Suggested reading

American College of Medical Genetics, 9650 Rockville Pike, Bethesda, MD 20814-3889, telephone (301) 571-1895.

American Society of Human Genetics, 9650 Rockville Pike, Bethesda, MD 20814-3889, telephone (301) 571-1825.

Briggs G: *Drugs in pregnancy and lactation,* ed 3, Baltimore, 1990, Williams & Wilkins.

Directory of National Genetic Voluntary Organizations and Related Resources, 1992: Alliance of Genetic Support Groups, Chevy Chase, MD, telephone 1-800-336-GENE or (301) 652-5553.

Jones KL: *Smith's recognizable patterns of human malformation,* Philadelphia, 1988, WB Saunders.

National Society of Genetic Counselors, Executive office, 233 Canterbury Drive, Wallingford, PA 19086-6617, telephone (610) 872-7608; fax (610) 872-1192.

Robinson A, Linden M: *Clinical genetics handbook,* Boston, 1993, Blackwell Scientific Publications.

23.5 HYPERTENSION IN PREGNANCY

John R. Barton, M.D., and Baha M. Sibai, M.D.

1. Hypertensive disorders are the most common medical complication of pregnancy, occurring in approximately 7% to 10% of all pregnancies.
2. Hypertensive disorders are associated with significant maternal and perinatal mortality and present as a wide spectrum of disorders, ranging from minimal elevation of blood pressure to severe hypertension with multiple organ dysfunction.
3. The Committee on Terminology of the American College of Obstetricians and Gynecologists (ACOG) defines hypertension in pregnancy as either:
   a. A systolic pressure of 140 mm Hg or more or an increment of 30 mm Hg or more from a baseline value established in the first half of pregnancy.
   b. A diastolic blood pressure of 90 mm Hg or more or an increment of 15 mm Hg or more from a baseline value established in the first half of pregnancy.
   c. The absolute blood pressure levels or threshold increments in pressure must be observed on at least two occasions, 6 hours apart.
   d. If blood pressure in the first half of pregnancy is unknown, readings of 140/90 mm Hg after 20 weeks gestation are considered diagnostic of pregnancy-induced hypertension (PIH).
   e. The committee also regards an increase in mean arterial blood pressure of 20 mm Hg or a mean arterial pressure of 105 mm Hg or more as diagnostic of PIH.
4. Classification guidelines for hypertension disorders of pregnancy by ACOG are as follows:
   - I. Pregnancy-induced hypertension
     - A. Preeclampsia
       - 1. Mild
       - 2. Severe
     - B. Eclampsia
   - II. Chronic hypertension preceding pregnancy (any etiology)
   - III. Chronic hypertension (any etiology) with superimposed PIH
     - A. Superimposed preeclampsia
     - B. Superimposed eclampsia
   - IV. Gestational or transient hypertension
5. The following definitions apply to the previously mentioned classifications:
   a. Preeclampsia: hypertension together with abnormal edema, proteinuria, or both
   b. Eclampsia: the development of convulsions or coma in patients with signs and symptoms of preeclampsia in the absence of other causes of convulsions
   c. Chronic hypertension: patients with a persistent elevation of blood pressure to at least 140/90 mm Hg on two occasions before 20 weeks gestation, and patients with hypertension that persists for more than 6 weeks postpartum

   d. Superimposed preeclampsia or eclampsia: the development of either preeclampsia or eclampsia in patients with diagnosed chronic hypertension
   e. Gestational hypertension: hypertension appearing in the second half of pregnancy or in the first 24 hours postpartum without edema or proteinuria and with a return to normotension within 10 days after delivery
6. The two most common forms of hypertension are as follows:
   a. PIH, a disorder that appears during pregnancy and is reversed by delivery
   b. Preexisting chronic hypertension, unrelated to but coinciding with pregnancy; may be detected for the first time in pregnancy and is not reversed by delivery

Preeclampsia

Etiology

Preeclampsia is a disorder of unknown etiology that is peculiar to human pregnancy. Many theories regarding its etiology have been suggested and include the following:

1. Abnormal placentation
2. Immunologic phenomena
3. Coagulation abnormalities
4. Abnormal cardiovascular adaptation
5. Dietary factors
6. Genetic factors
7. Vascular endothelial damage
8. Abnormal prostaglandin metabolism

Incidence

1. Preeclampsia is a disorder peculiar to human pregnancy.
2. Reported incidences range from 2% to 35%, depending on the diagnostic criteria and the population studied.
3. It is principally a disease of young primigravidas.
4. The incidence is about 6% to 7% of all pregnancies in the United States.

Risk factors

Although geographic and racial differences in incidence have been reported, several risk factors have been identified as predisposing to the development of preeclampsia.

1. Nulliparity
2. Multiple gestation
3. Family history of preeclampsia or eclampsia
4. Preexisting hypertension or renal disease
5. Diabetes
6. Nonimmune hydrops fetalis
7. Molar pregnancy
8. Previous preeclampsia, especially if remote from term

Prediction of preeclampsia

1. The fact that the etiology of preeclampsia remains unknown has made the prediction of preeclampsia very difficult.
2. More than 100 biophysical, clinical, and biochemical tests have been reported in the world's literature to predict the development of preeclampsia, but their overall prediction value remains poor.
3. Examples of clinical tests to predict preeclampsia include the following:
   a. Mean arterial pressure (MAP) at 20 weeks > 90 mm Hg
   b. Diastolic blood pressure in the midtrimester > 80 mm Hg
   c. Rollover test at 28 to 32 weeks
   d. Angiotensin II infusion test at 26 to 30 weeks
      (1) The angiotensin II test is an invasive procedure that requires infusions of this potent vasopressor at 26 to 30 weeks gestation and subsequent measurement of the diastolic blood pressure.
      (2) Whether the test is positive or negative depends on the amount of angiotensin II required to elicit an increase in diastolic pressure of 20 mm Hg or more.
      (3) Several investigators have studied the value of the angiotensin II test in predicting PIH.
      (4) It has a specificity of 90% to 95%, but the sensitivity is variable, with a high incidence of false-positive results.
      (5) The test is influenced by several factors, including gestational age, with different results obtained on serial testing.
      (6) In addition, it is a very invasive procedure and is not suitable for clinical use.

Diagnosis

1. Preeclampsia traditionally has been described as a triad of hypertension, proteinuria, and edema.
2. However, preeclampsia may present as a spectrum of clinical signs and symptoms, presenting either alone or in combination, often making the diagnosis difficult.
   a. Hypertension
      (1) Abnormal blood pressure elevation is the traditional hallmark for the diagnosis of the disease and the blood pressure criteria for preeclampsia have been presented earlier.
   b. Proteinuria
      (1) Protein excretion in the urine increases in normal pregnancy from approximately 5 mg/100 ml in the first and second trimesters to 15 mg/100 ml in the third trimester.
      (2) Significant proteinuria should be defined as a level greater than 300 mg per 24-hour urine sample.
      (3) When making a diagnosis of severe preeclampsia based on the criterion of proteinuria only, it is recommended that a 24-hour urine excretion of protein of greater than 5 g be documented.
   c. Edema
      (1) Excessive weight gain (more than 2 lb per week in the third trimester) may be the first sign of preeclampsia.

(2) Moderate edema is a feature of 80% of normotensive pregnancies.
(3) In addition, 40% of patients with eclampsia at the University of Tennessee-Memphis had no edema before the onset of convulsions.
(4) Moreover, the assessment of edema is highly subjective.

3. Early recognition of the development of preeclampsia can allow for more timely intervention to improve maternal and perinatal outcome.
4. This reinforces the reason for frequent antenatal visits late in pregnancy to allow early detection.
5. Figure 23-2 is a sample algorithm for the management of a normotensive patient that may be developing subtle signs and symptoms of preeclampsia.

Management of preeclampsia

1. Once the diagnosis of preeclampsia has been made, definitive therapy in the form of delivery is the desired goal, because it is the only cure for the disease.
2. The ultimate goals of the therapy must always be safety of the mother first, and then the delivery of a mature newborn that will not require intensive and prolonged neonatal care.
3. The decision is between expectant management and immediate delivery and is usually dependent on one or more of the following factors:
   a. Severity of the disease process
   b. Presence of labor
   c. Fetal gestational age
   d. Fetal condition
   e. Maternal condition
   f. Bishop cervical score

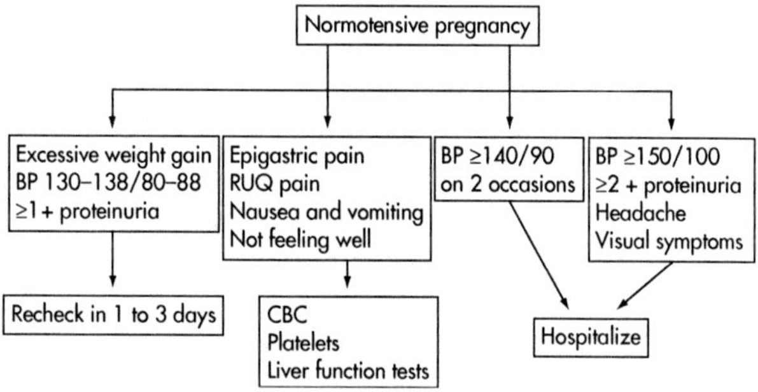

Figure 23-2
A sample algorithm for the management of a normotensive patient who may be developing subtle signs and symptoms of preeclampsia.

Mild preeclampsia

1. All patients with diagnosed preeclampsia should be hospitalized at the time of diagnosis for evaluation of maternal and fetal conditions.
2. These pregnancies usually are associated with reduced uteroplacental blood flow.
3. Thus, women with mild disease who have a favorable cervix at or near term should undergo induction of labor for delivery.
   a. Even if conditions for induction of labor are unfavorable, the pregnancy should not continue past term (beyond 40 weeks gestation), because uteroplacental blood flow is suboptimal.
   b. The optimal management of mild preeclampsia remote from term is very controversial.
   c. In general, there is considerable disagreement regarding the need for hospitalization versus ambulatory management, the use of antihypertensive drugs, and the use of sedatives and anticonvulsive prophylaxis.
   d. For a patient who has mild preeclampsia with an immature fetus, the goal of therapy should be to do the following:
      (1) Retard the hypertensive process so as not to endanger the mother or the fetus
      (2) Allow time for the fetus to mature and increase the potential for neonatal survival
      (3) Allow the cervix to ripen and therefore increase the probability for a vaginal delivery
   e. Therapy for these patients can be conducted by either ambulatory management or hospitalization.
      (1) Ambulatory management is acceptable for patients who are compliant, who can have frequent office visits including laboratory assessments, and who can perform some form of adequate blood pressure monitoring at home.
      (2) Hospitalization should be required for noncompliant patients and those who show unsatisfactory progress as outpatients.
      (3) In either situation, the following regimen is recommended for mild preeclampsia.
         I. Maternal evaluation
            A. Physical examination
               1. Blood pressure every 4 to 6 hours during the day
               2. Urine protein by dipstick daily
               3. Assessment of facial or pedal edema daily
               4. Weight daily
            B. Patient history

Symptoms of impending eclampsia or HELLP syndrome (hemolysis, elevated liver, low platelets) include the following:

               1. Persistent occipital or frontal headaches
               2. Visual disturbances
               3. Right upper quadrant or epigastric pain
            C. Laboratory evaluation
               1. Hematocrit and platelet count one or two times a week
               2. Liver function tests one or two times a week

3. 24-Hour urine collections at diagnosis and every 1 to 2 weeks

II. Fetal evaluation

1. Daily fetal movement assessment (kick counts)
2. NST twice weekly
3. BPP if nonreactive NST
4. Amniotic fluid volume assessment weekly
5. Ultrasound evaluation of fetal growth every 3 weeks

4. A patient is considered a candidate for induction of labor if she has reached 37 weeks gestation, the fetus is mature, and the condition of the cervix is favorable.
   a. She is also a candidate for induction if her diastolic blood pressure continues to rise despite conservative management.
5. A patient with mild PIH may be followed beyond 37 weeks of gestation if fetal evaluation is normal and the condition of the cervix is unfavorable.
6. Figure 23-3 is a sample algorithm for the management of a patient with mild preeclampsia.

Severe preeclampsia

1. The clinical course of severe preeclampsia is usually characterized by progressive deterioration in both maternal and fetal status.
2. These pregnancies are usually associated with increased rates of perinatal mortality and morbidity.
3. Most of the fetal or neonatal complications are related to intrauterine fetal growth retardation and prematurity.
4. The following represent the criteria for the diagnosis of severe preeclampsia:
   a. Blood pressure >160 mm Hg systolic or >110 mm Hg diastolic on two occasions at least 6 hours apart with the patient at bed rest
   b. Proteinuria >5 g in a 24-hour urine collection or >3 g on dipstick in at least two random clean-catch samples at least 4 hours apart
   c. Oliguria (<400 ml in 24 hours)
   d. Cerebral or visual disturbances
   e. Epigastric pain
   f. Pulmonary edema or cyanosis
   g. Thrombocytopenia
   (Adapted from ACOG Technical Bulletin No. 91)
5. Because the only cure for severe preeclampsia is delivery, there is universal agreement to deliver all patients if the disease develops beyond 34 weeks gestation or if there is evidence of fetal lung maturity or fetal jeopardy before that time.
6. In this situation, appropriate management should include the following:
   a. Parenteral medications to prevent convulsions
   b. Control of maternal blood pressure within a safe range
   c. Induction of labor to initiate delivery.
7. On the other hand, management of patients with severe disease remote from term (<34 weeks) is highly controversial.

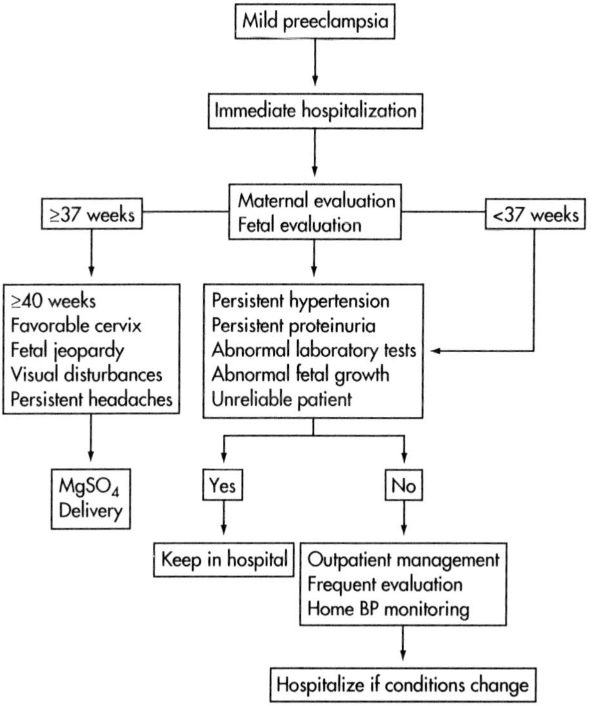

Figure 23-3
A sample algorithm for the management of a patient with mild preeclampsia.

a. Some institutions consider delivery as the definitive therapy for all cases, regardless of gestational age.
b. Others recommend prolonging pregnancy in all patients remote from term until one or more of the following is achieved:
   (1) Fetal lung maturity
   (2) Fetal jeopardy
   (3) Maternal jeopardy
   (4) 34 weeks gestation achieved

8. All patients with severe preeclampsia should be admitted to the labor and delivery area for close observation of the maternal and fetal condition.
9. All patients should receive intravenous magnesium sulfate to prevent convulsions.
10. Fig. 23-4 is a sample algorithm for the management of a patient with severe preeclampsia.

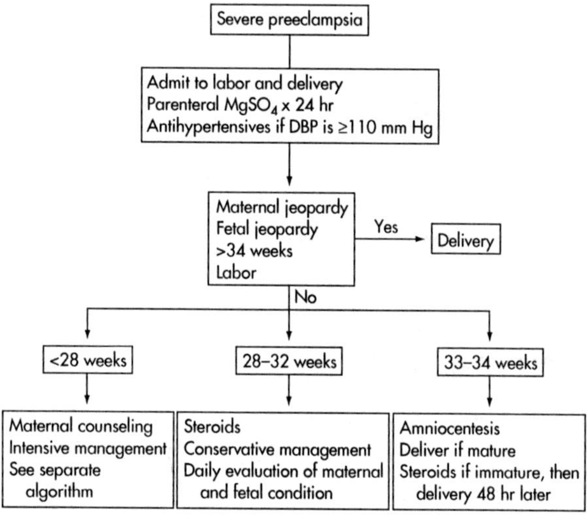

Figure 23-4
A sample algorithm for the management of a patient with severe preeclampsia.

Severe preeclampsia in midtrimester

1. Occasionally, a patient may develop severe preeclampsia at or before 28 weeks gestation.
2. These pregnancies are associated with high maternal and perinatal mortality and pose a difficult management decision for every obstetrician.
3. Immediate delivery will result in extremely high perinatal morbidity and mortality, whereas an aggressive attempt to delay delivery may cause severe maternal morbidity.
4. Fig. 23-5 is a sample algorithm for the management of a patient with severe preeclampsia in the midtrimester.

Prevention of preeclampsia

1. There are numerous reports and clinical trials describing the use of various methods to prevent or reduce the incidence of preeclampsia.
2. Methods used have included the following:
   a. Salt restriction or prophylactic diuretic therapy
   b. Low-dose aspirin
   c. Calcium supplementation
   d. Ingestion of fish or evening primrose oil.
3. Because the etiology of the disease is unknown, the reported methods have been used in an attempt to correct the pathophysiologic abnormalities of preeclampsia in the hope of preventing the disease or ameliorating its course.

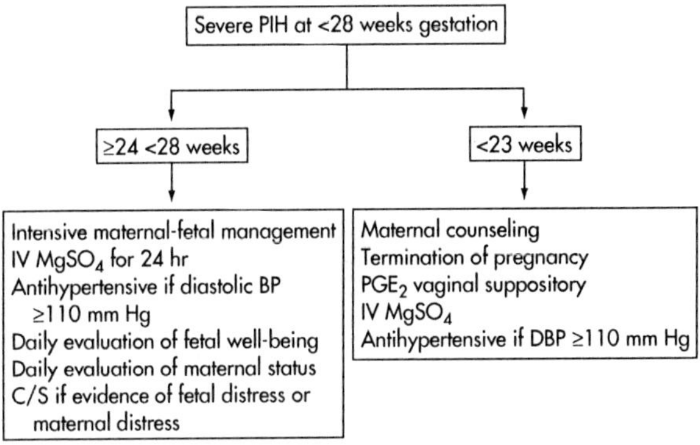

Figure 23-5
A sample algorithm for the management of a patient with severe preeclampsia in the mid-trimester.

4. Several multicenter studies are currently under way, but there is not yet a consensus on the optimal method for prevention or amelioration of this disease.

Eclampsia

1. Eclampsia is defined as the development of convulsions or coma unrelated to other cerebral conditions during pregnancy and the postpartum period in patients with signs and symptoms of preeclampsia.
2. The hazards of convulsions in pregnancy have been documented for centuries.
3. The reported incidence ranges from 1 in 100 to 1 in 3448 pregnancies.
4. The incidence is increased among nonwhite nulliparous women of low socioeconomic status.
5. At the University of Tennessee at Memphis, a tertiary referral center for several states, the incidence has remained stable at 1 in 300 pregnancies for the past 30 years.
6. However, considering the number of pregnancies in that area, the incidence actually is about 1 in 1600 pregnancies.
7. For patients obtaining prenatal care, the incidence is about 1 in 800 patients.
8. Eclamptic convulsions constitute a life-threatening emergency.
9. The basic principles in the management of eclampsia involve the following measures:
   a. Support of cardiorespiratory functions
      (1) Airway patency and ensuring maternal oxygenation should be assessed and established.
      (2) Suction should be used as needed and the patient protected from injury by making sure the bed side-rails are elevated and padded.

(3) Oxygen should be administered to improve maternal oxygen concentration and increase oxygen delivery to the fetus.

b. Control of convulsions and prevention of recurrent convulsions

(1) The natural tendency for those caring for an eclamptic patient is to provide therapy to immediately abolish the seizure activity.

(2) This philosophy is not only unwise, it is potentially dangerous to the patient.

(3) Parenteral magnesium sulfate is the drug of choice for convulsions resulting from eclampsia in the United States.

(a) Its major advantages include its relative maternal and fetal safety when used properly.

(b) The mother is awake and alert most of the time and laryngeal reflexes are intact, which helps protect against aspiration problems.

(c) There are several regimens of magnesium sulfate used to prevent convulsions. The two most commonly used are as follows:

i. Intravenous regimen popularized by Sibai at the University of Tennessee-Memphis

ii. The intramuscular regimen preferred by Pritchard used at Parkland Memorial Hospital in Dallas, Texas

(d) The Sibai regimen

i. An intravenous loading dose of 6 g of magnesium sulfate ($MgSO_4 .7 H_2O$) prepared as 6 g diluted in 150 ml D_5W is administered via infusion pump over 20 to 30 minutes.

ii. If the patient develops recurrent convulsions after the initial infusion of magnesium sulfate, a further dose of 2 to 4 g can be infused over 5 to 10 minutes.

iii. On completion of the magnesium sulfate loading infusion, a maintenance infusion of 2 to 3 g/hr is used.

iv. The infusion rate of magnesium sulfate should be adjusted on the basis of serial serum magnesium levels and physical examination.

(e) Pritchard's intramuscular regimen for severe preeclampsia and eclampsia includes the following:

i. Four g of magnesium sulfate IV over 3 to 5 minutes and 10 g IM is administered as a loading dose followed by a maintenance dose of 5 g IM every 4 hours.

ii. For mild preeclampsia, 10 g of magnesium sulfate IM is administered as a loading dose followed by a maintenance dose of 5 g IM every 4 hours.

(4) Clinical findings associated with increased maternal plasma levels of magnesium can be found in Table 23-11.

(5) Patients receiving magnesium sulfate therapy require monitoring for evidence of drug toxicity.

Table 23-11 Clinical findings associated with increased maternal plasma magnesium levels

Serum Magnesium Level (mg/dl)	Clinical Findings
1.5-2.5	Normal pregnancy level
4-8	"Therapeutic range for seizure prophylaxis"
9-12	Loss of patellar reflex
15-17	Muscular paralysis, respiratory arrest
30-35	Cardiac arrest

(6) Magnesium is excreted by the kidneys, and renal dysfunction may cause toxic accumulation. Magnesium toxicity can be avoided by doing the following:
   (a) Confirming adequate renal function with hourly urinary output assessment
   (b) Doing serial evaluation for presence of patellar deep tendon reflexes
   (c) Making close observation of respiratory rate
   (d) Monitoring serial serum magnesium levels

(7) If magnesium toxicity is suspected the following should be done:
   (a) The magnesium sulfate infusion should be discontinued immediately.
   (b) Supplemental oxygen should be administered.
   (c) A serum magnesium level should be assessed.

(8) If magnesium toxicity is recognized, 10 ml of 10% calcium gluconate is administered (1 g total) intravenously.
   (a) This medication must be given slowly (i.e., 2 to 5 ml/min) to avoid hypotension and bradycardia.
   (b) Calcium competitively inhibits magnesium at the neuromuscular junction, but its effect is only transient, because the serum concentration is unchanged.

(9) Symptoms of magnesium toxicity can recur following calcium gluconate if the magnesium level remains elevated.

(10) If respiratory arrest is identified, prompt resuscitative measures including intubation and assisted ventilation are indicated.

c. Correction of maternal hypoxemia and acidemia
   (1) Maternal hypoxemia and acidemia may result from the following:
      (a) Repeated convulsions
      (b) Respiratory depression from the use of multiple anticonvulsant agents
      (c) Aspiration
      (d) Or a combination of these factors
   (2) Supplemental oxygen may be administered by face mask or face mask with an oxygen reservoir at 8 to 10 L/min.

(a) At 10 L O_2/min, the oxygen concentration delivered approaches 100% using a face mask with an oxygen reservoir.

(3) Maternal oxygenation can be monitored noninvasively by transcutaneous pulse oximetry, whereas acid–base status may be assessed by arterial blood gas analysis.

d. Control of severe hypertension

(1) The objective of treating severe hypertension is to prevent maternal cerebrovascular accidents and congestive heart failure without compromising cerebral perfusion or jeopardizing uteroplacental blood flow, already reduced in eclampsia.

(2) Although the underlying causative factors are not completely delineated, hypertension in preeclampsia is clearly a consequence of a generalized arterial vasoconstriction.

(3) Desirable antihypertensive agent properties for the use in hypertensive emergencies in pregnancy include a rapid onset of action following administration and short duration of action in the event of overtitration.

(a) Labetalol

i. Labetalol is a competitive antagonist at both postsynaptic alpha-1-adrenergic and beta-adrenergic receptors.

ii. Labetalol is available in oral and intravenous form.

iii. Parenteral labetalol has a rapid onset of action and produces a smooth reduction in blood pressure with rare overshoot hypotension.

iv. Labetalol is contraindicated in patients with a greater than first-degree heart block.

v. Labetalol is administered in intermittent intravenous boluses of 20 to 80 mg.

(b) Hydralazine

i. Hydralazine is a direct arteriolar vasodilator.

ii. Intravenous hydralazine has an onset of action of 10 to 20 minutes with a peak effect in 60 minutes and a duration of action of 4 to 6 hours.

iii. Hydralazine is administered in intermittent bolus injections with an initial dose of 5 mg. Blood pressure should then be recorded every 5 minutes.

iv. If an adequate reduction in blood pressure is present 20 to 30 minutes after the initial dose, then a repeat dose or one increased to 10 mg in increments of every 20 to 30 minutes should be given.

(c) Nifedipine

i. Nifedipine is a calcium channel antagonist.

ii. Nifedipine improves renal function with a beneficial effect on urine output when treating preeclampsia in the postpartum period.

iii. Given sublingually, 10 mg of nifedipine has an onset of action within 3 minutes with a peak effect within 1 hour.

iv. Nifedipine is administered 10 to 20 mg orally every 3 to 4 hours.
v. Profound reductions in blood pressure with nifedipine can be partially reversed by the slow intravenous administration of calcium gluconate.

(d) Sodium nitroprusside
i. Sodium nitroprusside relaxes arteriolar and venous smooth muscle equally by interfering with both influx and the intercellular activation of calcium.
ii. Onset of action is immediate, and duration of action is very short (1 to 10 minutues).
iii. As preeclamptic patients have a propensity for depleted intravascular volume, they are especially sensitive to its effects. The initial infusion dose should therefore be 0.2 μg/kg/min, rather than 0.5 μg/kg/min as is standard in nonpregnant patients.
iv. Cyanide and thiocyanate are products of metabolism of this drug.

e. Initiation of the process for delivery
(1) Because evacuation of the uterus is the definitive treatment of preeclampsia and eclampsia, patients are evaluated for delivery, once stabilized.
(2) Vaginal delivery, unless obstetrically contraindicated, is the preferred method of delivery.
(a) An oxytocin infusion for induction or augmentation of labor may be administered simultaneously with the magnesium sulfate infusion.
(b) Total fluid intake is limited to 100 ml/hr.
(c) The protocol for oxytocin infusion for preeclampsia or eclampsia is the same as for routine patients; yet, because of fluid restrictions, oxytocin may need to be more concentrated and dosages per minute adjusted accordingly.
(d) Continuous fetal monitoring should be employed.
(3) At delivery, neonatal side effects of maternal administration of magnesium sulfate include the following:
(a) Hypotension
(b) Hypotonia
(c) Respiratory depression
(d) Lethargy
(e) Decreased suck reflex
(4) The pediatrician and newborn nursery should be informed of patients receiving magnesium sulfate.
(5) Calcium gluconate may also be administered to the newborn if magnesium toxicity is suspected.
(6) Following delivery, the patient should be monitored in the recovery room under close observation for a minimum of 24 hours.
(7) During this time, magnesium sulfate should be continued, and maternal vital signs and intake–output should be monitored hourly.

(8) Some of these patients may require intensive and invasive hemodynamic monitoring, because they are at increased risk of the development of pulmonary edema from fluid overload, fluid mobilization, and compromised renal function.
(9) Magnesium sulfate administration should continue until improvements in blood pressure, urine output, and sensorium are noted.

Postpartum eclampsia

1. Approximately 25% of eclampsia cases will occur during the postpartum period, most within the first 48 hours from delivery.
2. Late-onset postpartum eclampsia is defined as convulsions occurring more than 48 hours after delivery in patients with signs and symptoms of preeclampsia.
   a. If postpartum eclampsia is confirmed, the management is as previously noted for antepartum convulsions.
   b. More vigorous control of blood pressure is possible, however, because there is no longer a concern about compromising the uteroplacental circulation in the postpartum patient.
   c. Magnesium sulfate therapy should be continued for 24 to 48 hours from seizure onset.

Complications of eclampsia

1. There are several maternal complications with eclampsia convulsions including the following:
   a. Abruptio placentae
   b. Pulmonary edema
   c. Acute renal failure
   d. Aspiration pneumonia
   e. Intracerebral hemorrhage
   f. Retinal detachment
   g. Ruptured subcapsular liver hematoma
2. Abruptio placenta is the most frequent (5% to 10%) complication and intracerebral hemorrhage is the most serious.
3. Fortunately, most of the complications resolve after delivery with proper management.

HELLP syndrome

1. Hemolysis, abnormal liver functions tests, and thrombocytopenia have been recognized as complications of preeclampsia and eclampsia for many years.
2. In 1982, Weinstein described 29 cases of severe preeclampsia and eclampsia complicated by these abnormalities.
3. He suggested that this collection of signs and symptoms constituted an entity separate from severe preeclampsia and coined the term HELLP syndrome:
   a. *H* for hemolysis
   b. *EL* for elevated liver enzymes
   c. *LP* for low platelets

Criteria for the Diagnosis of HELLP Syndrome

HEMOLYSIS

Abnormal peripheral smear
Total bilirubin >1.2 mg/dl
Lactic dehydrogenase (LDH) >600 U/L

ELEVATED LIVER FUNCTIONS

Serum aspartate aminotransferase (AST) >70 U/L
Lactic dehydrogenase (LDH) >600 U/L

LOW PLATELETS

Platelet count <100,000/mm^3

From Sibai BM: The HELLP syndrome (hemolysis, elevated liver enzymes, and low platelets): much ado about nothing? *Am J Obstet Gynecol* 162:311-316, 1990.

4. There are considerable differences regarding the time of onset and the type and degree of laboratory abnormalities used to make the diagnosis of HELLP syndrome.
5. In an attempt to standardize the diagnosis of HELLP syndrome, investigators at the University of Tennessee-Memphis published criteria using cutoff values of more than three standard deviations above the mean to indicate abnormality. Their criteria for the diagnosis of HELLP syndrome are summarized in the box above.
6. The incidence of severe preeclampsia or eclampsia complicated by HELLP syndrome has been reported to range from 2% to 12%.
7. Patients with HELLP syndrome may present with a variety of signs and symptoms, including the following:
   a. Epigastric or right upper quadrant pain
   b. Nausea or vomiting
   c. Nonspecific viral syndrome-like symptoms
   d. History of malaise for the past few days before presentation
8. It is important to appreciate that severe hypertension (systolic blood pressure > 160 mm Hg, diastolic blood pressure >100 mm Hg) is not a constant or even a frequent finding in HELLP syndrome.
   a. In Weinstein's initial report of 29 patients, less than half (13) had an admission blood pressure >160/100 mm Hg.
9. As a result, these patients are often misdiagnosed as having various medical and surgical disorders, including appendicitis, gastroenteritis, pyelonephritis, or viral hepatitis.

Management of HELLP syndrome

1. Patients with HELLP syndrome who are remote from term should be referred to a tertiary care center and initial management should be as for any patient with severe preeclampsia.

2. The following is an outline of the management of antepartum HELLP syndrome:
   a. Maternal condition is assessed and stabilized.
      (1) If disseminated intravascular coagulopathy (DIC) present, coagulopathy is corrected.
      (2) Antiseizure prophylaxis is given with magnesium sulfate.
      (3) Treatment of severe hypertension is begun.
      (4) CT or ultrasound of the abdomen is done if subcapsular hematoma of the liver is suspected.
   b. Fetal well-being is evaluated.
      (1) NST
      (2) BPP
      (3) Ultrasonographic biometry
   c. If <35 weeks gestation fetal lung maturity is evaluated.
      (1) If mature → delivery
      (2) If immature → steroids → delivery
3. If the syndrome develops at or beyond 34 weeks gestation, or if there is evidence of fetal lung maturity or fetal or maternal jeopardy before that time, then delivery is the definitive therapy.
4. Without laboratory evidence of DIC and absent fetal lung maturity, the patient can be given two doses of steroids to accelerate fetal lung maturity and delivery then should be done 48 hours later.
5. However, maternal and fetal conditions should be assessed continuously during this time period.

Chronic hypertension

1. Management of the woman with chronic hypertension should begin before conception.
   a. If a patient with chronic hypertension is considering pregnancy, she should be advised to have her blood pressure checked several times to establish the cause and severity of her hypertension before pregnancy.
   b. In addition, her response to the antihypertensive drugs should be monitored and drugs with potential adverse effects on the fetus (angiotensin-converting enzyme inhibitors, diuretics) should be replaced by other drugs.
   c. The patient should then be instructed to seek prenatal care once pregnancy is confirmed.
   d. This will ensure accurate determination of the gestational age, as well as the severity of hypertension in the first trimester.
2. For patients who are seen for the first time during pregnancy, the first step in management should include a detailed evaluation and work-up to determine the etiology and severity of the hypertension.
   a. Attention should be paid to the renal disease, diabetes, thyroid disease, and the outcome in previous pregnancies (superimposed preeclampsia, preterm delivery, abruptio placentae, perinatal outcome).

Barton JR, Bronstein SJ, Sibai BM: Management of the eclamptic patient, *J Mat-Fet Med* 1:313-319, 1992.
Barton JR, Sibai BM: Care of the pregnancy complicated by HELLP syndrome, *Gastroenterol Clin North Am* 21(2):937-950, 1992.
Barton JR, Stanziano GJ, Sibai BM: Monitored outpatient management of mild gestational hypertension remote from term, *Am J Obstet Gynecol* 170:765-769, 1994.
Lubarsky SL et al: Late postpartum eclampsia revised, *Obstet Gynecol* 83:502-505, 1994.
Pritchard JA, Cunningham FG, Pritchard SA: The Parkland Memorial Hospital protocol for treatment of eclampsia: evaluation of 245 cases, *Am J Obstet Gynecol* 148:951-963, 1984.
Sibai BM: Magnesium sulfate is the ideal anticonvulsant in preeclampsia-eclampsia, *Am J Obstet Gynecol* 162:1141-1145, 1990.
Sibai BM: The HELLP syndrome (hemolysis, elevated liver enzymes, and low platelets): much ado about nothing? *Am J Obstet Gynecol* 162:311-316, 1990.
Sibai BM et al: Aggressive versus expectant management of severe preeclampsia at 28 to 32 weeks' gestation: a randomized controlled trial, *Am J Obstet Gynecol* 171:818-822, 1994.
Weinstein L: Syndrome of hemolysis, elevated liver enzymes, and low platelet count: a severe consequence of hypertension in pregnancy, *Am J Obstet Gynecol* 142:159-167, 1982.

23.6 HIV IN PREGNANCY

Stanley A. Gall, M.D.

Infection with human immunodeficiency virus type 1 (HIV-1) produces a chronic, progressive disease state resulting in acquired immunodeficiency syndrome (AIDS) and subsequent demise. The AIDS epidemic continues to be dynamic, with the first wave of patients being male homosexuals. This was followed by males and females infected because of intravenous drug abuse. During this phase of the epidemic, females were equally involved and 80% were in the reproductive age. The current phase of the epidemic features heterosexual transmission with females up to 20 times more likely to become infected. It is anticipated that by the year 2000 the sex ratio will be 1:1.

Epidemiology (See the box on p. 538.)

Perinatal transmission

1. Mechanisms of perinatal transmission include the following:
   a. Direct invasion of trophoblast and placental villi by HIV
   b. Passage of infected maternal lymphocyte into the fetal circulation
   c. Infection of cells with CD4 receptors in chorionic villi and villus endothelial cells (Tables 23-12 through 23-14).
2. Role of placenta in the transmission of HIV is not clear.
   a. *In vitro* studies have documented HIV-1 can infect human trophoblast and Hofbauer cells of different gestational ages.
   b. It is unknown whether HIV-1 infection of placenta can either facilitate fetal HIV-1 infection or inhibit fetal infection by sequestering virus.

Changing Epidemiology of AIDS

1. 1981-1992: Centers for Disease Control reported 253,448 cases of AIDS
   a. Male: 87%
   b. Female: 11%
   c. Children: 2%
2. Women were infected by the following routes during 1981-1992
   a. Intravenous drug abuse: 50%
   b. Heterosexual contact: 36%
   c. Other: 14%
3. Women were infected by the following routes 1989-1992
   a. Intravenous drug abuse: 43%
   b. Heterosexual contact: 39%
   c. Other: 18%
4. Racial distribution of women with AIDS
   a. African-American: 53%
   b. Hispanic: 21%
   c. Other: 26%
5. Annual case rate per 100,000 women
   a. Black: 27.2
   b. Hispanic: 13.1
   c. White: 1.8
   d. Other: 57.9
6. Seroprevalence rates (per 1000 women) using neonatal heel stick specimens from 1988 to 1990

State	Rate
New York	5.8
District of Columbia	5.5
New Jersey	4.9
Florida	4.5
Montana	0.0

From Gwinn M et al: Prevalence of HIV infection in childbearing women in the U.S., *JAMA* 265:1701, 1991.

Rate of transmission of HIV-1 from mother to fetus

Vertical transmission is dependent on a number of factors.

1. Factors that increase transmission
   a. Mother has AIDS
   b. Low CD4 counts, especially <200 cell/mm^3
   c. Presence of p24 antigenemia
   d. Presence of histologic chorioamnionitis
   e. Preterm delivery
2. Factors that decrease transmission
   a. Presence of antibody to HIV protein gp 120
   b. Prenatal care
   c. Taking Zidovudine (ZDV)

Table 23-12 Evidence for different times of vertical transmission

Intrauterine Transmission Probable	Intrapartum Transmission	Postpartum Transmission
Early onset of symptoms (<12 months old) ~30%	Later onset symptoms (>12 months old) ~70%	HIV isolation in breast milk
Neonatal period viral identification (<3 months old) ~30%-50%	Delayed viral identification (>4 months old) ~50%-70%	Cases of transmission via breast-feeding
HIV identifiable in fetal tissue (>13 weeks of gestation)	Intrapartum blood and secretion exposure	No evidence of transmission in households
Possible	"Acute primary infection"	
? HIV identified in placentas (≥8 weeks of gestation)	Viral/immunological pattern	
? *In vitro* infection of placenta-derived cells	HIV isolated from vaginal/cervical secretion	
Unlikely	Discordant twins	
? Dysmorphic syndrome		

From Mofenson LM et al: HIV pregnancy and effects on the fetus and infant, *Yearbk Obstet Gynecol* xiii-xlii, 1992.

3. European Collaborative Study transmission rate: 25%
4. The AIDS Clinical Trial Group (ACTG) 076 study: showed transmission rate to be 8% in group receiving ZDV antepartum or intrapartum and in the neonate receiving ZDV during the first 6 weeks of life

Pathogenesis of HIV infection

Viral replication and disease

1. Early studies into viral pathogenesis measured the amount of free culturable virus in peripheral blood and found that viral burden was low in the early stages of HIV infection (e.g., 0 to 10 infective doses per milliliter), rising to 100 to 1000 infective doses per milliliter in later stage disease.
2. Recent studies have shown a high level of ongoing viral replication during this period of latency.
3. Polymerase chain reaction (PCR) and branched DNA (bDNA) techniques have been used to measure significantly high levels of viral RNA in plasma after initial clearance of virus from peripheral blood.
   a. Viral burden is measured at 10^6 to 10^7 RNA copies per milliliter during the initial viremia, decreasing to 10^3 to 10^4 copies per milliliter during the latent period.

Table 23-13 Prevalence of vertically acquired HIV infection and AIDS: 1978-1993

Birth Year	Vertically Acquired HIV Infection	Vertically Acquired AIDS Cases	Deaths Among Vertically Acquired ARDS Cases
1978	70	50	40
1979	60	40	30
1980	120	70	50
1981	190	110	60
1982	270	150	100
1983	410	220	130
1984	660	290	190
1985	870	370	220
1986	1,100	460	260
1987	1,390	530	280
1988	1,360	610	320
1989	1,590	610	300
1990	1,690	610	270
1991	1,760	590	230
1992	1,750	440	150
1993	1,630	180	50
	14,920	5,330	2,680

From Davis SF et al: Prevalence and incidence of vertically acquired HIV infection in the United States, *JAMA* 274:952-955, 1995.
ARDS, Adult respiratory distressed syndrome.

4. Lymph nodes show replicating viruses and intense immunologic reaction in persons with early asymptomatic infection.
5. Antiretroviral treatment with Zidovudine (ZDV) shows a dramatic fourfold to fivefold decrease in plasma HIV RNA level within 1 week after the drug is initiated (Fig. 23-6).
6. When the drug is withdrawn the plasma level rapidly increases.

Care of the patient with HIV

1. Patients who present for prenatal care should be screened for HIV antibodies as a part of routine prenatal care.
2. The Centers for Disease Control and Prevention and the ACOG have recommended antenatal HIV testing be offered to women who admit to a history of risk-associated behavior.
   a. Targeted screening would miss a large segment of the population at risk (40%)
   b. Universal screening is recommended since publication of the ACTG 076 protocol, which showed a 67% reduction in vertical transmission with the use of Zidovudine.
   c. Initiation of HIV-1 screening programs in urban obstetric populations has been shown to be both cost effective and medically beneficial.

Table 23-14 Births to HIV-positive women and incidence of HIV infection in infants: estimates based on Survey of Childbearing Women (SCBW) United States 1988-1993

Year	Number of States in SCBW	Number Tested in SCBW	Percentage Vertically Acquired AIDS Cases	Estimated Number Births to HIV-positive Women	Estimated Incidence of HIV Infection in Infants*
1988	13	590,128	81.4	5,430	1,360
1989	35	1,747,561	94.1	6,370	1,590
1990	43	2,349,661	96.8	6,770	1,690
1991	44	2,386,430	99.7	7,040	1,760
1992	44	2,711,603	99.7	6,990	1,750
1993	44	2,743,767	99.5	6,530	1,630

Davis SF et al: Prevalence and incidence of vertically acquired HIV infection in the United States, *JAMA* 274:952-955, 1995.
*Estimates based on 25% transmission rate.

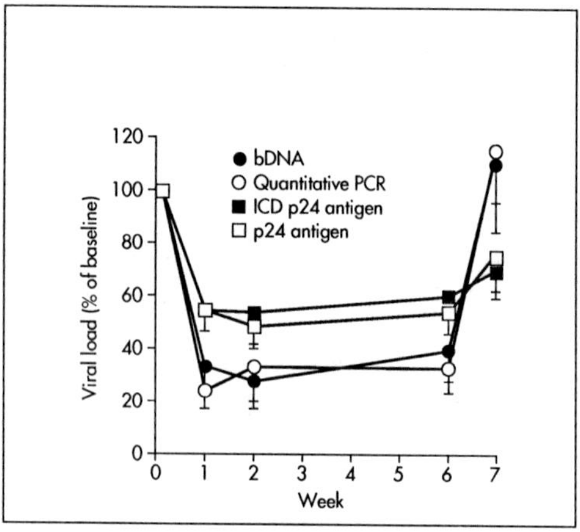

Figure 23-6
Changes in plasma viral RNA levels (bDNA and quantitative PCR assays) and plasma viral core antigen levels (standard and ICD p24 antigen assays) after the initiation of ZDV. The therapy was discontinued after 6 weeks. Values are means ±1 S.E.M. (Reproduced from Cao et al: Clinical evaluation of branched DNA signal amplification for quantifying HIV-1 21 in human plasma, *AIDS Res Hum Retroviruses* 11:353-360, 1995.)

Table 23-15 1993 revised classification system for HIV infection and expanded AIDS surveillance case definition for adolescents and adults

	Clinical Categories*		
CD4 Count	Asymptomatic or Lymphadenopathy	Symptomatic	AIDS-Indicator Conditions
>500/mm^3	A1	B1	C1
200-499/mm^3	A2	B2	C2
<200/mm^3	A3	B3	C3

From *MMWR* 41:1-9, 1992.

*Category A: Acute HIV infection, asymptomatic HIV, persistent generalized lymphadenopathy; Category B: persistent vulvovaginal candidiasis, severe cervical dysplasia or carcinoma, pulmonary TBC, pelvic inflammatory disease; Category C: includes conditions previously used as case definitions for AIDS.

3. Patients who are HIV-1 positive should be evaluated as follows (Table 23-15):
   a. Physician should determine risk category.
   b. Physician should determine stage of disease.
   c. Sexually transmitted diseases should be detected and treated.
   d. Appropriate vaccines and prophylactic medication should be administered.

Evaluations by the physician

1. Physical examinations
2. Laboratory evaluations
   a. CBC with platelets
   b. CD4 count each trimester
   c. Skin test for tuberculosis
   d. Papanicolaou smear
   e. Liver function tests
   f. p24 antigen levels
   g. Hepatitis B and C antibody levels
   h. Syphilis serology
   i. Cultures for *Neisseria gonorrhoeae* and *Chlamydia trachomatis*

Preventive care by the physician

1. Focus on prevention of sexually transmitted diseases (STDs).
2. Hepatitis B vaccine should be given.
3. "Safer sex" measures will reduce exposure to STDs, which may have an adverse effect on the mother and fetus.
4. Zidovudine, 100 mg, five times per day, should be started regardless of CD4 count.
5. Pneumovax vaccine should be given.
6. Trimethoprim-sulfa should be started if the CD4 count is $<200/mm^3$ as prophylaxis against *Pneumocystis carinii* pneumonia.
7. Influenza vaccine should be given (during September-March).

Prenatal care by the physician

1. The obstetrician must maintain a high index of suspicion for STDs and opportunistic infections.
2. IUGR is increased in this population; therefore periodic ultrasonic evaluation for growth is indicated.
3. CD4 counts should be performed each trimester.
4. Colposcopy should be performed if Papanicolaou smears are abnormal.
5. Other routine prenatal vitamins, maternal serum alpha-fetoprotein (MSAFP) triple screen, diabetes screening should be performed.

Intrapartum care by the physician

1. Zidovudine intravenously when labor starts: The dosage should be 200 mg IV over 1 hour, then 100 mg/hr until delivery.
2. Intrapartum procedures that expose the fetus to maternal blood and body fluids should be avoided if at all possible (see the box on p. 544).
3. There is no clear evidence that cesarean delivery reduces the incidence of maternal fetal transmission.
4. Evidence is present that suggests women with CD4 counts $<200/mm^3$ have a greater risk of transmission with longer labors (>12 hours) or prolonged range of motion (ROM) >12.

Postpartum care by the physician

1. A private room is desirable to decrease possible exposure of other patients to body secretions.

Invasive Obstetric Procedures That May Increase Fetal or Newborn Exposure to Maternal Blood and Secretions
1. Amniocentesis
2. Percutaneous umbilical cord sampling
3. Chorionic villus sampling
4. Fetal scalp sampling
5. Fetal scalp monitoring
6. Amnio-infusion

2. Patient should be fully counseled about contraceptive options and a reliable method advised.
3. Intrauterine devices should not be used because of the patient's immunosuppressive state and increased risk of pelvic inflammatory disease.
4. Forms of successful contraception include sterilization, oral contraceptives, Depo-Provera, Norplant, and barrier methods.
5. A condom should be used with every sexual encounter to reduce transmission of HIV-1 to partner and to reduce the risk of acquiring another sexually transmitted disease.
6. Physician should arrange for follow-up of mother and baby.

Pregnancy outcome and frequent complications

1. HIV-positive women began their prenatal care in the second trimester and 17% have no prenatal care.
2. HIV-positive women are more likely to have sexually transmitted diseases and medical complications such as diabetes and chronic hypertension.
3. There is an increased risk of bacterial pneumonia during pregnancy.
4. Women with CD4 counts $<300/mm^3$ are more likely to develop serious infections in pregnancy.
5. Vaginal candidiasis is a frequent problem and difficult to eradicate; topical antifungals are the treatment of choice.
6. Cervical dysplasia is a common finding and the patient should be managed in the usual manner.
   a. Colposcopy is necessary.
   b. Because abnormal genital cytology is a manifestation of human papilloma virus infection in an immunodepressed patient, therapy should be done.
7. The ACOG has presented statements of physician responsibility in caring for persons with HIV infections. They include the following:
   a. Learning about HIV and its associated conditions
   b. Awareness that although it is appropriate to consider physician risk in management decisions, "patient benefit should not be compromised in an effort to protect the physician"

c. Practice of "universal precautions"
d. Respect for the reproductive choices of every HIV-infected woman
e. Not allowing HIV infection to become a barrier to care
f. Providing care regardless of circumstances of infection
g. Providing patient education about the disease, including pretest and posttest counseling
h. Respecting patient confidentiality
i. Becoming familiar with local regulations regarding screening for HIV, reporting and disclosure of results, and confidentiality
j. Avoiding procedures that risk infecting a patient if the care provider is HIV-infected

Suggested reading

Cao Y et al: Clinical evaluation of branched DNA signal amplification for quantifying HIV-1 21 in human plasma, *AIDS Res Hum Retroviruses* 11:353-360, 1995.

Committee of Ethics, The American College of Obstetricians and Gynecology: Human immunodeficiency virus infection physician responsibilities, *Obstet Gynecol* 75:1043-1045, 1990.

Connor EM et al: Reduction of maternal-infant transmission of human immunodeficiency virus type I with Zidovudine treatment, *N Engl J Med* 331:1173-1180, 1994.

Davis SF et al: Prevalence and incidence of vertically acquired HIV infections in the United States, *JAMA* 274:952-955, 1995.

Piatok M Jr et al: High levels of HIV-1 in plasma during all stages of infection determined by competitive PCR, *Science* 259:1749-1754, 1993.

23.7 GROUP B STREPTOCOCCUS AND BACTERIAL VAGINOSIS

Michael P. Marcotte, M.D., and Louis Weinstein, M.D.

Group B Streptococcus (GBS) in pregnancy

Epidemiology and background

1. Synonyms: *Streptococcus agalactiae,* Lancefield group B *Streptococcus,* β-hemolytic *Streptococcus*
2. Not recognized as human pathogen until mid-1960s
3. Asymptomatic colonization present in the genital tract of 15% to 40% of pregnant women in the United States
   a. Highest rates in the lower third of the vagina and the rectum
   b. Lowest rates in the cervix and urinary tract
   c. Asymptomatic urinary tract colonization in 1% to 2% of pregnant women (may represent the highest inoculum size)
4. Presence of colonization dependent on multiple factors (see the box on p. 546)
   a. Ethnic group: highest in African-Americans, then Hispanics (Caribbean descent greater than Mexican), lowest in Caucasians
   b. Diabetics
   c. Older women
   d. Primigravidas
   e. Medically indigent
   f. Multiple gestations

High-Risk Factors for Colonization

Ethnic group: African-Americans > Hispanics > Caucasians
Diabetes
Older women
Primigravidas
Medically indigent
Multiple gestations

5. GBS infections: the most frequent cause of life-threatening infections in the newborn and a significant cause of morbidity in pregnant women in the United States
   a. 10,000 to 15,000 cases of neonatal sepsis annually (compared with 1000 cases of neonatal herpes simplex infections)
   b. Maternal morbidity: chorioamnionitis, endomyometritis, cystitis, and pyelonephritis (50,000 cases annually)
   c. Increased incidence of preterm deliveries with urinary tract colonization
6. Overall cost estimates of GBS-related infections in 1985 in the United States: $726 million

Diagnosis

1. Gold standard: selective culture media (Todd-Hewitt broth), a blood agar media containing gentamycin and nalidixic acid to inhibit gram negative bacterial overgrowth
   a. Increases the pickup rate by 50% over standard aerobic culture media
2. More rapid diagnostic testing (gram stain, immunofluorescent antibody test, antigen detection with coagglutination, latex particle agglutination, and nucleic acid probes): available but plagued with the problem of low sensitivity in identifying all patients with GBS colonization
3. Serotyping: type I_a, I_b, II, and III shown to be responsible for disease in humans

Clinical manifestations in the neonate

1. Early-onset neonatal sepsis (onset before 7 days of life)
   a. Early onset accounts for 66% of neonatal infection with GBS.
   b. Early onset occurs in 1 to 4/1000 live births in the United States.
   c. Attack rate is 10 to 40/1000 babies born to mothers with positive vaginal rectal colonization.
   d. Early onset neonatal sepsis presents as septicemia, pneumonia, and meningitis, with symptoms present at birth in 50% of neonates (mean age at onset of symptoms is 20 hours).
   e. If infection presents after first few days of life, meningitis predominates.

> **High-Risk Factors for Development of Early GBS Sepsis**
>
> Preterm delivery (less than 37 weeks)
> Prolonged rupture of membranes (greater than 18 hours)
> Maternal intrapartum fever or signs of chorioamnionitis
> Preterm premature rupture of membranes

(1) This accounts for 30% of early-onset disease.
(2) Permanent neurodevelopmental deficits occur in 50% with meningitis.

f. Mortality: Overall is 15%; in preterm infants it is 25% to 30%.
g. Vertical transmission (colonization of neonates without signs of infection) occurs in greater than 50% of neonates born to mothers with positive antenatal GBS cultures.
  (1) Only 1% of these infants develop early-onset disease.
  (2) Forty percent to 75% of GBS are caused by serotype III.
h. High-risk factors for development of early GBS sepsis include the following (see box above):
  (1) Preterm delivery (less than 37 weeks)
  (2) Prolonged rupture of membranes (greater than 18 hours)
  (3) Maternal intrapartum fever or signs of chorioamnionitis
  (4) Preterm premature rupture of membranes
  (5) Previous sibling affected by symptomatic GBS infection
i. Intrapartum chemoprophylaxis with ampicillin in mothers with GBS colonization and one or more high-risk factor has been shown to decrease occurrence of early-onset infection (see Intrapartum Treatment).

2. Late-onset neonatal infection (onset greater than 7 days of life)
  a. Presenting finding of meningitis is found in 85% of neonates.
  b. Overall attack rate is 0.5 to 1/1000 live births.
  c. Infection is not related to intrapartum vertical transmission.
  d. Intrapartum chemoprophylaxis is not effective at reducing the incidence of late-onset disease.
    (1) Transmission is postpartum by neonatal contacts: colonized family, friends, and nursing personnel (nursing personnel colonized 15% to 45% of time).
  e. Serotype III is responsible in greater than 90% of late-onset infections.
  f. Mortality is 10%, but 50% of neonates with meningitis have permanent neurodevelopmental abnormalities.
  g. Neonates may also develop other infections from GBS: middle ear, sinuses, conjunctiva, breasts, lungs, bones, joints, and skin.

Clinical manifestations in the mother

1. Urinary tract
  a. GBS is found in urine of pregnant women 1% to 2% of the time. Majority are asymptomatic.

b. Usually associated with heavy colonization of GBS in the genital tract.
c. The patient should be considered colonized with GBS in the genital tract.
d. If left untreated, GBS is associated with an increase in the rate of preterm deliveries and premature rupture of membranes.
e. Also associated with an increase in the rate of neonatal sepsis: 7/100 (whereas genital tract colonization alone associated with 1/100 cases of sepsis).
f. If left untreated, GBS is associated with a higher incidence of symptomatic maternal urinary tract infections: cystitis and pyelonephritis.
g. Treatment: Ampicillin or penicillin (aqueous PCN) is given.
   (1) PCN-allergic patients use erythromycin or clindamycin, for 7 to 14 days any time GBS is cultured from the urine tract.
   (2) Also plan intrapartum chemoprophylaxis in high-risk patients (see the box on p. 546).

2. Chorioamnionitis (intraamniotic infection)
   a. Defined as a maternal oral temperature greater than 37.8° C plus maternal tachycardia (>100 beats per minute), fetal tachycardia (>160 beats per minute), uterine tenderness, foul odor of amniotic fluid, or peripheral leukocytosis (>12,000/mm^3).
   b. If patient has GBS colonization of the genital tract there is a high rate of colonization (75%) of the intraamniotic cavity after rupture of membranes.
      (1) This amniotic colonization increases with internal monitoring and length of rupture of membranes.
      (2) The amniotic colonization is much higher than the incidence of intraamniotic infection (15%).
   c. If chorioamnionitis develops, there is a higher rate of neonatal infection (5 to 7/100).
      (1) Intraamniotic antibiotics may not decrease the rate of sepsis after the mother has signs of chorioamnionitis.
   d. Treatment: Immediate initiation of antibiotics is begun: ampicillin (or PCN) and gentamycin along with delivery.
      (1) Chorioamnionitis with GBS is almost always associated with other bacteria.
      (2) For PCN-allergic patients use gentamycin plus clindamycin or a first-generation cephalosporin.

3. Endomyometritis (synonyms: endometritis or endomyoparametritis)
   a. Endomyometritis is defined as a postpartum oral temperature greater than 37.8° C with localized uterine tenderness.
   b. GBS endomyometritis is usually associated with high fever within 12 hours of delivery, tachycardia, and abdominal distension.
      (1) Some patients are without localizing signs early in the course of the illness.
   c. Bacteremia is present in 35% of cases.
      (1) Most cases follow cesarean sections.
   d. Treatment: Endomyometritis is usually associated with multiple organisms.

(1) Broad-spectrum coverage indicated.
(2) Multiple regimens proposed with activity against GBS.

Prevention of GBS morbidity and mortality

1. Antepartum treatment
   a. Strategy
      (1) Ampicillin (or PCN) can be given at the time of positive GBS culture anytime during pregnancy.
      (2) Duration of treatment varies.
      (3) Shortcomings
         (a) Antepartum treatment is ineffective at preventing GBS infection in mother or neonate as well as preventing premature delivery.
         (b) GBS is transmitted between partners.
         (c) Impossible to eradicate GBS from the rectum because of presence of high concentrations of beta-lactamase producing bacteria, which inhibit the action of ampicillin and PCN.
         (d) Large numbers of patients need to be treated with long durations of PCN, which increases the chance of allergic reactions and promotes growth of resistant bacteria.
      (4) Only shown to be beneficial if a urine culture is positive for GBS
      (5) Reduces the incidence of preterm delivery, premature rupture of membranes, symptomatic urinary tract infections, and early neonatal GBS sepsis
2. Intrapartum treatment
   a. Strategy
      (1) Ampicillin (or PCN) given to patients with proven GBS colonization and one or more high-risk factors (see the box on p. 546)
         (a) Dosage: ampicillin 2 g IV then 1 to 2 g IV every 4 to 6 hours while in labor
         (b) Clindamycin or a first-generation cephalosporin given to PCN-allergic patients
   b. Controversy in determining the patients to be screened, when to screen them in pregnancy, and the diagnostic method to be used.
3. Several proposed methods to implement this strategy
   (1) Method 1
      (a) Patients who present to labor and delivery with a known high-risk factor (preterm premature rupture of the membranes or preterm labor) are cultured.
         i. Obtain prophylaxis of patients with positive cultures or patients who will deliver before culture results are available.
         ii. No prophylaxis for patients without risk factors and negative cultures.
      (b) Advantage
         i. It has been demonstrated that antibiotics initiated less than 1 hour before delivery are less effective at preventing transmission of GBS to the neonate.

ii. This method would allow many patients to receive antibiotics more than 1 hour before delivery (i.e., the neonate would have higher blood levels of the antibiotics).

(c) Shortcoming

i. A large number of women will be treated unnecessarily.

ii. This may increase the incidence of allergic reactions and promote the development of neonatal sepsis from bacteria resistant to ampicillin.

iii. This method has never been studied in a large, randomized, double-blind, controlled trial.

(2) Method 2

(a) Using a rapid diagnostic technique, patients who present in labor are tested for the presence of GBS.

i. Patients with a positive test and one or more high-risk factor receive prophylaxis.

(b) Advantage

i. GBS has been shown to be transiently present in genital cultures of one third or more of pregnant women throughout their gestation.

ii. This strategy would allow for identification of only women with GBS present at the time of delivery (the time when GBS will be vertically transmitted).

(c) Shortcoming

i. Some women presenting will deliver before the results of the rapid diagnostic tests are available.

ii. Most importantly, there are currently no tests available that have a high enough sensitivity to be used in clinical practice.

(3) Method 3

(a) In the mid-second trimester, culture for GBS.

i. When patients present in labor, prophylaxis for all patients with a positive culture and one or more high-risk factor.

(b) Advantage

i. This method is the only one that has been shown in large, randomized, double-blind, placebo-controlled studies to reduce the incidence of early-onset GBS neonatal sepsis.

ii. This method has also been shown to decrease the incidence of maternal postpartum febrile morbidity (endomyometritis).

(c) Shortcoming

i. Controversy exists in determining which women should have cultures in the second trimester.

ii. GBS is transiently present on genital cultures in more than one third of women and, therefore, a number of women who were culture negative earlier in pregnancy will be positive at delivery.

iii. Some cases of GBS sepsis occur before screening can be done (delivery before 26 weeks) when the mortality rate if infected may be increased.

(4) Method 4

(a) Screening with antepartum cultures is not done, and all women who have one or more high-risk factors are treated.

(b) Advantage: This method will prevent at least the same number of cases of GBS sepsis as method 3, without the cost of GBS screening.

(c) Shortcoming:

i. Many women will be given ampicillin who are not colonized with GBS.

ii. This method has not been studied in a randomized, double-blind, placebo-controlled study.

4. Neonatal therapy

a. Strategy: Prophylactic PCN is administered to all neonates at birth.

(1) Advantage

(a) Study has demonstrated a decreased incidence of GBS sepsis in neonates treated with PCN at birth for prevention of gonococcal ophthalmia.

(b) Eliminates the need for GBS screening.

(2) Shortcoming

(a) 40% to 50% of neonates who develop sepsis are symptomatic at birth, suggesting that prophylactic PCN after birth may not be adequate treatment and may increase the mortality.

(b) This treatment may select for sepsis from PCN-resistant bacteria.

(c) Also no randomized, double-blind, placebo-controlled studies have been done.

(d) This strategy will not reduce the incidence of GBS morbidity in the mother.

5. Recommendations

a. The ACOG recommends selective prophylaxis intrapartum of women with GBS colonization who have one or more risk factor (see the box on p. 546).

(1) ACOG does not recommend antenatal screening for all women.

(2) ACOG does recommend antepartum screening for women who have threatened or arrested preterm labor or premature rupture of membranes remote from term, and women who undergo cervical surgery in pregnancy.

(3) ACOG does recognize that if GBS colonization status is not known and delivery is imminent it may be beneficial to give intrapartum prophylaxis.

b. The American Academy of Pediatrics (AAP) recommends universal screening of all women at 26 to 28 weeks gestation.

(1) Intrapartum prophylaxis should be given to all patients with positive antepartum cultures and one or more risk factors (see the box on p. 546).

(2) AAP states that it may be appropriate to give intrapartum prophylaxis if GBS status is unknown with one of the above risk factors present.
(3) AAP further states that management of neonates of mothers who have received GBS prophylaxis while in labor should be based on clinical findings and gestational age of the neonate.

Summary

1. GBS early neonatal sepsis is the leading cause of mortality by infection in neonates in the United States. GBS is a significant source of maternal morbidity.
2. Controversy still surrounds the ideal way to screen for and prevent GBS morbidity and mortality.
3. Intrapartum chemoprophylaxis with ampicillin has been shown to reduce the incidence of early-onset neonatal GBS sepsis.
4. Selective media (Todd-Hewitt culture media) increases detection of GBS colonization by 50%.
5. Future: Rapid diagnostic tests for GBS that can be used when a patient presents in labor must have a high sensitivity and specificity; intrapartum treatment of those with a positive test and one or more high-risk factors (see the box on p. 546).
6. Active immunization of all pregnant women should be performed with a vaccine that stimulates development of protective antibodies of the IgG subtype, crosses the placenta, and protects the neonate in the intrapartum and immediate postpartum period.

Bacterial vaginosis

Epidemiology and background

1. Before 1955, vaginal discharge that was not caused by gonorrhea, trichomonads, or *Candida albicans* was referred to as nonspecific vaginitis.
2. Gardner and Duke, in 1955, isolated a new bacterium from patients with nonspecific vaginitis and called it *Haemophilus vaginalis.*
   a. They concluded that *H. vaginalis* caused nonspecific vaginitis.
   b. They also identified the clue cell as a diagnostic marker.
3. From 1960 to 1980, name changes occurred reflecting changing taxonomy of the bacterium originally identified by Gardner and Duke: The names included *Corynebacterium vaginalis* and *Gardnerella vaginalis.*
4. In the 1980s, it became clear that more than a single organism was responsible for bacterial vaginosis.
   a. It again went through several name changes: These included nonspecific vaginitis, anaerobic vaginosis, and finally in 1984 bacterial vaginosis (BV).
5. Data collected throughout this time showed that women with BV had an overgrowth of both aerobic and anaerobic bacteria and a loss of the normal flora of the vagina.
   a. Microbiology
      (1) Normal vaginal flora: *Lactobacillus* spp. predominate

(a) Usual concentration of bacteria $<10^7$ organisms per gram of tissue
(b) Can find *Gardnerella vaginalis* in up to 50% of patients without BV
(2) Flora in bacterial vaginosis: loss of *Lactobacillus* spp. and increased concentration of other bacteria up to 10^9 organisms per gram of tissue with an increase in anaerobic bacteria
(a) *Gardnerella vaginalis* isolated in 95% of women with BV concomitant with an increase in isolation of *Mycoplasma* spp. and *Mobiluncus* spp. in vaginal secretions of women with BV

b. Bacteria found in bacterial vaginosis
(1) Anaerobes: *Bacteroides* (now known as *Prevotella*) spp., *Peptostreptococcus* spp., *Mobiluncus* spp.
(2) Aerobes: *Gardnerella vaginalis, Mycoplasma* spp.

6. Risk factors: Race, sexually transmitted disease history, hormonal birth control methods, age, and number of life-time sexual partners are not associated with risk of developing BV.
a. Current intrauterine device (IUD) use is associated with an increased presence of BV.
b. Increased rates of BV are seen in women with multiple sexual partners within 1 month of the exam, compared to women in a monogamous relationship.

7. Etiology is unknown.
a. Some question whether BV is a sexually transmitted disease.
b. Evidence includes the following:
(1) Bacteria associated with BV seen in the urine and urethral scrapings of male partners of patients with BV.
(2) Higher rates of BV in women with multiple sexual partners.
(3) Decreased rate of BV in monogamous couples.
c. Evidence against it includes the following:
(1) Bacteria associated with BV that are found in male partners of women with BV do not persist in these men once they abstain from intercourse.
(2) No increase in cure rates when partners of women diagnosed with BV are treated.
(3) BV found in 12% of virginal women.

Diagnosis

1. Symptoms
a. Malodorous vaginal discharge is the most common presenting complaint.
b. More than 50% of women diagnosed with BV do not have any complaints.

2. Signs: gold standard: clinical findings
a. Diagnosis made if three of the four clinical findings are present.
(1) Vaginal pH greater than 4.5
(2) Wet preparation showing clue cells (squamous epithelial cells with so many bacteria attached to their surface that the cell borders become obscured)

Table 23-16 Diagnosis of bacterial vaginosis by gram stain

Reading	Normal	Intermediate	Abnormal
Grade	I	II	III
Predominant bacteria	*Lactobacillus*	Mixed	Anaerobes and *Gardnerella*

(3) A milky homogeneous vaginal discharge
(4) The release of an amine (fishy) odor after the addition of 10% potassium hydroxide to the vaginal fluid

b. Advantages
   (1) Sensitivity, 99.5%; positive predictive value, 98.8%
   (2) Easily and inexpensively performed in the office

c. Shortcomings
   (1) Vaginal discharge can appear normal; affected by recent douching and intercourse
   (2) pH of vagina increased by the presence of semen and menstrual blood

d. Other diagnostic aids: gram stain, cultures for *Gardnerella* and *Mobiluncus*, and rapid diagnostic tests used in research
   (1) Gram stain:
      (a) In BV the gram stain will show a loss of normal *Lactobacillus* species and an increase in gram positive cocci *(Peptostreptococcus)*, small gram negative rods (*Bacteroides* and *Gardnerella*), and curved gram negative rods (*Mobiluncus*).
      (b) Categorizes vaginal flora as normal (*Lactobacillus* predominates), intermediate (mixed flora), or bacterial vaginosis (Table 23-16).
   (2) Advantages
      (a) Standard method used in microbiology laboratories to evaluate bacteria.
      (b) Relatively inexpensive
   (3) Shortcomings
      (a) Not as sensitive or specific as the clinical criteria
      (b) Delays the diagnosis if gram stain equipment not in the office
   (4) Culture for *Gardnerella* and *Mobiluncus*
      (a) These are not used in clinical practice because women without symptoms or clinical criteria for BV have positive cultures 50% of the time.
   (5) Rapid diagnostic tests include gas–liquid chromatography, thin-layer chromatography, and enzyme analysis.

Natural history

1. In women who are pregnant, the incidence of BV is 10% to 30%.
   a. Approximately 50% of these women will be asymptomatic.

2. Persistent positive diagnosis of BV has been seen in 75% of women not treated.
3. Spontaneous resolution of BV seen in 25% of women.
   a. Reasons postulated include the promotion of *Lactobacillus* growth by the hormone milieu and the decreased frequency of intercourse as pregnancy progresses.
4. Treatment with metronidazole (500 mg, twice daily, for 7 days) or clindamycin (300 mg, twice daily, for 7 days) is shown to cure women in pregnancy of BV 85% of the time when cultures are repeated at 4 weeks.
5. BV is associated with preterm labor and delivery, premature rupture of membranes, LBW infants (<2500 g), chorioamnionitis, and postpartum endomyometritis.

Associated sequelae from bacterial vaginosis in pregnancy

1. Preterm labor
   a. Evidence suggests that women with BV are at a twofold to threefold increase in premature labor and delivery of a preterm low–birth weight infant.
   b. Pathophysiology
      (1) The bacteria present in BV have been shown to produce phospholipase A_2, an enzyme that liberates arachidonic acid, which may induce prostaglandin synthesis in the amnion, leading to premature labor.
      (2) Another proposed mechanism by which bacteria are thought to induce prostaglandin production is via direct invasion of the amniotic membranes adjacent to the cervix.
      (3) Lastly, the bacteria may stimulate migration of white blood cells that metabolize arachidonic acid leading to labor.
2. Premature rupture of membranes
   a. Studies have consistently demonstrated a twofold to threefold increased incidence of premature rupture of membranes (PROM) in women diagnosed with BV.
   b. Women with BV have been shown to have a much higher incidence of PROM prior to and at term.
   c. Pathophysiology: Bacteria associated with BV have been proved *in vitro* to produce protease that reduces the strength of the amnion.
   d. Uterine contractions increase intrauterine pressure, which may cause rupture of the already weakened membranes.
3. Chorioamnionitis and subclinical intrauterine infections
   a. Patients in premature labor with BV have a higher incidence of positive amniotic fluid culture for organisms associated with BV (i.e., anaerobic bacteria, *Gardnerella,* and *Mobiluncus*).
   b. These women are at higher risk for developing chorioamnionitis and delivering prematurely.
   c. These women are also less likely to respond to tocolytic therapy.
   d. Although causation has not been conclusively proved for BV and intraamniotic infections, the association is strong.
   e. Pathophysiology
      (1) The proposed mechanism for the development of chorioamnionitis is through direct ascending invasion of the amnion by

vaginal bacteria with proliferation in the amniotic fluid and release of phospholipase A_2.
(2) These bacteria attract white blood cells, which produce inflammatory mediators, leading to the systemic response.

4. Postpartum endomyometritis
   a. Few prospective reports are available to link the occurrence of intrapartum BV and postpartum endomyometritis.
   b. One study prospectively followed patients with the diagnosis of BV by gram stain made at the time of labor who subsequently underwent a cesarean section.
   c. Those who had BV had a sixfold increase in the rate of postpartum endomyometritis compared with women without BV.
   d. All patients received antibiotic prophylaxis at the time of surgery.
   e. The authors reported that one third of patients with the diagnosis of BV at the time of labor who had a cesarean section developed endomyometritis despite prophylactic antibiotics.
   f. These women grew twice the amount of bacteria on sensitive endometrial cultures than women without BV who developed endomyometritis.
   g. Pathophysiology
      (1) Bacteria gain access to the endometrial cavity by an ascending route.
      (2) Women with BV are shown to have a higher concentration of more virulent bacteria in the vagina than women without BV.
      (3) When a woman in labor undergoes a cesarean section these bacteria not only have access to the endometrial cavity, but also the myometrium, blood vessels, lymphatics, pelvic peritoneum, and the abdominal wound.
      (4) Sutures, which act as foreign bodies, result in a decrease in the bacterial inoculum necessary to establish an infection.

Treatment strategies

1. Historical perspective
   a. Gardner and Duke, in 1955, recommended using topical sulfonamides and oral tetracycline.
   b. They believed BV to be caused by a single organism, *Haemophilus vaginalis,* which is sensitive to these antibiotics.
   c. Elimination of this organism was thought to cure the disease.
   d. This was subsequently proved to be incorrect.
   e. Ampicillin was later recommended and has proved to be ineffective.
2. Treatment of the nonpregnant woman
   a. Standard treatment is oral metronidazole, 500 mg, twice daily for 7 days.
   b. The immediate cure rate is 98%, and long-term cure is expected in 60% to 95% of the cases.
3. Women with BV are encouraged to abstain from douching and some investigators recommend treating partners of patients with recurrent BV.

4. Douching may disrupt the normal *Lactobacillus* predominant microflora of the vagina and promote the overgrowth of organisms responsible for BV.
   a. No studies have conclusively shown a benefit to treating sexual partners.
      (1) New regimens shown to be as effective as metronidazole are intravaginal 0.75% metronidazole gel (one applicator full, 5 g, intravaginally, twice daily for 5 days), intravaginal clindamycin 2% cream (one applicator full, 5 g, intravaginally, once daily for 7 days), short-course oral metronidazole (2 g single dose) and oral clindamycin (300 mg, twice daily, for 7 days).
5. Treatment of the pregnant woman
   a. Multiple studies have examined the role of metronidazole and clindamycin to treat BV in pregnancy.
   b. The hope is that treatment of BV in pregnancy will reduce the incidence of associated morbidity.
      (1) Metronidazole
         (a) Full course: All studies to date have shown a 40% to 50% reduction in the incidence of preterm delivery, PROM, and delivery of a neonate weighing <2500 g.
         (b) Short course
            i. One study demonstrated that metronidazole, 400 mg, twice daily for 2 days effectively treated BV in pregnancy with an 85% response rate.
            ii. Cure was defined as resolution of the woman's symptoms, a negative clinical examination using a wet preparation and light or no growth of *Gardnerella* on culture.
            iii. Unfortunately, no information was supplied about the pregnancy outcome.
         (c) Intravaginal: No studies have been published.
         (d) Side effects
            i. A recent meta-analysis found no increased risk of fetal malformations of women who used metronidazole in the first trimester of pregnancy.
            ii. Gastrointestinal side effects are common, occurring in 15% to 20% of nonpregnant patients.
            iii. No major side effects have been reported in studies published with pregnant patients.
            iv. Metronidazole does not destroy the normal *Lactobacillus* and it is not associated with an increase in vaginal candidiasis.
      (2) Clindamycin
         (a) Oral therapy
            i. One study demonstrated that treating women with BV in pregnancy with oral clindamycin, 300 mg, twice daily for 7 days, resulted in a 50% reduction in the incidence of preterm births and PROM.

ii. This decrease was observed in both patients with a history of preterm births in preceding pregnancies and in women without such a history.

(b) Intravaginal therapy

i. Two well-designed studies demonstrated that in pregnant women with the diagnosis of BV, intravaginal clindamycin 2% cream was effective at curing BV but did not reduce the incidence of preterm birth or PROM.

ii. Cure was defined as both a negative clinical examination and a negative gram stain.

iii. These authors concluded that intravaginal treatment eliminated the BV-associated bacteria from the vagina but was unable to reach bacteria that had already ascended into the upper genital tract.

(c) Side effects

i. Both oral and intravaginal clindamycin are associated with an increase in the rate of subsequent vaginal candidiasis (15% to 20%).

ii. Oral clindamycin has been documented to cause pseudomembranous colitis.

Conclusions and recommendation

1. Bacterial vaginosis is present in 10% to 30% of pregnant women.
   a. Half of these women will be asymptomatic.
2. Clinical criteria for the diagnosis of BV have been established, are simple to perform, and are highly sensitive and specific.
3. Studies to date are in agreement that BV in pregnancy is associated with preterm labor, preterm birth, premature rupture of membranes, and LBW neonates.
   a. There also appears to be a relationship between BV and chorioamnionitis and postpartum endomyometritis.
4. Oral metronidazole has been shown to be highly effective and safe at eliminating the bacteria responsible for BV from the vagina in the pregnant and nonpregnant patient.
   a. There is also evidence demonstrating that metronidazole is effective at reducing the high incidence of preterm birth and PROM.
5. BV is likely to be part of the reason for the high incidence of premature birth and PROM.
   a. It is unlikely that treatment of women with BV in pregnancy will prevent all of these events.
6. Current evidence supports screening women in pregnancy for BV and treating infected women with oral metronidazole, 500 mg, twice daily for 7 days.
   a. In women who cannot tolerate oral metronidazole, oral clindamycin, 300 mg, twice daily for 7 days is an acceptable alternative.
   b. Clindamycin may be associated with a higher incidence of *Candida* vaginitis.
7. In the future, it must be determined whether all women will benefit from screening for BV or only those that are at high risk for

premature delivery (specifically, a history of premature birth in the past).
a. Currently, it seems prudent to screen all pregnant women for BV when they present for prenatal care, and if BV is present, treat them with a full course of oral metronidazole.
b. The benefit of treatment far outweighs the minimal risk.

Suggested reading

The American Academy of Pediatrics, Committee on Infectious Diseases and Committee on Fetus and Newborn: Guidelines for prevention of group B streptococcal (GBS) infection by chemoprophylaxis, *Pediatrics* 90:775-778, 1992.

The American College of Obstetricians and Gynecologists: *Group B streptococcal infections in pregnancy,* ACOG technical bulletin No. 170, Washington, DC, 1992, ACOG.

Burtin P, Safety of metronidazole in pregnancy: A meta-analysis, *Am J Obstet Gynecol* 172: 525-529, 1995.

Creasy, RK, Resnick, R: *Maternal-fetal medicine: principles and practice,* ed 3, pp. 655-657, Philadelphia, W.B. Saunders.

Greenspoon JS et al: Group B *Streptococcus:* the effectiveness of screening and chemoprophylaxis, *Obstet Gynecol Surv* 46:499-508.

McCoy MC et al: Bacterial vaginosis in pregnancy: an approach for the 1990s, *Obstet Gynecol Surv* 50:482-488, 1995.

Thomason JL, Gelbart SM, Scaglione NJ: Bacterial vaginosis: Current review with indications for asymptomatic therapy, *Am J Obstet Gynecol* 165:1210-1217, 1991.

23.8 PULMONARY DISEASE

Michael Parsons, M.D.

Physiologic changes of the lung during pregnancy have been outlined in Chapter 34. Pregnancy may also alter underlying pulmonary conditions. Several disease states deserve discussion for management, including appropriate medications.

1. Physiologic changes in normal pregnancy include the following:
   a. Increased
      (1) Vital capacity
      (2) Inspiratory capacity
      (3) Tidal volume
      (4) Minute ventilation
   b. Decreased
      (1) Expiratory reserve volume
      (2) Residual volume
      (3) Functional residual capacity
   c. Unchanged
      (1) Respiratory rate
2. These changes result in the following:
   a. Increased ventilation with increased basal oxygen consumption
   b. A decrease in arterial PO_2
   c. A slight increase in plasma pH to 7.45
   d. A decrease in bicarbonate

Dyspnea in pregnancy

Mechanism

Over half of all pregnant women report dyspnea at rest by midpregnancy. Proposed mechanisms include the following:

1. Alveolar hyperventilation, with the patient's subjective awareness
2. A response to decreased P_{CO_2}
3. Consequence of anatomic change in the thorax

Significance

Dyspnea may be a sign of decompensation of an underlying lung or heart disorder.

1. Physiologic dyspnea
   a. Tends to occur early in pregnancy and improves or plateaus in later pregnancy
   b. Is rarely extreme and does not usually interfere with daily activities
   c. Is not associated with specific disease indicators
2. Pathologic dyspnea
   a. May occur at rest or normal levels of activity
   b. May be acute, severe, progressive, intractable
   c. Is associated with signs and symptoms suggestive of pulmonary or cardiac disorders
      (1) Cough
      (2) Orthopnea
      (3) Paroxysmal nocturnal dyspnea
      (4) Syncope during exercise
      (5) Chest pain
      (6) Hemoptysis
      (7) Cyanosis and clubbing
      (8) Grade III or greater systolic murmur
      (9) Diastolic murmur
   d. Pulmonary causes (partial list)
      (1) Asthma
      (2) Pulmonary thromboembolism
      (3) Aspiration
      (4) Respiratory infections
      (5) Amniotic fluid embolism
      (6) Adult respiratory distress syndrome
   e. Cardiac causes (partial list)
      (1) Valvular heart disease
      (2) Arrhythmias
      (3) Ischemic heart disease
      (4) Cardiomyopathy

Diagnostic tests as appropriate

1. Echocardiogram
2. EKG
3. Exercise stress testing
4. Pulmonary exercise tests

Asthma

Asthma is a lung disease with the following:

1. Infiltration of the airway with inflammatory cells
2. Increased airway sensitivity and responsiveness
    a. Nonspecific stimuli, including cold air, exercise, strong odors, cigarette smoke
    b. Specific stimuli, including viral infection, F–series prostaglandins, ergonovine, aspirin, dust mites, molds
3. Reversible airway obstruction
    a. The reversibility of the obstruction is either spontaneous or with treatment, but in some cases is incomplete.

Incidence

1. The incidence of asthma during pregnancy is approximately 1%.
2. The incidence of status asthmaticus is about 0.2%.

Morbidity and mortality

1. Approximately one third of asthmatic women experience worsening of the disease at some time during pregnancy.
    a. Patients with severe asthma experience worsening of the disease more often.
    b. There is an 18-fold increased risk of exacerbation following cesarean delivery over vaginal delivery.
2. Adverse pregnancy outcomes in patients with severe asthma include the following:
    a. Spontaneous abortions
    b. Preterm labor
    c. LBW infants
    d. Neonatal hypoxia
    e. Maternal morbidity and mortality, including pneumothorax, pneumomediastinum, acute cor pulmonale, cardiac arrhythmias, and muscle fatigue with respiratory arrest

Pathophysiology

The cause of asthma remains unknown.

1. Bronchial smooth muscle constriction
2. Mucus hypersecretion with fluids within the airway lumen
3. Mucosal edema with thickening of the airway epithelium
4. Suspected mediators include the following:
    a. Histamine
    b. Leukotrienes
    c. Neuropeptides
    d. Prostaglandins
    e. Thromboxane
    f. Kinins
    g. Others.
5. The pathology includes mucosal edema and hyperemia with infiltration of mast cells, eosinophils, and lymphocytes.
    a. Interleukin is produced and IgE synthesized.
    b. The airway wall thickens and fluid within the lumen increases resistance to airflow.
    c. There is obstruction at all airway levels.

Clinical course

1. Maternal
   a. Acute bronchospasm results in airway obstruction and decreased airflow.
   b. Alterations in oxygenation results from ventilation perfusion mismatching.
   c. Clinical stages of asthma are as follows:
      (1) Hyperventilation compensates hypoxia with normal Po_2 and decreased Pco_2, resultant respiratory alkalosis.
      (2) The airways narrow and hypoxemia results.
      (3) CO_2 retention results from poor ventilation.
      (4) Respiratory failure may follow with hypercapnia and acidemia.
      (5) Pregnant patients are more susceptible to developing hypoxia and hypoxemia because of the smaller functional residual capacity.
2. Fetal
   a. Fetal hypoxemia with decreased umbilical blood flow
   b. Increased systemic and pulmonary vascular resistance
   c. Decreased cardiac output

Diagnosis

1. Clinical evaluation
   a. Cough
   b. Labored breathing
   c. Chest tightness
   d. Anxiety
   e. Breathlessness
   f. Prolonged expiration
   g. Wheezing unreliable in predicting severity
   h. Use of excessory respiratory muscles
   i. Tachypnea
   j. Tachycardia
   k. Pulses paradoxes
   l. Central cyanosis
   m. Altered level of consciousness
2. Laboratory tests
   a. Forced expiratory volume in 1 second (FEV-1) is the single best measure of pulmonary function for severity.
      (1) Peak expiratory flow rate (PEFR) reflects large airway function to monitor obstruction.
      (2) Of predicted baseline values, 80% or greater are normal for FEV-1 and PEFR.
   b. Arterial blood gas analysis provides objective assessment of moderate to severe asthma.
3. Other tests
   a. Sputum
      (1) Gram stain and Wright stain
      (2) Eosinophils
   b. Chest radiograph
      (1) Chest radiograph is often normal.

(2) Severe asthma may demonstrate hyperinflation and complications.

Management of asthma

1. Controlling asthma triggers
   a. Elimination of exposures to irritants
   b. Adjustment for anticipated events, such as pretreatment before exercise
   c. Desensitization
2. Pharmacologic therapy: The two main classes of medications are bronchodilators and antiinflammatories.
   a. Chronic treatment
      (1) Bronchodilator
         (a) The first-line agents are beta-2-adrenergic agonists.
         (b) They promote cyclic adenosine monophosphate (cAMP) synthesis and facilitate smooth muscle relaxation, mucociliary clearance, and decrease cell mediator release.
         (c) Inhaled beta-2 agonist puffs every 4 hours, prn, to relax constricted airway smooth muscle (e.g., albuterol, metaproterenol, terbutaline, isoproterenol).
      (2) Inhalational antiinflammatory therapy may be added if treatment with bronchodilators is necessary more than 3 times a week.
         (a) Choices include corticosteroids, 2 to 5 puffs, bid to qid (e.g., beclomethasone and/or cromolyn sodium), 2 puffs, qid (stabilizes mast cell membranes).
      (3) If asthma is not controlled by the combination in (2), a tapering dose of oral corticosteroids is indicated (e.g., prednisone, 40 mg, PO, qd for 1 week, then taper for 1 week).
         (a) Daily inhaled corticosteroids may be necessary.
      (4) Additional medications for control of nocturnal asthma may include evening dose of the following:
         (a) Theophylline
         (b) Sustained oral beta agonist
   b. Acute exacerbation
      (1) Lowered threshold for hospitalization during pregnancy
      (2) Intravenous hydration
      (3) Supplemental oxygen after a blood gas is obtained
      (4) Inhaled beta-2 agonists
      (5) If patient fails to respond, intravenous corticosteroids (e.g., hydrocortisone, 2 mg/kg, or methylprednisolone, 60 mg)
      (6) Additional treatments: intravenous aminophylline and subcutaneous epinephrine or terbutaline, 0.3 to 0.5 mg of 1:1000 solution

Assessment of fetus

1. Evaluation for appropriate fetal growth and fetal well-being during third trimester

Considerations in labor

1. Vaginal delivery should be planned for unless there is an obstetric contraindication.
2. Pulmonary status should be assessed by physical exam and expiratory flow measurements or oxygenation as necessary.
3. Fetal monitoring should be performed.
4. Routine inhaled asthma medications should be continued and oral medication transferred to the IV route.
5. Stress dose corticosteroids (e.g., hydrocortisone, 100 mg every 8 hours) if recent systemic steroids.
6. A non–histamine releasing narcotic (e.g., fentanyl) is preferable to meperidine or morphine.
7. PGF-2A uterotonics should be avoided.
8. Regional analgesia should be considered over general.
9. Oxygen to maintain O_2 saturation must be ≥95%.

Pneumonia

Pneumonia is an acute infection involving inflammation of the lung parenchyma distal to the larger airways.

Incidence

Bacterial and viral pneumonia occur in <0.5% of pregnancies.

Morbidity and mortality

1. Pneumonia is a major cause of nonobstetric maternal deaths, with a reported mortality of 3% in some series.
   a. Increased incidence of preterm labor
   b. Perinatal mortality rate: 40 per 1000

Etiology

1. Bacterial
   a. *Streptococcus pneumoniae (Pneumococcus pneumonia)* is the most common bacterial pneumonia in pregnancy, 30% to 50%.
   b. *Hemophilus influenzae* is more likely in a patient with a smoking history.
   c. *Staphylococcus aureus* is suspected with superimposed pulmonary infections.
   d. *Klebsiella pneumoniae* is seen in chronic alcoholics.
   e. Opportunistic infections include *Acinetobacter, Serratia, Pseudomonas,* increasing in immunocompromised patients.
   f. Overall gram-negative organisms are less common but nosocomial.
2. *Mycoplasma pneumonia* is most common atypical pneumonia.
3. *Chlamydia* pneumonia.
4. *Legionella pneumophila.*
5. Viral
   a. Influenza A during epidemics should be suspected if respiratory symptoms are present in patient recovering from flulike illness.
   b. *Varicella* is rare but may be life-threatening if a cause of pneumonia in pregnancy.

6. Fungal organisms are uncommon as a cause of pneumonia in pregnancy when compared with other organisms.
   a. Coccidiomycosis is the most common fungal cause in pregnancy.
      (1) Common in southwestern United States
   b. Other common causes include the following:
      (1) Histoplasmosis
      (2) *Blastomyces dermatitis*
      (3) Cryptococcoses
      (4) *Pneumocystis carinii* pneumonia (PCP) in immunocompromised patients, particularly with AIDS.
7. Aspiration
   a. Pregnant patients are at risk because of delay in gastric emptying and decreased gastroesophogeal sphincter tone.
   b. Aspiration is most associated with general anesthesia but can occur with any condition with decreased consciousness such as seizures, drug overdose, or alcoholism.
   c. Aspiration involves mixes of aerobic–anaerobic organisms and stomach contents.

Pathophysiology

1. The disease process may start by inhalation of organisms from the air or aspiration of organisms from the nasopharynx or oropharynx.
   a. Less common mechanisms are hematogenous spread or direct contagious spread.
2. The defense mechanisms of the lung, including ciliated lining epithelium, the cough reflex to expel material, and the immunologic system, are not always successful in preventing infection.
3. Other conditions, such as alteration of consciousness, surgery, or other physical impairments, may predispose to increased infection.
4. Pneumonia can lead to inadequate oxygenation.
5. The viral infections may progress to respiratory failure and acute respiratory distress syndrome.
6. Pregnancy is predisposed to more severe pneumonic infections.
   a. Altered maternal immune status
   b. Increased lung water

Diagnosis

1. Differential diagnosis: The diagnosis of pneumonia is usually evident from the signs, symptoms, physical examination, and laboratory studies. Other causes that should be considered include the following:
   a. Bronchitis
   b. Asthma
   c. Tuberculosis
   d. Tumor
2. History: Symptoms of pneumonia include cough, fever, dyspnea, sputum production, and chest pain; shaking chills may occur.
   a. *Mycoplasma* pneumonia has nonproductive cough.
3. Physical examination: Physical examination reveals fever, tachypnea, and tachycardia. There may be decreased respiratory excursion, and

dullness on percussion. If consolidation is present, bronchial breath sounds may be present.
   a. *Mycoplasma* pneumonia has low-grade fever.
   b. *Varicella* pneumonia presents 2 to 6 days after cutaneous eruptions.
4. Laboratory examination
   a. Leukocytosis with a marked left shift is common with bacterial infection. *Mycoplasma* pneumonia has only mild leukocytosis.
   b. Arterial blood gases may reveal hypoxemia, hypocarbia, and respiratory alkalosis.
   c. Roentgenographic examination is essential.
      (1) If a pregnant woman is suspected of having pneumonia, a chest x-ray film *must* be obtained.
      (2) It may provide a clue to the causative factor.
         (a) Homogeneous, nonsegmental consolidation in a lobe with air bronchogram suggests pneumococcal pneumonia.
            i. Pleural effusion may occur.
         (b) A reticular nonhomogeneous pattern suggests *Mycoplasma* pneumonia.
         (c) *Hemophilus influenzae* pneumonia has air bronchograms in upper lobes.
         (d) Influenza has bilateral lower lobe infiltrates.
   d. Identification of the specific organism is important.
      (1) Gram stain of sputum
      (2) Culture of sputum
      (3) Antigen testing of sputum
      (4) Blood cultures for bacteremia
      (5) Serum testing for *Mycoplasma* IgM

Management

1. Hospitalization
2. Hydration
3. O_2 at 3 L/min, nasal cannula, if hypoxia is present
4. Antipyretics
5. Evaluation for fetal well-being and preterm labor if appropriate
6. Antibiotic selection on basis of organism; initial dose empirical
7. Suggested therapy
   a. Penicillin G is given 1.2 to 2.4 million U/day to 1 to 2 million units, IV q4h in seriously ill patients, ampicillin, vancomycin, erythromycin, or cephalosporins for *Streptococcus* pneumonia.
   b. Erythromycin is given 500-1000 mg (not estolate), q6h for *Mycoplasma* pneumonia, *Streptococcus* pneumonia, or *Legionella* pneumonia.
   c. Serious *Hemophilus* infection is treated with third-generation cephalosporins.
   d. Most gram-negative organisms are treated with a third-generation cephalosporin or an aminoglycoside in conjunction with a beta-lactam agent.
   e. Fungal infections may require antifungal agents, such as amphotericin B.
   f. Amantadine hydrochloride is effective for influenza A.

(1) Influenza immunization is indicated in susceptible pregnant women and should be given after the first trimester.

g. Acyclovir is given 5 to 10 mg/kg, IV q8h as treatment for *Varicella* pneumonia.

h. If indicated, initial antibiotic therapy for aspiration pneumonia should include coverage for gram positive, gram negative, and anaerobes such as the following:
   (1) Third-generation cephalosporins
   (2) Penicillin or clindamycin and aminoglycoside

Tuberculosis

Incidence

The incidence of tuberculosis decreased in recent decades until the mid-1980s. Since 1986, there has been an increase in reported cases. In 1990, over 25,000 cases were reported in the United States, mostly in urban areas.

Pathophysiology

1. Tuberculosis is a systemic disease caused by *Mycobacterium tuberculosis,* a 0.5×4 μm aerobic, acid-fast, non–spore forming, nonmotile bacillus.
2. Infection is from the inhalation of droplet nuclei containing the organism.
3. Transmission is most often by close contact with those with cavitary pulmonary disease and productive sputum.
4. Bacteria reach terminal air spaces in the mid and lower air fields.
   a. The apical posterior portions of the lung favor growth.
   b. The infection may spread by lymphohematogenous spread.
   c. A granulomatous tissue reaction then develops, with activated macrophages, lymphocytes, fibroblasts, epithelial cells, and Langahans' giant cells.
   d. Healing usually occurs with calcification.
   e. Tissue necrosis from degenerating macrophages results in caseation necrosis.
5. Two to 8 weeks after the infection, cell-mediated hypersensitivity develops and there is a reactive tuberculin test and containment of the infection.
6. Some patients fail to contain the primary infection.

Clinical presentation

1. Pulmonary disease is the most common manifestation for over 80% of tuberculosis cases in the United States.
2. The primary pulmonary disease is apical cavitation in later childhood and early adulthood.
3. Chronic pulmonary tuberculosis is its most common disease manifestation in a pregnant woman.
   a. Through activation of bacterial colonies in subapical posterior portion of the upper lobe of the lung, caseous material may liquefy and drain into the bronchial tree, producing a cough.
   b. Early in the infection the patient can have minimal symptoms.

c. Later she may develop the following symptoms:
   (1) Anorexia
   (2) Fatigue
   (3) Weight loss
   (4) Chills
   (5) Fever
   (6) Night sweats
   (7) Hemoptysis
   (8) Chest pain
   (9) Dullness to percussion (revealed by physical examination)

Diagnosis

1. The Mantoux test is a quantitative use of purified protein derivative (PPD).
   a. This test is a delayed hypersensitivity response to microbacterial antigen.
   b. A 0.1-mg injection of PPD (5 TU strength) is injected intracutaneous, usually in the forearm.
   c. The skin should be read in 48 to 72 hours.
   d. The PPD is safe to give in pregnancy.
   e. Contrary to earlier data, pregnancy does not alter reactivity to the tuberculin skin testing.
      (1) 0 to 4 mm: negative
      (2) 5 to 10 mm: doubtful
      (3) >10 mm: reactive
2. A positive tuberculin skin test demonstrates that the patient has had a tuberculosis infection.
   a. If there is greater than a 5-mm induration, a chest x ray with shielding of the fetus should be performed.
   b. The chest x-ray film may show apical or subapical patchy infiltrates with cavitation.
   c. With a positive chest x-ray film, a sputum should be obtained in the early morning for AFB × 3 days.
   d. Bronchoscopy with endobronchial biopsy could help obtain a culture, which is the definitive diagnosis.
3. If there is a prior history of Bacille Calmette Guerin (BCG), administration guidelines are as follows:
   a. PPD placement is not contraindicated with history of BCG administration.
   b. Ten years after vaccination, a PPD should be interpreted in the usual manner.
   c. If there are concerning symptoms, findings on chest x-ray film, and known exposure history, a prior history of BCG administration should not influence the decision to treat.
4. A chest x-ray examination should be performed in the following:
   a. Tuberculin reactors with known prior negative reactions
   b. Tuberculin reactors in whom the time of conversion is unknown
   c. Patients with suggestive history or physical examination even if the skin test is negative

Tuberculosis and pregnancy

1. Pregnancy is not associated with the worsening or improvement of tuberculosis.
2. Symptoms are not altered during pregnancy.
3. There is no higher risk of acquiring tuberculosis during pregnancy.
4. Tuberculosis of the fetus is rare.
   a. Means of transmission to the fetus are as follows:
      (1) Hematogenous spread from placenta by umbilical vein.
      (2) Fetal aspiration of infected amniotic fluid *in utero* or at time of birth.
      (3) The major involvement in the fetus is in the liver and lung, but also dissemination to the CNS, bone, gastrointestinal tract, lymphatics, adrenal, skin, and kidney.
   b. For diagnosing congenital tuberculosis, lesions must be present plus one of the following:
      (1) Lesions in the first week of life
      (2) A primary hepatic complex or caseating granuloma
      (3) Documented primary infection of the placenta or endometrium
      (4) Exclusion of infection by a caretaker in postnatal period
   c. If congenital tuberculosis occurs, perinatal mortality approaches 40%.
5. Infants of mothers with tuberculosis: There is no need for routine separation of the mother if she is undergoing appropriate therapy. A PPD should be placed on the infant at 3 months.
6. Untreated, there is a higher rate of preeclampsia, vaginal hemorrhage, and fetal loss.
7. With chemotherapy, tuberculosis infection does not affect perinatal outcome except for the rare occurrence of congenital tuberculosis.

Less common presentations of tuberculosis

1. Miliary (disseminated)
2. Serofibrinous pleurisy with effusion
3. Female genital tuberculosis endosalpinx, ovaries, and endometrium

Medications for treatment of tuberculosis

1. The three medications most frequently used for treatment of tuberculosis during pregnancy are the following:
   a. Isoniazid (INH)
   b. Rifampin (RIF)
   c. Ethambutol (ETH)
2. All of these medications have been successfully used during pregnancy with little risk of teratogenicity.

INH prophylaxis for positive PPD

American Thoracic Society (ATS) and CDC recommendations are as follows:

1. For pregnant women less than 35 years old
   a. Greater than 15 mm not previously treated
   b. Greater than 10 mm and from high prevalence area or occupations or recent immigrants
   c. Greater than 5 mm if HIV positive or HIV contact

Table 23-17 Treatment of active tuberculosis

Drug	Duration
Isoniazid (INH), 5 mg/kg to a total of 300 mg/day	9 months
Pyridoxine, 50 mg/day	9 months
Rifampin (RIF), 10 mg/kg to a total of 600 mg/day	9 months
Ethambutol (ETH), 5 to 25 mg/kg to a total of 2.5 gm/day	8 weeks or until cultures are sensitive to INH/RIF
Pyrazinamide (PZA), 15 to 30 mg/kg to a total of 2 g/day. Start only if resistance to INH is likely or in HIV-infected patients	8 weeks or until cultures are sensitive to INH/RIF
Streptomycin, 15 mg/kg to a total of 1.5 gm/day	Generally contraindicated in pregnancy unless no alternative exists

From *MMWR* 42(RR-7):1, 1993.

2. For pregnant women 35 years of age or greater
   a. Less than 15 mm should not receive prophylaxis during pregnancy or immediate postpartum unless they have high-grade risk factors.
3. Chemoprophylaxis
   a. INH, 300 mg, every day for 9 months
   b. Pyridoxine, 50 mg a day, for 9 months
      (1) Pyridoxine is to decrease the incidence of peripheral neuropathy of INH.

Treatment of active disease in pregnancy

Tuberculosis is diagnosed by the culture of the tubercle bacillus from the skin or other bodily fluids. For treatment of active tuberculosis see Table 23-17.

Medication risks

1. INH can cause hepatitis, which has an incidence of 20/1000 with a 0.001% risk of death.
   a. It causes peripheral neuropathy by competition with pyridoxine.
2. Rifampin also has a risk of hepatitis.
   a. Rare adverse effects, including hydrops, have been reported to the fetus.
   b. Overall, teratogenicity with rifampin has not been shown.
3. Ethambutol side effects have included optic neuritis, with blurred vision and trouble with color discrimination.
4. Streptomycin can cause fetal defects from mild vestibular damage to bilateral deafness.
5. It is important to monitor for the response to therapy, and also for advanced reaction and drug toxicity.

Tuberculosis and HIV

1. HIV-positive individuals develop active tuberculosis by the following means:
   a. More rapid progression of new infections
   b. Reactivation of latent infections
   c. Reinfection with tuberculosis after adequate therapy.
2. The diagnosis may be complicated by anergy.
3. Preventive therapy is indicated for the following:
   a. Induration greater than or equal to 5 mm
   b. Anergy and from high-prevalence groups

Public health measures

The local health department should be notified of cases of tuberculosis so that contacts may be identified and follow-up provided.

Chronic respiratory disease

Tobacco smoking

1. Incidence
   a. It is estimated that over 25% of women are smoking when they become pregnant.
   b. Many will either stop smoking or smoke less frequently during pregnancy, but others will continue to smoke as usual (see the box on p. 572).
2. Morbidity and mortality
   a. The general effects of smoking, including increased risk of lung cancer, emphysema, chronic bronchitis, and cardiovascular disease, are well known.
   b. There are substantial risks to the fetus and neonate, and these are dose related.
   c. Obstetric problems that have been reported from smoking cigarettes include decreased mean birth weight of 200 g, increased incidence of placenta previa and abruptio placentae, prematurity, possible PROM, and possible long-term neurologic abnormalities in the infant.
   d. There is a decreased incidence of PIH.
3. Pathophysiology: The effects on the fetus in smokers have been attributed as follows:
   a. Nicotine causes uterine vasoconstriction and fetal hypertension.
   b. Carbon monoxide reduces fetal oxygen carrying capacity by combining with fetal hemoglobin.
   c. Benzopyrene and other polycyclic hydrocarbons are mutagens and carcinogens.
   d. Smoking is associated with poor nutrition.
   e. Nicotine increases cyanide in the bloodstream.
   f. It causes decreased density of fetal vessels in terminal villi of placenta.
4. Management
   a. Management consists of encouraging the pregnant woman to stop or decrease her cigarette smoking.

Surgeon General's Report on Health Benefits of Smoking Cessation in Pregnancy

1. Babies born to women who smoke during pregnancy weigh 200 g less on the average than their counterparts born to nonsmoking women.
2. There is a dose–response relationship between the amount of maternal smoking and reduced birth weight; the more a woman smokes during pregnancy, the greater the reduction in birth weight.
3. If a woman stops smoking by her fourth month of gestation, the risk of delivering a LBW baby approaches that of a nonsmoker.
4. Data indicate that maternal smoking during pregnancy may also affect a child's long-term development, intellectual development, and behavioral characteristics.
5. The risks of spontaneous abortion, fetal death, and neonatal death increase directly with increasing levels of maternal smoking during pregnancy.
6. Maternal smoking significantly increases the incidence of abruptio placenta, placenta previa, bleeding early or late in pregnancy, premature and prolonged rupture of membranes, and preterm delivery.

Data from U.S. Department of Health and Human Services: *The health benefits of smoking cessation: a report of the Surgeon General,* DHHS Publication No. (CDG) 90-8416, 1990.

(1) The importance of her infant's health as well as her own should be stressed.

b. If growth retardation is evident, appropriate monitoring should be performed.

c. Nicotine transdermal patch use should be individualized.
   (1) The benefit to heavy smokers (>20 cigarettes/day) may be greater than the risk.

Kyphoscoliosis

Kyphoscoliosis is a bony deformity of the spine that may have either excessive posterior (kyphosis) or lateral (scoliosis) curvature.

1. Incidence: The incidence is approximately 0.8 to 6/10,000 pregnancies.
2. Morbidity and mortality
   a. Kyphoscoliosis has been reported to be associated with increased rates of prematurity and possibly stillbirth.
3. Pathophysiology
   a. Causes of kyphoscoliosis include idiopathic factors (80%), neuromuscular disease, trauma, tuberculosis, connective tissue disease, and rickets.
   b. Physiologically, the maternal effect of this problem is an alteration of the rib cage configuration, which may lead to compression of the lungs, with emphysema and/or atelectasis.

c. This can cause decreased vital capacity and cardiopulmonary complications, including cor pulmonale.
4. Diagnosis: Careful physical examination should reveal the spinal deformity.
5. Prognosis
   a. Successful pregnancies can usually be achieved.
   b. Women with unstable scoliosis or with a curve of greater than 25% are at a greater risk of progressive disease during pregnancy.
   c. There is not an increase in cesarean deliveries.
6. Management
   a. The maternal status should be monitored for cardiopulmonary compromise, and the fetal status should be monitored for adequate growth and well-being and for preterm labor.
   b. Oxygen should be given if indicated for hypoxia.
   c. Antibiotics should be administered if indicated for pulmonary infection.
   d. Digitalis should be performed if indicated.

Sarcoidosis

1. Sarcoidosis is a systemic granulomatosis disease.
2. The etiology is unknown.
3. It occurs in 0.02% to 0.06% of pregnancies.
4. Morbidity and mortality
   a. Maternal
      (1) Sarcoidosis itself does not damage the pregnancy, but any disease that has compromised pulmonary or cardiac function may lead to deleterious effects in pregnancy.
      (2) Patients with more severe disease, including dyspnea and skin lesions, often have a worse prognosis.
      (3) Pregnancy does not worsen the clinical course of sarcoidosis, but there is a generalized improvement in disease in most patients, possibly caused by steroids; there is often a relapse postpartum.
   b. Fetal
      (1) Growth retardation and preterm labor have been reported.
      (2) Fetal surveillance may be indicated.
5. Pathophysiology
   a. A noncaseating granulomatous infiltration occurs in a perivascular pattern.
   b. The most common organs affected are the lungs.
      (1) They may be affected by pulmonary granulomas and alveolitis.
      (2) Progressive fibrosis with loss of volume results in a restrictive ventilatory defect.
   c. Other affected organs include lymph nodes, eyes, skin, bone, nerves, heart, kidneys, and liver.
6. Diagnosis
   a. Clinical manifestations include dyspnea, nonproductive cough, nonspecific chest pain, fever, fatigue, weakness.
   b. Clinical examination and pulmonary function tests revealing restrictive lung disease are suggestive.

(1) Noncaseating granulomas demonstrated by biopsy from the lung, lymph node, skin, conjunctiva, other organs are diagnostic.

c. Chest x-ray film may demonstrate bilateral hilar adenopathy, interstitial or alveolar infiltrates, or nodular lesions.
d. Hypercalcemia, hypergammaglobinemia, elevated liver enzymes in advanced disease.
e. Angiotensin-coverting enzymes have been used as a marker of disease activity but are not consistently helpful.

7. Management
   a. The goal is preservation of maternal pulmonary function and improvement of symptoms.
   b. Patients with mild, asymptomatic disease do not require treatment because the disease may resolve spontaneously.
   c. Corticosteroids suppress the granulomatous aspect of the disease in more severe cases.
   d. In hypercalcemic patients, prenatal vitamins should not include vitamin D.
   e. Oxygen may be needed during labor and delivery if hypoxia occurs.
8. Prognosis: Pregnancy is well tolerated if the following conditions are not present:
   a. Vital capacity <1 L
   b. Pulmonary hypertension
   c. Pao_2 <55 mm Hg
   d. Dyspnea
   e. High doses of steroids required

Suggested reading

Bass JB Jr et al: Treatment of tuberculosis and tuberculosis infection in adults and children, *Am J Respir Crit Care Med* 149:1359-1374.

Bennett JC, Plum F, editors: *Cecil textbook of medicine,* ed 20, Philadelphia, 1996, WB Saunders.

Cunningham FG et al, editors: *Williams' obstetrics,* ed 19, Norwalk, CT, 1993, Appleton & Lange.

Doucette JT, Bracken MB: Possible role of asthma in the risk of preterm labor and delivery, *Epidemiology* 4:143-150, 1993.

Ewald GA, McKenzie, CR, editors: *The Washington manual: Manual of medical therapeutics,* ed 28, St Louis, 1995, Department Medicine, Washington University School of Medicine.

Greenberger PA: Asthma in pregnancy, *Clin Chest Med* 13:597-605, 1992.

Hollingsworth HM, Irwin RS: Acute respiratory failure in pregnancy, *Clin Chest Med* 13:723-740, 1992.

King TE Jr: Restrictive lung disease in pregnancy, *Clin Chest Med* 13:607-622, 1992.

Maccato M: Respiratory insufficiency due to pneumonia in pregnancy, *Crit Care Obstet* 18:289-299, 1992.

McColgin SW, Glee L, Brian BA: Pulmonary disorders complicating pregnancy, *Med Compl During Pregn* 19:697-717, 1992.

Nolan TE, Hankins GDV: Acute pulmonary dysfunction and distress, *Obstet Gynecol Clin North Am* 22:39-54, 1995.

Review: Asthma in pregnancy, *Br J Obstet Gynaecol* 101:658-660, 1994.

Robinson CA, Rose NC: Tuberculosis: current implications and management in obstetrics, *Obstet Gynecol Surv* 51:115-124, 1996.

Rodriguez J, Niederman MS: Pneumonia complicating pregnancy, *Clin Chest Med* 13:679-691, 1992.
Zeldis SM: Dyspnea during pregnancy. Pulmonary disease in pregnancy, *Clin Chest Med* 13:567-585, 1992.

23.9 RENAL DISEASE

Helen Y. How, M.D.

Renal changes during normal pregnancy

Anatomic changes

1. Kidney length is increased 1 to 1.5 cm in late pregnancy.
2. Kidney weighs 50 g more in the pregnant state.
3. Dilation of the entire collecting system occurs; right more than left because of dextrorotation of the uterus, because rectosigmoid acts as a cushion for the left ureter, and because of compression of the right ureter by the engorged right renal vein.

Functional changes

1. Renal hemodynamics
   a. Glomerular filtration rate (GFR) achieves an incremental increase of 30% to 50% by the 12th week, which is sustained until term.
   b. Renal plasma flow (RPF) increases by 80% between conception and the second trimester and subsequently falls to a level of about 60% greater than the nonpregnant norm.
   c. Creatinine clearance (Cr Cl) of 150 to 170 ml/min/1.73 m^2 occurs by the end of the second trimester.
   d. Blood urea nitrogen (BUN) falls from 13 ± 3 mg/dl to 8.7 ± 1.5 mg/dl.
   e. Creatinine (Cr) falls from 0.67 ± 0.14 mg/dl to 0.46 ± 0.13 mg/dl.
   f. Increased excretion of amino acids, proteins (250 to 300 mg/24 hours), uric acid, glucose, and several water-soluble vitamins.
2. Volume regulation
   a. Total body water increases by 6 to 8 L by term.
   b. The bulk of this is concentrated in the extracellular compartment distributed between the plasma and interstitium.
   c. Plasma volume starts increasing early in the first trimester, accelerates in the second trimester, peaks at around 32 weeks, and stays elevated until term, with average gain of 1.1 to 1.3 L.
3. Sodium (Na^+) homeostasis
   a. Net Na^+ gain is 950 mEq, the majority of which is stored in the maternal compartment.
      (1) Factors increasing urinary Na^+ excretion are as follows:
         (a) Increased filtered load
         (b) Antinatriuretic hormone
         (c) Prostaglandins
         (d) Decreased renal vascular resistance
         (e) Progesterone
         (f) Arginine vasopressin

        (g) Decreased serum albumin
        (h) Increased RPF
    (2) Factors decreasing urinary Na^+ excretion are as follows:
        (a) Aldosterone
        (b) Increased filtration flow
        (c) Deoxycorticosteroid
        (d) Increased ureteral pressure
        (e) Exaggerated supine and upright position effects

4. Potassium (K^+) homeostasis
    a. Net K^+ gain is 350 mEq, which is primarily incorporated in the fetus.
    b. Progesterone blocks the effect of mineralocorticosteroids at the level of the renal tubules.
    c. Bartter's syndrome and primary hyperaldosteronism improve.
    d. Body tonicity
        (1) Plasma osmolality is decreased by 8 to 10 mOsm/kg (270 mOsm/kg H_2O).
        (2) Osmotic threshold is reset for both antidiuretic hormone (ADH) and thirst.
        (3) ADH secretion is increased in pregnancy and, together with increased water intake, results in a decrease of sodium by 5 mEq/L, which effectively decreases serum tonicity.

Effects of pregnancy on preexisting renal disease

Infection

1. Acute pyelonephritis
    a. The most common infectious complication of gestation and is more likely to lead to acute renal failure (ARF) in gravidas than in nonpregnant women.
    b. There are marked decrements of GFR and significant increases in their serum Cr levels.
    c. This can be because the vasculature of the gravidas may be more sensitive to the vasoactive effects of bacterial endotoxins.
    d. Acute pyelonephritis during pregnancy has been associated with hypotension and, on occasion, renal vein thrombosis.
2. Chronic pyelonephritis
    a. The prognosis of pregnancy in women with chronic pyelonephritis is similar to that of gravidas with glomerular disease.
    b. The outcome is favorable in normotensive patients with preserved renal function, but those with hypertension and renal insufficiency at conception do poorly.
    c. Bacteriuria in pregnancy can lead to exacerbation.

Glomerulonephritis (GN)

1. Acute GN
    a. Acute poststreptococcal GN is rare in pregnancy.
    b. It has been mistaken for preeclampsia when it does occur.
2. Chronic GN
    a. Usually no adverse effect if normotensive.
    b. Urinary tract infections (UTI) may occur more frequently.

Nephrotic syndrome

1. Defined by proteinuria, hypoproteinemia, and edema.
   a. The most common cause of these is membranous GN or membranous proliferative GN.
2. In the absence of azotemia or hypertension, pregnancy outcome is good and maternal morbidity low.
3. Infant birth weight was related to maternal serum albumin levels.
4. Steroid therapy has been beneficial for patients with nephrotic syndrome and should not be withheld because of pregnancy.
5. Other more common causes of nephrotic syndrome in pregnancy are as follows:
   a. Diabetic nephropathy
      (1) Glomerulosclerosis is part of a widespread angiopathy that involves small blood vessels throughout the body.
      (2) Thus renal involvement is uncommon in the absence of retinal changes.
      (3) The tubules may be affected by diabetes, most often by glycogen deposition in proximal tubules.
      (4) Chronic interstitial nephritis may also be present.
      (5) There is increased predisposition to preeclampsia and infection.
   b. Systemic lupus erythematosus (SLE)
      (1) Some, but not all, studies have demonstrated that lupus patients are more likely to experience a flare during pregnancy if the lupus is active at conception.
      (2) Although controversial, it is suggested that prognosis is most favorable if the disease is in remission 6 months or more before conception.
      (3) Most renal flares are temporary; however, some women will have a permanent decrease in renal function.
      (4) It is difficult to differentiate between lupus renal flare and preeclampsia.
      (5) It is possible that the two conditions can coexist.
      (6) Buyon and colleagues found that a lack of increase in complements C3 and C4 is more characteristic of lupus flare.
   c. Syphilis: Any organ system, including the kidneys, can be affected during the disseminated stage of secondary syphilis.

Polycystic disease

Functional impairment and hypertension are usually minimal in childbearing years.

Nephrolithiasis

1. Persistent pyelonephritis despite adequate antimicrobial therapy should prompt a search for nephrolithiasis.
2. When calculi are discovered, the possibility of hyperparathyroidism should also be considered.
3. Treatment depends on the symptoms and the duration of pregnancy.
4. In over half of the cases, the stone passes spontaneously, but about a third of the pregnant women with symptomatic stones will need

cystoscopy, percutaneous nephrostomy, basket extraction, or surgical exploration.

Severity of renal impairment and impact of pregnancy (excluding SLE)

1. Mild
   a. Plasma Cr ≤1.4 mg/dl (124 μmol/L)
   b. Usually a 95% successful obstetric outcome (82% if before 28 weeks)
   c. 20% pregnancy complication and < 5% long-term sequelae
2. Moderate
   a. Plasma Cr 1.5 to 2.5 mg/dl (133 to 265 μmol/L)
   b. Cr Cl 30 ml/min
   c. Usually a 90% successful obstetric outcome (56% if before 28 weeks)
   d. Accelerated renal deterioration with 44% pregnancy complication and 25% long-term sequelae (77% if before 28 weeks)
3. Severe
   a. Plasma Cr ≥3 mg/dl (265 μmol/L)
   b. Amenorrheic and anovulatory
   c. Decreased likelihood of conception
   d. Pregnancy vigorously discouraged with 47% successful obstetric outcome; 84% pregnancy complications (8% if before 28 weeks) and 58% long-term sequelae (92% before 28 weeks).
   e. Pregnancy reconsidered after renal rehabilitation by way of dialysis and a transplant program.

Chronic renal disease (antenatal care)

1. Follow-up every 2 weeks until 32 weeks gestation, then every week thereafter.
   a. Recommend induction of labor at 38 weeks.
2. Assess renal function, preferably by 24-hour Cr Cl and protein excretion (monthly).
   a. Near term, a 15% decrease in function that affects plasma creatinine minimally is permissible.
3. Early detection of asymptomatic bacteriuria or confirmation of UTI, if possible.
4. Carefully monitor blood pressure (BP) for early detection of hypertension (50%) and assess its severity (20% will develop diastolic pressure of 110 mm Hg).
   a. Diastolic pressure should be kept between 80 and 85 mm Hg.
5. Detect preeclampsia early, if possible.
6. Assess fetal size, development, and well-being.

Medical complications of renal insufficiency

1. Neurologic: as a result of water intoxication or electrolyte imbalance, patient seizures
2. Cardiovascular: circulatory congestion secondary to fluid overload, cardiac arrhythmia secondary to electrolyte disturbances, hypertension

3. Gastrointestinal: anorexia, nausea, vomiting, hemorrhage
4. Infections: at operative sites; urinary tract and respiratory system

Renal biopsy during pregnancy

1. Packham and Fairley report a series of 111 renal biopsies performed in preterm pregnant women:
   a. Transient gross hematuria: 0.9% (pregnant) vs. 3% to 5% (nonpregnant)
   b. Overall complication rate: 4.5%
   c. Conclusion: no increase in morbidity if BP is well controlled, normal coagulation, and an experienced hand
2. Rare indications are as follows:
   a. Sudden deterioration of renal function before 30 to 32 weeks gestation with no obvious cause
      (1) Certain forms of rapidly progressive GN may respond to aggressive treatment with steroid, chemotherapy, and perhaps plasma exchange, when diagnosed early.
   b. Symptomatic nephrotic syndrome before 30 to 32 weeks gestation
   c. When the patient fails to show signs of recovery within 3 weeks; when acute tubular necrosis (ATN) has been suspected clinically

Chronic dialysis in pregnancy

1. GFR ≤5 ml/min
2. Pregnancies in childbearing age: 0.5% to 0.9% (true frequency unknown)
3. Incidence of abortion: 50% with only 19% to 23% ending in live births
4. Dialysis strategy
   a. All will require a 50% increase in hours and frequency of dialysis.
   b. The aim of this is to do the following:
      (1) Maintain BUN less than 50 mg/dl (8 mmol/L) because intrauterine death is more likely if values exceed this mark.
      (2) Avoid hypotension during dialysis, which could be damaging to the fetus.
         (a) In late pregnancy, the enlarging uterus and supine posture may aggravate this by decreased venous return.
         (b) Continuous external fetal monitoring in the late second and third trimester is recommended.
      (3) Rapid fluctuations in intravascular volume are avoided by limiting interdialysis weight gain to approximately 0.5 to 1 kg.
      (4) Rigid control of BP must be ensured.
         (a) BP must be kept below 140/90.
         (b) First-line treatment is correction of volume overload by dialysis.
         (c) Conventional antihypertensive drugs should be used.
         (d) Phenobarbital or phenytoin should be used for seizure prophylaxis.
         (e) $MgSO_4$ may be given with caution.
         (f) Low-dose aspirin may be beneficial.
      (5) Physician should scrutinize carefully for preterm labor (40%) because dialysis and uterine contractions are associated.

   (a) Postulate progesterone removal.
   (b) This is also a result of increased incidence of abruptio placentae and polyhydramnios.
  (6) Plasma calcium should be watched closely to avoid hypercalcemia.
  (7) Correcting anemia:
   (a) Hematocrit (Hct) should be kept above 25%, and transfusion with packed red blood cells (RBCs) or erythropoietin therapy (50 to 160 U/g/wk, SC) may be necessary.
   (b) If erythropoietin therapy is used, iron and folic acid supplementation should be given simultaneously; Hct values are expected to increase at 0.6% to 2% per week.
   (c) Possible side effects of erythropoietin therapy are hypertension, coagulopathy, fetal polycythemia (? passage through the placenta), and polyhydramnios.
   (d) Weekly monitoring of maternal Hct and BP is required, with monthly evaluation of electrolytes, phosphate, Cr Cl, iron, and platelets.
  (8) Nutrition: A daily oral intake of 70 g protein, 1.5 g calcium, 50 mmol potassium, 80 mmol sodium, with supplements of dialyzable vitamins is advised.
  (9) Pregnant patients are in a state of chronic compensated respiratory alkalosis, and large drops in serum HCO_3 should be prevented.
   (a) Dialysates containing glucose and HCO_3 are preferred; those containing citrates should be avoided.

Chronic ambulatory peritoneal dialysis (CAPD)

1. Instillation of dialysate (1.5 to 3 L, four or more times daily and left in for 4 to 8 hours) through a permanent indwelling catheter inserted high in the abdomen under direct vision.
2. Advantages over hemodialysis include the following:
   a. No chronic requirement for chronic vascular access or regional heparinization
   b. Lesser degree of fluid and solute shift, more constant chemical and extracellular environment for the fetus
   c. Infrequent episode of hypotension
   d. Higher hematocrit levels
3. There are a total of eight reported cases of pregnancies treated with CAPD.
   a. These pregnancies resulted in six live births (one neonatal death) and two spontaneous abortions.

Pregnancy in the renal transplant recipient

1. The following are successful pregnancies:
   a. 1958: donor from twin sister
   b. 1966: living related donor
   c. 1970: cadaveric kidney
   d. 1990: >2000 pregnancies
      (1) 1/50 women of childbearing age with a functioning graft becomes pregnant.

(2) Forty percent had spontaneous abortions and elective termination of pregnancy.

2. Over 90% of pregnancies that do go beyond the first trimester end successfully (40% to 60% preterm delivery).
   a. Ectopic pregnancy: 0.5% of all conceptions
   b. Risk of preeclampsia: 25% to 30%
   c. Permanent decrement in kidney function: 15%
3. Allograft function
   a. A 30% decline in renal function in the third trimester is normal.
   b. Baseline renal ultrasound at 20 weeks gestation may assist in the evaluation of possible hydronephrosis later in pregnancy.
   c. UTIs are frequent and should be treated energetically as 50% of the transplanted ureters will reflux.
4. Allograft rejection
   a. Rejection occurs in 9% of patients.
   b. Rejection is difficult, especially in cases of occult chronic rejection with progressive subclinical course.
   c. Clinical hallmarks are present: fever, oliguria, deteriorating renal function, renal enlargement, and tenderness.
   d. Renal biopsy must be performed to distinguish rejection from acute pyelonephritis, recurrent glomerulopathy, possibly severe preeclampsia, and cyclosporine A nephrotoxicity.

Immunosuppressive therapy

1. Prednisone
   a. Active metabolite is prednisolone.
   b. Cord blood/maternal levels are 1:10.
   c. Two of the 44 live births with adrenal insufficiency.
   d. High dose is necessary to treat documented rejection episode.
2. Cyclosporine A
   a. Possibly less teratogenic potential than azathioprine (limited data)
   b. Adverse effects in nonpregnant patient: renal toxicity, liver dysfunction, tremor, convulsions, diabetogenic effects, hemolytic uremic syndrome, and neoplasia
3. Azathioprine
   a. Liver toxicity
   b. During organogenesis, cannot be activated in the fetus because of its lack of inosinate pyrophosphorylase
   c. May cause chromosomal aberrations in lymphocytes of infants exposed; cleared within 20 to 32 months
   d. Reports of thrombocytopenia and leukopenia in infants
   e. 20% to 50% incidence of intrauterine growth restriction
   f. ? Infertility, childhood malignancy
   g. Breast-feeding not recommended

Renal transplant

1. Antenatally, serial ultrasound and antenatal testing starting at 28 weeks is recommended.
2. Delivery and management in labor: Vaginal delivery should be the aim.

3. Obstructive problems and mechanical injury to the transplant are rare.
4. Cesarean section is performed for obstetric reasons or occasionally for cephalopelvic disproportion caused by osteodystrophy related to previous renal failure and dialysis or prolonged steroid therapy.

Maternal follow-up after pregnancy

1. Rejection postpartum may result from a return to a normal immune state (despite immunosuppression) or possibly from a rebound effect from altered gestational immunoresponsiveness.
   a. Five-year survival rate:
      (1) Living related donors: 70% to 80%
      (2) Cadaveric kidneys: 40% to 50%
   b. Threefold increase in cancers of the female genital tracts has been noted.
2. Contraception
   a. Birth control pills can cause or aggravate hypertension or thromboembolism and can also produce subtle changes in the immune system, but this does not contraindicate their use.
   b. IUD
      (1) Associated with bacteremia of vaginal origin in 13% of healthy women, so increased risk of pelvic inflammatory disease
      (2) Reduced efficacy in the presence of immunosuppressive and antiinflammatory agents
   c. Bilateral tubal ligation
      (1) Unwise to offer at the time of transplantation
   d. Norplant, Depo-Provera
      (1) Limited data

Idiopathic postpartum renal failure

1. Idiopathic condition is characterized by renal failure in association with microangiopathic hemolytic anemia and usually thrombocytopenia occurring within a few days to approximately 10 weeks after an apparently normal pregnancy and delivery.
   a. Etiology: unknown
   b. Pathophysiology: deposition of platelet thrombi in the microvasculature (? platelet aggregating factor)
   c. Prognosis: guarded
      (1) Most women who have succumbed required chronic dialysis or have survived with severely reduced renal function.
      (2) Only a few have recovered.
   d. Treatment: supportive
      (1) ? Plasmapheresis, platelet inhibitors

Acute obstetric renal failure

1. Incidence: less than 1:10,000 pregnancies: account for 9% of all episodes of ARF in women
2. Site of abnormality
   a. Prerenal
      (1) Renal ischemia is caused by hypoperfusion; it accounts for 75% of the pregnancy-associated ARF.

Table 23-18 Causes of obstetric acute renal failure

Volume depletion	Hemorrhage Antepartum Postpartum Ectopic pregnancy Abortion Dehydration Hyperemesis gravidarum Severe diarrhea
Disseminated coagulopathy	Preeclampsia or eclampsia Abruptio placentae Acute fatty liver of pregnancy Postpartm hemolytic uremic syndrome Drug or transfusion reactions
Sepsis	Septic abortion Acute pyelonephritis Puerperal sepsis Septicemia
Obstruction	Ureteric damage Bilateral pelviureteric obstruction Retroperitoneal hematoma
Renal parenchymal disease	Acute glomerulonephritis Renal involvement in multisystem disease

Adapted from Michael J: The management of renal disease in pregnancy, *Clin Obstet Gynecol* 13:319, 1986.

(2) Hemorrhage and hypotension are the most common precipitating factors.

b. Intrarenal: renal parenchymal disease

c. Postrenal: obstructive

Workup

To recognize and treat ARF appropriately, the clinician must rapidly identify the precipitating factors and correct them when possible (Table 23-18).

Clinical course

1. GFR declines rapidly toward a value that approaches zero.
2. Hallmark features include a linear increase in serum creatinine at a rate of 0.5 to 1.5 mg/dl/day; a progressive, rapid rise in serum urea nitrogen (BUN) at a rate of 10 mg/dl/day; and usually a fall in urine flow rate to less than 400 to 500 ml/day.
3. Twenty percent of the ARF cases are nonoliguric; therefore, using urine volume as an index of renal function may be misleading.
4. The next step after a careful history and physical examination is to evaluate urinary sediment.
   a. Prerenal azotemia or obstructive uropathy: normal findings
   b. Glomerular disease or vasculitis: protein or RBC casts

Table 23-19 Difference between bilateral renal cortical necrosis and acute tubular necrosis

	BRCN	ATN
Total anuria	2 to 7 days	Rare
Oliguria	Permanent	Oliguria phase: 10 to 14 days Polyuria phase: (>3 L/day) variable duration Recovery phase: 10 to 14 days
Hematuria	Generally at the beginning	Seldom initially
Renal biopsy	Cortical necrosis	Glomeruli are usually normal
Renal scan	↓ Perfusion ↓ Uptake ↑ Background activity	Normal perfusion ↑ Cortical retention

Adapted from Knuppel RA, Montenegro R, O'Brien WF: Acute renal failure in pregnancy, *Clin Obstet Gynecol* 28:288, 1985.

   c. ATN: epithelial or pigmented casts
   d. Interstitial nephritis: eosinophils
5. When ARF results from renal parenchymal injury, the prognosis will depend on the severity of renal ischemia.
   a. Quick recovery is expected with mild ischemia.
   b. Prolonged ischemia leads to reversible ATN.
   c. Severe ischemia leads to an irreversible bilateral renal cortical necrosis (BRCN).
   d. The differences between ATN and BRCN are summarized in Table 23-19.
6. Diagnostic indices (Table 23-20) to differentiate between prerenal and oliguria secondary to intrinsic renal disorder are helpful when there has been no recent administration of diuretics or sodium-containing solutions.
   a. The principle is that the underperfused kidney reabsorbs sodium and water in its glomerular filtrate (GF); thus, the small amount of urine is essentially devoid of sodium and is highly concentrated.
   b. In ARF, secondary to intrinsic renal disorder, the tubular function is lost, the limited GF that may be formed is altered minimally by the tubular system, and the values of the urine excreted closely resemble plasma composition values.

Treatment

1. The main goal of therapy is to eliminate the underlying cause of ARF.
2. Volume and electrolyte and acid–base maintenance are of primary concern.

Table 23-20 Diagnostic indices

	Prerenal Failure	ATN
Urine osmolality ($mosm/kg\ H_2O$)	>500	<350
Urine sodium (mEq/L)	<10-20	>40-60
Urine/plasma ratios		
Osmolality	≥1.5	<1.1
Urea	>8	<3
Creatinine	>40	<20
Fractional Na excretion $U/p_{Na}\ U/P_{Cr}$	<1%	>1%
Renal failure index $U\ Na\ U/P_{Cr}$	<1	>1

3. The "rule of 7" is a useful guide in fluid management:
   a. 50 to 200 ml of normal saline or lactated ringers solution can be infused over a 10-minute period.
   b. If the pulmonary capillary wedge pressure (PCWP) increases more than 7 mm Hg over baseline, infusion should be discontinued.
   c. If the PCWP increases less than 3 mm Hg, a second fluid challenge can be given using the same rule.
   d. If central venous pressure is used, the numbers are 5 cm H_2O and 2 cm H_2O.
4. Diuretics rarely help or harm the patient.
5. Diuresis after diuretic use in a previously oliguric patient probably indicates that the patient's renal failure is less severe.
6. In the presence of preeclampsia, these drugs are to be avoided because of hemoconcentration unless pulmonary edema is present.
7. In cases of metabolic acidosis, where the blood bicarbonate level is <15 mEq/L and the pH is below 7.2, the euvolemic patient may be treated with $NaHCO_3$ (desired increase in $HCO_3 \times 0.6 \times$ body weight).
8. The decision to dialyze usually depends on the following criteria:
   a. Serum K^+ over 6.5 mEq/L that does not respond to medical treatment (calcium gluconate, $NaHCO_3$ solution with insulin and glucose)
   b. Circulatory congestion secondary to fluid overload
   c. Presence of uremic symptoms such as anorexia and nausea, neuromuscular irritability, confusion, or a pericardial friction rub
   d. A BUN over 120 mg/dl or daily increments of 30 mg/dl in patients with sepsis or tissue necrosis
   e. Metabolic acidosis
   f. The presence of a dialyzable poison or toxic drug
9. ARF secondary to ureteral obstruction by a gravid uterus is a rare occurrence.
   a. Treatment consists of positional changes, delivery, and decompressive amniocentesis, because in some cases hydramnios, particularly

associated with multiple gestation, is a common complicating factor.

Nutrition

1. Nutritional recommendations for patients with ARF include a diet low in protein (40 g or 0.6 to 1.5/kg ideal body weight) and a minimum of 100 g of carbohydrates per day.
   a. Hyperalimentation is recommended for patients with catabolic ARF.
   b. This consists of 25 to 50 kcal/day with 70% as glucose, 20% to 30% as essential amino acids (1 to 1.5 g of protein/kg/day), and fat emulsion (a maximum lipid of 500 ml of a 10% intralipid solution).

Delivery management

1. Because fetal compromise results primarily from maternal cardiovascular decompensation, improvements in the maternal status will have positive effects on the fetal condition.
2. Furthermore, attempts to deliver the fetus in a hemodynamically compromised mother may lead to increased risks of fetal distress and the need for more aggressive obstetrical management.
3. In a mother who is already partially decompensated, such iatrogenic insults may produce disastrous results.
4. This of course, assumes that the fetal compartment is not the source of sepsis.
5. Under such circumstances, therapy would include attempts to initiate delivery while stabilizing the mother.

General guidelines

The guidelines listed below will help prevent ARF in pregnancy:

1. In cases of oliguria secondary to hypovolemia (hemorrhage, vomiting) prompt blood and fluid replacement is essential to avoid hypotension that may lead to renal ischemia, a known trigger mechanism of ATN.
2. Patients at risk to develop postpartum hemorrhage (multiple pregnancies, polyhydramnios, multiparity) should have their blood typed and screened for irregular antibodies.
   a. In addition the third stage of labor should be actively managed.
   b. The physician should be prepared to manage uterine atony aggressively.
   c. Other conditions such as soft tissue trauma, retained placenta, and blood dyscrasias should be considered and ruled out.
3. In patients with preeclampsia, the pregnancy should be terminated once there is deterioration of renal function, such as oliguria, marked decrease of creatinine clearance, or rarely azotemia.
4. Careful typing and cross-matching for blood transfusion should be done to minimize the risks of a reaction.
5. Patients with septic abortion, puerperal infection, chorioamnionitis, and pyelonephritis should be watched closely for signs of septic shock.
   a. In these cases, antibiotics and removal of the septic focus, when feasible, is the treatment of choice.
   b. The urine output should be monitored.

6. During pregnancy, as well as in gynecologic surgery, the possibility of obstructive uropathy should be considered as the cause of renal failure.
7. Early delivery should be planned in cases of intrauterine fetal death and abruptio placenta to avoid DIC.
8. The use of nephrotoxic drugs should be avoided in the presence of oliguria.
9. Renal function should be monitored when a potentially nephrotoxic drug is being used.

Suggested reading

Anderson RJ et al: Nonoliguric acute renal failure, *N Engl J Med* 296:1134-1138, 1977.

Asrat T, Nageotte MP: Renal failure in pregnancy, *Semin Perinatol* 14 (1):59-67, 1990.

Burrows DA, O'Neil TJ, Sorrells TL: Successful twin pregnancy after renal transplant maintained on cyclosporine A immunosuppression, *Obstet Gynecol* 72:459-461, 1988.

Cuddihee RE, Cavanagh D: Acute renal failure. In *Obstetric Emergencies,* ed 3, p. 92, Philadephia, 1982, Harper & Row.

Cunningham FG et al: Chronic renal disease and pregnancy outcome, *Am J Obstet Gynecol* 163:453-459, 1990.

Davison JM: Dialysis, transplantation, and pregnancy, *Am J Kidney Dis* 27(2):127-132, 1991.

Davison JM, Lindheimer MD: Chronic renal failure. In Gleicher N, Gall SA, Sibai BM, et al, editors: *Principles and practice of medicine therapy in pregnancy,* pp. 928-937, New York, 1992, Appleton & Lange.

Elliot JP et al: Dialysis in pregnancy: A critical review, *Obstet Gynecol Surv* 46(6):319-324, 1991.

Grunfeld JP, Pertuiset N: Acute renal failure in pregnancy, *Am J Kidney Dis* 9(4):359-362, 1987.

Hayslett JP: Current concepts in postpartum renal failure, *N Engl J Med* 3(2):1556-1559, 1985.

Hayslett JP: Pregnancy complicated by renal disorders. In Reece EA et al, editors: *Medicine of the fetus and mother,* pp. 1086-1096, Philadelphia, 1992, Lippincott.

Hou S: Acute and chronic renal failure in pregnancy. In Clark SL, et al, editors: *Critical care obstetrics,* ed 2, pp. 429-463, Boston, 1991, Blackwell Scientific.

Knuppel RA, Montenegro R, O'Brien WF: Acute renal failure in pregnancy, *Clin Obstet Gynecol* 28:288-297, 1985.

Lindheimer MD, Katz AI: Acute renal failure. In Gleicher N et al, editors: *Principles and practice of medicine therapy in pregnancy,* pp. 921-927, New York, 1992, Appleton & Lange.

MacCarthy EP, Pollak VE: Maternal renal disease: effect on the fetus, *Clin Perinatol* 8(2):307-319, 1981.

Michael J: The management of renal disease in pregnancy, *Clin Obstet Gynecol* 13(2):319-334, 1986.

Miller TR et al: Urinary diagnostic indices in acute renal failure: a prospective study, *Ann Intern Med* 89:47-50, 1976.

Nageotte MP, Grundy HO: Pregnancy outcome in women requiring chronic hemodialysis, *Obstet Gynecol* 72:456-458, 1988.

O'Shaughnessy R, Wesprin SA, Zuspan FP: Obstructive renal failure by an overdistended pregnant uterus, *Obstet Gynecol* 55:247-249, 1980.

Pertuiset N, Ganeval D, Grunfeld JP: Acute renal failure: an update, *Semin Nephrol* 4:232-239, 1984.

Redrow M et al: Dialysis in the management of pregnant patients with renal insufficiency, 67(4):199-208.

Samuels P: Renal disease. In Gabbe SG, Niebyl JR, Simpson JL, editors: *Obstetrics normal and problem pregnancies,* ed 2, pp. 1085-1096, New York, 1991, Churchill Livingstone.

Smith K et al: Renal failure of obstetric origin, *Br Med Bull* 24:49, 1968.

Stratta P et al: Pregnancy-related acute renal failure, *Clin Nephrol* 32:14-20, 1989.

Turney JH, Ellis CM, Parsons FM: Obstetric acute renal failure, *Br J Obstet Gynaecol* 96:679-687, 1989.

Yankowitz J et al: Erythropoietin in pregnancies complicated by severe anemia of renal failure, *Obstet Gynecol* 80:485-488, 1992.

Medical Complications of Pregnancy

24

24.1 PERINATAL VIRAL INFECTIONS

Anna K. Huang, M.D.

General considerations

1. Immunity during pregnancy
   a. Pregnancy is associated with a relative decrease in cell-mediated immune function, the peak occurring in the third trimester.
   b. Thus pregnant women have more severe viral infections, such as polio and primary varicella (chicken pox).
   c. Moreover, an immature immune system makes the fetus or neonate more susceptible to severe complications from viral infection.
2. Antiviral treatment
   a. Acyclovir is the antiviral agent most widely used in pregnancy and appears to be safe; however, it is not FDA approved for pregnant women.
   b. Acyclovir may be necessary in the treatment of severe primary infection of herpes simplex or varicella zoster virus occurring in the mother during pregnancy and in her infant.
   c. Dose size and frequency do not have to be adjusted during pregnancy.
   d. Most other antiviral agents have not been studied in pregnancy or are known teratogens, such as amantadine and ribavirin.
3. Prophylaxis, active and passive
   a. Live virus vaccines are contraindicated during pregnancy, including oral polio, measles-mumps-rubella, varicella, and yellow fever.
   b. Killed vaccines or those made of subunit components are safe, such as influenza, enhanced inactivated polio, hepatitis A, and hepatitis B.
   c. Immune globulins may be used in pregnant women after exposure to persons with specific acute viral illnesses; however, protection is not 100% effective.

Viral infections associated with perinatal complications

The viruses discussed here are those in which maternal infections occurring late in pregnancy and during the peripartum period often lead to medical complications or difficult management decisions. Table 24-1 summarizes the characteristics of these infections.

1. Herpes simplex virus (HSV)
   a. Epidemiology
      (1) In the United States, 5% of the general population have histories consistent with genital herpes; however, 15% to 32% of pregnant women are seropositive for herpes simplex virus type 2 (HSV-2), which is indicative of previous infection.
      (2) Asymptomatic shedding of HSV occurs in up to 4% of women during pregnancy or at time of delivery. Viral cultures obtained throughout pregnancy are not predictive for viral shedding during labor.
      (3) Untreated neonatal HSV infection is associated with a 70% mortality rate.
   b. Clinical disease
      (1) Symptomatic primary HSV-2 infection may include painful vesicular genital lesions often involving the cervix, fever, inguinal lymphadenopathy, and malaise.
         (a) In up to 25% of cases, patients can develop systemic disease, such as aseptic meningitis.
         (b) Viral shedding is prolonged.
      (2) Recurrent genital herpes infection is manifested by genital rash and nonspecific prodromal symptoms.
      (3) There are rare reports of fulminant hepatitis caused by disseminated HSV-1 or HSV-2 disease in pregnant women.
         (a) Even with aggressive antiviral and supportive therapy, most women do not survive their infection.
      (4) Intrauterine HSV-2 infection is rare (<5%) and manifested by skin lesions and scars, chorioretinitis, and central nervous system (CNS) abnormalities.
         (a) It may occur following primary or recurrent clinical maternal disease.
      (5) Neonatal HSV infection occurs in only 2% to 5% of infants whose mothers have known recurrent HSV-2 infection, even in the presence of asymptomatic shedding at the time of delivery.
      (6) In contrast, 41% of infants whose mothers had a first episode of HSV-2 close to term develop neonatal infection.
         (a) Symptoms include fever, vesicular skin lesions, lethargy, and poor feeding.
   c. Diagnosis
      (1) The standard for HSV diagnosis is viral culture and typing of the virus grown.
         (a) Samples may be obtained from vesicular fluid, open ulcer, or genital areas, such as the cervix and vagina, in persons suspected of having previous HSV-2 exposure.
      (2) With the Tzanck test, the base of a freshly unroofed vesicle can be swabbed and examined under the microscope with a Giemsa or Wright stain.
         (a) The presence of multinucleated giant cells gives a positive test result and confirms that this is either HSV or varicella zoster virus.

Table 24-1 Perinatal viral infections

Virus	Complications: Maternal	Complications: Fetal and Neonatal	Diagnosis	Treatments and Comments
Herpes simplex (HSV)	+ to +++	0 to +++	HSV IgM+ or culture biopsy or culture + in maternal dissemination; Tzanck test	Maternal: Consider acyclovir, 5 mg/kg, IV q8h for severe primary infection; cesarean section for active genital herpes Neonates: Culture for HSV if potentially exposed; start acyclovir for +HSV culture, abnormal CSF or signs of sepsis
Influenza	+		Culture from throat, sputum, or stool	Vaccinate all pregnant women
Measles	+ to ++		Rubeola IgM+, IgG–; rubeola culture from throat or sputum	Immune globulin (Ig), 0.02 ml/kg, IM for mother and child within 6 days of exposure to acute measles; give nonimmune women measles-mumps-rubella vaccine postpartum
Parvovirus B19		+++	Parvovirus B19 IgM+, IgG–; DNA hybridization; polymerase chain reaction	Consider fetal transfusion if evidence of fetal anemia or hydrops is present
Varicella (VZV)	+++	+ to ++	VZV IgM+; culture lesions or sputum; Tzanck test	Postexposure prophylaxis: VZIg 125 U/kg, IM, up to 625 U Acyclovir for severe infection Maternal: 10-15 mg/kg, IV q8h Neonates: 60 mg/kg, IV q8h

HSV, Herpes simplex virus; *IgM,* immune globulin; *CSF,* cerebrospinal fluid; *VZV,* varicella zoster virus; *VZIg,* varicella zoster immune globulin.

(b) The clinical syndrome would distinguish between these two viruses.

(3) Conventional (commercial) serologic testing cannot distinguish accurately between HSV-1 and HSV-2 infection because of a large number of cross-reacting antibodies.

(a) Therefore, a person with a positive HSV-1 and negative HSV-2 titer may have had previous HSV-2 infection.

(b) Negative titers for both HSV types is consistent with no previous HSV infection.

d. Management

(1) Before 36 weeks gestation

(a) For the pregnant woman with the first episode of suspected genital herpes, HSV cultures are done to confirm the diagnosis.

i. Serologic testing is done for HSV-1 and HSV-2 to determine whether this is recurrent infection.

(b) For the pregnant woman with recurrent genital herpes, episodes are monitored.

i. The box on p. 593 outlines the management of pregnant women with recurrent genital herpes.

(c) Acyclovir therapy should be considered only for suspected disseminated infection.

(2) During the perinatal period

(a) Viral cultures of the genital area in women with a history of HSV infection may be performed at the onset of labor.

i. The utility of these in assessing neonatal exposure risk is unclear.

(b) Prophylactic acyclovir or cesarean section are not indicated in the absence of visible lesions.

(c) For active genital herpes present at the onset of labor, cesarean section should be performed if labor cannot be postponed for several days or if membranes have ruptured.

(d) Vaginal delivery should be considered for women with active HSV lesions distant from the genital tract.

(e) The safety and efficacy of acyclovir therapy for active disease during labor is unknown.

(f) Neonates with potential HSV exposure (asymptomatic shedding, active lesions discovered after rupture of membranes, etc.) should have viral cultures performed on swabs of eyes and throats, and on urine, stool, and cerebrospinal fluid (CSF).

i. They should be monitored for signs of infection.

(g) Intravenous acyclovir therapy should be initiated in the neonate older than 48 hours who has positive HSV cultures, abnormal CSF studies, or suspected infection.

2. Influenza

a. Epidemiology

(1) There are some data that women in late pregnancy have an increased risk for infectious complications from influenza, such as serious pneumonia.

Considerations for the Management of Pregnant Women with Recurrent Genital Herpes

1. Sequential cultures during late gestation are not indicated unless they are done after clinically evident recurrent infection to document cessation of virus excretion.
2. Cesarean delivery should not be suggested as a "prophylactic" measure to women who do not have active genital lesions at delivery.
3. Symptomatic recurrences of genital herpes during the third trimester will be brief; vaginal delivery is appropriate if no active lesions are present at delivery.
4. Obtaining specimens for culture at delivery from women with a history of HSV infection may help in identifying exposed infants, but the clinical benefit of this procedure has not been established.
5. Options for the management of women with active genital herpes at onset of labor include the following:
   a. If the membranes have ruptured, the mother is afebrile, and the fetal lungs are immature, the following steps may be taken:
      (1) Delay delivery until betamethasone can be given, *or*
      (2) Proceed with cesarean delivery and give topical surfactant to the infant, *or*
      (3) Manage the patient expectantly with or without acyclovir therapy.*
   b. If term gestation or fetal lung maturity has been established and the membranes have ruptured, cesarean delivery is indicated.

From Prober CG et al: The management of pregnancies complicated by genital infections with herpes simplex virus, *Clin Infect Dis* 15(6):1031-1038, 1992.

*Because the value of acyclovir therapy is not known, its routine use is not indicated.

b. Clinical disease
   (1) Incubation period is 5 to 14 days.
      (a) Symptoms include fever, myalgias, headache, stomach upset, cough, and shortness of breath.
      (b) There is no associated fetal risk for abnormalities.
c. Diagnosis
   (1) Influenza may be identified by clinical syndrome and confirmed by viral culture of throat, sputum, or stool.
d. Management
   (1) Supportive treatment is recommended.
      (a) Amantadine for the prophylaxis and treatment of influenza type B is not indicated because of teratogenic effects.
   (2) Influenza vaccination of all pregnant women who will be in their third trimester during influenza season is now recommended.

3. Measles (rubeola)
   a. Epidemiology

(1) In a recent Los Angeles County measles epidemic, 60% of pregnant women with acute measles were hospitalized during their illness, twice as many as in the total infected population (Eberhart-Phillips JE et al: *Obstet Gynecol* 82:797-801, 1993).
(2) There was a 2½ times greater risk for pneumonia and 6.4-fold increase in death rate.
    (a) Complications occurred during all stages of pregnancy.
(3) A significant number of premature deliveries were noted within 2 weeks of rash onset.

b. Clinical disease
(1) Incubation period is 10 to 14 days.
(2) Classic presentation includes fever, generalized rash, coryza (rhinitis), cough, conjunctivitis, and Koplik spots in the mouth.
(3) Maternal infection may result in pneumonia, hepatitis, myocarditis, and encephalitis.
(4) No congenital abnormalities have been linked to *in utero* infection.
    (a) Exposure to acute maternal infection in the peripartum period can lead to neonatal infection with a higher risk for severe or fatal disease.

c. Diagnosis
(1) Rubeola serology (positive IgM titer) is diagnostic for acute infection.
(2) Nasal or throat swab or sputum for viral culture can confirm infection.

d. Management
(1) Treatment of maternal measles infection is supportive.
(2) A pregnant woman exposed to acute measles should be tested for immunity with measles IgG titer.
    (a) If she is nonimmune (IgG negative), consideration should be given to administering immune globulin, 0.02 ml/kg, IM, within 6 days of exposure.
    (b) Following delivery, she should receive measles-mumps-rubella vaccination if acute measles infection has not occurred.
(3) A healthy infant exposed to acute maternal measles infection in the perinatal period or up to the first 12 months of life should be given 0.25 ml/kg of immune globulin, IM, within 6 days of exposure.
    (a) Routine vaccination is begun at 1 year of life.

4. Human parvovirus B19

a. Epidemiology
(1) Parvovirus B19 causes erythema infectiosum (Fifth disease), transient aplastic anemia in patients with underlying hemolytic conditions, and chronic arthralgias.
(2) It may cause up to 30% of nonimmune hydrops fetalis because of viral infection of fetal erythroid stem cells.
(3) Fetal death can occur in the last trimester and perinatally, but it is most common between 10 and 20 weeks gestation. Fetal mortality rate has been estimated at 2% to 3%.

b. Clinical disease
   (1) Human parvovirus B19 is highly contagious and often presents in an epidemic form.
   (2) Incubation period is 5 to 14 days.
   (3) The classic presentation includes the facial rash with a "slapped cheek" appearance, reticular rash on the trunk and extremities, fever, myalgias, and arthralgias.
   (4) Maternal infection may be symptomatic or asymptomatic and is no worse than in normal hosts.
      (a) Fetal infection may present with a preeclampsia-like syndrome, abdominal pain, and polyhydramnios within 3 to 5 weeks of maternal symptoms.
c. Diagnosis
   (1) Parvovirus B19 is difficult to culture.
      (a) Serologic confirmation of recent maternal infection includes a positive B19 IgM titer or rising IgG titers over a 4-week period.
   (2) Fetal infection has been detected in fetal or amniotic fluids prenatally and in fetal tissues at postmortem examination using DNA hybridization and polymerase chain reaction (PCR) techniques.
d. Management
   (1) Pregnant women with acute parvovirus infection should be monitored with frequent serum alpha-fetoprotein determinations and weekly ultrasound examinations.
   (2) There have been anecdotal reports of intrauterine blood transfusion correcting hydrops fetalis with a successful fetal outcome.

5. Varicella zoster virus (VZV)
   a. Epidemiology
      (1) VZV is a highly contagious DNA virus in the human herpes virus family.
      (2) Of pregnant women, 95% are seropositive, although women from tropical or subtropical areas have lower rates of exposure.
      (3) Maternal VZV occurs in 5 of every 10,000 pregnancies.
         (a) Twenty percent to 30% of acute infections during pregnancy, especially during the third trimester, may disseminate and result in a 40% mortality rate.
      (4) Fetopathy in the form of a congenital varicella syndrome occurs in 2% to 3% of pregnancies following maternal VZV infection.
      (5) Neonates who have the chicken pox rash at birth or develop one during the first 4 days of life have a benign illness.
      (6) Rash that appears between the fifth and tenth days of life is associated with 30% mortality because of disseminated infection.
   b. Clinical disease
      (1) Incubation period is 7 to 21 days following exposure to the vesicular rash.
         (a) The most contagious period is the 24 hours preceding the appearance of rash in cases of acute VZV (chicken pox).

(2) Primary maternal varicella presents with the classic painless, scattered vesicular rash that may last for 5 to 10 days.
   (a) In late pregnancy, pneumonia complicates up to 20% of acute infections.
   (b) Other manifestations include encephalitis and hepatitis.
(3) Women who have a history of previous varicella infection may reactivate during pregnancy with herpes zoster (HZV, shingles), a painful vesicular rash presenting in a dermatomal distribution.
   (a) With the exception of severe disseminated herpes zoster, viremia, and therefore *in utero* infection, is unusual in shingles cases.
(4) Congenital abnormalities include dermatomal skin lesions (a hallmark of intrauterine infection), shortening of extremities exhibiting the skin lesions, and neurologic and ophthalmic anomalies.
(5) Neonates exposed in the perinatal period may demonstrate the chicken pox rash, then develop disseminated disease, including pneumonitis, hepatitis, and encephalitis.

c. Diagnosis
(1) Maternal primary varicella and herpes zoster will have the characteristic vesicular rashes for those infections.
   (a) Confirmation can be made with viral culture of vesicular fluid.
   (b) During primary infection, VZV IgM titers should be positive.
(2) Scraping of the base of a vesicular ulcer will reveal the characteristic multinucleated giant cell, giving a positive Tzanck preparation, on light microscopy.

d. Management
(1) Nonimmune women who are exposed to VZV during any stage of pregnancy should be evaluated with VZV IgG titers to confirm lack of previous infection.
   (a) If seronegative, she should be given varicella zoster immune globulin (VZIg) IM at a dose of 125 U/kg, with a maximum dose of 625 U, within 5 days of exposure.
   (b) Whereas acute maternal VZV may occur after VZIg administration, the risk of severe intrauterine infection is diminished.
   (c) VZIg may be obtained through local American Red Cross offices.
(2) Severe maternal VZV infection should be treated with acyclovir, 10 to 15 mg/kg, IV q8h.
(3) Intramuscular VZIg should be administered to neonates whose mothers present with chicken pox rash during the period 5 days before delivery through 2 days after delivery.
   (a) This may only be 50% effective in preventing acute VZV but will likely lessen the risk of fatal neonatal infection.
   (b) VZIg dose is 125 U/kg with a maximum dose of 625 U.
(4) Rarely, a pregnant woman will have perineal herpes zoster at the time of delivery.

(a) Cesarean section should be considered if this will avoid having the neonate in contact with actively shedding lesions.
(b) If contact cannot be avoided, the infant should be given VZIg as described previously.
(5) Neonates who exhibit VZV infection should be treated with intravenous acyclovir, 60 mg/kg, q8h.

Special cases in perinatal viral transmission

In the following section, viruses whose transmission during the perinatal period may be affected by medical intervention are discussed. These often are not associated with clinical perinatal disease.

1. Hepatitis B and hepatitis D (HBV, HDV)
   a. Epidemiology
      (1) Hepatitis B is transmitted via sexual contact, materials (such as needles) or tissues contaminated with blood, and perinatally.
         (a) Ten percent of infections will lead to a chronic carrier state and one half of these will progress to cirrhosis or hepatocellular carcinoma.
      (2) Perinatal transmission occurs in 10% to 90% of cases.
         (a) The highest rates are seen when the mother has chronic HBV with surface antigenemia (HBsAg+) and e antigenemia (HBeAg+) or has her acute infection during the third trimester of pregnancy.
         (b) These children have a greater risk for liver failure or carcinoma as adults than others with chronic HBV infection.
      (3) Hepatitis D (delta) is a virus dependent on HBV and can be transmitted only to someone who is a chronic HBV carrier or as simultaneous HBV and HDV infections.
         (a) Chronic hepatitis occurs in 80% of HDV infections.
         (b) Complication rates are much higher than for chronic HBV.
         (c) Perinatal transmission has been reported.
   b. Clinical disease
      (1) Incubation period of both HBV and HDV is 60 to 120 days.
      (2) Acute symptoms include nausea, malaise, abdominal pain, fever, and jaundice.
         (a) Fulminant hepatitis occurs in 1% of cases and is not increased during pregnancy.
         (b) Elevations in liver enzymes should resolve within 6 months of acute symptoms; otherwise, the patient has a chronic infection.
      (3) Patients with chronic HBV and HDV are often asymptomatic.
      (4) Children do not suffer increased rates of congenital abnormalities because of HBV and HDV.
   c. Diagnosis
      (1) Hepatitis B serology can distinguish acute from chronic disease states and can identify those chronic infections with the greatest risk of transmission.

(2) Hepatitis B core antibodies (HBcAb)
(a) IgM indicates acute infection.
(b) IgG indicates previous infection.
(3) Hepatitis B surface antigen (HBsAg)
(a) HBsAg is present only in acute infection or with chronic carrier state.
(b) It is not detectable if hepatitis B surface antibody (HBsAb) is present.
(4) Hepatitis B surface antibody (HBsAb)
(a) This antibody indicates prior resolved infection or post-vaccination status.
(b) Levels may fall over time or with immunosuppression, such as in infection with the human immunodeficiency virus (HIV).
(5) Hepatitis B e antigen (HBeAg) and antibody (HBeAb)
(a) The e antigen is present only with surface antigen.
(b) Persistent levels are consistent with the most contagious infections.
(c) Positive HBeAb confers less risk of transmission from a surface antigen–positive individual.
(6) Persons with HDV infection will have both HBsAg and delta antigen (hepatitis D Ag) detectable in blood.

d. Management
(1) *All* pregnant women should be screened for chronic HBV infection with a HBsAg test.
(2) Children born to HBsAg-positive mothers should receive hepatitis B immune globulin (HBIg), 0.5 ml, and hepatitis B vaccine, IM, in different extremities within 12 hours of birth.
(a) This regimen is 85% to 95% effective in protecting against hepatitis B transmission.
(3) In all other cases, neonates should receive routine immunization with hepatitis B vaccine alone before hospital discharge and at 1 and 6 months.
(a) Vaccine dosing varies by manufacturer.
(4) Perinatal transmission of hepatitis D is effectively prevented by the established immunoprophylaxis protocol for hepatitis B.
(5) Therapy for acute HBV infection is supportive.
(6) Alpha-interferon, which has been used to treat chronic HBV infection, has not been tested in large numbers of pregnant women.

2. Hepatitis C (HCV)
a. Epidemiology
(1) This RNA virus causes 90% of transfusion-associated non-A, non-B hepatitis.
(a) Other groups at risk for infection are intravenous drug users, HIV-infected individuals, and health care workers through occupational blood exposure.
(b) Sexual transmission is rare (0% to 14%).
(2) Perinatal transmission has been demonstrated in various studies but appears to be infrequent and may be associated with high levels of replicating virus in the mother.

(a) Vertical transmission of HCV is increased to 9% to 12% when the mother has concomitant HIV infection.

b. Clinical disease
   (1) Incubation period is 14 to 90 days.
   (2) Symptoms of acute infection are milder than in hepatitis B and include nausea, malaise, fever, abdominal pain, and jaundice.
      (a) Elevated serum chemistries may persist for 3 to 4 months.
   (3) Fifty percent of infected persons will develop chronic hepatitis, with one half of those progressing to cirrhosis.
   (4) There has been no observed increase in adverse pregnancy outcomes following acute infection.
   (5) Premature labor and intrauterine growth retardation have been linked to chronic active hepatitis.

c. Diagnosis
   (1) Newer enzyme linked immunosorbent assay (ELISA) antibody tests detect greater numbers of HCV infections, but there may be up to a 6-month delay in the appearance of antibodies.
   (2) Recombinant immunoblot assay (RIBA) is a confirmatory test.
   (3) PCR may be the most useful test in detecting perinatal transmission.
   (4) Liver biopsy is the only current diagnostic method able to determine the chronicity and severity of HCV hepatitis.
      (a) A measurement for contagiousness has not been developed.

d. Management
   (1) Alpha-interferon has been used in the treatment of chronic HCV infection, but controlled studies in pregnant women have not been conducted; otherwise, there is no therapy for acute infection.
   (2) Passive prophylaxis with immune globulin has not been tested in the prevention of vertical transmission.

3. Human T-lymphotropic virus I and II (HTLV-I, HTLV-II)
   a. Epidemiology
      (1) Both HTLV-I and HTLV-II are (RNA) retroviruses that can immortalize T-lymphocytes *in vitro*.
      (2) Transmission occurs via sexual contact, blood products, and mother to child through breast-feeding (25% of infants become infected).
      (3) In the United States, 16 of every 1000 blood donors are positive for HTLV-I or HTLV-II.
   b. Clinical disease
      (1) HTLV-I is associated with adult T-cell leukemia or lymphoma and HTLV-I-associated myelopathy or tropical spastic paraparesis, a chronic degenerative neurologic disease.
         (a) There is no associated neonatal disease.
      (2) HTLV-II has not been definitively linked to any diseases, although it was originally isolated from persons with hairy cell leukemia.

c. Diagnosis
   (1) Specific antibody tests for both viruses have recently been developed.
      (a) PCR testing may also be used.
d. Management
   (1) There is no specific therapy.
   (2) Routine screening is not recommended unless the patient or her sexual partner are from endemic areas.
   (3) Women who are seropositive for either HTLV-I or HTLV-II should be counseled against breast-feeding their infants.

Suggested reading

Centers for Disease Control and Prevention: Prevention and control of influenza, *MMWR* 44(4):RR-3, 1995.

Centers for Disease Control and Prevention and the U.S. Public Health Service Working Group: Guidelines for counseling persons infected with human T-lymphotropic virus type I (HTLV-I) and type II (HTLV-II), *Ann Intern Med* 118:448-454, 1993.

Eberhart-Phillips JE et al: Measles in pregnancy: a descriptive study of 58 cases, *Obstet Gynecol* 82:797-801, 1993.

Enders G et al: Consequences of varicella and herpes zoster in pregnancy: prospective study of 1739 cases, *Lancet* 343:1547-1550, 1994.

Hall CJ: Parvovirus B19 infection in pregnancy, *Arch Disease Child* 71:F4-F5, 1994.

Mandell GL, Bennett JE, Dolin R: *Principles and practice of infectious diseases,* ed 4, New York, 1995, Churchill Livingstone.

McIntosh D, Isaacs D: Varicella zoster virus infection in pregnancy, *Arch Disease Child* 68:1-2, 1993.

Prober CG et al: The management of pregnancies complicated by genital infections with herpes simplex virus, *Clin Infect Dis* 15:1031-1038, 1992.

Simms J, Duff P: Viral hepatitis in pregnancy, *Semin Perinatol* 17(6):384-393, 1993.

Spangler JG, Kirk JK, Knudson MP: Uses and safety of acyclovir in pregnancy, *J Fam Pract* 38:186-191, 1994.

24.2 TREATMENT OF EPILEPSY

Shirley K. Sawai, M.D.

Overview

Definition

1. *Epilepsy* is the predisposition to seizures caused by alterations in brain electrical activity, resulting in involuntary motor or sensory phenomena, with or without the loss of consciousness.
2. There is no one pathognomonic lesion of epilepsy because seizures can be induced by many etiologies including the following:
   a. Infection
   b. Metabolic
   c. Toxic poisons or drug overdose
   d. Trauma
   e. Vascular accidents or anomalies
   f. Drug withdrawal
   g. Degenerative disease of the CNS

h. Perinatal (trauma, asphyxia, anomalies)
i. Neoplastic
j. Genetic

3. Treatment is based on the correct diagnosis of the type of seizure and correction of any underlying precipitating factors.
4. Gestational epilepsy is seizures confined to pregnancy and the puerperium only; it is a rare and a retrospective diagnosis.

Pathogenesis

1. Seizures are marked by a rhythmic and repetitive hypersynchronous abnormal neuronal discharge in a localized area of the brain.
2. Seizures may be induced by the following:
   a. Decreases in inhibitory mechanisms caused by reductions in gamma-aminobutyric acid (GABA)
   b. Enhancement of excitatory synaptic mechanisms mediated by *n*-methyl-D-aspartate (NMDA)
   c. Enhancement of neuronal burst firing
3. Many environmental or circumstantial factors can precipitate seizures, such as fatigue, stress, hyperventilation, fever, or edema.

Classification of seizures

1. Several seizure type and epileptic syndrome classification systems have been used; seizures are generally classified based on electroencephalogram (EEG) characteristics and associated clinical findings.
2. The International Classification of Epileptic Seizures is given in the box on p. 602.
3. Recent nomenclature changes include the following:
   a. Petit mal seizures = absence seizures
   b. Focal motor or aura seizures = simple partial seizures
   c. Psychomotor or temporal lobe seizures = complex partial seizures
   d. Grand mal seizures = generalized tonic–clonic seizures
4. Incidence in general population[60] is as follows:
   a. Complex partial with secondary generalized seizures account for 60% of cases.
   b. Generalized tonic–clonic seizures account for 30% of cases.
   c. Generalized absence seizures account for 5% of cases.

Reproductive epidemiology

1. The incidence of seizure disorders in women of reproductive age is as high as 1% (includes seizures with any etiology, including epilepsy, head trauma, postinfectious, unclassified).
2. Seizure disorders affect 0.15% of all pregnancies.
   a. Approximately 0.33% of all infants born in the United States each year are born to women with seizures.
3. Family studies reveal that the risk of children having a seizure disorder if born to a parent with epilepsy is 3%.
4. A genetic component to seizure disorders is suggested by the fact that 41% of patients with epilepsy have a family history of seizure disorders compared with only 6.3% of the general population.

International Classification of Epileptic Seizures

I. Partial seizures (seizures beginning locally)
- A. Simple partial seizures (consciousness not impaired)
  1. With motor symptoms
  2. With somatosensory or special sensory symptoms
  3. With autonomic symptoms
  4. With psychic symptoms
- B. Complex partial seizures (with impairment of consciousness)
  1. Beginning as simple partial seizures and progressing to impairment of consciousness
     - a. With no other features
     - b. With features as in A.1-4
     - c. With automatisms
  2. With impairment of consciousness at onset
     - a. With no other features
     - b. With features as in A.1-4
     - c. With automatisms
- C. Partial seizures secondarily generalized

II. Generalized seizures (bilaterally symmetric and without local onset)
- A. 1. Absence seizures
  2. Typical absence seizures
- B. Myoclonic seizures
- C. Clonic seizures
- D. Tonic seizures
- E. Tonic–clonic seizures
- F. Atonic seizures

III. Unclassified epileptic seizures (inadequate or incomplete data)

From Commission of Classification and Terminology of the International League Against Epilepsy: Proposal for classification of epilepsies and syndromes, *Epilepsia* 26:268, 1981.

5. The recurrence risk of having a child with a seizure disorder is 3% and probably results from polygenic or multifactorial inheritance.
6. Fetal malformation
   - a. The rate of congenital malformations is 2.4 times that of the general population and may be attributed to genetic factors, frequency of seizures during pregnancy, or the use of anticonvulsant drugs (ACDs) during pregnancy.
   - b. Children of fathers with epilepsy have a higher incidence of fetal malformation than the control population.
   - c. Fetal malformation rates in women with trauma-induced seizures and with a family history of seizures is similar, suggesting that the genetic contribution to fetal malformation may be small.
7. Of women with epilepsy on ACDs, 90% have normal infants.

Effects of pregnancy on seizures

Effect on frequency and severity of seizures

1. Pregnancy has an unpredictable effect on the frequency of seizures as seen in varying reports in the literature.

Author:	Yerby[69]	Tanganelli[64]	Schmidt[57]	Bardy[2]
Increased:	17% to 24%	17%	37%	32%
Decreased:	5% to 25%	3%	13%	14%
No change:	60% to 83%	80%	50%	23%
Seizure free:				31%

   a. Schmidt and others[57] found that noncompliance was responsible for increased seizure frequency in 34 of 50 pregnancies and low drug levels were found in 47% of those who were poorly controlled. They concluded that the increase in seizure frequency was a result of noncompliance, sleep deprivation, and inadequate therapy.
   b. Tanganelli and Regent[64] found that seizures were more frequent in patients with focal epilepsy (38.8%) and with higher seizure frequencies before pregnancy (47.2%).
   c. Gjerde and others[21] compared the frequency and severity of seizures 9 months before and during pregnancy in the same patient and found no difference. There was also no relationship between the type of seizure and change in frequency.
   d. Bag reported that in those patients with an increase in frequency of seizures (n = 14) there was a significantly higher level of estrogen and lower level of progestesrone, as well as a lower level of ACD compared with those patients with no change in frequency (n = 15).
2. Prognosis for the course of seizure disorders in pregnancy is unrelated to age or age at onset.
3. Approximately half of patients follow a similar pattern in subsequent pregnancies.
4. The effects of pregnancy on epilepsy are temporary, with most patients after the puerperium returning to the pattern of frequency and severity they experienced before pregnancy.

Reasons for deterioration in seizure control during pregnancy

Physiologic changes of pregnancy and circumstances surrounding pregnancy may precipitate seizures in those who are susceptible.

1. Hormonal: increased serum estrogen and chorionic gonadotropin levels
2. Hyperventilation
3. Hyponatremia
4. Hypocalcemia
5. Expansion of extracellular fluid volume
6. Decreased ACD serum levels (see Monitoring ACD Levels)
7. Sleep deprivation, fatigue
   a. Schmidt[57] reported that sleep deprivation or noncompliance had a temporal relationship to seizure activity in 34 of 50 pregnancies and in five of six patients who experienced an increase in seizures during the puerperium.

8. Emotional stress (including financial or marital) and anxiety leading to sleep deprivation, hyperventilation, poor nutrition
9. Physical discomforts: nausea, back pain, entrapment neuropathies, pressure of fetus and movements, nocturia → → sleep deprivation

Effects of seizures on pregnancy

What the literature does agree on

1. Results of studies are difficult to evaluate because of the following:
   a. Limited number of cases
   b. Lack of comparative data on nonepileptic women
   c. Difference in severity of epilepsy and its treatment within studies
   d. Differences in medical background of women in the studies
   e. Differences in socioeconomic influences
   f. Lack of relevant information on social habits such as tobacco, alcohol, and drug use
2. More than 90% of women with epilepsy on ACDs can deliver normal infants without birth defects.
3. Six percent to 8% of fetuses exposed to ACDs *in utero* have an unequivocal risk for major malformations or minor anomalies.
4. It is difficult to distinguish the effects of epilepsy on pregnancy outcome from those of epileptic therapy because of the lack of data on the effects of multiple ACDs and the incidence of congenital malformations among untreated epileptics.
5. Untreated epileptic women may represent a mixed population of those with mild disease, noncompliant patients, and those with seizure disorders resistant to prior therapy.

Variations in the reports on effects of seizures on pregnancy (See the box on p. 605.)

1. Some report no increase in spontaneous abortion, prematurity, preeclampsia, low–birth weight (LBW) infants, multiple gestation, bleeding during pregnancy or delivery, or cesarean section rates.[30]
2. Complications of pregnancy reported in other studies include the following:
   a. Increase in incidence of first and third trimester bleeding in 7% to 10% of patients
   b. 50% to 250% increased risk of preeclampsia
   c. Increase in prematurity
   d. Increase in LBW infants by 2.8 times
   e. Six times increase in maternal herpes[72]
   f. Increase in breech presentation[54]
   g. Infants 2.5 times more likely to have low Apgar scores
3. Bjerkedal and Bahana[3] reported a twofold to threefold increase in preeclampsia, cesarean section, preterm delivery, LBW, congenital malformations, and perinatal mortality.
4. Nelson and Ellenberg[47] evaluated data from the Collaborative Perinatal Project and reported an increased incidence of cerebral palsy, seizures, and mental retardation in children of women with epilepsy.

Obstetric Complications Reported in Women with Epilepsy

Vaginal bleeding
Anemia
Hyperemesis gravidarum
Preeclampsia
Placental complications
  Placenta previa
  Placental abruption
Breech presentation
Stillbirth
Preterm delivery
Birth weight <2500 g
1-minute Apgar <5
5-minute Apgar <7
Maternal herpes exacerbation
(Induced labor)
(Cesarean section—primary and repeat)

5. Wilhelm and others[67] compared 98 women with epilepsy to controls and found a twofold to threefold increase in preeclampsia and preterm delivery and a congenital malformation rate of 14% as compared to 3% in the control group.
6. Teramo and others[65] described fetal heart rate (FHR) changes during a seizure episode with decelerations suggestive of hypoxia.
   a. This may be reflective of hypoxia or maternal metabolic changes.
   b. Prolonged or repetitive seizures could potentially lead to more prominent cardiac and systemic effects.
7. Perinatal complications were reported 1.5 to 4 times more often in women with epilepsy in older studies; however, more recent studies report more favorable rates of less than 2.5 times that of control groups.[70]

Effects of seizures on labor and delivery

1. The majority of women with epilepsy have a normal, spontaneous vaginal delivery.[29]
2. ACDs may weaken contractions and prolong labor.[43]
3. ACDs may cause a slight defect in coagulation factors or platelet number and function,[70] thereby slightly increasing the risk of bleeding at delivery.
4. Tonic–clonic seizures during labor and delivery may occur in <2% of epileptic women and in another 1% to 2% within the first 24 hours after delivery.[2]
5. Slightly greater numbers of labor inductions, amniotomies, forceps-assisted deliveries, and cesarean sections performed are reported in women with epilepsy; however, the indications for the procedures are questionable. A population-based Finnish study[28] reports no difference in the number of these procedures between epileptic and control pregnancies.

Effects of seizures on pregnancy outcomes

1. Decreased viability
   a. Lower Apgar scores
   b. Twofold increase in stillbirth, neonatal, and perinatal mortality rates (mostly caused by an increase in congenital malformations and neonatal hemorrhage; maternal trauma resulting from seizures could also predispose to PROM, preterm labor, and abruption)
   c. Higher mortality rate in the first year of life
2. Decreased growth parameters
   a. Lower birth weight with greater incidence of small for gestational age (SGA) infants
   b. 8.5% incidence of LBW (<2500 g) infants with 4% to 11% of those infants being premature
3. Neonatal complications
   a. Increased risk of neonatal hemorrhage within the first 24 hours of life (usually into internal body cavities) because of a deficiency in vitamin K–dependent clotting factors resulting from ACD use in pregnancy
      (1) There is approximately 10% prevalence among infants of epileptics.
      (2) Mortality rate may exceed 30%.[69]
   b. Neonatal withdrawal from barbiturates (see Phenobarbital)
4. Risk of epilepsy in offspring
   a. Children of mothers with epilepsy have a greater risk of developing epilepsy than children of fathers with epilepsy.
   b. Women whose age of onset of epilepsy was <18 years of age have twice the risk of having a child with epilepsy than those women with adult-onset disease.
   c. Women with epilepsy have a 1 in 30 chance of having a child with epilepsy.
   d. Seizures during pregnancy increase the risk of epilepsy in a child by twofold.[50]
5. Cognitive development
   a. Cognitive development may be affected by seizures during pregnancy, epilepsy itself, genetic tendencies, the side effects of maternal ACDs, from both *in utero* exposure and maternal–child interactions, and from psychosocial factors.
   b. Learning disabilities are more common in infants of women with epilepsy.
      (1) Hill and others[31] reported that 48% of 23 infants followed to age 4 had learning disabilities.
      (2) Leavitt and others[40] reported impaired language development at age 2; despite equivalent IQ scores with controls, children of mothers with epilepsy had half the vocabulary of controls.
   c. Gaily and others[20] reported in a prospective study that the prevalence of mental deficiency in infants of women with epilepsy was 1.4%, which was only slightly higher than that of the general population.
      (1) Mean IQ at 5.5 years of age was significantly lower in the ACD-exposed group.

(2) A lower IQ was associated with a higher number of minor anomalies.

6. Major congenital malformations: 1.25% to 11.5% reported risk (as compared to 2% to 3% risk in the general population)
   a. Seizures during the first trimester are associated with a greater incidence of fetal malformation (12.3% vs. 4% for other trimesters)[41]; however, this may be influenced by ACD use.
   b. Various studies report both an increase in and no change in the incidence of fetal malformations with seizures during pregnancy.[71]
   c. Incidence in infants of untreated women with epilepsy is 4.5% vs. 7.1% incidence in infants of treated women is 4.5%.[45]
   Note: Studies in the survey lacked a uniform definition of major malformation.
   d. Incidence in infants of epileptic mothers is 6.6% vs. 4.5% incidence in infants of epileptic fathers and 2.7% incidence in controls.[1]
7. Minor dysmorphic anomalies
   a. Nail and phalangeal hypoplasia and craniofacial hypoplasia tend to correct with growth in infancy.
   b. Except for hypertelorism, there is no statistically significant difference between affected children and controls by age 4.[36]

Adverse effects of ACDs

1. Congenital malformations (May also be related to genetic tendencies and a predisposition with epilepsy.)
   a. Koch and others[36] report a stronger association between maternal epilepsy and anomalies than ACD exposure and anomalies.
2. Altered maternal folate metabolism
3. Vitamin D deficiency
4. Neonatal coagulopathy
5. Neonatal depression
6. Neonatal drug withdrawal
7. Low neonatal thyroxine levels

Teratogenicity of anticonvulsant drugs

Definitions

1. *Major malformation:* a structural defect that occurs during the development of an organ or organ system that could result in significant dysfunction or threat to life
   a. Surgical intervention is usually required (e.g., neural tube defect [NTD], congenital heart disease, orofacial clefts, intestinal atresia, deformities of the urinary collecting system).
2. *Minor malformation:* a structural defect that occurs during the development of an organ or limb and that may impair function but does not result in a life-threatening condition if not treated (e.g., clubbed foot, equinovarus, hypospadias)
3. *Minor dysmorphic anomalies:* unusual morphologic features that affect the appearance of superficial aspects of the face or limbs but have no impact on function and are of no serious medical consequence (e.g.,

hypertelorism, epicanthal folds, broad flat nasal bridge, upturned nasal tip, long philtrum, distal digital hypoplasia)

Which ACD has the most teratogenic potential?

1. There are no good data on which ACD is the most teratogenic.
   a. Depending on the study cited, all four of the major ACDs (phenytoin, phenobarbital, valproate, and carbamazepine) have been reported as more teratogenic than the other three. Results are confounded by the following:
      (1) Use of polypharmacy in different combinations
      (2) Different dosages used
      (3) Different patient populations
      (4) Different genotypes exposed to ACDs
      (5) Insufficient numbers of women exposed to monotherapy in the studies
2. Many neurologists favor the use of carbamazepine in pregnancy because of earlier reports on the teratogenesis of phenytoin and the later reports on valproate.
   a. Koch and others[36] report valproate as "considerably teratogenic" and phenytoin, phenobarbital, and carbamazepine as "weakly teratogenic."
3. "Since no agreement has been reached regarding which AED (antiepileptic drug) is the most teratogenic, the present consensus opinion is that the AED that stops seizures in a given patient should be used." From the Consensus Guidelines established at the international symposium on Pregnancy, Teratogenesis, and Genetics in Epilepsy, July 1990.[14]
4. Many clinical teratologists believe there is a "fetal anticonvulsant syndrome" for phenytoin, carbamazepine, phenobarbital, and related compounds and, to a lesser extent, valproate, which produces a recognizable pattern of dysmorphogenesis previously termed the fetal hydantoin syndrome (Table 24-2).

True incidence of congenital malformations is difficult to measure

1. There is a 4% to 6% incidence on a single ACD at therapeutic levels.
2. Risk of congenital malformations increases as the number of ACDs increases: 6.5% on single therapy vs. 15.6% risk on multiple ACDs.[33]
3. Teratogenic effects differ between species; therefore, it is difficult to extrapolate animal data to humans.
4. Serum ACD levels are higher (and serum folate levels are lower) in those women with fetal anomalies.

Incidence of NTDs

1. Valproate
   a. 1% to 2%[42]
   b. 5.4%[48]: associated with higher daily valproate levels
2. Carbamazepine: 0.5%[55]

Table 24-2 Features of ACD-related teratogenic syndromes

Phenytoin	Valproic Acid	Primidone	Trimethadione
(7%-10% risk)	Postnatal growth retardation	Low–birth weight	IUGR
IUGR	Developmental delay	Developmental delay	Postnatal growth retardation
Postnatal growth retardation	Facial dysmorphism	Facial dysmorphism	Mild to moderate mental retardation
Hypotonicity	Inferior epicanthal folds	Thick nasal roots	Developmental delay
Motor delay?	Flat nasal bridge	Anteverted nostrils	Speech difficulties
Developmental delay	Upturned nasal tip	Long philtrum	Facial dysmorphism
Facial dysmorphism	Shallow philtrum	Thin vermillion border	V-shaped eyebrows
Midfacial hypoplasia	Thin vermillion border	Hirsute forehead	Hypertelorism
Hypertelorism	Inferior turned mouth	Distal digital hypoplasia	Strabismus
Long upper lip without well-developed philtrum	Limb anomalies	Cardiac anomalies	Inner epicanthal folds
Broad nasal bridge	Long, thin overlapping fingers and toes	Microcephaly	Visual impairment
Epicanthal folds	Hyperconvex nails		Low-set ears with anterior folded helix
Hirsutism	Cardiac anomalies		Hearing loss
Limb anomalies	Minor genital anomalies		Broad, depressed nasal bridge
Nail hypoplasia	Microcephaly		High-arched palate
Hypoplastic distal phalanges	Neural tube defects		Orofacial clefts
(3%-4% risk)			Irregular teeth
Congenital heart disease			Congenital heart defects
Microcephaly			Microcephaly
Diaphragmatic hernias			Tracheoesophageal anomalies
Inguinal hernias			Hypospadias
Abnormal genitalia			Inguinal hernias
Cleft lip or palate			Various GI and GU defects

IUGR, Intrauterine growth restriction; *GI*, gastrointestinal; *GU*, genitourinary.

Guidelines for anticonvulsant therapy in pregnancy

Objective

The objective for anticonvulsant therapy in pregnancy is to optimally reduce the frequency and severity of seizures with minimal maternal and fetal adverse effects. With appropriate therapy, seizure activity can be well controlled in 65% of patients, and the severity and frequency of seizures decreased in 20%.

1. The single drug that is most effective for the seizure type and has the "least" teratogenic potential is chosen.
   a. Addition of other drugs competes for degradative enzymes that detoxify ACD.
   b. Of cases involving polypharmacy, 36% can be controlled with a single ACD.
   c. Dosing is simplified to maximize compliance.
2. If possible, the ACD is selected and the lowest effective dose is determined *before* pregnancy (see Monitoring ACD Levels).
   a. Serum levels are checked and dose adjustments made after a steady state (three to four half-lives) is achieved.
   b. If toxicity develops before seizures are controlled, a different ACD should be used.
3. Drugs should be transitioned slowly.
   a. Changes should be made before pregnancy because an increase in seizure frequency may occur during the transition.
   b. The ACD should be tapered over 30 or more days overlapping with the new ACD; rapid changes can precipitate status epilepticus.
4. *The ACD should not be changed solely because pregnancy is diagnosed!*
   a. By the time an ACD transition has been made the period of teratogenesis may have passed and a more unstable seizure situation created, which may pose greater maternal and fetal risk.
5. Initiating ACD therapy in an untreated pregnant patient involves the following:
   a. Half of the usual maintenance dose is given and increased weekly until a full maintenance dose is achieved (except for phenobarbital, which can be given in the full 900-mg loading dose).
   b. Dose is increased until the following occur:
      (1) Seizures are well controlled.
      (2) Serum concentrations reach the upper end of the therapeutic range, *or*
      (3) Side effects limit further increments.
   c. If seizures continue despite optimal therapeutic levels, an alternative ACD should be substituted.
6. In a patient with an onset of seizure activity during pregnancy the following is done:
   a. Physician may or may not elect to start ACD after an isolated seizure: neurology follow-up should be obtained after delivery. (Patients with so-called gestational epilepsy may have only a single seizure episode and further treatment may not be necessary.)

b. With two or more seizures, treatment is prophylactic with ACD.
c. With a progressive clinical history of seizures, abnormal neurological findings, or focal EEG abnormality, an MRI should be obtained to exclude an underlying structural lesion.

Monitoring ACD levels

1. Low serum levels are caused by the following:
   a. Inadequate dosage
   b. Noncompliance (fear of teratogenesis, nausea and vomiting, inconvenience)
   c. Nausea and vomiting of pregnancy leading to decreased ingestion and absorption
   d. Dilutional effect of the expanded extracellular volume
   e. Increased hepatic and renal clearance (maximal in the third trimester)
   f. Induction of hepatic microsomal enzymes by increased level of steroid hormones (estrogen and progesterone) (If this were a significant factor in reduced serum levels, a rapid return to baseline ACD levels would be expected postpartum; however, it actually requires several weeks.)
   g. Decreased plasma protein binding and albumin concentration
   h. Displacement from protein binding sites
   i. Possible fetoplacental drug metabolism
   j. Alcohol and drug abuse
      (1) Excessive alcohol use can induce hepatic enzymes.
      (2) More than three or four drinks per occasion has been associated with an increase in seizure frequency over the subsequent days.
      (3) Intoxication predisposes to medication noncompliance and sleep deprivation and fatigue.
   k. Generic substitution
      (1) Difference in bioavailability and drug content may cause an effective dosage change of 10% or more.
      (2) Phenytoin has nonlinear kinetics; therefore, a small change in dose may cause a large difference in serum levels.
2. High serum levels are caused by the following:
   a. Improper dosage
   b. Impaired elimination
   c. Drug interactions
3. Monitor serum ACD levels in the following situations:
   a. After changing ACD therapy
   b. After adjusting doses
   c. In a patient with hepatic or renal disease
   d. Signs or symptoms of toxicity
   e. Other medications are added or withdrawn, because of the potential for drug interaction
   f. Recurrent seizure activity

Frequency of monitoring ACD levels

1. Baseline total and free levels obtained before pregnancy
2. Levels after four to five half-lives (Table 24-3)

Table 24-3 Dosages of commonly used anticonvulsants

Drug	Starting Daily Dose (mg)	Nonpregnant Total Daily Dose (mg)	Total Daily Dose (mg/kg)	Number of Divided Doses	Time Before Steady State (days)	Therapeutic Level (μg/ml)	Serum Half-Life (hr)	Protein Binding (%)
Phenytoin	900 (loading dose)	300-500	4-8	1 or more	5-10	10-20 (total) 1-2 (free)	22-40	88-92
Phenobarbital	30-60	90-250	2-5	2-3	14-21	10-40	100	50
Valproic acid	250	500-3000	10-60	3-4	2-4	50-120	7-17	90-95
Ethosuximide	250	200-2000	20-35	2-3	5-12	40-100	50-60	0
Primidone	50-125	750-1500	5-20	3	4-7	5-15	8-16	0-20
Carbamazepine	100-200	600-1200	5-25	3-4	3-6	4-10	Single dose: 40-50 Long-term dose: 8-19	67-81

3. Monthly free serum levels are followed when the following occur:
   a. Tonic–clonic seizures are uncontrolled in the year before pregnancy.
   b. Complex partial or other seizure types are uncontrolled in the year before conception, interfering with the ability to function in daily activities.
   c. Tonic–clonic seizures begin during pregnancy, although previously controlled.
   d. Seizures are controlled, but total ACD levels decline by >50%.
4. Serum levels are followed approximately every 2 months when the following occur:
   a. Complex partial, absence, myoclonic, or other seizure types do not interfere with activities of daily life.
   b. Epilepsy is well controlled.

Therapeutic range for ACD levels

The therapeutic range for ACD levels is that range of levels below which seizure control is unlikely and above which many experience symptoms of toxicity.

1. Different values within a "therapeutic range" are not necessarily equally effective in a given patient.
2. Some patients may need a level slightly above therapeutic range to achieve seizure control.
3. Some patients are effectively controlled with "subtherapeutic" levels.

Free levels

Because there is a difference in the amount of decline in total versus free ACD level in pregnancy, free levels should be obtained, if possible, and correlated with seizure control and medication side effects.

1. The decline in free serum ACD level is less than the decline in total level for all major ACDs except phenobarbital, which is approximately equal.[71]
2. The percentage of free ACD therefore increases for most ACDs.
3. Although the ratio of unbound to bound drug increases, the amount of free ACD actually declines for all ACDs except valproate, which increases by 25%, especially in the third trimester when symptoms of toxicity may occur.
4. The period of greatest decline in phenytoin and phenobarbital levels is in the first trimester.

Changing ACD dosage

1. Changes in ACD regimen should be avoided during pregnancy unless seizures are uncontrolled or there are medication side effects.
2. Reasons not to change ACD dosage are as follows:
   a. Decline in ACD level in a patient who is well controlled, unless there is a >30% decline in free level in a patient who has been poorly controlled before pregnancy.
   b. Pregnancy is diagnosed in a patient taking two or more ACDs.
      (1) Physician should not discontinue one of the medications unless the dose is very small and the serum level is insignificant.

(2) In many cases, the critical period for teratogenesis has passed and this only serves to increase the risk of seizure and does not lower the risk of congenital malformation.

3. Reasons to change ACD dosage are as follows:
   a. There is an increase in tonic–clonic seizures.
   b. Complex-partial or other seizure types interfere with daily activities.
   c. Decline of >60% in total level (75% for valproate) or decline of >30% in free level in a patient who had tonic–clonic seizures or other disabling seizure type in the year before pregnancy.
   d. Disabling side effects from medications.

Guidelines for the management of seizure disorders in pregnancy

Preconceptual counseling

1. Unless seizures are difficult to control and affect the ability to function in daily life (thereby also making responsible parenting difficult), women with seizures should not be discouraged from becoming pregnant.
2. The twofold to threefold increased risk of fetal anomalies on ACD, but >90% chance of normal pregnancy outcome, should be discussed with the patient.
3. A child of a woman with idiopathic epilepsy has a 2% to 3% or fivefold greater risk than the general population of also developing epilepsy.
4. If a patient seen preconceptually has been seizure free for several years and has a normal EEG, an attempt should be made to gradually withdraw the ACD over a period of several months before pregnancy is attempted. She should be advised of the following:
   a. Driving is to be avoided during the weaning period until stability is established.
   b. That there is a 25% to 40% chance of seizure recurrence even if she has been seizure free for at least 2 years on medications.[7]
      (1) Medical Research Council Antiepileptic Withdrawal Study reported the following:
         (a) A 12% relapse rate during the first 6 months of drug withdrawal
         (b) A 32% relapse during the first year
         (c) A 41% relapse during the first 2 years
      (2) Therefore, if an attempt is made to withdraw ACDs over 2 to 4 months before pregnancy, the patient may expect a 12% risk of relapse before and during the first trimester and at least a 28% risk of relapse sometime during the pregnancy.
5. If the patient is on combination therapy, the physician should attempt to control seizures with monotherapy.
   a. Trimethadione should be avoided during the reproductive years.
   b. Otherwise, use the first choice drug for the seizure type.
   c. Valproate and possibly carbamazepine should be avoided when there is a family history of NTDs.

d. If valproate is used, high plasma levels can be avoided by dividing daily dose into three or four administrations.
6. Good seizure control should be maintained with the lowest effective ACD levels.
7. Good nutrition and health and adequate sleep should be encouraged before conception.
8. Adequate folate levels should be maintained preconceptually. Folate supplementation (4 mg/day) should be begun before pregnancy to stabilize both folate and ACD levels.

Pregnancy management

1. If patient is seen first during pregnancy and is well controlled on current ACD regimen, physician *should not withdraw ACDs* because this can precipitate status epilepticus.
   a. Patient should be educated on the need for compliance: Uncontrolled seizures may have a greater adverse effect on the mother and fetus than the teratogenic potential of ACDs.
2. Status epilepticus should be treated aggressively (see Guidelines for Managing Status Epilepticus).
3. Folate supplementation should be maintained at least through the first trimester with careful monitoring of ACD levels if the patient is on phenytoin, phenobarbital, or primidone.
4. An early ultrasound should be obtained to confirm gestational age because there is a risk of later IUGR.
5. A level II ultrasound examination should be obtained at 16 to 18 weeks to rule out evidence of spina bifida, cardiac or limb anomalies, and facial clefts.
6. If an adequate level II examination cannot be obtained, an amniocentesis for amniotic fluid alpha-fetoprotein and acetylcholinesterase should be offered to rule out an open NTD.
7. A fetal echocardiogram is recommended if the patient is on phenytoin, phenobarbital, or primidone.
8. Serial ultrasound examinations should be obtained in the third trimester if there is a suspicion for IUGR (lagging fundal height).
   a. Antepartum fetal testing should be begun if IUGR is documented.
9. Patient should be warned that excessive weight gain and sudden fluid retention may increase the risk of seizures.
10. Patient should be advised of the 17% to 50% chance of worsening seizure activity during pregnancy (higher risk with more frequent seizures before pregnancy).
    a. This risk can be minimized with avoidance of sleep deprivation and ACD compliance.
11. Free ACD levels should be monitored if possible with frequency depending on clinical indications.
    a. A therapeutic free ACD level should be maintained in the last month to decrease the risk of seizures in labor.
    b. ACD levels should be followed postpartum to prevent toxicity.
       (1) A rise in serum level and a need to decrease dosage to prepregnancy levels should be anticipated.

12. If the patient is on phenytoin, phenobarbital, or primidone, oral vitamin K supplementation (20 mg/day) should begin at 36 weeks.

Labor and delivery

1. If ACD level has not been checked recently, a level should be obtained at the onset of labor.
2. The ACD should be administered parenterally in labor and immediately postpartum to prevent intrapartum or postpartum seizures.
   a. Use of phenytoin (500 mg, IV, q12h) is controversial because it may prolong labor via inhibition of myometrial contractions.
   b. Phenobarbital can be administered IM.
3. Epidural anesthesia may reduce the risk of stress-induced seizures.
4. Seizures during labor should be treated with IV lorazepam.
5. Cesarean section delivery should be reserved for obstetrical indications only unless there is a threat of fetal hypoxia from repetitive tonic–clonic seizures.
6. Physician should arrange for follow-up with patient's neurologist postpartum.

Neonatal care

1. Prevention of neonatal hemorrhage
   a. Coagulation studies on cord blood should be obtained.
   b. Infant should be given 1 mg vitamin K, IM, at birth.
   c. If any two neonatal coagulation factors are <5% of normal, infant will require fresh frozen plasma if bleeding.
   d. Infant's coagulation status must be checked before circumcision.
2. If the mother is on phenobarbital or primidone, the infant should be observed for signs of generalized depression or neonatal withdrawal symptoms: irritability, restlessness, tremulousness, hyperexcitability, voracious appetite, frequent vomiting after eating, poor weight gain despite increased appetite.
   a. Symptoms begin 7 days after delivery.
   b. Symptoms gradually increase in intensity, peaking in 2 to 6 weeks.
3. Special precautions should be taken in newborn care if its mother's seizure activity is poorly controlled.
4. Breast-feeding is not contraindicated in patients on ACDs as long as the infant does not display signs of generalized depression.
   a. If the infant suckles poorly or is somnolent, early weaning should be considered (more likely with phenobarbital and primidone).
5. Physician should evaluate regularly for developmental delay throughout early childhood.

Guidelines for managing status epilepticus

Definition

From Epilepsy Foundation of America's Working Group on Status Epilepticus, 1993. More than 30 minutes of the following:

1. Continuous seizure activity, *or*
2. Two or more sequential seizures without full recovery of consciousness between seizures

3. Status epilepticus can present as the following:
   a. Repeated generalized convulsive seizures
   b. Nonconvulsive seizures that produce a continuous or fluctuating "epileptic twilight" state
   c. Repeated partial seizures manifested as focal motor convulsions, focal sensory symptoms, or focal impairment of function not associated with altered consciusness

General statements

1. Prognosis depends on the following:
   a. General condition of the patient
   b. Interval between onset of seizures and the start of therapy
2. Mortality is high even with prompt treatment.
3. Most common precipitating factor is the abrupt cessation of ACDs.
4. Incidence of seizures is not more common in pregnancy.

Treatment protocol

Modified from New York Hospital-Cornell Comprehensive Epilepsy Center

1. Supportive care involves the following:
   a. Airway maintenance
   b. Vital signs assessment
      (1) During the first 30 to 45 minutes, status epilepticus usually produces hypertension; thereafter blood pressure returns to normal or below baseline.
      (2) Hypotension, which can lead to cerebral hypoperfusion and potentiate excitotoxic brain damage, should be avoided.
   c. Normal saline IV infusion should be started.
   d. EKG and FHR should be monitored.
   e. Bed rails should be padded.
2. Patient should be admitted to intensive care unit (ICU).
3. Initial laboratory studies include ACD level, glucose, electrolytes, arterial blood gas (ABG), toxicology screen, and CBC.
4. Any underlying causes should be treated.
5. Physician should give 50 ml of 50% glucose solution, IV, and thiamine, 100 mg, IM.
6. Physician should administer one of the following:
   a. IV lorazepam (0.1 mg/kg) at a maximal rate of 2 mg/min; may repeat in 4 hours and then as needed, in 8-hour intervals.
      (1) Duration of anticonvulsant action is up to 24 hours, making the addition of a longer acting agent less urgent.
   b. *Or* IV diazepam, 5 to 10 mg, over 2 to 5 minutes (not faster than 2 mg/min); may repeat at 10-minute intervals up to a total of 20 mg.
      (1) Duration of anticonvulsant action is 15 to 20 minutes, therefore, a long-acting agent should be started.
   c. *Or* diazepam drip: diluted 50 mg in 500 ml D_5W and run at a rate of 5 to 10 mg/hr, titrating the rate to control seizures.
   d. Should not be given with phenobarbital because of excessive respiratory depression.
   e. May need artificial ventilation.

7. Lumbar puncture should be performed for diagnostic studies if bacterial meningitis is seriously considered in the differential, and antibiotic therapy should be begun.
8. Administer phenytoin 1000 to 1150 mg (18 to 20 mg/kg), IV, load no faster than 50 mg/min.
   a. Phenytoin can cause hypotension, arrhythmias, and cardiac arrest if given faster.
   b. EKG and blood pressure (BP) should be monitored while loading.
   c. If hypotension develops, physician should give IV fluids and decrease the infusion rate.
   d. Phenytoin does not potentiate the depressant effects of diazepam.
   e. Phenytoin is effective in 50% of cases.
9. Patient should be intubated if status epilepticus persists.
10. IV phenobarbital (20 mg/kg) should be administered, no faster than 100 mg/min.
    a. When phenobarbital is used to treat status epilepticus from barbiturate withdrawal, physician should give 250 mg over 3 to 5 min; may repeat in 30 minutes.
    b. Onset of action is slow (15 to 30 minutes).
    c. Additive hypotensive and respiratory depressant actions are seen with diazepam.
11. An EEG should be obtained when convulsive activity ceases; if electrographic seizure activity persists or if convulsive status epilepticus persists, pentobarbital coma should be instituted with continuous EEG monitoring.
    a. Physician should give pentobarbital loading dose of 5 to 15 mg/kg with a continuous infusion rate of 1 mg/kg/hr.
    b. Infusion rate should be increased until a burst-suppression pattern is achieved.
    c. BP should be monitored closely, preferably with an intraarterial pressure transducer.
    d. Pentobarbital coma should be maintained for 24 hours.
    e. After a high level of phenytoin and phenobarbital is achieved, pentobarbital should be titrated downward and gradually discontinued over 24 hours.
       (1) Patient should be observed for recurrent status epilepticus.
       (2) If necessary, pentobarbital coma can be reinstituted for another 24 hours.
12. If seizures persist, a standing dose of carbamazepine should be administered via nasogastric tube, or valproate rectally or via nasogastric tube, or IV lorazepam (0.03 to 0.05 mg/kg) every 8 hours in addition to phenytoin, phenobarbital, and pentobarbital.
13. Paraldehyde and general anesthesia are used rarely when seizures persist.
    a. If they persist, halothane or another *inhalation* anesthetic should be given, along with a neuromuscular blocker.
    b. IV lidocaine, 50 to 100 mg, may be tried, followed by an infusion at 1 to 2 mg/min if it is effective.

Anticonvulsant drugs

Phenytoin

1. Pharmacokinetics
   a. Fifty percent of patients have more than 100% increase in clearance during pregnancy.[44]
   b. The usual standard doses (300 to 1200 mg/day), when used in pregnancy, produce a mean plasma level of 3.6 μg/ml (therapeutic level = 10 to 20 μg/ml).
   c. Phenytoin crosses the placenta rapidly, with fetal levels equaling maternal levels at steady state.
   d. Half-lives
      (1) Fetal = 60 hours.
      (2) Maternal = 24 hours.
      (3) Newborn elimination is complete by fifth day.
2. Teratogenicity
   a. In epidemiologic studies it is difficult to assess the exact risk from phenytoin and how much may be a result of the genetic contribution of epilepsy.
   b. Fetal hydantoin syndrome (FHS) (see Table 24-2)
      (1) Hanson and others[25] reported full manifestation of FHS in 11% of 35 children exposed in pregnancy and syndromic features of FHS in an additional 30%.
      (2) Gaily and others in a prospective study of 82 exposed infants reported no cases of FHS, although hypertelorism and distal digital hypoplasia associated with *in utero* exposure was found.
      (3) Many of the minor anomalies of FHS are seen in the mothers. Therefore, are they genetically linked to epilepsy rather than ACD exposure?
   c. More recently, a 3% to 4% risk of major anomalies (cleft lip or palate) has been reported, and a 7% to 10% risk of dysmorphic features, minor anomalies, and developmental delays reported when dilantin is used alone.[6]
      (1) Figures are higher when phenytoin is used in combination with other drugs.
   d. There are no consistent CNS malformations consistently associated with *in utero* exposure.
   e. A genetic defect in the arene oxide detoxification pathway that causes diminished epoxide hydrolase enzyme activity is proposed as the cause of teratogenesis.[6] This results in the accumulation of the reactive arene oxide intermediate of phenytoin (Fig. 24-1).
      (1) Infants with FHS have low levels of epoxide hydrolase.
      (2) Unaffected infants have intermediate to high levels of enzyme activity.
   f. ACD polypharmacy with phenytoin causes competition for the epoxide hydrolase enzyme and subsequent decreased rate of phenytoin detoxification and increased teratogenic potential.
   g. Epoxide hydrolase activity can be measured in fetal amniocytes, thereby possibly identifying those fetuses at increased risk for congenital malformations.

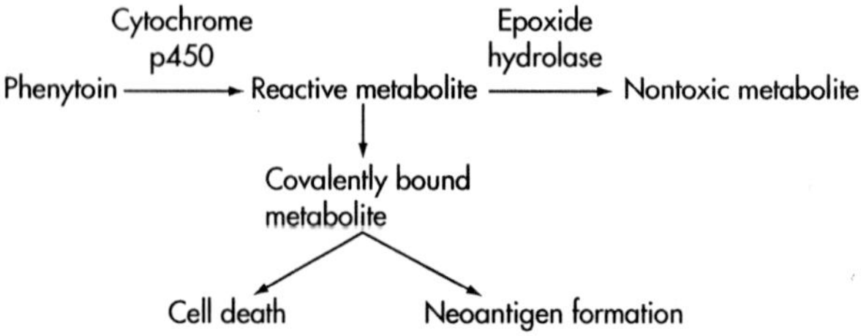

Figure 24-1
Phenytoin metabolism.

(1) Buehler and others[6] reported on 19 pregnancies exposed with phenytoin monotherapy.
(a) Four infants had low epoxide hydrolase activity
(b) All four had stigmata of ACD-induced dysmorphisms, two of which had a significant delay in motor development

h. Genetic variability in amount of available epoxide hydrolase may influence the susceptibility of the fetus to teratogenicity.
(1) Strickler and others[63] (1985) correlated the inability of a child's lymphocytes to detoxify phenytoin metabolites with the presence of major phenytoin-associated malformations as well as a similar abnormality in one of the parents' lymphocytes.

i. Studies of rat embryos exposed to ACD-containing serum in culture indicate that the relationship between ACDs and malformations is complex and may involve genetic factors, drug-related factors, nutritional factors, host factors, and species-specific issues.

j. There are conflicting reports on the possible effect on cognitive development after *in utero* exposure.[26,66]

3. Carcinogenicity
a. No controlled studies have been performed that establish the risk of transplacental carcinogenicity.
b. Eleven case reports suggest that phenytoin may be a transplacental carcinogen,[5] with the following tumors seen after *in utero* exposure.
(1) Neuroblastoma (five cases)
(2) Ganglioneuroblastoma (one case)
(3) Melanotic neuroexodermal tumor (one case)
(4) Extrarenal Wilms' tumor (one case)
(5) Mesenchymoma (one case)
(6) Lymphangioma (one case)
(7) Ependymoblastoma (one case)

4. Neonatal coagulopathy
a. A 10% risk of severe coagulopathy caused by deficiency in vitamin K–dependent clotting factors (II, VII, IX, and X) exists.
b. Neonates usually bleed within the first 24 hours, unlike hemorrhagic disease of the newborn in which bleeds occur during the second to fifth day.

c. Hemorrhages occur in unusual places: into pleural, pericardial, or peritoneal cavities, or into the retroperitoneal space or intracranially.
d. Hemorrhages are unrelated to prematury, hypoxia, or birth trauma.
e. Preventive measures include the following:
   (1) Prophylactic vitamin K during the final month of pregnancy is given because some infants bleed despite vitamin K therapy (10 to 20 mg/day).
      (a) Large doses are required because of questionable ability to cross the placenta.
      (b) Physician can also give patient 10 mg, IM, 4 hours before birth.
   (2) Neonate should be given 1 mg vitamin K, IM, at birth.
   (3) Cord blood clotting studies should be obtained.
      (a) If they are severely abnormal, the infant should be treated with additional vitamin K and fresh frozen plasma.
      (b) Some infants will die if therapy is delayed until clinical evidence of bleeding is detected.

5. Folate deficiency
   a. Deficiency can occur with phenytoin, phenobarbital, or primidone.
   b. A 33% to 91% risk depending on the following:
      (1) Population studied
      (2) Definition of normal
      (3) Particular test used
   c. Only a small number of patients demonstrate macrocytosis and even fewer experience megaloblastic anemia.
   d. Pathophysiology
      (1) Folate acts as a cofactor in hepatic reactions responsible for drug hydroxylation.
      (2) ACD induction of hepatic microsomal enzymes increases the demand for folate.
      (3) Phenytoin interferes with intestinal absorption of folate.
   e. Association with fetal malformation
      (1) Folate antagonists (aminopterin) are well-known teratogens.
      (2) Some retrospective studies show a relationship between folate deficiency and fetal malformations.[18,27]
         (a) Other studies have failed to confirm these findings.[51,58]
      (3) In a prospective study of 3000 patients, Hall[24] was unable to demonstrate a relationship between serum folate levels in early pregnancy and fetal anomalies.
   f. Some recommend prophylactic folate supplementation if on ACDs (1 to 4 mg/day).
      (1) Folate supplementation may increase hepatic drug hydroxylation, resulting in a decrease in serum phenytoin levels, but usually the drop is small and rarely results in exacerbation of seizures.
      (2) ACD levels should be monitored if on supplemental folate.
      (3) Physician should consider withholding folate supplementation if patient is experiencing more than one seizure per month.

6. Altered calcium metabolism
   a. Phenytoin induces enzymes that increase the metabolism of 25-hydroxycholecalciferol to inactive compounds (24,25-dihydroxycholecalciferol).[62]
   b. Phenytoin may interfere with calcium absorption.
   c. Some cases have been reported of severe prolonged neonatal hypocalcemia and tetany refractory to calcium therapy in infants exposed to phenytoin and phenobarbital.
   d. Some have suggested the use of supplemental vitamin D in patients on phenytoin and phenobarbital (the same amount found in prenatal vitamins).
7. Maternal side effects: nystagmus, ataxia, hirsutism, gingival hyperplasia, megaloblastic anemia, cardiovascular collapse after rapid IV injection, lymphadenopathy, skin rashes, Stevens-Johnson syndrome, lupus syndrome, osteomalacia, hepatic necrosis
8. Breast-feeding
   a. Crosses poorly into breast milk
      (1) Breast milk levels are one fourth to one third that of maternal serum.
   b. Not shown to be harmful despite slow neonatal elimination
   c. Considered compatible with breast-feeding by the American Academy of Pediatrics

Phenobarbital

1. Pharmacokinetics
   a. Phenobarbital crosses the placenta easily, reaching equilibrium between mother and fetus.
      (1) Cord blood levels equal 95% of maternal serum levels.
   b. Neonate clears drug slowly: only 1% to 20% every 24 hours.
   c. Phenobarbital is the drug of choice for grand mal or focal motor seizures.
2. Teratogenicity
   a. Relative risk of 3.5 for anomalies in Finnish data
   b. Possible fetal barbiturate syndrome[61]
      (1) Facial dysmorphism
      (2) Prenatal and postnatal growth deficiency
      (3) Developmental delay
      (4) Clinical features: resemble FHS and fetal alcohol syndrome
      (5) Phenytoin, phenobarbital, and alcohol: all can cause folate deficiency
         (a) Is this the common pathogenesis for related dysmorphisms?
   c. Conflicting reports on teratogenicity of maternal phenobarbital ingestion in nonepileptic patients[23,46,59] with lack of fetal malformation in nonepileptics in some reports suggesting a predisposition resulting from a genetic component of epilepsy
3. Neonatal coagulopathy
   a. Phenobarbital and primidone (which is partially metabolized to phenobarbital) are most commonly associated with neonatal coagulopathy (see 4. under Phenytoin).

4. Folate deficiency
   a. Phenobarbital and primidone are also associated with folate deficiency and occasionally megaloblastic anemia (see 5. under Phenytoin).
5. Neonatal depression
   a. Can occur after ingestion during the last few days of pregnancy
   b. Manifest by decreased alertness, respiratory depression, and hypotonia
   c. May cause a 48-hour lag in neonate's ability to adapt to breast-feeding
6. Neonatal withdrawal
   a. Withdrawal occurs in 10% to 20% of neonates exposed to as little as 60 mg/day during the last trimester.
   b. Symptoms begin between the fourth and seventh day of life, later than opiate withdrawal; some symptoms may persist for 2 to 6 months.
   c. Neonatal withdrawal syndrome (similar to opiate withdrawal symptoms) symptoms include the following:
      (1) Generalized neuromuscular excitability
      (2) Hyperactivity
      (3) Tremulousness
      (4) Hyperreflexia
      (5) Excessive crying
      (6) Sleep disturbances
      (7) Vomiting
      (8) Diarrhea
      (9) Hyperphagia
      (10) Occasional seizures
   d. Treatment
      (1) Infant stimulation should be minimized.
      (2) Infant is sedated with phenobarbital, phenothiazines, or paregoric if necessary.
7. Maternal side effects: drowsiness, ataxia, respiratory depression, sleep abnormalities, hypotension, allergic reaction, megaloblastic anemia, agranulocytosis, thrombocytopenia
8. Breast-feeding
   a. Breast milk concentration ranges from 10% to 40% of maternal serum.
   b. Half-life in the neonate is 40 to 300 hours (longer in premature infants).
   c. Free fraction can increase to greater than 90% of the total serum concentration in some infants, thereby increasing the sedative effects.
   d. Phenobarbital is not contraindicated unless the neonate exhibits signs of generalized depression; American Academy of Pediatrics advises use with caution because of potential to cause major adverse effects in nursing infants.

Carbamazepine

1. Carbamazepine is the only ACD that is a pregnancy category C drug (the others are pregnancy category D).

2. Carbamazepine is the drug of choice in children and young adults (less sedating) for clonic seizures.
3. Maternal and fetal serum levels are approximately equivalent at steady state.
4. Neonate eliminates drug at the same rate as adults with a half-life of 8 to 28 hours.
5. Twenty percent of patients develop leukopenia; therefore, WBC count should be monitored every 4 to 6 weeks.
6. Teratogenicity (see Table 24-2)
   a. Jones and others[32] reported minor malformations in 18% of exposed pregnancies (craniofacial defects, fingernail hypoplasia) and no significant increase in major malformations.
      (1) Although they reported a 20% association with developmental delay (5 of 25) there was lack of information on socioeconomic factors, lack of a control population and failure to allow for normal distribution of test scores in the drug-exposed children.
      (2) The study population, however, was self-referred, which may have introduced selection bias.
   b. Conflicting reports have come from studies that show no increased rate of congenital malformations and others that report a decrease in head circumference, birth weight, and length and isolated case reports of spina bifida, rib anomalies, optic nerve hypoplasia, and retardation.
   c. A 1% risk of spina bifida in infants of women taking carbamazepine alone was reported by Rosa[55] from the Michigan Medicaid cohort data; however, the adequacy of the data and conclusions have been strongly questioned.
      (1) A more recent large-scale study could not support these conclusions.[13]
   d. The proposed mechanism of teratogenicity is similar to that of phenytoin, involving epoxide hydrolase detoxification and arene oxide toxicity.
      (1) Combination therapy may predispose to increased accumulation of carbamazepine epoxide.
      (2) The association of this epoxide in monotherapy and fetal malformations has not been established.[49]
         (a) Valproate inhibits epoxide hydrolase: Increased epoxide accumulation?
         (b) Phenytoin and phenobarbital induce carbamazepine biotransformation.
         (c) The ratio of epoxide metabolite: Carbamazepine is lowest (<0.3) when taken alone and highest (0.52) in offspring of patients using polytherapy.
7. Maternal side effects: drowsiness, leukopenia, ataxia, mild hepatotoxicity, transient blurred vision, rash, disturbance of equilibrium, transient paresthesias, proteinuria, neutropenia, systemic lupus erythematosus, left ventricular failure, hypertension, hypotension, syncope and collapse, edema

8. Breast-feeding
   a. Carbamazepine crosses poorly into breast milk (levels are less than 40% of maternal serum levels, although reported up to 75%), but accumulation in nursing infants has been reported.
      (1) Milk to plasma ratios of 0.24/0.69 have been reported.
   b. Chronically exposed neonates are able to metabolize drug as efficiently as adults.
   c. Carbamazepine is not contraindicated by the American Academy of Pediatrics.

Valproic acid

1. Indicated in a variety of partial and generalized seizures
2. Pharmacokinetics
   a. Valproic acid crosses the placenta readily, with fetal levels equal to or slightly greater than that of the maternal serum.
   b. Half-life in newborns is four-fold longer than that of older patients.
3. May cause transient neonatal hyperglycinemia and a false-positive screen for aminoacidemia
4. Teratogenesis
   a. A 1% to 2% risk of NTD, usually spina bifida[8] compared with 0.35% risk with other ACDs.
   b. Risk for NTD is greatest from 17 to 30 days postconception.
   c. Odds ratio for valproate-associated NTD relative to other ACD-associated malformations ranges from 9.8 to 25.8.[37]
   d. A fetal valproate syndrome has been suggested by DiLiberti and others[15] (see Table 24-2); however, these observations were based on seven infants.
   e. Several reports describe a specific pattern of major malformations consisting of meningomyelocele, cardiovascular, and urogenital malformations with craniofacial, skeletal, and genital minor anomalies.[14]
   f. Six case reports of radial ray defects with *in utero* valproate exposure.[22]
5. Monotherapy recommended because of valproate's potential to enhance the teratogenicity of other ACDs
6. Maternal side effects: ataxia, drowsiness, alopecia, hepatotoxicity, thrombocytopenia
7. Breast-feeding
   a. Levels in breast milk are up to 15% of that of maternal serum (less than 2% in some reports).
   b. Valproic acid is considered compatible with breast-feeding by the American Academy of Pediatrics.

Primidone

1. Primidone is the only major ACD eliminated primarily by the kidney.
2. Phenobarbital is one of the major active metabolites; therefore, primidone is also associated with folate deficiency, neonatal coagulopathy, neonatal depression, and withdrawal.
3. There are reports of a possible primidone embryopathy[9,37,53] with features similar to FHS (see Table 24-3).

4. Primidone crosses the placenta to a variable degree.
5. Maternal side effects include drowsiness, ataxia, vertigo, headache, nausea, morbilliform rash, edema, nystagmus, impotence, leukopenia, megaloblastic anemia.
6. Breast-feeding
   a. A milk to plasma ratio of 0.8 has been reported.[35]
   b. Nursing should be avoided only if there are signs of generalized depression.
   c. Use is with caution because of potential to produce significant adverse effects in the nursing infant according to the American Academy of Pediatrics.

Trimethadione

1. Indications for use are absence seizures.
2. To be avoided during pregnancy: ethosuximide and clonazepam are preferred.
3. Of pregnancies exposed to trimethadione, 87% are complicated by either fetal anomaly or first-trimester loss.[17]
4. Teratogenicity: It is the most potent teratogen of the ACDs (see Table 24-2).[73]
   a. An 83% incidence of major fetal malformations has been reported.
   b. A 95% incidence of craniofacial anomalies has been reported.
      (1) 43% low-set ears
      (2) 28% cleft lip or palate
      (3) 10% to 20% high-arched palate, broad nasal bridge
   c. Fifty percent of affected children have mental retardation, developmental delay, or both.
   d. Twenty-five percent to 50% of affected children have speech, hearing, or vision impairment.
5. In rodent studies, dimethadione, the metabolite of trimethadione that accumulates in humans, was found to cause CNS malformations.
   a. In cultured rat embryos there was defective closure of the neural tube, abnormal segmentation of the mesoderm, cephalocaudal flexion, and abnormal brainstem development.

Ethosuximide

1. Far less teratogenic than trimethadione, which is the other drug of choice for absence seizures (which are usually rare after adolescence)
   a. Pregnancy category C
2. 6% risk of fetal malformation after *in utero* exposure[16]
3. Slow elimination by the neonate, with a half-life of 41 hours
4. Maternal side effects: nausea, hepatotoxicity, leukopenia, thrombocytopenia, aplastic anemia, pancytopenia, agranulocytosis, eosinophilia, morphologic and functional changes in the liver, diarrhea, hyperactivity or hypoactivity, behavioral changes, paranoid and suicidal ideations, Stevens-Johnson syndrome, systemic lupus erythematosus
5. Breast-feeding
   a. Breast milk levels are 90% that of the maternal serum.
   b. Toxicity has not been observed in nursing infants.

c. Ethosuximide is considered compatible with breast-feeding by the American Academy of Pediatrics.

Diazepam

1. Indications for use include status epilepticus.
2. Pharmacokinetics
   a. Diazepam crosses the placenta within seconds.
   b. Fetal serum level of the parent drug and its active metabolites is higher than maternal levels for the first 4 to 6 hours.
   c. Metabolism in the neonate is very slow, requiring greater than 1 week to eliminate.
3. Administration during labor causes depression of short-term and beat-to-beat variability of the fetal heart rate.
4. Neonatal effects from administration during labor (most pronounced when mother has received over 30 mg in the 15 hours before delivery) are as follows:
   a. Low Apgar scores
   b. Apneic spells
   c. Hypotonia
   d. Poor sucking
   e. Reluctance to feed
   f. Hypothermia and impaired metabolic response to cold
5. A withdrawal syndrome similar to that of narcotic withdrawal has been reported after prolonged exposure *in utero*.
   a. IUGR
   b. Tremors
   c. Irritability
   d. Hypertonicity
   e. Diarrhea and/or vomiting
   f. Vigorous sucking
6. Teratogenicity
   a. There is no evidence of teratogenic effects in high doses in rats.
   b. An association with oral clefts was reported after first-trimester exposure in four retrospective case control studies; however, the actual risk was only 0.2% for cleft palate and 0.4% for cleft lip.[56]
   c. Laegreid and others[38] described dysmorphic features, growth retardation, and CNS defects in eight infants after exposure to diazepam, 30 mg/day or more, or oxazepam, 75 mg/day or more, throughout pregnancy.
7. Maternal side effects: drowsiness, ataxia, confusion, depression, headache, syncope, constipation, hypotension, bradycardia, rash, paradoxical reactions, blurred vision, nystagmus
8. Breast-feeding
   a. Diazepam may accumulate in breast-fed neonates and cause lethargy and impaired suckling.
   b. Diazepam is not recommended because of slow neonatal elimination.

References

1. Annegers JF et al: Do anticonvulsants have a teratogenic effect? *Arch Neurol* 31:364, 1974.
2. Bardy AH: Incidence of seizures during pregnancy, labor and puerperium in epileptic women: a prospective study, *Acta Neurol Scand* 75:356, 1987.
3. Bjerkedal T, Bahana SL: The course and outcome of pregnancy in women with epilepsy, *Acta Obstet Gynecol Scand* 52:245, 1973.
4. Borchert LD, Labar DR: An organized approach to managing status epilepticus, *J Crit Illness* 8:965-972, 1993.
5. Briggs GG, Freeman RK, Yaffe SJ: *Drugs in pregnancy and lactation,* ed 4, Baltimore, 1994, Williams & Wilkins.
6. Buehler BA et al: Prenatal prediction of risk of the fetal hydantoin syndrome, *N Engl J Med* 322:22, 1990.
7. Chadwick D: The discontinuation of AED therapy. In Pedley TA, Meldrum BS, editors: *Recent advances in epilepsy,* vol 2, pp 111-124, Edinburgh, 1985, Churchill Livingstone.
8. Centers for Disease Control: Valproate: a new cause of birth defects—report from Italy and follow-up from France, *MMWR* 32:439, 1983.
9. Clericuzio CL: Fetal primidone effects, *Proc Greenwood Genet Ctr* 4:93, 1985.
10. Cole AP, Jailey DM: Diazepam and active metabolite in breast milk and their transfer to the neonate, *Arch Dis Child* 50:741-742, 1975.
11. Commission of Classification and Terminology of the International League Against Epilepsy: Proposal for classification of epilepsies and syndromes, *Epilepsia* 26:268, 1981.
12. Committee on Drugs, American Academy of Pediatrics: Transfer of drugs and other chemicals into human milk, *Pediatrics* 84:924-936, 1989.
13. Czeizel AE, Bod M, Halasz P: Evaluation of anticonvulsant drugs during pregnancy in a population-based Hungarian study, *Eur J Epidemiol* 8:122-127, 1992.
14. Delgado-Escueta A, Dieter J: Consensus guidelines: preconception counseling, management, and care of the pregnant woman with epilepsy; *Neurology* 42(suppl5):149–60, 1992.
15. DiLiberti JH et al: The fetal valproate syndrome, *Am J Med Genet* 19:473-481, 1984.
16. Fabro S, Brown NA: Teratogenic potential of anticonvulsants, *N Engl J Med* 300:1280, 1979.
17. Feldman GL, Weaver DD, Lovrien EW: The fetal trimethadione syndrome: report of an additional family and further delineation of this syndrome, *Am J Dis Child* 131:89-92, 1977.
18. Fraser JL, Watt HJ: Megaloblastic anemia in pregnancy and the puerperium, *Am J Obstet Gynecol* 89:532, 1964.
19. Gaily E et al: Minor anomalies in offspring of epileptic mothers, *J Pediatr* 112:520-529, 1988.
20. Gaily E, Kantola-Sorsa E, Granstrom ML: Intelligence of children of epileptic mothers, *J Pediatr* 113:667, 1988.
21. Gjerde IO, Strandjord RE, Ulmstein M: The course of epilepsy during pregnancy: a study of 78 cases, *Acta Neurol Scand* 78:198, 1988.
22. Graham JM Jr et al: Preaxial ray reduction defects valproate exposure during pregnancy (abstract), *Teratology* 43:441, 1991.
23. Greenberg G et al: Maternal drug histories and congenital abnormalities, *Br Med J* 2:853, 1977.
24. Hall MH: Folic acid deficiency and congenital malformation, *J Obstet Gynaecol Br Commonw* 79:159, 1972.
25. Hanson JW et al: Risks to the offspring of women treated with hydantoin anticonvulsants with emphasis on the fetal hydantoin syndrome, *J Pediatr* 8:662-668, 1976.

26. Hattig, H, Steinhausen H-Ch: Children of epileptic parents: a prospective developmental study. In Rauh H, Steinhausen H-Ch, editors: *Psychobiology and early development,* pp. 155-169 Amsterdam, 1987, Elsevier.
27. Hibbard ED, Smithells RW: Folic acid metabolism and human embryopathy, *Lancet* 1:1254, 1965.
28. Hiilesmaa VK: *A prospective study on maternal and fetal outcome in 139 women with epilepsy,* Dissertation, vol. 43, p. 55, Helsinki, 1982, University of Helsinki.
29. Hiilesmaa VK: Pregnancy and birth in women with epilepsy, *Neurology* 42(suppl 5):8-11, 192.
30. Hiilesmaa VK, Brady A, Teramo K: Obstetric outcome in women with epilepsy, *Am J Obstet Gynecol* 152:488-504, 1985.
31. Hill RM et al: Relationship of antiepileptic drug exposure of the infant and developmental potential. In Janz D et al: editors: *Epilepsy, pregnancy, and the child,* New York, 1982, Raven Press.
32. Jones KL et al: Pattern of malformations in the children of women treated with carbamazepine during pregnancy, *N Engl J Med* 320:1660-1666, 1989.
33. Kaneko S et al: Teratogenicity of antiepileptic drugs: analysis of possible risk factors, *Epilepsia* 29:459, 1988.
34. Kaneko S et al: Malformations in infants of mothers with epilepsy receiving antiepileptic drugs, *Neurology* 42(suppl 5):94-110, 1992.
35. Kaneko S, Sato T, Suzuki K: The levels of anticonvulants in breast milk, *Br J Clin Pharmacol* 7:624-627, 1979.
36. Koch S et al: Major and minor birth malformations and antiepileptic drugs, *Neurology* 42(suppl 5):83-88, 1992.
37. Krauss CM et al: Four siblings with similar malformations after exposure to phenytoin and primidone, *J Pediatr* 105:750, 1984.
38. Laegreid L et al: Teratogenic effects of benzodiazepine use during pregnancy, *J Pediatr* 114:126-231, 1989.
39. Lammer EJ et al: Teratogen update: valproic acid, *Teratology* 35:465, 1987.
40. Leavitt AM et al: Epilepsy and pregnancy: Developmental outcomes at 12 months, *Neurology* 42(suppl 5):141-143, 1992.
41. Lindhout D et al: Antiepileptic drugs and teratogenesis in two consecutive cohorts: changes in prescription policy paralleled by changes in pattern of malformations, *Neurology* 42(suppl 5):94-100, 1992.
42. Lindhout D, Omtzigt JGC, Cornel MC: Spectrum of neural-tube defects in 34 infants prenatally exposed to antiepileptic drugs, *Neurology* 42(suppl 5):111-118, 1992.
43. Medeiros YS, Calixto JB: Inhibitory effect of diphenylhydantoin on myometrium from pregnant women in vitro: a comparative study with nicardipine and trifluoperazine, *Pharmacol Res* 22:597-603, 1990.
44. Mygind KI, Dam M, Christiansen J: Phenytoin and phenobarbitone plasma clearance during pregnancy, *Acta Neurol Scand* 54:160, 1976.
45. Nakane Y et al: Multi-institutional study on the teratogenicity and foetal toxicity of anti-epileptic drugs: a report of a collaborative study group in Japan, *Epilepsia* 21:663, 1980.
46. Nelson AM, Forfar JO: Associations between drugs administered during pregnancy and congenital abnormalities of the fetus, *Br Med J* 1:523, 1971.
47. Nelson KB, Ellenberg JH: Maternal seizure disorder, outcome of pregnancy, and neurologic abnormalities in the children, *Neurology* 32:1247-54, 1982.
48. Omtzigt JCG et al: The risk of spina bifida apaerta after first-trimester exposure to valproate in a prenatal cohort, *Neurology* 42(suppl 5):119-125, 1992.
49. Omtzigt JGC et al: The 10,11-epoxide-10,11-diol pathway of carbamazepine in early pregnancy in maternal, serum, urine, and amniotic fluid: effect of dose, comedication, and relation to outcome of pregnancy, *Ther Drug Monit* 15:1-10, 1993.

50. Ottman R et al: Higher risk of seizures in offspring of mothers than fathers with epilepsy, *Am J Hum Genet* 43:357-364, 1988.
51. Pritchard JA et al: Infants of mothers with megaloblastic anaemia due to folate deficiency, *JAMA* 211:1982, 1970.
52. Ramsey RE et al: Status epilepticus in pregnancy: effect of phenytoin malabsorption on seizure control, *Neurology* 28:85, 1978.
53. Rating D et al: Teratogenic and pharmacokinetic studies of primidone during pregnancy and in the offspring of epileptic women, *Acta Paediatr Scand* 71:310, 1982.
54. Robertson IG: Breech presentation associated with anticonvulsant drugs, *J Obstet Gynecol* 4:174-177, 1984.
55. Rosa F: Spina bifida in infants of women treated with carbamazepine during pregnancy, *N Engl J Med* 324:674-677, 1991.
56. Safra MJ, Oakley GP Jr: Valium: an oral cleft teratogen? *Cleft Palate J* 13:198-200, 1976.
57. Schmidt D et al: Change of seizure frequency in pregnant epileptic women, *J Neurol Neurosurg Psychiatry* 46:751, 1983.
58. Scott DE, Whalley PJ, Pritchard JA: Maternal folate deficiency and pregnancy wastage, *Obstet Gynecol* 36:26, 1970.
59. Shapiro S et al: Anticonvulsants and parental epilepsy in the development of birth defects, *Lancet* 1:272, 1976.
60. Shorvon SD: Epidemiology, classification, natural history, and genetics of epilepsy, *Lancet* 336:93, 1990.
61. Smith DW: Teratogenicity of anticonvulsive medications, *Am J Dis Child* 1331:1337, 1977.
62. Stamp TCB et al: Plasma levels and therapeutic effect of 25-hydroxycholecalciferol in epileptic patients taking anticonvulsant drugs, *Br Med J* 4:9, 1972.
63. Strickler SM et al: Genetic predisposition to phenytoin-induced birth defects, *Lancet* 2:746, 1985.
64. Tanganelli P, Regesta G: Epilepsy, pregnancy, and major birth anomalies: An Italian prospective, controlled study, *Neurology* 42(suppl 5):89-93, 1992.
65. Teramo K et al: Fetal heart rate during a maternal grand mal epileptic seizure, *J Perinat Med* 7:3, 1979.
66. Vanoverloop D et al: The effects of prenatal exposure to phenytoin and other anticonvulsants on intellectual function at 4 to 8 years of age, *Neurotoxicol Teratol* 14:329-335, 1992.
67. Wilhelm J, Morris D, Hotham N: Epilepsy and pregnancy—A review of 98 pregnancies, *Aust NZ J Obstet Gynaecol* 4:290, 1990.
68. Working Group on Status Epilepticus. Treatment of convulsive status epilepticus, *JAMA* 270:854-859, 1993.
69. Yerby MS: Pregnancy and epilepsy, *Epilepsia* 32(suppl 6):S51, 1991.
70. Yerby MS, Devinsky O: Epilepsy in pregnancy, *Advan Neurol* 64:45-63, 1994.
71. Yerby MS, Friel PN, McCormick K: Antiepileptic drug disposition during pregnancy, *Neurology* 42(suppl 5):12-16, 1992.
72. Yerby M, Koepsell T, Daling J: Pregnancy complications and outcomes in a cohort of women with epilepsy, *Epilepsia* 26:631-635, 1985.
73. Zachai EH et al: The fetal trimethadione syndrome, *J Pediatr* 87:280-284, 1975.

24.3 **LUPUS ERYTHEMATOSUS AND ANTIPHOSPHOLIPIDS**

Stephanie Walton, M.D., and E. Nigel Harris, M.D.

Systemic lupus erythematosus (SLE)

Definition of SLE

1. American College of Rheumatology Epidemiologic Criteria (Table 24-4).
2. Clinical criteria may be used that at a minimum require one typical clinical sign (rash or arthritis), together with either anti-DNA or anti-Smith antibody and with exclusion of other rheumatic illnesses.
3. A lupus flare is a demonstration of inflammatory and immunologic abnormalities.

Effect of SLE on fertility

1. Disease
   a. Fertility is normal in patients without severe renal disease
   b. In patients with severe active disease, infertility results from the following:
      (1) Amenorrhea caused by chronic disease state
      (2) Drug therapy (Table 24-5)
2. Drug therapy (see Table 24-5)

SLE and pregnancy

1. When to become pregnant
   a. Well-controlled maternal SLE for >6 months is preferred.
   b. Successful pregnancy outcome is 85% even in patients with unplanned pregnancies.
2. Outcomes and risks
   a. Fetal outcome (effect of disease on pregnancy outcome)
      (1) Fetal loss occurs in 10% to 40% of SLE pregnancies.
      (2) Fetal loss in over 50% of SLE pregnancies with serum Cr >1.6 mg/dl and hypertension (HTN) present at time of conception.
      (3) Fetal loss risk factors
         (a) Maternal activity of lupus
         (b) Maternal renal disease: degree of impairment (moderate to severe)
            i. Proteinuria (nephrotic range = 3.5 g/day) *and*
            ii. Decreased creatinine clearance (Cr Cl <60 to 80 ml/min)
         (c) Antiphospholipid antibodies
            i. Anticardiolipin antibodies (IgG isotype >20 GPL units)
            ii. Positive lupus anticoagulant
         (d) Prior history of fetal losses
         (e) Maternal thrombocytopenia
            i. Decreases fetal survival
            ii. Treatment depends upon cause (Table 24-6)
      (4) Preterm birth (36-week gestation) occurs in 32% of pregnancies.
      (5) Preterm birth risk factors

Table 24-4 1982 revised criteria for the classification of systemic lupus erythematosus*

Criterion	Definition
1. Malar rash	Fixed erythema, flat or raised, over the malar eminences, tending to spare the nasolabial folds
2. Discoid rash	Erythematous raised patches with adherent keratotic scaling and follicular plugging; atrophic scarring may occur in older lesions
3. Photosensitivity	Skin rash as a result of unusual reaction to sunlight, by patient history or physician observation
4. Oral ulcers	Oral or nasopharyngeal ulceration, usually painless, observed by a physician
5. Arthritis	Nonerosive arthritis involving two or more peripheral joints, characterized by tenderness, swelling, or effusion
6. Serositis	a. Pleuritis—convincing history of pleuritis pain or rub heard by a physician or evidence of pleural effusion, *or* b. Pericarditis—documented by electrocardiogram (ECG) or rub or evidence of pericardial effusion
7. Renal disorder	a. Persistent proteinuria greater than 0.5 g/day or greater than 3+ if quantitation not performed, *or* b. Cellular casts—may be red cell, hemoglobin, granular, tubular, or mixed
8. Neurologic disorder	a. Seizures—in the absence of offending drugs or known metabolic derangements; e.g., uremia, ketoacidosis, or electrolyte imbalance, *or* b. Psychosis—in the absence of offending drugs or known metabolic derangements, e.g., uremia, ketoacidosis, or electrolyte imbalance

Table 24-4 1982 revised criteria for the classification of systemic lupus erythematosus—cont'd

Critcrion	Definition
9. Hematologic disorder	a. Hemolytic anemia—with reticulocytosis, *or* b. Leukopenia—less than 4000/ mm^3 total on two or more occasions, *or* c. Lympophenia—less than 1500/mm^3 on two or more occasions, *or* d. Thrombocytopenia—less than 100,000/mm^3 in the absence of offending drugs
10. Immunologic disorder	a. Positive lupus erythematosus (LE) cell preparation, *or* b. Anti-DNA: antibody to native DNA in abnormal titer, *or* c. Anti-Sm: presence of antibody to Smith (Sm) nuclear antigen, *or* d. False-positive serologic test for syphilis known to be positive for at least 6 months and confirmed by *Treponema pallidum* immobilization or fluorescent treponemal antibody absorption test
11. Antinuclear antibody	An abnormal titer of antinuclear antibody by immunofluorescence or an equivalent assay at any point in time and in the absence of drugs known to be associated with "drug-induced lupus" syndrome

*The proposed classification is based on 11 criteria. For the purpose of identifying patients in clinical studies, a person shall be said to have systemic lupus erythematosus if any four or more of the 11 criteria are present, serially or simultaneously, during any interval of observation.

(a) Maternal activity of lupus
   i. Clinical index
   ii. Prednisone dose >20 mg daily
(b) Maternal renal disease: moderate to severe renal impairment
(c) Antiphospholipid antibodies (IgG isotype >20 GPL units)

Table 24-5 Effects of antiinflammatory and immunosuppressive drugs on fertility

Acetylsalicylic acid (ASA)	No effect.
Nonsteroidal antiinflammatory drugs (NSAIDs)	No effect.
Glucocorticoids	No effect.
Hydroxychloroquine	No effect.
Azathioprine	Probably no direct effect. 1. Interferes with the effectiveness of IUDs.
Methotrexate	Reversible oligospermia reported in a few males but little effect on ovarian function.
Cyclophosphamide	Decreased fertility (ammenorrhea) 1. Decreased estradiol levels with subsequent increase in follicle stimulating hormone (FSH) and luteinizing hormone (LH) to cause amenorrhea. 2. Depletion of ovarian follicles may lead to sterility. 3. Dose (>15 months of therapy) and age (>25 years old) dependent. 4. Not always reversible when drug discontinued. 5. Spermatogenesis may be impaired in males.
Penicillamine	No data on fertility.
Chlorambucil	Amenorrhea and reversible azoospermia with high doses reported.

Table 24-6 Treatment of thrombocytopenia in SLE pregnancy

Time of Occurrence	Treatment
Before 25 weeks	
With anticardiolipin antibody	
No signs of active SLE	Aspirin
Clinical signs of active SLE or occurrence with prior flares	Steroid
After 25 weeks	
With anticardiolipin antibody	Aspirin
With hypertension or proteinuria	Antihypertensives
With liver function test abnormalities	Deliver
With fetal distress	Deliver
With placental abruption	Deliver

From Lockshin M: Pregnancy in SLE. In Harris EN, Exner T, Hughes GRV, editors: *Phospholipid-binding antibodies,* NIII, Boca Raton, FL, 1991, CRC Press.

(d) Hypertension (diastolic >88 mm Hg in second trimester or requirement of an antihypertensive agent)

b. Maternal outcomes (effect of pregnancy on disease)
  (1) Maternal lupus exacerbations
    (a) Relapse rates (flares) vary from 10% to 55%, although some investigators feel flares occur no more frequently during pregnancy.
    (b) Most flares are either cutaneous or musculoskeletal and are not in critical organ systems.
    (c) Flares are more common and more severe when conception begins during active disease.
    (d) Most flares occur in the third trimester or postpartum.
    (e) An increase in the corticosteroid dose in the postpartum period (6 weeks after pregnancy) does not affect the frequency of flares.
  (2) Renal disease
    (a) Permanent renal dysfunction, even in patients with a history of lupus nephritis, is uncommon if creatinine clearance >80 ml/min.
    (b) Majority of maternal deaths in lupus pregnancy are a result of renal disease.
    (c) Flares manifest as the following:
      i. Reversible and irreversible decline in renal function
      ii. Hypertension: reversible, irreversible, and worsening of preexisting
      iii. Increased proteinuria: rarely irreversible
    (d) Preeclampsia versus lupus nephropathy: see Peripartum and Postpartum Syndrome, p. 638
  (3) Thrombocytopenia: see SLE and Pregnancy, 2.e.

c. Neonatal outcome
  (1) The neonatal course is usually a function of gestational age and birth weight.
  (2) The risk of neonatal lupus confined to minority of children born to mothers positive for anti-Ro and anti-La antibodies (see Neonatal Lupus, p. 643).
  (3) Chance of a child of an affected parent to develop SLE as an adult is <10%.

3. Medical management
  a. When considering pregnancy
    (1) Drug effects: See Tables 24-5 and 24-7.
    (2) Prenatal vitamins should begin when a woman attempts conception.
    (3) Laboratory tests
      (a) Routine antepartum laboratory tests
      (b) Laboratory assessment of activity of SLE in addition to SLE and Pregnancy, 4.a.(3)(a)
        i. 24-hour urinary assessment of total protein and Cr Cl
        ii. C3, C4, anti-double-stranded DNA (dsDNA) (especially with renal disease) and erythrocyte sedimentation rate (ESR)

Table 24-7 Effects of antiinflammatory and immunosuppressive drugs on pregnancy

ASA	Low dose protective against PIH May prolong bleeding at delivery* May cause premature closure of patent ductus arteriosis (PDA) Pulmonary HTN in neonates May prolong labor* May cause intracranial hemorrhage near delivery* Hematological in neonates*
Indomethacin	Premature closure of PDA near term Teratogenicity in animals Avoid in third trimester unless specifically indicated for tocolysis Withdraw a few weeks before delivery for same reasons as outlined above for ASA
Other NSAIDs	Few studies No evidence of teratogenicity Concerns similar to above prostaglandin inhibitors
Glucocorticoids	Placental inactivation of prednisone and prednisolone Fluorinated steroids (dexamethasone and betamethsone) used for maturation of fetal lungs No evidence that low doses are teratogenic Attention to possibility of adrenal suppression in newborns Association of cleft plate in animals
Hydroxychloroquine or Chloroquine	Minimal data on hydroxychloroquine; toxicity reported based on chloroquine data Theoretical risk of fetal eye and ear impairment Consider discontinuation of drug unless required to suppress disease activity

*Withdraw a few weeks before delivery.

Table 24-7 Effects of antiinflammatory and immunosuppressive drugs on pregnancy—cont'd

Azathioprine	Crosses the placenta and is metabolized to 6-thioguanine 20% of infants small for gestational age (renal transplant data) Rare report of neonatal immunosuppression Continuation of drug dependent upon effectiveness of suppression of disease activity
Methotrexate	Induces abortions Congenital anomalies associated with first trimester administration include multiple skeletal anomalies, hydrocephalus, ear anomalies, cleft palate, anencephaly, cardiac anomalies, meningoencephalocele Teratogenicity alleviated if drug discontinued > 1 year before conception Drug should be avoided during pregnancy Occupational exposure precautions should be used
Cyclophosphamide	Congenital anomalies reported if used in first trimester and include multiple skeletal anomalies, facial anomalies, imperforate anus, hemangioma, umbilical hernia, single coronary artery Occupational exposure precautions should be used Minimal data on paternal use Risk to benefit ratio must be considered as this drug used in life-threatening emergencies
Penicillamine	Doses >500 mg/day have been associated with cutis laxa, inguinal hernia, hypotonia, growth retardation
Chlorambucil	Data scanty but suggest renal anomalies may occur; occupational exposure precautions should be used Drug should be avoided during pregnancy

*Withdraw a few weeks before delivery.

Continued.

Table 24-7 Effects of antiinflammatory and immunosuppressive drugs on pregnancy—cont'd

Coumadin	Not the treatment of choice during pregnancy, although normal pregnancies do occur in up to 70% if fetus is not exposed during the first trimester; associated defects include embryopathy (fetal warfarin syndrome), CNS defects, spontaneous abortion, stillbirth, prematurity, hemorrhage
Heparin	Treatment of choice if anticoagulation required Some studies suggest possible associations with malformations and cardiac defects Maternal osteopenia needs be discussed before institution of therapy

b. During pregnancy
   (1) Counseling
      (a) Patients should be advised of maternal and fetal outcomes.
      (b) If life-threatening disease occurs, therapeutic abortion may need to be considered.
   (2) Maternal and fetal assessment
      (a) See Table 24-8.
      (b) Other testing (i.e., chorionic villus sampling, umbilical artery waveforms) is done for obstetric purposes.
   (3) Drug therapy
      (a) Medications not essential for disease suppression or that are teratogenic should be discontinued (Table 24-7).
      (b) Although there is debatable evidence that exacerbations are more frequent in the third trimester and postpartum periods, the use of prophylactic steroids is not indicated.
      (c) Corticosteroids remain the mainstay of therapy for active SLE during pregnancy.
      (d) Intravenous methylprednisolone may be needed for severe flares of SLE.
   (4) Monthly evaluation by rheumatologist

Peripartum and postpartum syndromes

Differentiating between SLE nephropathy, preeclampsia, and HELLP syndrome (Table 24-9)

Table 24-8 Monitoring SLE pregnancy

Week	-4	-8	-12	-16	-20	-24	-28	-32	−36	-40
Platelets	+	+	+	+	+	+		+	+	+
aCL	+			+		+				
LA	+			+		+				
anti-Ro/La	+									
Urine protein	+	+	+	+	+	+	Weekly ----------			
Cr Cl	+			+			As indicated -----			
AFHRT						+	Weekly ----------			
Sonogram		+		+		+	As indicated -----			

Lockshin M: Pregnancy in SLE. In Harris EN et al, editors: *Phospholipid binding antibodies*, Boca Raton, FL, 1991, CRC Press.

aCL, Anticardiolipin antibody; *LA*, lupus anticoagulant; *Cr Cl*, creatinine clearance; *AFHRT*, antepartum fetal heart rate test.

Table 24-9 Differentiating SLE nephropathy from preeclampsia (pregnancy-induced hypertension)

Abnormality	SLE	Preeclampsia
Urine protein	High*	High*
Cr Cl	Low	Low
Blood pressure	Normal to high†	High†
Complement	Low	Normal
Hemolytic anemia	May occur	Occurs with HELLP‡
Urine blood	Microscopic with casts	Microscopic without casts
Platelets	Low or normal	Low or normal
	Responds to steroids	No response to steroids
Liver enzymes	Rarely elevated	High with HELLP* or severe preeclampsia
Uric acid	High or normal§	High§
Anti-DNA antibody	Rising or high	Normal or stable
Other SLE symptoms	Present	Absent

*High urinary protein = >300 mg/day.

†In general, BP >140/90.

‡*HELLP*, hemolysis, elevated liver enzymes, low platelet count. HELLP may or may not be associated with elevated blood pressure and/or proteinuria.

§Uric acid >5 mg/dl.

Contraception and SLE

1. Use of effective contraception is required for women taking immunosuppressive agents.
2. Use of estrogen-containing oral contraceptives is controversial but not absolutely contraindicated. Other methods should be considered first (see the box on p. 640).

Methods of Contraception for Patients with SLE (Excluding Estrogen-Containing Oral Contraceptives)
Irreversible
Tubal ligation
Vasectomy
Reversible
IUD*
Barrier methods (condom, diaphragm) used with spermicidal creams†
Natural family planning†
Withdrawal†
Abstinence
Progestin-only agents‡

*Efficacy rate = 97% to 99.9%.
†Efficacy rate = 80% to 91%.
‡Efficacy rate = 97.5% to 99.75%.

Antiphospholipid syndrome (APS)

Definition

1. Clinical and laboratory features (Table 24-10)
2. Pathophysiology
   a. Most likely, pregnancy loss results from uteroplacental insufficiency caused by microvascular thrombosis, vasoconstriction, and necrotizing decidual vasculopathy.
3. Occurrence
   a. APS may occur as an isolated disorder (primary antiphospholipid syndrome) or in association with SLE or other autoimmune diseases.

Effect of APS on fertility

1. There is no effect on fertility other than that associated with use of immunosuppressive agents (see Table 24-5).
2. Successful pregnancy outcome (at least one live birth) occurs in fewer than 50% of patients with APS, and particularly if there is a previous history of pregnancy loss.

APS and pregnancy

1. Up to 10% of patients referred for recurrent pregnancy loss will have lupus anticoagulant or antiphospholipid antibodies.
2. Outcomes: Percentages given are approximations because of the relative recent recognition of this disease entity and the limited number of prospective studies.
   a. Fetal: untreated
      (1) Pregnancy losses may occur in as many as 70% of patients with high levels of antiphospholipid (aPL) antibodies or a positive lupus anticoagulant test.

Table 24-10 Clinical and laboratory features of APS

Clinical	Laboratory
Major Features*	
Venous thrombosis	Lupus anticoagulant test
Arterial thrombosis	Anticardiolipin test (medium to high positive,† IgG, IgM, or IgA)
Thrombocytopenia	
Recurrent pregnancy loss	
Other (Proposed) Features	
Endocardial valvular vegetations	
Livedo reticularis	
Migraine headaches	
? Transverse myelopathy	
? Chorea	
? Leg ulcers	

*A diagnosis of APS should be based on a history of one major clinical feature (preferably not explainable by any other predisposing condition) and a positive laboratory test (which has remained positive for several weeks to months).
†Medium to high positive values are 20 to 80 GPL, MPL, APL.

(2) Fifty percent of untreated pregnancies end in preterm delivery, most commonly because of preeclampsia.

b. Fetal: treated
   (1) With therapy, pregnancy loss decreases to less than 40%.
   (2) With therapy, newborn survival rate is greater than 60%.
   (3) Preterm delivery rate is improved somewhat with treatment.
   (4) Small for gestational age (<10th percentile by weight) occurs in about 30% of babies.
   (5) Preeclampsia still occurs in up to 50% but is often delayed in onset.
   (6) Severe preeclampsia occurs in under 30% and frequently < 34 weeks gestation.
   (7) Fetal distress occurs in approximately 50%.
   (8) PROM occurs in less than 15%.
   (9) An increased number of previous fetal deaths puts one at higher risk for unsuccessful pregnancy despite therapy.

c. Maternal
   (1) There is an increased risk (up to 30%) of vascular events in pregnancy and postpartum period, in both primary and secondary APS.
   (2) Maternal outcomes should be considered if another autoimmune illness present.
   (3) There are case reports of an "autoimmune postpartum syndrome."
      i. No previous autoimmune disease other than APS
      ii. Thrombosis
      iii. Pleuropulmonary or cardiac disease
      iv. Unexplained fever
      v. Requires initiation of steroids when infection ruled out

Indications To Test For aPL Antibodies

Recurrent pregnancy loss
  Unexplained second or third trimester
  Two or more first trimester losses
Thromboembolic disease (arterial or venous)
Severe preeclampsia
SLE or other autoimmune disease
False-positive test for syphilis
Thrombocytopenia (platelet count <150,000)
Abnormal PTT or PT test

d. Neonatal risk is based on gestational age at delivery and complications of prematurity.

3. Medical management
   a. When considering pregnancy
      (1) Drug effects (see Table 24-7)
      (2) Anticoagulant therapy (see Table 24-7)
      (3) Prenatal vitamins as soon as one contemplates pregnancy
      (4) Laboratory tests
         (a) Who is to check for aPL antibodies? (See the box above.)
         (b) See Systemic Lupus Erythematoses, SLE and Pregnancy, 4.a.(3).
         (c) The anticardiolipin test is more predictive of pregnancy loss when IgG isotype is present at medium to high levels (20 to 80 GPL).
   b. During pregnancy
      (1) Counseling
         (a) Maternal and fetal risks should be discussed.
         (b) Risks of therapy must be discussed.
      (2) Monitoring patient
         (a) Table 24-8
         (b) Prothrombin time or partial prothrombin time (PT or PTT) for anticoagulation status

Treatment

1. Low-dose aspirin (LDA) or no treatment
   a. First pregnancy, low (+) aPL (< 20 GPL), history of thrombosis
   b. Recurrent first trimester Ab, low (+) aPL
2. Heparin + LDA
   a. Medium/high (+) aPL *and*
   b. History of thrombosis, three first trimester losses or one or more second or third trimester loss
3. IV immunoglobulin (0.4 mg/kg/day × 5 days/month + LDA, ± low-dose heparin)

a. Definite APS
b. Failed prior therapy
4. Prednisone (20 to 40 mg/day) + LDA
   a. Active SLE + definite APS
   b. Failed heparin and IV immunoglobulin

Contraception and APS

1. See the box on p. 640. No data are available for APS patients only.
2. Estrogen is procoagulant and absolutely contraindicated.

Neonatal lupus erythematosus (NLE)

Definition

A disease of the newborn defined by the demonstration of maternal autoantibodies and characteristic transient and permanent clinical features in the newborn period

Anti-Ro/SSA antibodies and risk of NLE

1. Anti-Ro/SSA positive mothers with SLE have a 1% to 5% chance of having a child with NLE.
2. Subsequent pregnancy risk, however, is up to 25%.
3. NLE accounts for 90% of isolated congenital heart block.

Outcomes

1. Effect on child (transient)
   a. Cutaneous: 40%
      (1) Plaques are described as erythematous, scaly, nonindividual round or elliptical occurring in the scalp or face (Fig. 24-2).
      (2) Time frame: Lesions appear from birth (2 to 3 weeks of age + last 6 months).
      (3) Residual: Plaques are nonscarring with mild telangiectasis at the involved site.
   b. Other
      (1) Increased liver function testing
      (2) Noninfectious hepatitis
      (3) Thrombocytopenia
      (4) Myocarditis
      (5) Pericarditis
2. Effect on child (permanent)
   a. Cardiac
      (1) Congenital heart block (CHB): 50% of infants with NLE
      (2) CHB with other cardiac anomalies
         (a) Patent ductus arteriosus
         (b) Transposition of the great vessels
         (c) Myocardial fibroelastosis
      (3) CHB with congestive heart failure (CHF)
      (4) Outcomes
         (a) Most survive
         (b) Few die of CHF

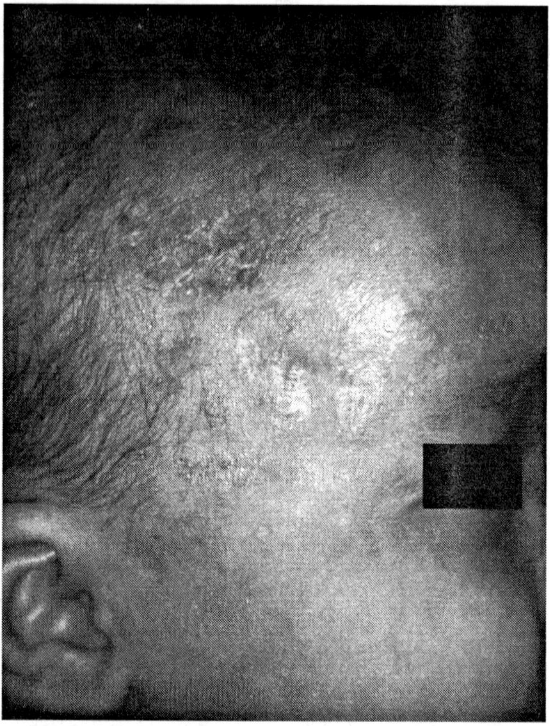

Figure 24-2
Appearance of neonatal lupus erythematous plaques. (Photograph compliments of Dr. Jeffrey Callen, Chief, Division of Dermatology, Department of Medicine, University of Louisville.)

   b. CHB
      (1) Associated with HLA-DR3, Anti-SSA, Anti-SSB, and Anti-U1RNP in mother
3. Maternal
   a. Half of mothers of children with NLE will have SLE, Sjögren's syndrome, or other connective tissue disease (CTD).
   b. Asymptomatic mothers of children with NLE (50%) often develop symptoms of a connective tissue disease.
   c. Mothers at risk for NLE should be monitored from 18 to 20 weeks gestation by fetal echocardiography.

Treatment

1. Rash
   a. Avoidance of sunlight
   b. Topical corticosteroids

2. Cardiac
   a. Pacemakers are required by 50% postnatally.
   b. Maternal administration of fluorinated glucocorticosteroids has been shown to decrease the inflammatory response in the fetus in some cases of heart block and pericardial or pleural effusions.
3. Indications for postnatal therapy with glucocorticosteroids
   a. CHF despite pacemaker
   b. Severe thrombocytopenia
   c. Severe hepatitis

Suggested reading

Bobrie G et al: Pregnancy in lupus nephritis and related disorders, *Am J Kidney Dis* 9(4):339-343, 1987.

Branch DW et al: Outcome of treated pregnancy in women with antiphospholipid syndrome: an update of the Utah experience, *Am J Obstet Gynecol* 80(4):614-620, 1992.

Briggs G, Freeman RK, Yaffe SJ: *Drugs in pregnancy and lactation,* Baltimore, 1994, Williams & Wilkins.

Cecere FA, Persellin RH: The interaction of pregnancy and the rheumatic diseases, *Clin Rheum Dis* 7(3):747-768, 1981

Cowchock FS et al: Repeated fetal losses associated with antiphospholipid antibodies: A collaborative randomized trial comparing prednisone with low dose heparin treatment, *Am J Obstet Gynecol* 166(5):1318-1323, 1992.

Derksen RHWM: Systemic lupus erythematosus and pregnancy, *Rheumatol Int* 11:121-125, 1991.

Harris EN: *Rheumatic disease and reproduction,* MKSAP in the subspecialty of rheumatology, ACP (Pending).

Harris EN: Syndrome of the black swan, *Br J Rheumatol* 26:324-326, 1987.

Harris EN et al: *Phospholipid binding antibodies,* Boca Raton, FL, 1991, CRC Press.

Harris EN, Spinnato JA: Should anticardiolipin tests be performed in otherwise healthy pregnant women? *Am J Obstet Gynecol* 165(5);1272-1277, 1991.

Lockshin MD et al: Lupus pregnancy: case control prospective demonstrating absence of lupus exacerbation during or after pregnancy, *Am J Med* 77:893-898, 1984.

Petri M: Lupus and pregnancy, *Bull Rheum Dis* 44 (2):1-3, 1995.

Petri M: Systemic lupus erythematosus and pregnancy, *Rheum Dis Clin North Am* 20 (1):87-117, 1994.

Preston S, Needs C: Guidelines on the use of antirheumatic drugs in women during pregnancy and child-bearing age, *Bailliere's Clin Rheum* 4(3)687-698, 1990.

Schumacher HR, Klippel JH, Koopman WJ: *Primer on the rheumatic diseases,* Atlanta, GA, 1993, Arthritis Foundation.

Spinnato JA et al: Intravenous immunoglobulin therapy for the antiphospholipid syndrome, *Am J Obstet Gynecol* 172(2):690-694, 1995.

Sibai BM et al: Prevention of pre-eclampsia with low dose aspirin in healthy, nulliparous pregnant women, *N Engl J Med* 329(17):1213-1218, 1993.

Weinstein L: Syndrome of hemolysis, elevated liver enzymes, and low platelet count: a severe consequence of hypertension in pregnancy, *Am J Obstet Gynecol* 112(2):159-167, 1982.

White PH: Pediatric lupus erythematosus and neonatal lupus, *Rheum Dis Clin North Am* 20(1):119-127, 1994.

24.4 GASTROINTESTINAL DISEASE IN PREGNANCY

Ronald L. Richardson, M.D.

Gastrointestinal (GI) disorders are among the most common problems encountered during pregnancy. A wide variety of physiologic changes occur in the body associated with pregnancy that may account for increased problems such as heartburn and gallbladder disease, whereas other problems may arise that are unrelated to the pregnancy itself. Diagnosis may be more difficult to establish because of the obvious reluctance to use the usual radiologic and nuclear scanning techniques employed if the patient were not pregnant. Once a diagnosis is reached, treatment often must be altered because of the concern about fetal effects of medications. Fortunately, most of the GI problems encountered in pregnancy are self-limiting or respond to therapy; however, problems such as some of the acute hepatic syndromes or acute surgical abdominal conditions may be life-threatening. Delay in making a diagnosis in these situations often occurs, because of multiple factors and leads to an increase in the mortality rate.

This chapter deals with the most commonly encountered GI problems seen in the pregnant patient, including comments on diagnostic studies used, and including a discussion of the therapeutic regimens employed with particular attention to safety issues regarding the fetus.

Esophageal disorders during pregnancy

Esophageal disorders, such as gastroesophageal reflux disease (GERD) manifested as heartburn, are quite common during pregnancy, whereas infectious esophagitis is unusual and problems such as achalasia are quite rare in pregnancy. Clinical diagnoses are often possible, however, when the patient's symptoms of heartburn are refractory or are associated with significant odynophagia, dysphagia, or chest pain, invasive studies such as endoscopy or manometry may be necessary. The issue of risk versus benefit must always be raised whenever invasive studies are being considered. The same question must also be addressed whenever medications are prescribed since safety of the fetus is always a foremost concern.

Gastroesophageal reflux disease in pregnancy

1. Incidence
   a. Heartburn occurs in 30% to 50% of all pregnancies and up to 80% in some populations.
   b. In most cases, symptomatic GERD begins in pregnancy and ceases after delivery, often to recur in subsequent pregnancies (see the box on p. 647).
   c. Symptoms may occur at any time during pregnancy but are most severe during the third trimester.
   d. The risk of heartburn increases with increasing gestational age, prepartum heartburn, and parity.
2. Pathogenesis: The pathogenesis of heartburn of pregnancy is thought to involve both factors intrinsic to the lower esophageal sphincter pressure (LESP) and mechanical factors.
   a. The LESP is abnormal during pregnancy.

Suggested Algorithm for Diagnosis and Treatment of GERD in Pregnancy

Clinical History

↓

Diagnosis

- History usually classical
- Endoscopy safe
- pH studies for atypical cases

↓

Treatment

- Lifestyle changes
- Nonsystemic drugs
- H2 blockers

From Baron TH, Richter J: Gastroesophageal reflux disease in pregnancy, *Gastroenterol Clin North Am* 21(4):777, 1992.

(1) There is a decrease in the absolute resting pressure at all stages of pregnancy, gradually decreasing as the pregnancy progresses.

(2) The effects are secondary to high female sex hormones, with progesterone mediating LES smooth muscle relaxation.

b. Mechanical factors

(1) The enlarging uterus may increase intraabdominal pressure and delay gastric emptying and thus enhance GER.

(2) An increase in intragastric pressure is usually accompanied by an increase in LESP; however, this adaptive response does not occur in pregnant patients with heartburn.

3. Clinical features

a. Heartburn and regurgitation are the most typical symptoms.

b. Castro reported that 78% of patients had symptoms aggravated by eating, often causing them to restrict their food intake with resultant weight loss.

c. Of patients, 81% experience recumbent reflux symptoms, causing them to sleep in an upright position.

d. Complications of GER, such as bleeding or stricture formation, are rare in pregnancy.

4. Diagnosis

a. Complete history is usually all that is necessary to make a diagnosis of GERD.

b. Barium studies are usually not necessary and are best avoided during pregnancy because of the radiation risks to the fetus.

c. Endoscopy is usually not necessary but is safe to do if symptoms of heartburn persist despite medical therapy.

d. Ambulatory 24-hour pH studies are rarely needed but on those occasions may be helpful in evaluation of atypical symptoms such as cough, chest pain, wheezing, or hoarseness.

5. Treatment
   a. Lifestyle modifications should include the following:
      (1) Elevating the head of the bed 6 inches on blocks
      (2) Avoiding oral intake 3 hours before bedtime
      (3) Eating several small meals
      (4) Avoiding postural changes such as stooping or bending
      (5) Eating diet low in fats and acidic foods
      (6) Avoiding chocolate, caffeine, and peppermints
   b. Nonsystemic drug therapy
      (1) When lifestyle modifications above do not control symptoms of heartburn, use of nonsystemic drug therapy is recommended with antacids or alginic acid (Gaviscon) being the drugs of choice.
         (a) Both usually give symptomatic relief.
         (b) Sodium bicarbonate should be avoided because it may lead to fluid overload or metabolic alkalosis in both the mother and fetus.
         (c) Antacids may interfere with iron absorption and magnesium-containing antacids may cause diarrhea.
      (2) Sucralfate (Carafate) also appears to be safe, because almost none of the drug is absorbed. At a dose of 1 g, tid, it has been shown to relieve heartburn in up to 90% of cases. This may be the ideal drug for mild heartburn of pregnancy.
   c. Systemic drug therapy
      (1) H2 blockers, which include cimetidine (Tagamet), ranitidine (Zantac), famotidine (Pepcid), and nizatidine (Axid), are frequently used in pregnancy, although no controlled studies are available.
         (a) Animal studies show that these drugs cross the placenta and are excreted into breast milk.
         (b) The usual treatment dosages are ranitidine, 150 mg, bid, or cimetidine, 400 mg, bid.
      (2) Teratologic studies have not shown problems with cimetidine, ranitidine, or famotidine, but, at high doses, nizatidine given to rats has been shown to have teratogenic effects.
         (a) Most data in humans are with cimetidine, where no teratogenic effects have been noted.
      (3) Omeprazole (Prilosec), a potent inhibitor of acid secretion, has produced dose-related increases in embryo lethality, fetal resorption, and pregnancy interruptions in rabbits and developmental toxicity in the offspring of rats treated at high doses.
      (4) Metoclopramide (Reglan), a prokinetic agent, crosses the placenta but has not been shown to have toxic effects on the fetus.
         (a) Cisapride (Propulsid) is another prokinetic agent that has been shown to have fetotoxic effects in rabbits and rats.

6. Summary
   a. A stepwise approach of treatment using lifestyle modifications and reassurance is usually all that is necessary in mild cases.
   b. Antacids, alginic acid, or sucralfate may be added in more moderate cases.
   c. Addition of H2 blockers may be necessary in more refractory cases, with cimetidine or ranitidine the drugs of choice.
   d. Metoclopramide may rarely be needed for the more refractory cases not responsive to the other measures.
   e. It would be best to avoid nizatidine and omeprazole in the pregnant patient under normal circumstances.

Achalasia

1. Incidence
   a. Achalasia is the most common motor disorder of the esophagus with an incidence of 1 to 2/200,000 per year.
   b. The onset of achalasia is usually in the third to fifth decade, affecting both sexes equally.
   c. This condition rarely occurs in pregnancy, but early reports suggested poor fetal outcome in some patients. More recent reports refute these claims.
2. Pathogenesis
   a. The pathogenesis is poorly understood, but there is an underlying abnormality of the innervation of the LES and the esophageal smooth muscle.
   b. The end result is loss of the peristaltic wave of the esophagus with swallowing and hypertension and incomplete relaxation of the LES.
3. Symptoms
   a. The primary symptom of achalasia is dysphagia, with nausea and vomiting, regurgitation, chest pain, and weight loss being other symptoms.
   b. In early cases, these symptoms may be confused with hyperemesis gravidarum.
   c. This diagnosis needs to be considered if nausea and vomiting and dysphagia begin in the latter stages of pregnancy.
4. Diagnosis
   a. Endoscopy may show features that suggest the diagnosis; however, esophageal manometry is the test that gives the most definitive diagnosis.
   b. Barium swallow contrast studies should be avoided in early pregnancy but can be done safely in the late pregnancy with proper shielding of the fetus.
      (1) Typical findings on x-ray film include esophageal dilatation, aperistalsis, and distal tapering.
5. Therapy
   a. Medical therapy involves using medications such as calcium channel blockers, long-acting nitrates, or anticholinergics, all of which have been shown to have at least some benefit on the LES tone.

(1) Nifedipine has been the most studied medication and appears to be the most effective, although it has been shown to be teratogenic and is best avoided in pregnancy.

(2) Because the response to medical therapy is suboptimal as compared with the more definitive surgical approaches, they should be reserved for the patients who cannot tolerate surgical therapy.

b. Surgical treatment of achalasia includes both pneumatic dilation or surgical myotomy.

(1) The pneumatic dilation should be considered as the initial treatment because it can be done with conscious sedation and is generally effective.

(2) There is a perforation rate of 2% to 5% with this treatment.

(3) The potential risks to the fetus must be considered before undertaking a surgical myotomy.

Peptic ulcer disease

1. Incidence

a. Although peptic ulcer disease (PUD) is a common medical problem, the true incidence in pregnancy is unknown and probably underestimated.

b. Because the symptoms of indigestion, nausea and vomiting, and heartburn are common in pregnancy, it is difficult to know which cases result from other causes such as GERD or hyperemesis gravidarum.

c. Refractory dyspepsia or gastrointestinal bleeding are the primary indications for further investigation and upper endoscopy is the preferred test to establish the diagnosis.

2. Epidemiology

a. The prevalence of ulcer disease has changed very little in recent decades.

(1) Although hospitalizations for ulcer disease have markedly decreased, the complications of GI bleeding and perforation have not lessened.

b. Risk factors for ulcers include cigarette smoking, nonsteroidal antiinflammatory drug (NSAID) use, genetic predisposition, and *Helicobacter pylori* gastritis.

c. There is no evidence that certain foods, such as spicy foods, cause ulcers, although GERD may be aggravated by fatty foods, caffeine, or chocolate.

(1) Alcohol may predispose to gastric mucosal damage by disrupting the gastric mucosal barrier.

d. Because most pregnant patients are not on NSAIDs, stopping smoking and abstaining from alcohol are the most important lifestyle changes that may impact ulcer disease.

e. The most enlightening discovery regarding peptic ulcer has been the establishment of the association between ulcer disease and *H. pylori* gastritis.

(1) The spiral bacteria can be found in the gastric mucosa of 85% to 100% of patients with PUD.

(2) Many experts, however, would dissuade vigorous searches for the infection during pregnancy if the patient is responding to therapy because of the hesitancy to treat the infection while the patient is pregnant.

3. Symptoms
   a. There is a wide variety of symptoms, but 60% to 85% of patients with ulcers have some form of abdominal pain, occasionally penetrating into the back.
   b. Classic symptoms are pain when the stomach is empty with relief with eating, although eating may aggravate the symptoms in some patients.
   c. Of patients, 20% to 60% have only nausea and vomiting that may be dismissed as nausea of pregnancy if it occurs in the first trimester, and 20% to 50% have predominantly heartburn, which may be attributed to heartburn of pregnancy if it occurs in the third trimester.
   d. Unfortunately, a small percentage of patients have no symptoms before complications such as GI bleeding or perforation.
4. Treatment (Table 24-11)
   a. When PUD is associated with *H. pylori* infection, the general recommendation is to treat the ulcer process with conventional therapy and defer treatment of the infection until after delivery.
      (1) The ulcer can usually be controlled without eradication of the infection, and best treatment of the infection requires antibiotics that are potentially teratogenic.
      (2) It is wise, however, to attempt to control the infection after delivery in an effort to reduce the risk of recurrent ulcer disease.
   b. Antacids are usually the first line of therapy and will control most symptoms if used frequently enough, usually 1 hour after meals and at bedtime.
      (1) Sodium bicarbonate antacids may lead to fluid overload and metabolic alkalosis in both the mother and fetus and should not be used.
      (2) Antacids containing calcium, aluminum, and magnesium appear to be safe, although the frequent dosing schedule and the diarrhea often associated with the magnesium-containing antacids makes compliance a problem.
   c. Histamine-2 receptor antagonists, or H2 blockers, which now include cimetidine, ranitidine, famotidine, and nizatidine, are frequently needed to control ulcer disease.
      (1) Because of ethical concerns, no controlled trials have been done in pregnant patients; however, a large experience has been gained with these medicines, particularly cimetidine and ranitidine.
      (2) Although both are felt to be safe, the potential antiandrogen effects of cimetidine may make ranitidine the better choice.
      (3) Because of teratogenic effects seen in animal studies with nizatidine, it should not be used, and although no adverse effects have been noted with famotidine, must less experience has been gained with this medicine.

Table 24-11 Recommendations* for use of antiulcer drugs during pregnancy and lactation

Antiulcer Drug	FDA Pregnancy Category	First Trimester	Second or Third Trimester	Nursing†
Antacids	B	R vs. B?	B > R	II
Cimetidine	B	R vs. B?	B > R	IV
Ranitidine	B	R vs. B?	B > R	IV
Sucralfate	B	B > R	B > R	IIIA
Famotidine	B	B vs. R?	B > R	IV
Lansoprazole	B	B vs. R?	R ? R	IV
Nizatidine	C	B vs. R?	B ? R	IV
Omeprazole	C	B vs. R?	B ? R	IV
Gaviscon	C2	B > R	B > R	IIIA
Misoprostol	X	R > B	R > B	IV
Phenothiazines	C1	R vs. B	R vs. B	IV
Pepto-Bismol	C1	R vs. B	R vs. B	IIIB
Simethicone	C2	R vs. B	R vs. B	IIIA

Modified from Michaletz-Onody PA: Peptic ulcer disease in pregnancy, *Gastroenterol Clin North Am* 21:817, 1992.

*Recommendations are defined as follows: R vs. B = Implies risk : benefit profile has not been determined and caution is advised for systemically active drug. R > B = Implies potential risks outweighs potential benefits and the use of the drug is not recommended. B > R = Implies that the potential benefits outweigh the potential risks.

†Breast-feeding categories are defined as follows: Group I = Drug does not enter breast milk. Group II = Drug enters breast milk but is not thought to effect the neonate when used in therapeutic doses. Group III: Not known whether the drug enters breast milk. A = No adverse neonatal effects are suspected. B = Breast-feeding is not recommended, because the drug is systemically absorbed. Group IV = Drug enters breast milk and is not recomnmended while nursing because of potential risk to neonate.

(4) Patients usually respond well to a single bedtime dose of medication, cimetidine 800 mg or ranitidine 300 mg, and will usually heal their ulcers in 3 to 6 weeks.

d. Omeprazole, a proton pump inhibitor, is the most potent acid blocking agent available, but because some fetal toxicity changes have been noted with this drug, its use should be when the benefits clearly outweigh the risks to the fetus.

e. Lansoprazole (Prevacid), another proton pump inhibitor, has not been shown to have teratogenic effects but much less experience has been gained with this medication.

f. Misoprostol is a prostaglandin normally produced by the gastroduodenal mucosa which may inhibit gastric secretion.

(1) The drug has been marketed primarily to enhance mucosal resistance in patients taking NSAIDs.

(2) Unfortunately it is abortifacient and is clearly contraindicated in females of childbearing age.

g. Sucralfate is a sulfated disaccharide complex with aluminum hydroxide that works primarily as a topical agent by forming an ulcer-adherent complex, which protects the ulcer base from the gastric acid.
   (1) The drug is thought to be minimally absorbed and has not been found to have any teratogenic effects.

5. Summary
   a. In general, PUD is relatively rare in pregnancy, being much less common than GERD and hyperemesis gravidarum.
   b. Since symptoms of each of these problems are similar, specific diagnosis is sometimes difficult.
   c. Endoscopy is safe to perform in pregnancy and often helps establish the correct diagnosis.
   d. Patients who smoke and those with prior history of ulcers are at highest risk for ulcers during pregnancy.
   e. Multiple medications are available for treatment of ulcers, with antacids and sucralfate being the initial therapies of choice; however, H2 blockers are becoming the mainstay of therapy because of their effectiveness, ease of use—and therefore better compliance, and apparent safety.

Gallstone disease in pregnancy

1. Incidence
   a. The suggestion of an epidemiologic link has been made between pregnancy and gallstone disease, although evidence for this association is extremely weak.
   b. In a study using ultrasonography, Marginghini demonstrated that biliary sludge develops frequently in pregnancy, in up to 45% of patients, but is generally not associated with symptoms and resolves in two thirds of patients after delivery.
      (1) Gallstones developed much less frequently, in about 6% of patients, but are more likely to be associated with biliary colic.
   c. Some studies have suggested an increased incidence of gallstone formation in pregnancy becomes significant only with the fourth pregnancy.
2. Alterations in biliary physiology in pregnancy
   a. Seventy percent to 80% of gallstones are composed of at least 50% cholesterol.
      (1) Gallstones are formed when bile becomes supersaturated with cholesterol, followed by crystallization and growth of the stone.
      (2) Alterations of gallbladder function and biliary composition which favor gallstone formation are noted in pregnancy.
   b. Alterations in biliary physiology during pregnancy include:
      (1) Increased bile acid pool size
      (2) Decreased enterohepatic circulation
      (3) Decreased percentage of chenodeoxycholic acid
      (4) Increased percentage of cholic acid
      (5) Increased secretion of cholesterol
      (6) Stasis of bile in the gallbladder

3. Manifestations of gallstone disease
   a. Symptoms of gallstone disease tend to be similar in the nonpregnant and pregnant patient.
   b. Epigastric or RUQ pain, often radiating into the back or shoulder, is the most typical.
      (1) Unrelenting nausea and vomiting, fever, and leukocytosis suggest acute cholecystitis.
   c. Fatty food intolerance is not thought to occur any more frequently in patients with stones as compared with those without stones.
   d. Abnormal laboratory studies may include liver dysfunction, but significant elevations of the liver studies, particularly the bilirubin and alkaline phosphatase are suggestive of choledocholithiasis.
   e. Pancreatitis may complicate gallstone disease and suggest passed or retained common duct stones.
4. Diagnosis
   a. If a patient has symptoms suggestive of gallstone disease, an ultrasound of the gallbladder should be performed and is usually diagnostic if stones are present.
   b. In certain situations, ultrasonography may not be definitive and further investigation is felt warranted.
      (1) There is a general admonition against x-ray examination, particularly in early pregnancy, as there has been with radionuclide scanning techniques.
      (2) The dose of ionizing radiation is considerably less with hepatobiliary scanning as compared with conventional x-ray films.
      (3) If a patient has symptoms that are suggestive of acute cholecystitis and has a normal ultrasound of the gallbladder, particularly in late pregnancy, radionuclide scanning could probably be done with minimal risk, although the risks and benefits of the study should be carefully discussed with the patient.
5. Differential diagnosis
   a. Acute viral hepatitis
   b. Acute alcohol hepatitis
   c. Duodenal ulcer
   d. Acute pancreatitis
   e. Pulmonary embolus
   f. Right lower lobe pneumonia
   g. Acute myocardial infarction
   h. Acute appendicitis
   i. Acute fatty liver of pregnancy
   j. Preeclampsia
   k. HELLP syndrome
6. Management
   a. If a routine ultrasound detects gallstones in an asymptomatic patient, no therapy is necessary or recommended.
   b. Biliary colic should be treated with hydration, analgesics, nasogastric tube if vomiting is persistent, and antibiotics if felt indicated.

(1) If possible, surgery should be deferred until the postpartum period.
(2) However, if complications of gallstone disease occur and are not diagnosed early, the maternal and fetal mortality rises significantly.
(3) The requirement for cholecystectomy during pregnancy is less than 0.1%.

c. Surgical dogma states that abdominal surgery of any type in the first trimester is associated with fetal loss and the rate with cholecystectomy has been estimated at 5%.
   (1) Cholecystectomy in the second and third trimesters does not seem to be associated with an increased fetal loss.
d. The ideal timing for surgery is in the second trimester when fetal risk is less than in the first trimester and when the uterine size is still small enough to not compromise the surgery.
e. Open cholecystectomy has been the surgery of choice and laparoscopic cholecystectomy has been felt to be contraindicated in the pregnant patient.
   (1) However studies recently reported have shown apparent safety using this technique in selected patients.
   (2) It has been suggested this procedure be considered for use in the first and early second trimesters.
   (3) Modifications of the technique in pregnant patients include an initial open approach or with a needle through an upper abdominal approach.
   (4) Lower insufflating pressures are also used.
   (5) There are medicolegal issues with this relatively new approach, and the risks and benefits of laparoscopy must be carefully explained to the patient.
f. There is a special concern in the pregnant patient with jaundice secondary to choledocholithiasis in that cholecystectomy and common bile duct exploration, particularly in patients with pancreatitis, is associated with a 15% maternal mortality and a 60% fetal loss.
   (1) The use of endoscopic retrograde cholangiopancreatography (ERCP) and papillotomy is a logical option in this group of patients, and seemingly can be done safely with uterine shielding, minimal fluoroscopy, and no radiography.
g. There are no recommended medications available for dissolution of gallstones during pregnancy.
   (1) Ursodiol (Actigall) has been used inadvertently in a few patients during the first trimester without ill effects.
   (2) Chenodiol has been shown to be teratogenic and is contraindicated.

7. Summary
   a. Gallstone disease is not uncommon during pregnancy and can usually be diagnosed with ultrasonography.
   b. It is preferable to manage the patient with a conservative medical approach if possible and defer surgery until after delivery.
   c. However, if complications such as choledocholithiasis or pancreatitis occur, prompt surgery may be necessary to lessen maternal and fetal mortality.

d. Open cholecystectomy would be considered the operation of choice; however, laparascopic cholecystectomy may play a larger role in therapy in the future, particularly in the first and early second trimesters. ERCP appears to be a logical option in the management of choledocholithiasis.

Pancreatitis and pregnancy

1. Incidence
   a. Pancreatitis occurs relatively infrequently in pregnancy, occurring in about 1 of 1400 pregnancies.
   b. It may occur at any stage of pregnancy but seems to be more frequent in the third trimester.
   c. There is no clear relation to parity.
   d. The fetal loss associated with pancreatitis is between 10% and 20%.
2. Etiology
   a. The causes of pancreatitis during pregnancy are similar to those in the general population, except alcoholism is less frequently a problem is pregnant patients.
   b. Gallstones are the most common cause.
   c. Drug-induced pancreatitis, especially with thiazide diuretics, occurs occasionally.
   d. Viral pancreatitis occurs infrequently in pregnancy.
   e. Hyperlipidemia seems to predispose to pancreatitis, and in pregnant patients the triglyceride level may increase threefold secondary to high circulating estrogen levels.
   f. Pancreatitis secondary to pancreatic carcinoma occurs occasionally but is very rare in pregnancy.
   g. There is a large group of patients with idiopathic pancreatitis in both pregnancy and in the general population.
3. Diagnosis
   a. Typical symptoms of abdominal pain into the back, nausea and vomiting, and fever suggest the possibility of pancreatitis.
   b. Serum amylase and lipase levels are typically elevated; however, some investigators have suggested that the amylase level may be elevated slightly in some pregnant patients normally.
   c. Elevation of the amylase to creatinine clearance ratio is suggestive of pancreatitis, with this ratio not being altered by pregnancy.
   d. Ultrasonography may be of benefit if the pancreas can be well visualized, showing changes of edema.
   e. Complicated pancreatitis may occur in pregnancy and, significantly, is associated with a maternal mortality of 3.4%.
4. Differential diagnosis
   a. Acute cholecystitis
   b. Penetrating duodenal ulcer
   c. Ruptured spleen
   d. Perinephric abscess
   e. Acute cardiopulmonary event (embolus or infarction)
   f. Acute appendicitis
   g. Ruptured ectopic pregnancy

h. Hyperemesis gravidarum
i. Preeclampsia

5. Management
   a. Management of pancreatitis is supportive, using IV fluids, nothing by mouth (NPO), nasogastric suction if there is prolonged nausea and vomiting, and meperidine for analgesia.
   b. Gallstone pancreatitis is often managed supportively with elective cholecystectomy after delivery, although the operation can be done safely after the first trimester if necessary.
   c. Choledocholithiasis may present a special problem and should be handled with ERCP and papillotomy for stone extraction.
   d. Patients with a protracted course should be managed with total parenteral nutrition (TPN).
      (1) Elimination of intravenous lipids is necessary if the serum triglycerides are elevated.
6. Summary
   a. Pancreatitis occurs infrequently in pregnancy, usually in association with gallstone disease.
   b. Supportive care is recommended although ERCP with papillotomy for common duct stones or exploration for complicated pancreatitis is occasionally necessary.

Irritable bowel syndrome, constipation, and diarrhea during pregnancy

1. Definition
   a. Irritable bowel syndrome (IBS) has been defined as continuous or recurrent symptoms of abdominal pain relieved with defecation or associated with change of frequency or consistency of stool or disturbed defecation (straining, urgency or sensation of incomplete defecation) as well as passage of mucus and a feeling of bloating or distension.
   b. Constipation and diarrhea may accompany IBS or may be separate entities with causes other than IBS to be considered in each case.
2. Incidence
   a. IBS is a common problem in the general population and presumably in pregnancy as well, although no specific studies in pregnancy have been reported.
   b. Levy and Lemberg, studying a group of 1000 Israeli women before, during, and after pregnancy, reported no changes in bowel habits in 55%, an increase in bowel habits in 34%, and a decrease in bowel habits in 11%. Anderson, however, reporting on a group of English women, found that 38% developed constipation during pregnancy with 20% of these during the third trimester.
   c. There have not been studies documenting the prevalence of diarrhea in pregnancy reported in the literature.
3. Pathogenesis
   a. IBS
      (1) The exact cause of IBS is not clear.
      (2) Wald demonstrated that the GI transit time was significantly prolonged in the luteal phase of menstruation, when proges-

terone levels were increased, leading to the speculation that progesterone served as a smooth muscle relaxant responsible for intestinal hypomotility during pregnancy.

(3) Elevated prostaglandin levels have also been implicated in changes in bowel symptoms, suggesting that patients with IBS might have an exaggerated colonic motility response to prostaglandin stimulation.

b. Constipation

(1) Studies have shown a reversible prolongation of GI transit time in the pregnant female, most prolonged in the second and third trimesters, correlating with the rise of progesterone levels.

(2) Lower concentrations of motilin, a stimulant, may also be a factor in prolongation of transit time.

(3) Other factors, including an enlarging uterus applying pressure on the muscles used in defecation, pressure of the fetal head and uterus on the rectum, and painful anorectal lesions, including hemorrhoids, may play a role in constipation.

c. Diarrhea

(1) The most common causes of diarrhea in pregnancy are infectious agents, including pathogenic bacteria, parasites, and viruses. *Clostridium difficile* enterocolitis is not an infrequent cause, particularly if the patient has been on antibiotic therapy in the preceding 6 weeks.

(2) Diarrhea may also be a signal of a pregnancy at risk. Relaxin, a substance released by the placenta to quiet smooth muscle contractions affects the intestinal smooth muscle as well.

(3) Diarrhea and vaginal discharge may suggest preterm labor.

4. Treatment

a. IBS

(1) Conservative therapy with stool-bulking agents and high-fiber diet is recommended.

(2) Dietary changes to eliminate offensive foods are helpful, including sorbitol, caffeine, and gas-producing foods.

(3) Behavioral treatments, such as biofeedback, passive muscle relaxation, and supportive psychotherapy, may also be used safely during pregnancy.

(4) Medications traditionally used to treat IBS, including anticholingerics, antidepressants, and anxiolytics, are contraindicated in pregnancy because of possible teratogenic effects.

b. Constipation

(1) Elimination of medications, such as aluminum-containing antacids, detection and treatment of anorectal lesions including hemorrhoids, and diagnosis and treatment of thyroid dysfunction may help with the constipation.

(2) Increase in dietary fiber may be very helpful, with Anderson showing that constipation was reduced with an increase of the daily fiber intake from 20 to 27 g.

(3) Processed hydrophilic stool-bulking agents (Metamucil, Fiberall, and PerDiem) appear safe, with onsets of action of 12 to 24 hours.

(a) Fluid intake should also be increased with these agents.

(4) Emollient laxatives, such as Colase and Surfak, decrease the surface tension of the liquid contents of the stool, allowing more liquid to stay in the stool.

(a) These agents have an onset of action of 24 to 48 hours and appear to be safe in pregnancy.

(5) Lubricants, such as mineral oil, are comparable to emollients in action but are not recommended for routine use because they have been noted to cause decreased absorption of fat-soluble vitamins with resultant neonatal hypothrombinemia and hemorrhage.

(6) Hyperosmotic laxatives, including lactulose, sorbitol, and saline, act by increasing osmolar tension, creating an increase in water collection, distension, peristalsis, and evacuation, generally acting in 24 to 48 hours.

(a) Lactulose has not been shown to be teratogenic.

(b) Saline hyperosmotics, such as Milk of Magnesia, citrate of magnesia, magnesium sulfate, and Fleet's Phospho-Soda, act within 30 minutes to 3 hours but may cause sodium retention in the mother.

(7) Stimulant laxatives cause colonic contraction and result in cramping.

(a) Dulcolax, Ex-Lax, and Correctol appear to be safe but should not be used routinely because of the possibility of dependency.

(b) Castor oil is contraindicated because it may initiate premature contractions.

(c) Cascara has been noted to cause loose stools in neonates.

(8) In the 1940s, Arnold Kegel developed a series of exercises for strengthening the pelvic floor muscles to treat stress urinary incontinence.

(a) These exercises more recently have been combined with biofeedback to treat constipation, urinary and fecal incontinence, and pelvic floor dyssyngeria.

c. Diarrhea

(1) Acute diarrhea usually responds to symptomatic therapy in 24 to 96 hours; however, if symptoms persist, stools for ova and parasites, culture and sensitivity, and possibly *C. difficile* toxin should be obtained.

(a) Flexible sigmoidoscopy is usually safe to do to evaluate for inflammatory bowel disease, and on rare occasions, esophagogastroduodenoscopy (EGD) may be necessary to evaluate for celiac disease.

(2) Treatment of specific infections may be required.

(a) Metronidazole, used to treat *Giardia* and *Entamoeba* infestations, has teratogenic effects and should be avoided, at least in the first trimester.

(b) Sulfa, tetracycline, and quinolones also have deleterious effects and must be avoided.

(3) Kaolin and pectin, which act by absorbing water and reducing stool frequency, may be used for moderate to severe diarrhea.

(4) Opiates generally should be avoided because of the possibility of bacterial overgrowth and superinfections.
(5) Addition of *Lactobacillus* may help diarrhea by replacing normal bowel flora.
(6) Antibiotics, such as erythromycin and ampicillin, are safe to use if necessary.
(7) Fluid replacement is the mainstay of treatment as is fetal monitoring for signs of premature labor.

5. Summary
   a. IBS
      (1) A careful history should be done to determine whether the symptoms are acute or longstanding.
      (2) Conservative treatment is recommended and may include stool-bulking agents, a high-fiber diet, avoiding offensive foods, and behavioral therapy.
   b. Constipation
      (1) This is usually a self-limited problem, but sometimes requires treatment with high-fiber diet, stool-bulking agents, and pelvic muscle exercise.
      (2) Laxatives should be used very cautiously.
   c. Diarrhea
      (1) Infectious problems may require specific therapy with safe antibiotics.
      (2) Mild antidiarrheal agents may be used safely for symptomatic control.
      (3) Fluid replacement is the mainstay of therapy for the well-being of both the mother and the fetus.

Inflammatory bowel disease

1. Epidemiology
   a. Inflammatory bowel disease (IBD) refers to chronic ulcerative colitis (CUC) and Crohn's disease, diseases with unknown cause but distinct pathology.
   b. Estimates of the prevalence of IBD range from 1 to 2 million patients, with about 25,000 new cases yearly.
   c. Peak incidence of the disease is between the years 15 and 35, coinciding with the most fruitful childbearing years.
2. Fertility
   a. Patients with CUC have normal fertility.
   b. Fertility is reduced in patients with Crohn's disease in proportion to the activity of the disease.
   c. Fertility seems to be more reduced in Crohn's colitis than in Crohn's ileitis.
   d. Reduced fertility is often of the patient's choice and not because of disease-related impairment, with the patients being afraid of pregnancy because of fear of the disease worsening and fear of fetal complications related to the disease or the medications used for treatment.

3. Inheritance of IBD
   a. It has long been recognized that genetic factors play a role in the etiology of IBD, with complex non-Mendelian patterns of inheritance.
   b. In Jewish populations, the lifetime risk of developing IBD is 7.8% if the proband has Crohn's disease and 4.5% if the proband has CUC.
   c. The lifetime risk of developing IBD in non-Jewish populations is 5.2% if the proband has Crohn's disease and 1.6% if the proband has CUC.
   d. If both parents have IBD, the risk of the offspring developing IBD may be substantially increased.
4. Effects of IBD on pregnancy
   a. CUC
      (1) In pregnant patients with CUC there are healthy offspring in 76% to 97%, congenital abnormalities in 0% to 3%, spontaneous abortions in 1% to 13%, and stillbirths in 0% to 3%, not dissimilar from the results in the normal population.
      (2) Birth weights of babies born to mothers with CUC were slightly lower than normal but not statistically significant.
      (3) CUC did not influence the mode of delivery (vaginal vs. cesarean section) or the incidence of preeclampsia or eclampsia during pregnancy.
   b. Crohn's disease
      (1) Healthy offspring were noted in 70% to 93% of mothers with Crohn's disease, with congenital abnormalities in 0% to 1%, stillbirths in 1% to 4%, and spontaneous abortions in 3% to 9%, similar to the normal population.
      (2) Baiocco and Korelitz reported that among patients with Crohn's disease whose pregnancy was complicated by developmental defects, stillbirths, or spontaneous abortions, 62% had active Crohn's disease.
      (3) Although patients were taking multiple medications to control symptoms, case analyses revealed that disease activity and not drug treatment was responsible for the increase in complications.
      (4) The cesarean section rate in women with severe Crohn's disease or CUC was similar to that of a normal population, with most patients having vaginal deliveries.
         (a) Cesarean section may be the preferred route of delivery for patients with perirectal Crohn's disease, because of the possibility of complications of the episiotomy scar when fistulous tracts are present.
5. Influence of pregnancy on the course of IBD
   a. The course of IBD during pregnancy usually correlates with the activity of the disease at the time of conception.
   b. The risk of exacerbation of CUC is 32% per year in both nonpregnant and pregnant women, with exacerbation usually in the first two trimesters.

c. In women with active CUC at conception, approximately half will remain equally active or even worsen, whereas some may improve or even enter a complete remission, usually in the first trimester.
d. The impact of pregnancy on the course of Crohn's disease is similar to that of CUC, with 27% of patients having a relapse during the course of the pregnancy.
e. In Crohn's disease patients with active disease at conception, one third of patients will remain the same, one third will improve, and one third will worsen; 15% of patients will experience an exacerbation in the postpartum period.

6. Management of IBD during pregnancy
   a. There is no contraindication to flexible sigmoidoscopy or gastroscopy during pregnancy.
      (1) Colonoscopy should be avoided, unless essential for management, in that safety of colonoscopy has not been firmly established during pregnancy.
   b. X-ray examinations should be avoided except for plain films to evaluate suspected toxic megacolon or small bowel obstruction.
   c. CT scans, which expose the fetus to less irradiation than traditional barium x-ray examinations, may be used in the diagnosis of complications of Crohn's disease but abdominal ultrasonography may also be of use in the evaluation of abdominal abscesses.
   d. MRI, which appears to be safe when used in pregnancy, has been used to evaluate the terminal ileum in patients with suspected Crohn's disease with some success and may play a larger role in the evaluation of this group of patients.
   e. Surgical intervention may be necessary for complications such as severe bleeding, perforation, or toxic megacolon refractory to intensive medical therapy.
      (1) Total colectomy and ileostomy done during pregnancy carries a 60% overall risk of postoperative spontaneous abortion.
      (2) Therefore aggressive medical treatment to induce remission as early as possible is indicated.
   f. Patients with preexisting ileostomies generally tolerate pregnancy well; however, one report suggests a 10% rate of bowel obstruction in patients with an ileostomy during pregnancy.
      (1) Patients with an ileal pouch–anal anastomosis for CUC appear to tolerate pregnancy and delivery well.
      (2) Delivery, whether vaginal or cesarean section, did not affect the pouch or the pregnancy.
7. Drug therapy of IBD in pregnancy
   a. Sulfasalazine, or the newer 5-ASA compounds mesalamine or olsalazine, are the first-line drugs of choice in IBD.
      (1) These medications do not appear to have any adverse effects on the neonate.
      (2) Because sulfasalazine interferes with folate absorption, supplemental folate should be given.
   b. Corticosteroids are indicated for treatment of moderate to severe disease.

(1) Crohn's disease patients treated with corticosteroids experienced a slightly higher rate of fetal complications; however, this is attributed to the activity of the disease and not the drug therapy.
(2) Although defects such as cleft palate have been noted in laboratory animals treated with corticosteroids, these defects have not proved to be problematic in humans.

c. Antibiotics are often used in IBD, especially in treating abscesses and fistulae.
(1) Metronidazole, the usual drug of choice, is teratogenic and should be avoided except perhaps in patients with severe perirectal disease in the second and third trimesters.
(2) Ciprofloxacin has recently been used for treatment of fistulae, but its chronic use in pregnancy has not been proved safe as yet.

d. Immunosuppressive therapy with 6-mercaptopurine (6-MP) or azathioprine has an established role for patients with refractory CUC or Crohn's disease, often allowing for reduction of the steroid dose or its elimination.
(1) These agents are also useful in maintaining remissions.
(2) Questions of safety have been raised in that laboratory animals treated with immunosuppressive drugs show low birth weights, congenital abnormalities, and small litter size.
(3) These drugs have shown relative safety in that over 1000 renal transplant patients have become pregnant and the only birth anomalies have been in patients on a higher dose of drug used for allograft rejection than is used for IBD.
(4) Although these agents are generally felt to be safe in pregnancy, their use cannot be encouraged until their safety is better established.
(5) Cyclosporine has recently been shown to be of benefit in severe CUC; however, it is contraindicated in pregnancy because of nephrotoxicity, hypertension, and hepatic toxicity.

8. Breast-feeding
a. IBD does not usually interfere with the mother's ability to breast-feed.
b. Although sulfasalazine and corticosteroids are secreted into the breast milk, their concentration is quite small and not thought to be of harm to the infant.
c. Because the safety of breast-feeding for patients on immunosuppressive therapy is not known, women should be discouraged from breast-feeding while on these agents.

9. Summary
a. IBD is a relatively common problem encountered in pregnant patients and in general should be treated as in the nonpregnant.
b. Poor outcomes are generally related to activity of the disease; therefore, the goal of intensive medical management should be to induce and maintain a remission.
c. Surgical intervention may be necessary for complications such as obstruction, abscess, or bleeding; however, definitive surgical

therapy, with its attendant high fetal loss, should be reserved for toxic megacolon if at all possible.

Surgical management of complications of pregnancy

Acute general surgery problems are uncommon in the pregnant patient but potentially may have devastating effects on both the mother and the fetus, particularly if there is any delay in diagnosis. These patients should, in general, be approached as a nonpregnant one would be.

1. Incidence
   a. Complications during pregnancy that require surgery occur in 0.5% to 1% of pregnancies
2. Reasons for delay in diagnosis
   a. Symptoms of abdominal pain, nausea and vomiting, and heartburn occur normally in many pregnancies.
   b. There is often difficulty making the correct diagnosis in a pregnant patient.
   c. There is often hesitation in ordering appropriate diagnostic tests.
   d. There is often a fear of anesthesia.

Acute appendicitis

1. Incidence
   a. This is the most common surgical problem of pregnancy, occurring in about 0.1%.
   b. The perforation rate is higher in pregnant patients, reported in up to 38% of cases.
   c. Fetal mortality correlates with the incidence of perforation, with 10% or more for perforating appendicitis.
2. Diagnosis
   a. Pain is the most common symptom, either with the classic pattern of midabdominal pain that settles in the RLQ or it may occur in atypical locations.
   b. The hallmark of diagnosis is signs of localized peritoneal inflammation, often displaced by the uterus to the RUQ.
   c. Laboratory studies may show an elevated WBC; however, this may occur normally in pregnancy.
   d. The differential diagnosis may include Crohn's disease, diverticulitis, cholecystitis, or mesenteric adenitis as well as pyelonephritis, renal stone, or pneumonia.
      (1) Gynecologic problems such as ectopic pregnancy, rupture of the corpus luteum, or torsion of an ovarian cyst need also be considered.
   e. The accuracy of making a correct diagnosis has been reported at 60% to 80%.
3. Treatment
   a. The treatment is the same as for a nonpregnant patient, with immediate surgery.
   b. Prophylactic antibiotics are recommended.
   c. Tocolytic drugs have been recommended.

d. Retraction of the uterus during surgery should be avoided as much as feasible.

Biliary tract disease

Biliary tract disease is the second most common surgical problem during pregnancy, occurring in 0.03% to 0.09% of pregnancies.

Pancreatitis

Pancreatitis is usually secondary to gallstones.

Peptic ulcer disease

1. PUD is an uncommon problem in pregnancy.
2. Perforation is the most likely complication diagnosed by peritoneal signs on physical examination and free air on plain abdominal irradiation.
3. Plication of the ulcer is usually the procedure of choice, but definitive surgery may be necessary for chronic symptoms or for technical reasons.
4. GI bleeding is handled in the traditional fashion with ligation of the bleeding vessel, vagotomy, and a drainage procedure, usually a pyloroplasty.

Inflammatory bowel disease

1. CUC: The indications for surgery are fulminant colitis, toxic megacolon, and hemorrhage, with colectomy and ileostomy the procedure of choice.
2. Crohn's disease: The indications for surgery are obstruction, perforation, abscess or fistula formation, or rarely, intractability.

Intestinal obstruction

1. Intestinal obstruction is a rare complication of pregnancy, often difficult to diagnose because nausea and vomiting are common in pregnancy and distension may be difficult to distinguish in late pregnancy.
2. The most common cause of obstruction is volvulus with adhesions, occurring in 25% of cases.
   a. Sigmoid volvulus occurs more frequently than cecal volvulus.
   b. Surgery is the best approach but endoscopic decompression may be tried initially if there are no signs of peritonitis.
3. Incarcerated hernias rarely cause obstruction, usually in the first trimester when intra-abdominal pressure increases.
   a. Known hernias should be repaired electively before the patient becomes pregnant if possible.
4. Intussusception is the cause of about 5% of obstructions, usually secondary to benign causes.

Splenic and hepatic disorders

The most common cause for splenic and hepatic rupture is trauma, although spontaneous rupture of the liver has been reported in pregnancy.

Summary

Although uncommon, acute surgical problems arising in pregnancy may be catastrophic to the mother and fetus, with the principle of management being to treat the pregnant as a nonpregnant one, keeping a high degree of suspicion for the possibility of acute surgical problems and ordering the appropriate diagnostic tests in a timely fashion.

Liver disease and pregnancy

Jaundice may occur during pregnancy from several causes, some related to the pregnancy and others unrelated. The most common cause of jaundice is viral hepatitis, usually hepatitis A, B, or C; however, other viruses such as cytomegalovirus (CMV), Epstein-Barr, or herpes simplex virus may occur. Drug-induced liver disease is uncommon because pregnant patients usually are on few medications. Alcoholic hepatitis may occasionally occur. Biliary obstruction secondary to gallstones occurs infrequently. Pregnancy-related causes of jaundice include intrahepatic cholestasis of pregnancy, acute fatty liver of pregnancy, hyperemesis gravidarum, preeclampsia or eclampsia, and spontaneous rupture of the liver.

When evaluating liver functions, it must be remembered that some laboratory studies vary secondary to the pregnancy. Laboratory studies that are increased during pregnancy include alkaline phosphatase, triglycerides, cholesterol, fibrinogen, transferrin, and ceruloplasmin. The albumin is often decreased in pregnancy. The hepatic enzymes (ALT and AST), LDH, bilirubin, and prothrombin time usually remain normal in pregnancy (Table 24-12).

Viral hepatitis

The viral agents responsible for viral hepatitis include hepatitis A (HAV); hepatitis B (HBV); hepatitis C (HCV); hepatitis D (HDV), formerly known as delta agent; hepatitis E (HEV), formerly known as epidemic hepatitis; and the recently described hepatitis G (HGV).

1. Incidence: The overall incidence of hepatitis in pregnancy is 0.03% to 0.1%, similar to the nonpregnant population, with 75% to 80% HBV and 10% HAV.
2. Pathophysiology
   a. HAV, the classic short-incubation, infectious hepatitis, is a small 27-nm RNA picornavirus that is spread by the fecal–oral route.
      (1) The incubation period is 2 to 6 weeks.
      (2) Epidemics are not rare.
   b. HBV, a double-stranded, 44-nm DNA virus in the family Hepdnaviridae, contains a 7-nm hepatitis B surface antigen in the outer coat and a hepatitis B e antigen (HbeAg) in the core.
      (1) It is spread through contact with infected blood and body fluids, parenterally and by sexual contact.
      (2) The incubation period ranges from 2 to 26 weeks, with a mean of 12 weeks.
   c. HCV, a small enveloped 50-nm to 60-nm RNA virus in the family Flavivirus, is predominantly spread parenterally or from contact with infected blood products, but may also be spread sexually.

Table 24-12 Hepatitis panel testing

Type	Profile	Markers	Purpose
Diagnostic	Acute	HbsAg Anti-HBc IgM Anti-HAV IgM Anti-HCV HCV-RNA by PCR	To differentiate between HBV, HAV and HCV infection Retest for anti-HCV if negative but clinical signs or symptoms suggest hepatitis C
Screen	Hepatitis C	Anti-HCV	To evaluate for late seroconversion in recent HCV infection and to identify HCV-infected individuals
	Perinatal	HbsAg HbeAg	To diagnose for HbsAg-positive pregnant women who may transmit HBV to their newborn infants; if the HbsAg-positive mother is HbeAg positive, her infant will have a 90% chance of acquiring chronic hepatiits B infection (e.g., Southeast Asians, Alaskans, health care workers)
	Immunity	HbsAg Anti-HBc Anti-HBs	1. Test blood for infection with HbsAg 2. Test exposed person for immunity with anti-HBc and anti-HBs (in particular, dialysis patients, health care workers, recipients of frequent transfusions, and illicit drug users 3. Also test sexual partners of individuals with acute or chronic HBV to minimize the spread of infection by the application of prophylaxis 4. To determine whether an individual is currently infected or has antibodies to HBV

Continued.

Table 24-12 Hepatitis panel testing—cont'd

Type	Profile	Markers	Purpose
Monitor	Chronic hepatitis B	HbsAg HbeAg Anti-HBe	To evaluate for late seroconversion and/or disease resolution in known HBV carrier
	Infant follow-up	HbsAg Anti-HBs	To monitor the success of treatment for perinatal transmission of HBV (12 to 15 months after birth)
	Postvaccination	Anti-HBs	To ensure that immunity has been achieved after vaccination

(1) The incubation period span is similar to HBV but the mean is only 8 weeks.

d. HDV, a defective RNA virus that requires the presence of HBV for infection and replication to occur, is most often spread parenterally or by blood products.

(1) In the United States this disease is largely confined to drug addicts and hemophiliacs.

(2) It may appear as a coinfection with HBV or superimposed on HBV.

e. HEV, a single-stranded linear RNA virus, is spread by fecal–oral route and is predominantly found in Africa and eastern Europe.

(1) Rare cases have been seen in travelers to the United States.

(2) The incubation period is slightly longer than that of HAV.

f. HGV, the most recently described form of viral hepatitis, is in the same family as HCV and they share about 25% of their genomes.

(1) They probably have a similar route of spread and incubation periods.

3. Clinical course

a. There is a wide range of manifestations of hepatitis, from asymptomatic to fulminant hepatitis.

b. The prodromal period, which lasts from a few days to 2 weeks, is characterized by "flulike" symptoms with nausea and vomiting, myalgias, arthralgias, low-grade fever, and fatigue.

c. The icteric phase is associated with the development of dark urine and acholic stools, jaundice and fatigue, with pruritus and anorexia and weight loss common.

d. Hepatomegaly and liver tenderness are common.

e. The serum enzymes may become markedly elevated, particularly in HAV, HBV, and HEV.

f. The illness usually runs its course in a few weeks with complete resolution in 3 to 6 months.

g. One percent to 10% of HBV patients enter a chronic phase, whereas the majority of HCV and HGV become chronic.

h. HAV and HEV do not appear to have chronicity.

4. Morbidity and mortality

a. HAV has a low maternal mortality (<0.1%), because it does in the general population, and the risk of vertical transmission to the fetus is low because of the brief viremia.

(1) The incidence of preterm labor may be increased with HAV.

b. HBV has a similar course in the pregnant as in the nonpregnant patient with a mortality <0.1%.

(1) Vertical transmission to the fetus, either *in utero* or at the time of delivery, is a definite risk to the fetus.

(2) Perinatal transmission accounts for about 10% of the new HBV cases.

(3) Fetal infection is more likely if the mother develops the illness in the third trimester and much more likely if she is HbeAg positive (80%) as compared to HbeAg negative (25%).

c. HCV has a course in pregnancy similar to the nonpregnant patient.

(1) It tends to be a milder illness than HBV but is more likely to enter a chronic phase.

(2) Vertical transmission may occur but is much less likely than in HBV.

d. HDV acute infection may be associated with fulminant hepatitis or severe hepatitis.

(1) Vertical transmission is extremely rare, requiring transmission of HDV and HBV simultaneously.

(2) Because most carriers of HBV with superimposed HDV are anti-Hbe positive, transmission of HBV to the infant is less likely to occur.

e. HEV is clinically similar to HAV but may have a 10% to 20% maternal mortality rate, possibly reflecting the socioeconomic conditions of the affected countries.

(1) The rate of vertical transmission is not clear at this point.

f. HGV morbidity and mortality has not been fully defined but is probably similar to that of HCV.

5. Diagnosis: The typical clinical syndrome with nausea, vomiting, headache, and anorexia along with physical findings of jaundice, tender liver, and elevated liver enzymes raise the suspicion of acute hepatitis. Testing the blood for specific antibodies will usually define the type of hepatitis present.

a. The diagnosis of HAV is established by detecting IgM antibodies (IgM anti-HAV), which are present early in the illness and persist for up to 6 months.

(1) IgG anti-HAV also develops early in the illness and persists for life.

b. The diagnosis of HBV is established by demonstrating HbsAg 30 to 50 days after exposure.

(1) HBcAg and HBeAg follow and antibodies to the hepatitis antigens B, c, and e develop as the patient recovers from the disease.

(2) The development of HbsAb indicates recovery from the illness.

c. HCV is diagnosed by detecting anti-HCV antibodies.

(1) These antibodies have limitations in that they develop as late as 6 months after exposure.

(2) They do not appear to be protective antibodies but probably represent ongoing infection.

(3) Detection of HCV-RNA by polymerase chain reaction (PCR) technique gives a measure of active viral load and is the best test for detecting acute HCV.

d. HDV can be diagnosed by anti-HDV antibodies of the IgM and IgG classes.

e. HEV can be diagnosed by solid-phase immune electron microscopy; however, this method is not commercially available.

f. HGV can be diagnosed by HGV-RNA by PCR but this method is not yet available commercially.

6. Management

a. Treatment

(1) Patients with uncomplicated acute hepatitis are treated with supportive care, usually at home, with hospitalization necessary

only if the patient is unable to keep hydrated or maintain nutrition, or is having signs of deteriorating liver function.

(2) Progressive rising bilirubin levels are worrisome but prolongation of the prothrombin level to >3 seconds over control is the best indicator of serious liver dysfunction.

(3) Rest is essential but mandated bed rest is not usually necessary.

(4) No special dietary restrictions are usually needed unless the patient develops hepatic encephalopathy, where protein intake may need to be restricted, or if the patient develops edema, where sodium restriction may be helpful.

(5) There are no specific medications for treatment of acute hepatitis.

(6) Interferon alpha-2b is used to treat chronic HCV and HBV but is marginally effective at best (15% to 25% cure rate).

(7) It is a pregnancy category C drug and it would generally be recommended that it be avoided during pregnancy.

b. Prevention

(1) HAV: Immunoglobulin administration, 0.02 ml/kg, IM, is effective in the prevention of HAV and should not be withheld from the pregnant patient.

(2) HBV

(a) All pregnant women should be screened for HBV with HbsAg on the initial visit.

(b) Identification of maternal infection and prophylaxis of the newborn can reduce neonatal infection and reduce the sequelae of chronic viral hepatitis, which include cirrhosis and hepatocellular carcinoma.

(c) Both hepatitis B vaccine and HBV immunoglobulin (HBIg, 5 ml) should be given within 48 hours of delivery to infants of HBsAg-positive women.

(d) Deliveries by cesarean section may reduce vertical transmission from some high-risk mothers with high HBV DNA levels.

(e) Pregnant patients at high risk for contracting HBV should be vaccinated with HBV recombinant vaccines.

(f) HBIg should be given to susceptible women within 48 hours of exposure to HBV.

(3) At the present time there is no form of passive or active immunity for HCV.

Intrahepatic cholestasis of pregnancy (ICP)

ICP is characterized by skin pruritus and biochemical cholestasis, which appear late during a pregnancy, persist until delivery, and disappear after parturition.

1. Incidence

a. The incidence of cholestasis of pregnancy is less than 0.1% of all pregnancies.

b. It is the second most common cause of jaundice in pregnancy.

c. It usually occurs in the third trimester and recurs in subsequent pregnancies.

2. Morbidity and mortality
   a. Pregnant women with ICP have pruritus and occasionally coagulation defects because of decreased vitamin K absorption, but it is otherwise a benign disease in the mother.
   b. It may, however, be associated with fetal distress, with premature delivery, and stillbirths.
3. Pathogenesis
   a. The cause of ICP is unknown although clinical observations suggest an increased sensitivity to estrogens.
   b. There appears to be an autosomal dominant pattern of inheritance.
   c. The histologic changes on liver biopsy are those of cholestasis without inflammation with bile plugging of the canaliculi.
4. Diagnosis
   a. History: The history is of generalized pruritus usually beginning in the third trimester, occasionally accompanied by fatigue, jaundice, steatorrhea, and dark urine.
   b. Physical examination: The patients may be mildly icteric and may have excoriations as a result of scratching from the pruritus.
   c. Laboratory findings
      (1) Serum bilirubin ranges from 1.2 to 5.0 mg/dl but rarely reaches 10 mg/dl.
      (2) Serum levels of bile salts may reach 100 times normal.
      (3) The alkaline phosphatase levels are elevated up to 10 times the usual found in pregnancy.
         (a) The GGTP and 5′-nucleotidase, other markers of cholestasis, are generally not particularly elevated.
      (4) Serum aminotransferase levels are usually increased from 2 to 10 times.
      (5) Steatorrhea may be present.
5. Treatment
   a. Antipruritics provide a partial and irregular benefit.
      (1) Diphenhydramine HCl (Benadryl), 25 to 50 mg, PO, q4-6h up to 400 mg/day, or hydroxyzine HCl (Vistaril), 50 to 100 mg, IM, q4-6h or 25 to 50 mg, PO, q6h are often tried.
   b. Cholestyramine has been used to increase fecal excretion of bile salts at a dose of 4 g PO, tid, but with limited success.
   c. Phenobarbital, given at a low dose of 90 mg qhs for 2 to 3 weeks, has been shown to reduce the bilirubin level and pruritus in patients with ICP and may be tried if cholestyramine is ineffective.
   d. Ursodeoxycholic acid, given orally at a dose of 15 mg/kg/day for 3 weeks has been shown to alleviate pruritus and reduce serum bile salt and enzyme levels.
   e. Plasmapheresis may also provide relief for a few to several weeks.

Acute fatty liver of pregnancy (AFLP)

AFLP is characterized by microvesicular fatty infiltration of the liver, hepatic failure, and encephalopathy developing in the third trimester of pregnancy.

1. Incidence
   a. The incidence of AFLP is estimated at 1/13,000 pregnancies, with patients with multiple gestations at higher risk.

   b. Pregnant patients with male fetuses are two to three times more likely to be affected.
2. Morbidity and mortality
   a. Fetal and maternal mortality up to 85% has been reported in the past.
   b. However a more recent study reports fetal and maternal mortality of 23% and 18%, respectively.
3. Pathogenesis
   a. The cause of AFLP is unknown.
   b. Histologic examination of the liver shows microvesicular fatty infiltrate, when stained with oil red O stain.
   c. There is usually little in the way of inflammation in the liver.
   d. These changes are quite similar to those seen in Reye's syndrome in children and with tetracycline toxicity.
4. Diagnosis: The combination of the history, physical examination, and laboratory should suggest the diagnosis.
   a. History: The patient develops symptoms of nausea, vomiting, headache, and abdominal pain during the third trimester.
   b. Physical examination: Signs of liver dysfunction with jaundice and fever appear, often followed by signs of liver failure with mental confusion, coma, and signs of multiple organ failure.
   c. Laboratory findings
      (1) The serum transaminase levels may range from 100 to 1000 U/L with the SGPT being greater than the SGOT.
      (2) The bilirubin level is variable but usually is between 5 and 10 mg/dl.
      (3) The alkaline phosphatase level is usually three to four times normal.
      (4) Amylase values may be elevated because of concomitant pancreatitis.
      (5) The protime, PTT, and fibrinogen are abnormal and disseminated intravascular coagulation (DIC) may be present.
      (6) The glucose level is often less than 60 mg/dl.
   d. Liver biopsy
      (1) The key to the diagnosis is demonstration of the typical changes on frozen section of liver biopsy.
      (2) Caution must be exercised in the decision to perform a liver biopsy in that the prothrombin must be within 3 seconds of the control and the platelet count should be above 60,000/mm^3.
      (3) If the coagulation studies will not allow safe percutaneous liver, a biopsy may be performed under direct visualization.
5. Differential diagnosis: The major illness to be considered in the differential diagnosis is severe preeclampsia, with drug-induced liver injury, biliary tract disease, acute rupture of the liver, and viral hepatitis also to be considered.
6. Management: Care is supportive but must be aggressive, usually requiring intensive care unit (ICU) treatment. Issues to be addressed include the following:
   a. Correction of the coagulation defects with fresh frozen plasma to keep the prothrombin time <15 seconds
   b. Close monitoring of the electrolytes and glucose levels

c. Respiratory support as necessary
d. Nutritional support including TPN: often necessary
e. Monitoring for multiple organ failure
f. Delivery of the fetus: may be helpful in shortening the disease state

Suggested reading

Alstead EM et al: Safety of azathioprine in pregnancy in inflammatory bowel disease, *Gastroenterology* 99:443-446, 1990.

Anand S, Van Thiel DH: Prenatal and neonatal exposure to cimetidine results in gonadal and sexual dysfunction in adult males, *Science* 218:493-494, 1982.

Anderson AS: Dietary factors in the aetiology and treatment of constipation during pregnancy, *Br J Obstet Gynaecol* 93:245-249, 1986.

Anderson AS, Whichelow MJ: Constipation during pregnancy: dietary fibre intake and the effect of fibre supplementation, *Hum Nutr Appl Nutr* 39A:202-207, 1985.

Anderson JB, Turner GM, Williamson RC: Fulminant ulcerative colitis in late pregnancy and the puerperium, *J R Soc Med* 80(8):492-494, 1987.

Armantaro G, Bracco PL, DiSilverio C: Ranitidine in the treatment of reflux esoophagitis, *Clin Obstet Gynecol* 13:335-346, 1986.

Bailey LE et al: Acute appendicitis during pregnancy, *Am Surg* 52:218-221, 1986.

Baille J et al: Endoscopic management of choledocholithiasis during pregnancy, *Surg Gynecol Obstet* 171:1, 1990.

Baiocco PH, Korelitz BI: The influence of inflammatory bowel disease and its treatment on pregnancy and fetal outcome, *J Clin Gastroenterol* 6:211-216, 1984.

Baird DD, Narendranathan M, Sandler RS: Increased risk of preterm birth for women with inflammatory bowel disease, *Gastroenterology* 99(4):987-994, 1990.

Baron TH, Richter J: Gastroesophageal reflux disease in pregnancy, *Gastroenterol Clin North Am* 21(4):777-791, 1992.

Basso L et al: A study of cholelithiasis during pregnancy and its relationship with parity, menarche, breast-feeding, dysmenorrhea, oral contraception and a maternal history of cholelithiasis, *Surg Gynecol Obstet* 175(1):41-46, 1992.

Bennion LJ, Grundy SM: Risk factors for the development of cholelithiasis in man, *N Engl J Med* 299:1221, 1978.

Berk JE, Smith BH, Akrawi MM: Pregnancy pancreatitis during pregnancy and the postpartum period, *Surg Gynecol Obstet* 168:426, 1989.

Bleijenberg G, Kuijpers HC: Treatment of spastic pelvic floor syndrome with biofeedback, *Dis Colon Rectum* 30:108-111, 1987.

Block P, Kelly TR: Management of gallstone pancreatitis during pregnancy and the postpartum period, *Surg Gynecol Obstet* 168(5):426-428, 1989.

Brucker MC: Management of common minor discomforts in pregnancy, *J Nurse Midwifery* 33:67-73, 1988.

Burns PA et al: Treatment of stress incontinence with pelvic floor exercises and biofeedback, *J Am Geriatr Soc* 38:693-698, 1990.

Calhoun BC: Gastrointestinal disorders in pregnancy, *Obstet Gynecol Clin North Am* 19(4):733-744, 1992.

Castro L de P: Reflux esophagitis as the cause of heartburn of pregnancy, *Am J Obstet Gynecol* 98:1-10, 1967.

Centers for Disease Control: Prevention of perinatal transmission of hepatitis B virus: prenatal screening of all pregnant women for hepatitis B surface antigen, *MMWR* 37:341-351, 1988.

Chen CP et al: Acute pancreatitis in pregnancy, *Acta Obstet Gynecol Scand* 74(8):607-610, 1995.

Ching CK, Lam SK: Antacids. Indications and limitations, *Drugs* 47(2):305-317, 1994.

Ching MS et al: Placental transfer of omeprazole in maternal and fetal sheep, *Dev Pharmacol Ther* 9:323-331, 1986.

Christofides ND et al: Decreased plasma motilin concentration in pregnancy, *Br Med J* 285:1453-1454, 1982.
Clemendor A, Sanford S, Harbilas E: Achalasia and nutritional deficiency during pregnancy, *Obstet Gynecol* 33:106-113, 1969.
Dayan A et al: 6-mercaptopurine in inflammatory bowel disease patients of childbearing age: No increase in congenital anomalies—a case controlled study, *Gastroenterology* 100:A824, 1990.
De Vore GR, Bracken M, Berkowitz RL: The amylase/creatinine clearance ratio in normal pregnancy and pregnancies complicated by pancreatitis, hyperemesis gravidarum, and toxemia, *Am J Obstet Gynecol* 136:747, 1980.
Dixon NP, Faddis DM, Silberman H: Aggressive management of cholecystitis during pregnancy, *Am J Surg* 154:292, 1987.
Dreiling DA et al: Pregnancy and pancreatitis, *Am J Gastroenterol* 64:23, 1975.
Duane WC: Pathogensis of gallstones: implications for management, *Hosp Pract* 25:65, 1990.
Elerding SC: Laparoscopic cholecystectomy in pregnancy, *Am J Surg* 165:625-627, 1993.
Fagan EA: Disorders in obstetric practice. In de Sweet M, editor: *Medical disorders in obstetric practice,* Oxford, 1989, Blackwell Scientific Publications.
Farmer RG et al: Hyperlipoproteinemia and pancreatitis, *Am J Med* 54:161, 1973.
Fiest TC, Foong A, Cholhavatia S: Successful balloon dilation of achalasia during pregnancy, *Gastrointest Endosc* 29:810-812, 1993.
Friedman GD, Kannel WB, Dawber TR: The epidemiology of gallbladder disease: observations in the Framingham study, *J Chronic Dis* 19:273, 1966.
Friedman GD, Sieglaub AB, Seltzer CC: Cigarettes, alcohol, coffee, and peptic ulcer, *N Engl J Med* 290:469, 1974.
Gadacz TR, Talamini MA: Traditional versus laparoscopic cholecystectomy, *Am J Surg* 161:336, 1991.
Goldschmiedt M, Wolf L, Shires T: Treatment of symptomatic choledocholithiasis during pregnancy, *Gastrointest Endosc* 39:812-813, 1993.
Graaf J, Pijpers PM: Spontaneous rupture of the spleen in the third trimester—Report of a case and review of the literature, *Eur J Obstet Gynecol Reprod Biol* 25:2243-2247, 1987.
Grandien M et al: Management of pregnant women with diarrhea at term and of healthy carriers of infectious agents in stools at delivery, *Scand J Infect Dis Suppl* 71:9-18, 1990.
Graham DY: Helicobacter pylori: Its epidemiology and its role in duodenal ulcer disease, *J Gastroenterol Hepatol* 6:97-105, 1991.
Habal FM, Hiu G, Greenberg GR: Oral 5-aminosalicylic acid for inflammatory bowel disease in pregnancy: safety and clinical course, *Gastroenterology* 105:1057-1060, 1993.
Halvorsen A, Brandt B, Andreasen JJ: Acute appendicitis in pregnancy: complications and subsequent management, *Eur J Surg* 158:603-606, 1992.
Hanan IM, Kirsner JB: Inflammatory bowel disease in the pregnant woman, *Clin Perinatol* 12:682-699, 1985.
Harer WB, Jarrer WB Sr: Volvulus complicating pregnancy and the puerperium, *Obstet Gynecol* 12:399-406, 1958.
Hill LM, Symmonds RE: Small bowel obstuction in pregnancy, *Obstet Gynecol* 49:170-173, 1976.
Homan WP, Thorbjarnarson B: Crohn's disease and pregnancy, *Arch Surg* 111:545, 1976.
Hould FS et al: Progesterone receptors regulate gallbladder motility, *Am J Obstet Gynecol* 122:283, 1975
Hudson CN: Ileostomy in pregnancy, *Proc R Soc Med* 65:281-285, 1972.
Juhasz ES et al: Ileal pouch-anal anastomosis function following childbirth: An extended evaluation, *Dis Colon Rectum* 38(2):159-165, 1995.

Kaplan M: Acute fatty liver of pregnancy, *N Engl J Med* 33:367-370, 1985.
Klein KB: Pancreatitis in pregnancy. In Rustgi VK, Cooper JN, editors: *Gastrointestinal and hepatic complications of pregnancy,* p. 138, New York, 1986, John Wiley and Sons.
Knudsen A, Lebech M, Hansen M: Upper gastrointestinal symptoms in the third trimester of the normal pregnancy, *Eur J Obstet Gynecol Reprod Biol* 60(1):29-33, 1995.
Korelitz BI: Inflammatory bowel disease in pregnancy, *Gastroenterol Clin North Am* 21(4):827-834, 1992.
Korelitz BI: Pregnancy and IBD, *Semin Colon Rectal Surg* 4:48-54, 1993.
Korelitz BI: Immunosuppressive therapy of inflammatory bowel disease: a historical perspective. *Gastroenterologist* 3(2):141-152, 1995.
Lawson M, Kern F, Everson GT: Gastrointestinal transit time in human pregnancy: prolongation in the second and third trimesters followed by postpartum normalization, *Gastroenterology* 89:996-999, 1985.
Lee SD, Chan CY, Wang YJ: Mother to infant transmission of hepatitis C virus infection, *J Med Virol* 30:178-180, 1990.
Levy N, Lemberg E: Bowel habit in pregnancy, *Digestion* 4:216-222, 1971.
Lewis JH, Weingold AB: The use of gastrointestinal drugs during pregnancy and lactation, *Am J Gastroenterol* 80:912-923, 1985.
Lewis JH, Weingold AB, the Committee of FDA-related matters, American College of Gastroenterology: The use of gastrointestinal drugs during pregnancy and lactation, *Am J Gastroenterol* 80:912-923, 1985.
Liddle C, Craig PI, Farrell GC: The A, B, C, D and E of viral hepatitis: new agents for old diseases, *Aust NZ J Med* 20:3-4, 1990.
Lind JF, Smith AM, McKiver DK: Heartburn in pregnancy—A manometric study, *Can Med Assoc J* 98:571-574, 1968.
Mabie WC: Obstetric management of gastrointestinal complications of pregnancy, *Gastroenterol Clin North Am* 21(4):923-935, 1992.
Mabie WC: Acute fatty liver of pregnancy, *Gastroenterol Clin North Am* 21(4):951-960, 1992.
Marchand P: The gastroesophageal sphincter and the mechanism of regurgitation, *Br J Surg* 42:504-513, 1955.
Maringhini A et al: Biliary sludge and gallstones in pregnancy: incidence, risk, and natural history, *Ann Intern Med* 119(2):116-120, 1993.
Mayberry JF, Atkinson M: Achalasia in pregnancy, *Br J Obstet Gynaecol* 94:812-814, 1987.
Mayberry JF, Weterman IT: European survey of fertility in women with Crohn's disease: a case controlled study by European collaborative group, *Gut* 27:821-825, 1986.
Michaletz-Onody PA: Peptic ulcer disease in pregnancy, *Gastroenterol Clin North Am* 21:817-826, 1992.
Mishra L, Seeff LB: Viral hepatitis, A through E, complicating pregnancy, *Gastroenterol Clin North Am* 21(4):873-887, 1992.
Mogadam M et al: Effects of sulfasalazine and corticosteroids on fetal outcome, *Gastroenterology* 80:72-76, 1981.
Nagler R, Spiro HM: Heartburn in late pregnancy: manometric studies of esophageal motor function, *J Clin Invest* 40:954-970, 1961.
Nathan L, Huddleston JF: Acute abdominal pain in pregnancy, *Obstet Gynecol Clin North Am* 22(1):55-68, 1995.
Nelson H et al: The effect of pregnancy and delivery on the ileal pouch and anal anastomosis functions, *Dig Dis Sci* 40:472-479, 1995.
Nelson OH et al: Pregnancy in ulcerative colitis, *Scand J Gastroenterol* 18:735-742, 1983.
Ostenson H et al: Smoking, alcohol, coffee and familial factors: any associations with peptic ulcer? A clinically and radiologically prospective study, *Scand J Gastroenterol* 20:1227, 1985.

Pietrantoni M, Sanfilippo J: Endoscopic surgical procedures during pregnancy. In Levine R, Sanfilippo JS, editors: *Operative gynecologic endoscopy,* New York, 1995, Springer-Verlag.
Pietrantoni M, Sanfilippo J: Operative laparoscopy and pregnancy. In Hankins G et al, editors: *Operative Obstetrics,* Norwalk, CT, 1995, Appleton & Lange.
Pietrantoni M, Sanfilippo J: Operative laparoscopy during surgery. In Vitale G, Sanfilippo JS, editors: *Atlas of laparoscopic general surgery,* Philadelphia, 1995, Lippincott.
Pietrantoni M, Sanfilippo J: Operative laparoscopy during surgery. In Vitale G, Sanfilippo JS, editors: *Atlas of laparoscopic general surgery,* ed 1, Philadelphia, 1995, Lippincott.
Porter RJ, Stirrat GM: The effects of inflammatory bowel disease on pregnancy: a case-controlled retrospective analysis, *Br J Obstet Gynaecol* 93:1124-1131, 1986.
Present DH et al: Treatment of Crohn's disease with 6-mercaptopurine: a long-term randomized double study, *N Engl J Med* 302:981-987, 1980.
Printen KJ, Ott RA: Cholecystitis during pregnancy, *Am Surg* 44:432, 1978.
Rabe T et al: Action of PGE methyl analogue misoprostol on the pregnant human uterus in the first trimester, *Geburtshilfe Frauenheilkd* 47:324-331, 1987.
Ranchet G, Gangemi O, Petrone M: Sucralfate in the treatment of gravidic pyrosis, *G Ital Ostret Ginesol* XXII:1-16, 1990.
Reyes H: The spectrum of liver and gastrointestinal disease seen in cholestasis of pregnancy, *Gastroenterol Clin North Am* 21(4):905-921, 1992.
Robertson CS, Hardy JG, Atkinson M: Quantitative assessment of the response to therapy in achalasia of the cardia, *Gut* 30:768-773, 1989.
Rosenberg V et al: Pancreatic exocrine secretion during and after pregnancy, *Am Surg* 181:47, 1975.
Rubin SD, Korelitz BI: Considerations regarding fertility and pregnancy in the management of inflammatory bowel disease, *Pract Gastroenterol* 20(1):12-23, 1996.
Scott LD: Gallstone disease and pancreatitis in pregnancy, *Gastroenterol Clin North Am* 21(4):803-815, 1992.
Shaked G, Twena M, Charuzi I: Laparoscopic cholecystectomy for empyema of gallbladder during pregnancy, *Surg Laparosc Endosc* 4:65-67, 1994.
Shoenut JP et al: MRI in the diagnosis of Crohn's disease in two pregnant women, *J Clin Gastroenterol* 17(3):244-247, 1993.
Slater G: Complications of pregnancy: Surgical aspects, *Pract Gastroenterol* 19(10):15-26, 1995.
Smoleniec JS, James DK: Gastrointestinal crises during pregnancy, *Digestive Dis* 11(4-5):313-324, 1993.
Snydman DR: Hepatitis in pregnancy, *N Engl J Med* 33:1398-1401, 1985.
Soll AH: Duodenal ulcer and drug therapy. In Sleisinger MH, Fordtran JS editors: *Gastrointestinal Disease,* ed 4, pp. 814-879, Philadelphia, 1989, W.B. Saunders.
Swisher SG et al: Biliary disease during pregnancy, *Am J Surg* 168(6):576-579, 1994.
Thompson WG et al: Irritable bowel syndrome: Guidelines for the diagnosis, *Gastroenterol Int* 2:92-95, 1989.
Torbey CF, Richter JE: Esophageal disorders during pregnancy, *Pract Gastroenterol* 19(9):22-34, 1995.
Trallori G et al: 5-Aminosalicylic acid in pregnancy: clinical report, *Ital J Gastrol* 26(2):75-78, 1994.
Traube M, McCallum RW: Calcium-channel blockers and the gastrointestinal tract, *Am J Gastroenterol* 79:892-896, 1984.
Van Thiel DH et al: Heartburn of pregnancy, *Gastroenterology* 72:666-668, 1977.
Wald A et al: Gastrointestinal transit: the effect of the menstrual cycle, *Gastroenterology* 80:1497-1500, 1981.
Watson R, Quayle AR: Intussusception in pregnancy: case report and review of the literature, *Br J Obstet Gynaecol* 93:1093-1096, 1986.

Watson WJ, Gaines TE: Third trimester colectomy for severe ulcerative colitis: a case report, *J Reprod Med* 32:869-872, 1987.

West L, Warren J, Cutts T: Diagnosis and management of irritable bowel syndrome, constipation, and diarrhea in pregnancy, *Gastroenterol Clin North Am* 21(4):793-802, 1992.

Whitehead WE et al: Evidence for exacerbation of irritable bowel syndrome during menses, *Gastroenterology* 98:1485-1489, 1990.

Wilkenson EJ: Acute pancreatitis in pregnancy: A review of 98 cases and a report of 8 new cases, *Obstet Gynecol* 28:281, 1973.

Willoughby CP, Truelove SC: Ulcerative colitis and pregnancy, *Gut* 21:469-474, 1980.

Yang H, Rotter JI: The genetics of inflammatory bowel disease. In *Inflammatory bowel disease, from bench to bedside,* pp. 32-64, Baltimore, 1992, Williams & Wilkins.

Zeldis JB: Pregnancy and inflammatory bowel disease, *Western J Med* 151(2):168-171, 1989.

Premature Labor

25

25.1 **PREMATURE LABOR**

Kathy B. Porter, M.D.

Definition

Progressive dilation or effacement of the cervix in the presence of regular uterine contractions; or cervical dilation greater than or equal to 2 cm or cervical effacement of greater than 80% between 20 and 37 weeks gestation with intact membranes

Background

1. Incidence is 5% to 10% of deliveries.
2. Preterm deliveries result in 60% to 85% of perinatal mortality.
3. Complications of pregnancy result in 20% of preterm births.
4. Consequences of preterm birth are listed in the box on p. 680.
5. Clinicians should know the institution's statistics on preterm infant survival rates and national data (Tables 25-1, 25-2, and 25-3).
   a. Respiratory distress syndrome (RDS) is unlikely to occur after 37 weeks.
   b. Patent ductus arteriosus and intraventricular hemorrhage are usually unlikely after 32 weeks.

Symptoms

1. Menstrual cramps
2. Rhythmic low back pain
3. Rhythmic pelvic pressure
4. Change in vaginal discharge
5. Diarrhea

Risk factors

1. Low socioeconomic status (17% to 20%)
2. Urinary tract infections (20%)
3. Hypertensive disorders
4. Heavy smoking
5. History of preterm delivery (50%)
6. Poor nutrition

Consequences of Preterm Birth

Neonatal complications
Respiratory distress syndrome
Patent ductus arteriosus
Necrotizing enterocolitis
Apnea
Bradycardia
Bronchopulmonary dysplasia
Temperature instability
Hyperbilirubinemia
Retinopathy of prematurity
Neurologic deficits
Handicaps
Death

Table 25-1 Neonatal survival by gestational age and birth weight

	Mean (%) Survival Rates (Range) Reported	
Factor	1987-1988	1989-1990
Age (wk)		
23	23 (0-33)	15 (0-29)
24	34 (10-57)	54 (27-100)
25	54 (30-72)	59 (47-74)
Weight (g)		
501-600	21 (0-44)	20 (0-33)
601-700	33 (9-50)	41 (25-56)
701-800	53 (31-73)	65 (38-83)

Data from Hack M et al: Very low birth weight outcomes of the National Institute of Child Health and Human Development Neonatal Network, *Pediatrics* 87:587-597, 1991, and Hack M, Wright LL, Shankaran S: Very-low-birth-weight outcomes of the National Institute of Child Health and Human Development Neonatal Network, November 1989 to October 1990, *Am J Obstet Gynecol* 172:457-464, 1995.

*Rates were reported by the National Institute of Child Health and Human Development neonatal centers.

7. Maternal age <16 or >35 years
8. Premature rupture of membranes
9. History of incompetent cervix
10. Uterine anomalies (3% to 40%)
11. Overdistension of uterus
12. Antepartum bleeding
13. Retained intrauterine device
14. Acute or chronic systemic illness
15. Fetal anomalies (25%)

Table 25-2 Serious morbidities in infants with birth weights <750 g experienced by the NICHD neonatal centers, 1989-1990*

Condition	Frequency (%)	Range (%)
Respiratory distress syndrome	86	80-100
Ventilator support at 28 days†	72	23-100
Chronic lung disease‡	35	8-82
Necrotizing enterocolitis	9	2-19
Septicemia	34	13-50
Grade III intraventricular hemorrhage	13	5-20
Grade IV intraventricular hemorrhage	17	0-24
Seizures	10	2-14
Periventricular leukomalacia	11	7-20

Data from Hack M, Wright LL, Shankaran S: Very-low-birth-weight outcomes of the National Institute of Child Health and Human Development Neonatal Network, November 1989 to October 1990, *Am J Obstet Gynecol* 172:457-464, 1995.

*NICHD indicates the National Institute of Child Health and Human Development.

†Data are for infants alive at 28 days.

‡Data are for survivors.

Table 25-3 The birth weight–specific neonatal mortality for inborn neonates at Tampa General Hospital from July 1, 1993, to June 30, 1994

Weight (g)	<500	500-749	750-999	1000-1499	1500-1999	2000-2499	>2500
Number of newborns	12	27	21	44	83	276	3215
Percentage died	100	56	14	4.5	4.8	0	0.1

16. Abdominal surgery
17. Repeated second trimester abortions
18. Multiple gestations

Prenatal laboratory risks

1. An elevated maternal serum alpha-fetoprotein is associated with increased rate of preterm delivery.
2. Lupus anticoagulant being present increases the risk for preterm delivery and abruption.

Management

Physicians should search for treatable conditions and be aware of the contraindications to labor inhibition.

1. Expectant management
   a. Observation with bed rest, intravenous fluid hydration, and sedation will result in 50% success rate. NOTE: All clinical studies

would require greater than 50% success to perform better than placebo.

b. Continuous external fetal monitoring is indicated.

c. Physician should establish there is no evidence of premature rupture of the membranes by sterile speculum examination.
   (1) Delay of digital cervical examination is indicated until membrane status is confirmed to be intact.
   (2) If rupture of membranes has occurred, digital examination is not performed because infection increases after such an examination.

d. Cervical-vaginal cultures and probes for group B *Streptococcus*, gonorrhea, and *Chlamydia* are performed.

e. Baseline complete blood count (CBC) and urinalysis are performed to evaluate for infectious etiology and to assess maternal hydration status.

f. Chorioamnionitis should be ruled out by looking for maternal and fetal signs or symptoms of infection such as the following:
   (1) Maternal or fetal tachycardia
   (2) Foul or purulent discharge from vagina
   (3) Uterine tenderness
   (4) Maternal fever
   (5) Elevated WBC or a shift in the peripheral smear in the number of polymorphonuclear cells
   (6) Elevation of C-reactive protein on a maternal blood sample

g. Ultrasound is indicated to evaluate gestational age and to rule out anomalies incompatible with tocolysis.

2. Tocolytic management

a. Tocolytic efficacy is usually only 1 to 3 days with the present agents available to clinicians. Thus, tocolytic therapy has not decreased the rate of preterm births or morbidity, but allows for adjunctive therapy such as steroids and thyroid-releasing hormone.

b. Before a tocolytic therapy is begun, absolute contraindications to treatment should be reviewed by the provider:
   (1) Severe pregnancy-induced hypertension
   (2) Severe abruptio placentae
   (3) Severe bleeding
   (4) Chorioamnionitis
   (5) Fetal death
   (6) Fetal anomaly incompatible with life (anencephaly and bilateral renal agenesis are examples)
   (7) Severe intrauterine growth retardation (IUGR)
   (8) Advanced cervical dilation (> 5 cm)
   (9) Gestational age of 37 weeks or greater

c. If the patient is assessed to be in preterm labor then close supervision is warranted in a facility familiar with this form of obstetric management.
   (1) A neonatal intensive care unit should be readily available to accept the newborn if medical treatment fails because tocolytics only delay the delivery, not prevent it.

(2) Recent changes in delivery sites of low–birth-weight infants in Washington have resulted in detrimental effects with increasing preventable mortality at centers not equipped to handle premature infants.

d. When expectant management fails, tocolytic treatment should be considered. All the steps listed under Management, 1, (a through g) should have been completed by the time tocolytic therapy is considered.

e. Ancillary treatments with tocolytics

(1) Glucocorticosteroids benefit the fetus by reducing RDS, necrotizing enterocolitis, intraventricular hemorrhage (IVH), and neonatal morbidity and mortality.

(a) Mechanism is by accelerating lung maturation.

(b) They are indicated between 24 and 34 weeks gestation.

(c) They are equally effective in all races and sexes.

(d) Partial treatment may be helpful to give as soon as possible. The preferred treatment period is 48 hours from the first injection.

(e) Tocolytics are contraindicated if mother is septic or if there is evidence of an intrauterine infection.

(f) Multiple gestations should be treated.

(g) Dose of betamethasone is 12 mg intramuscularly every 24 hours for two doses or dexamethasone, 6 mg, every 6 hours × 8 doses per os.

(h) In summary, fetuses eligible for therapy with tocolytics should also be eligible for treatment with antenatal corticosteroids.

(i) Surfactant therapy is routinely used in the neonatal period and has significantly reduced RDS.

(j) Animal models are promising concerning administering surfactant in utero.

(2) Antibiotics: It is controversial whether adjunctive antibiotics improve tocolytic efficacy.

(a) Dosage for adjunctive antibiotics is, for group B *Streptococcus* prophylaxis, either ampicillin, 2 g every 6 hours, or penicillin, 5 million units, every 6 hours intravenously.

(b) Other organisms and conditions associated with infection risks include *N. gonorrhoea,* bacterial vaginosis, and *Mycoplasma.*

(3) Amniocentesis may be warranted if tocolysis with a single agent fails or if the clinical presentation is suspicious for intraamniotic infection.

(a) Ultrasound guidance is used to obtain amniotic fluid for gram stain, glucose concentration, lung maturity studies, and culture and sensitivity for bacterial organisms. If there is evidence of IUGR or anomalies compatible with life, then karyotype is indicated.

(4) Fetal fibronectin is a protein found in amniotic fluid, placental tissue, or after mechanical or inflammatory mediated damage occurs to membranes.

(a) A swab of the vaginal area is performed to predict delivery.
(b) If the test is negative, the chance for delivery within 7 to 14 days of testing is under 1%.
(c) Thus, those that test positive may need special intervention.

f. Tocolytic agents
(1) Beta-agonists work through the cyclic adenosine monophosphate (AMP) system by inhibiting smooth muscle contraction.
(a) Ritodrine is mixed in D_5W and is given intravenously with 50 μg/min as the initial dose and is increased every 20 minutes until desired response is achieved (maximum rate 350 μg/min). After 60 minutes, effective reduction is begun by 50 μg/min every 30 minutes until the lowest effective dose is achieved.
(b) The following maternal laboratory parameters should be obtained for a baseline and followed subsequently: CBC, electrocardiogram (EKG), potassium levels, glucose concentrations, and urine output.
(c) Total maternal input should be limited to 1500 to 2500 ml/24 hours to reduce iatrogenic pulmonary edema.
(d) Signs of maternal toxicity should be followed: Tachycardia of 130 beats/min, cardiac arrhythmia, myocardial ischemia, hypotension, and pulmonary edema. If these signs or symptoms are noted the beta-agonist should be discontinued.
(e) The contraindications to beta-agonist encompass those listed in 2.b.(1) through (9), and the following:
i. Maternal cardiac disease
ii. Uncontrolled diabetes mellitus
iii. Hyperthyroidism
iv. Hypovolemia
(f) Potential fetal and neonatal side effects
i. Tachycardia, hypoglycemia, hypocalcemia, hypotension, and ileus are common.
ii. A questionable increase in fetal weight and lung maturation acceleration has been reported.
iii. Infants have been followed up to 6 years of age with normal anthropometric measurements, neurologic tests, and general behavior after exposure to beta-agonists.
iv. However, others have reported decreased school performance, which may be related to prematurity and not actually the tocolytic therapy.
v. Further developmental follow-up is indicated.
(g) Once tocolysis is successful, transition to oral therapy is not beneficial based on two randomized trials. These studies demonstrated no significant difference in gestational ages achieved.

(h) Terbutaline, a beta-agonist, is given subcutaneously 250 μg every 3 to 4 hours or can be administered via a pump for long-term tocolysis.
   i. The minimed pump infusion requires demand doses of 0.002 to 0.720 ml with a continuous rate of 0.002 to 0.720 ml/hr.
   ii. The use of the pump is controversial concerning effectiveness.

(2) Magnesium sulfate alters nerve transmission by affecting acetylcholine release and sensitivity at the motor endplate. It is also a known competitive antagonist of calcium.
   (a) Dose: 4 to 6 g loading is given over 20 minutes; then 2 g/hour or more. The lowest effective dose is maintained for 12 hours.
   (b) Common side effects: Chest pain (1.1%), pulmonary edema (1% to 10%), severe nausea or flushing (3.6%), headache, nystagmus, lethargy, dry mouth, diplopia, hypothermia, urticarial reaction, and transient ischemia are seen.
   (c) Following clinical parameters such as maternal reflexes, respiratory rate, and urine output are indicated. If toxicity is suspected then a serum magnesium level is necessary. A therapeutic level is 5 to 8 mg/dl.
   (d) Contraindications include recent myocardial infarction, myasthenia gravis, heart block, and severe renal disease.
   (e) Long-term treatment will decrease maternal and fetal bone density by suppressing the parathyroid gland.
   (f) Perinatal effects include respiratory and motor depression, reduced muscle tone, weakness, decreased fetal variability and respirations, and the potential for long bone demineralization after exposure of 7 days or more to magnesium sulfate. Recent reports have noted a decreased incidence of developmental handicaps in infants exposed to magnesium sulfate.
   (g) If tocolysis fails with magnesium sulfate, the drug is stopped. The serum levels will be reduced to half by 30 minutes, which minimizes perinatal effects.
   (h) Transition to oral magnesium tocolytic therapy has been shown to be ineffective.

(3) Calcium channel blockers inhibit calcium influx into the cell.
   (a) Two types of channels exist, L-type and T-type. The commonly used calcium channel blockers, dihydropridines, operate via the L-type (slow channels); examples include nifedipine, nicardipine, and nitrendipine. Initial dosing may begin with 30 mg orally and be repeated 20 mg every 5 to 8 hours for 3 days.
   (b) The sublingual dose of nifedipine is 10 mg initially, followed by 10 mg every 20 minutes until contractions

cease (up to 40 mg in first hour). Then 20 mg orally is given every 4 to 6 hours. The long-acting forms may be used once inhibition is effective. Nifedipine's effects are reversible after the drug is stopped and it does not induce tachyphylaxis.

(c) Side effects include flushing (5% to 100%), headache, (5% to 40%), nausea, hypotension, hepatotoxicity, transient increase in maternal heart rate, heartburn, fatigue, dyspnea, nervousness, dizziness, tremor, constipation, diarrhea, chest pain, nasal congestion, and potential neuromuscular blockade, and enhanced cardiac toxicity when used in conjunction with magnesium sulfate.

(d) Early work in animal models demonstrated fetal peripheral vasodilation and impaired oxygenation secondary to reduced pulmonary vascular resistance. Human studies have not shown this description.

(e) Elimination of calcium channel blockers occurs through the renal and gastrointestinal, (GI) systems. The clinician should be aware of this to prevent toxicity or lack of effectiveness in those patients when these systems are diseased.

(4) Prostaglandin synthetase inhibitors: Mechanism of action is through inhibition of cyclooxygenease, which reduces myometrial gap junctions and decreases intracellular calcium concentrations.

(a) Indomethacin was the original inhibitor and was given either orally or rectally. The rectal route peaked sooner. A loading dose per rectum was 100 mg with 25 mg, orally, every 6 hours for 48 hours.

(b) Maternal side effects of the inhibitors include postpartum hemorrhage, GI discomfort, and headache. Perinatal side effects include ductus arteriosus constriction, oligohydramnios, and potentially increased incidence of IVH. The half-life of indomethacin is longer in the preterm neonate and is predominantly protein bound (90%).

(c) Studies of prostaglandin synthetase inhibitors to date demonstrate equivalency to beta-agonists.

(d) Sulindac has been reported not to result in oligohydramnios or ductus arteriosus constriction. The dose is 200 mg, orally, every 12 hours for 48 hours.

(e) Ketorolac may also be a promising inhibitor because placenta crossing is less than 25% in animal models. Oral and injectable forms exist, but further research is indicated before this drug is implemented in the clinical setting.

(f) The contraindications to using inhibitors are drug-induced asthma, coagulation disorders, and hepatic or renal insufficiency.

(5) Oxytocin antagonist
   (a) Mechanism: Blockade of oxytocin receptors by binding competitively to the receptors. The resulting effect is a decrease in uterine contractions.
   (b) Oral and infusion forms are available. Limited information is available with contemporary controls.
   (c) No major side effects were noted in preliminary trials.
(6) Lidocaine in an experimental animal model has been reported to inhibit uterine contractions via voltage-gated sodium channels. Research studies are in development in humans. Class 1 cardiac antiarrhythmic agents, such as lidocaine, affect these sodium channels. With some available in oral forms, they are under investigation.
(7) Nitric oxide donors have been reported to relax the uterine smooth muscle but their use remains investigational to date.
   (a) Nitric oxide (NO) donors: Mechanism is uterine smooth muscle relaxation via L-arginine–NO–cyclic glucose monophosphate (cGMP) pathway.
   (b) Limited information on infusion L-arginine in humans in threatened preterm labor demonstrated a decrease in myometrial activity with elevation in serum nitrites and growth hormone levels, indicating NO is involved in the effect. Others have reported using glyceryl trinitrate (a NO donor) with 13 pregnant women, inhibiting and prolonging pregnancy for a mean of 34 days.
   (c) Side effects include headache, hypotension, and uterine atony.
   (d) Acute tocolytic therapy has been reported with nitroglycerin sublingually and intravenously. The dose ranges from 50 to 500 μg. The intravenous dose is 50 to 100 μg. The onset of action is 15 to 90 seconds, with a duration of 120 seconds. Nitroglycerin is unstable and requires sealed dark containers, and skin absorption can occur with direct contact to the tablets.
   (e) Further research is indicated with NO donors; thus these are considered investigational drugs as tocolytics.
(8) Multiple tocolytics
   (a) Caution with the use of multiple tocolytics is indicated secondary to the compounding of complications with the addition of tocolytic agents.
   (b) Indications include gestational ages less than 28 to 30 weeks with the opportunity to administer glucocorticosteroids.
   (c) Combined use of ritodrine (beta-agonist) and magnesium sulfate has been reported in 20- to 35-week gestations with success rates of 59%, versus 34% in those pregnancies exposed to multiple agents and a single agent, respectively ($p < 0.05$).

(d) Meticulous fluid restriction and evaluation of clinical signs and symptoms of infection are mandatory to prevent maternal morbidity. Total fluid administration of 100 ml/hr with either D_5W or 0.25% normal saline are required to prevent maternal pulmonary edema. Amniocentesis should be considered to rule out infection before multiple tocolytics are initiated.

(9) Consideration by clinicians of any tocolytic require detailed maternal and fetal surveillance in a center experienced in managing the consequences of a preterm birth. Neonatal long-term follow-up is needed to provide clinicians with information on final outcomes in those fetuses exposed to tocolytics.

Other concerns

1. Maternal prenatal stress
   a. Maternal stress has been reported to result in a 55.3-g reduction in fetal weight.
   b. Maternal stress has an odds ratio of affecting low birth weight by 1.32.
   c. An increase in prenatal pregnancy anxiety may be associated with a 3-day decrease in gestational age at birth, which would be important when using glucocorticoids for lung maturation.

Successful management

1. Limited information is available on the effectiveness and safety of repetitive steroid dosing.
   a. Clinical studies are in process and will provide insight into this management.
   b. The decision to administer steroids every 7 days is at the discretion of the provider until these studies are completed.
2. Long-term use of supplemental antibiotics has not been proved effective based on the NICHD and maternal-fetal medicine (MFMU) Network.
   a. However, use of adjunctive antibiotics for group B beta-hemolytic *Streptococcus* prophylaxis is effective in reducing perinatal complications of streptococcal infection.
   b. Long-term use of antibiotics is not indicated.
3. The administration of vitamin K and phenobarbital to the mother has been shown to be ineffective in preventing the consequences of prematurity such as IVH.
   a. However, magnesium sulfate appears to be protective against IVH in very low–birth weight infants (< 1500 g), resulting in lower rates of cerebral palsy.
   b. Further studies are indicated in this exciting area.
4. Thyrotropin-releasing hormone, in the largest prospective randomized trial to date, was not effective in reducing RDS and the other consequences of prematurity.
5. Primary prevention has not been effective when using risk screening protocols.

a. Secondary prevention includes home uterine activity monitoring (HUAM), serial cervical sonography, and antepartum fetal fibronectin [2.e.(4)].
b. HUAM does not work effectively based on numerous studies
c. HUAM is expensive and is not indicated until further trials prove otherwise.
d. The ACOG contends that HUAM should remain investigational based on the difficulty of identifying suitable candidates and the lack of supporting clinical data.
e. Serial cervical sonography remains investigational.

6. Preparing the family for a preterm delivery is necessary. Opportunities for the family to consult with a neonatologist before delivery often allay anxiety.
7. Limiting maternal activity is commonly recommended, but not uniformly by all providers. The benefits of long-term bedrest are questionable.

When preterm birth is inevitable

1. The physician should stop tocolytic therapy to reduce perinatal side effects of the agents.
2. Continuous fetal electronic monitoring should be maintained because preterm infants have inadequate reserves and are susceptible to hypoxia. Umbilical cord gas studies after delivery are often obtained because Apgar scores may be reduced secondary to prematurity.
3. Plan for a vaginal delivery (26 to 32 weeks) unless in the breech presentation; then cesarean section is indicated because of the concerns of head entrapment, nuchal arms, hyperflexed heads, and inexperience with vaginal breech deliveries.
   a. At gestational ages less than 26 weeks, the route of delivery may be vaginal because these risk factors are less likely to occur.
4. The neonatologist should be notified of the imminent delivery.
5. Antibiotic prophylaxis should be continued for group B *Streptococcus* as described earlier.
6. Analgesic pain relief with epidurals and narcotics must be closely monitored because deliveries may be rapid.
7. Routine use of outlet forcep and episiotomy are not justified.
8. Emotional support to the mother and her family members are especially needed.

Summary

The patient who presents in preterm labor requires extensive evaluation and surveillance. The early involvement of the neonatologist in the team often reduces maternal concerns. Innovative therapies are continually being developed to reduce maternal and fetal risks and improve neonatal outcomes.

Suggested reading

ACTOBAT Study Group: Australian collaborative trial of antenatal thyrotropin-releasing hormone (ACTOBAT) for prevention of neonatal respiratory disease, *Lancet* 345:877-882, 1995.

Allen MC, Donohue PK, Dusman AE: The limit of viability—neonatal outcome of infants born at 22 to 25 weeks' gestation, *N Engl J Med,* 329:1597-1601, 1993.

American College of Obstetricians and Gynecologists: *Ethical decision-making in obstetrics and gynecology,* ACOG Technical Bulletin 136, Washington, DC, 1989, ACOG.

Benisty A et al: Constriction of the fetal ductus arteriosus during prenatal betamethasone therapy, *Obstet Gynecol* 85:874-876, 1995.

Canadian Preterm Labor Investigators Group: Treatment of preterm labor with the beta-adrenergic agonist ritodrine, *N Engl J Med* 327:308-312, 1992.

Carlan SJ et al: Outpatient oral sulindac to prevent recurrence of preterm labor, *Obstet Gynecol* 85:769-774, 1995.

Carlan SJ et al: Randomized comparative trial of indomethacin and sulindac for the treatment of refractory preterm labor, *Obstet Gynecol* 79:223-228, 1992.

Childress CH, Katz VL: Nifedipine and its indications in obstetrics and gynecology, *Obstet Gynecol* 83:616-624, 1994.

Committee on Obstetric Practice, American College of Obstetricians and Gynecologists: *Antenatal corticosteroid therapy for fetal maturation,* ACOG Committee Opinion No. 147, December 1994.

Creasy RK: Preterm labor and delivery. In Creasy RK, Resnik R, editors: *Maternal-fetal medicine: principles and practice,* ed 3, Philadelphia, 1994, WB Saunders.

Dyson DC, Crites YM, Ray DA: Prevention of preterm birth in high risk patients: the role of education and provider contact versus home uterine monitoring, *Am J Obstet Gynecol* 164:756-762, 1991.

Eden RD, Boehm FH, editors: *Assessment & care of the fetus: physiological, clinical and mediocolegal principles,* Norwalk, CT, 1990, Appleton & Lange.

Ehrenhaft PM, Wagner JL, Herdman RC: Changing prognosis for very low birth weight infants, *Obstet Gynecol* 74:528-535, 1989.

Elliott JP, Radin TG: The effect of corticosteroid administration on uterine activity and preterm labor in high-order multiple gestations, *Obstet Gynecol* 85:250-254, 1995.

Gabbe SG, Niebyl Jr, Simpson JL, editors: *Obstetrics: normal and problem pregnancies,* New York, 1986, Churchill Livingstone.

Galan HL et al: Surfactant replacement therapy in utero for prevention of hyaline membrane disease in the preterm baboon, *Am J Obstet Gynecol* 169:817-824, 1993.

Gardner MO et al: Predicting low Apgar scores of infants weighing less than 1000 grams: the effect of corticosteroids, *Obstet Gynecol* 85:170-174, 1995.

Goodwin T et al: The effect of the oxytocin antagonist atosiban on preterm uterine activity in the human, *Am J Obstet Gynecol* 170:474-478, 1994.

Gray SE et al: Effect of intravenous magnesium sulfate on the biophysical profile of the healthy preterm fetus, *Am J Obstet Gynecol* 170:1131-1135, 1994.

Hack M, Fanaroff AA: Outcomes of extremely-low-birth-weight infants between 1982 and 1988, *N Engl J Med* 321:1642-1647, 1989.

Hack M et al: Very low birth weight outcomes of the National Institute of Child Health and Human Development Neonatal Network, *Pediatrics* 87:587-597, 1991.

Hack M et al: School-age outcomes in children with birth weights under 750 g, *N Engl J Med* 331:753-759, 1994.

Hack M et al: Very-low-birth weight outcomes of the National Institute of Child Health and Human Development Neonatal Network, November 1989 to October 1990, *Am J Obstet Gynecol* 172:457-464, 1995.

Hadlock FP et al: Estimation of fetal weight with the use of head, body and femur measurements—a prospective study, *Am J Obstet Gynecol* 151:333-337, 1985.

Hatjis CG et al: Efficacy of combined administration of magnesium sulfate and ritodrine in the treatment of premature labor, *Obstet Gynecol* 69:317-322, 1987.

Hauth JC et al: Reduced incidence of preterm delivery with metronidazole and erythromycin in women with bacterial vaginosis, *N Engl J Med* 333:1732-1736, 1995.

Hedegaard M et al: Psychological distress in pregnancy and preterm delivery, *Br Med J* 307:234-239, 1993.
Higby K, Xenakis EM, Pauerstein CJ: Do tocolytic agents stop preterm labor? A critical and comprehensive review of efficacy and safety, *Am J Obstet Gynecol* 168:1247-1259, 1993.
Hill WC et al: Home uterine activity monitoring is associated with a reduction in preterm birth, *Obstet Gynecol* 76:13S-18S, 1990.
Hillier SL et al: Association between bacterial vaginosis and preterm delivery of a low-birth-weight infant, *N Engl J Med* 333:1737-1742, 1995.
Iams JD, Johnson FF, O'Shaughnessy RW: A prospective random trial of home uterine activity monitoring in pregnancies at risk of preterm labor, *Am J Obstet Gynecol* 159:595-603, 1988.
Janke J: Use of terbutaline sulfate in a subcutaneous infusion pump to treat preterm labor, *Nurse Practitioner* 18:33-40, 1993.
Kao C, Wang S: Effects of lidocaine on rat myometrial sodium channels and implications for the management of preterm labor, *Am J Obstet Gynecol* 171:446-454, 1994.
Kitchen W et al: Cesarean section or vaginal delivery at 24 to 28 weeks' gestation: Comparison of survival and neonatal and two-year morbidity, *Obstet Gynecol* 66:149-157, 1985.
Knight DB, Liggins GC, Wealthall SR: A randomized, controlled trial of antepartum thyrotropin-releasing hormone and betamethasone in the prevention of respiratory disease in preterm infants, *Am J Obstet Gynecol* 171:11-16, 1994.
Lamm CI et al: Congenital rickets associated with magnesium sulfate infusion for tocolysis, *J Pediatr* 113:1078-1082, 1988.
Lantos JD et al: Providing and forgoing resuscitative therapy for babies of very low birth weight, *J Clin Ethics* 3:283-287, 1992.
Lockwood CJ et al: Fetal fibronectin in cervical and vaginal secretions as a predictor of preterm delivery, *N Engl J Med* 325:669-674,1991.
Macones M, Berlin M, Berlin JA: Efficacy of oral beta-agonist maintenance therapy in preterm labor: A meta-analysis, *Obstet Gynecol* 85:313-317, 1995.
Malloy MH, Onstad L, Wright E: The effect of cesarean delivery on birth outcome in very low birth weight infants. National Institute of Child Health and Human Development Neonatal Research Network, *Obstet Gynecol* 77:498-503, 1991.
Malloy MH et al: Increasing cesarean section rates in very low-birth weight infants. Effect on outcome, *JAMA* 262:1475-1478, 1989.
Martin RW et al: Oral magnesium and the prevention of preterm labor in a high-risk group of patients, *Am J Obstet Gynecol* 166:144-147, 1992.
Melsen NC, Noreng MF: Epidural blockade in the treatment of preterm labour, *Anesthesia* 43:126-127, 1988.
Moise KJ et al: Continuous subcutaneous terbutaline pump therapy for premature labor: safety and efficacy, *So Med J* 85:255-260, 1992.
Morales WJ et al: Fetal lung maturation: the combined use of corticosteroids and thyrotropin-releasing hormone, *Obstet Gynecol* 73:111-116, 1989.
Morales WJ et al: Efficacy and safety of indomethacin versus ritodrine in the management of preterm labor: a randomized study, *Obstet Gynecol* 74:567-572, 1989.
Mou SM et al: Multicenter randomized clinical trial of home uterine activity monitoring for detection of preterm labor, *Am J Obstet Gynecol* 165:858-866, 1991.
Neri I et al: Impact of the L-arginine/nitric oxide system in pregnancy, *Obstet Gynecol Surv* 50:851-858, 1995.
NIH Consensus Development Panel on the Effect of Corticosteroids for Fetal Maturation on Perinatal Outcomes: Effect of corticosteroids for fetal maturation on perinatal outcomes, *JAMA* 273:413-418, 1995.
Nuwayhid B, Rajabi M: Beta-sympathomimetic agents: use in perinatal obstetrics. *Clin Perinatol* 14:757-782, 1987.

Parilla BV et al: The efficacy of oral terbutaline after intravenous tocolysis, *Am J Obstet Gynecol* 169:965-969, 1993.
Parsons MT, Wilson L: Oxytocin antagonists. In *Clinical consultations in obstetrics & gynecology,* vol 3, pp. 255-259, Philadelphia, 1991, WB Saunders.
Powell SL et al: Recent changes in delivery site of low-birth-weight infants in Washington: impact on birth weight-specific mortality, *Am J Obstet Gynecol* 173:1585-1592, 1995.
Rauk PN, Laifer SA: The prostaglandin synthesis inhibitor ketorolac blocks ritodrine-stimulated production of prostaglandin $F_{2\alpha}$ in pregnant sheep, *obstet Gynecol* 81:323-326, 1993.
Rhoden NK: Treating Baby Doe: the ethics of uncertainty, *Hastings Cent Rep* 16 (4):34-42, 1986.
Ricci JM et al: Oral tocolysis with magnesium chloride: a randomized controlled prospective clinical trial, *Am J Obstet Gynecol* 165:603-610, 1991.
Smith LG, Burns PA, Schanler RJ: Calcium homeostasis in pregnant women receiving long-term magnesium sulfate therapy for preterm labor, *Am J Obstet Gynecol* 167:45-51, 1992.
Stanton RJ: Comanagement of the patient on subcutaneous terbutaline pump therapy, *J Nurse Midwifery* 36:204-208, 1991.
Stein HM et al: The effects of corticosteroids and thyrotropin-releasing hormone on newborn adaptation and sympathoadrenal mechanisms in preterm sheep, *Am J Obstet Gynecol* 171; 17-24, 1994.
Thorp JA et al: Antepartum vitamin K and phenobarbital for preventing intraventricular hemorrhage in the premature newborn: a randomized double-blind, placebo-controlled trial, *Obstet Gynecol* 83:70-76, 1994.
Worthington D et al: Factors influencing survival and morbidity with very low birth weight delivery, *Obstet Gynecol* 62:550-555, 1983.

25.2 PREMATURE RUPTURE OF MEMBRANES

Jonathan W. Weeks, M.D.

Definitions

1. The terms *premature rupture of membranes* (PROM) and *premature amniorrhexis* describe the disruption of the chorioamniotic membrane before the onset of labor.
2. When disruption of the chorioamniotic membrane occurs before 37 weeks gestation, the terms *preterm PROM* (PPROM) or *preterm premature amniorrhexis* are used.
3. When the duration of premature amniorrhexis exceeds 24 hours, the term *prolonged rupture of membranes* is used.
4. The term *latency period* refers to the time interval from amniorrhexis to the onset of labor.

Prevalence

1. Premature rupture of membranes complicates 10% of term gestations and 4% of preterm gestations.
2. Preterm PROM causes approximately one third of all premature deliveries and is a leading cause of perinatal morbidity and mortality.
3. Economically disadvantaged women, unwed women, teenagers, and cigarette smokers are disproportionately affected.

4. Other risk factors include a history of sexually transmitted disease, bacterial vaginosis, and a history of vaginal bleeding during the antenatal period.
5. A history of PPROM in a previous pregnancy is an important, but often overlooked, risk factor.
6. Asrat and others[2] found that 32% of patients with histories of PPROM in the past had a recurrence in subsequent pregnancies.
7. It is important to note that the absence of risk factors does not confer absolute protection.

PROM and PPROM

1. The fetal membranes and amniotic fluid serve several critical functions during normal fetal growth and maturation.
   a. The fluid-filled enclosure provides an environment for fetal movement and musculoskeletal development.
   b. Fetal respiratory efforts produce a "to and fro" movement of amniotic fluid within the fetal respiratory tract, promoting the development of the alveolar sacs.
   c. The membranes also serve as a barrier to separate the sterile environment of the fetus from the polymicrobial vaginal flora.
2. Hence, whether PROM occurs at term or preterm, the risk of adverse perinatal outcome is high because of the unfavorable mechanical and microbiological effects on the products of conception.

Complications

1. PROM is associated with an increased likelihood of premature labor (if PPROM occurs), chorioamnionitis, endometritis, and fetal stress or asphyxia.
2. The first three complications are the result of microbial invasion of the amniotic cavity and inflammation of the chorioamniotic membranes.
   a. The incidence of chorioamnionitis is inversely related to gestational age.
   b. Hillier[8] found histologic chorioamnionitis in 100% of cases at ≤26 weeks, 70% of cases at ≤30 weeks, and 60% of cases at ≤32 weeks.
3. The rate of positive amniotic fluid cultures in women who are evaluated by amniocentesis shortly after admission is 15% to 40%. The yield is highest when the fluid is sent for anaerobic cultures, *Mycoplasma,* and *Ureaplasma* as well as the usual aerobic cultures.
4. Fetal stress or asphyxia may result from prolonged or repeated umbilical cord compression in association with oligohydramnios or cord prolapse.
5. Moreover, when very preterm PROM occurs and oligohydramnios is prolonged, fetal deformations can occur, including pulmonary hypoplasia, Potter's facies, and limb deformities.

Initial evaluation

1. Whenever a patient reports "a gush of fluid," persistent or repeated vaginal leaking, or unusual vaginal dampness, the diagnosis of PROM must be considered.

Table 25-4 Initial evaluation of patients with suspected PPROM

Evaluation Goal	Tests/Methods
Confirm amniorrhexis	Speculum examination for pooling of fluid in the posterior fornix, sample from posterior fornix to be tested for pH (nitrazine) and ferning
Rule out active labor	Speculum examination for cervical dilation, tocodynamometry
Evaluate fetal status	Fetal heart rate (FHR) monitoring, sonogram for gestational age, presentation, estimated weight, and amniotic fluid volume
Rule out infection and group B *Streptococcus* (GBS) colonization	Collection of cervical swabs for gonorrhea and *Chlamydia,* lower vaginal swab for GBS, CBC, amniocentesis

2. The general goals of the initial evaluation are to do the following:
   a. Confirm the diagnosis
   b. Assess the fetal status
   c. Determine whether the patient is in active labor
   d. Rule out infection (Table 25-4).
3. A digital vaginal examination should not be a part of the initial evaluation.
   a. Recent studies have shown that a digital vaginal examination before the onset of active labor is associated with an increased incidence of neonatal infection and shortening of the latency period.
   b. Over 10 years ago Schutte[15] reported an association between the interval from vaginal examination to delivery and the risk of neonatal infection. He reported that infants delivering more than 24 hours after a vaginal examination were infected in 33% of cases.
   c. Adoni and others[1] randomized PPROM patients to initial evaluation by speculum or digital vaginal examination. They found that the latency period was significantly longer when digital examination was avoided (9.5 vs. 3.1 days).
   d. Lewis and others[10] in a recent prospective study also demonstrated a prolongation of gestation (11.3 vs. 2.1 days) when digital examinations were avoided.
4. A speculum examination should be done instead of a digital examination, even if the patient is felt to be in early labor.
   a. Speculum examination is clearly sufficient to rule out advanced cervical dilation.

b. In fact, adequate correlation of speculum to digital examination for assessment of cervical dilation has been reported[5,12] in patients with PPROM.

5. Because subclinical intraamniotic infection is common and a major source of morbidity for the mother and fetus, it is important to evaluate the patient for signs and symptoms of infection.
   a. Overt infection with maternal fever, tachycardia, uterine tenderness, and purulent, foul-smelling vaginal discharge indicates late-stage, advanced infection.
   b. In an attempt to make an earlier diagnosis, several other tests have been advocated.
      (1) A steady upward trend in white blood cell count or C-reactive protein may occur in the early stages of infection.
      (2) However, these laboratory tests are relatively nonspecific.
      (3) They may also increase under the influence of antenatal steroids.
6. Amniocentesis remains the most direct and sensitive way to detect intraamniotic infection.
   a. Many level III perinatal centers have implemented routine amniocentesis in cases of PPROM to rule out microbial invasion of the amniotic cavity before expectant management or tocolysis is employed.
   b. The fluid is sent for cell count, glucose level, gram stain, *Ureaplasma, Mycoplasma,* and aerobic and anaerobic cultures.
   c. Amniotic fluid can be successfully retrieved in 49% to 96% of cases.
   d. The lower success rates are reported by clinicians who do not attempt sampling in patients with anterior placentas or oligohydramnios.
   e. Complications attributable to amniocentesis are low (1%) and no investigators have experienced a fetal loss or significant injury secondary to the procedure when used for evaluation of PROM.[4,6,7,13,14]

Management near term (> 36 weeks)

1. Spontaneous labor will begin by 12 hours in 50%, by 24 hours in 70%, and by 48 hours in 90% of cases.
2. Unfortunately, the risk of chorioamnionitis is also proportional to the duration of the latency period (from 2% at <12 hours to 24% at 24 hours).
3. Although some investigators have advocated expectant management to avoid the increased risk of cesarean delivery associated with labor induction, expectant management should generally be limited to 12 hours or less.
4. The initial cervical examination should be limited to an inspection by speculum when expectant management is anticipated.
5. In such cases, Leopold maneuvers should be performed to ensure a vertex presentation, followed by a limited sonogram when there is uncertainty.

6. Patients with a vertex presentation and a reactive admission nonstress test may be allowed to ambulate.
7. Expectant management is ill advised in patients with GBS colonization, meconium-stained amniotic fluid, hypertension, fetal compromise (e.g., abnormal fetal heart rate, IUGR), or immunocompromise.
8. When a patient is known to be GBS colonized, prophylaxis should be started at admission. Otherwise, prophylaxis should be started by 6 hours after amniorrhexis if labor has not ensued and by 12 hours for patients who are in labor, but have not yet delivered.

Management of preterm gestations (< 36 weeks)

1. Management of PPROM requires a circumspect evaluation of mother and fetus to balance the risks of prematurity against the risks of infection (Table 25-5).
2. Generally, pregnancies of 34 weeks gestation or less should be transferred to a level III perinatal center unless pulmonary maturity can be documented by one of several rapid tests (e.g., foam stability index > 47, PG slide test).
3. In cases where the fetal lung maturity is absent, several medical interventions have been advocated.
   a. Antenatal steroids have been extensively studied and a recent NIH consensus conference recommended their use in patients with PPROM at less than 32 weeks in the absence of chorioamnionitis.
4. Prophylactic antibiotics have consistently been shown to extend the latency period.
   a. Ampicillin and erythromycin have been used most frequently.
   b. Most studies have shown only a modest increase in gestational age (3 to 4 days) and little or no improvement in neonatal morbidity or mortality.
   c. Broader spectrum antibiotics such as ampicillin-sulfactam may be more efficacious.
   d. The most cost effective prophylaxis regimen has yet to be established.
5. Tocolysis has proved to be ineffective at extending gestation or improving neonatal outcome.
   a. At the University of Louisville, How and others[9] conducted a prospective randomized study of aggressive $MgSO_4$ tocolysis versus no tocolysis for PPROM.
      (1) All patients received prophylactic antibiotics and glucocorticoids.
      (2) Over 130 patients were studied.
      (3) No improvement in gestational age at delivery or perinatal outcome was found.
   b. Given the potential for severe maternal complications with aggressive tocolysis and the trend toward an increase in chorioamnionitis it is my opinion that aggressive tocolysis has no place in the routine management of PPROM.
   c. Aggressive tocolysis may be appropriate in cases where amniocentesis has been used to rule out microbial invasion of the amniotic cavity.

Table 25-5 Management of PROM (level II perinatal center)

Term	32 to 36 wk	24 to 31 wk	<24 wk
Speculum examination, electronic fetal monitoring, pitocin induction if not in labor in 6 to 12 hours or immediately, GBS prophylaxis if not in labor in 6 hours or delivered in 12 hours	Speculum examination and cultures, inpatient care through delivery, electronic fetal monitoring, amniocentesis for maturity and infection studies (vaginal pool studies if amniocentesis is not an option), deliver if mature or MIAC, steroids if immature, prophylactic antibiotics	Speculum examination and cultures, inpatient care through delivery, electronic fetal monitoring, amniocentesis for maturity and infection studies (vaginal pool studies if amniocentesis is not an option), deliver if mature; if MIAC without overt infection or labor, consider delivery 48 hours after steroids if fetus is >1500 g, or aerobic and anaerobic antimicrobials with repeat amnio in 48 to 72 hours, deliver if labor or overt infection	Speculum examination and cultures, discuss termination versus expectant management, 24 hours observation for infection, weekly outpatient follow-up (examination, AFI, CBC), readmission at >24 weeks, begin prophylactic antibiotics after viability

Management of PPROM in patients with a cervical cerclage

1. On occasion, patients who have undergone cervical cerclage in the late first or early second trimester experience preterm amniorrhexis the early third trimester.
2. The timing of cerclage removal in such cases has been somewhat controversial.
   a. Theoretically, early removal could result in a decreased latency period.
   b. However, because the suture is a foreign body in a colonized milieu, delayed removal could result in an increased risk of chorioamnionitis.
   c. Two studies[3,16] have shown that when the cerclage is promptly removed after PPROM, the latency period is similar to that of patients without a cerclage who experience PPROM.
   d. Moreover, Ludmir and others[11] found that neonatal sepsis and perinatal mortality was increased when cerclage removal was delayed.
3. The aforementioned studies notwithstanding, the benefit of mechanical reinforcement of the cervix would be of little benefit once the patient is admitted and at bed rest.
4. Prompt removal after PPROM seems to be the best course of action.

References

1. Adoni A et al: Prolongation of the latent period in patients with premature rupture of the membranes by avoiding digital vaginal examination, *Int J Gynecol Obstet* 32:1921, 1990.
2. Asrat T et al: Rate of recurrence of preterm premature rupture of membranes in consecutive pregnancies, *Am J Obstet Gynecol* 165:1111-1115, 1991.
3. Blickstein I, Katz Z, Lancet M: The outcome of pregnancies complicated by preterm rupture of membranes with and without cerclage, *Int J Gynaecol Obstet* 28:237-242, 1989.
4. Broekhuizen FF, Gilman M, Hamilton PR: Amniocentesis for gram stain and culture in preterm premature rupture of the membranes, *Obstet Gynecol* 66: 316, 1985.
5. Brown C et al: Cervical dilation: accuracy of visual and digital examinations, *Obstet Gynecol* 81:215-216, 1993.
6. Cotton DB et al: Use of amniocentesis in preterm gestation with ruptured membranes, *Obstet Gynecol* 63:38, 1984.
7. Feinstein SJ et al: Amniocentesis with premature rupture of membranes, *Obstet Gynecol* 68:147, 1986.
8. Hillier SL et al: A case-control study of chorioamniotic infection and histologic chorioamnionitis in prematurity, *N Engl J Med* 131:972-978, 1988.
9. How H et al: Preterm premature rupture of membranes: aggressive tocolysis versus expectant management, *Am J Obstet Gynecol* 174:306, 1996.
10. Lewis D et al: Effects of digital vaginal examinations on latency period in preterm premature rupture of membranes, *Obstet Gynecol* 80:630-634, 1992.
11. Ludmir J et al: Poor perinatal outcome associated with retained cerclage in patients with premature rupture of membranes, *Obstet Gynecol* 84:823-826, 1994.
12. Munson L et al: Is there a need for digital examination in patients with spontaneous rupture of the membranes? *Am J Obstet Gynecol* 153:562-563, 1985.
13. Romero R, Emamian M, Quintero R: The value and limitations of the gram stain examination in the diagnosis of intra-amniotic infection, *Am J Obstet Gynecol* 159:114, 1988.

14. Romero R, Quintero R, Oyarzun E: Intra-amniotic infection and the onset of labor in preterm rupture of the membranes, *Am J Obstet Gynecol* 159:661, 1988.
15. Schutte M et al: Management of premature rupture of membranes: the risk of vaginal examination to the infant, *Am J Obstet Gynecol* 146:395-400, 1983.
16. Yeast J, Garite T: The role of cervical cerclage in the management of preterm premature rupture of membranes, *Am J Obstet Gynecol* 158:106-110, 1988.

26 Genetics

26.1 ABNORMAL TRIPLE MARKER SCREENING

Brad Angle, M.D., and Gail Williams, M.D.

The object of a screening test is to identify, among a large population, a small group that is at sufficiently increased risk for certain disorders to warrant offering specific diagnostic tests. Maternal serum marker screening has become a routine component of modern obstetric management as a noninvasive method of identifying pregnancies at risk for a variety of fetal disorders.

Maternal serum alpha-fetoprotein (MSAFP) testing has been used to identify pregnancies at increased risk for fetal neural tube defects (NTDs) since the 1970s. The use of MSAFP screening expanded in the 1980s to include identification of pregnancies at risk for Down's syndrome. More recently, additional serum markers, unconjugated estriol (uE_3) and human chorionic gonadotropin (HCG), have been included in a "triple marker" screening test to improve the detection rate of chromosome abnormalities and possibly to identify other pregnancies at risk for adverse outcomes.

Physiology of alpha-fetoprotein (AFP)

1. AFP is synthesized in the fetal liver and yolk sac.
2. AFP is the major serum protein early in fetal life.
3. Functional role during fetal development is uncertain.
4. Concentration in fetal serum peaks at the end of the first trimester (Fig. 26-1, *a*).
   a. Fetal liver continues to produce AFP at a constant rate.
   b. Increasing fetal blood volume results in dilution and decrease in concentration after the first trimester.
5. AFP is filtered by the fetal kidney and appears in amniotic fluid, which is largely composed of fetal urine.
   a. Peak concentration of amniotic fluid AFP (AFAFP) occurs at about 12 weeks gestation.
   b. It decreases by approximately 10% per week during the second trimester (Fig. 26-1, *b*).
6. Some fetal AFP may reach maternal circulation by the following:
   a. Diffusion across the placenta (70%)
   b. Diffusion across the amnion (30%)

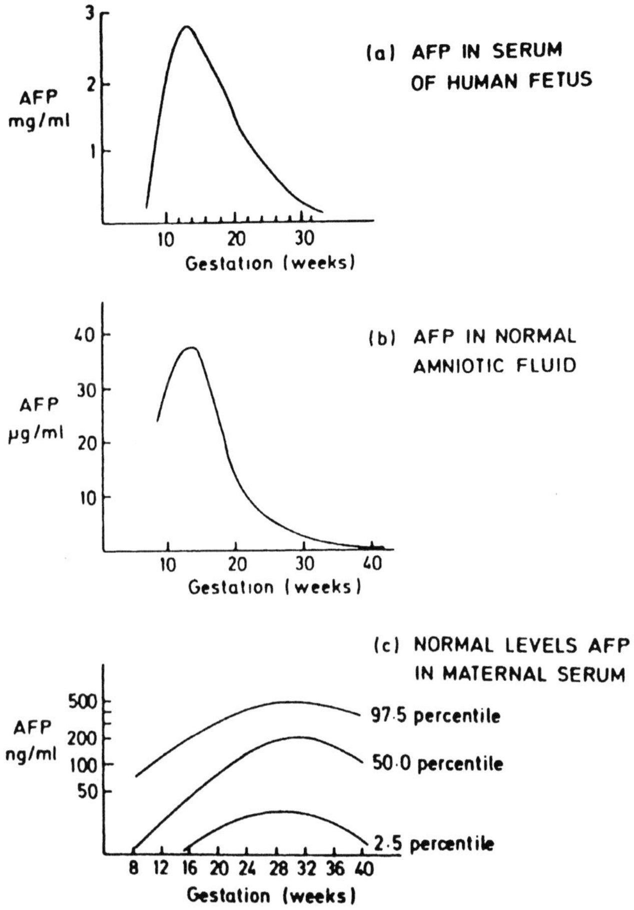

Figure 26-1
The relationship between alpha-fetoprotein levels in **(a)** fetal serum, **(b)** amniotic fluid, and **(c)** maternal serum. (From Milunsky A, editor: *Genetic disorders of the fetus,* Baltimore, 1992, Johns Hopkins University Press.)

7. MSAFP concentration (0.02 μg/ml) is approximately five orders of magnitude lower than fetal serum (2000 μ/ml).
   a. Placental and amniotic barriers between fetus and mother allow only a small fraction of fetally derived AFP to reach maternal circulation.

   b. Greater volume of maternal blood further dilutes the AFP concentration.
8. MSAFP levels increase approximately 15% per week during the second trimester and fall after the 30th week (Fig. 26-1, *c*)
9. Paradoxical rise in maternal serum as levels decrease in fetal serum and amniotic fluid results from increased diffusion caused by the following:
   a. Enlarging placental and amniotic surface areas
   b. Increasing placental permeability

Clinical aspects of MSAFP measurements

1. Patient sampling
   a. MSAFP screening may be obtained between 15 and 20 completed weeks of pregnancy.
   b. Optimal time of testing is at 16 to 18 weeks for greatest sensitivity.
   c. MSAFP testing should not be performed after invasive procedures (e.g., amniocentesis), which may give rise to MSAFP elevations.
2. Reporting of measurements
   a. Results are expressed as a multiple of the unaffected population median.
   b. The absolute concentration of MSAFP is converted to a multiple of median (MoM), which relates it to the median in normal pregnancies at the same gestational age.

$$\text{MoM} = \text{Measured MSAFP} \div \text{Median MSAFP for gestational age}$$

   c. The median MSAFP value for each week of gestation is designated as 1.0 MoM (e.g., MSAFP concentration twice that of population median = 2.0 MoM)
   d. Accuracy of gestational dating is critical because MSAFP levels normally rise during the second trimester.
      (1) If actual gestational age is further advanced than estimated, then MSAFP MoM will appear higher than the true value.
      (2) If actual gestational age is less advanced than estimated, then MSAFP MoM will appear lower than the true value.
3. MoM values are adjusted to account for several factors that affect MSAFP levels.
   a. Race
      (1) MSAFP levels in African-Americans are approximately 15% higher than in Caucasians.
      (2) Lack of correction results in falsely elevated MSAFP MoM values in the African-American population.
   b. Weight
      (1) MSAFP levels decrease with increasing maternal weight as a result of dilutional effects of larger maternal blood volumes.
      (2) Lack of correction results in falsely low MSAFP MoM values in heavier women.
   c. Maternal diabetes
      (1) Insulin-dependent diabetes mellitus is associated with MSAFP levels 20% to 40% lower than nondiabetic women.

(2) Lack of correction results in falsely low MSAFP MoM values in diabetic women.

MSAFP screening for neural tube defects

1. Neural tube defects result from the failure of fusion of the neural tube at 20 to 24 days after fertilization.
2. Population incidence of NTDs is 1/1000 to 2/1000 in the United States.
3. The severity of the defects range from anencephaly (absence of forebrain and cranial bones) to spina bifida (myelomeningocele).
4. "Open" neural tube defects are associated with exposed membrane and blood vessels, allowing AFP to leak into amniotic fluid and subsequently diffuse into the maternal circulation.
   a. Anencephaly and 90% of cases of spina bifida are open defects, with complete exposure of neural tissue to amniotic fluid or separation by only a thin membrane.
   b. The larger the exposed surface area, the more AFP diffuses.
      (1) Anencephaly, which has a larger exposed surface, on average, than open spina bifida (OSB), results in higher amniotic fluid AFP and MSAFP levels.
      (2) Median MSAFP approximately 6.5-fold higher than normal with anencephaly and 3.8-fold higher with OSB (Fig. 26-2).
5. Ten percent of spina bifida lesions are "closed" (covered by a thick membrane) and not identifiable by MSAFP screening.
6. Considerable overlap between MSAFP levels in affected and unaffected pregnancies (see Fig. 26-2).
7. No level of MSAFP can be selected as a screening cutoff that will completely separate unaffected from affected pregnancies.
8. Most screening programs use MSAFP cutoff point of 2.0 or 2.5 MoM (MSAFP level 2 or 2.5 times higher than normal median values).
   a. Each cutoff point represents a compromise between maximizing detection rate and minimizing false-positive rate.
      (1) Cutoff of 2.0 MoM detects 93% of anencephaly and 85% of OSB with a 4% false-positive rate.
      (2) Cutoff of 2.5 MoM detects 89% of anencephaly and 75% of OSB with a 2% false-positive rate.
9. Individual risks based on MSAFP MoM values are commonly reported and used to counsel patients in decision-making process concerning options for further diagnostic evaluation (Table 26-1).
10. MSAFP concentrations are usually higher in multiple gestation pregnancies than in singleton pregnancies, approximately in proportion to the number of fetuses (e.g., median MSAFP MoM in twin pregnancies is approximately 2.0).
    a. Data are available to estimate individual risks for women with twin pregnancies.

Other fetal anomalies associated with elevated MSAFP

1. Ventral wall defects
   a. Elevated MSAFP levels may be associated with open ventral wall defects that allow increased diffusion of fetal AFP into amniotic fluid and maternal serum.

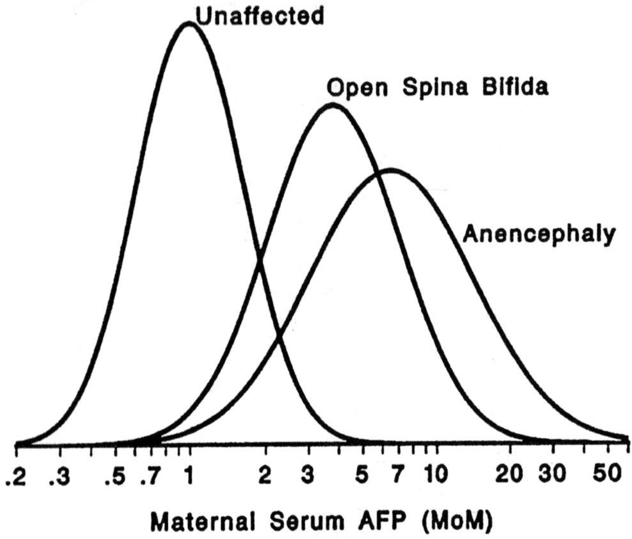

Figure 26-2
Distribution of maternal serum AFP concentrations, expressed as multiple of median (MoM), in normal fetuses, fetuses with open spina bifida, and fetuses with anencephaly.

Table 26-1 Individual odds for having a fetus with an open neural tube defect based on specific MSAFP MoM values

	Odds at a Given Population Incidence	
Serum AFP (MoM)	1 per 1000	2 per 1000
2.0	1 : 800	1 : 400
2.5	1 : 290	1 : 140
3.0	1 : 120	1 : 59
3.5	1 : 53	1 : 27
4.0	1 : 26	1 : 13
4.5	1 : 14	1 : 7
5.0	1 : 7	1 : 4

Data from Fourth Report of the O.K. Collaborative Study on Alpha-Fetoprotein in Relation to Neural Tube Defects, *J Epidemiol Community Health* 36:87-95, 1982.

b. Omphalocele is a midline defect of the abdominal wall with herniation of abdominal organs into a membrane-covered sac from which the umbilical cord arises.
c. Gastroschisis is a defect of the right side of the abdominal wall and is not membrane covered.

d. Because gastroschisis is not membrane covered, higher levels of MSAFP are found, on average, as compared with omphalocele.
   (1) Median MSAFP values with gastroschisis is 7.0 MoM.
   (2) Median MSAFP values with omphalocele is 4.0 MoM.
e. MSAFP screening detects almost 100% of cases of gastroschisis and 70% to 80% of omphaloceles at commonly used screening cutoffs.

2. Renal abnormalities
   a. Congenital nephrotic syndrome
      (1) Rare autosomal recessive condition in which increased filtration of AFP through fetal kidney into amniotic fluid causes very elevated (>10 MoM) MSAFP levels
   b. Some urinary tract malformations
3. Congenital skin disorders
   a. Epidermolysis bullosa and cutis aplasia are rare conditions in which normal skin barriers are disrupted, resulting in increased diffusion of fetal AFP into maternal circulation.
4. Chromosome abnormalities
   a. Some fetuses with chromosome abnormalities, most commonly trisomies 13 and 18, have an increased MSAFP because of the presence of open fetal defects (e.g., neural tube defects, omphalocele).
   b. Women with elevated MSAFP levels without identified anomalies may be at increased risk for a variety of other chromosome abnormalities, including triploidy, sex chromosome anomalies, and structural anomalies.
   c. The overall risk of a fetal chromosome abnormality in women with elevated MSAFP levels is approximately 1%.
5. Unidentified fetal anomalies
   a. There is a higher incidence of congenital malformations identified at birth in infants whose mothers had elevated MSAFP levels.

Evaluation of the patient with an elevated MSAFP level

Approximately 5% of women who have MSAFP screening have elevated levels. These women should be offered genetic counseling and the option of further diagnostic testing to evaluate for fetal anomalies. With careful follow-up testing, most abnormal MSAFP results can eventually be explained. The following is an example of a protocol for follow-up testing for an elevated MSAFP level (Fig. 26-3).

1. High-resolution ultrasonography is the primary follow-up of elevated MSAFP levels.
2. First priority of ultrasound examination is to confirm estimated gestational age.
   a. Because MSAFP levels vary with gestational age, inaccurate dating used to determine MSAFP MoM may result in a falsely low or high value.
   b. Underestimation of gestational age is the most common reason for an elevated MSAFP level.
   c. If estimated gestational age used for calculating MSAFP MoM differs by greater than 10 days from gestational age determined by

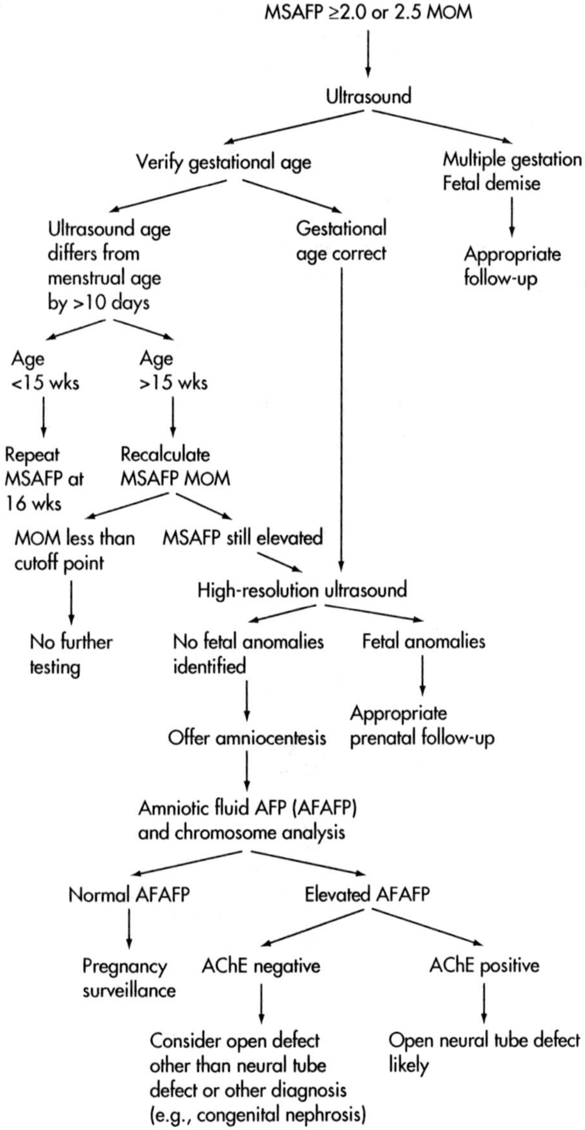

Figure 26-3
Algorithm for evaluation of elevated MSAFP levels.

ultrasound examination, then the MoM is recalculated using the ultrasound dating.

d. If ultrasound gestational age is less than 15 weeks, then a repeat MSAFP test must be obtained after 15 weeks.

3. If gestational dating is correct, then a high-resolution ultrasonogram is performed to evaluate for fetal anomalies.
   a. Detection rate of neural tube defects is 70% to 100%; many centers achieve detection rates of 90% or better.
   b. Detection rate of gastroschisis and omphalocele is 80% to 95%.
4. Some centers provide individual adjusted risks for open neural tube defects based on a normal ultrasound examination.
   a. Prior risk based on the MSAFP test alone may be reduced by 90% to 95%.
   b. Tables for calculating adjusted risks are available (Thornton JG, Lilford RJ, Newcombe RG: Tables for estimation of individual risks of fetal neural tube and ventral wall defects, incorporating prior probability, maternal serum alpha-fetoprotein levels, and ultrasonographic examination results, *Am J Obstet Gynecol* 164:154-160, 1991).
5. Amniocentesis is an option for further evaluation of an elevated MSAFP that remains unexplained by ultrasonography.
   a. An elevated AFAFP level suggests the presence of an open defect.
   b. Additional test for presence or absence of acetylcholinesterase (AChE) in amniotic fluid is used to differentiate neural tube defects from other fetal defects.
      (1) AChE is an enzyme contained in blood cells and neural tissue.
      (2) Both AFAFP and AChE are elevated in the presence of an open neural tube defect (95% to 98% detection rate).
      (3) Elevated AFAFP and normal AChE suggest the presence of other open defects (gastroschisis, omphalocele).
   c. If a normal AFAFP is obtained after a normal ultrasound examination, the likelihood of an open fetal defect is very low.
   d. Chromosome analysis should be performed on fetal cells obtained by amniocentesis to evaluate for chromosome abnormalities.
6. The detection rate of open neural tube defects using a combination of MSAFP screening and high-resolution ultrasound is comparable with that achieved by amniotic fluid studies.
7. Until more data are available, women with true elevated MSAFP levels and normal ultrasound examinations should continue to be offered the option of amniocentesis for AFAFP, AChE, and chromosome analysis.

Elevated MSAFP in the absence of fetal anomalies

In approximately 50% of pregnancies with elevated MSAFP levels, ultrasonography and amniocentesis do not identify a cause. The majority of patients with unexplained MSAFP elevations have no complications. However, unexplained elevated MSAFP levels are associated with an increased risk (20% to 38%) for adverse pregnancy outcomes. Findings associated with elevated MSAFP levels include the following:

1. Fetal death
   a. Approximately 3% to 5% of all patients with MSAFP elevations and 20% of those with MSAFP levels greater than 5.0 will be found to have experienced fetal demise at the time of ultrasonography.
   b. Patients with elevated MSAFP levels who have a viable fetus at ultrasonography are at increased risk for later fetal loss or stillbirth; the higher the MSAFP elevation, the greater the risk.
      (1) A 2.5-fold increased risk for MSAFP MoM in the range of 2.0 to 2.9
      (2) A 10-fold increased risk for MSAFP MoM greater than 3.0
2. Placental anomalies
   a. Transient fetomaternal hemorrhage
   b. Tumor
   c. Infarction
3. Intrauterine viral infections
   a. Cytomegalovirus (CMV)
   b. Parvovirus
   c. Herpes simplex
4. Premature delivery, low birth weight, or intrauterine growth retardation (IUGR)
   a. Significantly higher risk with MSAFP MoM greater than 5.0
5. Other pregnancy complications
   a. Preeclampsia
   b. Placental abruption

Management of the patient with unexplained MSAFP elevations

It has been suggested that the presence of an unexplained elevated MSAFP level should be considered an indication of a high-risk pregnancy warranting increased surveillance because of the known increased risk of adverse pregnancy outcome. There is currently neither consensus on an appropriate management protocol for such pregnancies nor clear evidence that specific interventions improve pregnancy outcomes. Each pregnancy should be considered on an individual basis.

Individual serum markers used in screening for chromosome abnormalities

1. Low MSAFP levels are associated with an increased risk for fetal Down syndrome.
   a. Reduced MSAFP levels may result from decreased fetal hepatic AFP production.
   b. Detection rate for Down syndrome is 20% to 25% with MSAFP levels <0.5 MoM.
   c. Patient-specific risks for Down syndrome are based on a combination of MSAFP MoM values and maternal age.
   d. An assigned risk of ≥1:270 (the age-related risk for a 35-year-old woman at midtrimester) is considered abnormal.
   e. Findings other than fetal Down syndrome that may be associated with low MSAFP levels include the following:

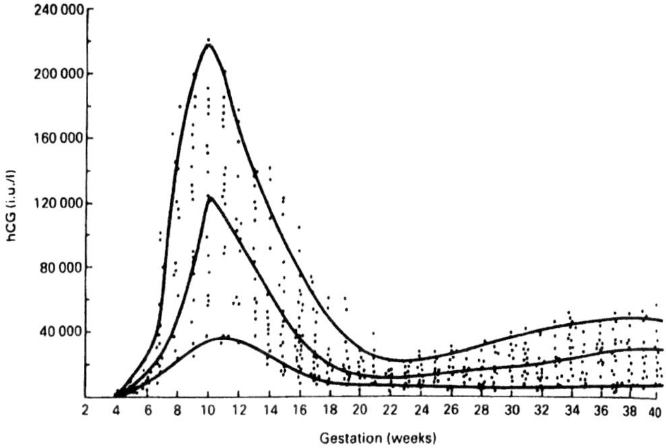

Figure 26-4
The relationship between human chorionic gonadotropin (HCG) levels and gestational age, showing 5th, 50th, and 95th centiles. (From Hay DL: Placental histology and the production of human chorionic gonadotropin and its subunits in pregnancy, *Br J Obstet Gynecol* 95:1270, 1988.)

(1) Other chromosome abnormalities (most commonly trisomy 18 and Turner syndrome)
(2) Fetal demise
(3) Hydatidiform mole
(4) Overestimated gestational age
(5) Normal variant

2. Elevated maternal serum human chorionic gonadotropin (MSHCG) levels ≥2.0 MoM are associated with an increased risk for fetal Down syndrome.
   a. HCG is a placental glycoprotein composed of two nonidentical subunits (alpha and beta).
   b. Intact (total) HCG and free beta-HCG levels peak at 8 to 10 weeks gestation (Fig. 26-4).
   c. As with MSAFP, MSHCG MoM values are adjusted to account for factors that affect MSHCG levels (gestational age, maternal weight, race, diabetes).
   d. Most laboratories measure intact (total) HCG, although it has been suggested that beta-HCG may be a more sensitive marker.
   e. MSHCG is the best single serum marker for the detection of Down syndrome.
   f. Findings other than fetal Down syndrome that may be associated with an elevated MSHCG level include the following:
      (1) Fetal hydrops
      (2) IUGR
      (3) Placental disruption

(4) Pregnancy-induced hypertension
(5) Overestimated gestational age

3. Low levels of maternal serum unconjugated estriol ($MSuE_3$) are associated with an increased risk for fetal Down syndrome.
   a. $MSuE_3$ is a steroid derived from dehydroepiandrosterone sulfate (DHEAS) produced in the fetal adrenal glands, converted to alphahydroxy DHEAS in the fetal liver, and metabolized in the placenta.
   b. As with MSAFP and MSHCG, $MSuE_3$ MoM values must be adjusted to account for factors that affect levels (gestational age, maternal weight, race, diabetes).
   c. The median $MSuE_3$ value for pregnancies affected with Down syndrome is 0.78 MoM.
   d. $MSuE_3$ is the second best single indicator for the detection of Down syndrome.
   e. Other findings associated with low uE_3 values include the following:
      (1) Placental pathology
      (2) Fetal demise
      (3) IUGR
      (4) Maternal chronic hypertension
4. The use of other serum markers for the detection of chromosome abnormalities, including pregnancy-specific beta-glycoprotein and neutrophil alkaline phosphatase, have been considered; however, only the three markers discussed are currently used in clinical settings.

Maternal serum triple marker screening for detection of chromosome abnormalities

1. A maternal serum triple marker screening test should be offered to all pregnant women under age 35 as a screen for chromosome abnormalities and neural tube defects.
2. The maternal serum triple marker screen consists of the concurrent measurements of MSAFP, MSHCG, and $MSuE_3$.
3. A computerized formula based on Gaussian multivariate analysis is used to derive a specific numerical risk for fetal Down syndrome that is based on the combination of a woman's age-related risk and the three biochemical marker values.
   a. A calculated risk of ≥1:270 (midgestational age-related risk for a 35-year-old woman) is considered abnormal.
   b. The detection rate is 60% to 65% in pregnant women under age 35 with a calculated risk of ≥1:270.
   c. Detection rate increases to 85% to 90% in women over age 35 because of the effect of maternal age in the calculated risk.
4. In addition to Down syndrome, the maternal serum triple marker test is also useful as a screen for trisomy 18.
   a. Approximately 60% of fetal trisomy 18 will be identified on the basis of combined low levels of MSAFP, MSHCG, and $MSuE_3$.
   b. Although no calculated numerical risk is reported with concurrent low values, it has been estimated that the odds of having an affected fetus given a positive test result are 1 in 15.

Table 26-2 Patterns of abnormal maternal serum triple marker screen results

MSAFP	MSHCG	$MSuE_3$	Differential
Low	High	Low	Down syndrome Hydropic Turner syndrome
Low	Low	Low	Trisomy 18 (without ventral wall defect)
High	Normal	Normal	Open neural tube defect or ventral wall defect

5. Other chromosome abnormalities have been identified in pregnancies with abnormal triple marker results.
   a. A pattern of low MSAFP, low uE_3, and elevated MSHCG levels may be associated with hydropic Turner syndrome.
   b. Pregnancies with various other chromosome abnormalities may be identified by subsequent amniocentesis for abnormal triple marker results; however, there have been an insufficient number of cases to confirm a true association with specific chromosome anomalies.
   c. Triple marker screening results are currently reported and interpreted only as to the risk for Down syndrome and trisomy 18.
6. Although it has been suggested that inclusion of $MSuE_3$ in the serum marker screen may not add significantly to the detection rate of fetal Down syndrome, it is useful in the detection of trisomy 18 and most laboratories offer the triple marker combination.
7. Triple marker screening cannot be interpreted for multiple-gestation pregnancies because of a lack of normative values for this population.
8. The risk for a neural tube defect is reported as part of the triple marker screen result using the MSAFP MoM value alone (see MSAFP Screening for Neural Tube Defects).
9. Based on the correlation of increased or decreased levels of individual biochemical markers with chromosome abnormalities and neural tube defects, certain patterns of multiple marker values may be associated with increased risks for specific anomalies (Table 26-2).

Evaluation of the patient with an abnormal triple marker screening test for chromosome abnormalities

The following is an example of a protocol for follow-up testing for an abnormal triple marker screening test (Fig. 26-5).

1. If the screening test indicates a risk >1:270 for Down syndrome or concurrent low levels indicating an increased risk for trisomy 18, high-resolution ultrasonography is performed to confirm gestational age and evaluate for fetal anomalies.
2. If the estimated gestational age is correct, genetic counseling is provided and the patient is offered the option of amniocentesis.
3. If the estimated gestational age used to calculate triple marker results differs by more than 10 days from that determined by ultrasound,

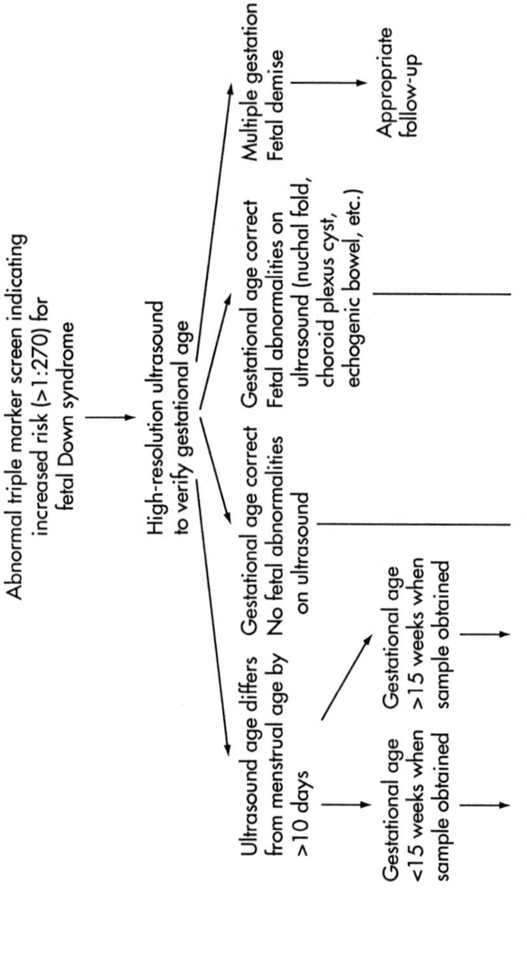
Abnormal triple marker screen indicating increased risk (>1:270) for fetal Down syndrome
High-resolution ultrasound to verify gestational age
Ultrasound age differs from menstrual age by >10 days
Gestational age correct No fetal abnormalities on ultrasound
Gestational age correct Fetal abnormalities on ultrasound (nuchal fold, choroid plexus cyst, echogenic bowel, etc.)
Multiple gestation Fetal demise
Appropriate follow-up
Gestational age <15 weeks when sample obtained
Gestational age >15 weeks when sample obtained

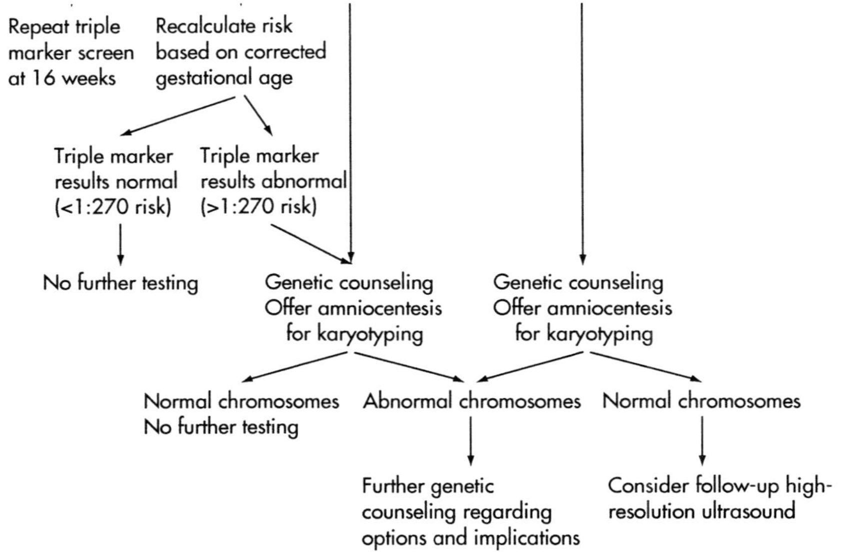

Figure 26-5
Algorithm for evaluation of abnormal maternal serum triple marker screening test indicating an increased risk for Down syndrome.

results are recalculated by the laboratory performing the study or the sample is redrawn if the specimen has been obtained before 15 weeks gestation.

4. If the patient elects to proceed with amniocentesis and results are abnormal, the patient receives additional genetic counseling regarding the findings and available options.

Issues regarding the use of the triple marker screen

1. Benefits include cost effectiveness and potential for identifying fetal chromosome abnormalities and neural tube defects.
   a. Of Down syndrome infants, 80% are born to women under age 35, who are not routinely offered the option of amniocentesis.
   b. Maternal screening is a noninvasive method for identifying pregnancies with an increased risk for fetal anomalies in a low-risk population.
2. Whereas amniocentesis is offered to women 35 years of age or older for diagnosis of chromosome abnormalities, triple marker screening should be offered to these women to provide individual risks for Down syndrome (which may be higher or lower than their age-related risk alone) and to assist in the decision-making process regarding the options for further testing.
3. Concerns have been raised regarding unnecessary anxiety resulting from false-positive results.
   a. It is estimated that 5% to 10% of screening results will be positive for an increased risk for a chromosome abnormality or neural tube defect.
   b. Of those positive screening tests, only 3% will represent an actual neural tube defect or chromosome abnormality.
4. Screening should be offered with an explanation as to its purposes and limitations.
5. Test results should be provided in a timely fashion to assist in the patient's decision process.
6. It is essential that triple marker screening results be used in conjunction with ultrasound findings and appropriate genetic counseling.

Suggested reading

Canick JA, Saller DN Jr: Maternal serum screening for aneuploidy and open fetal defects, *Obstet Gynecol Clin North Am* 20(3):443-454, 1993.

Elias S, Simpson JL, editors: *Maternal serum screening for fetal genetic disorders,* New York, 1992, Churchill Livingstone.

Haddow JE, Palomaki BS, Knight GJ: *Prenatal screening for major fetal disorders—The Foundation for Blood Research handbook,* Scarborough, ME, 1990, Foundation for Blood Research.

Milunsky A: Maternal serum screening for neural tube and other defects. In Milunsky A, editor: *Genetic disorders and the fetus: diagnosis, prevention and treatment,* ed 3, Baltimore, 1992, Johns Hopkins University Press.

Milunsky A: The use of biochemical markers in maternal serum screening for chromosome defects. In Milunsky A, editor: *Genetic disorders and the fetus: diagnosis, prevention and treatment,* ed 3, Baltimore, 1992, Johns Hopkins University Press.

26.2 DOWN SYNDROME

Joseph Hersh, M.D.

In 1866, John Langdon Down described a condition in which affected individuals had mental retardation and a characteristic facial appearance.[27] Although later it was hypothesized that the disorder described by Langdon Down may have resulted from a chromosomal abnormality, convincing evidence that chromosomal abnormalities occurred in humans was lacking. However, in 1959, after techniques were developed to analyze human chromosomes, Lejeune and others[54] identified the presence of 47 rather than 46 chromosomes in affected individuals, and the extra chromosome was designated as human chromosome number 21.

Down syndrome is the most common genetic cause of mental retardation, occurring in approximately 1 in 800 live births. Its incidence increases with advanced maternal age, and especially in pregnant women 35 years of age or older. However, approximately 90% of cases are born to younger women, because of the significantly greater number of births in this age group.

Although serious and potentially life-threatening medical complications are observed in Down syndrome, in contrast to 25 years ago, the infant with this chromosomal abnormality has significantly greater opportunities to live a longer, healthier, and more productive life. These changes reflect greater opportunities in the area of education, employment, and community living. Although institutionalization was a frequent recommendation after the birth of an affected infant as recently as 15 years ago, institutionalization is no longer considered an option. Even in those infrequent instances when a couple is overwhelmed by the diagnosis and unable to bring an affected infant into their home, adoption of a child with Down syndrome is readily available by other families.

Access to health care has dramatically improved for children with Down syndrome. In 1965, 50% of affected children did not survive beyond 5 years of age, primarily because of the lack of surgical intervention for congenital heart disease. However, with more aggressive medical and surgical intervention for structural abnormalities and medical diseases, especially in the last two decades, survival has improved dramatically and is in excess of 80% at 30 years of age. This figure, in fact, may actually be an underestimate of survival rates now, because a portion of adults did not receive optimum medical care earlier in their lives. Therefore, today, no difference in health care provision exists in the child with Down syndrome when compared with an unaffected population.

Two important federal laws have increased the availability of early developmental and educational programming, beginning in early infancy, after establishment of a diagnosis. Public Law 94-142, legislated in 1977, guaranteed free, equal, and appropriate educational opportunities in the least restrictive environment for all individuals with disabilities from the age of 3 to 22 years. In 1986, Public Law 99-457 enabled an extension of services to include a population of children from birth to 3 years. The recognition of benefits achieved by integrating children with disabilities into regular academic classroom settings has enhanced learning experiences for school-age children with Down syndrome, and in adulthood, greater acceptance of individuals with disabling conditions has led to employment opportunities in the community.

The neonate with Down syndrome

Down syndrome is usually diagnosable at, or shortly after, birth, based on a distinctive clinical phenotype, and especially facial characteristics. In fact, the term *mongolism,* originally used by Langdon Down to describe an affected child, was coined because of the resemblence of the face to Asiatic individuals; however, this term no longer is regarded as an appropriate one to describe an affected child.

Facially (Fig. 26-6 and the box on p. 718) the palpebral fissures are upslanting and frequently shortened. The bridge of the nose is flattened, and the ears are small with overfolded helices. Epicanthal folds are present, and brushfield spots around the margin of the iris are commonly found. There is facial flattening, with a depressed nasal bridge, and brachycephaly. Tongue protrusions may be observed. Redundant skin over the posterior aspect of the neck is common and, occasionally during pregnancy, can be recognized on ultrasonography in the first and second trimesters. The hands of an infant with Down syndrome tend to be broad and short, and clinodactyly of the fifth fingers is often seen. Frequently, a single palmar crease is identified (i.e., simian crease) and there is evidence of a wide space between the first and second toes with a deep hallucal groove on the plantar surface of the foot, running longitudinally. Muscular hypotonia is a constant feature and may be the first finding identified in the neonate that raises suspicion of the diagnosis. In addition, low muscle tone leads to joint hypermobility and an increased risk for hip dislocation.

Major structural defects are common in Down syndrome and may lead to medical complications shortly after birth or in early infancy if not recognized promptly. The most common structural abnormality is congenital heart disease, which is present in approximately 40% of cases. Although the lesion is frequently asymptomatic at birth and a murmur may not be heard as a result of increased pulmonary vascular resistance, early diagnosis and treatment are critical because of a significant risk for morbidity and mortality resulting from early development of irreversible pulmonary hypertension. In approximately 40% of cases with congenital heart disease, an atrioventricular (AV) canal (i.e., AV communis) is present. Ventricular septal defect is found in about 31% of cases, with approximately 9% of infants having an atrial septal defect, or patent ductus arteriosus, and with teratology of Fallot being present in about 6% of cases. Rarely, a more complex heart lesion is identified. For instance, I have seen a few infants that have had both an AV communis and tetralogy of Fallot. Therefore, in view of the significant risk for morbidity and mortality resulting from congenital heart disease, echocardiography should be performed routinely in all neonates after a diagnosis of Down syndrome is established.

Gastrointestinal (GI) anomalies are found in up to 12% of newborns with Down syndrome. Duodenal atresia and stenosis are the most common defects identified, and these obstructive lesions are found in about 2.5% of patients with Down syndrome. In addition, Down syndrome is found in about 25% to 30% of cases of duodenal atresia. Annular pancreas occasionally is present as an associated feature. *In utero,* diagnosis of duodenal atresia may be suspected

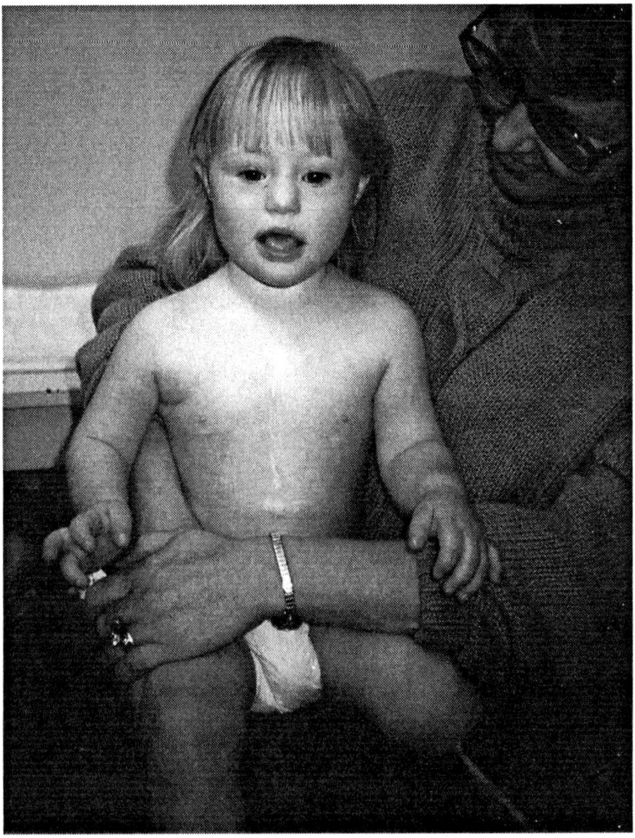

Figure 26-6
Two-year-old female with Down syndrome. Note the incisional scar from a previously repaired heart lesion.

on ultrasound in the presence of polyhydramnios, or evidence of a double bubble on examination of the fetal abdomen. Following the infant's birth, bilious vomiting after initiation of feeding should raise suspicion of the diagnosis and the need for further medical intervention. Other GI lesions that occur with increased frequency in Down syndrome include imperforate anus, seen in about 1% of cases; Hirschsprung disease in 0.56% of cases; and tracheoesophageal fistula in 0.43% of affected infants. Feeding difficulties unrelated to an anatomic GI lesion are not uncommon and result from an inefficient suck resulting from decreased oral muscle tone. The emotional stress of parents dealing with the diagnosis may amplify feeding

Clinical Features in the Neonate with Down Syndrome

CRANIOFACIAL

- Flat face
- Brachycephaly
- Upslanting and occasionally short palpebral fissures
- Epicanthal folds
- Brushfield spots
- Flat nasal bridge
- Small ears
- Overfolded ear helices
- Tongue protrusions
- Excessive posterior nuchal skin

EXTREMITIES

- Short, broad hands
- Clinodactyly fifth fingers
- Proximal thumbs
- Single palmar crease
- Gap between first and second toes
- Deep hallucal groove on foot
- Hypermobile joints

NEUROLOGIC

- Hypotonia

difficulties, leading to poor weight gain initially. These problems combined with poor growth related to a congenital heart lesion, that may eventually require surgical correction, can result in significant failure to thrive, increasing the risk for postoperative complications in the affected infant. Therefore, intervention from a feeding specialist may be indicated, with patience and support of family members to facilitate adequate growth, especially when surgery to correct a cardiac lesion may be anticipated in infancy.

Congenital cataracts occur in approximately 3% of infants with Down syndrome. Early recognition and surgical extraction are extremely important to retain adequate vision to facilitate growth and development in the future.

In addition, in the neonatal period, an increased risk for developing transient myeloproliferative disorder (i.e., transient acute leukemia) results in a significant elevation of peripheral white blood cells and may include the presence of blast cells. However, unlike leukemia, there are normal numbers of granulocytes and macrophage stem cells in the bone marrow, and ultrastructural differences between leukemoid and leukemic blast cells can be recognized. This disorder is so commonly associated with Down syndrome that its presence, even in the absence of a typical Down syndrome phenotype, should signal the need to search for mosaicism. Although the condition generally is regarded as benign, resolving spontaneously in infancy, an increased risk for developing myeloid leukemia or myelofibrosis later in life exists, warranting closer monitoring of the hematologic status in affected children manifesting this hematologic abnormality.

The young child with Down syndrome

Cognitive deficits represent the greatest long-term disability in Down syndrome. Although development may appear to be normal in early infancy, developmental delay is usually apparent by the latter part of the first year of life. At that time, delays in cognitive and motor development are evident.[12] By school age, most affected children demonstrate a moderate degree of mental retardation on standardized tests of intelligence. Although variability in intellectual abilities exists, including some affected children functioning in an educable range, a progressive decline in IQ is commonly observed. Controversy exists whether there is a relationship between parental educational level or IQ and those observed in affected children, and it has been suggested in one study that a correlation between mothers with 16 or more years of education and higher IQ scores in their affected child exists. Children with Down syndrome have relative delays in the development of language skills, even when compared with children of comparable mental ages. Communication difficulties may be further complicated by significant speech articulation problems. Use of a total communication approach, including both verbal and augmentative therapy, therefore, may facilitate communication abilities in the affected child. An area of strength that is often seen in Down syndrome is the acquisition of social and adaptive skills, and successes in these areas frequently enhance an affected individual's potential to procure some form of meaningful employment in adulthood and to be able to function adequately in a semi-independent living setting. Initiation of early intervention services with motor, cognitive, and speech and language stimulation has had a beneficial effect on development in Down syndrome. Although long-term impact on intellectual functioning may not be great, clear benefits have been seen in the acquisition of social and adaptive skills. Initiation of early services also has provided an important source of support for families dealing with their child's disability.

In addition to surgical correction of anatomic abnormalities, early detection and treatment of several medical problems commonly observed in Down syndrome are critical. Children with Down syndrome have an increased susceptibility to infections, particularly involving the upper respiratory tract. Sinusitis is probably more common than suspected. In my experience, the presence of chronic purulent rhinorrhea frequently is associated with sinusitis that can be demonstrated on computerized tomography. Hearing loss is observed in over 75% of young children with Down syndrome, and this usually is conductive in nature, resulting from persistent middle ear effusions. Treatment of this problem is necessary to maintain normal hearing to facilitate language development. Audiologic evaluations, therefore, should be initiated in the first year of life and performed, at least, on a yearly basis.

Results of immunologic studies in Down syndrome have been conflicting. Studies have demonstrated both decreased T and B lymphocyte numbers and function. T-cell abnormalities appear to be most consistently present, and in one study, the number of T-helper cells (CD4+) was decreased, resulting in a decreased ratio of T-helper to T-suppressor (CD8+) cells. In addition, an increased risk for autoimmunity is observed in Down syndrome with antithyroid antibodies and alopecia areata being present in about 10% to 15% of cases, and in rare instances there is an association of the latter finding with diabetes mellitus and hypoparathyroidism.

A variety of different ocular abnormalities are common in children with Down syndrome. In addition to congenital cataracts and occasionally glaucoma, congenital nystagmus is observed in about 35% of infants. This finding is not necessarily associated with visual deficits and may resolve spontaneously in childhood. However, refractive errors occur in up to 70% of children with Down syndrome and frequently result from myopia. Strabismus is observed in 60% of cases, and in 20% of affected children, there is evidence of nasolacrimal duct obstruction. The high-frequency association of ocular abnormalities, therefore, necessitates routine ophthalmological evaluation with determination of whether cataracts are present in early infancy, and subsequently followed by ophthalmologic reevaluation in the second year of life, again at about 5 years of age, and in midadolescence.

Thyroid dysfunction, and especially hypothyroidism, is an occasional manifestation of Down syndrome. Congenital hypothyroidism is present in 1.1% of Down syndrome cases. A risk for acquired thyroid disease also exists. In a retrospective study of 49 children with Down syndrome between the age of 4 months and 3 years, in addition to congenital hypothyroidism being present in three cases, two others either had acquired hypothyroidism or hyperthyroidism. In addition, in 13 of the 49 children, there was a mild elevation of thyroid stimulating hormone level in the face of a normal thyroxin level. It has been estimated that thyroid dysfunction may be present in as high as 15% of cases. Because hypothyroidism can further compromise central nervous system function in the child with a developmental disability, prompt recognition and treatment are necessary. However, because early clinical symptoms may be misinterpreted as representing features of Down syndrome, this may not be possible. Therefore, routine screening of thyroid function on a yearly basis until school age is indicated.

In addition to transient myeloproliferative disease that is unique to Down syndrome, an increased incidence of leukemia is also observed and is 10 to 18 times more common than that found in chromosomally normal individuals up to 16 years of age. In addition, in adults with Down syndrome, there is also an increased risk for hematologic malignancies, but not to the same magnitude as that seen in younger individuals. Acute nonlymphoblastic leukemia is the type primarily observed in children who develop this malignancy before a year of age. However, in affected children 3 years of age or older, the distribution of leukemic types is similar to that seen in a chromosomally normal population of children. Survival in children with Down syndrome who have leukemia is lower, in all likelihood, as the result of a lower frequency of remission and increased risk for life-threatening infections. One type of leukemia that is observed up to 200 to 400 times more frequently in Down syndrome is acute megakaryoblastic leukemia. Although not seen frequently, this form of leukemia can be a later manifestation in children who had transient myeloproliferative disorder as a neonate.

Seizures are seen more frequently in Down syndrome, and it has been estimated that the incidence ranges from 2.6% to 8.8%. An increased risk for infantile spasms also exists, and Pueschel reported infantile spasms in 5 of 89 affected children under one year of age. Autism also occurs with greater frequency in Down syndrome.

Hypermobility of the joints can result in an increased risk for cervical instability that could lead to spinal cord compression and permanent neurologic sequelae. Radiologically, atlantoaxial instability is observed in approximately 15% of young children with Down syndrome. Although in most instances, the abnormality is asymptomatic, a small percentage have symptoms secondary to spinal cord compression. Risk for neurologic sequelae may be heightened by the presence of bone abnormalities of the cervical spine as well, which are observed on occasion. Therefore, it is generally recommended that radiographs of the cervical spine, including views in flexion and extension, be performed in all affected children between 2½ and 3 years of age, and again before participation in Special Olympics at school age. In the presence of cervical instability, it is generally recommended that participation in competitive sports that could lead to a traumatic neck injury be avoided.[3,14] In addition to the increased risk for atlantoaxial instability, atlanto-occipital instability has been found in up to 30% of Down syndrome children as well. Even in the absence of radiographic evidence of cervical instability, the presence of symptoms suggestive of spinal cord compression, such as chronic neck pain, newly developed deficits in motor abilities and bladder and bowel function, pyramidal tract signs, and loss of sensation should necessitate further investigation for the possible presence of this problem. Finally, because a potential risk for spinal cord injury may exist with extreme hyperextension of the neck for intubation, radiographic investigation of the cervical spine before an operative procedure may be indicated.

Problems related to the oral airway and dental development are common in Down syndrome. Upper airway obstruction leading to obstructive apnea may be insidious and potentially life threatening. The presence of a small airway that lacks musculature and connective tissue support, and enlarged tonsils and adenoids, can result in increased airway resistance, leading to hypoxia, pulmonary hypertension, and cor pulmonale. Obesity, a common problem in Down syndrome, may further increase the risk for airway obstruction. Altered sleep habits, such as restlessness, wakefulness with agitation, snoring, daytime fatigue, and apnea should signal the need for further investigation of this potentially serious medical complication. Tonsillectomy and adenoidectomy may be indicated to remedy this problem effectively, but the potential risk must be recognized for vocal resonance problems, with hypernasality developing as a result of velopharangeal incompetence postoperatively. Delayed dental eruption, altered tooth size and morphology, and hypodontia may be observed in up to 50% of Down syndrome cases. Malocclusion is frequent, and although periodontal disease was common in institutionalized patients, the risk for this problem is not felt to be increased in those children reared in a home setting. Macroglossia is observed in Down syndrome, although in some instances, the macroglossia is relative, resulting from a small oral cavity. Both factors plus oral hypotonicity contribute to frequent tongue protrusions. Fissuring of the tongue also is commonly observed. Although tongue protrusions frequently represent a concern of parents, in many instances, they tend to decrease in frequency with age and growth of the oral cavity.

Beginning in early infancy, programming to facilitate neurodevelopmental status should be emphasized. Enrollment in an early intervention program, combined with services provided in the area of occupational, physical, and speech and language therapy are ideal. At 3 years of age, enrollment in a regular preschool with continued provision of ancillary services is important in continuing to optimize an affected child's developmental potential and strengthening social and adaptive skills. Once school age is reached, the child's enrollment in a regular school classroom, for at least part of the day, is mandatory; additional services should be provided by a special educational teacher either by integrating them in the classroom or in a separate setting on an individual basis. Continued efforts at maximizing speech and language development should be pursued on an intensive basis, again incorporating a variety of different modes of communication, if necessary. Occupational and physical therapy, to enhance fine and gross motor development, should be included as part of the academic curriculum. Many children with Down syndrome have demonstrated the ability to learn basic reading, writing, and mathematics skills, and the opportunity to achieve successes in these areas should be readily available.

The adolescent with Down syndrome

Adolescence brings on its own unique challenges in Down syndrome. In addition to continuing to enhance developmental skills, programming must begin to be directed at developing vocational competency, to function in society as an adult. Coping with the desire for independence represents a new challenge for parents and school personnel. In males, pubertal changes occur at an age similar to that of males without Down syndrome. In addition, no differences are noted in the size of external genitalia or gonadotropin levels; however, sterility is present in almost all cases, and there has been only one instance in which reproduction by a male with Down syndrome has been reported. In females, menarche occurs slightly later than an unaffected female with a mean age at menarche of 12 years 6 months, in contrast to 12 years 1 month. The development of pubertal changes is not strikingly different, and menstrual periods are similar. The potential for reproduction in a female with Down syndrome is considerably greater than that in an affected male. In a study by Tricomi et al,[99] it was found that 39% of affected females ovulated, 15% probably ovulated, 15% possibly ovulated, and 30% were not ovulatory. There have been numerous reports of affected females giving birth to offspring and in about 50% of cases the infant was similarly affected.

Adolescence is also a time when most individuals with Down syndrome enjoy good health. However, the risk for obesity increases, necessitating close monitoring of dietary intake, and stressing the importance of participating in a regular exercise program. Dry skin is present in about 90% of cases and skin can become thick and cracked, particularly over the surfaces of the hands, feet, wrists, and elbows. Premature aging from exposure to ultraviolet light is a risk; therefore, protecting skin against excessive sun exposure with sunscreen and protective clothing is important. Beginning in adolescence, follicular skin infections develop in 50% to 60% of affected individuals; these can result in abscess formation if not treated promptly, particularly around the buttocks and thighs. Benign sweat gland tumors (i.e., syringoma) can also develop in the periorbital area, neck, thoracic, and axillary regions and in the periumbilical and pubic areas.

Emotional stresses in the home and at school need to be dealt with in an open, patient, and supportive manner to minimize the risk for abnormal emotional adjustment and behavioral disorders. These problems appear to be seen less frequently in a supportive family setting, where the developmental problems that can adversely impact an individual's self-image can be dealt with promptly in a positive and caring manner.

Growth in Down syndrome

At birth, a neonate with Down syndrome may be slightly smaller than a chromosomally normal infant, although the difference in size is not significant. Delayed growth velocity occurs in infancy and, even to a greater degree, in the presence of significant congenital heart disease. Adolescent growth spurt is less than that observed in chromosomally normal teenagers, ultimately resulting in a mild degree of short stature. Growth hormone studies in Down syndrome have not revealed growth hormone deficiency. Although growth hormone therapy in this group has been advocated by some, and one study has demonstrated increased mean growth velocity to greater than twice that observed with pretreatment values, the significance of this short-term finding is uncertain and efficacy from growth hormone use has not been proved. Growth charts ranging from 1 month to 18 years of age are available to monitor linear growth after the birth of an infant with Down syndrome.

Survival in Down syndrome

In the first decade of life, and especially in the first 5 years, the presence or absence of congenital heart disease and surgical correction of the lesion, if one is present, has been a major determinant of survival. Compared with a background population at any point in time, life expectancy in Down syndrome is about 10 to 20 years shorter. Major causes of death in decreasing order of frequency include pneumonia (23% to 41%), congenital heart disease (30% to 35%), other infections (2% to 15%), malignancy (2% to 9%), and senility and stroke (0% to 9%). In a Canadian study, major causes of death up to 30 years of age were complications related to major organ malformations, infection, and leukemia.

More recently, with improved medical and surgical care of individuals with Down syndrome beginning in the neonatal period, life expectancy has increased, and it is anticipated that these figures will continue to improve in the future. Nearly half of Down syndrome patients survive to 50 years of age, with ⅐ still alive at 68 years of age.

The adult with Down syndrome

With survival well into adulthood, physicians caring for individuals with Down syndrome must become aware of the medical needs of this aging population. Ocular problems are frequent, with cataracts occurring in 30% to 60% of cases, but rarely dense enough to require surgery. Other ocular complications such as glaucoma, blepharitis, and keratoconus occur more frequently and must be monitored for. Hypothyroidism becomes a much more significant problem than in childhood, being present in up to 50% of adults, and yearly monitoring of thyroid function is indicated. Cardiovascular disease is seen more commonly, with an increased risk for mitral valve prolapse and aortic regurgitation. Periodic evaluation of an affected adult's cardiac status appears to be warranted, and in the presence of a cardiac lesion, prophylaxis for subacute bacterial endocarditis should be initiated in the event that instrumentation, such as in the case of dental intervention, is pursued. High-frequency hearing loss is common and may necessitate amplification; therefore periodic audiologic testing is recommended.

The greatest concern associated with the aging process in Down syndrome is the risk for Alzheimer's disease. It has long been recognized that there is a relationship between Down syndrome and dementia, and that the pathologic changes of Alzheimer's disease develop in the brains of middle-age adults with this chromosomal abnormality. Alzheimer changes begin to develop in the fourth decade of life and, by 40 years of age, nearly all Down syndrome adults have evidence of the pathologic hallmarks of Alzheimer's disease, including granulovacuolar changes, senile plaques, neurofibrillary tangles, and neuronal loss. The earliest anatomic change of Alzheimer's disease is the preplaque, which is diffuse deposition of amyloid protein adjacent to cell bodies of morphologically normal neurons. Granular deposition of oligosaccharide is also present. It has been proposed that amyloid progressively accumulates around the cell body until the neuron degenerates with the appearance of tangles and plaques. Therefore, deposition of amyloid protein is presumed to be an early and progressive phenomenon and is possibly a result of overexpression of the amyloid precursor protein gene that is located on the long arm of chromosome 21 at band q21. This gene is also known to be responsible for one familial form of Alzheimer's disease. Although the pathologic changes in Down syndrome brains are identical to those seen in Alzheimer's disease, a significant portion of adults with Down syndrome do not develop dementia, although it is seen in about 25% of cases. It has been proposed that the number of tangles and plaques must exceed a threshold before there is actual evidence of clinical regression in previously acquired cognitive skills, and in Down syndrome it may be higher than in a chromosomally normal adult population, thus lowering the risk for development of dementia.

Regardless of whether or not there is evidence of frank dementia, there is progressive loss of a variety of intellectual functions and receptive language skills that are not simply attributable to mental retardation in the majority of older Down syndrome individuals. Other potentially treatable causes for dementia unrelated to Alzheimer's disease should be searched for, such as depression, which is not an uncommon occurrence, and hypothyroidism.

Allelic variation in apolipoprotein E isoforms has been recognized as being a risk factor for Alzheimer's disease in the general population. The presence of the episilon 4 isoform has been associated with an increased risk for amyloid deposition in the brain, leading to Alzheimer changes. However, van Gool et al. [103] demonstrated that apolipoprotein E allele frequency was similar in Down syndrome individuals with and without Alzheimer's disease, demonstrating that apolipoprotein E does not play a role in the pathogenesis of Alzheimer changes in this patient population. Schupf et al.[83] have shown that the risk of dementia in mothers that have given birth to a child with Down syndrome before the age of 35 years is increased fivefold, while a similar risk is not present when maternal age is greater than 35 years at the time of an affected infant's birth. It has been postulated that the increased risk for

Alzheimer's disease in young mothers that have given birth to a child with Down syndrome may be the result of an accelerated aging process that also plays a contributing role in the development of nondysjunction.

Chromosomal basis of Down syndrome

Down syndrome results from the presence of an extra chromosome 21. In approximately 95% of cases, the karyotype will reveal trisomy 21 (Fig. 26-7). It has been demonstrated that the extra 21 is maternal in origin in up to 95% of cases of trisomy 21, and the nondysjunctional event occurs in meiosis I in about 77% of cases, and in meiosis II in approximately 23% of cases. A Robertsonian translocation accounts for approximately 3% to 4% of Down syndrome, resulting from fusion of an extra chromosome 21 to another acrocentric chromosome, either in the D group, i.e., chromosome 13, 14, or 15, or in the G group (i.e., chromosomes 21 or 22). The most commonly observed Robertsonian translocation involves chromosome 14, resulting in a translocated chromosome that contains both a 21 and a 14 chromosome (Fig. 26-8). In contrast to trisomy 21, which is associated with advanced maternal age, age does not appear to play a role in the development of a Robertsonian translocation, and the risk may actually decrease with advancing maternal age. Rarely, Down syndrome can result from a reciprocal translocation, and in one instance, I have seen a child with Down syndrome that was the result

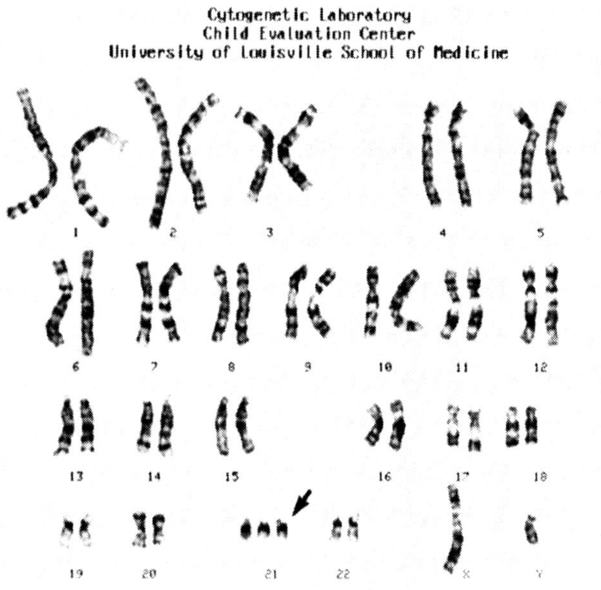

Figure 26-7
Trisomy 21 karyotype.

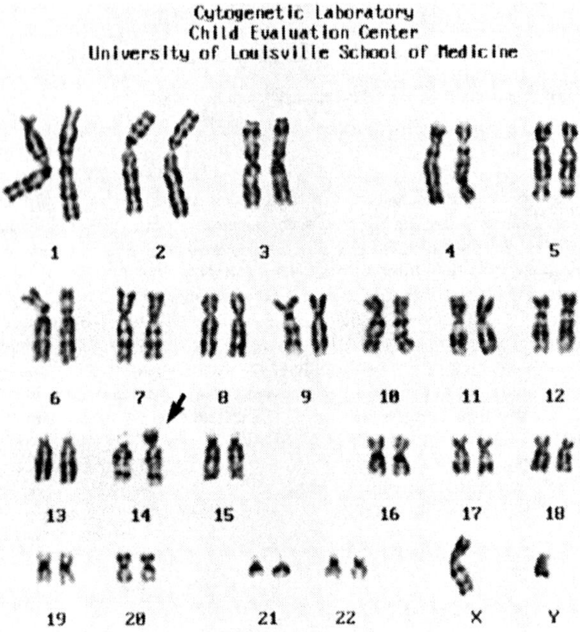

Figure 26-8
14 solids/21 Robertsonian translocation Down syndrome karyotype.

of a reciprocal translocation involving one chromosome 6, which was paternally derived. About 1% to 2% of Down syndrome results from mosaicism, in which two populations of cells can be identified, one with a diploid number (i.e., 46 chromosomes) and the other with a trisomic number (i.e., 47 chromosomes). Mosaicism can occur in the presence of either meiotic or mitotic nondysjunction, although the former is probably the more frequent mechanism, with a normal cell line being derived postconceptionally and the monosomic cell line being lost early in embryogenesis. The clinical phenyotype in mosaic Down syndrome is somewhat more variable than that seen in classic Down syndrome with the potential for higher cognitive functioning; however, if the child is ascertained because of a suspected clinical diagnosis of Down syndrome based on physical findings or the presence of mental retardation, little difference in outcome usually is observed, even in the face of mosaicism.

In women under 35 years of age who have given birth to an infant with trisomy 21, an increased risk for recurrence is observed and it is in the range of 1%. There have been rare instances in which multiple family members have had trisomy 21, or a couple has had multiple affected children. This phenomenon may result from two mechanisms: the first is low-grade mosaicism unrecognized in one of the parents, and the second is germ line mosaicism, in which a subpopulation of trisomic germ cells is present only in a reproductive organ.

When Down syndrome results from a Robertsonian translocation, parental karyotyping is important since a balanced Robertsonian translocation can be identified in one of the parents 40% to 45% of the time. In the case of a 14/21 Robertsonian translocation, the presence of a carrier parent increases the risk for recurrence in a subsequent pregnancy, and especially if the mother is identified as the carrier. Risk for recurrence of a maternally derived translocation is 10% to 15%, and in the case of a paternally derived Robertsonian translocation, in the range of 1% to 2%. In the presence of 21/21 translocation Down syndrome, a parent is found to be a carrier in about 4% of cases. In this situation, only two conceptions can be formed (i.e., 21/21 translocation Down syndrome or monosomy 21). All pregnancies surviving to term will have Down syndrome because the latter chromosomal abnormality will result in spontaneous loss. Recurrence risk in the group in which neither parent is identified as being a carrier is approximately 2.6%, probably the result of mosaicism in a germ line in one of the partner's reproductive organs.

Prenatal diagnosis of Down syndrome

It has long been recognized that the risk for Down syndrome increases with advanced maternal age. A similar risk has not been demonstrated with advanced paternal age, on the other hand.

Prenatal diagnostic techniques have been established that either can screen a pregnancy for Down syndrome or provide definitive diagnosis of the chromosomal abnormality. The availability of these tests has become extremely valuable for those couples who have an affected child, or who are considering a pregnancy and the woman is 35 years of age, or older, but would not have pursued the option of childbearing without the availability of chromosomal testing *in utero*. Procedures capable of karyotyping fetal cells include chorionic villus sampling (CVS), amniocentesis, and percutaneous umbilical blood sampling (PUBS). CVS is performed between 10 and 12 weeks' gestation. A sample of chorionic villus tissue, which is fetal in origin, is obtained either transcervically, or transabdominally, for the purpose of performing a chromosome analysis. Amniocentesis, on the other hand, is generally offered between 15 and 16 weeks gestation, and fetal cells are cultured from a sample of amniotic fluid that is removed transabdominally. After fetal cells are cultured, chromosome analysis from both procedures is usually available in 8 to 14 days. Risk of miscarriage from the CVS procedure is slightly higher than that of amniocentesis but appears to vary based on experience. Risk of miscarriage from the CVS procedure ranges from approximately 1% to 2%, in contrast to amniocentesis, in which the risk for miscarriage is 0.5%. It has also been suggested that an increased risk for limb reduction defects, and possibly for oromandibular abnormalities as well, may be associated with the CVS procedure. Numerous reports from Europe earlier this decade highlighted this association, although it appears that the greatest risk lies with a procedure that is performed before 10 weeks gestation. Although results of follow-up studies on CVS procedures performed in the United States after 10 weeks gestation are conflicting, it has been suggested that risk for limb reduction defects exceeds that of the background risk in the general population, but is probably somewhere in the range of 1/1000 to 1/3000.

PUBS generally is not offered before 20 weeks gestation because of the technical difficulty of performing the procedure. Late in the second trimester, in instances when a chromosome abnormality is suspected based on ultrasound findings, successful sampling of fetal blood enables more rapid karyotyping, with a result that can be obtained in 3 to 5 days. However, the success rate of the procedure varies from approximately 25% to 75% depending on placental position, and the risk for miscarriage probably is in the range of 1%.

In the early 1970s, in the United Kingdom, measurement of MSAFP was developed as a noninvasive diagnostic tool to screen pregnancies in the second trimester for open NTDs. In 1984, Merkatz et al. demonstrated that approximately 20% to 25% of fetuses with Down syndrome were diagnosable using this screening technique. Low levels of MSAFP were detected. Subsequently, their results were confirmed by other investigators, and in combination with advanced maternal age, measurement of MSAFP also became a method for screening low-risk pregnancies in women under 35 years of age for this chromosomal abnormality. Lower MSAFP levels have been attributed to decreased AFP production or AFP content in the liver of a Down syndrome fetus. More recently, it was discovered that by combining the measurement of AFP with human chorionic gonadotropin and unconjugated estriol levels in maternal serum between 15 and 20 weeks gestation from pregnant women under 35 years of age, 60% to 65% of fetuses with Down syndrome could be detected without increasing the percentage of false-positive results obtained when serum AFP was measured alone, which is in the range of 6% to 8%. It has been suggested that triple marker screening may also represent a valuable tool in a population of pregnant women 35 years of age or older, and particularly in those instances when the couple is uncertain whether they are interested in pursuing invasive prenatal diagnostic testing. It has been demonstrated that close to 90% of Down syndrome fetuses, and close to 50% of a few other forms of aneuploidy are detectable by triple marker screening, although 25% to 30% of this population will test positive, meaning that the risk for Down syndrome based on the results are equal to or greater than the empiric risk for Down syndrome at midgestation of a 35-year-old woman, which is 1/270.

Approximately 75% of Down syndrome conceptions survive to term. The majority of fetal loss occurs in the first trimester. However, in instances in which a Down syndrome fetus is recognized in the second trimester, there is still a risk for fetal loss during the remainder of the pregnancy, which is approximately 20% to 25%. Although the majority of couples seeking prenatal diagnosis opt to terminate a pregnancy in which the fetus has Down syndrome, couples should be given the option of pursuing invasive prenatal diagnosis if results of the test will provide them with valuable information that will help them prepare for the birth of an affected infant, even if termination is not an option.

Alternative therapy in Down syndrome

No definitive treatment is available in Down syndrome. However, because the condition results in a chronic disability and can be associated with significant medical complications, a variety of unconventional therapeutic interventions have been attempted, although typically these have not undergone careful scientific scrutiny before being marketed. The use of a variety of high-dose vitamin and mineral supplements, occasionally in combination with hormones and enzymes, has been advocated as improving both physical characteristics and cognitive functioning in children with Down syndrome. However, several controlled trials in the early 1980s were not able to demonstrate the efficacy of these preparations. More recently, it has been suggested that administration of the drug Piracetam may improve cognitive functioning and physical appearance in Down syndrome, although there have been no scientific studies to corroborate these ancedotal reports.

In Europe, injection of lyophilized or freeze-dried cells from vertebrate animal fetuses has been advocated as a successful intervention in Down syndrome to improve intellectual abilities, and to normalize the physical characteristics of Down syndrome in an affected child. No measurable benefits have been demonstrated from such treatment, and in addition, an increased risk for hypersensitization and the introduction of slow viruses with this procedure also exists. Currently, cell therapy is not available in the United States.

Anecdotal success in improving outcome in Down syndrome has been suggested with the use of patterning and craniosacral manipulation, although outcomes claimed by this form of intervention have been challenged as well.

Finally, reports from both Germany and Israel have suggested that performing plastic surgery on children with Down syndrome to normalize the facial appearance through procedures such as a partial glossectomy; lateral canthoplasty to remove epicanthal folds; nose, cheek, and chin augmentation; and otoplasty could lead to normalization of the affected child's functional abilities. These procedures are occasionally performed in this country, but clearly positive benefits have not been demonstrated with follow-up of children undergoing this surgical intervention.

Molecular insights into trisomy 21

With rapid advances in molecular genetics, it is feasible to envision that the genetic structure of chromosome 21 eventually will be completely defined, and that the pathogenetic relationship between the presence of an extra set of genes on chromosome 21 and features of Down syndrome will be understood. To date, the mechanism leading to the phenotype in Down syndrome is not known, although it has been suggested that it may be a nonspecific disturbance of chromosomal balance or a gene dosage effect with an increase in the production of certain proteins encoded by normal genes on the extra number 21 chromosome that alters the delicate balance of several biochemical pathways important in proper development and organ function.[12] Rare instances of translocations involving chromosome 21 leading to a triplication of a portion of the long arm and resulting in a Down syndrome phenotype have helped in narrowing down the region of the chromosome that appears to be critical for developing the phenotype. Currently, band q22 appears to be the candidate for this critical region, and as few as 50 to 100 genes on this portion of the chromosome may be responsible for most of the characteristics typical of Down syndrome. However, identifying a Down syndrome–critical region on chromosome 21 does not provide a complete explanation for the phenotype, since the amyloid precursor protein thought to be involved in Alzheimer changes in the brains of Down syndrome adults lies outside this region, at band q21 (Fig. 26-9).

Studying animal models that share biologic similarities with humans also may provide insights into the effects of aneuploidy. Investigations performed on the trisomy 16 mouse, and other mutant strains homologous to regions of the long arm (q) of human chromosome 21 have helped facilitate a better understanding of the pathogenesis of Down syndrome.

The prognosis for an infant born with Down syndrome in 1996 is considerably brighter than it was previously (Table 26-3). Longer and healthier survival with greater access to successful experiences in the areas of education, employment, and community life are now realistic expectations. Learning of the diagnosis shortly after giving birth to an affected infant is usually overwhelming for a couple and fraught with a great deal of sadness. However, establishing a diagnosis promptly, sharing accurate information in an optimistic and sensitive manner, and being supportive of family members in crisis after learning of the diagnosis can lay down the groundwork for many positive experiences that will occur in the lifetime of the affected individual. The physician can play a critical role in serving as an advocate for the child, to maximize the potential for growth and development. If provided with optimal medical care and developmental intervention, it is anticipated that children with Down syndrome will have an enhanced quality of life and make a substantial contribution to society.

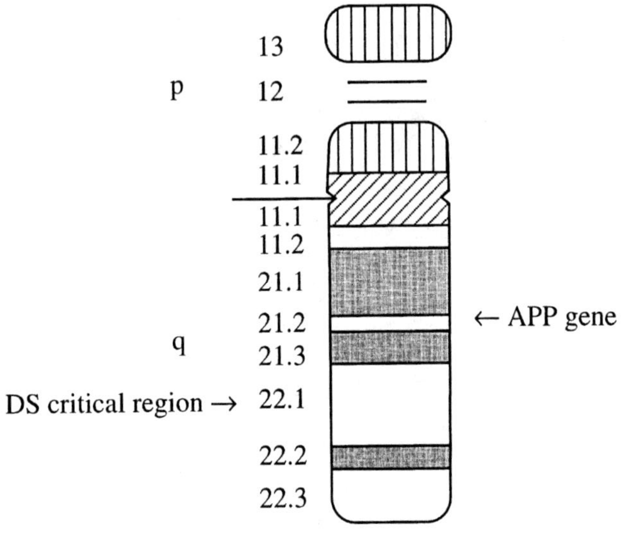

Figure 26-9
Idiogram of chromosome 21 demonstrating presumed Down syndrome critical region and gene locus for the amyloid precursor protein (APP) gene.

Table 26-3 Medical and neurodevelopmental issues to be addressed in the lifecycle of Down syndrome

Neonate	Child	Adolescent	Adult
Congenital heart disease	Frequent upper respiratory infections	Dry skin and skin infections	Dementia
Gastrointestinal obstructive lesion	Hearing loss	Obesity	Visual deficits
Congenital cataracts	Visual deficits	Pubertal changes	Hypothyroidism
Transient myeloproliferative disorder	Thyroid dysfunction	Mental retardation, behavioral concerns	Cardiovascular disease
Hypothyroidism	Leukemia		Hearing loss
Hypotonia	Cervical instability		Emotional concerns
Feeding difficulties	Upper airway obstruction		
Parental reaction	Dental abnormalities		
	Seizures		
	Growth deficiency		
	Delayed development		

References

1. Adams MM et al: Down's syndrome: recent trends in the United States, *JAMA* 246:758-760, 1981.
2. Allsop D et al: Early senile plaques in Down's syndrome brains show a close relationship with cell bodies of neurons, *Neuropathol Appl Neurobiol* 15:531-542, 1989.
3. Antonarakis SE: Down syndrome collaborative group: paternal origin of the extra chromosome in trisomy 21 as indicated by analysis of DNA polymorphisms, *N Engl J Med* 324:872-876, 1991.
4. Antonarakis SE et al: The meiotic stage of nondisjunction in trisomy 21: determination using DNA polymorphisms, *Am J Hum Genet* 50:544-558, 1991.
5. Baird PA, Sadovnick AD: Life expectancy in Down syndrome, *J Pediatr* 110:849-854, 1987.
6. Baird PA, Sadovnick AD: Life tables for Down syndrome, *Hum Genet* 82:291-292, 1989.
7. Barak Y et al: Transient acute leukaemia in a newborn with Down's syndrome: prediction of its reversibility by bone marrow cultures, *Acta Paediatr Scand* 71:699-701, 1982.
8. Bell JG, Weiner S: Has percutaneous umbilical blood sampling improved the outcome of high risk pregnancies? *Clin Perinatol* 20:61-80, 1993.
9. Bennett FC et al: Vitamin and mineral supplementation in Down's syndrome, *Pediatrics* 72:707-713, 1983.
10. Bogart MH: Current and future modes of prenatal diagnosis. In Lott IT, McCoy EE, editors: *Down syndrome: advances in medical care,* p. 13, New York, 1992, Wiley-Liss.
11. Brock DJ: Screening for fetal neural tube defects: rationale and experience, *Prog Clin Biol Res* 103:461-472, 1982.
12. Buckley LP: Congenital heart disease in infants with Down syndrome. In Pueschel SM, editor: *A study of the young child with Down syndrome,* p. 351-364, New York, 1983, Human Sciences Press.
13. Burger PC, Vogel FS: The development of pathologic changes of Alzheimer's disease and senile dementia in patients with Down's syndrome, *Am J Pathol* 73:457-475, 1973.
14. Burton BK, Schulz CJ, Burd LI: Limb anomalies associated with chorionic villus sampling, *Obstet Gynecol* 79:726-730, 1992.
15. Capute AR et al: Down syndrome: clinical review of ocular features, *Clin Pediatr* 28:355-358, 1989.
16. Chumlea WC, Cronk CE: Overweight among children with trisomy 21, *J Ment Defic Res* 25:275-280, 1981.
17. Clapp S et al: Down syndrome, complete atrioventricular canal, and pulmonary vascular obstructive disease, *J Thorac Cardiovasc Surg* 100:115-121, 1990.
18. Jackson-Cook CK et al: Nucleolar organizer region variants as a risk factor for Down syndrome, *Am J Hum Genet* 37:1049-1061, 1985.
19. Cooley WC, Graham JM: Down syndrome—an update and review for the primary pediatrician, *Clin Pediatr* 30:233-253, 1991.
20. Cowie VA: *A study of early development of Mongols,* London, 1970, Pergamon.
21. Cronck C et al: Growth charts for children with Down syndrome: 1 month to 18 years of age, *Pediatrics* 81:102-110, 1988.
22. Cronck C, Pueschel SM: Arthropometric studies. In Pueschel SM, editor: *A study of the young child with Down syndrome,* p. 105, New York, 1983, Human Sciences Press.
23. Cutler AT, Benezra-Obeiter R, Brink SJ: Thyroid function in young children with Down syndrome, *Am J Dis Child* 140:479-483, 1986.
24. Cutress TW: Periodontal disease and oral hygiene in trisomy 21, *Arch Oral Biol* 16:1345-1350, 1971.
25. Cuckle HS, Wald NJ, Lindenbaum RH: Maternal serum alpha-fetoprotein measurement: a screening test for Down syndrome, *Lancet* 1:926-929, 1984.

26. Dalton AJ, Crapper-McLachlan DR: Clinical expression of Alzheimer disease in Down syndrome, *Psychiatr Clinic North Am* 9:659-670, 1986.
27. Down JLH: Observations on an ethnic classification of idiots, *London Hospital. Clinical Lectures and Reports* 3:259-262, 1866.
28. Dupont A, Vaeth M, Vedebech P: Mortality and life expectancy of Down syndrome in Denmark, *J Med Defic Res* 30:111-120, 1986.
29. Epstein CJ: Down syndrome (Trisomy 21). In Scriver CR et al, editors: *The metabolic bases of inherited disease,* pp. 757-794, New York, 1995, McGraw-Hill.
30. Evan DIK, Steward JK: Down's syndrome and leukemia, *Lancet* 2:1322, 1972.
31. Firth HV et al: Limb abnormalities and chorionic villus sampling (letter), *Lancet* 338:1091-1092, 1991.
32. Fishler K, Koch R, Donnell GN: Comparison of mental development in individuals with mosaic and trisomy 21 Down's syndrome, *Pediatrics* 58:744-748, 1976.
33. Fort P et al: Thyroid function in young children with Down syndrome, *J Pediatr* 104:545-549, 1984.
34. Fowler A: Language abilities in children with Down syndrome: evidence for a specific syntactic delay. In Cicchetti D, Beeghly M, editors: *Children with Down syndrome—A developmental perspective,* p. 302, New York, 1990, Cambridge University Press.
35. Gardiner K et al: Analysis of human chromosome 21: correlation of physical and cytogenetic maps; gene and CpG island distribution, *EMBO J* 9:25-34, 1990.
36. Gibbs ED et al: Total communication for children with Down syndrome (Abstract). Annual Convention, American Speech-Language-Hearing Association, November, 1990.
37. Giraud F, Mattei JF: Aspects epidemiologiues de la trisomie 21, *J Genet Hum* (Suppl)23:1-30, 1975.
38. Golden GS: Controversies in therapies for children with Down syndrome, *Pediatr Rev* 6:116-120, 1984.
39. Haddow JE et al: Maternal serum unconjugated estriol are lower in the presence of fetal Down syndrome, *Am J Obstet Gynecol* 163:1372-1374, 1990.
40. Haddow JE et al: Reducing the need for amniocentesis in women 35 years of age or older with serum markers for screening, *N Engl J Med* 330:1114-1118, 1994.
41. Harris DJ et al: Parental trisomy 21 mosaicism, *Am J Hum Genet* 34:125-133, 1982.
42. Hershey DW, Crandall BF, Schroth PS: Maternal serum alpha-fetoprotein screening for fetal trisomies, *Am J Obstet Gynecol* 153:224-225, 1985.
43. Hook EB: Epidemiology of Down syndrome. In Pueschel S, Rynders JE, editors: *Down syndrome, advances in biomedicine and the behavioral sciences,* p. 11, Cambridge, MA, 1982, Ware Press.
44. Howlin P, Wing L, Gould J: The recognition of autism in children with Down syndrome—Implications for intervention and some speculations about pathology, *Dev Med Child Neuro* 37:406-414, 1995.
45. Iselius L, Jacobs P, Morton N: Leukemia and transient leukemia in Down syndrome, *Hum Genet* 85:477-485, 1990.
46. Karttunen R et al: Cell mediated immunodeficiency in Down syndrome: Normal IL-2 production but inverted ratio of T cell subsets, *Clin Exp Immunol* 55:257-263, 1984.
47. Katz S, Kravetz S: Facial plastic surgery for persons with Down syndrome: Research findings and their professional and social implications, *Am J Ment Retard* 94:101-110, 1989.
48. Knox GE, Bensel RW: Gastrointestinal malformations in Down syndrome, *Minn Med* 55:542-544, 1972.

49. Korenberg JR, Bradley C, Disteche CM: Down syndrome: Molecular mapping of the congenital heart disease and duodenal stenosis, *Am J Hum Genet* 50:294-302, 1992.
50. Korenberg JR et al: Molecular definition of a region of chromosome 21 that causes features of the Down syndrome phenotype, *Am J Hum Genet* 47:236-246, 1990.
51. Kronquist KE et al: Reduced fetal hepatic alpha-fetoprotein levels in Down syndrome, *Prenat Diagn* 10:739-751, 1990.
52. Kuliev AM, Modell B, Jackson L: Limb abnormalities and chorionic villus sampling (letter), *Lancet* 340:1034, 1992.
53. Lee SL, Rosner F: Down's syndrome and acute leukemia, *Lancet* 1:110, 1973.
54. Lejeune J, Gauthier M, Turpin R: Etude des chromosomes somatiques de neuf enfants mongoliens, *CR Acad Sci* 248:1721-1722, 1959.
55. Levy J: The gastrointestinal tract in Down syndrome. In Epstein CJ, editor: *The morphogenesis of Down syndrome,* p. 245, New York, 1991, Wiley-Liss.
56. Locke PA et al: Apolipoprotein E4 allele and Alzheimer disease: examination of allelic association and effect on age at onset in both early- and late-onset cases, *Genetic Epidemimology* 12:83-92, 1995.
57. Ludlow JR, Allen LM: The effect of early intervention and preschool stimulus on the development of the Down's syndrome child, *J Ment Defic Res* 23:29-44, 1979.
58. Malamud N: Neuropathology. In Steven HA, Herber R, editors: *Mental retardation: A review of research,* pp. 126-135, Chicago, 1964, University of Chicago Press.
59. Mann DMA, Esiri MM: The pattern of acquisition of plaques and tangles in the brains of patients under 50 years of age with Down's syndrome, *J Neurol Sci* 89:169-179, 1989.
60. Martin RH, Rademaker RA: The effect of age on the frequency of sperm chromosome abnormalities in normal men, *Am J Hum Genet* 39:123A, 1986.
61. Matroiacovo P et al: Limb anomalies following chorionic villus sampling: A registry based case-control study, *Am J Med Genet* 44:856-864, 1992.
62. Melyn MA, White DT: Mental and developmental milestones of noninstitutionalized Down's syndrome children, *Pediatrics* 52:542-545, 1973.
63. Merkatz IR et al: An association between low maternal alpha-fetoprotein and fetal chromosomal abnormalities, *Am J Obstet Gynecol* 148:886-894, 1984.
64. Meyers LF: Using computers to teach children with Down syndrome spoken and written skills. In Nadel L, editor: *The psychology of Down syndrome,* pp. 247-265, Cambridge, MA, 1988, MIT Press.
65. Miller JF: The developmental asynchrony of language development in children with Down syndrome. In Nadel L, editor: *The psychobiology of Down syndrome,* pp. 167-198, Cambridge, MA, MIT Press.
66. Motte J, Williams RS: Age-related changes in the density and morphology of plaques and neurofibrillary tangles in Down syndrome brain, *Acta Neuropathol* 77:535-546, 1989.
67. Olney RS et al: Increased risk for transverse digital deficiency after chorionic villus sampling: Results of the United States Multistate case-control study, 1988-1992, *Teratology* 51:20-29, 1995.
68. Parrenchuck TA et al: Posterior occipito-atlantal hypermobility in Down syndrome, *J Pediatr Orthop* 14:304-308, 1994.
69. Petersen MB et al: Clinical, cytogenetic, and molecular genetic characterization of two unrelated patients with different duplications of 21q, *Am J Med Genet Suppl* 7:104-109, 1990.
70. Phillips DE, Rogers JH: Down's syndrome with lingual tonsil hypertrophy producing sleep apnoea, *J Laryngol Otol* 102:1054-1055, 1988.
71. Pueschel SM: Cardiology. In Pueschel SM, Rynders JE, editors: *Down syndrome: advances in Biomedicine and the Behavioral Sciences,* p. 203, Cambridge, MA, 1982, Ware Press.

72. Pueschel SM: Clinical aspects of Down syndrome from infancy to adulthood, *Am J Med Genet Suppl* 7:52-56, 1990.
73. Pueschel SM: Growth, thyroid function, and sexual maturation in Down syndrome, *Growth, Genetics and Hormones* 6:1-5, 1990.
74. Pueschel SM, Louis S, McKnight P: Seizure disorders in Down syndrome, *Arch Neurol* 48:318, 1991.
75. Pueschel SM et al: Adolescent development in males with Down syndrome, *Am J Dis Child* 139:236-238, 1985.
76. Pueschel SM, Pezzullo JC: Thyroid dysfunction in Down syndrome, *Am J Dis Child* 139:636-639, 1985.
77. Pueschel SM, Rynders J: *Down syndrome: Advances in biomedicine and the behavioral sciences.* Cambridge, MA, 1982, Ware Press.
78. Pueschel SM, Scola FH: Atlantoaxial instability in individuals with Down syndrome: epidemiologic, radiographic, and clinical studies, *Pediatrics* 80:555-560, 1987.
79. Ridgway D et al: Transient myeloproliferative disorder of the Down type in the normal newborn, *Am J Dis Child* 144:1117-1119, 1990.
80. Robinson LL et al: Down syndrome and acute leukemia in children: a 10 year retrospective survey from the Children's Cancer Study Group, *J Pediatr* 105:235-242, 1984.
81. Rumble B et al: Amyloid A4 protein and its precursor in Down's syndrome and Alzheimer's disease, *N Engl J Med* 320:1446-1452, 1989.
82. Sara VR et al: Somatomedins in Down's syndrome, *Biol Psychiatry* 18:803-811, 1983.
83. Schupf N et al: Increased risk of Alzheimer's disease in mothers of adults with Down's syndrome, *Lancet* 344:353-356, 1994.
84. Schwartz DM, Schwartz RH: Acoustic impedance and otoscopic findings in young children with Down syndrome, *Otolaryngol* 104:652-656, 1978.
85. Seibel NL, Sommer A, Miser J: Transient neonatal leukemia reactions in mosaic trisomy 21, *J Pediatr* 104:251-254, 1984.
86. Shapiro MB, France TO: The ocular features of Down syndrome, *Am J Ophthalmol* 99:659-663, 1985.
87. Sharav T, Collins R, Shlomo L: Effect of maternal education on prognosis of development in children with Down syndrome, *Pediatrics* 76:387-391, 1985.
88. Sheridan R et al: Fertility in a male with trisomy 21, *J Med Genet* 26:294-298, 1989.
89. Smith GF, Berg JM: *Down's anomaly,* Edinburgh, 1976, Churchill Livingstone.
90. Smith GF et al: Use of megadoses of vitamins with minerals in Down syndrome, *J Pediatr* 105:228-234, 1984.
91. Southall DP et al: Upper airway obstruction with hypoxemia and sleep disruption in Down syndrome, *Dev Med Child Neurol* 29:734-742, 1987.
92. Stark AM: Dentistry. In Pueschel SM, Rynders JE, editors: *Down syndrome: Advances in biomedicine and the behavioral sciences,* pp. 199-202, Cambridge, MA, 1982, Ware Press.
93. Steinberg C et al: Recurrence rate for de novo 21q21q translocation Down syndrome: a study of 112 families, *Am J Med Genet* 17:523-530, 1984.
94. Stiller CA, Kinnier Wilson LM: Down syndrome and leukemia, *Lancet* 2:1343, 1981.
95. Storme M: Obstructive sleep apnea in Down syndrome children: A surgical approach, *Laryngoscope* 96:1340-1342, 1987.
96. Strittmatter WJ, Roses AD: Apolipoprotein E and Alzheimer disease, *Proc Natl Acad Sci* 92:4725-4727, 1995.
97. Thase ME: Longevity and mortality in Down's syndrome, *J Ment Defic Res* 26:177-192, 1982.
98. Torrado C et al: Treatment of children with Down syndrome and growth retardation with recombinant human growth hormone, *J Pediatr* 119:478-483, 1991.

99. Tricomi V, Valenti C, Hall JE: Ovulatory patterns in Down's syndrome, *Am J Obstet Gynecol* 89:651-656, 1964.
100. Uchida IA, Freeman VCP: Trisomy 21 Down syndrome—parental mosaicism, *Hum Genet* 70:246-248, 1985.
101. Ugazi OAG et al: Immunology in Down syndrome: A review, *Am J Med Genet Suppl* 7:204-212, 1990.
102. Van Dyke DC et al: Cell therapy in children with Down syndrome: a retrospective study, *Pediatrics* 85:79-84, 1990.
103. van Gool WA, Evenhuis HM, van Duijn CM: A case-control study of apolipoprotein E genotypes in Alzheimer's disease associated with Down's syndrome. Dutch study group on Down's syndrome and aging, *Ann Neurol* 38:225-230, 1995.
104. Wegman M: Annual survey of vital statistics, *Pediatrics* 86:835-847, 1990.
105. Wexler M et al: Rehabilitation of the face in patients with Down syndrome, *Plast Reconstr Surg* 77:383-393, 1986.
106. Wiesniewski KE, Miezejeski CM, Hill AL: Neurological and psychological status of individuals with Down syndrome. In Nadel L, editor: *Psychobiology of Down syndrome,* pp. 315-343, Cambridge MA, 1988, MIT Press.
107. Williams JP et al: Atlantoaxial subluxation and trisomy 21: Another perioperative complication, *Anesthesiology* 67:253-254, 1987.
108. Wisniewski HM, Rabe A: Discrepancy between Alzheimer-type neuropathology and dementia in people with Down syndrome, *Ann NY Acad Sci* 477:247-260, 1986.
109. Wisniewski KE et al: Alzheimer's disease in Down's syndrome: clinicopathologic studies, *Neurology* 35:957-961, 1985.
110. Wong KY et al: Transient myeloproliferative disorder and acute nonlymphoblastic leukemia in Down syndrome, *J Pediatr* 112:18-22, 1988.
111. Zipursky A, Peeters M, Poon A: Megakaryocytic leukemia and Down's syndrome—a review. In McCoy EE, Epstein CJ, editors: *The oncology and immunology of Down syndrome,* p. 19, New York, 1987, Liss.

Amniocentesis and Chorionic Villus Sampling

27

Vernon Cook, M.D.

27.1 AMNIOCENTESIS

History

1. Tissue karyotype technology originated in mid-1960s.
2. Before the ultrasound era (approximately 1980), amniocentesis (amnio) site was selected by palpation.
3. By 1980, amnio site selection was done by ultrasound. Subsequently, needle insertion guidance and observation of needle tip location (relative to fetus and placenta) throughout amniocentesis procedure has become common.
4. Before ultrasound, amnio was not technically feasible before 15 weeks gestation
   a. The traditional 15-week lower limit for amnio was defined by this limitation.
   b. The 1 in 200 procedure-related pregnancy loss rate data came from the preultrasound era.
5. Since 1990, early amnio (EA), defined by less than 15 weeks gestation, has received additional attention.
   a. EA is associated with a higher, 1% to 4%, loss rate and probable increased incidence of inability to retrieve fluid.
   b. > 10,000 EA procedures have been reported in literature.
   c. For each week of gestation (up to 15 weeks), 1 ml of amniotic fluid is removed.

Indications

1. Screening: Karyotype is based on maternal age or other prenatal diagnosis indication.
2. Diagnostic
   a. Spina bifida
      (1) Amniotic fluid alpha-fetoprotein AFAFP (vs. maternal serum AFP, MSAFP)
      (2) Acetyl cholinesterase
   b. Rh isoimmunization: liley curve, delta optical density (OD) 450 measurement

(1) Quantitative evaluation is done for bilirubin.
(2) Bilirubin is present in proportion to intensity of hemolysis.
(3) Liley curve zones
(a) Zone 1: not affected or mildly affected
(b) Zone 2: affected; serial observations are required to establish trend; may need fetal transfusion
(c) Zone 3: intense hemolysis, fetal transfusion required or hydrops will develop

c. Isoimmunization: fetal antigen status (Rh or irregular antigen) determination by polymerase chain reaction (PCR) (e.g., CDE, Kell antigens)
d. Single-gene disorders
e. Ultrasound abnormality
f. Other (e.g., cytomegalovirus [CMV] culture, PCR viral testing)
g. Pulmonary maturity: lecithin/sphingomyelin (L/S) ratio, foam stability index (FSI), phosphatidyl glycerol (PG)

3. Therapeutic: reductive amniocentesis
a. Removal of up to 5 L has been reported.
b. Indications include symptomatology (dyspnea, discomfort) and preterm labor complicated by polyhydramnios.
c. There is little if any association with abruptio placentae; it is not related to volume removed.
d. It is most frequently performed in twin–twin transfusion syndrome.

Relative and absolute contraindications

1. Absence of satisfactory amniotic fluid (AF) pocket away from placenta and fetus; increased risk of fetal hemorrhage
a. Oligohydramnios or anhydramnios
b. Complete anterior placenta in third trimester
(1) Transplacental amnio is relatively contraindicated because of potential fetal hemorrhage from vessel on placental surface.
(a) Umbilical cord has Wharton's jelly, which stops hemorrhage.
(b) Placental surface vessels have no jelly and may slowly (or rapidly) hemorrhage until vascular collapse occurs perhaps 2 to 3 hours later.
2. Absence of consent

Patient counseling

1. Reasonable patient concept: Physician is obligated to explain to patient anything and everything a reasonable person might want to know.
2. Generally all risks and potential complications should be explained before the amniocentesis.
3. Alternatives to amniocentesis include the following:
a. Explain consequences of not having amniocentesis.
b. Can information be obtained by another method, such as waiting until delivery to determine karyotype, biometry (biparietal diameter, femur length) for pulmonary maturity, maternal serum alpha-fetoprotein triple screening.

4. Benefit to having amniocentesis: Patient should understand rationale for performing amniocentesis.

Risks

1. Second trimester
   a. A 1/200 (0.5%) procedure-related pregnancy loss rate, in excess of gestational age-related loss
   b. Amniotic fluid leakage 1/100 (1%)
   c. Controversial increased incidence of neonatal respiratory complications related to gestational age at amnio and amount of fluid withdrawn
   d. Chorioamnionitis: 1/1000 incidence
   e. Inability to retrieve fluid: more than one needle insertion for approximately 5% of amnios
   f. Failure of cell growth: 1/800
2. Third trimester
   a. Fetal hemorrhage and exsanguination: There is a remote possibility.
      (1) Umbilical cord laceration and acute, massive hemorrhage: obvious streaming on ultrasound
      (2) Laceration of placental surface vessel
         (a) Relatively slow hemorrhage; exsanguination is reported though risk is remote; streaming may or may not be observed.
         (b) Wharton's jelly prevents exsanguination from umbilical cord; placental surface vessels lack this protection.
   b. Emergency cesarean section: Incidence is 1/1000 amnios.
   c. Fetal demise has been reported; possibility is remote.
3. Risks not dependent on gestational age
   a. Isoimmunization: Rh immune globulin prophylaxis is indicated for Rh-negative women.
   b. Fetal injury has been reported; possibility is remote.
4. Amnio: not cause of preterm labor, although contractions may be noted after procedure

Complications

1. Isoimmunization: fetal maternal hemorrhage with maternal sensitization to fetal antigen
   a. Rh immune globulin (anti D) prophylaxis is indicated to prevent Rh isoimmunization.
2. Umbilical cord laceration: sudden fetal (or maternal) movement with needle tip laceration of cord vessel
   a. Emergency cesarean section may be warranted in third trimester.
3. Amnion tenting and prevention of fluid retrieval
   a. Amnion seals to chorion at 13 to 15 weeks. Membrane separation usually can be observed on ultrasound examination.
   b. Amnion is tough; before amnion–chorion fusion, needle penetration of amnion may be difficult because amnion will simply be indented by needle (i.e., tenting) until needle contacts an object (e.g., opposite uterine wall).

c. Alternatives
   (1) Persist in present attempt: Stylet replacement and needle repositioning usually will achieve fluid retrieval.
   (2) Reattempt procedure in 1 to 2 weeks when membrane separation cannot be seen on both transabdominal and transvaginal ultrasound.

Procedure description

1. Informed consent process: Physician explains risks, benefits, and alternatives so that patient understands them.
2. Ultrasound localization of placental and amniotic fluid pocket: Physician selects site away from fetal face (eye injury prevention) and placenta and documents fetal viability.
3. Procedural instructions: Patient is told to minimize body motion during the procedure (no laughing, talking, moving suddenly or unexpectedly).
4. Physician talks to patient during procedure (e.g., play-by-play narrative).
5. Antiseptic precautions are used.
6. Local anesthesia is given if patient desires.
7. Ultrasound guidance and observation occur during (20 or 22 gauge) needle insertion.
8. Aspiration, dye insertion, and needle withdrawal are done.
9. Ultrasound (U/S) transducer is not moved after needle withdrawal to facilitate observation for streaming (blood movement through AF) from needle puncture site.
10. Postprocedural demonstration is given to patient of fetal heart action.
11. Nonstress test × 30 to 60 minutes is performed (if > 25 weeks).
12. Explanation and copy of postprocedural instructions (see next section) are given to patient.

Postamniocentesis patient instructions

1. For the first 24 hours following the amniocentesis, the patient will need to limit her activities to exclude heavy lifting or strenuous exercise.
2. Patient should refrain from sexual intercourse for the next 48 hours.
3. Patient may eat a regular diet unless restricted by the physician.
4. Patient should report to her physician any of the following:
   a. Moderate to severe cramping or pain continuing for longer than 2 hours following the amniocentesis.
   b. *Any* unsuspected leakage of amniotic fluid from the vagina.
   c. *Any* vaginal bleeding.
   d. A temperature elevation of greater than or equal to 100.4°F within 1 week after the procedure.
5. If not allergic to Tylenol, patient can take two regular Tylenol every 6 hours for mild cramping
6. If patient has had a genetic amniocentesis, the final results will not be available for approximately 2 to 3 weeks. The results will be given to patient by her private physician.
7. If patient is having amniocentesis to determine fetal lung maturity or Delta OD 450, her results will be available later in the day or the next day. The physician will notify patient of the results.

8. If the patient's blood type is A negative, B negative, O negative, or AB negative, she may require Rh immune globulin before leaving the unit.
9. Patient certifies that she has read the above information, she understands her instructions, and has received a copy.

Suggested reading

Cunningham FG et al: *William's obstetrics,* ed 19, Norwalk, CT, 1993, Appleton & Lange.

Hobbins JC, Reece EA: First-trimester prenatal diagnosis. In Reece EA et al, editors: *Medicine of the fetus and mother,* Philadelphia, 1992, JB Lippincott.

Jackson L, Wapner RJ: Amniocentesis. In Simpson JL, Elias S, editors: *Essentials of prenatal diagnosis,* New York, 1993, Churchill Livingstone.

Lynch L, Berkowitz RL: Amniocentesis, skin biopsy, and umbilical cord sampling in the prenatal diagnosis of genetic disease. In Reece EA et al, editors: *Medicine of the fetus and mother,* Philadelphia, 1992, JB Lippincott.

Simpson JL: Genetic counseling and prenatal diagnosis. In Gabbe SG, Niebyl JR, Simpson JL, editors: *Obstetrics normal and problem pregnancies,* New York, 1991, Churchill Livingstone.

Simpson JL, Elias S: Prenatal diagnosis of genetic disorders. In Creasy RK, Resnik R, editors: *Maternal-fetal medicine, principles and practice,* ed 3, Philadelphia, 1994, WB Saunders.

27.2 CHORIONIC VILLUS SAMPLING

Chorionic villus sampling overview

The main advantage of chorionic villus sampling (CVS) is the time (10 to 12 weeks gestation) at which it is performed. This first-trimester diagnostic procedure offers couples an opportunity to evaluate the normalty of the pregnancy during the first trimester. With CVS, those who would not carry an affected pregnancy could have a safer first-trimester termination rather than a mid or late second-trimester procedure.

CVS indications and contraindications

1. First trimester
   a. CVS is appropriate for any patient in whom second-trimester amniocentesis would be indicated to exclude aneuploidy, such as the following:
      (1) Maternal age ≥35 years
      (2) Prior affected child
      (3) Family history of a specific disorder (e.g., hemophilia)
   b. Alternative viewpoint: Because CVS has a higher risk than amniocentesis, CVS may be restricted to conditions with higher risk (e.g., age ≥40 years).
   c. Postmortem CVS is used for evaluation of recurrent pregnancy loss.
      (1) CVS may be performed at diagnosis of demise.
      (2) Placental tissue remains viable.
      (3) Only 1 in 23 specimens gave normal karyotype.
      (4) 100% of CVS tissue grew in culture; in other tissues (skin, products of conception, amniotic fluid), 36% to 96% failed to grow.

2. Second-trimester CVS
   a. Indications: Amniocentesis or percutaneous umbilical blood sampling (PUBS) is not feasible (e.g., oligohydramnios); rapid karyotype is needed.
   b. Sampling success rate is 91% (200/220).
   c. Complication rate appears similar to PUBS, although data are limited.
3. CVS contraindications
   a. Vaginal bleeding (CVS may exacerbate bleeding)
   b. Cervical infection: gonorrhea, *Chlamydia,* herpes
   c. Vaginal infection
   d. Gestational age <10 weeks
   e. Twins
   f. Rh isoimmunization (CVS may exacerbate isoimmunization)
4. CVS limitations
   a. CVS *cannot* check for spina bifida or anencephaly; MSAFP screening is recommended.
   b. CVS does not evaluate for anatomic abnormalities; ultrasound anatomic survey is suggested.

CVS history

1. Initial report
   a. 4-mm transcervical endoscopic biopsies of chorion were done.
   b. Of 95 patients, all planned elective termination.
   c. Twenty-one patients maintained pregnancy 8 days.
   d. Forty-seven percent of procedures retrieved chorionic villi.
   e. Problems included bleeding and puncture or biopsy of amnion.
2. Subsequent report
   a. Similar endoscopic technique was done with 38 patients.
   b. Nineteen patients were observed 7 to 48 days before termination.
   c. Two patients developed significant infections.
   d. Subsequently there was little further interest in CVS in U.S. or European medicine until the Chinese reported.
3. CVS success in China
   a. A 3-mm transcervical metal cannula aspiration with no optical guidance was done.
   b. Of 100 pregnancies, 99 were successfully sexed with six errors (three male, three female errors).
   c. Four fetal losses occurred.
4. CVS to date
   a. By 1995, 200,000 cases were reported in literature.
   b. Five national trials were completed.
   c. Several series of 10,000 to 20,000 cases were reported from a single center.

Procedure description

1. Procedural prerequisites
   a. At 10 to 12 weeks gestation: Gestational sac fills uterine cavity (at 12 to 14 weeks, amnion fuses to chorion).

   b. Technically, CVS can be performed earlier but is not because of the increased risk of limb reduction defect (see CVS Complication, 3.).
   c. Genetic counseling is provided.
   d. Ultrasound is done for the following:
      (1) Crown rump length (gestational age ±3 day accuracy)
      (2) Placental site that determines the sampling route
         (a) Fundal placenta often requires transabdominal CVS.
         (b) Posterior or anterior placentas can often be accessed transcervically.
         (c) Lowest complication rates are reported from operators who perform CVS by either approach.
      (3) Placental cord insertion
2. Transcervical CVS
   a. Bladder filling may facilitate passage of sampling catheter through cervical canal if uterus is anteverted or anteflexed.
   b. Ultrasound guidance: Assistance from technologist is crucial in guiding catheter into placenta.
   c. Cervix and vagina are prepped with betadine. Aseptic technique is observed.
   d. Uterine sound is slowly passed through cervical canal to locate internal os by ultrasound observation.
   e. Uterine sound is removed and replaced by Portex catheter, which should readily advance without force or obstruction.
   f. Catheter is guided into placenta, stylet is removed, and specimen is aspirated. Catheter is removed under suction.
3. Transabdominal CVS
   a. Fundal placenta or anterior placenta with anteverted uterus
   b. Local anesthesia of skin and uterine serosa for needle insertion site
   c. Ultrasonic guidance of needle into placenta
   d. Several needle passes through placenta during aspiration
   e. From 3% specimens retrieved <10 mg tissue, 93% >20 mg ($n = 325$)
4. Specimen evaluation
   a. Aspiration syringe contents are inspected; white villi are usually visible.
   b. Petri dish examination is done in cytotechnology laboratory.
   c. Single good aspiration yields 10 to 25 mg of wet tissue.
   d. Some DNA studies require up to 50 mg of wet tissue.
   e. Specimen is reviewed with cytotechnologist to confirm adequacy of specimen before patient leaves.
5. Specimen processing
   a. Direct method
      (1) Trophoblast cells are analyzed in spontaneous metaphase.
      (2) Karyotype is available in 4 to 12 hours.
      (3) Placental mosaicism and false negatives are about 1% higher than with culture.
   b. Coverslip culture
      (1) Collagenase enzyme releases mesenchymal cells from villi for traditional cell culture in Chang medium.
      (2) Karyotype is available in 10 to 14 days.

6. CVS registry
   a. All patients are contacted by telephone 2 weeks after procedure.
   b. Karyotype results are explained.
   c. Complications are elicited.

CVS complications

1. General
   a. Bleeding: 2% is transabdominal, 10% is transcervical.
   b. Cramps: 10% is transabdominal, 2% is transcervical.
   c. Infection: Septic abortion is a remote possibility.
   d. Rupture of the amniotic membrane is a remote possibility.
   e. Rh sensitization: Rh immune globulin prophylaxis is indicated.
   f. Procedure-related pregnancy loss: 1% to 2% above background 2% loss rate.
   g. Limb reduction defect (LRD): See next section.
2. LRDs
   a. Following CVS, LRDs occur 1/3000 to 1/1000, "generally increased over background rates."
   b. Background population incidence of LRD is 5 to 6 per 10,000 or approximately 1/2000.
   c. Timing of CVS is related to the rate and severity of LRD; LRD from CVS at ≥70 days has been limited to fingers or toes.
   d. Proposed LRD mechanism
      (1) Early gestational age
      (2) Placental trauma and vascular disruption
      (3) Limb ischemia before or after digit formation
      (4) Transient MSAFP elevation post-CVS
   e. LRD model of Quintero et al.
      (1) Before elective abortion, intrauterine fiberscope was placed for observation.
      (2) Placenta was detached or a subchorionic hematoma formed after blunt instrumentation.
      (3) Ecchymotic lesions of scalp, face, head, and thorax were observed.

Patient counseling

1. Initial counseling session with medical geneticist
   a. Family history
   b. Pregnancy history
   c. Education regarding risks and alternatives
2. Subsequent preprocedural counseling with CVS physician
   a. Indications are reviewed.
   b. Procedural risks are reviewed in detail, including photographs of infants with an LRD.
   c. Alternatives are reviewed.
      (1) Noninvasive screening consisting of ultrasound for nuchal sonolucency (50% sensitivity for trisomy 21) and MSAFP-3 screening (60% sensitivity for trisomy 21)

(2) Amniocentesis to avoid LRD risk
    (a) Early amnio at 13 to 15 weeks (1% fetal loss rate)
    (b) Traditional amnio at 15 weeks (1/200 fetal loss rate)

3. Postprocedural counseling
   a. Spina bifida MSAFP screening is explained and recommended.
   b. Ultrasound anatomic survey at 18 to 20 weeks is recommended with emphasis on digits.
   c. Postprocedural instructions are reviewed.

Post-CVS patient instructions

1. If patient's blood type is A negative, B negative, O negative, or AB negative, she may need an injection of Rh immune globulin before leaving the unit.
2. Following the CVS procedure, patient may experience spotting or bleeding.
3. Clinician will be concerned if the following occur:
   a. Patient has heavy bleeding like a period.
   b. Patient develops a fever and chills like the flu.
4. If patient has any of these symptoms or any other concerns, she should contact clinician or call her own physician.
5. As a precaution, patient should refrain from sexual intercourse for 3 to 4 days or while bleeding persists. It is also recommended that patient avoid strenuous activity such as jogging, swimming, or tennis during this time.
6. Patient may eat a regular diet unless restricted by her physician.
7. Clinician will call patient as soon as the test results are available.
8. Clinician recommends a follow-up ultrasound and blood test at 17 weeks of pregnancy. The blood test, called AFP is used to screen for neural tube defects (openings in the baby's brain or spine). CVS does not check for this abnormality. Whereas the AFP test can be scheduled through her physician's office, the clinician suggests the ultrasound be performed at the Reproductive Testing Center to permit an examination targeted on the fetal extremities and face.
9. Patient certifies she has read the above information, understands her instructions, and has received a copy. (Signature) Copy is kept in patient's chart.

Suggested reading

Center for Disease Control and Prevention: Chorionic villus sampling and amniocentesis: recommendations for prenatal counseling, *MMWR* 44(RR-9):1-12, 1995.

Chieri PR, Aldini AJR: Feasibility of placental biopsy in the second trimester for fetal diagnosis, *Am J Obstet Gynecol* 160:581-583, 1989.

Copeland KL et al: Integration of the transabdominal technique into an ongoing chorionic villus sampling program, *Am J Obstet* 161:1289-1294, 1989.

Cunningham FG et al: *William's obstetrics,* ed 19, pp. 948-950, Norwalk, CT, 1993, Appleton & Lange.

Evans MI et al: Transabdominal chorionic villus sampling for rapid karyotyping in advanced gestation, *J Reprod Med,* 36:416-418, 1991.

Hahneman N, Mohr J: Genetic diagnosis in the embryo by means of biopsy from extraembryonic membrane, *Bull Eur Soc Hum Genet* 2:23-29, 1968.

Hobbins JC, Reece EA: First-trimester prenatal diagnosis. In Reece EA et al, editors: *Medicine of the fetus and mother,* pp. 630-640, Philadelphia, 1992, JB Lippincott.

Jackson L, Wapner RJ: Chorionic villus sampling. In Simpson JL, Elias S, editors: *Essentials of prenatal diagnosis,* pp. 45-51, New York, 1993, Churchill Livingstone.

Johnson MP et al: Postmortem chorionic villus sampling is a better method for cytogenetic evaluation of early fetal loss than culture of abortus material, *Am J Obstet Gynecol* 163:1505-1510, 1990.

Kullander S, Sandahl B: Fetal chromosome analysis after transcervical placental biopsies during early pregnancy, *Acta Obstet Gynecol Scand* 52:355-359, 1973.

Quintero RA et al: Embryoscopic demonstration of hemorrhagic lesions on the human embryo after placental trauma, *Am J Obstet Gynecol* 168:756-759, 1993.

Simpson JL: Genetic counseling and prenatal diagnosis. In Gabbe SG, Niebyl JR, Simpson JL, editors: *Obstetrics normal and problem pregnancies,* pp. 269-298, New York, 1991, Churchill Livingstone.

Simpson JL, Elias S: Prenatal diagnosis of genetic disorders. In Creasy RK, Resnik R, editors: *Maternal-fetal medicine, principles and practice,* ed 3, pp. 61-88, Philadelphia, 1994, WB Saunders.

Smidt-Jensen S et al: Implications of maternal serum alpha-fetoprotein elevation caused by transabdominal and transcervical CVS, *Prenatal Diagnosis* 14:35-45, 1994.

Teitung Hospital of Anshan Iron and Steel Co: Fetal sex prediction by sex chromatin studies of chorionic villi cells during early pregnancy, *Chin Med J* 11:117-126, 1975.

Biochemical Monitoring

28

28.1 **FETAL LUNG MATURITY**

Deward H. Voss, M.D.

Fetal lung development

1. Fetal lung development begins on approximately embryonic day 26 as a laryngotracheal groove that subsequently differentiates into the laryngotracheal diverticulum and laryngotracheal tube.
2. Lung buds develop at the caudal end of the laryngotracheal tube.
   a. The glands of the larynx, trachea, bronchi, and pulmonary lining epithelium are derived from the endodermal lining.
   b. The splanchnic mesenchyme gives rise to connective tissue, cartilage, and smooth muscle.
3. Eight to 10 branchings of each secondary lung bud are present by 7 weeks, and by 24 weeks gestation, 15 to 17 branches are noted along with respiratory bronchioles.
4. After term birth, an additional seven orders of airways develop.
5. Lung development can be divided into four stages.
   a. Pseudoglandular period (5 to 17 weeks)
   b. Canalicular period (13 to 25 weeks)
   c. Terminal sac period (24 weeks to birth)
   d. Alveolar period (late fetal to 8 years)
6. During the pseudoglandular period the airways are lined with simple cuboidal cells and the architecture of the developing lung resembles a gland.
   a. By 17 weeks gestation, all major elements of the lung have formed; however, those elements that allow gas exchange are not present.
7. With the canalicular period the lumina of the bronchi and bronchioles increase and the lung tissue becomes much more vascular.
   a. By 24 weeks, two or more respiratory bronchioles have developed from each terminal bronchiole.
   b. At this same time, some thin-wall saccules and terminal sacs (primitive alveoli and alveolar ducts) can be seen and the production of surfactant is noted in some type II pneumocytes.

8. During the terminal sac phase there is proliferation of terminal sacs; the epithelium of the terminal sacs are lined with thin type I pneumocytes; and capillaries start to bulge into the terminal sacs.
   a. By 25 to 28 weeks gestation, the development of terminal sacs is adequate to permit survival of the infant.
9. Alveolar ducts develop from the terminal sacs.
   a. Characteristic mature alveoli do not form until some time after birth.
   b. The increase in lung size after birth is primarily from an increase in the number of primitive alveoli, with only 12% to 15% of the adult number of alveoli present at term.

Pulmonary surfactant

Surfactant lowers the potential for atelectasis by lowering the surface tension at the air–alveolar interface.

1. The primary surface-active component of surfactant is dipalmitoylphosphatydylcholine (lecithin).
2. The second most surface-active glycerophospholipid component is phosphatidylglycerol (PG).
3. Ninety percent of surfactant is lipid, and 80% of the glycerophospholipids are phosphatidylcholines (lecithins).
   a. Lecithin (dipalmitoylphosphatidylcholine, disaturated phosphatidylcholine, or disaturated choline) represents approximately 50% of the glycerophospholipids.
4. PG represents approximately 10% to 15% of the lipid component of surfactant.
5. Three surfactant specific proteins have also been identified: SP-A, SP-B, and SP-C.
   a. These proteins are critical for the regulation of the biophysical effects of surfactant and for lipid organization.
6. Surfactant is synthesized by the type II pneumocytes and secreted by exocytosis as lamellar bodies into the alveolus, where it is incorporated into a tubular myelin pool to maintain a surface film.
   a. Newly synthesized surfactant constantly enters the surface film.
7. The concentration of sphingomyelin serves as a reference for the synthesis of glycerophospholipid and remains relatively constant throughout gestation.
   a. The concentration of lecithin in amniotic fluid increases with advancing gestational age and fetal pulmonary maturity.

Pulmonary maturation

There are several maternal and fetal conditions that influence fetal pulmonary maturation and the pulmonary function of the neonate.

1. For the fetal lung to develop properly, the fetus must show appropriate frequency and amplitude of fetal breathing movements and must maintain a critical volume of fetal lung fluid during the early development.
   a. If the fetal lung fluid volume is decreased for a prolonged period of time before the canalicular stage there is a significant risk of pulmonary hypoplasia.

Clinical Syndromes Associated with Pulmonary Hypoplasia

Thoracic compression
- Renal agenesis
- Urinary tract outflow obstruction
- Prolonged oligohydramnios before 28 weeks
- Extraamniotic fetal development

Decreased intrathoracic space
- Diaphragmatic hernia
- Pleural effusions
- Abdominal distension sufficient to limit chest volume
- Thoracic dystrophies

Decreased fetal breathing
- Intrauterine central nervous system damage
- Fetal Werdnig-Hoffmann syndrome
- Other neuropathies and myopathies

Other associations
- Primary pulmonary hypoplasia
- Trisomy 21
- Multiple congenital anomalies
- Erythroblastosis fetalis

   b. The fluid volume may be diminished by either external compression or space occupying lesions in the fetal chest.
   c. Clinical syndromes that may be associated with pulmonary hypoplasia are listed in the box above.
2. Several conditions have been associated with alterations in fetal lung maturation and are listed in the box on p. 750.

Assessment of fetal pulmonary maturity

Fetal pulmonary maturity can be evaluated by multiple tests as shown in the box on p. 750.

1. The semiquantitative assessment of the lecithin/sphingomyelin ratio (L/S) was first introduced by Gluck and others in 1971 and remains the "gold standard" for fetal pulmonary maturity testing.
   a. The sphingomyelin concentration of the amniotic fluid remains relatively constant throughout pregnancy.
   b. The lecithin concentration rises rapidly at about 34 weeks gestation.
   c. An L/S ratio of ≥ 2 was not associated with neonatal respiratory distress syndrome (RDS).
   d. Determination of the L/S has disadvantages in that assessment of the L/S may require amniocentesis and is a labor-intensive and skill-intensive test that may require 3 to 4 hours for completion.
   e. The sensitivity and specificity are approximately 80% to 85%.
2. PG determination has an advantage as a test of fetal pulmonary maturity in that its presence in amniotic fluid is uniquely from surfactant.

Conditions Associated with Alterations in Fetal Lung Maturation

Accelerated maturation
- Chronic maternal hypertension
- Maternal cardiovascular disease
- Placental infarction
- Intrauterine growth retardation
- Severe pregnancy-induced hypertension
- Prolonged rupture of membranes
- Hemoglobinopathies

Delayed maturation
- Diabetes mellitus
- Rh isoimmunization with hydrops fetalis

Tests of Fetal Lung Maturity

Biochemical test
- Lecithin/sphingomyelin ratio
- Phosphatidylglycerol

Biophysical test
- Shake test (bubble stability test or foam test)
- Foam stability index
- Tap test
- Fluorescent polarization assay

Lamellar body counts

Ultrasound

a. The test is positive when 3% or more of the total phospholipids are from PG.
b. However if even a trace of PG is present, it is very unlikely that neonatal RDS will develop.
c. Two-dimensional thin-layer chromatography is used to detect PG and is labor and skill intensive.
d. The presence of PG can be assessed by the use of commercially available kits using latex agglutination or enzymatic testing.
e. Assessment for PG is 100% sensitive and about 75% specific for RDS.

3. The shake test assesses the biophysical capability of pulmonary surfactant to generate a stable foam in the presence of ethanol, which eliminates the contributions of protein, bile salts, and salts of free fatty acids to the foam stability.
   a. An ethanol concentration of 47.5% is required.
   b. If blood or meconium contaminate the amniotic fluid, falsely mature results may be obtained.

c. A positive test (i.e., a complete ring of bubbles at the meniscus with a 1:2 dilution of amniotic fluid) is rarely associated with RDS.
d. Approximately 75% of negative tests are falsely immature.

4. Tests of the foam stability index (FSI) are conducted using graded concentrations of ethanol.
a. Commercially available kits in which testing wells are provided with predispensed volumes of ethanol are available and the addition of 0.5 ml of amniotic fluid to each well will result in final ethanol concentrations of 44% to 50%.
b. Once these dilutions have been made, the fluid–ethanol mixture is shaken and the FSI value is established as the highest value concentration producing a stable ring of foam.
c. Contamination of the amniotic fluid with blood or meconium may invalidate the test.
d. Neonatal RDS is unlikely with an FSI ≥47.

5. The tap test is a semiquantitative assessment of pulmonary surfactant function.
a. Contaminated fluid must be centrifuged before the test can be performed.
b. One milliliter of amniotic fluid is mixed with 1 drop of 6 *N* hydrochloric acid, followed by the addition of 1.5 ml of diethyl ether in a 6 × 150 mm test tube.
c. The test tube is briskly tapped to create an estimated 200 to 300 bubbles in the ether (top) layer.
d. With pulmonary maturity, the bubbles formed rise quickly to the top and break; however, with immaturity, the bubbles are stable or break down slowly.
e. The test is read at 2, 5, and 10 minutes.
f. The cutoff value for maturity is ≤5 bubbles.

6. The optical absorbance of amniotic fluid at 650 nm can be used for assessment of pulmonary maturity.
a. The large size of lamellar bodies in amniotic fluid results in an intense scattering of light, and the turbidity of the amniotic fluid is quantified at a wavelength of 650 nm to avoid the interference of other chromagens.
b. Maturity is generally 0.15.
c. Polyhydramnios or the presence of other absorbing pigments may alter the accuracy of the test.

7. The relative lipid content of amniotic fluid, microviscosimetry, can be assessed by fluorescent depolarization.
a. In original assessments, the amniotic fluid was incubated with a lipid-soluble dye (1,6-diphenyl-1,3,5-hexatriene) for 30 minutes, during which time some dye would be absorbed into the phospholipid membranes.
b. The degree of dye absorbed was then determined by measuring the fluorescence of polarized light (*P*) via the microviscosimeter.
c. With an increasing L/S, the *P* value falls.
d. Because the cost of microviscosimeters was high, fluorescence polarization assays were developed using a different fluorescent probe and the TDx Analyzer (an automated fluorescence polarimeter utilized for therapeutic drug monitoring in most laboratories).

   e. This assay now determines the relative amount of surfactant phospholipid by measuring the portioning of dye between albumin (high polarization) and surfactant lipid (low polarization).
   f. There is low risk of RDS if the $P < 0.260$.
   g. Contamination with blood may invalidate the test.
8. The lamellar body number density can be used for assessment of fetal pulmonary maturity.
   a. The volume of small platelets and lamellar bodies are approximately the same, and lamellar bodies can be counted by electronic cell counters (e.g., Coulter counters).
   b. The lamellar body number density count has a high concordance with other measurements of fetal lung maturity.
   c. Criteria for maturity are different for centrifuged and noncentrifuged specimens.
      (1) A lamellar body number density of 26,000/μl is mature if the specimen was centrifuged (5 min at $500 \times g$).
      (2) Alternatively, a count of 40,000 to 60,000/μl in the unspun specimen is considered mature.
   d. Using a sample that has not been centrifuged saves time and removes the greatest factor in lab-to-lab variation.
   e. The cell counter is able to discriminate large cells and debris from lamellar bodies; however, the lamellar body number density will be significantly lowered by even 1% contamination with blood.
9. Assessment of fetal lung maturity by ultrasound can eliminate the need for assessment of amniotic fluid.
   a. Multiple ultrasonic parameters have been evaluated as potential markers of fetal pulmonary maturity, including the following:
      (1) Biparietal diameter (BPD)
      (2) Femur length
      (3) Placental grade
      (4) Lung texture
      (5) Epiphyseal ossification centers
      (6) Free-floating particles in the amniotic fluid
   b. While some controversy remains, Golde and others reported that a BPD ≥92 mm in the nondiabetic patient predicted pulmonary maturity by both L/S and neonatal clinical performance.
   c. Likewise, in the nondiabetic patient, a fetal femur length of ≥72 mm enhanced the specificity of the BPD and the placental grade in predicting pulmonary maturity.
   d. Placental grade alone and other ultrasonic markers are less predictive of the absence of neonatal respiratory distress.

Pharmacologic enhancement of pulmonary maturation

Multiple agents are known to alter fetal lung maturity. Both corticosteroids and thyrotropin-releasing hormone (TRH) have received considerable attention recently.

1. The National Institutes of Health (NIH) released recommendations regarding the antepartum administration of corticosteroids, noting that the benefits of such therapy vastly outweigh the potential maternal and neonatal risks.

   a. The benefits of antenatal steroids to the preterm fetus include:
      (1) Reduced risk of RDS
      (2) Decreased mortality
      (3) Decreased incidence of intraventricular hemorrhage
2. The NIH recommendations suggest that all women between 24 and 34 weeks gestation who are at risk for preterm delivery are at risk and should be considered candidates for antenatal corticoid therapy if they are candidates for tocolytic therapy.
   a. Fetal race, gender, and the availability of surfactant therapy should not be used as factors in the decision to administer antenatal corticosteroids.
3. Antenatal corticoid therapy should consist of either:
   a. Betamethasone 12 mg, IM, two doses 24 hours apart, *or*
   b. Dexamethasone 6 mg, IM, four doses 12 hours apart
   c. These agents are recommended in that they cross the placenta in a biologically active form, have a prolonged half-life, and have minimal mineralocorticoid activity.
4. Optimal benefit to the fetus or neonate is seen at approximately 24 hours after therapy is initiated and lasts approximately 7 days.
   a. Treatment of less than 24 hours is of benefit and, therefore, antenatal corticosteroid therapy should be given unless delivery is imminent.
   b. Although there is not any proven improvement in pulmonary maturity following preterm premature spontaneous rupture of membranes (PPROM), antenatal corticosteroid therapy is recommended in patients with PPROM at less than 30 to 32 weeks gestation in the absence of clinical chorioamnionitis to reduce the incidence of intraventricular hemorrhage.
5. Antenatal TRH has been shown to be of benefit in early animal studies and human trials by stimulating fetal thyroid hormone production, an endogenous stimulant of fetal pulmonary maturation.
   a. TRH has been used in conjunction with antenatal corticosteroid therapy to enhance fetal lung maturity.
   b. The usual dose of TRH is 400 μg, IV, q8-12h, for four to six doses.
   c. Each injection is given slowly over at least 4 minutes.
6. Antenatal TRH has the following potential maternal side effects:
   a. Hypertension
   b. Rash
   c. Dyspnea
   d. Nausea
   e. Dizziness
   f. Blurred vision
   g. Suppression of the fetal or neonatal pituitary–thyroid axis with neonatal rebound at approximately 10 days has been reported as well.
7. The Australian Collaborative Trial of Antenatal Thyrotropin-Releasing Hormone (ACTOBAT) reported the results of 1234 women treated with 200 μg of TRH, IV, q12h for four doses versus placebo at 24 to 31$\frac{6}{7}$ weeks gestation.

a. All patients also received antenatal corticosteroids.
b. The frequencies of RDS and the need for ventilation were higher in the treatment group, with the excess risk greater in infants delivered more than 10 days after treatment.

Surfactant

Surfactant became clinically available in the United States in 1990 and can be used to improve the pulmonary function of the neonate.

1. There are two preparations of surfactant currently available in the United States.
   a. Exosurf: composed of synthetic lipids and an emulsifying agent
   b. Survanta: bovine surfactant extract containing lipids and the surfactant proteins SP-B and SP-C
2. Two clinical indications have been suggested.
   a. Rescue treatment for the neonate with RDS
   b. Prophylactic treatment for the preterm infant at risk for RDS, provided immediately following birth
3. Multiple trials have demonstrated the mortality secondary to RDS is decreased by approximately 30% with surfactant therapy.
   a. There is a decreased incidence of pneumothorax, oxygen requirements, and the need for ventilator support.
   b. Survivors of RDS, however, have not shown any significant decrease in the incidence of bronchopulmonary dysplasia.

Prevention of respiratory deficiency syndrome

1. By ACOG committee opinion, fetal maturity may be assumed if:
   a. Fetal heart tones have been documented for 30 weeks by Doppler or 20 weeks by fetoscope.
   b. A positive serum or urine HCG was noted 36 weeks earlier.
   c. An ultrasound measurement of the crown–rump length obtained at 6 to 11 weeks gestation indicates a gestational age of ≥39 weeks.
   d. The gestational age of ≥39 weeks, as established by history and physical, is confirmed by an ultrasound at 12 to 20 weeks.
2. RDS may or may not be surfactant-dependent RDS, and many clinical situations may mandate premature delivery, but decreasing the incidence of RDS begins with decreasing premature delivery.
   a. Accurate dating of the pregnancy is essential, as is decision making regarding the necessity of delivery.
   b. If delivery is urgent but elective, multiple tests of fetal pulmonary maturity are available.
   c. The risks of fetal lung maturity testing include the following:
      (1) Falsely immature test (30% to 90%)
      (2) Unnecessary delay of delivery
      (3) Risk of prolonged gestation
      (4) Hazards of repeat testing
   d. Although antenatal corticosteroid therapy may be of benefit, the role of TRH to enhance fetal pulmonary maturity remains controversial.
   e. Surfactant therapy can be used to reduce the morbidity of RDS.

Suggested reading

ACTOBAT Study Group: Australian collaborative trial of antenatal thyrotropin-releasing hormone (ACTOBAT) for prevention of neonatal respiratory disease, *Lancet* 85:877-882, 1995.

American College of Obstetricians and Gynecologists: *Fetal maturity assessment prior to elective repeat cesarean delivery,* ACOG Committee Opinion 98, Washington, DC; 1991, ACOG.

Ashwood ER, Oldroyd RG, Palmer SE: Measuring the number of lamellar body particles in amniotic fluid, *Obstet Gynecol* 75:289-292, 1990.

Ashwood ER et al: Lamellar body counts for rapid fetal lung maturity testing, *Obstet Gynecol* 81:619-624, 1993.

Ashwood ER et al: Improved fluorescence polarization assay for use in evaluating fetal lung maturity. III. Retrospective clinical evaluation and comparison with the lecithin/sphingomyelin ratio, *Clin Chem* 32:260-264, 1986.

Ballard RA et al: TRH Study Group: Respiratory disease in very-low-birthweight infants after prenatal thyrotropin-releasing hormone and glucocorticoid, *Lancet* 339:510-515, 1992.

Bayer-Zwirello LA et al: Amniotic fluid surfactant-albumin ratio as a screening test for fetal lung maturity—two years of clinical experience, *J Perinatol* 13:354-360, 1993.

Carson PL, Meyer CR, Bowerman RA: Prediction of fetal lung maturity with ultrasound, *Radiology* 155:533, 1985.

Cavalieri RL, Woodling S: Purification of lamellar bodies from human amniotic fluid, *Am J Obstet Gynecol* 150:409-414, 1984.

Cayea PD et al: Prediction of fetal lung maturity: Inaccuracy of study using conventional ultrasound instruments, *Radiology* 155:473-475, 1985.

Chen C et al: Clinical evaluation of the NBD-PC flourescence polarization assay for prediction of fetal lung maturity, *Obstet Gynecol* 80:688-692, 1992.

Cunningham FG et al: The morphological and functional development of the fetus. In *Williams obstetrics,* ed 19, pp. 186-194, Norwalk, CT, 1993, Appleton & Lange.

Dewhurst CJ et al: Prediction of respiratory-distress syndrome by estimation of surfactant in the amniotic fluid, *Lancet* 301:1475-1457, 1973.

Dubin SB: Characterization of amniotic fluid lamellar bodies by resistive-pulse counting: Relationship to measures of fetal lung maturity, *Clin Chem* 35:612-616, 1989.

Dubin SB: Assessment of fetal lung maturity by laboratory methods, *Reprod Med* 12:603-620, 1992.

Fakhoury G et al: Lamellar body concentrations and the prediction of fetal pulmonary maturity, *Am J Obstet Gynecol* 170:72-76, 1994.

Foerder CA et al: Improved fluorescence polarization assay for use in evaluating fetal lung maturity. II. Analytical evaluation and comparison with the lecithin/sphingomyelin ratio, *Clin Chem* 32:255-259, 1986.

Gluck L, Kulovich MV: Lecithin/sphingomyelin ratios in amniotic fluid in normal and abnormal pregnancy, *Am J Obstet Gynecol* 115:539-546, 1973.

Golde SH et al: Fetal lung maturity: The adjunctive use of ultrasound, *Am J Obstet Gynecol* 142:445-447, 1982.

Gross TL et al: When is an amniocentesis for fetal maturity unnecessary in nondiabetic pregnancies at risk? *Am J Obstet Gynecol* 149:311-319, 1984.

Hadlock FP et al: Ultrasound prediction of fetal lung maturity, *Radiology* 155:469-472, 1985.

Herbert WNP, Chapman JF, Schnoor MM: Role of the TDx FLM assay in fetal lung maturity, *Am J Obstet Gynecol* 168:808-812, 1993.

Ivie WM et al: Modified lamellar body phospholipid assay compared with L/S ratio and phosphatidylglycerol assay for assessment of fetal pulmonary status, *Clin Chem* 33:24-31, 1987.

Kassanos D et al: The tap test: a simple and inexpensive method for the diagnosis of fetal pulmonary maturity, *Int J Gynecol Obstet* 41:135-138, 1993.
Kjos SL et al: Prevalence and etiology of respiratory distress in infants of diabetic mothers: Predictive value of fetal lung maturation tests, *Am J Obstet Gynecol* 163:898-903, 1990.
Knight DB, Liggins GC, Wealthall SR: A randomized, controlled trial of antepartum thyrotropin-releasing hormone and betamethasone in the prevention of respiratory disease in preterm infants, *Am J Obstet Gynecol* 171:11-116, 1994.
Liggins GC et al: Synergism of cortisol and thyrotropin-releasing hormone in lung maturation in fetal sheep, *J Appl Physiol* 65:1880-1884, 1988.
Lockitch G et al: Prediction of fetal lung maturity by use of the Lumadex-FSI test, *Clin Chem* 32:361-363, 1986.
Mahony BS et al: Epiphyseal ossification centers in the assessment of fetal maturity: Sonographic correlation with the amniocentesis lung profile, *Radiology* 159:521-524, 1986.
Moore KL: The respiratory system: larynx, trachea, bronchi, and lungs. In *The Developing Human,* ed 2, pp. 188-196, Philadelphia, 1977,
Morales WJ et al: Fetal lung maturation: the combined use of corticosteroids and thyrotropin-releasing hormone, *Obstet Gynecol* 73:111-116, 1989.
Mullin TJ, Gross TL, Wolfson RN: Ultrasound screening for free-floating particles and fetal lung maturity, *Obstet Gynecol* 66:50-54, 1985.
Nguyen H, Golde SH: The amniostat immunologic slide test for phosphatidylglycerol: a comparison of efficacy among screening tests for fetal lung maturity, *J Perinatol* 7:16-20, 1987.
Papageorgiou et al: Antenatal prevention of the neonatal respiratory distress syndrome: Benefits and potential risks for the mother and the infant, *J Perinat Med* 14:75-86, 1986.
Pearlman ES et al: Utility of a rapid lamellar body count in the assessment of fetal maturity, *Am J Clin Pathol* 95:778-780, 1991.
Petrucha RA, Golde SH, Platt LD: The use of ultrasound in the prediction of fetal pulmonary maturity, *Am J Obstet Gynecol* 144:931-934, 1982.
Russell JC et al: Multicenter evaluation of TDx test for assessing fetal lung maturity, *Clin Chem* 35:1005-1010, 1989.
Schwartz RM et al: Effect of surfactant on morbidity, mortality, and resource use in newborn infants weighing 500 to 1500 g, *N Engl J Med* 330:1476-1480, 1994.
Socol ML: The tap test: confirmation of a simple, rapid, inexpensive, and reliable indicator of fetal pulmonary maturity, *Am J Obstet Gynecol* 162:218-222, 1990.
Steinfeld JD et al: The utility of the TDx test in the assessment of fetal lung maturity, *Obstet Gynecol* 79:460-464, 1992.
Tahilramaney M, Platt LD, Golde S: Ultrasound in evaluation of fetal pulmonary maturity, *P-N* Jan/Feb:9-13, 1986.
Tahilramaney MP, Platt LD, Golde SH: Use of femur length measured by ultrasonography to predict fetal maturity, *J Perinatol* 11:157-160, 1991.
Tait JF et al: Prospective clinical evaluation of an improved fluorescence polarization assay for predicting fetal lung maturity, *Clin Chem* 33:554-558, 1987.
Tait JF et al: Improved fluorescence polarization assay for use in evaluating fetal lung maturity. I. Development of the assay procedure, *Clin Chem* 32:248-254, 1986.
Thurlbeck WM: Prematurity and the developing lung, *Clin Perinatol* 19:497-519, 1992.
Verder H et al: Surfactant therapy and nasal continuous positive airway pressure for newborns with respiratory distress syndrome, *N Engl J Med* 331:1051-1055, 1994.
Ward RM: Pharmacologic enhancement of fetal lung maturation, *Clin Perinatol* 21:523-542, 1994.

28.2

FETAL SCALP SAMPLING

Bryan J. DeMarco, M.D.

1. Background
   a. Fetal scalp sampling was introduced by Saling in 1962.
   b. It is the "gold standard" against which biophysical indications of fetal distress are judged (Fig. 28-1).
   c. Fetal scalp sampling is 85% to 90% (pH > 7.20) accurate with Apgar score of > 7.
   d. Fetal distress is falsely predicted 35% to 78% (pH < 7.20).
2. Indications and utility of method
   a. Assessment of fetal well-being
   b. Assessment of fetal platelet count
   c. Interpretation of fetal heart rate patterns that are unclear (Table 28-1)

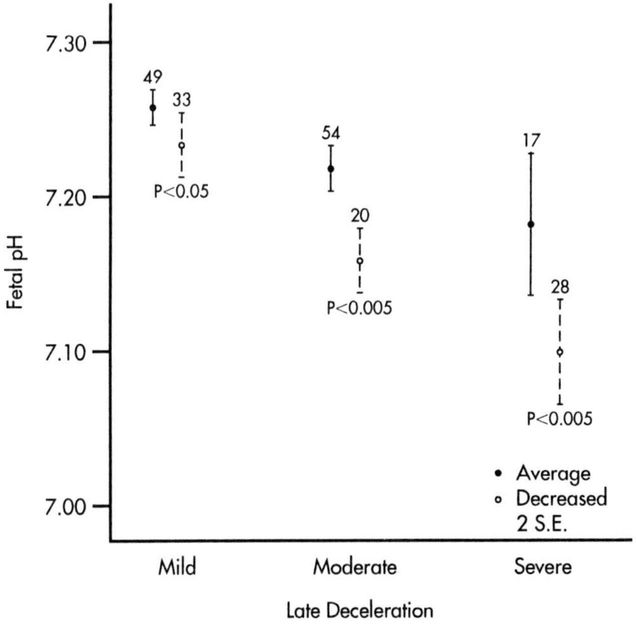

Figure 28-1

Relationship between fetal blood pH and severity of late decelerations at time of blood sampling. Each fetal heart rate (FHR) classification is further divided into average (> 5 beats per minute) or decreased (< 5 beats per minute) FHR variability. (From Paul RH et al: Clinical fetal monitoring: VII. The evaluation and significance of intrapartum baseline FHR variability, *Am J Obstet Gynecol* 123:206, 1975.)

Table 28-1 Fetal scalp blood sampling—indications and outcome

Indications for Sampling	No. of Fetuses	No. with Scalp pH < 7.20
Later Decelerations		
Good variability		
Normal baseline rate	3	0
Tachycardia	4	0
Diminished variability		
Normal baseline rate	12	3
Tachycardia	9	6
Total	28	9
Moderate to Severe Variable Decelerations		
Good variability		
Normal baseline rate	6	2
Tachycardia	2	1
Diminished variability		
Normal baseline rate	5	1
Tachycardia	4	3
Total	17	7
No Periodic Changes		
Good variability		
Normal baseline rate	0	0
Tachycardia	4	0
Diminished variability		
Normal baseline rate	26	1
Tachycardia	15	1
Total	45	2
Baseline bradycardia	5	3
Other (sinusoidal, fetal arrhythmia)	5	0

3. Technique
   a. Illuminated endoscope is inserted through a dilated cervix with ruptured membranes.
   b. Fetal scalp or buttock is cleaned and a small incision is made to a depth of 2 mm with a long-handled scalpel.
   c. Drops of blood are collected in a heparinized capillary tube and the pH is measured.
4. Contraindications
   a. Fetus known to have a blood dyscrasia (e.g., hemophilia or von Willebrand's disease)
   b. Amnionitis: considered a relative contraindication
   c. Suspected herpes genitalis

Table 28-2 Total births, cesarean births, and rate of fetal scalp blood sampling*

	1986	1987	1988	1989	1990	1991	1992
Live births	16,947	16,193	16,288	17,947	17,878	14,659	14,398
Fetal scalp blood sampling	242	351	276	134	42	14	4
	(1.43%)	(2.17%)	(1.69%)	(0.75%)	(0.23%)	(0.10%)	(0.03%)
Total cesarean births	2465	3086	2621	2400	2267	1999	1911
	(14.5%)	(19.1%)	(16.1%)	(13.4%)	(12.7%)	(13.6%)	(13.3%)
Cesarean for fetal distress	430	534	477	438	509	330	319
	(2.54%)	(3.30%)	(2.93%)	(2.44%)	(2.85%)	(2.25%)	(2.22%)

*%, Percentage of live births.

Table 28-3 Indirect indicators of perinatal asphyxial morbidity*

	1986	1987	1988	1989	1990	1991	1992
Live births	16,947	16,193	16,288	17,947	17,878	14,659	14,398
5-min Apgar score ≤5	130 (0.77%)	143 (0.88%)	114 (0.70%)	92 (0.51%)	72 (0.40%)	60 (0.41%)	7 (0.50%)
Perinatal asphyxia	36 (0.21%)	36 (0.22%)	33 (0.20%)	21 (0.12%)	21 (0.12%)	13 (0.09%)	1 (0.07%)
Meconium aspiration	136 (0.80%)	136 (0.84%)	172 (1.06%)	150 (0.84%)	118 (0.66%)	124 (0.85%)	13 (0.94%)

*%, Percent of live births.

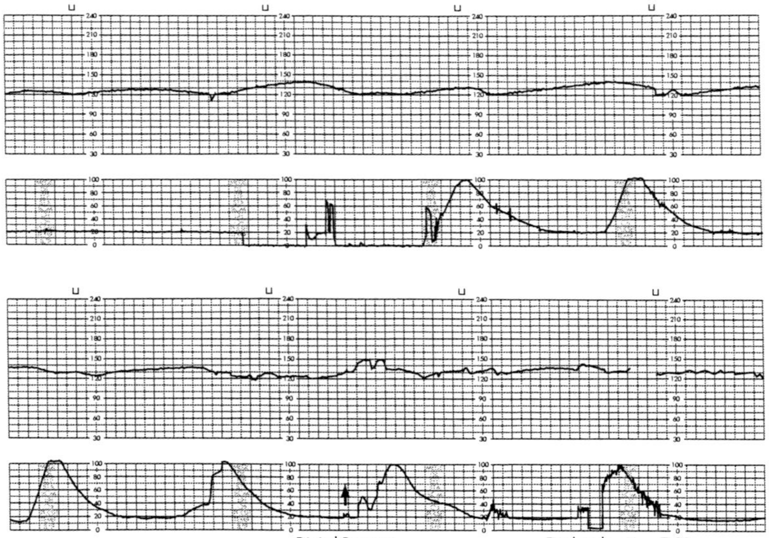

Figure 28-2
Fetal heart rate tracing exhibiting diminished variability and repetitive late decelerations. Scalp stimulation *(arrow)* was followed by an acceleration of fetal heart rate as previously defined. Scalp pH was 7.28.

5. Interpretation of results
   a. If pH is > 7.25, labor should be observed.
   b. If pH is between 7.25 and 7.20, pH sampling should be repeated within 20 to 30 minutes.
   c. If pH is < 7.20, delivery should be considered.
   d. If pH is ≤7.15, expeditious delivery should be considered.
6. Practical problems
   a. Unavailabity of technical personnel and equipment for pH analysis
   b. Technical difficulty in performing the procedure
   c. Time delay in obtaining results
   d. Misinterpretation of pH data
   e. Need for repetitive sampling
   f. Falsely elevated scalp pH possible because of collection technique
7. Factors contributing to the decline in use of pH sampling
   a. There is no agreement on scientific grounds on an appropriate threshold for intervention.
   b. The literature is unable to demonstrate what degree of acidosis from scalp pH is associated with predictable fetal harm.
   c. Cost of maintaining a pH analysis machine is high.
   d. Recent studies have revealed that a decrease in use of fetal scalp sampling has not shown an increase in cesarean section rates or perinatal asphyxia (Tables 28-2 and 28-3).
   e. The use of a fetal scalp stimulation technique that evokes a fetal heart rate acceleration of 15 bpm for 15 seconds will assure a nonacidotic fetus (Fig. 28-2).
   f. It is not considered a standard of obstetric care.

Suggested reading

Clark S: The scalp stimulation: a clinical alternative to fetal scalp blood sampling, *Am J Obstet Gynecol* 148:274, 1984.

Clark S: Intrapartum fetal surveillance: the role of fetal scalp blood sampling, *Am J Obstet Gynecol* 153:717, 1985.

Creasy, Resnik: *Maternal fetal medicine, principles and practice,* 1994.

Cunningham F: In *Williams obstetrics,* ed 19, Norwalk, CT, 1993, Appleton & Lange.

Goodwin T: Elimination of fetal scalp blood sampling on a large clinical service, *Obstet Gynecol* 83:971, 1994.

Nieto A: Intrauterine growth retardation fluctuation of fetal pH measured between beginning and at the completion of labor, *J Perinat Med* 22:329, 1994.

Sherman D: The effect of sampling technique on measurement of fetal blood pH and gases—An in vitro system, *Am J Obstet Gynecol* 171:1125, 1994.

Spencer J: Predictive value of a fetal heart rate acceleration at the time of fetal blood sampling in labour, *J Perinat Med* 19:207, 1991.

Viscarello R: Is the risk of perinatal transmission of human immunodeficiency virus increased by intrapartum use of spiral electrodes or fetal scalp pH sampling? *Am J Obstet Gynecol* 170:740, 1994.

Antenatal Assessment

29

29.1 ANTENATAL ASSESSMENT

Stephen J. Carlan, M.D.

Antepartum fetal surveillance is performed in identified high-risk pregnancies to reduce both perinatal mortality and morbidity. The overall perinatal mortality rate in the United States in 1992 was 7.2 per 1000. These were fetal deaths that occurred from 28 weeks to birth. Up to two thirds of these antenatal deaths may be associated with chronic processes that might be detected with antepartum surveillance. Thus, antenatal fetal assessment is an important component of modern obstetric care.

Although a variety of tests have been proposed, there are six main tests in current use in the United States that are discussed in this chapter:

Nonstress test (NST)
Contraction stress test (CST)
Biophysical profile
Modified biophysical profile
Umbilical artery Doppler velocimetry
Fetal movement

The indications for the tests originally were limited to hypertension and other severe medical complications. However, with the introduction of more sophisticated testing methods, the clinical application has expanded and now includes any pregnancy condition at risk for developing either decreased uteroplacental function or other disorders associated with stillbirth, (see the box on p. 764).

1. Background
   a. There are variations in technique, timing, frequency, test preference, and interpretation among centers.
   b. The time in gestation to initiate surveillance reflects the severity of the condition and the risk of intrauterine fetal death, as well as the likelihood that *in utero* therapy or delivery would result in a better chance for survival.
   c. The more serious or more unpredictable the condition, the sooner testing should begin.
   d. The frequency of testing depends on the type of test, but typically tests are repeated one or two times per week.

Indications for Antenatal Surveillance

1. Maternal disease
   - Diabetes mellitus—insulin
   - Connective tissue disease
   - Antiphospholipid syndrome
   - Hypertension—all forms
   - Hyperthyroidism
   - Anemia
   - Preterm premature ruptured membranes
   - Unexplained vaginal bleeding
   - Cyanotic heart disease
   - Advanced maternal age
2. History of poor obstetric outcome
3. Postdate pregnancy
4. Fetal indications
   - Intrauterine growth retardation
   - Decreased fetal movement
   - Nonimmune hydrops fetalis
   - Irregular or abnormal fetal heart rate tracing
   - Isoimmunization
   - Multiple gestation

e. Changes in the patient's clinical condition may warrant more frequent studies.
f. Antenatal surveillance cannot prevent most cord accidents, abruptios, or acute fetal compromise.
g. Although most clinicians feel that the use of antepartum surveillance in selected patients provides information that may change obstetric management and lead to improved perinatal outcome, all studies have not demonstrated a uniform improvement in perinatal outcome as a result of antepartum testing.
h. One study concluded that by the time the fetal compromise is diagnosed with antepartum testing, fetal damage may have already occurred.[37]
i. A normal test implies that the fetus is not significantly compromised, and the pregnancy can be extended until either the clinical condition deteriorates or the next scheduled test.
j. Although a normal test accurately predicts a well fetus, an abnormal test does not always mean a sick fetus.
k. Abnormal results, in fact, are seldom reliable and the recommended management of an abnormal test is usually either to repeat the test or to add a backup test rather than to initiate immediate delivery.
l. Antenatal surveillance is more useful in documenting fetal wellness than in determining fetal illness.

Nonstress test

1. Background
   a. In 1976, the association of fetal heart rate (FHR) acceleration with fetal movements was reported to signify fetal health.[38]
   b. Although a normal test result can accurately predict a healthy fetus, an abnormal test result is difficult to interpret.
   c. The presence of accelerations is more predictive of health than the absence of accelerations is predictive of compromise.
   d. In late pregnancy, normal, healthy fetuses exhibit 34 accelerations per hour and they average 20 to 25 beats per minute (bpm) in amplitude, lasting 40 seconds.[23]
   e. Between 24 and 28 weeks, about 50% of NSTs are nonreactive.[1]
   f. Between 28 and 32 weeks, 15% of NSTs are nonreactive.[5]
   g. After 32 weeks, the incidence of reactive and nonreactive NSTs is comparable with that seen at term.
   h. At term, fetal movements are associated with accelerations at least 90% of the time.
2. Description
   a. The NST is a noninvasive method of evaluating the immediate condition of the fetus by observing the response of the FHR to fetal movement.
3. Instrumentation
   a. External FHR monitor
4. Contraindications
   a. None
5. Procedure
   a. The patient should be in a high semi-Fowler's position in a recliner or left lateral decubitus position.
   b. Blood pressures are recorded before the test and every 15 minutes during the test.
   c. Continuous wave Doppler ultrasound is used to record FHR, and the tocodynamometer is placed and adjusted to detect uterine contractions and fetal movement.
   d. The patient or health care provider records fetal movement with an event marker.
   e. The patient is observed up to 120 minutes until the criteria for a reactive test are met, and the patient is rescheduled for follow-up tests if results are normal and tests are clinically indicated.[3]
   f. If the test is read as nonreactive, either plan for additional testing or attempt stimulation with sound (vibroacoustic stimulation [VAS]).
   g. Maintain a permanent record and hard copy of the patient's visit and test.
6. Test modification
   a. VAS may change a fetus from quiet to active sleep and result in a reactive NST.
      (1) Most studies have used an artificial larynx to produce the sound stimulus.
   b. A reactive NST after VAS is a reliable indication of fetal well-being.

7. Interpretation
   a. There are many different definitions of a reactive NST that vary in number, duration, and amplitude of acceleration.[12]
   b. Reactive test: The most widely accepted definition of a reactive NST is two or more FHR accelerations of at least 15 bpm and 15 seconds duration in a 20-minute observation period with no decelerations[14] (Fig. 29-1).
   c. Nonreactive test is when there is a failure to meet reactive criteria.
   d. Unsatisfactory test is when tracing is not satisfactory for interpretation.
   e. A test may be reactive with decelerations.
      (1) Mild decelerations, defined as a ≤15 bpm decrease and a ≤15-second duration are commonly encountered[26] and are not associated with poor perinatal outcome.[18]
      (2) Prolonged decelerations predict intrapartum fetal distress in 50% of cases and are ominous.[6]
8. Management
   a. Reactive NST: Repeat the test twice weekly unless clinical condition requires daily or more frequent evaluations. The ideal interval between testing has not been determined.
   b. Nonreactive NST: Perform backup evaluation with biophysical profile, CST, or multiparameter surveillance, or extend test up to 120 minutes.
   c. Unsatisfactory NST: Perform a repeat NST or backup evaluation within 24 hours.
   d. Reactive with variable deceleration: Perform an ultrasound and, if low amniotic fluid, consider delivery based on gestational age and nursery.
9. Predictive value of NST
   a. A reactive NST is associated with a fetal death within 1 week at a rate of 4 to 5 per 1000 patients tested[36] and a 10-fold lower risk for intrapartum intervention for fetal distress.

Contraction stress test

1. Background
   a. The CST was developed in 1972 by Ray and colleagues[29] and was originally called the oxytocin challenge test (OCT). Historically it was one of the first forms of fetal testing.
   b. The concept of the CST is based on the belief that FHR changes seen intrapartum and associated with a compromised fetus can also be seen antepartum in a fetus evolving into a compromised state when sufficient stress (uterine contractions) is applied.
   c. Studies have shown that this is a sound concept and that the stress of uterine contractions can uncover an evolving uteroplacental insufficiency.
   d. Because the CST could effectively detect diminished fetal oxygen reserve, it became the standard for fetal testing, replacing urinary estriol and human placental lactogen.
   e. The CST is still the only form of antepartum fetal surveillance to use a principle of induced stress to reveal marginal uteroplacental insufficiency.

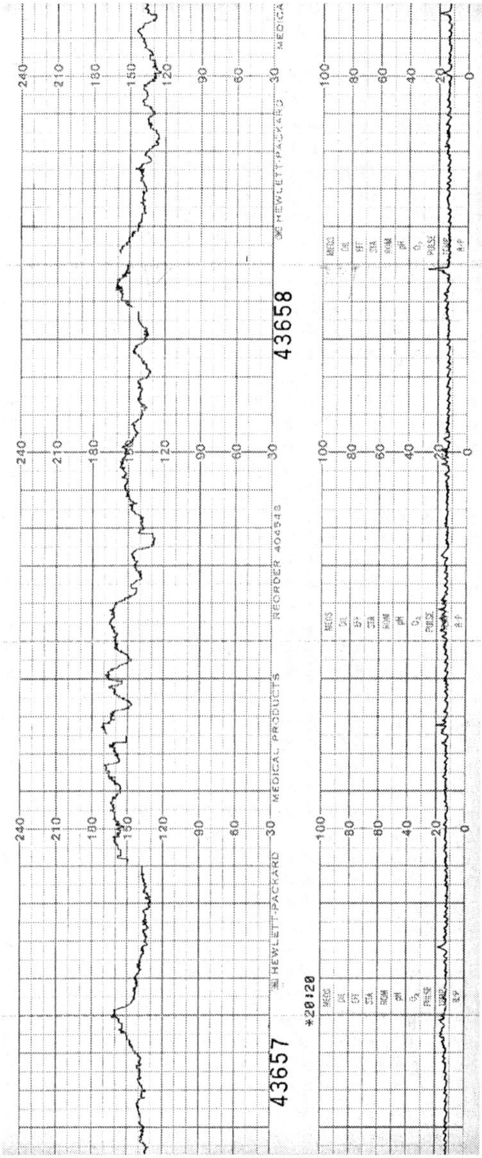

Figure 29-1
Reactive NST.

f. A negative CST has been consistently associated with good fetal outcome; therefore, a negative CST allows the health care provider to prolong a high-risk pregnancy safely.[10,11]
g. Fetal death within 1 week of a negative CST is under 1 per 1000.[8,9]
h. Therefore, although arbitrary, a negative CST is usually repeated in 1 week. The exceptions to the weekly rule are women with diabetes or a changing clinical condition.
i. A positive CST has been associated not only with stillbirths, but also with an increased incidence of low 5-minute Apgar scores, intrauterine growth retardation (IUGR), and late decelerations in labor.
j. The false-positive rate of a positive CST (i.e., calling a healthy fetus sick) is 30%.[4]
k. The CST can be performed as early as 26 weeks and the results used to manage pregnancy.

2. Instrumentation
   a. Electronic FHR monitor
3. Description
   a. The CST is a method of assessing the placental respiratory function by observing the response of FHR to uterine contractions.
4. Contraindications
   a. See the box below.
5. Procedure
   a. When the CST is used as a backup for a nonreactive NST, always perform the test in the hospital, preferably in the labor and delivery area.
   b. Place the patient in the semi-Fowler's or left lateral recumbent position.
   c. Baseline blood pressures are determined at the start of and every 15 minutes during the test.

Contraindications to the CST

Absolute contraindications:

Previous classic cesarean delivery
Placenta previa, abruptio, or unexplained vaginal bleeding
Premature ruptured membranes
Funic presentation or vasa previa
Any factor considered to be a contraindication to labor

Relative contraindications:

Preterm labor
Multiple gestation at < 36 weeks
Incompetent cervical os

d. Attach the monitor belts for both FHR and tocodynamometer in an area on the patient's abdomen where the signals are acceptable.
e. Baseline FHR and uterine activity should be reported for 20 minutes before the uterine contractions are initiated with oxytocin.
f. If there are three contractions (each ≥40 seconds in duration) in a 10-minute period, the test can be stopped.
g. If baseline uterine activity is insufficient, oxytocin is begun by IV infusion pump at 0.5 mU/min via piggyback into main IV and the rate is increased 1 to 2 mU/min in 15- to 20-minute interval until three contractions lasting 40 to 60 seconds over a 10-minute period occur.
h. Discontinue the oxytocin if the following occur:
   (1) The test is positive.
   (2) Hyperstimulation occurs.
   (3) The test is negative.
   (4) Variable decelerations occur.
   (5) Spontaneous rupture of membranes.
i. After the test, observe the patient until uterine activity has returned to baseline.
j. Ninety minutes may be required to perform the CST.

6. Interpretation
   a. See Table 29-1.

Table 29-1 Interpretation of CST

CST Result	Definition
Reactive	Two accelerations of 15 sec with maximal increase of 15 bpm above baseline
Nonreactive	Fewer than 2 accelerations of 15 sec with maximal increase of 15 bpm above baseline
Negative	No decelerations noted after any contractions
Suspicious	Under 50% of the contractions have late decelerations, no hyperstimulation
Positive	Over 50% of contractions have an associated late deceleration, no hyperstimulation
Unsatisfactory	Either the quality of the recording is insufficient to assure that no later decelerations are present or the contraction frequency is <3 in 10 minutes

7. Management
   a. Positive CST
      (1) Nonreactive positive CST
         (a) Over 32 weeks: Deliver by cesarean delivery.[2]
         (b) Under 32 weeks: Evaluate the tracing for long-term variability and, if present, manage as though the result were reactive positive.
      (2) Reactive positive CST: individualize
         (a) Over 37 weeks: Induce labor.
         (b) Preterm fetus
            i. Assess fetal maturity
            Immature: Survey daily.
            Mature: Induce labor.
   b. Suspicious CST: requires further evaluation with either repeat or backup tests
      (1) Reactive suspicious: Repeat in 24 hours.
      (2) Nonreactive suspicious: Repeat in 24 hours and evaluate for cause of nonreactive tracing, for example, prematurity, medications, and CNS abnormality.
   c. Hyperstimulation
      (1) If there are no decelerations, the test should be classified as hyperstimulation.
      (2) If hyperstimulation is associated with late decelerations, repeat the test in 24 hours or use a backup test.
   d. Unsatisfactory CST: requires further evaluations by using backup test
   e. Negative CST (Fig. 29-2)
      (1) Reactive negative: Repeat in 7 days.
      (2) Nonreactive negative: Repeat in 24 hours; evaluate for cause of nonreactive tracing (i.e., prematurity, medication, central nervous system [CNS] abnormality).
   f. Observable variable deceleration (a decrease in FHR to 90 bpm, or a decrease 40 beats below the baseline for > 15 seconds)
      (1) Perform sonography and, if oligohydramnios, consider immediate delivery.
8. Modification of CST
   a. Nipple stimulation test[13,21]
      (1) Adequate uterine activity can be obtained in 80% to 100% of cases.
      (2) Repeat steps 1 through 6 for the CST.
      (3) Apply warm, moist towel to each breast for 5 minutes.
      (4) If uterine activity is not adequate, massage one nipple for 10 minutes.
      (5) Once contractions begin, the nipples are stimulated only intermittently.
      (6) Note the starting and stopping time of nipple stimulation on the monitor strip.
      (7) Observe carefully for hyperstimulation.
      (8) Interpret CST (see Table 29-1).

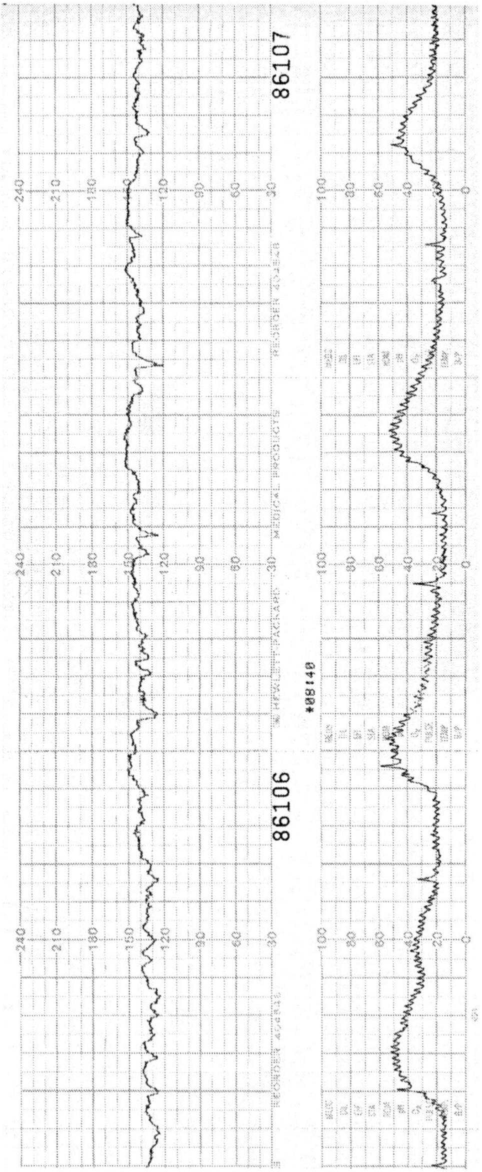

Figure 29-2
Negative CST.

Biophysical profile (BPP)

1. Background
   a. The test was introduced in 1980 and added real-time ultrasound to the NST to evaluate dynamic functions that reflect the integrity of the fetal CNS.[17]
   b. Five biophysical variables are assessed, and the test has a total of 10 points possible, with 0 or 2 points being assigned for the presence or absence of reactivity in the NST, fetal breathing, fetal movement, fetal tone, and amniotic fluid volume (Table 29-2).

Table 29-2 Components and their scores of the biophysical profile

Variable	Score 2	Score 0
Fetal breathing movements	The presence of at least 30 sec of sustained fetal breathing movements in 30 min of observation	Less than 30 sec of fetal breathing movements in 30 min of observation
Fetal movements	Three or more gross body movements in 30 min of observation; simultaneous limb and trunk movements	Less than three gross body movements in 30 min of observation
Fetal tone	At least one episode of motion of a limb from position of flexion to extension and rapid return to flexion	Fetus in position of semi-limb extension or full-limb extension with no return or slow return to flexion with movement; absence of fetal movement counted as absent tone
Fetal reactivity	Two or more fetal heart rate accelerations of at least 15 bpm and lasting at least 15 sec and associated with fetal movement within 20 min	No acceleration or less than two accelerations of fetal heart rate in 20 min of observation
Qualitative amniotic fluid volume	Pocket of amniotic fluid that measures at least 2 cm in two perpendicular planes	Largest pocket of amniotic fluid measures <2 cm in two perpendicular planes

   c. Clinical trials report favorable outcomes in a large series using the BPP for primary surveillance.[16]
   d. The correlation between abnormal scores and poor outcomes increases as the score decreases from 6 to 0.[15]
   e. Scores of 8 and 10 are almost always associated with a good outcome, and the false reassuring (negative) rate is comparable to the CST of 1 to 2 per 1000 fetuses dying within 7 days of a reassuring test.
   f. The testing interval is 7 days with all conditions except postdate pregnancies, insulin-dependent diabetes, and IUGR, which are two times per week.
   g. In addition to evaluating the fetus for uteroplacental insufficiency, the BPP has also been reported to increase the detection of anomalies and also the probability of diagnosing fetal infection in patients with ruptured membranes if there is absence of fetal breathing.
2. Description: A prenatal physical examination of the fetus using the NST and combination with real-time ultrasound equipment.
3. Contraindications
   a. None
4. Procedure
   a. An NST is performed as described previously.
   b. Real-time ultrasound is used to assess for four fetal variables (see Table 31-2).
   c. The duration of the ultrasound observation period is extended until normal criteria have been met for each biophysical variable or a maximum 30-minute period has been reached.
5. Interpretation and management (Table 29-3)

Modified biophysical profile (NST and amniotic fluid index)[7,20,39]

1. Background
   a. Amniotic fluid volume is a reliable marker of placental perfusion, especially chronic conditions.
   b. When the amniotic fluid index is <5 cm, the frequency of nonreactive NST is increased.
   c. This is a noninvasive test designed to assess acute as well as chronic changes in fetal well-being by using the amniotic fluid index and NST.
2. Contraindications
   a. None
3. Procedure
   a. The NST is performed as previously described with the patient in the semi-Fowler's position.
   b. The amniotic fluid index (AFI)[25,27] is found by first dividing the maternal abdomen into quadrants, with the umbilicus as a reference point and the linea nigra dividing the abdomen into right and left halves.
   c. The ultrasound transducer is held perpendicular to the floor in the longitudinal axis.

Table 29-3 Biophysical profile score, interpretation, and pregnancy management

Biophysical Profile Score	Interpretation	Recommended Management
10	Normal non-asphyxiated	No fetal indication for intervention; repeat test weekly except in diabetic patient and postterm pregnancy (twice weekly)
8/10 normal fluid 8/8	Normal non-asphyxiated fetus	No fetal indication for intervention; repeat testing per protocol
8/10 decreased fluid	Chronic fetal asphyxia suspected	Deliver
6	Possible fetal asphyxia	If amniotic fluid volume abnormal, deliver If normal fluid at >36 weeks with favorable cervix, deliver If <36 weeks or lecithin–sphingomyelin <2/1 or cervix unfavorable, repeat test in 24 hr If repeat test ≥4, deliver If repeat test >6, observe
4	Probable fetal asphyxia	Repeat testing same day; if biophysical profile score ≤6, deliver
0 to 2	Almost certain fetal asphyxia	Deliver

   d. The largest vertical diameter without fetal parts or cord in each quadrant is measured.
   e. The total sum of the measurements in centimeters is the amniotic fluid index.
4. Interpretation: Oligohydramnios is defined as an amniotic fluid index either less than fifth percentile for gestational age (7.0 to 9.8 cm),[19] or less than 5 cm at term.[27]
5. Management
   a. Patients who have decreased amniotic fluid index, nonreactive NSTs, late decelerations during the NST, or variable decelerations during the nonstress test receive a backup test, either a CST or a biophysical profile.
   b. Depending on gestational age, the patient may be a candidate for obstetric intervention.

Doppler velocimetry

1. Background
   a. Doppler assessment of the umbilical artery was first reported in 1977, and this vessel remains the most commonly investigated fetal structure in antenatal surveillance schemes using Doppler velocimetry.
   b. The shift in frequency of sound waves between the emitted and returning signals is called the Doppler shift.
   c. The electronics of the Doppler instrument convert the reflected sound into electrical voltage and analyze the shift in frequency between the transmitted and reflected beam.
   d. This is displayed on a screen by a waveform and reflects downstream placental resistance.
   e. Because of the influence of the angle of the sound beam when it strikes the moving column of fetal red blood cells, the diastolic component was added to act as an internal standard, resulting in the commonly used systolic-diastolic (S/D) ratio.
   f. Because of the decreasing resistance to flow during fetal diastole in the normal pregnancy, as the gestation advances, the umbilical artery S/D ratio progressively falls.
   g. Certain pregnancy disorders are associated with poor placental perfusion, which has been shown to be associated with increased downstream resistance during diastole or decreased flow that results in a progressively higher S/D ratio in these compromised pregnancies.
   h. When there is no flow into the placenta during diastole, there is absent end-diastolic velocity (AEDV), a serious clinical condition when it occurs after viability.
   i. If there are progressive placental arterial changes, there may even be reversed end-diastolic velocity (REDV), which is almost always associated with other poor surveillance tests and poor perinatal outcome.
   j. Umbilical artery Doppler results appear to be most helpful in managing pregnancies complicated by hypertension, IUGR, or both.
   k. Clinical action guided by Doppler has been shown to reduce the odds of perinatal mortality by 38%.[33]
   l. The beneficial effect of umbilical artery Doppler depends on the incidence of AEDV and not as much on the type of high-risk pregnancy factor.
2. Description
   a. Umbilical artery Doppler velocimetry is a noninvasive method of evaluating placental resistance to flow using sound waves. In most centers, it is not a primary method of fetal surveillance but is used most often to supplement information obtained in pregnancies complicated by IUGR and hypertension.
3. Contraindications
   a. None
4. Instruments: The following two types of Doppler machines are in common use:

a. Continuous wave Doppler, which uses a continuous wave with a frequency of 2 to 10 MHz
b. Pulsed wave duplex Doppler, which allows a directed beam to reflect off a specific target

5. Procedure
   a. Continuous wave Doppler is a "blind" procedure because concurrent real-time images are not performed; therefore, the umbilical artery is identified by its characteristic sound signal.
   b. The pulsed wave duplex Doppler is performed with a real-time ultrasound machine that allows coordinated real-time images and a Doppler signal with a range gate that can be placed over the specific vessel.
   c. Both machines will display the velocity information as waves and the S/D ratios as calculated off the display screen.
6. Pitfalls of Doppler include the following:
   Maternal obesity hinders ability to obtain waveform.
   Oligohydramnios hinders ability to obtain waveform.
   Breathing results in a false abnormal result.
   Doppler angle can lose lower peak frequency shifts if >60 degrees.
   Fetal tachycardia decreases the S/D ratio.
   Bradycardia increases the S/D ratio.
7. Interpretation
   a. The most clinically ominous umbilical artery waveforms that can occur after viability are AEDV and REDV (Fig. 29-3).
   b. Natural history of AEDV and REDV is as follows:

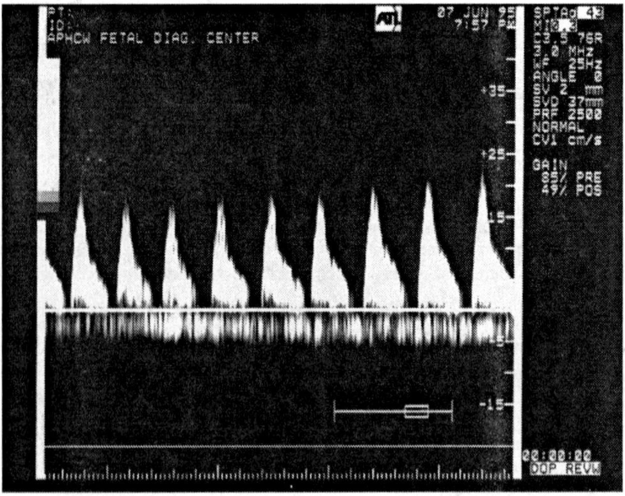

Figure 29-3
Absent end-diastolic velocity of umbilical artery.

(1) Once present, AEDV usually persists and may even deteriorate into REDV.
(2) Without intervention this usually leads to fetal distress or possibly demise.
(3) The more immature the fetus, the longer the time interval between the appearance of AEDV and fetal distress.
(4) An improvement in AEDV has occasionally been reported.

8. Management
   a. The management of patients with umbilical artery AEDV is controversial.
   b. In general, patients are admitted to the hospital for bed rest with treatment of any underlying associated maternal conditions such as hypertension, and intensive fetal monitoring is employed.
   c. Monitoring could be in the form of daily NSTs or even continuous electronic fetal monitoring with biophysical profile testing as often as necessary.
   d. Delivery is indicated when there is acute fetal distress, worsening maternal condition, or severe IUGR with no interval growth over a reasonable time period.
   e. REDV is the most extreme form of increased vascular resistance in the placental bed, and by the time this finding occurs, severe fetal compromise is evident using most of the standard tests of fetal well-being.
   f. It is not clear whether REDV by itself is an indication for early delivery, although this finding practically never occurs in isolation.

Fetal movement charting

Assessment of fetal movement in the second half of pregnancy is one of the oldest and simplest methods of monitoring fetal well-being. The "movement alarm signal" was introduced in 1973[35] after the observation that fetal movements decreased before fetal death in pregnancies complicated by placental insufficiency caused by preeclampsia. It is now felt that fetal movement monitoring is especially useful as a surveillance tool for clinical conditions associated with long-standing placental insufficiency. Although several different methods of charting have been proposed, the most commonly used for routine assessment involves a "count to 10" system based on the recognition that most women feel more than 10 movements in a 12-hour period.[24] Of importance, regardless of the method used, the reports of subjective decreases in fetal movement often are inaccurate. Therefore, rigorous methods using graphs with consistent start time and possibly a formal quiet time for counting should be used by the mother to record truly objective fetal movement.

1. Background
   a. The third-trimester fetus makes 30 gross body movements per hour.[22]
   b. The mother percieves 80% of the movements.[31]
   c. Fetal movement peaks between 9:00 PM and 1:00 AM and may be related to decreasing maternal glucose levels.[22]
   d. The longest period of inactivity in the normal fetus is 75 minutes.[22]
   e. Factors that influence maternal perception of fetal movement include the following:

Anterior placental location
Polyhydramnios
Maternal activity
Obesity
Medications (narcotics and barbiturates)

f. Decreased fetal movement is shown by 26% of fetuses with major birth defects.[32]
g. No monitoring method consistently distinguishes between twin fetuses; therefore, fetal movement charting is inadequate to assess the well-being of multiple gestations.
h. Although the application to low-risk pregnancies has appeal, especially considering that 50% of term stillbirths occur without obvious cause,[28,30] a large study failed to show a reduction of unexplained stillbirths when using routine fetal movement charting.

2. Contraindications
   a. None
3. Method[24,34]
   a. Fetal movement should be counted beginning in the morning, and they should be recorded.
   b. The time of day at which the tenth movement is perceived should be recorded.
4. Interpretation
   a. If there are greater than 10 movements per 12-hour period, the test is reassuring.
   b. If the mother has fewer than the required movements, further evaluation of fetal condition must be made.

References

1. Bishop E: Fetal acceleration test, *Am J Obstet Gynecol* 141:905-909, 1981.
2. Braly P, Freeman RK: The significance of fetal heart rate reactivity with a positive oxytocin challenge test, *Obstet Gynecol* 50:689-693, 1977.
3. Brown R, Patrick J: The nonstress test: how long is enough? *Am J Obstet Gynecol* 141:646-651, 1981.
4. Collea J, Holls W: The contraction stress test, *Clin Obstet Gynecol* 25:707-717, 1982.
5. Druzin ML et al: The relationship of the nonstress test to gestational age, *Am J Obstet Gynecol* 153:386-389, 1985.
6. Druzin ML et al: Antepartum fetal heart rate testing: VII. The significance of fetal bradycardia, *Am J Obstet Gynecol* 139:194-198, 1981.
7. Eden RD et al: A modified biophysical profile for antenatal surveillance, *Obstet Gynecol* 71:365-369, 1988.
8. Everston L, Gauthier R, Collea J: Fetal demise following negative contraction stress tests, *Obstet Gynecol* 51:671-673, 1978.
9. Freeman R, Anderson G, Dorchester W: A prospective multiinstitutional study of antepartum fetal heart rate monitoring. I. Risk of perinatal mortality and morbidity according to antepartum fetal heart rate test results, *Am J Obstet Gynecol* 143:771-777, 1982.
10. Freeman RK et al: The significance of a previous stillbirth, *Am J Obstet Gynecol* 151:7-13, 1985.
11. Freeman R et al: Postdate pregnancy: Utilization of contraction stress testing for primary fetal surveillance, *Am J Obstet Gynecol* 140:128-135, 1981.

12. Hage ML: Interpretation of nonstress tests, *Am J Obstet Gynecol* 153:490-495, 1985.
13. Keegan KA et al: A prospective evaluation of nipple stimulation techniques for contraction stress testing, *Am J Obstet Gynecol* 157:121-125, 1987.
14. Lavery J: Nonstress fetal heart rate testing, *Clin Obstet Gynecol* 25:689-705, 1982.
15. Manning FA et al: Fetal assessment based on fetal biophysical profile scoring, IV: an analysis of perinatal morbidity and mortality, *Am J Obstet Gynecol* 162:703-709, 1990.
16. Manning FA et al: Fetal assessment based on fetal biophysical profile scoring: experience in 12,620 referred high-risk pregnancies, I. Perinatal mortality by frequency and etiology, *Am J Obstet Gynecol* 151:343-350, 1985.
17. Manning FA, Platt LD, Sipos L: Antepartum fetal evaluation: development of a fetal biophysical profile, *Am J Obstet Gynecol* 136:787-795, 1980.
18. Meis P et al: *Variable decelerations during non-stress tests (NST): a sign of fetal compromise?* Society of Perinatal Obstetricians, Fourth Annual Meeting, San Antonio, TX, 1984.
19. Moore TR: Superiority of the four-quadrant sum over the single-deepest-pocket technique in ultrasonographic identification of abnormal amniotic fluid volumes, *Am J Obstet Gynecol* 163:762-767, 1990.
20. Ocak V, Sen C, Madazil R: Is fetal biophysical profile with all parameters needed? *J Matern Fetal Invest* 4:37, 1994.
21. Oki EY et al: The breast-stimulated contraction stress test, *J Reprod Med* 32:919-923, 1987.
22. Patrick J et al: Patterns of gross fetal body movements over 24-hour observation intervals during the last 10 weeks of pregnancy, *Am J Obstet Gynecol* 142:363, 1982.
23. Patrick J et al: Accelerations of the human fetal heart rate at 38 to 40 weeks' gestational age, *Am J Obstet Gynecol* 148:35-41, 1984.
24. Pearson JF, Weaver JB: Fetal activity and fetal well-being, *Br Med J* 1:1305-1307, 1976.
25. Phelan JP et al: Amniotic fluid index measurements during pregnnacy, *J Reprod Med* 32:601-604, 1987.
26. Phelan JP, Lewis PE: Fetal heart rate decelerations during a nonstress test, *Obstet Gynecol* 57:288, 1981.
27. Phelan JP et al: Amniotic fluid volume assessment using the four-quadrant technique in the pregnancy between 36 and 42 weeks' gestation, *J Reprod Med* 32:540-542, 1987.
28. Picquadio K, Moore T: A prospective evaluation of fetal movement screening to reduce the incidence of antepartum fetal death, *Am J Obstet Gynecol* 160:1075-1080, 1989.
29. Ray M et al: Clinical experience with the oxytocin challenge test, *Am J Obstet Gynecol* 114:1-9, 1972.
30. Rayburn WF: Antepartum fetal assessment: monitoring fetal activity, *Clin Perinatol* 9:1-14, 1982.
31. Rayburn WF: Clinical significance of perceptible fetal motion, *Am J Obstet Gynecol* 138:210, 1980.
32. Rayburn W, Barr M: Activity patterns in malfored fetuses, *Am J Obstet Gynecol* 142:1045, 1982.
33. Recent metanalysis of randomized controlled trials, *Am J Obstet Gynecol* 172:1379-1387, 1995.
34. Sadovsky E et al: The definition and the significance of decreased fetal movements, *Acta Obstet Gynecol Scand* 62:409, 1983.
35. Sadovsky E, Yaffe H: Daily fetal movement recording and fetal prognosis, *Obstet Gynecol* 41:845, 1973.

36. Schneider EP, Hutson JM, Petrie RH: An assessment of the first decade's experience with antepartum fetal heart rate testing, *Am J Perinatol* 5:134-141, 1988.
37. Todd AL et al: Antenatal tests of fetal welfare and development at age 2 years, *Am J Obstet Gynecol* 167:66-71, 1992.
38. Trierweiler MW, Freeman RK, James J: Baseline fetal heart rate characteristics as an indicator of fetal status during the antepartum period, *Am J Obstet Gynecol* 125:618-623, 1976.
39. Vintzileos AM et al: The use and misuse of the fetal biophysical profile, *Am J Obstet Gynecol* 156:527-533, 1987.

29.2 ULTRASOUND AND FETAL ANEUPLOIDY

Luanna Lettieri, M.D.

Obstetric ultrasound is used to assess the well-being of the fetus and the pregnancy. Technologic advances in high-resolution ultrasound have made the ultrasonic detection of fetal chromosomal abnormalities or aneuploidy possible.

1. Frequency of aneuploidy in liveborn infants
   a. Trisomy 21 (Down's syndrome): 1/800
   b. Trisomy 18 (Edward's syndrome): 1/8000
   c. 45X (Turner's syndrome): 1/10,000
   d. Trisomy 13 (Pateau's syndrome): 1/20,000
   e. Triploidy: very rare
2. Methods of prenatal detection of fetal aneuploidy
   a. Advanced maternal age and history
   b. Maternal serum screening tests (maternal serum alpha-fetoprotein [MSAFP], estriol, human chorionic gonadotropin [HCG]) known as AFP-3
   c. Ultrasound

Ultrasound detection of fetal aneuploidy

1. Abnormal biometry
   a. Nuchal fold
      (1) Measurement
         (a) Obtain between 15 and 21 weeks gestation (transverse axial scan of fetal head at level of cavum septum pellucidum, cerebral peduncles, cerebellar hemispheres, and cisterna magna); measure from outer skull table to outer skin surface
      (2) Abnormal: ≥6 mm (early second trimester)
      (3) Associated with: trisomy 21; 80% of babies with trisomy 21 will have excess nuchal skin
      (4) Sensitivity: 35% to 40%
      (5) False positive rate: 0.5%
   b. Femur length
      (1) Measurement
         (a) Obtain measurement between 15 and 23 weeks gestation.
         (b) Measure only the ossified femoral diaphysis.
         (c) Do not include nonossified cartilage of distal epiphysis or greater tuberosity.

(2) Abnormal: biparietal diameter/femur length (BPD/FL) ratio >1.5 standard deviation (SD); FL < fifth percentile for gestational age (GA)
(3) Associated with: trisomy 21
(4) Sensitivity: 35%
(5) False-positive rate: 6%

c. Humerus length
(1) Measurement
(a) Obtain between 15 and 23 weeks gestation.
(b) Measure only ossified diaphysis
(2) Abnormal: BPD/HL >1.5 SD; HL < fifth percentile for GA
(3) Sensitivity: 40%
(4) False-positive rate: 7%
(5) Associated with trisomy 21

d. Ear length
(1) Measurement
(a) Measurement can be obtained at any gestational age.
(b) Nomograms are available only for 14 to 25 weeks gestation.
(c) Measure from the helix to the end of the lobe.
(2) Abnormal: ≤10th percentile for GA
(3) Sensitivity: 70%
(4) False positive rate: 8%
(5) Associated with all types of aneuploidy (Abnormally short ears are the most sensitive indicators of trisomy 21 in newborn infants.)

e. Hypoplasia of middle phalanx of fifth digit
(1) Measurement: length of the middle phalanx of the fifth digit as compared with the middle phalanx of the fourth digit
(2) Abnormal: middle phalanx (MP) 5th/4th <0.7 or <0.5
(3) Sensitivity: 37% for <0.7; 75% for <0.5
(4) False-positive rate: 18% <0.7; 8% <0.5
(5) Associated with trisomy 21; 60% of neonates with trisomy 21 have hypoplasia of middle phalanx of fifth digit.

f. IUGR
(1) Early onset, second trimester symmetric IUGR—trisomy 18
(2) Severe asymmetric IUGR—triploidy

Structural abnormalities

Risk of aneuploidy in presence of structural anomalies detected in the following:

Fetus 11% to 35%
Neonate 6% to 7%

1. CNS lesions
a. Isolated hydrocephaly
(1) Measurement
(a) Distance from the lateral wall of the lateral ventricle to the midline compared with the hemispheric width (LV/HW)
(b) Amount of choroid plexus within the lateral ventricle
(c) Diameter of lateral ventricular atrium

(2) Abnormal
(a) LV/HW: dependent on GA
(b) Choroid plexus does not fill the lateral ventricle—"Dangling choroid plexus sign"
(c) Ventricular atria >10 mm
(3) Associated with: trisomy 21, trisomy 18, and triploidy, 3% to 8%

b. Meningomyelocele
(1) Sonographic features: separation of the posterior ossification centers on both transverse and longitudinal scans
(2) "Lemon sign": lemon-shaped skull
(3) Associated with: trisomies 13, 18, and 21 and triploidy, 33% to 50%

c. Hydrocephaly and meningomyelocele: associated with trisomies 13, 18, and 21 and triploidy, 8% to 15%

d. Dandy-Walker syndrome
(1) Definition: range of disorders resulting from abnormal development of cerebellum and fourth ventricle
(2) Sonographic features: separation of cerebellar hemispheres by enlarged fourth ventricle
(3) Associated with: trisomies 18 and 13 and triploidy, 29% to 50%

e. Holoprosencephaly
(1) Definition: three disorders (lobar, semilobar, alobar) caused by failure of normal forebrain development
(2) Sonographic features: varying degrees of a monoventricle with fused thalami
(3) Facial abnormalities frequent: proboscis, cyclopia, cebocephaly, median cleft lip, ethmocephaly
(4) Associated with: trisomies 13 and 18 and triploidy in 43% to 59% of alobar and semilobar types

f. Agenesis of corpus callosum
(1) Definition: absence of commissural fibers that radiate to cerebral cortex bilaterally
(2) Sonographic features
(a) Lateral ventricles are displaced laterally and superiorly.
(b) Frontal horn is indented.
(c) Third ventricle elevated producing an "interhemispheric cyst."
(3) Associated with: trisomies 13 and 18 and and triploidy, 14% to 20%

g. Choroid plexus cysts
(1) Sonographic features: cysts within choroid plexus of lateral ventricles; usually seen between 16 and 21 weeks gestation and regress by 23 to 25 weeks
(2) Associated with: trisomies 21 and 18

2. Cystic hygroma
a. Definition: nuchal edema resulting from lymphatic obstruction
b. Sonographic features: circumferential edema of the head and neck; may contain septation caused by nuchal ligament

c. Associated with: prenatally diagnosed
66% 45X
25% normal
5% trisomy 21
5% trisomy 18
1% other
d. Also associated with parvovirus
3. Facial abnormalities
a. Cleft lip/palate
(1) Sonographic features: flattened nose, displaced upper lip, disruption of maxilla; not possible to diagnose cleft in soft palate prenatally
(2) Associated with: trisomies 13 and 18 and triploidy, 40% to 75%
b. Common ocular abnormalities
(1) Holoprosencephaly
(2) Trisomy 13 or 18
c. Micrognathia
(1) Associated with: trisomies 13 and 18
d. Small, deformed ears
(1) Associated with: trisomies 13, 18, and 21 and triploidy, 23%
4. Hydrothorax
a. Definition: fluid in pleural cavity
b. Sonographic features: anechoic fluid collection in fetal chest
(1) Usually there is return of normal shape and contour of chest; however, with large fluid collections there can be bulging of chest, flattening of diaphragm, and cardiac axis shift.
(2) Associated with 45X (most frequent), trisomy 21 and triploidy, 9% to 12%.
5. Diaphragmatic hernia
a. Definition: failure of fusion of the four structures comprising the muscular diaphragm:
(1) Septum transversum
(2) Pleuroperitoneal membranes
(3) Dorsal mesentery of esophagus
(4) Body wall
Occurs in $\frac{1}{2000}$ to $\frac{1}{5000}$ live births.
b. Sonographic features: visualization of abdominal organs in chest cavity
(1) Definitive sign is fluid-filled mass behind left side of heart in a transverse scan.
(2) Associated features include polyhydramnios, absence of stomach or other abdominal organs in the abdominal cavity, mediastinal shift, and decreased abdominal circumference.
c. Associated with the following:
(1) Prenatal studies: trisomy 18 and 21, 4% to 25%
(2) Neonatal studies: trisomy 18 and 13, 6%
6. Congenital heart disease
a. Definition: structural abnormality of the heart or valves or cardiac arrhythmia

(1) Most frequent congenital anomaly (occurs in 8/1000 live births)
(2) Numerous abnormalities, the most common being septal defects.

b. Sonographic features: depends on type of cardiac anomaly
(1) Recent studies indicate that with prenatal scan, a normal four-chamber view can rule out most cardiac defects.

c. Associated with the following:

Chromosome Abnormality	CHD frequency	Type of Defect*
Trisomy 21	50%	VSD, ECD
Trisomy 18	99%	VSD, ECD, DORV
Trisomy 13	90%	VSD, ASD, dextrocardia
45X	20%	coarc

**VSD, ECD, DORV, ASD, coarc,* ventricular septal defect; endocardial cushion defect; double-outlet right ventricle; atrial septal defect; coarctation of aorta.

7. Esophageal malformations
   a. Definition: malformation or absence of esophagus; can range from simple esophageal atresia to tracheoesophageal fistula
      (1) Blind proximal esophageal pouch with a tracheoesophageal fistula of the distal esophagus is the most common malformation.
      (2) Esophageal atresia occurs in 1/2500 live births.
   b. Sonographic features: difficult to diagnose
      (1) Nonvisualization of stomach in 50% of fetuses
      (2) Polyhydramnios in third trimester
      (3) Rarely, visualization of proximal esophageal pouch
   c. Associated with the following:
      (1) Prenatal detection 20%—aneuploidy, most commonly trisomy 18
      (2) Neonatal detection—3% to 4% aneuploidy
8. Duodenal atresia
   a. Definition: absence of duodenum, most likely caused by failure of recanalization of duodenum; most common type of small bowel atresia (occurs in 1/10,000 live births)
   b. Sonographic features: dilated stomach and proximal duodenum—"double-bubble sign"—two fluid-filled cystic structures in upper abdomen seen on transverse scan; may not be sonographically evident until after 24 weeks gestation
      (1) Polyhydramnios—45% of cases
      (2) Other anomalies—50%
      (3) Cardiac anomalies—20% to 30%
      (4) Symmetric growth retardation—50%
   c. Associated with: if diagnosed prenatally, 20% to 30% will have trisomy 21
9. Omphalocele
   a. Definition: extrusion of the abdominal contents through an anterior abdominal wall defect into the amniotic cavity

(1) The extraabdominal organs are covered by a sac and the umbilical cord inserts into the omphalocele itself, also called exomphalos.

b. Sonographic features
   (1) Midline anterior abdominal mass outside of the abdominal cavity containing abdominal organs—stomach, bowel, liver
   (2) Contained within a sac, although sac may rupture, allowing abdominal contents to float freely within the amniotic cavity, resembling gastroschisis
   (3) May see ascites

c. Associated with the following:
   (1) Risk of aneuploidy dependent on the following:
      (a) Associated anomalies (especially cardiac, genitourinary [GU])
      (b) Size
      (c) Contents (liver vs. small bowel)
   (2) Prenatal detection: 30% to 40%, trisomies 13, 18, and 21
   (3) Neonatal detection: 12%, trisomies 13 and 18

10. Echogenic bowel
   a. Definition: most likely represents small bowel that is impacted with meconium
   b. Sonographic features: echogenic masses in fetal abdomen
   c. Associated with: normal variant, cystic fibrosis, and aneuploidy (trisomies 18 and 21)

11. GU anomalies
   a. Definition: Spectrum of congenital malformations of GU tract can occur.
      (1) Pyelectasis
         (a) Definition: mild dilation of renal pelvis
         (b) Sonographic features: increased diameter of renal pelvis
         (c) Associated with the following:
            i. 17% to 25% of fetuses with trisomy 21 have pyelectasis.
            ii. More severe hydronephrosis can be associated with trisomies 13 and 18.
      (2) Multicystic/dysplastic kidneys
         (a) Definition: Renal parenchyma contains numerous cysts of varying sizes.
         (b) Sonographic features: Multiple cysts of different sizes are seen. Cysts may be so small that they cannot be delineated; instead large echogenic parenchyma is seen. Larger cysts may distort shape of the kidney. Oligohydramnios often occurs.
         (c) Associated with trisomies 13 and 18.
      (3) Horseshoe kidney: rarely able to diagnose prenatally; associated with trisomy 18

12. Limb anomalies
   a. Definition: deformities of extremities, particularly hands and feet
      (1) Limb reduction: trisomy 18
      (2) Radial, thumb aplasia: trisomy 18

(3) Overlapping fingers (clinodactyly): trisomies 13 and 18
(4) Flexion deformities: trisomy 18
(5) Polydactyly: all aneuploidies, especially trisomy 13
(6) Hypoplasia of middle phalanx of fifth digit: trisomy 21
(7) Wide space between first and second toe: trisomy 21

13. Nonimmune hydrops
    a. Definition: excessive extravascular fluid accumulation
    b. Sonographic features: skin thickening > 5 mm, ascites, pleural/pericardial effusions, polyhydramnios, placentamegaly > 4 cm
    c. Associated with: trisomies 18 and 21, Turner's syndrome, triploidy, 14% to 18%
14. Single umbilical artery
    a. This occurs in up to 1% of deliveries. If another anomaly is not present, the fetus is not at an increased risk for aneuploidy.
15. First-trimester ultrasound
    a. Recent studies indicate that an increased nuchal translucency is associated with an increase in the maternal age-related risk for trisomies 13, 18, and 21.

Useful ultrasound findings in the detection of fetal aneuploidy

1. Major anomaly: all aneuploidies
2. Combined biometry: all trisomies
3. Early onset severe IUGR: trisomy 18, triploidy

Suggested Reading

Callen PW, editor: *Ultrasonography in obstetrics and gynecology,* ed 3, Philadelphia, 1994, WB Saunders.

Hammerton JL et al: A cytogenetic survey of 14,069 newborn infants: I. Incidence of chromosome abnormalities, *Clin Genet* 8:223-245, 1975.

Lettieri L et al: Ear length in second-trimester aneuploid fetuses, *Obstet Gynecol* 81:57-60, 1993.

Pandya PP et al: First-trimester fetal nuchal translucency thickness and risk for trisomies, *Obstet Gynecol* 84:420-423, 1994.

29.3 NUTRITION IN PREGNANCY

Patricia Harris, R.N., R.D., L.D., and Marcello Pietrantoni, M.D.

Maternal nutrition

The goal of nutrition during pregnancy is to nourish the mother while including the additional nutrients necessary to support fetal growth. The need for nutrients increases more than the need for additional calories (Table 29-4).

1. Principles of diet
    a. The mother should be encouraged to eat regularly and to eat a sufficient amount of food to satisfy her appetite. She should avoid skipping meals, especially breakfast, because hypoglycemia and ketonuria can result from an extended fast.
    b. Energy requirements are greatest at gestational weeks 10 to 30, when large amounts of maternal fat are deposited (Fig. 29-4).

Table 29-4 Dietary recommendations for pregnancy

Food Group	Ideal Number of Daily Servings
Milk/cheese/dairy	At least 6
Meat/protein	2 to 3
Vegetables/fruits	At least 5
Cereals/breads/starches	At least 6

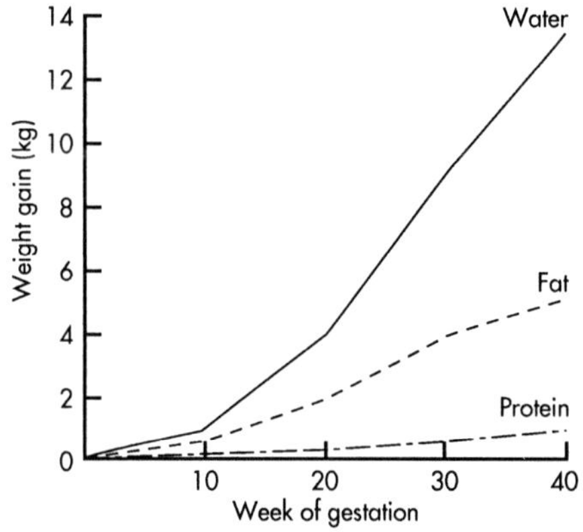

Figure 29-4
Composition of weight gain during pregnancy. (Redrawn from National Academy of Sciences: *Nutrition during pregnancy and lactation: an implementation guide,* Washington, DC, 1992, National Academy Press.)

c. An additional 300 calories during the second and third trimesters are needed for optimal weight gain and may be achieved by two additional servings of dairy products and an additional 1 to 2 ounces of meat.

2. Weight gain during pregnancy
   a. A positive linear relationship has been shown between maternal weight gain and newborn weight, and pregnancy outcome (Fig. 29-5).
   b. A positive linear relationship has also been shown between prepregnancy maternal weight and newborn weight (Fig. 29-6).
   c. Low prepregnancy maternal weight and inadequate gestational weight gain have been shown to contribute to decreased intrauterine growth and low birth weight.
   d. Gestational weight gain, especially in the second and third trimesters, is an important determinant of fetal growth (Table 29-5).

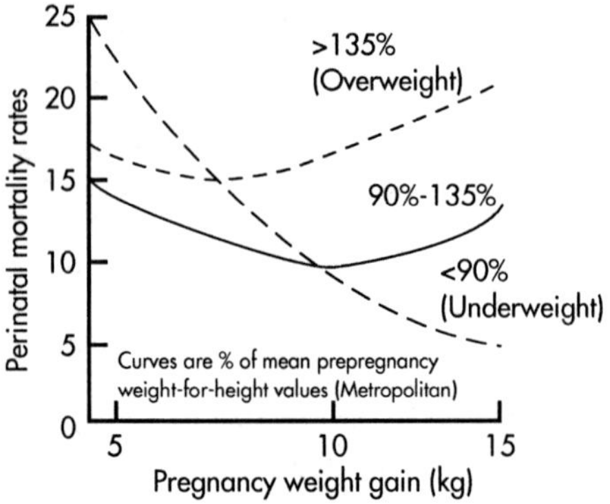

Figure 29-5
Perinatal mortality as a function of maternal weight gain. (Redrawn from National Academy of Sciences: *Nutrition during pregnancy and lactation: an implementation guide,* Washington, DC, 1992, National Academy Press.)

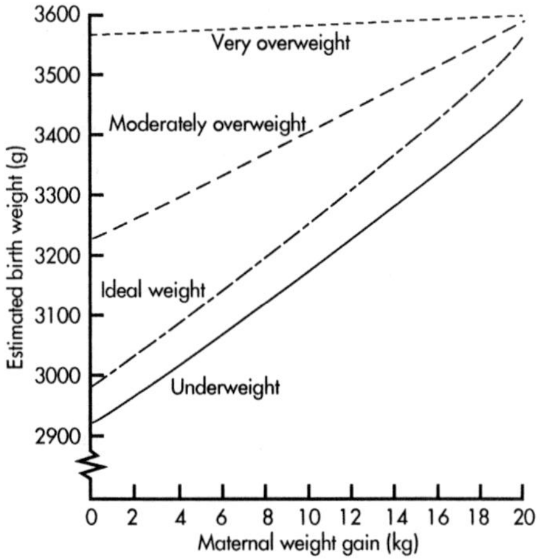

Figure 29-6
Birth weight as a function of maternal weight and prepregnancy weight for height. (Redrawn from National Academy of Sciences: *Nutrition during pregnancy and lactation: an implementation guide.* Washington, DC, 1992, National Academy Press.)

e. The only anthropometric measures of clinical value at this time are prepregnancy weight-for-height, or body mass index (BMI), and serial measurements of gestational weight gain.
f. Height, without shoes, should be measured at the first prenatal office visit.
g. BMI = wt. (kg)/ht. (m) squared.
h. Standard weight-for-height = 100 pounds for the first 5 feet plus 5 pounds for each inch taller than 5 feet or minus 4 pounds for each inch shorter than 5 feet.
i. Women generally gain 2 to 4 pounds during the first trimester and about 1 pound per week during the second and third trimesters (Fig. 29-7).
j. The accumulation of some fluid during pregnancy is physiologic as expansion of maternal blood volume may account for 10% of total weight gain. Large shifts of fluid, indicated by sudden large weight gains (8 pounds or more per month), may indicate preeclampsia, especially after 20 weeks gestation.
k. The components and rate of weight gain are more important than the actual number of pounds gained.

3. Nutrients of interest during pregnancy
   a. Folic acid is necessary for closure of the neural tube during early fetal development.
      (1) Physiologic needs for folate can be met through a healthy diet that includes dark green, leafy vegetables and enriched cereals.
      (2) Supplementation with low doses (0.8 mg/day) is recommended from preconception through the first trimester if there is any question of diet adequacy.
   b. Iron needs greatly increase during pregnancy because of the increased production of blood cells.
      (1) Although iron is found in meats and enriched grain products, the increased requirement is very difficult to obtain through diet, especially during the second and third trimesters.
      (2) Low-dose iron supplements (30 mg/day) are recommended and pose no danger to mother or fetus.
      (3) Higher doses (60 to 120 mg/day, in divided doses bid or tid) are recommended in cases of documented iron deficiency anemia.
      (4) Iron supplements may be better tolerated if taken at bedtime.
      (5) Iron absorption is inhibited if taken with food, prenatal vitamins, or calcium supplements.
   c. Zinc is necessary for protein production, bone building, and DNA and RNA production.
      (1) The increased requirement for zinc during pregnancy can generally be met through a balanced diet containing meat, fish, and dairy products.
      (2) Zinc is a component of prenatal vitamins.
   d. Vitamin A is essential to tissues lining the lungs, digestive organs, and GU tract.
      (1) Birth defects may be caused at much lower doses than previously thought. Research has shown that women who took more than 10,000 IU of preformed vitamin A were five times more likely to have a baby with birth defects than those women

Table 29-5 Weight gain recommended for pregnancy

Classification	Standard Prepregnancy Body Weight-for-Height (%)	Prepregnancy BMI	Recommended Gestational Weight Gain			
			Singleton		Twin	
			kg	lb	kg	lb
Underweight	<90	<19.8	12-18	28-40	18-23	40-50
Normal weight	90-120	19.8-26	11-16	25-35	16-20	35-45
Overweight	120-135	26-29	7-11	15-25	11-16	25-35
Obese	>135	>29	7	15	7-16	15-25

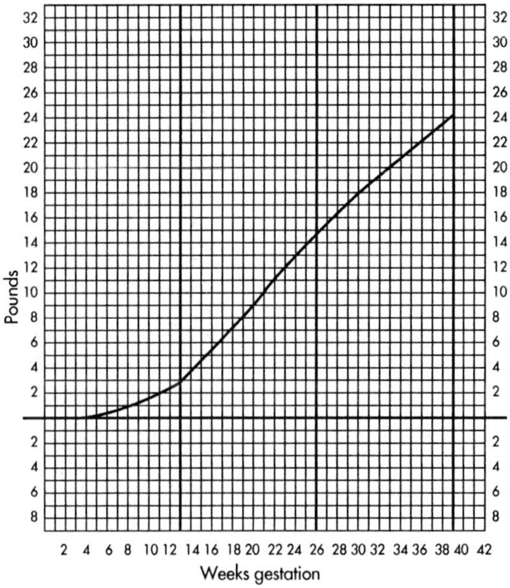

Figure 29-7
Gestational weight gain grid.

who took less than 5000 IU. Therefore, supplementation with preformed vitamin A should be avoided, especially during the first trimester.

(2) Vitamin A requirement is *not* increased in pregnancy.

(3) Beta carotene, which is found in yellow and dark green leafy vegetables and yellow fruits, need not be restricted.

e. Sodium is needed in increased amounts during pregnancy because of the increased fluid volume in the mother, the requirements of the fetus, and the level of sodium in amniotic fluid. Salt restriction in pregnant women is *not* recommended.

4. Nutrition-related laboratory values of interest

a. Generally, it is impractical and expensive to use laboratory or function tests to assess nutrient status in normal prenatal care. However, nutrient status can be assessed using hematocrit (Hct), hemoglobin (Hgb), complete blood count (CBC) and, possibly, serum ferritin.

(1) Hematocrit (Hct)

(a) Decreased secondary to bleeding, iron deficiency anemia, or water overload

(b) Elevated because of dehydration

(2) Hemoglobin (Hgb)
(a) Decreased secondary to bleeding, iron deficiency anemia, or protein–calorie malnutrition
(b) Elevated because of dehydration
(3) Transferrin
(a) Decreased secondary to protein malnutrition, pernicious anemia, or iron overload
(b) Elevated because of iron deficiency, blood loss, or pregnancy
(4) Albumin
(a) Decreased secondary to overhydration, decreased protein intake, or impaired digestion or absorption
(b) Elevated because of dehydration
(5) Prealbumin
(a) Decreased secondary to protein malnutrition, stress, or inflammation
(6) Mean corpuscular volume (MCV)
(a) Decreased secondary to advanced iron-deficiency anemia, or vitamin B_6 or copper deficiency
(b) Elevated because of folic acid, vitamin B_{12}, or vitamin C deficiency
(7) Mean corpuscular Hgb concentration (MCHC)
(a) Decreased secondary to advanced iron-deficiency anemia

b. Cholesterol levels in pregnant women may be elevated. This may be secondary to the normal decreased intestinal secretion rate, which allows more circulating exogenous cholesterol for the synthesis of estrogens.

5. Alimentary changes during pregnancy
   a. Increased appetite, usually in the second and third trimesters
   b. Decreased motility because of the increase in progesterone, which may lead to the following:
      (1) Esophageal regurgitation
      (2) Nausea and vomiting
      (3) Delayed emptying of the stomach
      (4) Reverse peristalsis, which may result in heartburn
   c. Decreased intestinal secretion for enhanced absorption of nutrients
   d. Increased water absorption from the colon, which may lead to constipation
   e. An altered sense of taste, which may lead to PICA or irregular dietary intake
   f. An intensified sense of smell, which may contribute to nausea and vomiting

Complications of pregnancy

1. Multiple fetuses
   a. Ten pounds additional total maternal weight gain is recommended for a twin pregnancy. This recommendation may be adapted for additional fetuses.
   b. As the number of fetuses increases, the duration of pregnancy may decrease. It is therefore essential that nutrition counseling

occur early in pregnancy to ensure the most nutrient-dense diet possible.

c. Additional requirements include the following:
   (1) Folic acid
      (a) 0.4 to .8 mg, twins
      (b) 0.8 to 1 mg, triplets, quadruplets, etc.
   (2) Zinc
      (a) 15 mg, twins
      (b) 20 to 25 mg, triplets, quadruplets, etc.
   (3) Iron
      (a) 30 to 60 mg, twins
      (b) 60 mg, triplets, quadruplets, etc.

2. Anemia
   a. Hgb ≤11.0 g/dl (WHO criteria)
   b. Need increased dietary intake of protein, iron-rich foods, and vitamin C–rich foods
   c. Need iron supplementation

3. Diabetes
   a. Preexisting diabetes
      (1) The normal prepregnancy diet should provide the following:
         (a) 30 kcal/kg current weight for active women
         (b) 20 kcal/kg current weight for sedentary and obese women
      (2) The normal nonpregnant woman of average height and stable weight may consume approximately 2200 kcal per day.
      (3) An additional 300 kcal/day in the second and third trimesters are needed for optimal weight gain and prevention of starvation ketosis, indicated by trace or small amounts of urinary ketones.
      (4) Calorie needs should be determined on an individual basis.
   b. Gestational diabetes (GDM)
      (1) GDM is defined as glucose intolerance with onset or first recognition during the current pregnancy.
      (2) Glucose monitoring is important because the criteria for initiating insulin should be based on fasting (fasting blood sugar [FBS]) and postprandial responses to the prescribed diet. The American Diabetes Association recommends the following guidelines:
         (a) Premeal or fasting, ≤105 mg/dl
         (b) 1 hour postprandial (pp), ≤140 mg/dl
         (c) 2 hour pp, ≤120 mg/dl
      (3) Nutrition management is successful if the following occur:
         (a) Necessary nutrients for maternal and fetal health and growth are provided.
         (b) Normoglycemia is maintained.
         (c) Ketonuria is prevented.
         (d) Weight gain is appropriate.
      (4) The 1995 American Diabetes Association recommendations for pregnancy include the following:
         (a) If prepregnancy weight was less than 90% ideal body weight (IBW), 36 to 40 kcal/kg current weight per day.

(b) If prepregnancy weight was 90% to 120% IBW, 30 kcal/kg current weight per day.
(c) If prepregnancy weight was 120% to 150% IBW, 24 kcal/kg current weight per day.
(d) If prepregnancy weight was >150% IBW, 12 to 18 kacal/kg current weight per day.
(e) Keep calories and carbohydrates low at breakfast because of morning insulin resistance.

(5) Elevated fasting triglycerides in GDM are more strongly associated with macrosomia than FBS or pp glucose.
(6) Postpartum women should monitor glucose for 1 week and report any elevations
(a) Six to 8 weeks postpartum or shortly after breast-feeding cessation, give patient a 75 g 2 hour oral glucose tolerance test (OGTT).
(b) Check blood glucose at her annual examination.

c. Monitoring
(1) Urinary ketones
(a) Trace or small amounts may indicate starvation ketosis.
(b) Moderate or large amounts may suggest existing or impending diabetic ketoacidosis.
(2) Urine glucose levels imprecisely represent blood glucose concentrations because of varying renal thresholds for glucose excretion resulting from long-standing diabetes or pregnancy.

4. Pregnancy-induced hypertension (PIH)
a. Increased calcium intake may counteract the effects of sodium in the development of hypertension in salt-sensitive individuals.
b. The presence of hypocalciuria is a diagnostic aid in differentiating preeclampsia from other forms of gestational hypertension.
c. There is sufficient recent evidence to support supplementation with large amounts of calcium (2000 mg/day) as a means of preventing PIH/preeclampsia in susceptible women.
d. Calcium competes with copper, iron, zinc, and magnesium for absorption and is best used if obtained from dietary sources or if supplemented in doses of 500 mg qid between meals.

5. "Morning sickness"
a. Because of varying levels of estrogen, HCG, and progesterone, women may have any or all of the following symptoms, with different intensities, at any time of the day.
(1) Nausea, vomiting, and retching
(2) Aversion to odors, bright lights, loud noises, or tight clothes
(3) Sensitivity to invasion of her personal space
b. Different things may trigger an episode of "morning sickness" in different women.
(1) Odors, even those that previously were pleasant
(2) Abrupt motion
(3) Bright lights
(4) Loud noises
c. Ptyalism, the excessive production of saliva, may alter the sense of taste and increase nausea.

d. Dietary treatment may include the following:
   (1) Drink liquids 1 hour before or after eating solid foods.
   (2) Avoid water, caffeine, and carbonated beverages.
   (3) Keeping a cut lemon handy to sniff may help to neutralize offensive odors.
   (4) Tart candies, lemonade, etc., may be tolerated.
   (5) Whatever works, eat it.

6. Diarrhea may occur because of iron supplementation or lactose intolerance. Dietary treatment should include the following:
   a. Increase fluids by mouth, excluding caffeine and milk products.
   b. Decrease fiber foods, such as raw fruits (except bananas) and vegetables.
   c. Avoid milk products. Gradually add into diet in small amounts (¼ cup) as tolerated.
7. Constipation may occur because of normal alimentary changes during pregnancy or from iron supplementation. Dietary treatment should include the following:
   a. High-fiber foods such as raw fruits and vegetables, beans, legumes, nuts, and whole-grain breads and cereals
   b. Increased fluids by mouth, excluding caffeine
8. PICA
   a. PICA is defined as the craving of nonfood items.
   b. Acting on these cravings may limit nutrient intake or absorption and have adverse hematologic and gastrointestinal effects.
   c. Depending on the craving, this can be extremely harmful to the mother and the fetus.
   d. Any unusual cravings should be discussed with a registered dietitian to assess whether they are associated with short-term or long-term nutrition problems.
9. Starvation ketosis
   a. Indicated by ketonuria
   b. Causes
      (1) Inadequate carbohydrate intake
      (2) Inadequate calorie intake
      (3) Skipped meals or snacks
      (4) Greater than 10 hours between hour of sleep (hs) snack and breakfast
      (5) Vomiting
10. Vegetarianism
   a. Most vegetarian diets meet or exceed the RDA for protein.
   b. A lower protein intake than in a nonvegetarian diet may be associated with better calcium retention.
   c. Western vegetarians generally have adequate intakes of iron (because of fortification) and consume greater amounts of ascorbic acid (vitamin C), which enhances the absorption of non-heme (plant) iron.
   d. Vegans (those who eat no animal products) may require vitamin B_{12} supplementation.
   e. Vegans who have limited exposure to the sun may require vitamin D supplementation.

   f. Vegetarian diets tend to be lower in calories and higher in fiber.
   g. For the additional calories needed in the second and third trimesters of pregnancy, add two between meal snacks rich in calories and nutrients, including nuts, nut butters, and dried fruits.
   h. The vegetarian woman who becomes pregnant should be referred to a registered dietitian to assure that she is informed about a proper diet.
11. Dietary inadequacy
   a. Poor hygiene may be suggestive of life circumstances interfering with adequate nutrient intake.
   b. Untreated dental disease, depression, domestic violence, etc., may interfere with adequate dietary intake.
   c. Signs of eating disorders include the following:
      (1) Dental enamel erosion
      (2) Little subcutaneous fat
      (3) Swollen parotid glands (rare)
      (4) Callouses on the knuckles
   d. Refer to the registered dietitian for assessment and counseling or further referral.
   e. Refer to social services for assistance with housing, food stamps, WIC, commodities, etc.
12. Smoking, alcohol, and drugs (SAD)
   a. The use of substances such as tobacco, alcohol, caffeine or coffee, marijuana, and cocaine may affect maternal nutrition as well as have teratogenic effects on the fetus.
   b. Substance abuse may increase the need for one or more nutrients through malabsorption or increased urinary excretion.
   c. Substance abuse may also lead to undesirable changes in food and nutrient intake.

Suggested reading

American Diabetes Association: *Medical management of pregnancy complicated by diabetes,* 1995, Author.

Belzian JM et al: Calcium supplementation to prevent hypertensive disorders of pregnancy, *N Engl J Med* 325(20):1399, 1991.

Dimperio D: Nutritional management of multiple pregnancy. In *The perinatal nutrition report,* Fall 1994, The American Dietetic Association, p. 6.

Erick M: *No more morning sickness: a survival guide for pregnant women,* New York, 1993, Penguin Books.

Guyton AC: *Textbook of medical physiology,* Philadelphia, 1976, WB Saunders.

Havala S, Dwyer J: Position of the American Dietetic Association: vegetarian diets, *J Am Dietetic Assn,* 93(11):1317-1319, 1993.

Institute of Medicine: *Nutrition during pregnancy and lactation: an implementation guide,* 1992, National Academy Press.

Nutrition during pregnancy, 1990, National Academy Press.

Orten J, Neuhaus O: *Human biochemistry,* St Louis, 1975, Mosby.

Vitamin A, pregnancy don't mix. *Environ Nutr* 18(11):1, 1995.

Worthington-Roberts B, Williams SR: *Nutrition in pregnancy and lactation,* 1989, Times Mirror/Mosby College.

Isoimmunization

30

Joseph A. Spinnato, M.D.

Isoimmunization, in a context pertinent to obstetrics, refers to a woman's antibody response (sensitization) to red cell antigens that are foreign to her and that, during pregnancy, may place her fetus at risk for red blood cell (RBC) hemolysis, anemia, hydrops fetalis, and even death. This syndrome, characterized by the presence of erythroblasts in the fetal circulation (erythroblastosis fetalis), was described well before the modern science of immunology existed and is classically noted among Rh(D) negative women sensitized by Rh(D) antigen exposure during a pregnancy episode (fetal-maternal hemorrhage [FMH]). In most centers, the availability of passive immunization (anti-Rh(D) antibody, e.g., Rhogam) against this particular sensitization has resulted in a relative increase in sensitizations to antigens other than Rh(D). Approximately two thirds of hemolytic disease of the fetus is the result of ABO incompatibility whose mild antenatal course does not require obstetric surveillance.

30.1 POSSIBLE MODES OF SENSITIZATION

1. Pregnancy episode
   a. Spontaneous FMH (almost always observed after the first trimester)
      (1) Partial placental separation/abruptio placentae
      (2) Placenta previa
   b. Induced FMH
      (1) Second-trimester or third-trimester abdominal trauma
      (2) Invasive obstetric procedures
         (a) Amniocentesis
         (b) Umbilical vein blood sampling
         (c) Chorionic villus sampling (CVS)
2. Blood transfusion: particularly true for non-Rh(D) antigen sensitization
3. Maternal to fetal hemorrhage *in utero* (grandmother theory) (Table 30-1)

30.2 IMMUNOLOGY AND PATHOPHYSIOLOGY

1. The mother is negative for the RBC antigen.
2. The father possesses the antigen.

Table 30-1 Non Rh(D) antigens and hemolytic disease (HDF) (partial list)

Antigen	Designator	Severity of disease
Lewis	Le^a, Le^b	Does not cause HDF
I	I	Does not cause HDF
Kell	K	Mild to severe
	k	Generally mild
Duffy	Fy^a	Mild to severe
Kidd	Jk^a	Mild to severe
	Jk^b	Mild to severe
MNSs	M	Generally mild
	N	Generally mild
	S,s	Mild to severe
P	P	Mild to severe

Modified from Weinstein L: Irregular antibodies causing hemolytic disease of the newborn: a continuing problem, *Clin Obstet Gynecol* 25:321-332, 1982.

3. The fetus inherits the antigen from the father.
4. Antigen-positive RBCs pass into the maternal circulation (unnecessary if previously sensitized).
5. Maternal immune response (IgG, IgM) occurs within 8 to 10 weeks.
6. Antibody (IgG) transfers back into the fetal circulation.
7. Hemolysis of fetal RBCs occurs.
8. Fetal anemia prompts extramedullary erythropoiesis and hepatic congestion that results in hydrops fetalis and congestive heart failure.
9. Fetal death occurs.

30.3 PREVENTION OF AND SURVEILLANCE FOR ISOIMMUNIZATION DURING PREGNANCY

Every pregnant patient should be considered at risk for hemolytic disease of the fetus. Therefore, during the first prenatal visit, every patient should be typed for Rh(D) and ABO status. In addition, an antibody screen (indirect Coomb's test) should be performed. The subsequent management is outlined in Fig. 30-1.

Patients who are Rh(D) positive and have a negative antibody screen require no further testing. Although these patients are at some risk for atypical antigen sensitization during pregnancy, this risk is low, and the risk of serious fetal disease is very low. Among Rh(D) negative patients, at 28 to 30 weeks gestation, a repeat antibody screen is performed and Rh immunoglobulin prophylaxis (300 μg, IM) is offered to antibody screen negative patients. A positive indirect Coomb's test to an antigen other than Rh(D) (e.g., anti-Kell) does not preclude Rh prophylaxis.

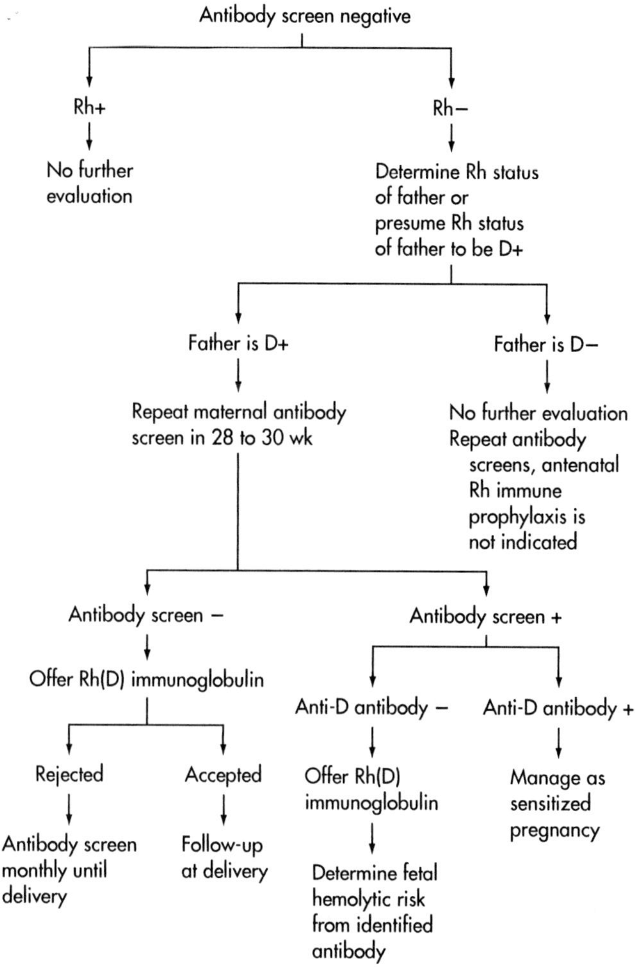

Figure 30-1
Prenatal care when the initial antibody screen is negative.

30.4 OTHER ANTENATAL USES OF Rh IMMUNE GLOBULIN

1. Second and third trimester maternal abdominal trauma
2. Second and third trimester vaginal bleeding
3. Following amniocentesis, CVS, or umbilical vein blood sampling
4. Following external cephalic version

If delivery occurs within 21 days of antenatal prophylaxis, a repeat dose may be unnecessary if the indirect Coomb's test continues to be positive (from the administration). At delivery, Rh immune globulin is repeated if the blood type of the infant is unknown or is Rh(D) positive.

30.5 CRITERIA FOR RH IMMUNE GLOBULIN ADMINISTRATION AT DELIVERY

1. The mother must be both D and Du antigen negative.
2. The infant must be either D or Du positive.
3. Mother must be unsensitized (negative indirect Coomb's) to D.*
4. Infant must have a negative direct Coomb's test.*
5. IM is the only acceptable route of administration.
6. Immune globulin should be administered within 72 hours of delivery.

30.6 SENSITIZED PREGNANCIES

The management of maternal sensitization to fetal red cell antigens has undergone a revolution in recent years because of the ability to (1) sample directly and transfuse the fetal circulation and (2) determine (for most antigens) the fetal blood type from amniocytes obtained from amniocentesis using DNA amplification techniques.

A sensitized pregnancy is heralded by a positive indirect Coomb's test (Fig. 30-2). Regardless of Rh status, if the indirect Coomb's test is positive, the offending antigen must be identified. In most laboratories, this is done automatically if the patient is known to be pregnant. In a first sensitized pregnancy, the severity of the antibody response, as measured by the antibody titer, is predictive of the severity of fetal disease.

Paternal zygosity testing

For most of the red cell antigens known to cause hemolytic disease of the fetus, paternal testing can be performed to assess zygosity for the antigen. For example, red cells from a father who is heterozygous for E would carry both the E and e antigens, indicating a 50% risk that his offspring would inherit the E antigen. Although this is true for most antigens associated with HDF, it is not true for Rh(D) because an elaborated antigen for Rh(D) has not been identified. For Rh(D), however, there exists a probability table, based on the presence or absence of C, c, E, and e, that can be used to predict the probability of heterozygosity for the antigen. When paternal heterozygosity for an offending antigen is known or suspected, the ability to separate the antigen-positive from the antigen-negative fetus would allow the clinician to avoid the risks of serial invasive procedures when there is no risk of HDF (antigen-negative fetus). In these cases, fetal blood typing at the first amniocentesis or at umbilical vein blood sampling could eliminate the need for further testing if the fetus is antigen negative.

*A low positive titer (<1:4) may be observed after antenatal Rh immunoglobulin administration and does not preclude administration.

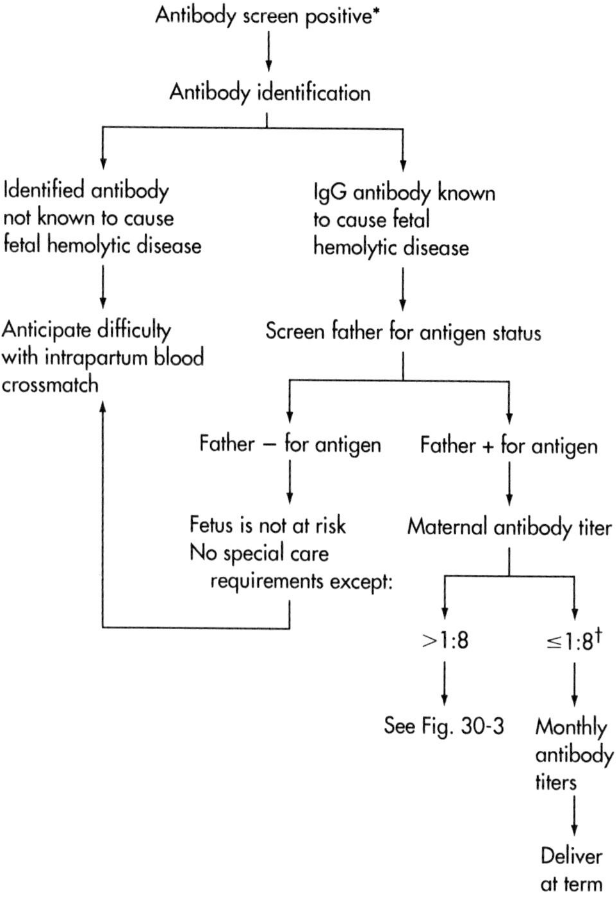

*If an Rh− patient has an antibody screen positive for an antigen other than Rh(D), she remains a candidate for Rh immunoglobulin and should be evaluated as outlined in Fig. 30-3.

†First sensitized pregnancy only. If other than first sensitized pregnancy, manage as though titer >1 : 8.

Figure 30-2
Initial prenatal care when the antibody screen is positive.

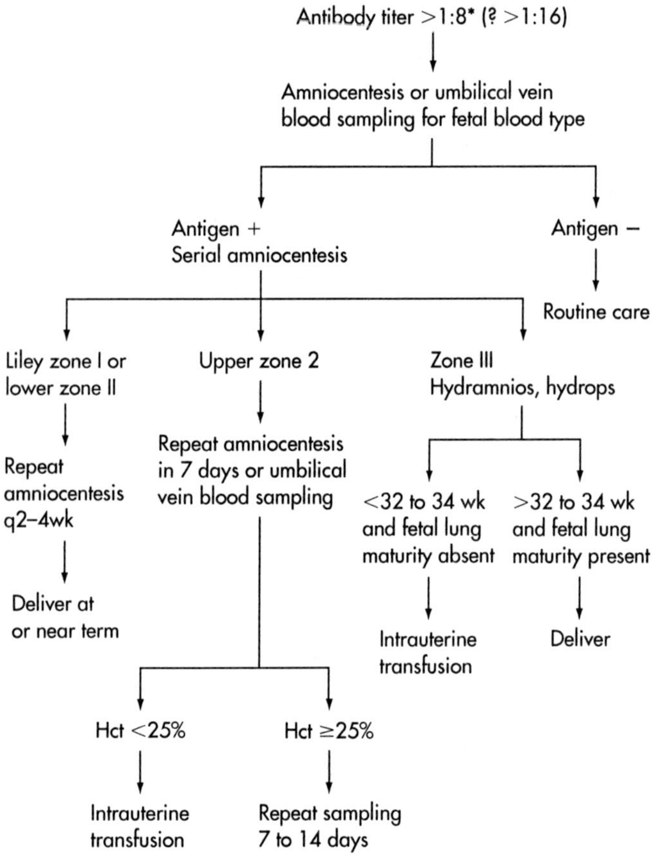

*Or previously sensitized pregnancy, without regard to titer.

Figure 30-3
Management scheme for sensitized pregnancies; father is antigen positive.

Using the indirect Coombs' titer

The available data suggest that there is no risk of intrauterine death if the titer remains ≤1:16. Despite these data, the American College of Obstetricians and Gynecologists (ACOG) has adopted more stringent recommendations by setting the threshold for invasive testing at values exceeding 1:8 (rather than 1:16). This issue, as well as issues of timing of first invasive test and type of invasive test, are beyond the bounds of this chapter. The management scheme herein presented is acknowledged to represent one of several accepted approaches. Suffice it to say, the initial management

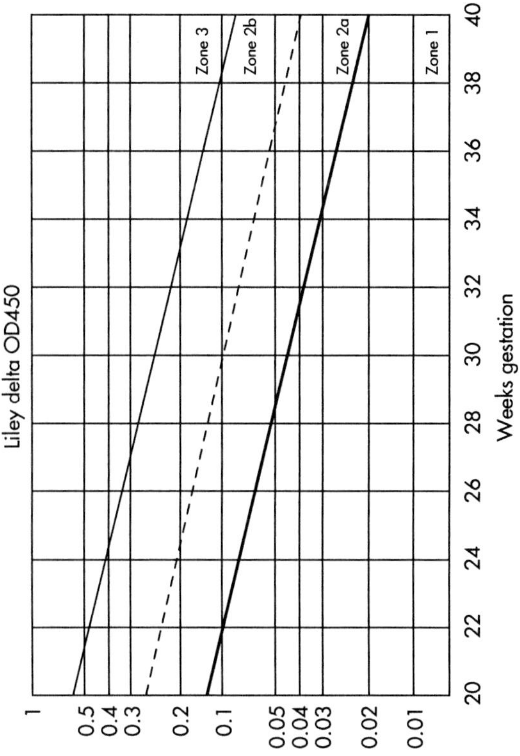

Figure 30-4
Liley delta OD 450 versus weeks gestation.

of the first sensitized pregnancy is based on the indirect Coomb's titer (see Fig. 30-2).

When the indirect Coomb's titer exceeds 1:8 (? exceeds 1:16), most authorities recommend some type of invasive testing (Fig. 30-3). The recently introduced ability to determine fetal blood type from DNA amplification of amniocytes obtained from amniocentesis has permitted selection of patients requiring continued testing. For example, if the fetus is Rh(D) negative by DNA amplification testing, there is no risk of HDF regardless of the antibody titer.

Amniotic fluid bilirubin determination

With the possible exception of anti-Kell sensitization (where the reliability of bilirubin as a marker for anemia has been challenged), management based on the measurement of amniotic fluid bilirubin remains the cornerstone of management of sensitized pregnancies. Measuring the change from expected for the optical density of amniotic fluid at 450 mU as a measure of bilirubin (the delta OD 450), the risk of severe anemia warranting possible fetal transfusion or early delivery can be determined. The most commonly used method is the Liley curve, shown in an extended form in Fig. 30-4.

The ability to sample the fetal circulation directly via ultrasonographically direct umbilical vein blood sampling permits the determination of fetal hematocrit, reticulocyte count, and bilirubin level to direct the need for and the frequency of fetal blood transfusion. In most centers, in the absence of fetal lung maturity, fetal intrauterine transfusion is preferred to delivery. The particulars of this management are beyond the scope of this chapter and interested readers are encouraged to consult other texts and references.

Suggested reading

American College of Obstetricians and Gynecologists: *Prevention of D isoimmunization,* ACOG Technical Bulletin 147, Washington DC, 1990, ACOG.

Bowman JM: Suppression of Rh isoimmunization: a review, *Obstet Gynecol* 52:385-393, 1978.

Lighten AD et al: Accuracy of prenatal determination of RhD type status by polymerase chain reaction with amniotic cells, *Am J Obstet Gynecol* 173:1182-1185, 1995.

Spinnato JA: Hemolytic disease of the fetus: a plea for restraint, *Obstet Gynecol* 80:873-877, 1992.

Spinnato JA et al: Amniotic fluid bilirubin and fetal hemolytic disease, *Am J Obstet Gynecol* 164:1030-1035, 1991.

Postpartum Hemorrhage

31

John M. O'Brien, M.D.

31.1 IMPORTANCE AND PERSPECTIVE

1. Postpartum hemorrhage is a leading cause of maternal death; an obstetric emergency.
   a. Hemorrhage accounts for 16% of all maternal deaths, and postpartum hemorrhage accounts for greater than 50% of these cases.
   b. Significant hemorrhage occurs in 6% of all cesarean deliveries and 3% of all vaginal births. Therefore, this clinical problem likely will be experienced by all practitioners.
2. Recognition and prompt evaluation can reduce the need for transfusion and its associated morbidities.
3. Algorithm for management must be memorized. When a patient is exsanguinating, there is no time to look up treatments or learn steps of proper evaluation.
4. Diagnosis of postpartum hemorrhage is arbitrarily defined as an estimated blood loss of >500 ml. This definition overestimates the population at risk. A more useful estimate may be an estimated blood loss of >1000 ml, which more commonly alters hemodynamics.
5. Hemorrhage may occur either immediately after delivery or be delayed for more than 24 hours. The differential diagnosis differs between immediate and delayed postpartum hemorrhage.

31.2 ETIOLOGIES

Uterine atony

1. Uterine atony is the most common etiology for postpartum hemorrhage.
2. Predisposing factors are those factors that either overdistend the uterus, overwork the muscle, or inhibit it from contracting.
   a. Labor arrest or protraction disorder
   b. Prolonged use of higher dose oxytocin
   c. Chorioamnionitis
   d. Multiple gestations
   e. Polyhydramnios

f. Pharmacologic agents used during labor or delivery
   (1) Magnesium sulfate
   (2) Betamimetics
   (3) General anesthetics
g. Multiple or large uterine leiomyomas
h. Uterine distension by large clot in lower segment or other mass
3. Physical examination notes "boggy" uterus.
4. Other etiologies such as lower genital tract lacerations or retained products of conception must be ruled out, especially if the uterus is firm and continued hemorrhage is noted.

Obstetric trauma

1. Iatrogenic
   a. Forcep or vacuum incorrectly applied or rotation performed
      (1) Vaginal lacerations
      (2) Cervical lacerations
   b. Laceration of pudendal artery at time of pudendal block
   c. Extension of incision during cesarean delivery into uterine vessels
2. Precipitous delivery
   a. May result in cervical or vaginal lacerations
3. Vulvar hematoma
   a. May extend into ischiorectal fossa with potential for extension along the psoas muscle and into retroperitoneum
   b. More common in vaginal deliveries with macrosomic fetus and maternal hematologic or hypertensive disorders

Retained placenta

1. Manual extraction attempted before appropriate analgesia, not allowing successful removal, or improper technique
2. Unrecognized succenturiate lobe or bilobed placenta
3. Abnormal placentation with difficulty creating a plane for removal at time of manual extraction
4. May be cause for either immediate or delayed hemorrhage

Placentation abnormalities—accreta, increta, or percreta

1. Do not allow separation of placenta from uterus because of ingrowth of placenta to varying degrees into or through myometrium
2. Most common in patients with placenta previa and a history of cesarean delivery
3. May be recognized antepartum by elevated alpha-fetoprotein or ultrasonography

Uterine rupture

1. Almost exclusively limited to women with a history of a previous uterine incision (i.e., cesarean delivery, hysterotomy, or myomectomy)
2. Fetal bradycardia most common clinical sign
3. Maternal symptom of persistent rather than intermittent abdominal pain
4. Uterine exploration after successful VBAC with postpartum hemorrhage.

Uterine inversion

1. Abnormalities in vital signs may be out of proportion to blood loss.
2. Physical examination demonstrates "mass" in vagina or at introitus.

Maternal coagulation defect or medical disorders

1. Uterine bleeding hemostasis is primarily the result of uterine contractions; therefore it is rarely the result of coagulation defect.
2. Vaginal or vulvar hematoma or excessive bleeding at cesarean delivery may be the result of factor deficiency such as von Willebrand's disease.
3. Other medical conditions such as Marfan's syndrome or Ehlers-Danlos syndrome may not allow sufficient vasoconstriction within the uterus or may result in hemorrhage at other sites involving major vessels because of a defect in connective tissue synthesis.

Subinvolution of the placental site

1. Cause for delayed postpartum hemorrhage, which is defined as excessive bleeding occurring greater than 24 hours after delivery
2. May be associated with abnormal placental function such as growth restriction or preeclampsia

31.3 TREATMENTS

General principles

1. Get help
   a. Anesthesia, nursing, and other physicians experienced in treatment protocols and surgical procedures should be called if they become necessary.
   b. Blood bank should be contacted for type and cross early in evaluation or O negative blood called for if emergency transfusion is necessary.
2. Intravenous access must be obtained: Two large bore intravenous lines are started.
3. Foley catheter is placed to minimize potential trauma to the lower urinary tract and urine output is followed.

Manipulations

1. Uterine massage for atony
2. Bimanual compression of uterine arteries for temporary control of blood loss
3. Uterine packing for uncontrolled atony
   a. Uterine packing should be considered only after failed pharmacologic therapies.
   b. Patient should desire future fertility or be hemodynamically unstable.
   c. Sterile gauze is packed tightly into the uterus must be removed within 24 hours of placement.
   d. Prophylactic antibiotics should be considered because of the presence of the internal foreign body.
   e. Packing soaked in thrombin may enhance clot formation.

Pharmacologic and medical therapies

1. Agents for uterine atony
   a. Oxytocin, up to 40 U/L
      (1) Too rapid IV infusion, which can lead to hypotension, is to be avoided.
   b. Ergot alkaloids, Methergine, 0.2 mg is given through IM injection.
      (1) Relatively contraindicated in patients with hypertensive disorders
   c. Prostaglandin F2-alpha, Carboprost, 250 μg, is given IM.
      (1) Relatively contraindicated in asthmatics, hypertensives, and women with history of cardiac dysfunction
      (2) Dose repeated at 15- to 20-minute intervals in refractory cases, but adverse reactions have been reported in patients receiving numerous doses
2. Blood products and volume expansion
   a. Intravenous crystalloid
      (1) Ringer's lactate or normal saline at a ratio of 2 to 3:1 for each milliliter of estimated blood loss
   b. Packed red blood cells
      (1) Transfusion if hemodynamically unstable, uncontrolled bleeding with estimated blood loss of 2000 ml, or bleeding controlled and patient symptomatic
   c. Fresh frozen plasma
      (1) Patient should be transfused if consumptive coagulopathy is present or if dilutional coagulopathy is detected.
   d. Calcium gluconate
      (1) Not compatible in IV solution with magnesium sulfate
      (2) Consider if greater than 5 U packed red cells transfused
   e. Platelets
      (1) Transfuse if profound dilutional anemia is present or persistent bleeding occurs with thrombocytopenia
   f. Cryoprecipitate or specific factor replacement
      (1) Cryoprecipitate is necessary for treatment of von Willebrand's disease.
      (2) Other factors may be indicated on diagnosis of preexisting hematologic disorder.
   g. Cell savers
      (1) Have been used in patients with massive blood loss once the risk of collection and transfusion of amniotic fluid is eliminated
   h. For patients who are identified as being at significant risk for obstetric hemorrhage
      (1) Self-donation and directed donation of blood products should be discussed and arranged if applicable.

Surgical

1. For retained placenta or subinvolution of placental site
   a. Perform sharp or suction curettage.
   b. Beware of uterine perforation of the gravid uterus.
   c. Consider use of ultrasound for guidance during the procedure.

2. For uterine atony
   a. Bilateral uterine artery ligation: O'Leary stitch
   b. Stepwise devascularization of the uterus with ligation of the vaginal branches of the uterine artery and subsequent ligation of the utero-ovarian pedicles
   c. Bilateral internal iliac artery ligation
      (1) It reduces pulse pressure by 85% to the uterine vasculature but may not be effective in stopping hemorrhage in up to 50% of cases because of extensive pelvic collateral circulation.
      (2) Ligation of posterior branch and superior gluteal artery, which can lead to necrosis of gluteus maximus, is to be avoided.
      (3) Ligation of external iliac by assessing pedal or femoral pulses is to be avoided. Inappropriate ligation may result in loss of lower extremity.
      (4) Ligation is not appropriate if the physician is inexperienced with procedure.
   d. Hysterectomy
      (1) Hysterectomy may be considered earlier in the evaluation of postpartum hemorrhage, depending on family planning desires and amount of active blood loss.
      (2) Most common indications for cesarean hysterectomy are as follows:
         (a) Uterine atony: 43%
         (b) Abnormal placentation: 30%
         (c) Uterine rupture: 13%
         (d) Extension of uterine incision: 12%
         (e) Fibroid uterus: 4%
      (3) Major morbidity is associated ureteral tract injury.
         (a) Obstructed ureter presents as flank pain 2 to 3 days postoperatively.
         (b) Consider intraoperative stenting or other evaluation of ureteral patency.
   e. Abdominal packing
      (1) Abdominal packing may be necessary to perform abdominal mushroom pack with life-threatening bleeding during laparotomy.
      (2) Gauze pads are stuffed inside sterile Mayo stand (plastic bag), which is placed in the abdomen and brought out through the vagina with the end tied to a liter of saline draped off the end of the bed for weight.
3. For abnormal placentation
   a. Accreta
      (1) Oversewing of placental bed (conservative, i.e., retain uterus), or
      (2) Hysterectomy if bleeding persists
   b. Increta
      (1) Hysterectomy, or
      (2) Hysterotomy with placenta left *in situ* if strong desire for future fertility and placental bleeding not active
      (3) Adjuvant postoperative methotrexate

c. Percreta: Assistance from an experienced pelvic surgeon or gynecologic oncologist is needed.
    (1) Hysterectomy with bladder, ureter, or bowel repair if necessary
    (2) Option of hysterotomy with placenta left *in situ* if no active bleeding
    (3) Postoperative adjuvant methotrexate

4. For uterine rupture
    a. Repair of uterine defect is primarily with trimming back of incision edges for improved healing.
    b. Hysterectomy may also be required if extensive uterine damage occurs.
5. For uterine inversion
    a. Uterine relaxation is initiated with halogenated anesthetic, intravenous nitroglycerin, or magnesium sulfate.
    b. Pressure is gently applied circumfrentially to the edge of fundus where the inversion is present.
        (1) Fundus is kneaded back into normal position.
    c. Other maneuvers to replace fundus include the following:
        (1) Hydrostatic pressure: Vagina is filled with saline under pressure, while egress of fluid from the introitus is blocked.
        (2) Laparotomy
            (a) Traction is placed on the round ligaments from above.
            (b) A figure of eight suture is placed in the fundus and traction is applied.
            (c) Hysterectomy for intractable inversion is performed.
6. For vulvar hematoma
    a. Foley catheter is placed to allow for bladder drainage.
    b. This is followed with serial hematocrit determinations every 6 hours.
    c. Intervention for intractable bleeding or evidence of retroperitoneal extension is considered.
        (1) Angiographic embolization is the treatment of choice.
        (2) Surgical exploration and vulvar packing may allow for identification of bleeding vessel.
    d. Observe closely for infected hematoma, which may require drainage and intravenous antibiotics.
        (1) Drainage procedure consists of stab incision in vagina and "milking" hematoma.
        (2) Word catheter may be desired if purulent drainage is persistent.

Catheterization and embolization

1. For refractory postoperative hemorrhage
    a. Excellent for bleeding from vessels of the pelvic floor
    b. May not be possible if prior internal iliac artery ligation has been performed
2. Performed under fluoroscopic guidance by interventional radiologist
3. Gelfoam or glue commonly used
4. For patients with anticipated obstetric hemorrhage, such as from a case of placenta percreta diagnosed antepartum
    a. Prophylactic catheterization before delivery may minimize blood loss because embolization can be performed intraoperatively.

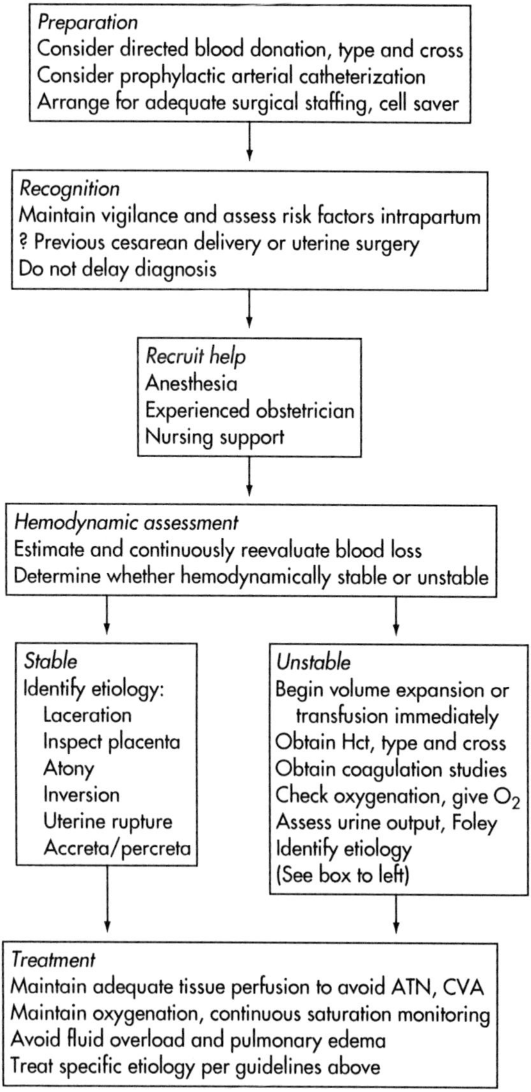

Figure 31-1
Algorithm for management of postpartum hemmorrhage.

31.4 ALGORITHM FOR MANAGEMENT

Fig. 31-1 shows management for postpartum hemorrhage.

Suggested reading

Bobrowski RA, Jones TB: A thrombogenic uterine pack for postpartum hemorrhage, *Obstet Gynecol* 85:836-837, 1995.

Clark SL et al: Emergency hysterectomy for obstetrical hemorrhage, *Obstet Gynecol* 64:376-380, 1984.

Combs CA, Murphy EL, Laros RK: Factors associated with postpartum hemorrhage with vaginal birth, *Obstet Gynecol* 77:69-76, 1991.

Combs CA, Murphy EL, Laros RK: Factors associated with hemorrhage in cesarean deliveries, *Obstet Gynecol* 77:77-82, 1991.

Gilstrap LC, Ramin SM: Postpartum hemorrhage, *Clin Obstet Gynecol* 37:824-830, 1994.

Hallak M et al: Transvaginal pack for life threatening pelvic hemorrhage secondary to placenta accreta, *Obstet Gynecol* 78:938-940, 1991.

Khong TY, Khong TK: Delayed postpartum hemorrhage: a morphological study of causes and their relation to other pregnancy disorders, 82:17-22, 1993.

Maier RC: Control of postpartum hemorrhage with uterine packing, *Am J Obstet Gynecol* 169:317-323, 1993.

Mitty HA et al: Obstetric hemorrhage: prophylactic and emergency arterial catheterization and embolotherapy, *Radiology* 188:183-187, 1993.

32 The Abnormal Papanicolaou Smear in Pregnancy

Dennis M. O'Connor, M.D., and Catherine Sewell, M.D.

Details regarding the Papanicolaou smear can be found in Chapter 5; changes in management due to pregnancy are detailed in this chapter.

32.1 MANAGEMENT OPTIONS

1. Intraepithelial lesions: Biopsy proven L SIL and H SIL are best managed expectantly. Papanicolaou smears and colposcopic examinations are repeated once each trimester. Treatment, if necessary, is postponed until 2 to 3 months after delivery.
2. Invasive lesions: The patient should undergo LEEP or CKC for the following conditions:
   a. Any lesion that cannot be completely assessed because of extension into the endocervical canal
   b. Any lesion that might potentially be invasive

32.2 TRIAGE AND MANAGEMENT SCHEMES

1. Benign cell changes: See Fig. 32-1.
2. Epithelial cell abnormalities: See Figs. 32-2 and 32-3.

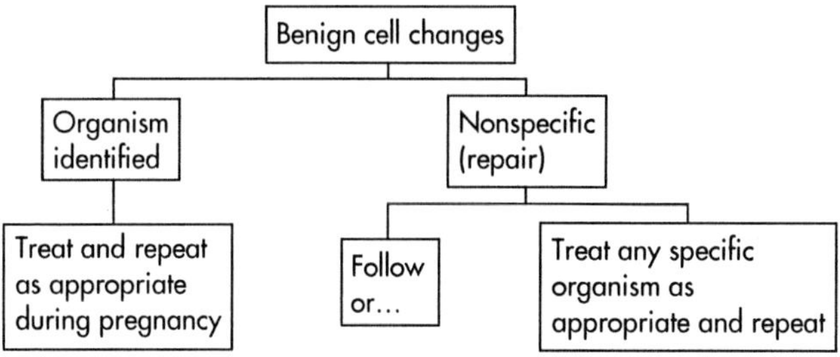

Figure 32-1
Triage options for a cytologic diagnosis of benign cell changes.

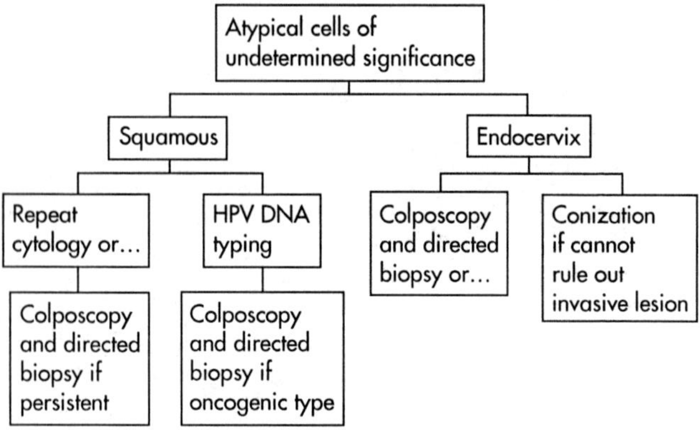

Figure 32-2
Triage options for a cytologic diagnosis of atypical cells of undetermined significance.

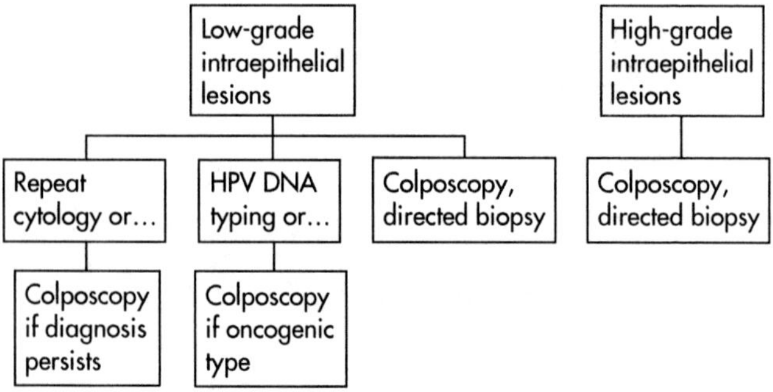

Figure 32-3
Triage options for a cytologic diagnosis of L SIL or H SIL.

Suggested reading

Paraiso MF et al: Evaluation of the endocervical Cytobrush and Cervex-Brush in pregnant women, *Obstet Gynecol* 84:539-543, 1994.
Rivlin ME et al: Comparison of cytobrush and cotton swab for Papanicolaou smears in pregnancy, *J Reprod Med* 38:14-50, 1993.

Antibiotics in Pregnancy

33

Barb Fingar, R.Ph.

The reader is referred to the Appendices for complete comparative information on prescribing antibiotics in pregnancy. This chapter focuses on three commonly prescribed regimens that must be used with special care in the pregnant patient.

33.1 GENTAMICIN AND TOBRAMYCIN AND DOSING GUIDELINES

1. In an average weight female with normal serum creatinine: A loading dose of 2 mg/kg is given, then 1.5 mg/kg q8h.[1] Dose should be to nearest 10 mg.
2. In obese patients, the following is done:
   a. Ideal body weight (IBW) is calculated: IBW = 45 + 2.3 (number of in. > 5 ft).
   b. Adjusted body weight (ABW) is calculated: ABW = IBW + 0.4 (TBW – IBW).
   c. In obese patients with normal serum creatinine: A loading dose of 2 mg/kg (ABW) is given, then 1.5 mg/kg (ABW) q8h.
   d. In obese patients with elevated creatinine: A loading dose of 2 mg/kg (ABW) is given, then 1.5 mg/kg (ABW). Dose is rounded to nearest 10 mg. Dosing interval is determined by calculating the estimated creatinine clearance (Cr Cl) as described in 3.a. and by comparing this to the guidelines shown in 3.b.
3. In patients with elevated creatinine clearance, the following is done:
   a. Estimated Cr Cl[5] is calculated: $\text{Cr Cl (ml/min)} = \frac{(140 - \text{age})(\text{TBW})}{(72 \times \text{serum creatinine})}$ (IBW instead of TBW is used if patient is obese.)
   b. Select dosing interval[7] for Cr Cl is as follows:
      (1) > 70 ml/min: q8h
      (2) 40 to 69 ml/min: q12h
      (3) 20 to 39 ml/min: q24h
   c. A 2 mg/kg loading dose is given, then 1.5 mg/kg at the selected dosing interval. Round dose to the nearest 10 mg.
4. The peak and trough levels should be checked with the third or fourth dose. Therapeutic peaks are 5 to 10 μg/ml and troughs should be <2 μg/ml.

5. Dose is adjusted based on levels and clinical response. Some patients will respond to therapy even when the peak is <5 μg/ml.[2,6]

33.2 VANCOMYCIN DOSING GUIDELINES

1. For patients with normal serum creatinine: 15 mg/kg (1.5 g max) is given q12h.[2] Dose is rounded to the nearest 250 mg.
2. For patients with elevated creatinine clearance, the following is done:
   a. Estimated Cr Cl is calculated[5]: $\text{Cr Cl (ml/min)} = \dfrac{(140 - \text{age})(\text{TBW})}{(72 \times \text{serum creatinine})}$ (IBW is used instead of TBW if patient is obese.)
   b. Select dosing interval for Cr Cl is as follows:
      (1) > 80 ml/min:~q12h
      (2) 50 to 79 ml/min:~q24h
      (3) < 50 ml/min:~> q24h
3. The peak and trough levels should be checked with the third or fourth dose. Therapeutic peaks are 25 to 40 μg/ml and troughs should be <10 μg/ml. Dose is adjusted based on levels and clinical response.

33.3 AMPICILLIN COMPARED WITH PENICILLIN FOR INTRAPARTUM CHEMOPROPHYLAXIS OF EARLY-ONSET NEONATAL GROUP B *STREPTOCOCCUS* INFECTIONS

1. The American Academy of Pediatrics recommends that select patients receive intrapartum antibiotic therapy with either ampicillin (2 g initially; 1 to 2 g q4-6h) or penicillin G (5 million U, IV, q6h) until delivery to prevent group B streptococcal infections in their neonate.[4]
2. There may be some advantages to using ampicillin instead of penicillin for this indication.
   a. Ampicillin has a broader spectrum of antimicrobial activity.
   b. In addition to its activity against group B streptococci, ampicillin is also active against *E. coli, H. influenzae,* and other organisms that can cause early-onset neonatal sepsis.[3]
   c. Compared with penicillin, ampicillin has more favorable pharmacokinetics in pregnant patients.
   d. Ampicillin fetal sera concentrations are comparable with the maternal levels 60 to 90 minutes after administration.
   e. Penicillin G levels are only one third of the maternal levels 120 minutes later.

References

1. Anderson PO: Drug use during breast-feeding, *Clin Pharmacol* 10:594-624, 1991.
2. Bourget P et al: Transplacental passage of vancomycin during the second trimester of pregnancy, *Obstet Gynecol* 78:908-909, 1991.
3. Boyer KM, Gotoff SP: Prevention of early-onset neonatal group b streptococcal disease with selective intrapartum chemoprophylaxis, *N Engl J Med* 314:1665-1669, 1986.
4. Committee on Infectious Disease, American Academy of Pediatrics: Guidelines for prevention of group b streptococcal (GBS) infection by chemoprophylaxis, *Pediatrics* 90:775-778, 1992.

5. Crockcoft DW, Gault MH: Prediction of creatinine clearance from serum creatinine, *Nephron* 16:31, 1976.
6. McNeeley SG et al: Delayed gentamicin elimination in patients with severe preeclampsia, *Am J Obstet Gynecol* 7:793-796, 1985.
7. Sarubbi FA, Hull HJ: Amikacin serum concentrations: prediction of levels and dosage guidelines, *Ann Intern Med* 89:612-618, 1978.

34 Physiology in Pregnancy

Marcello Pietrantoni, M.D.

The biochemical, physiologic, and anatomic adaptations that occur during the 9 months of pregnancy are profound. Many of these changes begin soon after fertilization and continue throughout gestation. An equally astounding fact is that a pregnant woman returns almost completely to her prepregnancy state following delivery and lactation.

Emotional changes occur early in pregnancy. Starting with the first trimester, the patient experiences easy fatigability and has a desire to spend much of her time sleeping. During the second trimester, the patient frequently experiences a period of euphoria and extreme well-being. Last, in the third trimester, there are again some elements of depression and chronic fatigue, probably a result of the increased weight gain.

34.1 MATERNAL NUTRITION

In the United States the average body mass index (BMI) among women is increasing. BMI is calculated by weight (kg)/height $(m)^2$, using the prepregnancy weight.

The accumulation of body fluid during pregnancy is physiologic; expansion of maternal blood volume may account for 10% of the weight gain.

Nutrition

1. Adequate nutrition is paramount for optimal fetal growth.
2. Serum markers to measure long-term and short-term protein nutrition in nonpregnant individuals are not valid during pregnancy because of an increased maternal plasma volume.
   a. Prealbumin, albumin, retinol-binding protein.
   b. Decreased serum albumin may also reflect on maternal circulating alpha-fetoprotein.
3. The recommended dietary allowance suggests an additional caloric intake of 300 kcal/day during pregnancy.
4. Increases in caloric intake should be encouraged with teenagers and in women with increased physical activity.

Maternal weight gain

1. Weight gain during pregnancy and birth weight outcome differ by the prepregnancy weight for height status.

a. Patient self-reported weight is reliable within a standard deviation of about 1.5 kg as opposed to actual measurements.
b. An additional 10 lb of maternal weight gain is recommended for multiple gestations.
c. With increased weight gain over what is recommended (24 to 35 lb) during pregnancy, the following may occur:
(1) Increased incidence of high birth weight (HBW)
(a) HBW is defined as >4500 g.
(2) Decreased incidence of growth restriction
(a) Low birth weight (LBW) is defined as <2500 g.

2. HBW infants are at 66% or three times more likely to die within the first 28 days of life than are normal–birth weight infants.
3. Underweight women (BMI <19.8 kg/m^2) are recommended to gain between 28 and 40 lb.
4. Average weight women (BMI is 19.8 to 26 kg/m^2) should gain between 25 and 35 lb.
5. Overweight women (BMI >26 to 29 kg/m^2) are suggested to gain between 15 and 25 lb.
6. Very overweight women (BMI >29 kg/m^2) guidelines are set at 15 lb which account for the weight of the fetus, placenta, and amniotic fluid.
   a. A gestational weight gain in this group of over 15 lb is associated with increased perinatal morbidity.
7. The best reproductive outcomes are associated with a weight gain of approximately 20 lb in the last half of pregnancy.
   a. A weekly mean rate of gain from the 20th week of gestation to delivery of 1.0 lb/week is recommended.

34.2 MATERNAL SKIN CHANGES

Hair and nails

1. The normal ratio of actively growing hair (anagen phase) to resting (telogen) hairs is approximately 9 to 1.
   a. The increased estrogen and progesterone levels during pregnancy stimulate a greater percentage of hairs to enter the anagen phase.
   b. If vellus hairs are also stimulated to become terminal hair, the patient will become aware of increased facial hair and sometimes generalized hirsutism.
   c. After delivery, hair-cycle ratios are reversed and many scalp hairs fall out (telogen effluvium).
   d. The patient should be reassured that this condition is temporary and that hair cycles will return to normal.
   e. Iron and thyroid deficiency should also be considered if scalp hair loss continues for more than a few months.
2. The nails may become more brittle and show signs of dystrophy, including transverse and longitudinal ridging and onycholysis (elevation of the distal nail plate from the nail bed).
   a. Changes lasting beyond a few months postpartum should prompt an investigation for thyroid disease and iron deficiency.
3. Pruritus itching is the most common skin complaint during pregnancy.

a. It often originates in the abdominal area and occasionally becomes generalized.
b. Pruritus without skin lesions is usually attributed to cholestasis of pregnancy.
c. During pregnancy, the skin has an increased sensitivity, and pruritus may be easily caused by external factors such as body soap, laundry detergent, and radiation.
d. Relief is obtained by eliminating any irritant and use of mild glycerine cleansing bars, bland lotions with aloe vera, and oils.

4. Vascular skin changes are demonstrated by vessel distension, proliferation, and instability during pregnancy.
   a. Palmer erythema, "spider angiomas" (telangiectasias with a central punctum), and a mottled venous pattern to the skin, particularly on exposure to cold, occur frequently and are usually reversible.
   b. Marginal gingivitis, a condition caused by hyperemia and edema of the gums, occurs in many pregnant women and should be managed by good oral hygiene.
5. Striae (stretch marks) are linear, atrophic, light-red to violaceous lesions and commonly develop over the abdomen, breast, and inguinal areas.
   a. Postpartum, the color of the striae will fade; however, they will remain permanently.
6. Melasma is a bilaterally symmetric, lacelike, facial hyperpigmentation often known as chloasma.
   a. Chloasma has a predilection for the malar area, temples, forehead, and the neck region.
   b. Progesterone, estrogen, and melanocyte-stimulating hormone (MSH) play a part in the pigment deposition.
   c. The axillae, pubic skin, and areola show varying degrees of slowly progressing hyperpigmentation.
   d. The linea alba when pigmented is termed the linea nigra.

34.3 MATERNAL BLOOD VOLUME

Hematocrit

1. The hematocrit at the end of pregnancy is usually within the normal range (38% to 45%) in well-nourished women.
2. However, a value less than 34% is highly suspect for true anemia.
3. Maternal red cell mass expansion occurs mostly during the last 8 to 10 weeks.
4. Diluational anemia (first 24 weeks) during pregnancy arises from the increased maternal plasma volume, which occurs before the rise in total erythrocyte mass.
5. Postpartum, the hematocrit will rise approximately 3% to 5% as a result of physiologic diuresis.
6. In high-altitude areas (>3300 ft), there is a greater rise in erythrocyte volume to increase oxygen transport.
7. A hemoglobin less than 11 g/100 ml or a hematocrit less than 33% during pregnancy implies anemia.
8. Changes in hemoglobin and hematocrit values are induced by altitude and smoking.

   a. Because of the lower oxygen partial pressure in high-altitude areas, women will have a reduced oxygen saturation with a compensatory increase in red blood cell production.
   b. Similarly this is also seen with smokers; however, this is a result of the increased carboxyhemoglobin, a poor carrier of oxygen.

Plasma volume

1. There is approximately a 50% increase in maternal plasma volume (equivalent to 2600 ml) over nonpregnant women, and it plateaus at about 30 to 34 weeks.
2. Larger increases are associated with multiple pregnancies and larger fetuses.
3. In tropical climates there is an increase in maternal plasma volume over climates that are cold.
   a. This is because of the greater loss in body heat and fluid in tropical climates.

Uterine blood flow

1. As the result of the increase in maternal cardiac output there is also a substantial increase in uterine blood flow.
2. Approximately 50 ml/min in early pregnancy to 500 ml/min at term.
3. The main blood supply to the uterus (approximately 80%) originates from the uterine arteries.
4. Therefore, the progressive increase in uterine arterial blood flow measured by pulsed Doppler ultrasonography is approximately a fourfold increase in flow rate as compared with nonpregnant values.
5. The cardiac output that is distributed to the uterine vessels is approximately 3.5% in early pregnancy and 12% near term.
6. Also, placental perfusion continues to rise until term, when it accounts for 80% to 90% of the total uterine blood flow, which accommodates the exponential growth of the fetus.

34.4 MATERNAL VASCULAR CHANGES

Arterial circulation

1. The integrity of the maternal vascular arterial circulation is proposed as the primary determinant of body fluid volume regulation.
2. Peripheral arterial vasodilation with relative underfilling of the arterial circulation occurs in early gestation.
   a. This causes a decrease in the systolic and diastolic blood pressures, increased cardiac output secondary to afterload reduction, nonosmotic stimulation of thirst and vasopressin release, stimulation of the renin–angiotensin–aldosterone axis, and renal sodium and water retention.
   b. This results in extracellular fluid and plasma volume expansion.

Renal blood flow

1. In early pregnancy, there is an increase in renal blood flow and glomerular filtration rate of 30% to 50%, secondary to arterial

vasodilation, the latter occurring before maternal plasma volume expansion.
2. Also, during pregnancy the sodium-retaining effect of aldosterone is not seen, and similarly in the vascular resistance to angiotensin.
3. Approximately 85% of the total blood volume resides in the venous circulation, as only 15% of the total blood volume circulates in the arterial system.
4. In early pregnancy renal vasodilation with arterial underfilling leads to sodium and water retention.
5. Hence, the observed increased renal and glomerular filtration rates during pregnancy of 30% to 50%, respectively.
6. The maternal increase in progesterone may account for the aldosterone escape in pregnancy, because progesterone is known to counteract the tubular sodium transport effects of aldosterone.

34.5 FETAL AND PLACENTAL PHYSIOLOGY

Placenta

1. The placenta regulates maternal–fetal interactions for physiologic exchange and acts as a selective barrier between mother and fetus.
2. It also participates in the immunity of the fetus by actively transporting IgG antibodies for fetal and neonatal use.
3. The fetus obtains maternal IgG for its *in utero* immunologic protection, and before 22 weeks gestation the IgG is transported via simple diffusion.
4. After 22 weeks gestation, IgG is transported across the placental membranes by pinocytosis.

Fetus

1. The fetus directs about 50% of its cardiac output through the umbilical arteries.
2. This translates to approximately 500 to 600 ml/min.
3. Therefore, the fetal blood pressure and cardiac output are obvious determinants of umbilical artery flow.
4. Hence, fetal heart failure, arrhythmias, and cord compression could adversely affect umbilical artery blood flow.
5. The fetus contributes to the amniotic fluid volume by urinating approximately 800 ml/day or 5 ml/hr.
6. Also, some of the amniotic fluid is reabsorbed by fetal swallowing and the mechanism of *in utero* breathing.
7. There is always additional fluid exchange at the chorionic plate between mother and fetus.
8. The fetal skin (keratinized at 24 weeks gestation), chorion–amnion, and umbilical cord contribute little to the amniotic fluid exchange after 24 weeks.

Physiologic functions of the placenta

1. Respiratory: exchange of oxygen and carbon dioxide; acts as a lung
2. Nutrition: acts as the gastrointestinal tract with transfer of sugars, amino acids, protein, and lipids

3. Excretion: acts as a kidney in disposing of waste (bilirubin)
4. Protective: acts like the skin by moderating heat transfer; protects against bacterial invasion
5. Endocrine function: produces human chorionic gonadotropin (HCG), luteinizing releasing factor, thyrotropin releasing factor, progesterone, cortisol, estriol, and human placental lactogen (HPL)

Placental transport

Transport of H_2O

1. Transfer of water takes place by what is called "bulk flow."
2. This refers to a process by which small transient changes in hydrostatic and osmotic pressure across the placental membrane result in movement of water.
3. Because water is extremely responsive to such changes, these gradients are transient and difficult to measure.
4. There is a large movement of water in both directions.
5. The net transfer is in favor of the fetus with an accumulation of water of approximately 0.14 ml/min or 20 ml/day.
6. This large movement of fluid exchange also probably produces a substantial amount of other solutes by "solvent drag."

Transport of electrolytes

1. The placental membrane is permeable to sodium, potassium, and chloride.
2. So far, no sodium or potassium pump has been discovered in the placental membrane.
3. Transport of these ions occurs by simple diffusion through water-filled "pores" lying between cells.
4. Concentrations of these electrolytes are the same in the fetus as in the mother, and the permeability of the membrane to these electrolytes increases by 70-fold from as early as 9 weeks to 35 weeks, then drops off slightly near term.
5. Calcium, phosphate, iodine, and probably magnesium, as well as many of the trace elements and minerals, are present in higher concentrations in the fetus than in the mother and are transported by active transport mechanisms across the placental membrane.
6. The same can be said of iron.
7. Receptors for iron have been found on the placental membrane and its active transport system increases in efficiency as gestation progresses.

Vitamins

1. Water-soluble vitamins such as thiamine (B_1), pyridoxine (B_6), and B_{12}, as well as vitamin C (ascorbic acid) and folic acid, all have higher concentrations in the fetus and require active transport systems.
2. The concentrations of fat-soluble vitamins (A, D, E, K) are the same or slightly lower in the fetus and these probably traverse the placenta by passive diffusion.

Carbohydrates

1. Glucose is the major metabolic fuel of the fetus and fetal levels are approximately 15% lower in the fetus as compared with the mother's.
2. It is estimated that about two thirds of the glucose uptake is used for placental metabolism, with only the remaining third being transferred for fetal use.
3. Transfer of glucose to the fetus occurs by facilitated diffusion, with glucose being transferred more rapidly than fructose or other sugars of similar molecular weight, which cross by simple diffusion.
4. This transport is not energy dependent but is carrier mediated by a protein carrier in the syncitiotrophoblastic cell membrane.
5. This transport system is very much stereospecific since only D-glucose is facilitated, whereas L-glucose is not.
6. Glycogen storage takes place in the liver, skeletal muscle, and placenta.
7. Near term, the glycogen storage shifts quantitatively from the placenta to the liver.
8. Pyruvate and lactate also cross the placenta by simple diffusion.

Free fatty acids

1. Free fatty acids (FFA) are bound to albumin, making them water soluble.
2. They also traverse the placenta by simple diffusion.
3. FFA are used not for energy but for fetal complex lipid synthesis.
4. Both saturated and unsaturated FFA cross the placenta equally as well, but the rate of transfer is inversely proportional to the fatty acid chain length.
5. As the transplacental supply of FFA falls short of fetal requirements for fat deposition in the third trimester, some of the fetal free FFA are probably made *de novo* by the fetus.

Complex lipids

1. Complex lipids (triglycerides, cholesterol, and phospholipids) are transported in the mother as lipoproteins and are characterized as low or high density.
2. Cholesterol, as well as many of these more complex lipids, is probably used by the placenta for its own needs.
3. In addition, transport of these large molecules, if it occurs at all, is probably very small.
4. For these reasons, the fetus synthesizes much of its lipids *de novo* from precursors.
5. There is a suggestion that the placenta may break down complex lipids for fetal use, but this is unproven.

Amino acids

1. Amino acids have a fourfold higher concentration in the fetus as compared with the mother's.
2. This transport is effected by an active transport mechanism.
3. This mechanism is stereospecific, with the naturally occurring L-forms or isomers crossing more rapidly than the D-isomers.

4. The receptor site, however, is nonspecific, with all of the amino acids competing for the same sites on an equal basis.
5. The fetus synthesizes almost all of its proteins from those amino acids that cross the placenta.
6. In addition, it is felt that the fetus may use these amino acids as a metabolic fuel, deriving as much as 25% of its energy requirements from their degradation in some studies.

Proteins

1. Most of the fetal protein requirements come from the fetal synthesis of proteins from amino acids that are actively transported across the placenta.
2. Polypeptides and larger proteins cross the placental membrane slowly, if at all.
3. They cross generally by one of two mechanisms:
   a. Simple diffusion: more important earlier in gestation
   b. Pinocytosis: more important later in gestation
4. Plasma proteins, notably albumin, and the beta-globulins such as transferrin and fibrinogen, cross in very small quantities by simple diffusion and the amounts transferred are not significant.
5. Protein hormones such as thyroid-stimulating hormone (TSH), adrenocorticotropic hormone (ACTH), T_4, and T_3 cross the placenta little if at all.
6. Insulin diffuses only in micro amounts, so the fetus must manufacture almost all of its own insulin.
7. The fetus does not manufacture IgG in any appreciable quantities and, indeed, does not attain this ability until well into the newborn period.
   a. The fetus obtains its IgG from the mother.
   b. This sustains the fetus into the newborn period and protects it *in utero*.
   c. Before 22 weeks, this IgG transfer occurs via simple diffusion.
   d. After 22 weeks, IgG of maternal origin traverses the placental membrane by pinocytosis, an energy-requiring mechanism of "cell drinking."
   e. This transfer is specific only for antibodies of the IgG class and receptors for the Fc portion of the IgG molecule have been located on the syncitiotrophoblastic cell membrane.
   f. Unfortunately, this transfer is not specific among the IgG antibodies types, and IgG antibodies that may be harmful to the fetus are transferred with the same efficiency as those that are not harmful.
   g. This occurs in Rh disease, maternal immune thrombocytopenia (ITP), and myasthenia gravis.
   h. In the latter two diseases, the antibodies cross the placenta and induce the same disease in the fetus.

Nucleic acids

Nucleic acids are synthesized from maternal precursors that cross the placenta by simple diffusion: ATP, ADP, AMP, and purine and pyrimidine bases.

Bilirubin

1. Unconjugated bilirubin rapidly traverses the placenta by simple diffusion; conjugated bilirubin does not.
2. As a result of the ductus venosus through which vena caval and umbilical blood bypass the liver, as well as the immaturity of the liver enzymes, the bilirubin is kept predominantly in the unconjugated form favorable for placental transfer.
3. This explains the absence of jaundice in some neonates who have suffered hemolytic disease *in utero.*

Nitrogenous compounds

1. Nitrogenous waste products cross the placenta by simple diffusion and include creatinine, blood urea nitrogen (BUN), and uric acid.
2. If the maternal levels of any of these substances are high, as occurs in maternal renal failure, this will be reflected in the fetus and in the fetal urine.
3. This is important to keep in mind because amniotic fluid creatinine levels (derived from the fetal urine) are often used in lung maturity studies.

Temperature

The placenta functions as a heat exchange unit, with the temperature of the fetus usually 1° C higher than the mother.

34.6 MATERNAL RESPIRATORY SYSTEM

Antepartum pulmonary changes begin in the fourth week of gestation. The earliest changes to elicit symptoms are related to mucosal capillary engorgement, resulting in swelling and congestion of the nostrils and throat. The diaphragm becomes elevated because of the enlarging uterus. The subcostal angle is increased from 68° to 103°, causing an increase of approximately 2 cm in the transthoracic diameter. Also, the respiratory rate is usually unchanged.

The increased respiratory effort and concomitant reduction of P_{CO_2} is caused in large part by progesterone by a central direct stimulatory effect on the respiratory center.

Anatomic changes

1. There is 4-cm rise from the diaphragm.
2. Subcostal angle widens as the transverse thoracic diameter increases by 2 cm.

Changes in pulmonary function

1. Physiologic increase occurs in (not pregnant/pregnant = percentage change) the following:
   a. Tidal volume (487 ml/678 ml = +39% change).
      (1) The tidal volume (TV) lowers P_{CO_2}, causing a mild respiratory alkalosis and a decreased HCO_3.
      (2) Volume increases by about 200 ml.

(3) This is the volume of air breathed in and out during normal respiration.

b. Minute O_2 uptake (201/266 = +32% change).

c. Minute ventilation (7270 ml/10,340 ml = +42%).

d. Increased airway conductance is caused by a decrease in bronchomotor tone secondary to a progesterone effect.

e. Inspiratory capacity appears to increase progressively throughout pregnancy, reaching a matrix of approximately 300 ml above nonpregnant levels at term.

2. Physiologic decrease occurs in (not pregnant/pregnant = percentage change) the following:

a. Functional residual capacity.

b. Residual volume (965 ml/770 ml = –20% change).

(1) Decreased by some 300 ml (volume of air remaining in the lung spaces after normal expiration)

c. Decrease in total pulmonary resistance.

d. A decrease in the difference between the arterial–venous oxygen content.

e. Expiratory reserve volume is decreased by approximately 200 ml.

(1) This is the maximum air volume exhaled after normal resting respiration.

f. Pulmonary diffusion capacity decreases by approximately 4 ml/min/mm H_2O.

3. No physiologic pulmonary changes occur in the following:

a. Maximum breathing capacity (102/97 = –5%).

b. No change in forced vital capacity.

c. Vital capacity (3260 ml/3310 = +1%).

(1) May be increased but earlier reports suggest no change.

(2) This is the maximum total volume of air that can be breathed out after maximal forced inspiration.

d. No change in lung compliance.

e. No significant change in the respiratory rate (15/16).

f. Forced expiratory volume appears to be unaffected.

g. Peak expiratory flow rate appears not to be affected.

4. Changes in air requirements

a. Maternal adaptations to pregnancy in cardiac, renal, and respiratory performance account for approximately two thirds of the extra oxygen need during pregnancy.

b. The fetus also has an oxygen demand, but its needs are relatively modest because it does not need to regulate its own temperature.

c. It may be calculated that the extra metabolic activity of pregnancy requires oxygen in the amount of 30 to 40 ml/min or 15% above nonpregnant needs.

d. The developing fetus must off-load its CO_2 into the mother.

(1) The mother could reduce her basal P_{CO_2} status.

(2) The mother "overbreathes" to wash out her P_{CO_2}: This leads to alkalosis, but she compensates by excreting more bicarbonate into the renal system, excreting with it some obligatory sodium.

(3) Unfortunately, sodium is a major determinant of plasma osmolality, so this decreases.

(4) Lowering osmolality normally causes a diuresis so that the mother's hypothalamic osmoreceptor centers must be reset to accept and guard this lower value.

(5) Thus the primary need to lower P_{CO_2} initiates a series of events that affect the respiratory and renal systems, as well as significantly altering plasma biochemistry.

(a) Carbon dioxide pressure (P_{CO_2})

i. This is dramatically decreased from the nonpregnant range of 35 to 40 mm Hg to 28 to 30 mm Hg during pregnancy.

ii. This pregnancy reduction is almost certainly an effect of progesterone.

(b) Oxygen pressure (P_{O_2})

i. As would be anticipated from the decrease in P_{CO_2}, there is an increase in P_{O_2} during gestation.

ii. This increase is small, from 85 mm Hg to approximately 92 mm Hg.

(c) pH

i. Maternal arterial pH is unaltered from the normal average of 7.4.

ii. The implication is that the decrease in P_{CO_2}, which leads to respiratory alkalosis, is matched by a decrease in the bicarbonate.

34.7 MATERNAL URINARY SYSTEM

Kidney

1. The mean kidney length was found to increase in size by approximately 1 to 1.5 cm, and the enlargement probably reflects the increase in renal blood flow and renal vascular volume, with perhaps a degree of hypertrophy.
2. Earliest physiologic renal change occurs with dilation of the renal pelvis and ureters (physiologic hydroureter of pregnancy).
   a. These become evident in the first trimester and persist to term and until approximately 6 weeks postpartum.
   b. The proposed mechanisms are as follows:
      (1) External compression of the ureters from the uterus with fetus, iliac arteries, and ovarian veins.
      (2) Hormonal changes are caused by the increases in the levels of progesterone, gonadotropins, and estrogens.
      (3) Ureteral hypertrophy is caused by hyperplasia of the connective tissue, hypertrophy of the longitudinal smooth muscles (Waldeyer's sheath), and edema.
   c. The hydroureter is more prominent on the right.
   d. The maternal renal calyces and ureters dilate and may contain 40 to 100 ml of urine in total.
   e. Contrary to popular belief, the ureteral muscular tone is not reduced and may indeed be slightly increased during pregnancy, secondary to the compression and obstruction of the ureter at the pelvic inlet by the pregnant dextrorotated uterus.
   f. The dextrorotation is caused by the sigmoid colon.

Bladder

1. Because of the atonic effects of pregnancy on smooth muscle the tone of the bladder is progressively decreased and its capacity increased, retaining double its normal volume by term.
2. The trigone area undergoes moderate hyperplasia and muscular hypertrophy, giving a concave appearance to the base of the bladder.
3. As the uterus enlarges hyperemia of the pelvic organs occurs, and the bladder is displaced anteriorly and superiorly, which makes cystoscopy, if necessary, difficult.
4. Near term, the bladder mucosa becomes more edematous and easily traumatized and therefore more susceptible to bacterial infection.
5. Because of the fetal presenting part toward the end of pregnancy, an impairment of the emptying of the venous blood and lymph flow from the base of the bladder often causes edema and more susceptibility for trauma and infection.
6. Urinary tract infections are therefore more common in pregnancy because bacteria can then be transmitted to the ureters via vesicoureteral reflux.
7. The increase in urinary volume in the ureteropelvic system enhances the growth of organisms and hence the observed increase in pyelonephritis in pregnancy.
8. In addition, the maternal bladder vessels tend to increase in size and become tortuous.

Renal physiology

1. Renal blood flow increases markedly during pregnancy, with midpregnancy increments attaining 60% to 80% followed by a significant fall in the third trimester from 480 to 890 ml/min.
2. The glomerular filtration rate (GFR) is increased by approximately 50% throughout pregnancy.
   a. This is increased from the nonpregnant state average of 97 ml/min to 128 ml/min by the 10th week of gestation; also, there may be a small decrease between 36 weeks of gestation and term.
   b. Urinary flow and sodium excretion decrease by half in the supine position, and the BUN and creatinine decrease because of the increased GFR.
   c. However, the creatinine clearance is not affected by pregnancy.
   d. As a test of renal function, dye excretion urinary tests may be misleading because during daylight pregnant women tend to accumulate water in the form of dependent edema and at night, while the patients are recumbent, they mobilize and excrete fluid (nocturia).
3. Homeostatic control during pregnancy causes women to retain some 2 L of water, 290 mEq sodium, 155 mEq of potassium, and the corresponding anions. The normal kidney has an almost unlimited ability to control water and electrolytes; during pregnancy the kidney resets to achieve a new balance.
   a. Acid–base physiology
      (1) During pregnancy, the mean arterial P_{CO_2} decreases from approximately 39 to 30 mm Hg.
      (2) The blood levels of hydrogen ions are also slightly decreased, as is the bicarbonate (HCO_3) by some 4 mEq/L.

(3) The effect of the these changes is that the arterial pH averages 7.44 during pregnancy vs. 7.40 in nonpregnant women.
(4) The majority of maternal acid (about 1300 mEq_2 of H^+ per day) is produced from the reaction of CO_2 and H_2O to form H_2CO_3, which dissociates into H^+ and HCO_3^-.
(5) This acid is eliminated by the lung, where the reverse reaction takes place and CO_2 is liberated.
(6) In the fetus, this respiratory elimination of acid takes place at the placental membrane.
(7) A smaller amount of fixed, nonvolatile acids are produced by metabolic processes (about 80 mEq/day).
(8) This is eliminated to some degree by the fetal kidneys and to a lesser degree by the transfer of H^+ across the placental membrane.
(9) Because of its ionic charge, however, this transfer is very slow and probably contributes little to overall acid–base balance.
(10) As in the adult, the major buffers of the fetal blood are HCO_3^- and hemoglobin.
(11) The minor buffers are inorganic and organic phosphates, and plasma proteins.
(12) The buffering capacity of the fetus is the same as in the adult (buffer base) and, because the fetus is not in metabolic acidosis, has the same base deficit as the adult.

b. Potassium
(1) Approximately 350 mEq is retained in the course of pregnancy.
(2) This resistance for choleresis has been ascribed to the action of progesterone.

c. Sodium
(1) Renal sodium is the prime determinant for the maintenance of volume homeostasis.
(2) Despite an increase of about 47% in the amount of sodium presented to the renal tubules every 24 hours, their reabsorption efficiency is maintained at better than 99%.
(3) Approximately 950 mEq of sodium is accumulated throughout pregnancy.

d. Urinary output
(1) The 24-hour urine volume is largely unchanged.
(2) The increased filtered load of water is reabsorbed with equal efficiency when required.

e. Posture
(1) Changes in maternal posture cause only a short-term effect on the kidneys' ability to handle water and sodium.

f. Excretion of nutrients
(1) Glucose
(a) Glucose is excreted in increasing amounts; but the pattern of glycosuria and amount excreted per 24 hours appear to be random.
(b) Therefore it is apparent that testing or screening for glycosuria during the antenatal period for diabetes mellitus is not appropriate.

(c) Other sugars are also excreted in increased amounts, except arabinose.

(2) Amino acids

(a) The total amount of amino acids excreted is increased, but there is a variation among individual amino acids.

(3) Vitamins

(a) Water-soluble vitamins are excreted in greater amounts.

(4) Proteins

(a) Proteins are unchanged over a 24-hour period and up to 200 mg/dl is considered normal.

(5) Creatinine clearance

(a) The creatinine clearance is taken as an index of the GFR.

(b) By the eighth week of pregnancy, a mean increment of 45% has occurred in a 24-hour creatinine clearance.

(c) Throughout the second trimester, it remains elevated, but during the weeks preceding delivery there is a consistent decrease down to the nonpregnant levels.

	Plasma	
	Creatinine	BUN
1st trimester	0.73/100 ml	11
2nd trimester	0.58/100 ml	9
3rd trimester	0.53/100 ml	10

(d) Values of 0.8 mg/100 ml and 14 mg/100 ml should alert the clinician to investigate renal function.

(6) Uric acid

(a) During normal pregnancy, there is a relative hypouricemia.

(b) Plasma uric acid concentrations decrease by 25% as early as the eighth week of pregnancy and begin to increase once more during the third trimester, reaching a concentration equivalent to the nonpregnant mean.

(c) Uric acid concentration and renal reabsorption are significantly higher in pregnancies complicated by preeclampsia or intrauterine growth restriction.

(d) Above a critical level of 580 mg/100 ml, there is a significant perinatal mortality in hypertensive patients.

(7) Renin–angiotensin system

(a) During normal pregnancy, the level of the circulating renin begins to increase during the early first trimester and continues to increase progressively until term, achieving values 5 to 10 times greater than nonpregnant concentrations.

(b) Like most globulin fractions, angiotensin also increases, and it rises from a mean nonpregnancy values of 0.7/L to a mean peak of 3.6 mg/L.

(c) As might be anticipated, the concentrations of angiotensin I and II also increase, but the anticipated effects, vasoconstriction and consequent rise in blood pressure, do not occur.

(d) Indeed, pregnant women are remarkably resistant to the pressor effects of the infused angiotensin from as early as 10 weeks gestation.

34.8 MATERNAL GASTROINTESTINAL SYSTEM

Appetite

1. Pregnant women appear to have a significant increase in appetite.
2. In some cases, this tends to take bizarre forms.
3. These few peculiar habits in themselves are unlikely to cause any adverse effects.
4. Such things as coal and clay have a significant absorption and buffering capacity and could, if taken in excess, reduce the absorption of minerals and vitamins from the gastrointestinal system.
5. In a few women, appetite may be decreased secondary to nausea or reflux esophagitis, and attention to these symptoms usually improves appetite.

Gastric reflux

1. Gastric reflux is probably caused by a combination of the esophageal (cardiac) sphincter laxity and the anatomic displacement of the lower esophageal sphincter, increased intraabdominal pressure, and even a hiatal hernia.
2. Management with an antacid preparations is usually effective in improving appetite.

Gastric secretion

1. Gastric secretion decreases in terms of acidity during early and midpregnancy.
2. However, it increases late in pregnancy, although the amount of mucus production may also be increased.

Gastric motility

1. Gastric motility almost certainly decreases, and with a delay in complete emptying time, this is probably further reduced during labor.
2. Gastric emptying is double in time in pregnant women compared with nonpregnant women.

Intestinal absorption

1. Efficiency of gastric absorption may be increased, either by specific mechanisms or by a delay in transit time that allows more time for digestion and absorption.

Large intestine

1. Absorption efficiency appears to be greater (more water absorption) during pregnancy, and intestinal transit time is probably slower, which may also explain constipation.

Liver

1. In functional terms, liver function tests are probably unchanged, with normal levels of serum bilirubin.
2. Also, nonspecific alkaline phosphatase increases in pregnancy are attributable to the alkaline phosphatase isoenzymes from the placenta.

Gallbladder

1. Gallbladder may be passively dilated and hence larger in size; however, the composition of the bile itself appears to be unchanged.
2. There is anecdotal evidence that gallstones are more frequent during pregnancy with the decreased motility of the gallbladder and incomplete emptying, causing the large residual volume of bile causing cholesterol crystals to be formed and retained.

34.9 MATERNAL REPRODUCTIVE SYSTEM

Most of these changes result from an increase in the hormones estrogen and progesterone.

Breasts

1. Size and nodularity are increased (soon after missed period).
2. Superficial veins are more prominent because of increased blood supply and blood vessels.
   a. This causes the feelings of fullness and tingling (end of second month).
3. Striae (stretch marks) may appear.
4. Pigmentation usually increases.
5. There is an increase in sebaceous glands in areola (Montgomery's tubercles), which lubricate the nipple.
6. Precolostrum starts the 16th week; colostrum is noted in the third trimester.

Ovaries

1. No ovulation occurs during pregnancy because necessary hormones are suppressed.
2. Blood vessels to ovaries enlarge.

Fallopian tubes

1. Fallopian tubes elongate but otherwise experience few changes.
2. Blood vessels to fallopian tubes enlarge.

Uterus

1. Enlarges from solid organ (approximately 2 oz) to a thin-walled muscular sac (2.2 lb) for gestation as a result of hormones that do the following:
   a. Provide new muscle fibers
   b. Increase blood supply and enlarge blood vessels
   c. Enlarge preexisting fibers
   d. Develop the lining of the uterus

2. Braxton-Hicks contractions
   a. Begin at fourth month
   b. Painless; stimulate blood flow through placenta
3. Blood flow
   a. One sixth of maternal blood flow in the uterine system
   b. Affected by hemorrhage, malnutrition, maternal position, uterine contractions

Vagina and vulva

1. Increase in size and number of cells
2. Increase in secretions
   a. Acidic to prevent growth of microorganisms (except yeast)
3. Increase in blood vessels and blood supply
   a. Increased sensitivity
      (1) Increased sexual interest

Cervix

1. Endocervical glands enlarge.
2. Glandular activity increases.
   a. Secretion of thick, tenacious mucus: mucus plug
      (1) Seals the cervix preventing bacteria and other organisms from entering the uterus
      (2) Leads to much vaginal discharge

Table 34-1 shows the Bishop scores for evaluating changes in the cervix.

34.10 COMMON DISCOMFORTS OF PREGNANCY: CAUSES AND RELIEF

See the box on p. 836.

Ache in back, hips, or thighs

1. Cause
   a. Pressure of baby on small nerves on inside of vertebrae and pelvis
2. Relief
   a. Pelvic rock on all fours or creeping on all fours; this may encourage fetus to readjust its position

Backache

1. Causes
   a. Poor posture
      (1) This is more common in multiparas whose muscle tone is poor.
      (2) Lax abdominal muscles let uterus fall forward; this leads to lordotic posture for maintenance of balance.
   b. Softening effect of hormone action on spinal discs and sacroiliac joints
   c. Obesity
2. Relief
   a. Careful attention to correct posture and body mechanics
   b. Pelvic rock, especially on all fours

Table 34-1 Bishop prelabor cervical score

	0	1	2	3
Dilation (cm)	Closed	1-2	3-4	5 or greater
Effacement (%)	0-30	40-50	60-70	80 or greater
Station	−3	−2	−1, 0	1+ or greater
Consistency	Firm	Medium	Soft	—
Position	Posterior	Midposition	Anterior	—

The Discomforts of Pregnancy

First Trimester	Second Trimester	Third Trimester
Ambivalence	Ankle edema	Ankle edema
Backache	Backache	Anxiety
Breast tenderness	Changing body image	Backache or hip pain
Changing body image	Constipation	Changing body image
Depression	Depression	Constipation
Emotional lability	Emotional lability	Depression
Fatigue	Fainting or dizziness	Emotional lability
Fearfulness	Fearfulness	Fatigue
Gingival hyperplasia	Gingival hyperplasia	Fearfulness
Headache	Headache	Fetal movements
Increased urinary frequency	Heartburn	Gingival hyperplasia
Increased or decreased libido	Increased or decreased libido	Headache
Increased sensitivity	Increased fetal movements	Heartburn
Indecisiveness	Increased sensitivity	Hemorrhoids
Irritability	Increased vaginal discharge	Increased sensitivity
Ligament pain	Indecisiveness	Increased or decreased libido
Morning sickness	Irritability	Increased urinary frequency
Nasal congestion	Leg cramps	Increased vaginal discharge
Skin changes	Ligament pain	Indecisiveness
	Nasal congestion	Insomnia
	Shortness of breath	Irritability
	Skin changes	Leg cramps
	Varicose veins	Ligament pain
	Weight gain	Nasal congestion
		Shortness of breath
		Skin changes
		Slight nausea
		Varicose veins
		Weight gain

c. Kneeling in a crawling position several times a day
d. When standing, lifting one foot and placing it on an object so it is higher than the other foot; or standing with one foot in front of the other and rocking back and forth slightly
e. Firm mattress on bed

f. CAUTION
   (1) Not all backaches can be classified as to the same cause.
   (2) Each patient must be dealt with privately to find the exact location and type of pain.
   (3) Backache high and to one side may indicate kidney problems.
   (4) Ache in the middle of a buttock with muscle cramping may be caused by a sacroiliac problem.
   (5) Manipulative exercises can help but must be done by an operant with expertise in this area.

Breast tenderness

1. Causes
   a. Exaggerated sebaceous glands (Montgomery glands)
   b. Hyperplasia of the breast
2. Relief
   a. Wearing a good support bra (during sleep as well)

Constipation

1. Causes
   a. Diminished peristalsis caused by pressure of the enlarged uterus and the relaxing effect on muscle coat of intestines
   b. Decreased physical activity
   c. Impaired tone of stretched abdominal muscles
2. Relief
   a. Drinking three glasses of cool water at 5-minute intervals on rising, then a glass of fruit juice with breakfast
   b. Making sure diet includes plenty of vitamin B, found in wheat germ, liver, whole grains, and Brewer's yeast
   c. When sitting on toilet, assuming a semisquatting position by putting feet up on a stool; relaxes pelvic floor

Diaphragm pressure (cramp or stitch under ribs)

1. Cause
   a. When baby is high in abdomen, diaphragm is compressed against the base of the lungs.
2. Relief
   a. Lifting rib cage by raising arms sideways and upward above head, then stretching

Dizziness, fainting, and lightheadedness

1. Causes
   a. Vasomotor changes
   b. Pressure of gravid uterus on greater abdominal vessels
   c. Anemia
   d. Decreased blood sugar
2. Relief
   a. Avoiding sudden changes in posture, especially after practice of conscious release
   b. After lying down, getting up slowly, rolling to side, then pushing up to sitting position (using arms)

c. Avoiding standing or lying flat on back for long periods
d. Following physician's advice for treatment of anemia
e. Not skipping meals; eating properly
f. Avoiding hot, stuffy rooms

Dyspnea (shortness of breath)

1. Causes
   a. When baby is high in abdomen, diaphragm is compressed against the base of the lungs.
   b. Dyspnea may indicate anemia.
2. Relief
   a. Sleeping well propped up with pillows or spending first 10 minutes in bed lying on back with arms extended above head and resting on the bed
   b. Lightening during late pregnancy

Edema

1. Causes
   a. Peripheral arterial vasodilation with a resultant decreased filling of arterial circulation
   b. Sodium and water retention
   c. Pressure on the iliac vein and inferior vena cava caused by an enlarging uterus increases capillary pressure in the lower extremities, with a resulting filtration of fluid into the interstitial spaces
2. Relief
   a. Lying on left side for 30 minutes three to four times daily
   b. Getting regular exercise
   c. Increasing fluid intake
   d. Eating three servings of protein daily

Emotional discomforts (anxiety, depression, and emotional lability)

1. Causes
   a. Perceived lack of control during childbirth experience
   b. Fear of the "unknown" (labor, etc.)
   c. Physical discomforts (nausea, vomiting, backache, fatigue)
   d. Changing body image
   e. Unresolved conflicts, ambivalence about pregnancy and its subsequent changes, emotional turmoil, poor coping skills, and genetic predisposition
   f. External pressures, such as finances
   g. Physical and hormonal changes of pregnancy
2. Relief
   a. Maintenance of physical health
   b. Encouragement, positive reinforcement, and communication therapy
   c. Pharmacologic treatment with SSRIs such as Prozac or Paxil

Fatigue

1. Causes
   a. Significant hormonal increases
   b. Poor nutrition, anemia, and slowed circulation
   c. Sleep disturbances caused by urinary frequency, leg cramps, respiratory difficulties, vomiting, or other problems
2. Relief
   a. Daily exercise to improve circulation
   b. Toward term, lying down at least once daily

Fingers (tingling, numbness, and a feeling of swelling)

1. Causes
   a. Enlargement of breast tissue high in armpit, resulting in pressure on nerves and blood vessels
   b. May indicate need for more iron
2. Relief
   a. Placing hands on shoulders and rotating elbows in a circle

Flatulence

1. Cause
   a. Decreased motility of intestinal tract
2. Relief
   a. Avoiding gas-forming foods: parsnips, beans, cabbage, corn, fried foods, pastry, very sweet desserts, and any food known by patient to cause problems
   b. Encouraging regular bowel habits (see constipation treatment)
   c. Eating bulky foods; drinking plenty of liquids

Foot pain

1. Cause
   a. Excessive weight gain (40 to 60 lb) and lordotic curvature of the spine may affect stability of foot, causing a breakdown of the arch.
2. Relief
   a. Inverting foot (i.e., turning it in when walking barefoot to hold arch up)
   b. Wearing shoes with arch supports

Groin ache or pain

1. Causes
   a. Poor posture
   b. Standing too long
   c. Pressure of baby
   d. Spasm of round ligaments
2. Relief
   a. Doing light effleurage (small circular massage) in groin area, giving a slight lift as hands come upward gives relief. Pressure should not be used on the down stroke.
   b. Pulling up leg on same side as spasm, as if tying a shoe; or lying down on affected side with leg drawn up will provide relief for a sudden spasm.

Heartburn

1. Causes
    a. Enlarged uterus displaces stomach upward.
    b. Progesterone relaxes cardiac sphincter of stomach.
    c. Nervous tension, worry, and fatigue intensify problem.
2. Relief
    a. Eating several small meals a day instead of three large ones
    b. Avoiding greasy or highly spiced foods and coffee
    c. Chewing gum
    d. Breathing slowly and deeply
    e. Taking a tablespoon of cream one-half hour before meals (This will not help if heartburn is already present.)
    f. Avoiding over-the-counter remedies, especially baking soda and Alka-Seltzer, because of their high sodium content
    g. If problem is especially bad at night, sleeping propped up with pillows

Hemorrhoids (varicose veins of the lower bowel and rectum)

1. Causes
    a. Relaxing effect of progesterone and pressure of heavy uterus on lower part of large bowel
    b. Obesity
    c. Lack of exercise, excessive sitting
    d. Constipation
    e. Failure to empty bowel when urge is felt
    f. Straining to move bowels
2. Relief
    a. As for constipation
    b. Doing Kegel exercise regularly to stimulate circulation in the pelvic area
    c. Applying cold compresses (e.g., ice, witch hazel, epsom salt)

Increased vaginal discharge

1. Causes
    a. Prevention of the growth of microorganisms (except yeast)
    b. Irritations or allergic reactions
2. Relief
    a. Bathing vaginal area frequently with cool water and unperfumed soap
    b. Wearing cotton underwear
    c. Avoiding pantyhose and tight fitting pants
    d. Avoiding vaginal sprays, powders, feminine hygiene products, and colored or scented toilet tissues

Leg cramps

1. Causes
    a. Pressure of gravid uterus on blood vessels, lessening the flow of blood to legs
    b. Overextension of the foot

(1) This occurs with pointing of the toes (e.g., when bedcovers are too heavy, with tightly made beds, or when exercises are improperly done).

c. Sudden stretching
d. Fatigue or chilling
e. Lack of calcium in diet
f. Excessive amounts of phosphorus absorbed from milk and milk products

2. Relief
   a. The object is to stretch the cramped muscle, thus improving circulation.
   b. For a foot cramp, standing on affected foot will provide relief.
   c. For cramp in calf, straightening knee, pulling foot toward head, holding, then relaxing and repeating if necessary gives relief.
   d. For cramp in front of thigh, stretching leg backward helps.
   e. For cramp in buttock, stretching leg forward helps.
   f. A cramped muscle should never be massaged. Massage enhances rather than relieves the cramp and may cause tenderness that can last for days.
      (1) Because phlebitis could be present, the leg should be examined before massage is used for any reason.
      (2) If the physician feels inadequate calcium or excessive phosphorus intake is the cause, he or she will probably suggest various dietary adjustments.
      (3) An instructor may be in a good position to help a woman replan her dietary habits.
      (4) For this, some background information on nutrition and foods containing calcium and phosphorus is needed.

Nausea

1. Causes
   a. Increased estrogen or HCG levels
   b. Combination of hormonal, psychologic, and neurologic factors
2. Relief
   a. Consuming dry crackers, toast, or cereal before getting out of bed or whenever nausea begins
   b. Eating five or six small meals each day so that the stomach does not get empty
   c. Avoiding greasy or spicy foods
   d. Limiting fluid intake during meals but drinking water freely between meals
   e. Avoiding strong food smells

Varicose veins of vulva

1. Cause
   a. Same as varicose veins of legs
2. Relief
   a. Lying with hips elevated several times a day, either on back or in Simms lateral position
   b. Or putting entire body in slant position by lying on a slant board

c. Wearing firmly applied perineal pad for support
(1) Special pads are available from surgical supply companies.

Varicose veins or leg ache

1. Causes
   a. Hereditary predisposition
   b. Relaxing effect of progesterone on walls of veins
   c. Pressure of enlarged uterus on abdominal veins (slows blood return from lower limbs)
   d. Fatigue
   e. Standing with knees locked, causing a muscular constriction, preventing proper venous return
2. Relief
   a. Avoiding round garters, thigh highs, or any clothing that causes pressure on any part of the body
   b. Changing positions frequently; avoiding long standing or sitting
   c. Doing Kegel exercises regularly
   d. Taking long walks
      (1) The massaging action of muscles close to veins is good for stimulating circulation.
   e. Crawling on hands and knees several times a day; doing pelvic rock
   f. Elevating legs and hips several times a day; keeping knees flexed and supported by pillows
   g. Wearing support hose or stockings made of elastic
      (1) These should be put on while lying down, ideally before getting up in the morning.
   h. Cautions
      (1) Patients should never stand "at attention" with knees locked. Knees should always be slightly flexed.

34.11 ENDOCRINOLOGY AND PHYSIOLOGIC CHANGES

Thyroid

Thyroid disorders are much more common in women than in men.

Normal adult thyroid function

1. Thyrotropin-releasing hormone (TRH) is synthesized in the supraoptic and paraventricular nuclei of the hypothalamus and is stored in the median eminence.
2. TRH stimulates the anterior pituitary to both release and synthesize TSH.
3. TSH stimulates both synthesis and release of thyroid hormones: (T_4) and triiodothyronine (T_3).
4. T_4 and T_3 have feedback control of TSH at the pituitary level and, possibly, at the hypothalamus level.
5. Thyroid hormone synthesis and release
   a. Trapping
      (1) Iodide accumulates within the thyroid gland from plasma by active transport via iodide pump.
      (2) Pump is stimulated by TSH and iodide deficiency within thyroid.

Table 34-2 Alterations in thyroid function during pregnancy

Measure of Function	Status
Protein-bound iodine	Increased
T_4 (total)	Increased
T_3 (total)	Increased
TBG	Doubled
Resin T_3 uptake (RT_3U)	Decreased
T_4 (free)	No change
T_3 (free)	No change
Free thyroxine index (FTI)	No change
TSH	No change

(3) Pump is inhibited by perchlorate and thiocyanate.

b. Iodination
   (1) Glandular iodide reacts with a peroxidase and the thiouracil groups of thyroglobulin to create monoiodotyrosine (MIT) and diiodotyrosine (DIT).
   (2) This step is inhibited by propylthiouracil (PTU) and methimazole (TAP).

c. Coupling
   (1) Previously formed iodotyrosines oxidatively couple to create thyroxine (T_4 by DIT + DIT) and triiodothyronine (T_3 by DIT + MIT).

d. Release
   (1) Thyroglobulin bound T_4 and T_3 are released into the circulation by the action of a protease.
   (2) This step is stimulated by TSH.
   (3) This step is inhibited by iodine and lithium.

e. Peripheral conversion
   (1) Circulating T_4 is converted to T_3 (active) and rT_3 (reverse T_3; inactive).
   (2) This step is inhibited by PTU and is decreased by propranolol.

6. Pregnancy normally results in certain physiologic alterations that influence clinical and laboratory evaluation of thyroid function.
   a. Increased iodine renal clearance
   b. Increased thyroid clearance of iodine
   c. Possible role of placental thyrotropins (HCT, HCG)
   d. Increased synthesis of thyroxine binding globulin (TBG)
      (1) TBG doubles by 8 to 12 weeks gestation.
   e. Decreased thyroxine binding prealbumin (TBPA)
7. Laboratory evaluation of thyroid function during pregnancy (Table 34-2) should be done.
8. Normal ranges for laboratory tests of thyroid function are listed in Table 34-3.
9. The FTI is a mathematic expression without units used to compensate for pregnancy-related changes in total T_4 and RT_3U.
   a. Its normal range approximates that of total T_4 in nonpregnant patients.

Table 34-3 Normal ranges for laboratory tests of thyroid function

Test	Nonpregnant	Pregnant
T_4 (total)	5-12.5 μg/dl	6-15 μg/dl
T_3 (total)	50-175 ng/dl	125-275 ng/dl
T_4 (free)	2.5 ng/dl	2.5 ng/dl
T_3 (free)	0.3 ng/dl	0.3 ng/dl
TSH	1.9-5.9 μU/ml	1.9-5.9 μU/ml
FTI	4.5-12	4.5-12
RT_3U	25%-35%	15%-25%

b. It is calculated by the following equation:

$$FTI = \frac{T_4 \text{ total} \times RT_3U}{\text{Mean NL } RT_3U = 30}$$

Normal fetal thyroid function

1. Like other fetal tissues, the fetal thyroid gland shows progressive maturational changes as gestation advances.
   a. By 11 to 12 weeks, fetal thyroid can produce iodotyrosines and iodothyronines.
   b. Fetal thyroid concentrates iodine by 12 to 14 weeks.
   c. TSH appears at 10 weeks.
      (1) Increases between weeks 20 and 30 and then declines
   d. Total T_4 and free T_4 rise in response to an increase in TSH.
   e. Amniotic fluid T_4 increases to peak at 25 to 30 weeks gestation and then declines.
   f. Amniotic fluid T_3 increases progressively.
   g. Amniotic fluid rT_3 increases to peak at 17 to 20 weeks and then declines.
2. The role, if any, of maternal thyroid hormones in fetal development, especially in the first 12 weeks, remains unclear and is highly disputed.
   a. Placental passage from mother to fetus is shown in Table 34-4.

Normal neonatal thyroid function

1. Following birth, very rapid changes in thyroid function occur.
   a. Thyroid iodine uptake increases at birth to peak at about 48 hours of life.
   b. Uptake normalizes by the fifth day of life.
   c. Cord serum T_3 values are low at birth.
   d. Cord serum rT_3 values are elevated at birth.
   e. TSH rises sharply minutes after birth and peaks within 3 hours.
   f. Following the rise in TSH is an increase in total T_4 and free T_4.
   g. Serum T_3 rises and rT_3 decreases as a result of alterations in peripheral conversion of T_4.

Table 34-4 Placental passage of maternal thyroid hormones

Hormone	Passage
TSH	Negligible
T_4	Very poor
T_3	Poor
TRH	Good
Thyronine analogues (Dimit)	Good
Thyroid-stimulating immunoglobulins (TSIg)	Good
Iodine	Rapid

Hyperthyroidism

1. Etiology
   a. There are three major causes of hyperthyroidism in pregnancy.
      (1) Toxic diffuse goiter (Graves' disease)
         (a) T_3 thyrotoxicosis
      (2) Toxic nodular goiter (Plummer's disease)
      (3) Gestational trophoblastic disease
2. Indications for hyperthyroidism
   a. These can present with a wide range of severity.
   b. In their milder forms, they can mimic normal symptoms of pregnancy as illustrated in the box on p. 846.
3. Therapeutic modalities for thyrotoxicosis can be considered in the following five categories:
   a. Radioactive iodine (^{131}I)
      (1) ^{131}I is contraindicated in pregnancy because ^{131}I will destroy fetal thyroid gland.
         (a) Fetal thyroid concentrates iodide after 12 weeks.
      (2) ^{131}I frequently causes maternal hypothyroidism.
   b. Surgery
      (1) Surgery is an increasingly less common approach during pregnancy.
      (2) There is a high incidence of hypothyroidism postoperatively.
      (3) Surgical morbidity includes hypoparathyroidism and recurrent laryngeal nerve palsy.
      (4) There is a small risk of surgical and anesthetic mortality.
      (5) Surgery is reserved for failures of medical management.
   c. Iodides
      (1) Older mode of therapy
      (2) Limited in modern practice to immediate preoperative use
      (3) High incidence of fetal goiter and hypothyroidism
      (4) Does not result in adequate control of thyrotoxicosis
      (5) "Escape" common occurrence
   d. Beta-blockers: propranolol
      (1) Indications are as follows:
         (a) Symptomatic relief for toxic patients beginning thioamide therapy

Indication of Hyperthyroidism that May Mimic Pregnancy

Abnormal glucose tolerance test	Increased appetite with weight loss
Bouts of atrial fibrillation	Increased total T_4
Diarrhea	Insomnia
Diffuse erythema	Nervousness
Emotional instability	Osteoporosis
Emotional lability	Persistent vomiting
Excessive perspiration	Proximal myopathy
Exophthalmos: 25% of patients with stare, lid lag, and pretibial myxedema	Systolic flow murmurs
Heat intolerance	Tremulousness
Hypercalcemia	Unusual tachycardia: ectopic beats
Increased RT_3U	Varying degrees of tachycardia
Increased FTI	Warm extremities: peripheral vasodilation

(b) Patients unable to take (or poorly responsive to) thioureas
(c) Thyroid storm

(2) Propranolol controls only autonomic (sympathetic) symptoms of hyperthyroidism.
(3) Peripheral conversion of T_4 to T_3 is reduced.
(4) Possible adverse effects on fetus (intrauterine growth restriction [IUGR], neonatal bradycardia, neonatal hypoglycemia) require risk and benefit consideration.

e. Thioureas
(1) Thioureas is the mainstay of hyperthyroid therapy.
(2) PTU and TAP are agents used.
(3) Synthesis is blocked but not the release of thyroid hormone.
(4) PTU is preferred over TAP because of additional inhibition of peripheral conversion of T_4 to T_3.
(5) Side effects (in fewer than 2% to 3% of patients) are as follows:
(a) Skin rash, pruritus
(b) Drug fever
(c) Nausea, vomiting, or diarrhea
(d) Cholestatic jaundice
(e) Granulocytopenia (5%)
(f) Agranulocytosis (0.2%)
(6) Side effects do not usually occur with both drugs.
(a) Reaction to one drug will permit changing to an alternate drug.
(7) Agranulocytosis requires cessation of all thioamide therapy.

4. Fetal effects of thioamide therapy
a. As with any drug therapy during pregnancy, risk and benefit ratios with respect to fetal effects must be considered.
b. Thioamides cross the placenta and block fetal thyroid gland.
c. Risk of fetal goiter is reported to be as high as 10%.

d. Risk may be higher with doses of 300 to 800 mg, but there is no consistent dose relationship.
e. Transient hypothyroidism may be seen in neonatal period (1% to 5%).
f. Aplasia cutis may occur (TAP more than PTU).
g. Onset (10 to 14 days) of neonatal thyrotoxicosis may be delayed because of TSIg.
h. No long-term developmental effects have been found with PTU exposure *in utero*.

5. Therapy
   a. Thioamide therapy can be approached in one of the following two controversial ways:
      (1) Antithyroid–thyroid therapy
         (a) Consists of PTU, 150 to 300 mg/day, or TAP, 15 to 30 mg/day, plus desiccated thyroid, 120 to 180 mg/day, or equivalent dose of liotrix (Euthyroid)
            i. Avoids drug-induced hypothyroidism in mother
            ii. Inhibits goitrogenic effects of antithyroid drugs as euthyroidism is achieved
            iii. Provides a source of thyroid hormone for the fetus
            iv. Achieves good fetal outcome (95% normal infants)
      (2) Antithyroid therapy alone
         (a) Consists of PTU, 150 to 300 mg/day, or TAP, 15 to 30 mg/day
            i. Single-drug therapy
            ii. Avoids theoretic need for higher doses of antithyroid drugs to cover exogenous hormone
            iii. Available evidence indicates maternal thyroid hormone is not available to fetal compartment
               - Irreversible developmental abnormalities are seen in athyreotic offspring of euthyroid mothers.
               - Normal offspring are seen with hypothyroid mothers.
            iv. Permits accurate laboratory assessment of response to therapy
            v. Achieves good fetal outcome (95% normal infants)

6. Management plan
   a. Initiate therapy with PTU, 100 to 150 mg, or TAP, 10 to 15 mg, q8h.
   b. Some improvement is seen after 1 week.
   c. Four to 6 weeks may be needed for full effect.
   d. Monitor FTI or T_4 (free) to avoid overshoot and development of maternal hypothyroidism.
   e. As FTI or T_4 (free) begins to decrease, decrease dosage by one fourth to one third over 3 to 4 week intervals.
   f. Seek lowest dose possible for FTI in 14 to 18 range or T_4 (free) in upper normal range.
   g. Anticipate amelioration as pregnancy progresses (30% to 40% of patients).
   h. Anticipate worsening postpartum and consider increasing dosage immediately.

7. Thyroid storm
   a. A medical emergency with a mortality as high as 25%, even with appropriate management
   b. Diagnosis
      (1) History of hyperthyroidism is the most common feature, with storm precipitated by infection or stress (labor, cesarean section) and it is characterized by the following:
         (a) Hyperpyrexia: can be more than 105° F (40.5° C)
         (b) Diarrhea
         (c) Dehydration: hypovolemic shock
         (d) Tachycardia and arrhythmias: high output failure
         (e) Central nervous system (CNS) abnormalities: coma
   c. Therapy
      (1) IV fluids, electrolytes, and vasopressor agents as needed
      (2) Cooling blanket for hyperthermia
      (3) Hydrocortisone, 200 to 500 mg daily
      (4) Digitals for congestive heart failure
      (5) Sodium iodide, IV, slowly for 1 to 2 g/24 hours
      (6) Lithium, 300 mg, tid
      (7) PTU, 600 to 1000 mg, or TAP, 60 to 100 mg, as loading dose
      (8) Followed by PTU, 100 to 200 mg, or TAP, 10 to 20 mg, q8h for maintenance
      (9) Propranolol, 40 to 80 mg, PO, q6h, or 1 mg/min, IV, for total of 2 to 10 mg
8. Fetal consequences of maternal hyperthyroidism
   a. Possible increase in first-trimester spontaneous abortions
   b. Increased incidence of stillbirth (8% to 15%)
   c. Increased preterm delivery (11% to 25%)
   d. Decrease in mean birth weight
   e. Intrauterine fetal or neonatal thyrotoxicosis caused by TSIg
9. Neonatal thyrotoxicosis
   a. Incidence is 1% in offspring of mothers with Graves' disease.
   b. Neonatal thryrotoxicosis is usually transient, lasting 2 to 3 months.
   c. Mortality rate can be as high as 16%.
   d. Premature craniosynostosis can result.
   e. Thyrotoxicosis results from transplacental passage of TSIg.
   f. Maternal long-acting thyroid stimulatory (LATS) activity is a poor predictor.
   g. Alternate measures of TSIg may show better correlation (e.g., LATS protector).
   h. Maternal thioamide therapy may mask symptoms at birth and cause delayed onset (10 to 14 days)
   i. Diagnosis
      (1) Maternal history of Graves' disease
         (a) Need not be active and mother may be euthyroid or hypothyroid
      (2) Goiter
      (3) Exophthalmos
      (4) Tachycardia
      (5) Hyperirritable newborn
      (6) Cardiac failure

(7) Hepatosplenomegaly
(8) Jaundice
(9) Thrombocytopenia
(10) Elevated serum T_4

Hypothyroidism

1. Etiology
   a. Primary
      (1) Nongoitrous: idiopathic atrophy, thyroiditis, postoperative, postirradiation
      (2) Goitrous: hereditary, acquired
   b. Secondary
      (1) Anterior pituitary insufficiency
   c. Tertiary
      (1) Hypothalamic insufficiency
2. Diagnosis
   a. History: Certain historical factors may suggest the diagnosis, such as the following:
      (1) History of Hashimoto's thyroiditis
      (2) Previous thyroid surgery
      (3) Previous radioiodine therapy
      (4) History of significant thyroid replacement in past, even if indication is unclear
      (5) History of suppressive therapy for any length of time
   b. Signs and symptoms
      (1) Goiter or nodular thyroid tissue
      (2) Cold intolerance
      (3) Dry skin
      (4) Coarse hair
      (5) Constipation
      (6) Paresthesias (75% of patients)
      (7) Delayed relaxation of Achilles tendon reflex
      (8) Low total T_4 and free T_4
      (9) Low FTI
      (10) Elevated TSH
      (11) Elevated antimicrosomal antibodies
      (12) Elevated antithyroglobulin antibodies
3. Therapy
   a. An initial diagnosis of hypothyroidism during pregnancy is unusual.
   b. More often, patients who are already taking or are supposed to be taking thyroid replacement are seen.
   c. Replacement can be accomplished with one of the following preparations:
      (1) Desiccated thyroid: T_4/T_3, 90 to 180 mg/day
      (2) Levothyroxine (Synthyroid): T_4, 0.20 to 0.40 mg/day
      (3) Liothyronine (Cytomel): T_3, 0.075 to 0.125 mg/day
      (4) Liotrix (Euthyroid): T_4/T_3, 0.15/0.0375 to 0.3/0.075 mg/day
   d. Adequacy of replacement needs to be monitored because, in as many as one third of patients, pregnancy-related increase in TBG and expansion of plasma volume may necessitate an increase in daily dosage.

(1) TSH <5 mU/ml
(2) T_4 (total) in normal pregnant range: 6 to 15 μg/dl

4. Fetal consequences of maternal hypothyroidism
   a. Documentation in the literature is sparse and conflicting.
      (1) Increase in spontaneous abortions
      (2) Increase in stillbirths
5. Fetal or neonatal hypothyroidism: mandatory newborn screening
   a. Incidence
      (1) Primary hypothyroidism
         (a) Thyroid dysgenesis, 1/4000
         (b) Inborn errors of thyroid function, 1/30,000
         (c) Drug induced, 1/10,000
         (d) Endemic hypothyroidism, 1/7
      (2) Secondary and tertiary hypothyroidism, 1/60,000
   b. Diagnosis: difficult clinically, but suggested by the following:
      (1) Prolonged gestation resulting in large for gestational age (LGA) baby
      (2) Feeding and respiratory difficulties
      (3) Constipation
      (4) Abdominal distension (may see vomiting)
      (5) Hyperbilirubinemia
      (6) Epiphyseal dysgenesis (distal femoral or proximal tibial)
      (7) Low serum T_4
      (8) High TSH

Pituitary

The pituitary gland is not essential after 12 weeks gestation; however, pituitary mass increases by 50%, primarily because of increased prolactin from the anterior pituitary.

1. Prolactin levels increase from 10.5 to 250 ng/ml.
   a. Function is uncertain.
   b. Lactation requires the basal metabolic level.
   c. Episodic nature of release continues.
   d. Present in amniotic fluid: Not under the influence of dopamine.
   e. Questionable role in Na^+/H_2O homeostasis.
2. FSH is suppressed.
   a. Suppression is primarily secondary to increased estrogen levels.
   b. Increased HCG also suppresses FSH.
3. LH is suppressed.
4. Growth hormone (GH) is suppressed.
   a. Paradoxical because E_2 normally increases GH
5. ACTH is increased.
   a. Paradoxical because elevated cortisol seen with pregnancy is not associated with negative feedback
6. TSH level is unchanged.
7. Melanin-stimulating hormone is increased.
   a. Function = hyperpigmentation (linea nigra, chloasma, areola, etc.)
8. Vasopressin level is unchanged.
   a. This is paradoxical because the hypoosmolality associated with pregnancy causes no change.
   b. Osmoreceptors are reset at lower level.

9. Oxytocin level is increased.
   a. Function = milk letdown; has no correlation with strength of contractions.

Adrenal

The adrenal glands are not significantly altered during pregnancy; however, there is an expansion of the zona fasciculata (glucocorticoid production).

1. Corticosteroid binding globulin (CBG) increases from 33 mg/dl in nonpregnant women up to 70 mg/dl during pregnancy.
   a. This increase results from increased hepatic synthesis, which is secondary to elevated maternal estrogen levels.
   b. The estrogen-mediated increase in CBG elevates plasma cortisol levels.
2. Free cortisol is also elevated during pregnancy and progressively increases from the first trimester until term.
   a. The increase in free cortisol results from its increased production and delayed clearance.
3. Desoxycorticosterone (DOC) is elevated; however, plasma levels of DOC during pregnancy do not respond to ACTH stimulation or to dexamethasone suppression.
   a. The increase is secondary to a possible second site of production, which is fetoplacental.
   b. Mineralocorticoid activity is weak.
4. Dehydroepiandrosterone sulfate levels are decreased during pregnancy because of the increased metabolical clearance.
5. Aldosterone (ALD) levels are increased because of increased production.
6. Androstenedione levels are increased.
7. Testosterone levels are increased.
   a. However because of increased SHBG, free testosterone decreases.
8. Dehydroepiandrosterone/dehydroepiandrosterone sulfate (DHEA/DHEAS) are decreased.

Pancreas

Pancreatic hypertrophy and hyperplasia of the pancreatic beta cells occurs during pregnancy.

1. Insulin (beta cells)
   a. Fasting: small increase by change 3
   b. Fed: slower response to rise/peak; higher peak; longer duration
2. Glucagon (alpha cells)
   a. Basal levels are increased.

Ovary/placenta

1. Source of progesterone
   a. Corpus luteum until 8 to 12 weeks
   b. Placenta after 8 to 12 weeks
2. Source of estradiol
   a. Placenta from DHEA (maternal and fetal origin)
3. 17-OHP
   a. Source is corpus luteum.
   b. Graph peaks at 12 weeks, then declines.

4. Estriol
   a. Source is placenta 16-hydroxy DHEAS.
   b. Graph is increased.
5. HPL
   a. Source is placenta.
   b. Function is unknown but it has a metabolic role.
6. HCG
   a. Structure
      (1) Alpha subunit: >LH, TSH, FSH
      (2) Beta subunit: >LH
   b. Graph
      (1) Initial peak at 8 to 10 weeks
      (2) Second peak at 32 to 38 weeks
   c. Function
      (1) To maintain corpus luteum

34.12 BIOCHEMICAL CHANGES DURING PREGNANCY

1. Protein levels decrease overall because of decreased albumin.
   a. AFP: Role is unknown but similar to albumin.
      (1) First change = one-third total protein.
      (2) Term = 1% total protein.
2. Enzyme levels vary; some increase, some decrease, others are unchanged.
3. Lipid levels are generally increased.
   a. Cholesterol increases 100%; it is unaffected by diet.
4. Nonprotein nitrogen
   a. BUN and creatinine are decreased.
   b. Uric acid decreases until 24 weeks, then increases to nonpregnancy levels at term.
5. Clotting factors
   a. Increased risk of clotting
      (1) 1 × nonpregnant
      (2) 1.8 × pregnant
      (3) 5.5 × puerperium
   b. Increased factors
      (1) FBG
      (2) VII
      (3) VIII
   c. Decreased factors
      (1) XI
      (2) XIII
      (3) Antithrombin-3
6. All electrolyte concentrations are decreased except copper, which increases.

34.13 REVIEW: ANATOMIC CHANGES IN NORMAL PREGNANCY

1. Uterine changes
   a. Macroscopic: weight, capacity, size, and shape
   b. Microscopic: muscular, elastic and fibrous tissues, vessels, lymphatics, and nerves

c. Contractibility
d. Uterine blood flow (concept of perfusion)
e. Cervical: vascularization, edema, gland proliferation, "mucus plug" formation, and cervical "erosion"

2. Ovarian changes
   a. Anatomy and physiology of the corpus luteum of pregnancy
   b. Concept of luteoma of pregnancy
   c. Morphologic changes of the ovarian pedicle
3. Vaginal and perineal changes
   a. Connective tissue of the perineum
   b. Microscopic vaginal changes: vascular and muscular
   c. Vaginal secretion (change in pH)
   d. Vaginal cytology: navicular cells and "naked nuclei"
4. Abdominal wall and skin changes
   a. Striae gravidarum
   b. Diastasis recti
   c. Linea nigra-chloasma: melanocyte-stimulant hormone and estrogen effect (relationship with oral contraceptives)
   d. Vascular spiders: palmar erythema
5. Breast changes
   a. Macroscopic: size, nodularity, nipple hypertrophy and pigmentation, areolar hypertrophy and pigmentation, and colostrum
   b. Microscopic: histology of the breast during pregnancy (hormonal effect)
6. Metabolism changes
   a. Weight gain (responsible factors)
   b. Water metabolism (normal distribution of water in the pregnant patient), dependent edema
   c. Protein metabolism: increment and fetomaternal distribution
   d. Carbohydrate metabolism
   e. Maternal "accelerated starvation" state
      (1) Fasting blood sugar levels response to oral glucose load
      (2) Lipolysis, maternal levels of free fatty acids
      (3) Insulin "blocking" effect
         (a) Role of HPL
         (b) Placental "insulinase" activity
         (c) Placental steroids (estrogen, progesterone)
         (d) Corticosteroid and thyroxin
      (4) Insulin response to carbohydrate intake in pregnancy
   f. Fat metabolism
      (1) Hyperlipemia: degree of total and specific lipids
      (2) Starvation effect in pregnancy
7. Hematologic changes
   a. Increase in total blood volume (cell and plasma components)
   b. Degree of increase in each trimester
   c. Plasma and red cell mass ratio of increment
   d. Mechanism of increment of red cell mass (erythropoietin)
   e. Normal average Hb level in pregnancy
   f. Total body iron content in the female
   g. Iron storage as related to total content

h. Average iron content of fetus at birth
i. Average maternal red cell mass increase
j. Total iron needed
k. Excretion average
l. Daily iron requirement
m. Iron content and absorption in commonly used ferrous compounds
n. Maternal blood loss in vaginal and cesarean section deliveries
o. Maternal blood volume and plasma concentrations during labor and early and late puerperium
p. Leukocytes
   (1) During pregnancy, labor, and puerperium
   (2) Alkaline phosphatase activity
q. Coagulation factors
   (1) Fibrinogen (sedimentation rate)
   (2) Other clotting factors and changes
   (3) Fibrinolytic activity

8. Cardiovascular system changes
   a. Heart rate
   b. Cardiac silhouette
   c. Increased cardiac volume
   d. Heart sounds (heart murmurs)
   e. Cardiac output
   f. Arterial blood pressure
      (1) Changes according to trimester
      (2) Changes according to maternal posture: criteria of abnormality (uterine artery pressure as related to brachial artery pressure), venous pressure
      (3) Upper and lower extremities
9. Respiratory tract changes
   a. Anatomic (chest) changes
   b. Respiratory rate and tidal volume
   c. Minute ventilation
   d. Minute O_2 uptake
   e. Vital capacity
   f. Force expiratory volume
   g. Residual volume
   h. Functional residual capacity
   i. Lung compliance
   j. Total pulmonary resistance
   k. Airway conductance
   l. Pco_2-pH: respiratory alkalosis
10. Urinary system changes
   a. Increased glomeruli filtration rate (degree and possible HPL effect)
   b. Increased renal plasma flow
   c. Importance of maternal position in renal function at term, i.e., sodium excretion
   d. Renal function tests in pregnancy

   e. Glycosuria of pregnancy (despite normal glucose level)
   f. Ureters: anatomic changes, reasons
   g. Bladder: trigonal changes
11. Gastrointestinal tract changes
   a. Displacements: appendix
   b. Pyrosis (esophagitis gastritis)
   c. Increased motility in stomach
   d. Gastric emptying in labor
   e. Gums: epulis of pregnancy
   f. Hemorrhoids and constipation
12. Liver and gallbladder changes
   a. Liver laboratory studies in pregnancy
   b. Alkaline phosphatase activity
   c. Serum albumin
   d. Serum globulins
   e. ALB/globulin ratio
   f. Cholinesterase in serum
   g. Leucine-aminopeptidase in serum
   h. Gallbladder function and propensity to stone formation
13. Endocrine gland changes
   a. Pituitary: enlargement; role in pregnancy, labor, and delivery
      (1) Pituitary growth hormone
      (2) Pituitary prolactin
         (a) Serum levels in pregnancy
         (b) Serum levels in puerperium
         (c) Serum levels in lactating mothers
         (d) Serum levels in nonlactating mothers
      (3) Progesterone effect
      (4) Fetal serum and amniotic fluid levels of prolactin
   b. Thyroid
      (1) Enlargement
      (2) Basal metabolic rate
      (3) Thyroid hormone concentration in pregnancy
         (a) Protein-bound iodine (PBI)
         (b) Butanol-extractable iodine (BEI)
         (c) Free thyroxine
      (4) Triiodothyronine resin uptake (estrogen effect)
      (5) Placental permeability to T_4
      (6) Placental permeability to LATS
   c. Adrenal
      (1) Circulating cortisol
      (2) Non–protein bound cortisol
      (3) Metabolic rate of cortisol in pregnancy
      (4) Aldosterone
      (5) Renin–angiotensin system
14. Musculoskeletal system changes
   a. Lordosis
   b. Pelvic joint relaxation

Suggested reading

1. American Academy of Pediatrics and American College of Obstetricians and Gynecologists: *Guidelines for perinatal care,* p.166, Washington, DC, and Elk Grove Village, IL, 1983, ACOG and AAP.
2. Brown MA et al: Measuring blood pressure in pregnant women: a comparison of direct and indirect methods, *Am J Obstet Gynecol* 171:661-667, 1994.
3. Clark SL et al: Position change and central hemodynamic profile during normal third-trimester pregnancy and post partum, *Am J Obstet Gynecol* 164:883-887, 1991.
4. Cogswell ME et al: Gestational weight gain among average-weight and overweight women—what is excessive? *Am J Obstet Gynecol* 172:705-712, 1995.
5. Institute of Medicine (United States): *Nutrition during pregnancy,* Report of the Committee on Nutritional Status During Pregnancy and Lactation, Food and Nutrition Board, Washington, DC, 1990, National Academy Press.
6. Joffe GM et al: Diagnosis of cervical change in pregnancy by means of transvaginal ultrasonography, *Am J Obstet Gynecol* 166:896-900, 1992.
7. Kimura M et al: Physiologic thyroid activation in normal early pregnancy is induced by circulating hCG, *Obstet Gynecol* 75:775-778, 1990.
8. Lopez MC et al: The measurement of diastolic blood pressure during pregnancy: which Korotkoff phase should be used? *Am J Obstet Gynecol* 170:574-578, 1994.
9. Maher JE et al: Indicators of maternal nutritional status and birth weight in term deliveries, *Obstet Gynecol* 81:165-169, 1993.
10. Schrier RW, Briner VA: Peripheral arterial vasodilation hypothesis of sodium and water retention in pregnancy: implications for pathogenesis of preeclampsia-eclampsia, *Obstet Gynecol* 77:632-639, 1991.
11. Thaler I et al: Changes in uterine blood flow during human pregnancy, *Am J Obstet Gynecol* 162:121-125, 1990. *Am J Obstet Gynecol* 162:121-125, 1990.

35 Anemia and Pregnancy

Marcello Pietrantoni, M.D.

Iron-deficiency anemia

1. Traditionally, anemia is defined as a hemoglobin value of less than 10 mg/dl.
2. Iron-deficiency anemia (IDA) is the most common medical complication of pregnancy (95%).
   a. Not uncommonly, iron deficiency is the result of an increased need for iron (e.g., during infancy, childhood, or pregnancy).
   b. Anemia also is commonly a result of the depletion of the bodily reserves of iron (e.g., during hemorrhage, menometrorrhagia, or multiple gestation).
3. The diagnosis and appropriate therapy of anemia in pregnancy is essential for maternal and fetal well-being.
4. The compounding factor during pregnancy is the large rise in maternal plasma volume relative to the increase in red blood cell mass (i.e., hemoglobin).
   a. The maternal plasma volume usually expands by 40% to 50% (1000 ml) near term, whereas the red blood cell mass increases by approximately 25% (300 ml).
   b. This relationship is often termed "the physiologic anemia of pregnancy."
   c. The physiologic anemia of pregnancy is actually a misnomer because the red blood cell increases during pregnancy (albeit less than total plasma volume).
5. Anemia may be either acquired or inherited; therefore, a thorough history and physical examination along with laboratory evaluations are necessary to identify the cause of anemia and to provide appropriate treatment.
6. Proper assessment of anemia during pregnancy is outlined in Tables 35-1 and 35-2.
7. Assessment of anemia during pregnancy (Table 35-3 and the box on p. 860)
   a. Complete blood cell count (CBC)
   b. Serum iron
   c. Total iron-binding capacity

Table 35-1 Iron compartments in iron sufficient individuals

	Iron Content (mg)		
	Male	Nonpregnant Female	Percent (%)
Hemoglobin iron	2500	1700	67.0
Storage iron	1000	700	27.0
Myoglobin iron	130	130	3.5
Labile pool	80	80	2.2
Other tissue iron	8	8	0.2
Transport iron	3	3	0.08

Table 35-2 Iron demands during pregnancy

Increased maternal hemoglobin	500 mg
Fetus	275 mg
Placenta	25 mg
Delivery loss	230 mg
Basal loss	190 mg
Total iron needed for pregnancy	1220 mg

d. Ferritin-to-folate level
e. Hemoglobin electrophoresis
f. Reticulate count
g. Peripheral smear

8. Nutritional requirements of iron and its absorption
   a. Acquired anemia is usually IDA; however, it may be caused by malnutrition, chronic disease states, or autoimmune disorders.
   b. The average daily American diet consists of the consumption of 2000 kcal providing 50 mg of elemental iron, of which 5% to 10% is absorbed.
      (1) During the first trimester and early second trimester, approximately 13 mg of iron is adequate.
      (2) Iron absorption is increased by approximately 10% during the first trimester.
      (3) After 20 weeks gestation, iron requirements increase because of the increase in maternal red blood cell mass.
      (4) Iron absorption is increased by up to 25% during the second trimester.
      (5) Iron absorption is increased by up to 30% (over nonpregnant levels) during the third trimester.
      (6) Maximal iron absorption occurs with 550 mg of dietary iron.
      (7) The total iron requirements of pregnancy is approximately 800 to 1200 mg.
      (8) Serum ferritin levels during pregnancy range from 55 to 70 µg/dl.
      (9) Serum ferritin levels in nonpregnant patients range from 30 to 50 µg/dl.

Table 35-3 Normal screening and specific test values

	Nonpregnant	Pregnant
General Screening Assays		
Hemoglobin	12-16 g/dl	10-13 g/dl
Packed cell volume	37%-45%	30%-39%
Red blood cell count	4.2-5.4 million/mm^3	3.8-4.4 million/mm^3
Mean corpuscular volume	80-100 U^3/cell	70-90 U^3/cell
Mean corpuscular hemoglobin	27-34 pg/cell	23-31 pg/cell
Mean corpuscular concentration	32-35 g/dl/RBC	Unchanged
Reticulocyte count	0.5%-1.0%	1.0%-2.0%
Specific Diagnostic Tests		
Serum iron	50-110 g/dl	30-100 μg/dl
Unsaturated iron-binding capacity	250-300 g/dl	280-400 μg/dl
Transferrin saturation	25%-35%	15%-30%
Iron stores (bone marrow)	Adequate ferritin	Unchanged
Serum folate	4-16 ng/ml	4-10 ng/ml
Serum B_{12}	70-85 ng/dl	70-500 ng/dl

RBC, Red blood cell.

(10) Serum ferritin levels under 10 μg/dl are indicative of iron deficiency.

(11) Serum iron levels under 30 μg/dl are reflective of iron deficiency.

(12) Hemoglobin contains approximately 0.34% iron by weight, and the average nonpregnant woman has approximately 1700 mg of iron contained in her hemoglobin.

(a) Approximately 0.1% of total body iron is lost per day.

i. Menstruating women lose approximately 0.7 to 1.4 mg of iron per day.

ii. Mothers who breast-feed may lose up to 1.0 mg of iron per day as lactoferrin.

(b) Iron stores are divided between ferritin and hemosiderin.

i. Ferritin contains approximately 20% iron by weight and is insoluble in water.

ii. Ferritin is found in the maternal plasma and in cells.

iii. Hemosiderin is found in the reticuloendothelial system of the bone marrow, liver, and spleen.

(c) Iron is transported from the intestinal mucosal cell by transferrin.

i. Transferrin transfers the iron (ferritin) from the mucosal cell to the normoblast.

(13) The lifespan of the erythrocyte (red blood cell) is approximately 120 days.

Approach to a Patient with Anemia

I. History
- A. Symptoms of anemia
  1. Chest pain on exertion (angina)
  2. Dizziness and syncope (fainting)
  3. Fatigue and weakness
  4. Rapidity of onset of symptoms
  5. Response of anemia to therapy
  6. Shortness of breath
- B. Blood loss
  1. Gastrointestinal: hematemesis (vomiting blood), melena (black stools), hemorrhoidal bleeding, hematochezia (red blood in stools)
  2. Bleeding at operation or delivery
  3. Respiratory: hemoptysis (coughing blood), epistaxis (nosebleed)
  4. Uterine: menorrhagia (excessive bleeding), metrorrhagia (irregular bleeding)
  5. Other: hematuria (blood in urine), purpura (black and blue marks)
- C. Bleeding tendency
  1. Bleeding after trauma, operations (circumcision, tonsillectomy), deliveries, tooth extractions
  2. Bleeding into joints
  3. Menstrual bleeding
  4. Petechiae (capillary hemorrhages appearing as red splinters)
  5. Spontaneous purpura
- D. Iron-deficiency anemia
  1. Blood loss (see I.B.)
  2. Glossitis (sore or inflamed tongue)
  3. Pregnancies and iron supplementation
- E. Megaloblastic anemia
  1. Foul-smelling diarrhea with greasy stools
  2. Glossitis
  3. Paresthesias (tingling toes or fingers), difficulty with gait
- F. Drugs and toxins
  1. Alcohol
  2. Occupational exposures
  3. Therapeutic medications
  4. Toxins
- G. Miscellaneous
  1. Bone pain
  2. Jaundice (yellow skin)
  3. Weight loss
- H. Family history
  1. Anemia
  2. Racial and geographic derivation
  3. Recurrent jaundice
  4. Splenomegaly

Approach to a Patient with Anemia—cont'd

II. Physical examination
   A. Vital signs
      1. Blood pressure, pulse, temperature
      2. Orthostatic hypotension (lowered blood pressure upon standing or sitting)
   B. Skin
      1. Leg ulcers
      2. Nail beds: koilonychia (spoon-shaped nails)
      3. Pallor (pale skin)
      4. Purpura, petechiae
      5. Spider angioma (spider-shaped capillaries), other signs of chronic liver disease
   C. Conjunctivae
      1. Jaundice
      2. Pallor
      3. Petechiae
   D. Fundi
      1. Papilledema
      2. Petechiae, hemorrhage
   E. Mouth
      1. Lips: cheilosis (split lips), angular stomatitis (sores at angles of lips)
      2. Mucous membranes: pallor, petechiae
      3. Tongue: redness, atrophy of papilla
      4. Uremic breath
   F. Lymph nodes
      1. Enlargement in cervical (neck), axillary, inguinal (groin), epitrochlear (near elbow), or other areas
   G. Bones
      1. Tenderness over sternum, ribs, or vertebrae
   H. Cardiorespiratory system
      1. Cardiac gallop
      2. Heart murmurs
      3. Peripheral edema
      4. Pulmonary rales
   I. Abdomen
      1. Hepatomegaly
      2. Splenomegaly
      3. Masses
      4. Ascites
   J. Neurologic examination
      1. Loss of vibratory or position sense
      2. Positive Romberg sign (inability to stand upright with eyes closed)
      3. Peripheral neuritis
   K. Pelvic and rectal examinations
      1. Bleeding
      2. Tumors

Continued.

Approach to a Patient with Anemia—cont'd

III. Laboratory data
  A. Hematocrit and hemoglobin
  B. Wintrobe indices
  C. Reticulocyte count
  D. White cell count and differential
  E. Platelet estimation
  F. Peripheral blood smear
  G. Bone marrow aspirate or biopsy
  H. Special tests
    1. Schilling test for vitamin B_{12} absorption
    2. Serum iron and total iron-binding capacity
    3. Vitamin B_{12} and folic acid serum levels
    4. Others as determined by patient's problem

(a) Approximately 80% of iron contained in an erythrocyte is reused for hemoglobin synthesis.
(b) The remaining 20% of iron is returned to the iron stores.

(14) During the early pregnancy state, there is a progressive rise in blood volume (40% to 50%) that is greater than the respective increase in red cell mass (25% to 30%), which contains the hemoglobin (both measurements are per kilogram of body mass).

(15) The expansion of the hemoglobin mass by 25% requires at least 500 mg/day of iron; additionally, 300 to 500 mg/day of iron are consumed by the fetal–placental unit and are eliminated as waste.
(a) The maternal red cell mass increase occurs because of the pregnancy-related increase in erythropoietin, a glycoprotein with a molecular weight of 46,000.
  i. Erythropoietin is produced in the kidney and is released into the bloodstream when there is decreased oxygenation of the blood.
  ii. Erythropoietin increases during the early second trimester up to the 20th week of gestation.
  iii. Erythropoietin may be stimulated by adrenocorticotropic hormone (ACTH), thyroid-stimulating hormone (TSH), growth hormone, prolactin, and androgens.
(b) The average increase in the red cell mass during pregnancy is between 300 and 350 ml.
(c) However, during pregnancy, the red blood cell itself (mean cell volume) shows a progressive decrease in size, thought to occur for its passage through the small placental vessels.

Table 35-4 Diagnostic values in the nonpregnant, pregnant, and iron-deficient woman

	Nonpregnant	Pregnant	IDA
General Screening Assays			
Hemoglobin	12.5-14 g/dl	10-13 g/dl	<11 g/dl
Packed cell volume	34%-45%	33%-38%	<35%
Red blood cell count	4.2-5.4 million/mm^3	3.8-4.4 million/mm^3	Unaltered
Mean corpuscular volume	80-100 U^3/cell	70-90 U^3/cell	Unaltered
MCHC	31.4-35.8 g/dl	31.4-35.8 g/dl	<30 g/gl
Reticulocyte count	0.5%-1.0%	1.0%-2.0%	<1%
Specific Diagnostic Tests			
Serum iron	50-110 μg/dl	30-100 μg/dl	30 μg/dl
Unsaturated iron-binding capacity	250-300 μg/dl	280-400 μg/dl	>400 μg/dl
Transferrin saturation	25%-35%	15%-30%	<15%
Serum ferritin	10-100 μg/L	55-70 μg/L	10 μg/L
Free erythrocyte	25 μg/L	35 μg/L	Increased 5-fold
ESR	0-15 mm/hr	40-50 mm/hr	40-50 mm/hr

MCHC, Mean corpuscular hemoglobin concentration.

i. As a result, red blood cells are thicker and more spherical.

ii. This alteration in form of the red blood cell explains the increase in agility of the erythrocyte in pregnancy.

9. Secondary to the physiologic anemia of pregnancy, there is an increase in 2,3-diphosphoglycerate (2,3-DPG).
   a. 2,3-DPG binds to the beta chain of the deoxyhemoglobin, which thereby increases the affinity for oxygen.
      (1) Fetal oxygenation is facilitated by this increase in 2,3-DPG found in the maternal hemoglobin.
   b. With an arterial Po_2 of 100 mm Hg, the hemoglobin of a nonpregnant patient carries approximately 20 ml O_2 per deciliter whole blood.
   c. The venous Po_2 is approximately 40 mm Hg, carrying an oxygen content of 15 ml/dl of whole blood; hence, there is a 5 ml/dl difference in oxygen released to the maternal and fetal tissues.

The diagnosis and management of anemia in pregnancy

1. Approximately 75% of all women with abnormally low hemoglobins are confirmed to have IDA (Table 35-4).

Table 35-5 Morphologic classification of anemia

Type of Anemia	Red Blood Cell Indices
Microcytic–Hypochromic	MCV <80 U^3, MCHC <30%
Iron deficiency	
Thalassemia	
Sideroblastic	
Macrocytic	MCV >94 U^3, MCHC >30%
Megaloblastic	
Vitamin B_{12} deficiency	
Folate deficiency	
Normoblastic	
Increased reticulocytosis as seen in acute blood loss and some hemolytic anemias	
Liver disease	
Hypothyroidism	
Normochromic–Normocytic	MCV 80-94 U^3, MCHC >30%
Marrow failure	Low reticulocyte count
Aplastic anemia	
Refractory anemia	
Marrow fibrosis	
Secondary to endocrinopathies	
Renal failure	
Hemolysis	Elevated reticulocyte count
Hereditary hemolytic anemia	
Acquired hemolytic anemia	

MCV, Mean corpuscular volume; *MCHC,* mean corpuscular hemoglobin concentration.

2. A diagnosis of anemia is made when the hemoglobin concentration is less than 10% or when the hematocrit is less than 30%.
   a. The Centers for Disease Control and Prevention (CDC) recommend the following cutoff values for diagnosis of anemia:
      (1) During the first and second trimesters, hemoglobin less than 11 g/100 ml or a hematocrit less than 33%
      (2) During the second trimester, hemoglobin less than 10.5 g/100 ml or a hematocrit less than 32% (Table 35-5)
3. IDA is calculated by measuring the maternal serum iron (SI) concentration and total iron-binding capacity (TIBC).
   a. When the SI concentration is divided by the TIBC, the result is the transferrin saturation.
   b. If the transferrin saturation is less than 60%, then it can be presumed that IDA is present.
   c. During pregnancy, approximately two thirds of the available transferrin and its binding sites are unoccupied because of a secondary increase caused by the elevated estrogen levels.

(1) Consequently, the transferrin saturation is decreased from 25% to 30% during the nonpregnant state to 15% to 30% during pregnancy.

4. IDA can also be assessed by measuring the maternal plasma ferritin level: A value of less than 10 μg/L indicates iron-deficiency anemia.
5. Although rarely used, during severe iron-deficiency states, zinc may replace iron in the protoporphyrin ring; therefore measurements of red cell zinc per protoporphyrin may be diagnostic of IDA.
6. Decreased hemoglobin hematocrit values are at their lowest between gestational weeks 20 and 30.
7. Laboratory assessment should be undertaken with a full blood count (CBC), a white blood cell count (WBC), a peripheral blood smear, a platelet count, and the mean corpuscular volume (MCV).
   a. On the peripheral smear during IDA, poikilocytosis (pear-shaped cells), schistocytes (red cell fragments), and occasional basal cell stippling can be seen (Table 35-6).
8. The specific etiology of the anemia should be addressed by identifying and classifying the mechanism that triggers it (Table 35-7).
   a. It is necessary to assess the reticulate count, which should be corrected for the degree of anemia.
      (1) For example, if the reticulate count is low (<3%) then its cause is the lack of erythropoiesis.
         (a) If the anemia is caused by a decrease in erythropoiesis, which is reflected by the decreased red blood cell count, then further investigation is needed by assessing the MCV.
            i. If the MCV is less than 80 mEq, it is then considered to be microcytic and a hypoproliferative anemia.
            ii. If the MCV is greater than 80 mEq, then it is a normocytic, hypoproliferative anemia.
            iii. In addition, the mean corpuscular hemoglobin concentration will be less than 30%.
      (2) If the reticulate count is greater than 3%, then the anemia may result from hemolysis or acute blood loss.
9. Microcytic, hypochromic anemias are seen with IDA, thalassemia, and sideroblastic anemia.
   a. The majority of microcytic, hypoproliferative anemias occur secondary to iron deficiency.
   b. A second cause of microcytic, hypoproliferative anemia is thalassemia.
      (1) Using the hemoglobin electrophoresis and an elevated level of the hemoglobin A2 (HbA2; normal is under 3.5%) establishes the diagnosis of beta-thalassemia minor.
      (2) If the ratio of alpha-chain to beta-chain synthesis is decreased, this indicates alpha-thalassemia.
      (3) Thalassemias are often encountered in patients of either Mediterranean, African, or Southeast Asian origin.
      (4) All patients with thalassemia should have genetic counseling to assess the fetal risks.
      (5) In the differential diagnosis of the thalassemic patient, there

Table 35-6 Peripheral blood (red cell) abnormalities

Abnormality	Description	Associated Diseases
Anisocytosis diameter	Abnormal variation in size (normal diameter = 6-8 μm)	Any severe anemia (e.g., iron deficiency, megaloblastic)
Microcytosis	Small cells, less than 6 μm (MCV <80 fl)	Iron-deficiency and iron-loading (sideroblastic) anemia, thalassemia, lead poisoning
Macrocytosis	Large cells, greater than 8 μm (MCV >100 fl)	Megaloblastic anemia, liver disease, hypothyroidism, hemolytic anemia (reticulocytes), multiple myeloma, physiologic macrocytosis of newborn, myelophthisis
Macroovalocytosis	Large (>8 μm) oval cells	Megaloblastic anemia
Hypochromia	Pale cells with decreased concentration of hemoglobin (MCHC <30 g/dl)	Iron-deficiency and iron-loading (sideroblastic) anemia, thalassemia, lead poisoning, transferrin deficiency, anemia of chronic disease (inflammatory diseases, e.g., rheumatoid arthritis, collagen diseases, malignancies)
Poikilocytosis	Abnormal variation in shape	Any severe anemia: megaloblastic, iron deficiency, myeloproliferative syndrome, hemolytic; certain shapes are diagnostically helpful (see following, Spherocytosis through Teardrop cells)
Spherocytosis	Spherical cells without pale centers; often small (i.e., microspherocytosis)	Hereditary spherocytosis, Coombs'-positive hemolytic anemia, small numbers are seen in any hemolytic anemia and after transfusion of stored blood
Ovalocytosis	Oval cells	Hereditary elliptocytosis or iron deficiency

Table 35-6 Peripheral blood (red cell) abnormalities—cont'd

Abnormality	Description	Associated Diseases
Stomatocytosis	Red cells with slit-like, instead of circular, areas of central pallor	Congenital hemolytic anemia, thalassemia, burns, lupus erythematosus, lead poisoning, liver disease, artefact
Sickle cells	Crescent-shaped cells	Sickle cell hemoglobinopathies
Target cells	Cells with a dark center and periphery and a clear ring in between	Liver disease, thalassemia, hemoglobinopathies (S, C, SC-thalassemia)
Schistocytes	Irregularly contracted cells (severe poikilocytosis)	Uremia, carcinoma, hemolytic–uremic syndrome, disseminated intravascular coagulation, microangiopathic hemolytic anemia, toxins (lead, phenylhydrazine), burns, thrombotic thrombocytopenic purpura
Helmet cells	A type of schistocyte shaped like a military helmet	Uremia, hemolytic–uremic syndrome, disseminated intravascular coagulation, microangiopathic hemolytic anemia, burns, thrombotic thrombocytopenic purpura

MCV, Mean corpuscular volume; *MCHC,* mean corpuscular hemoglobin concentration.

tends to be an increase in target cells and frequent basal-cell stippling.

(6) Also, the MCV is less than 65 in patients with thalassemia; this is not seen in patients with severe IDA.

(7) The erythrocyte count in patients with thalassemia is fewer than 5 million/mm^3 despite a low hemoglobin level.

c. Differential diagnoses

(1) A normal serum iron concentration and transferrin saturation lean toward a diagnosis of thalassemia, whereas both these levels are reduced in IDA.

(2) Red blood cell distribution width (RDW) is found to be elevated with IDA; however, it is normal in patients with thalassemia minor.

(3) Differential diagnosis of hemoglobinopathies is made by either the family history or hemoglobin electrophoresis by assessing the quantity of hemoglobin A2.

Table 35-7 Features of differential diagnosis in iron-deficiency anemia*

RBC Morphology		Hemoglobin	MCV	MCHC	Reticulocytic Count	Serum Iron	Transferrin Saturation	Unsaturated IBC	Serum Ferritin	ESR	Free Erythrocyte Protoporphyrin
IDA	Hypochromic–microcytic	D	D	D	D	D	D	I	D	U	I
Hemoglobinopathies	Hypochromic–microcytic 1 target cells 1 basal cell stippling	D	D	U	I	U	D	U	I	D	U
Inflammatory process	Normal red cells	D	U	U	D	D	D	I	I	I	II

Malignancies	Normal red cells	D	U	U	D	D	I	D	I	I	I
Chemical toxicity	Hypochromic–normocytic 1 large cells ring sideroblasts	D	D	U	I	I	I	D	I	I	I
Pyridorine responsive anemia	Hypochromic–microcytic 1 ring sideroblasts Prominent target cells	D	I	D	D	I	I	D	I	U	D

D, decreased; *I*, increased; *U*, unaltered.
MCV, Mean corpuscular volume; *MCHC*, mean corpuscular hemoglobin concentration; *IBC*, iron-binding capacity; *ESR*, erythrocyte sedimentation rate.

(4) Ingestion of alcohol isoniazid and other agents that cause deficiency in porphyrin synthesis may lead to reversible sideroblastic anemia.
   (a) Unlike IDA, with sideroblastic anemia, target cells or ovalocytes are seen on the peripheral smear.
   (b) Also, the sideroblastic anemia elevated serum iron levels are seen, and transfer and saturation are also increased.

10. The primary cause of IDA in nonpregnant patients is excessive iron loss (usually caused by chronic intestinal or uterine bleeding) that is greater than the amount absorbed by the patient.
11. Other causes of IDA include the following:
    a. Multiple gestations (particularly nonspaced)
    b. Pregnancy during adolescence
    c. Chronic blood loss
    d. Intravascular hemolysis
    e. Poor intestinal iron absorption
12. Symptoms of IDA
    a. Clinically, patients with anemia present with symptoms of tachycardia, dyspnea, skin pallor, and heart palpitations, fatigue, irritability, headache, paresthesias, and malaise.
    b. Patients with IDA not uncommonly may complain of menometrorrhagia before conception, bleeding during pregnancy, and rectal bleeding.
    c. In patients with an inadequate amount of tissue iron in the oral mucosa cells, pica (which may include ingestion of dirt [geophagia], clay, ice [pagophagia], or starch [emulophagia]) may be seen.
    d. In patients with severe IDA, stomatitis chelitis, koilonychia, retinal hemorrhages, and splenomegaly may be encountered when the hemoglobin is less than 5 g/dl.
    e. In the last stages of IDA, a loss of myoglobin is seen.
13. Iron therapy
    a. Dietary iron is generally sufficient during the first 20 weeks of pregnancy.
       (1) However, during the second half of the pregnancy, iron should be supplemented.
       (2) The average woman has approximately 300 to 500 mg of stored iron; therefore, she only requires 30 mg/day of elemental iron to meet her daily requirements.
          (a) Hematologic assessment is prudent before 30 weeks gestation to ensure that the patient's hematologic demands are met (i.e., iron stores have not been depleted).
    b. In known iron-deficient women, iron therapy should be instituted as soon as possible to replenish the iron stores.
    c. Normally, 30 to 60 mg of iron per day are supplemented; however, 200 to 300 mg may be necessary in iron-deficiency states.
    d. Supplemental iron is prescribed in the ferrous form, which is absorbed through the intestinal wall; however, it is converted to the ferric form for hemoglobin utilization.

(1) The absorption capacity of the intestinal tracts is maximal every 8 to 10 hours.

e. With iron supplementation, a hemoglobin rise of at least 1 g/dl per month should be expected (initially 6 to 8 weeks after therapy has begun).

f. Calcium and vitamin C have been shown to enhance the absorption of iron, and consumption of citrus juices, because of their high acidity, is often recommended during iron ingestion.

(1) Consumption of iced tea should be avoided because of its inhibitory effects on absorption.

g. Iron should be taken with meals (or postprandially) because of its gastric side effects.

(1) The most common side effects of iron supplementation are nausea, vomiting, diarrhea, abdominal cramps, and constipation.

14. If the patient fails to respond to a trial of iron therapy, the physician should proceed next to hemoglobin electrophoresis.

15. Maternal patients with severe iron deficiency who demonstrate an MCV of under 30% or a hemoglobin concentration of under 10 g/dl and who must undergo a repeat cesarean section or any other surgical procedure should undergo a blood transfusion.

16. Fetal complications of IDA in pregnancy

a. Fetal compromise caused by intrauterine growth restriction or stillbirth may take place when hemoglobin levels are under 6.5 g/dl.

Suggested reading

Carr MC: Managing iron deficiency in pregnancy, *Contemp Obstet Gynecol* 4:15, 1974.

Cook JD et al: Serum ferritin as a measure of iron stores in normal subjects, *Am J Clin Nutr* 27:681, 1974.

Disler PB et al: The effect of tea on iron absorption, *Gut* 16:193, 1975.

Garn SM et al: Maternal hematologic levels and pregnancy outcomes, *Semin Perinatol* 5:155-162, 1981.

Monsen ER: Iron nutrition and absorption: dietary factors which impact iron availability, *J Am Diet Assoc* 88:786-790, 1988.

National Academy of Sciences: *Recommended dietary allowances,* ed 9, Washington, DC, 1980, NAS.

Pritchard JA, Scott DE: Iron demands during pregnancy. In Hallberg L, Harwerth HG, Vannotti A, editors: *Iron deficiency: pathogenesis, clinical aspects, therapy,* New York, 1970, Academic Press.

Scott DE, Pritchard JA: Anemia in pregnancy, *Clin Perinatol* 1:491, 1974.

36 Obstetric Ultrasound Scanning

Asim Kurjak, M.D., and Milan Kos, M.D.

Basic physics and instrumentation

1. Definition
   a. Ultrasound is defined as the range of sound waves with frequencies >20,000 Hertz (Hz), which are undetectable by the human ear.
   b. An ultrasound is produced when transmitted pulses of sound from the transducer cross body structures and reflect energy back to the transducer from the interfaces of organs, from vessel walls, or from differences in tissue density and structure of an organ.
   c. The same transducer transmits and receives sound waves.
2. Obstetric clinical practice
   a. The most commonly employed frequencies of diagnostic ultrasound are 3.5 MHz and 5 MHz.
   b. The basic type of imaging mode in obstetrics is B mode (brightness modulation).
   c. The amplitude of B-mode ultrasound is represented by a spot of light on the monitor screen.
   d. When the spots of all received amplitudes are combined, a real-time tomogramic picture is produced.
   e. Obstetric ultrasound scanning can be performed either transabdominally (TAS) or transvaginally (TVS).
   f. For routine or basic scanning, an instrument with high resolution, real-time imaging, and one 3.5-MHz convex, transabdominal transducer, is the minimal but sufficient requirement.
   g. A 5.0- to 7.5-MHz vaginal transducer is obligatory in hospital practice and perinatal centers, because of high-level expertise needed in early pregnancy.
   h. The 3.5 MHz beam penetrates deeper into the body than the 5.0 beam; however, higher frequencies provide better resolution for detailed examination.
   i. Transvaginal scanning is performed primarily in the first trimester of pregnancy and generally enables visualization of the targeted structure 1 to 2 weeks earlier than transabdominal scanning.

3. Guidelines for ultrasound scanning in obstetrics
   a. Indications
      (1) Confirmation of an intrauterine pregnancy
      (2) Biometric estimation of gestational age
      (3) Biometric evaluation of fetal growth
      (4) Evaluation of fetal and placental morphology
      (5) Follow-up of fetal anomalies
      (6) Follow-up of fetal condition (biophysical profile)
      (7) Interventional ultrasonographic procedures
      (8) Abnormal maternal serum alpha-fetoprotein (MSAFP)
      (9) Multiple gestation assessment
      (10) Estimation of fetal presentation and birth weight
4. Ultrasonographic examinations
   a. Obstetric ultrasound studies are defined as either basic (routine survey) or targeted (selected).
   b. Basic obstetric scanning includes the components of examination to confirm the normal developing of pregnancy and detection of major abnormalities (see the box on p. 874).
   c. Targeted examinations are done for suspected disorders in pregnancy and should be performed by an operator experienced in more sophisticated ultrasound practice.
      (1) A targeted evaluation is performed to search for fetal anomalies; it should be considered for every patient who is suspected of carrying a physiologically or anatomically defective fetus.
      (2) The success of ultrasonographic detection of abnormalities in high-risk pregnancies is examiner dependent.
      (3) Progressive improvements in ultrasound equipment have permitted its diagnostic capacity to determine the presence of structural defects within a sensitivity range of 90% to 95% and a specificity range of 95% to 98%.
   d. Appropriate management must include a system of rational levels.
      (1) There is a consensus to classify ultrasound into three levels that take into consideration the preparation and ability of the operator and the purpose of the explorations (see the box on p. 874).

First trimester

Confirmation of an intrauterine pregnancy

1. Landmarks by transvaginal scanning
   a. 4 weeks: choriodecidual thickening
   b. 5 weeks: gestational sac 5 to 10 mm, yolk sac
   c. 6 weeks: yolk sac, embryo, heart rate
   d. 7 weeks: yolk sac, embryonic movements
   e. 8 weeks: physiologic bowel herniation, extremities
2. Transvaginal landmarks and beta-human chorionic gonadotropin (beta-HCG) levels
   a. Gestational sac visible by 1000 to 1200 mIU/ml
   b. Yolk sac visible by 7200 mIU/ml
   c. Embryo with heart rate visible by 10,000 to 11,000 mIU/ml

Obstetric Ultrasound Scanning

LEVEL 1: BASIC ULTRASOUND EXAMINATION

First trimester	*Second and third trimesters*
1. Gestational sac location	1. Fetal life and number
2. Embryo identification	2. Fetal presentation
3. Gestational age estimation	3. Fetal heart action
4. Fetal heart action	4. Amniotic fluid volume
5. Fetal number	5. Placental location
6. Uterus and adnexal structures	6. Gestational age estimation
	7. Fetal growth estimation
	8. Basic survey of fetal anatomy

LEVEL 2: SELECTED EXAMINATIONS

Echography of fetal anatomy performed by an expert and to study fetal anatomy, which permits diagnosis of major malformations

LEVEL 3

Ultrasonographic expertise in fetoplacental morphology, biometry, and function, including functional doppler measurements and sonographically-guided invasive procedures

Biometric measurements and gestational age estimation

1. Early in pregnancy, embryonic crown–rump length (CRL) is the basic biometric evaluation (Figs. 36-1 and 36-2).
2. The CRL is the longest length of the embryo, excluding the limbs.
3. Its determination is part of the most accurate sonographic technique for establishing gestational age.
4. After 12 weeks, the fetus is no longer easily measurable in a straight line because it is more likely to flex or extend.

Sonoembryology

1. Transvaginal probes that employ high frequencies significantly increase image resolution and early detection of embryonic and extraembryonic structures.
2. At the fifth week the intrauterine gestational sac is visible and its diameter is about 5 mm.
3. One week later, at 6 completed weeks of pregnancy, the developing embryonic plate is visible, measuring about 5 to 6 mm (CRL) within the greater gestational sac.
   (1) In this period, the embryo normally grows 1 mm per day.
   (2) The yolk sac, which is located in the extraembryonic coelom, is visible as a small circular structure smaller than 5 mm between the amnion and chorion (Figs. 36-1 and 36-3).
   (3) At this gestational age, the fetal heart rate (FHR) should be clearly detectable within the embryonic pole.

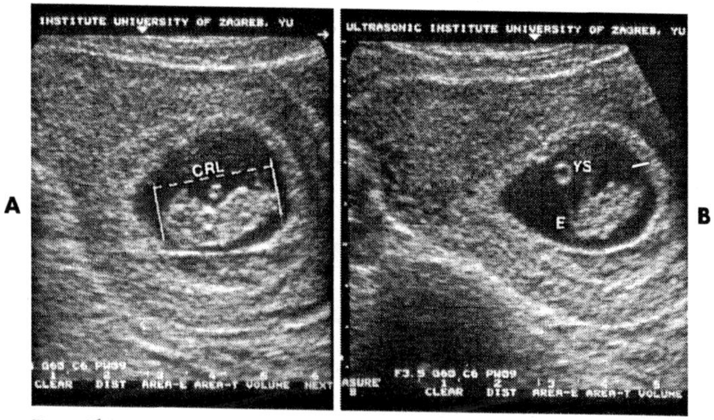

Figure 36-1
Fetal biometry, transabdominal scan. **A,** crown–rump length (*CRL*) measured in ninth week of gestational age. **B,** Embryo (*E*) in seventh week of gestational age, normal yolk sac is visible (*YS*).

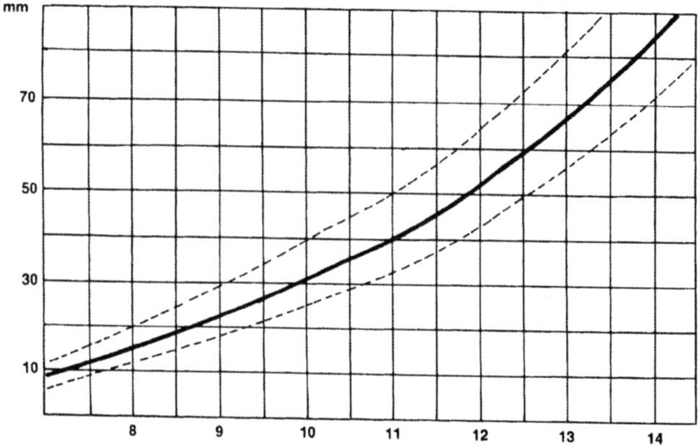

Figure 36-2
Growth curve: Crown–rump length (*CRL*) vs. gestational age.

(4) The embryo should be normally identified in all pregnancies when the gestational sac is greater than 18 mm.

4. From the seventh week, the embryonic head can be distinguished, the spine and lower limb buds can be imaged; the upper limb buds are visible a week later.

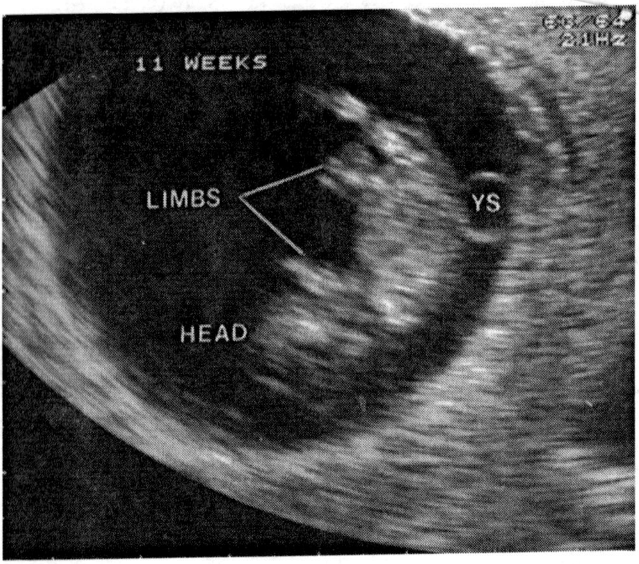

Figure 36-3
Transvaginal scan: At the 11th week of gestational age, the emrbyo is positioned adjacent and tangential to the visible yolk sac (*YS*).

5. After the ninth week, the entire upper and lower extremities are visible throughout their entire sagittal length.
   (1) At this age, CRL is about 25 mm, and within the embryonic head, lateral brain ventricles became detectable because of the clearly visible choroid plexus tissue.
6. All embryos at 10 weeks and beyond have visible midline echo, the falx, and two lateral ventricles containing the prominently echogenic choroid plexuses.
7. Other landmarks
   a. One of the most important landmarks for defining the developing processes is the physiologic midgut herniation.
      (1) Because of its extensive length, the embryonic midgut fills most of the abdominal cavity during the sixth week, but a portion of the intestine protrudes into the umbilical cord, creating a physiologic midgut herniation.
      (2) This finding exists from the seventh until the end of the 11th week, but it is detectable by transvaginal approach starting at the eighth week.
      (3) After the 12th week it should not be detectable.
      (4) These findings are very important for the early detection of umbilical herniation and ventral wall defects.

Table 36-1 Sonographic (TVS) appearance of embryonic structures

Structure	Gestational age 5 6 7 8 9 10 11 12
Gestational sac	I--->
Yolk sac	I------------------------I
Embryonic pole	I------------------------->
Heart action	I---------------------->
Spine	I------------------>
Lower extremities	I----------------->
Upper extremities	I---------------->
Midgut herniation	I------------I
Choroid plexus	I------------->
Kidneys	I---->

b. It has been clearly established that the sequential appearance of embryonic anatomic landmarks is in very close temporal relationship to the gestational age (Table 36-1).

First trimester abnormalities

1. Blighted ovum or anembryonic gestation is sonographically recognizable by the following:
   a. Gestational sac smaller than expected of normal size
   b. Absent embryonic pole and viability
   c. Angular or crenated shape of gestational sac
      (1) The cited gestational age is not always accurate and it is therefore advisable to repeat the examination within 1 week to avoid any misinterpretation.
      (2) Early diagnosis of blighted ovum is very important because it prevents the development of trophoblastic disease, which results from the trophoblastic hydropic degeneration of anembryonic pregnancy.
2. Molar pregnancy (hydatidiform mole) is represented by the following sonographic findings:
   a. The uterus is larger than expected for gestational age.
   b. Hyperechoic appearance of many fluid-filled vesicles of different sizes.
   c. Ovarian theca lutein cysts of different sizes may be scanned in about 50% of the cases.
3. Impending (imminent) abortion is mainly a clinical diagnosis based on bleeding in early pregnancy. The features of an impending abortion as visualized on ultrasound include the following:
   a. Poorly formed or collapsed gestational sac
   b. Various amounts of blood in the uterine cavity between chorioamniotic membrane and decidua
   c. A clot between gestational sac and internal os
   d. Sometimes even the absence of fetal viability
4. Uterine abnormalities that can be detected by ultrasound are more easily diagnosed in early pregnancy.

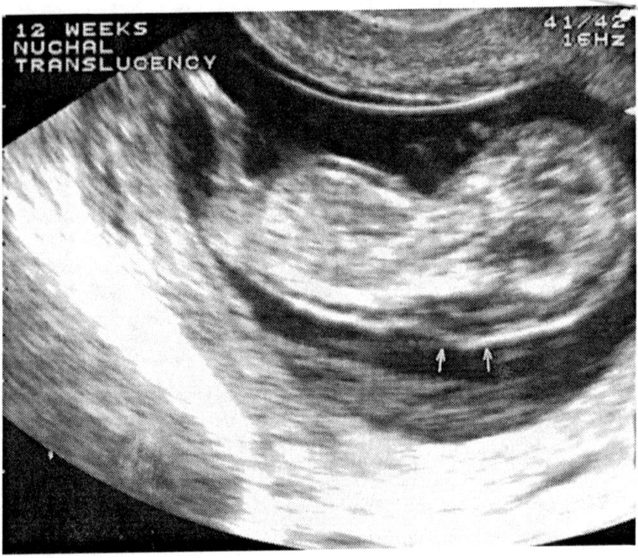

Figure 36-4
Transvaginal scan, 12th week of gestational age, embryo with generalized hydrops and nuchal edema (arrows). Both of these findings are markers for fetal chromosomal disorders.

   a. In cases of uterus duplex or bicornis the early gestational sac occupies one horn, while decidual reaction can be imaged in the nonpregnant horn.
   b. Uterine septum can be clearly visualized by transvaginal examination.
5. Early detection of embryonal and early fetal malformations
   a. Routine application of high-frequency vaginal transducers enables detection of fetal malformations even during the late first trimester and early second trimester.
   b. Nonimmune fetal hydrops, nuchal edema, cystic hygroma, omphalocoelae, and multicystic kidneys are disorders with the possibility for the earliest diagnosis (Fig. 36-4).

Second and third trimesters

Biometric measurements and gestational age estimation

1. BPD (biparietal diameter) (Figs. 36-5 and 36-6)
   a. Gestational age estimation is done between the 12th and 28th weeks.
   b. The distance between the outer table of the proximal fetal skull and the inner table of the distal side should be measured.
   c. Reference plane involves a cross-section through the falx, the thalamus, and the cavum septum pellucidum.

A

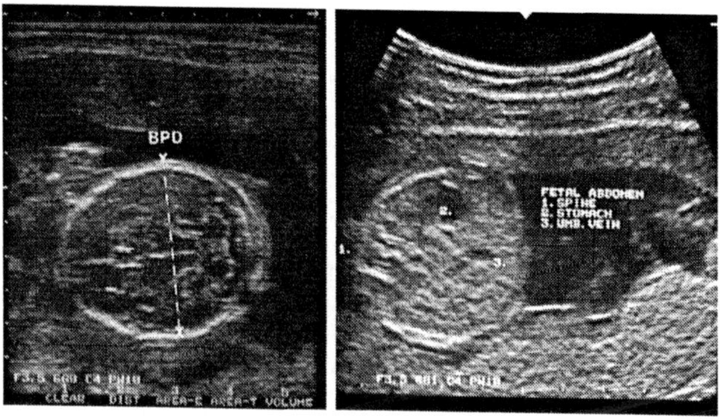

B

Figure 36-5

A, Transabdominal scan, 20 weeks of gestational age; biparietal diameter (BPD) measurement. **B,** Transabdominal scan, 20 weeks gestational age, transverse section of fetal abdomen suitable for measurement of abdominal circumference (AC). Fetal spine (*1*), fetal stomach (*2*), and intrahepatic portion of umbilical vein (*3*) are the landmarks of referral section.

d. The diameter has to be measured vertically to the midline echo at the point of the greatest width.
   (1) Occasionally, the fetal head can be compressed laterally and appear dolichocephalic.
   (2) The same phenomenon can also be observed in cases of breech presentation.
   (3) To check for this the biparietal diameter should be compared with the fronto-occipital diameter, which can be measured in the same section.
   (4) The ratio of the biparietal to fronto-occipital diameter has to be greater than 0.75 (cephalic index [CI] greater than 0.75).
   (5) If it is smaller, the biparietal diameter is not reliable for gestational age.

2. Abdominal circumference (AC) (see Figs. 36-5 and 36-6)
   a. Measurement is used for estimating gestational age and for detecting growth disturbances.
   b. Transverse section plane has to be at right angles to the fetal spine at the level of the fetal liver.
   c. An important criterion is to obtain the abdominal section as round as possible.
   d. The anteroposterior and laterolateral diameters are measured.
   e. The abdominal circumference is calculated by multiplying the sum of the diameters (*D*) by 1.57.

$$AC = (D_1 + D_2) \times 1.57$$

(Measurements are obtained from one outer to the other outer edge.)

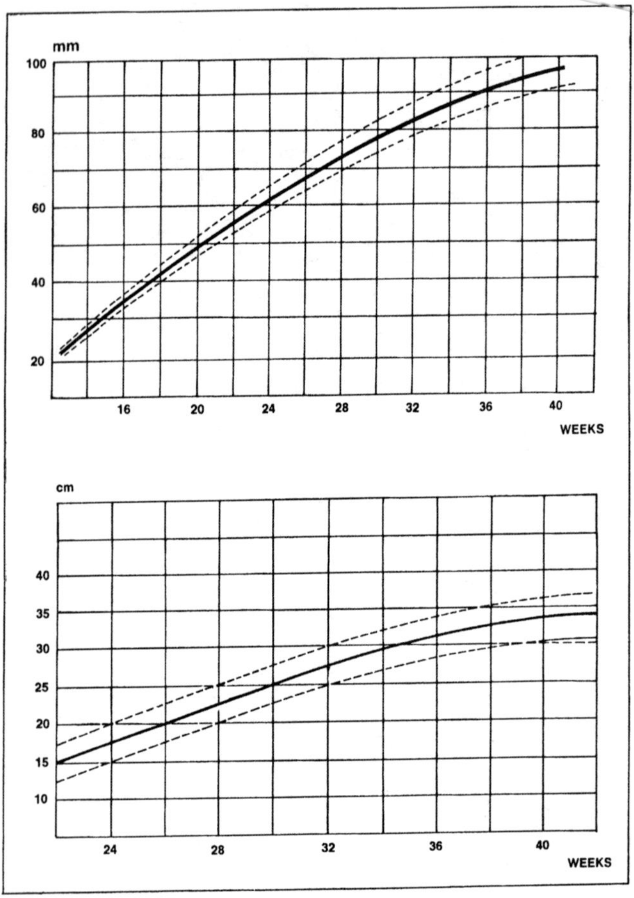

Figure 36-6
Growth curves of biparietal diameter (BPD) (*top*) and fetal abdominal circumference (AC) (*bottom*) vs. gestational age.

3. Femur length
   a. The central diaphysis of the shaft of the femur should be measured in a longitudinal section.
   b. Measurements are performed by placing the calipers at the lateral edges of the ossified diaphysis.
   c. Fetal long bone measurements were originally developed to detect skeletal disorders, but recently, femur length has also been found to be a useful parameter for better estimation of gestational age (Fig. 36-7).

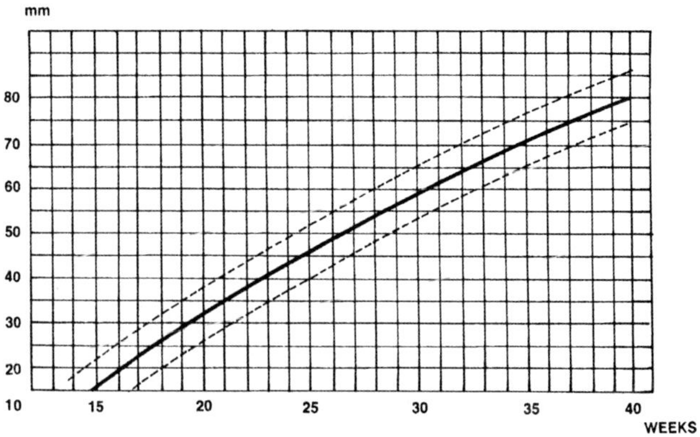

Figure 36-7
Growth curve of fetal femur length (FL) vs. gestational age.

4. Fetal body ratios
   a. The CI can be used to screen for cranial shape abnormalities.
      (1) It is calculated from the ratio of BPD/OFD (occipitofrontal diameter).
      (2) The CI is constant throughout pregnancy, ranging around 0.75.
   b. Fetal head to abdominal circumference ratio (HC/AC) begins at a maximal value of 1.29 at 12 weeks gestation, then falls to 1.00 at 36 weeks, and is less than 1.00 after 37 weeks.
      (1) Conditions that decrease the ratio include microcephaly, anencephaly, and fetal abdominal enlargement (e.g., ascites, maternal diabetes, fetal intestinal obstruction, hydronephrosis).
      (2) Conditions associated with increased ratio are hydrocephaly, asymmetric intrauterine growth retardation (IUGR), fetal triploidy, intracranial cysts, and fetal abdominal pathology associated with smaller AC.

Ultrasonic imaging of fetal anatomy

1. Neural tube (fetal head and spine)
   a. Fetal head
      (1) Lateral brain ventricles filled with a hyperechoic choroid plexus are the main anatomic landmarks within the fetal head.
         (a) The midline cerebral echo (falx) divides the fetal head into two symmetric portions.
      (2) Between the 20th week and term, there is little structural change of the fetal brain.
      (3) Neuroanatomy is most often evaluated in the transverse or transaxial plane.
         (a) Beginning at the vertex of the cranium, the first structure to be identified is the falx cerebri, which appears as a midline echogenic line (Fig. 36-8, Section 1).

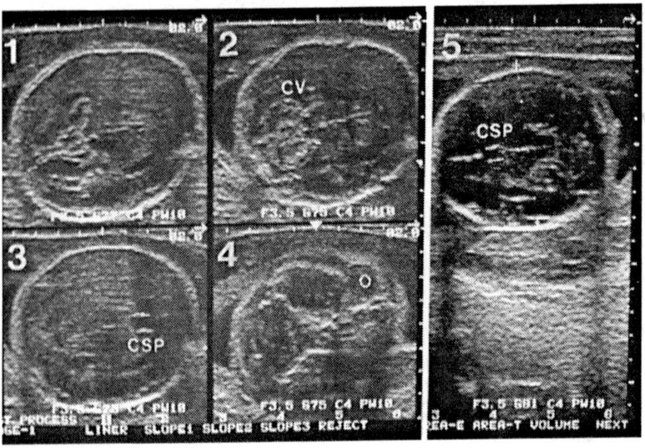

Figure 36-8
Transabdominal scan. Different sections of fetal head. The main biometric landmark is cavum septi pellucidi (*CSP*); cerebellum with vermis (*CV*) is clearly visible in section 2.

(b) Progressing caudally, the bodies of the lateral ventricles are seen as two lines parallel to the midline echo (Fig. 36-9).

(c) The anterior and posterior horns of the lateral ventricles may be visualized in the occipital and frontal portion of the head as bilateral parallel lines to the midline.

(d) At the level caudal to the lateral ventricles, the brain stem is visible.

(e) Beginning at the highest level of the brain stem, the thalami are seen as bilateral hypoechoic structures very close to the midline.

(f) Anteriorly, between the frontal and medial third of the midline echo, the cavum septi pellucidi are visible (Fig. 36-8, Section 5).

(g) The third brain ventricle is slightly posterior to and lower than the cavum septi pellucidi.

(h) The third ventricle is narrower than the cavum septi pellucidi and is positioned between two hypoechoic thalami continuing posteriorly and caudally with aqueductus sylvii.

(i) The posterior fossa is recognizable because of the paired, echogenic cerebellar hemispheres.

(j) The vermis can be recognized in the middle because of its strong echogenicity (Fig. 36-8, Section 2).

(k) The low axial scan of the fetal head shows the hyperechoic base of a skull, which appears as an X-shaped structure (Fig. 36-8, Section 4).

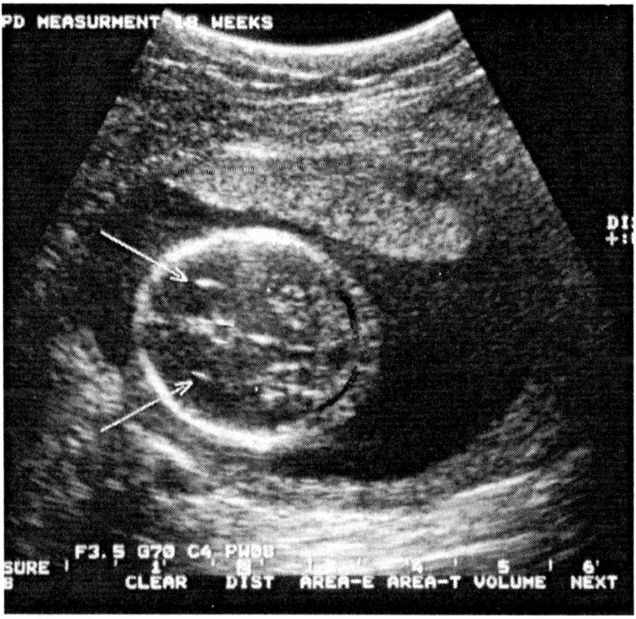

Figure 36-9
Transabdominal scan, 18th week of gestational age. Anterior (frontal) horns of lateral ventricles are depicted (*arrows*).

(l) The anterior branches correspond to the sphenoid wings, with the orbits in front of them.
(m) The posterior branches of the skull base correspond to the petrous pyramids of the temporal bones.
(n) Fetal orbits are easy to identify and the ocular lenses appear as bright dots in the anterior portion of each orbit.

b. Fetal spine
(1) Fetal spine is visible during the late first trimester by transvaginal examination.
(2) However, detailed examination of morphology and segmentation is possible from the 16th week onward.
(a) In the longitudinal plane the spine appears as double hyperechogenic, parallel lines with mild cervical widening and gradual sacral tapering (Fig. 36-10).
(b) On the transverse scan three ossification centers, in triangular formation, are seen in a dorsal part of the abdominal plane (Fig. 36-11).
(c) The anterior center is within the vertebral body, and two posterior centers represent the interarticular parts (lami-

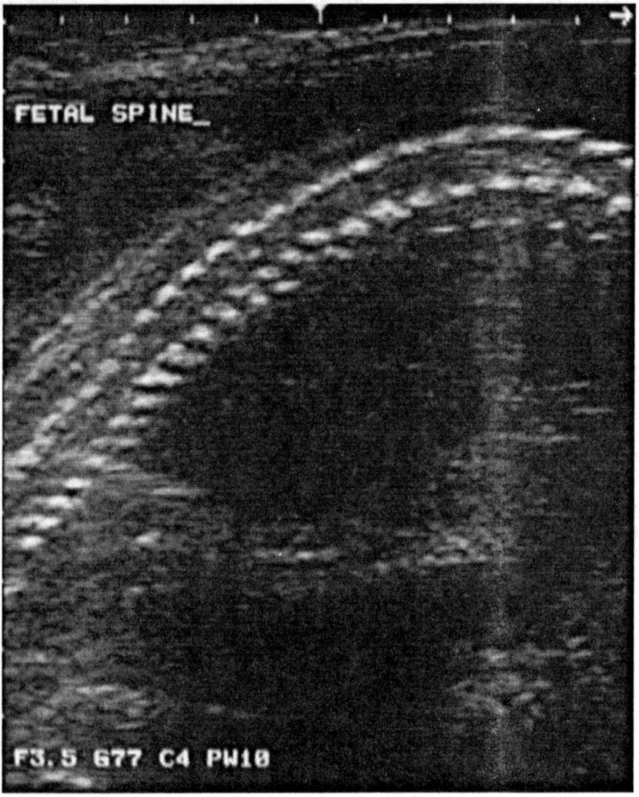

Figure 36-10
Transabdominal scan: normal longitudinal appearance of fetal spine.

nae). The dorsal part of the fetal spine has to be covered with a continuous, intact layer of fetal back skin along the entire spinal length.

2. Fetal thorax
   a. Examination of the fetal thorax should include a demonstration of FHR, the position of the heart within the thorax, a "four-chamber" view of the fetal heart, and a demonstration of the lungs and breathing motions.
   b. An image of the fetal heart long axis can be obtained by a transverse scan through the fetal chest.
      (1) This is the so-called four-chamber view, demonstrating the right and left ventricles and atria, interventricular septum, the tricuspid and mitral valves, the interatrial septum, and the foramen ovale (Fig. 36-12).

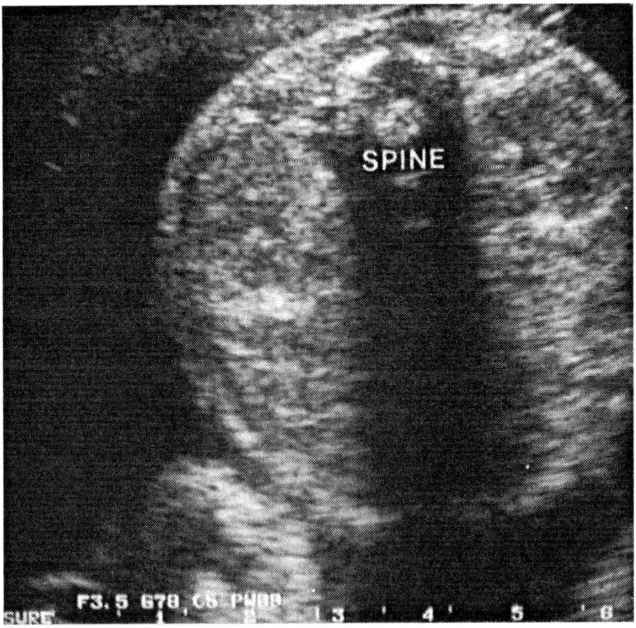

Figure 36-11
Transabdominal scan: normal fetus in transverse section.

(2) This section is easy to obtain and should be considered an obligatory diagnostic minimum during a routine ultrasound examination.

c. The fetal aorta is easily recognized on longitudinal scan, and its different portions can be identified.
d. The vena cava can be recognized as a large vessel entering the right atrium.
e. The fetal lung is fluid filled and collapsed so it has an echogenicity that is similar to other organs, such as the liver and spleen.
f. In the longitudinal section, the diaphragm is recognized between the lungs and the liver as a relatively transonic sliver moving during respiratory excursions.

3. Fetal abdomen
   a. The upper portion of the fetal abdomen is occupied by the liver, which has a homogeneous echogenicity higher than that of the lungs.
   b. The most commonly obtained section through the fetal abdomen is the transverse section through the liver at the level of the intrahepatic portion of the umbilical vein.

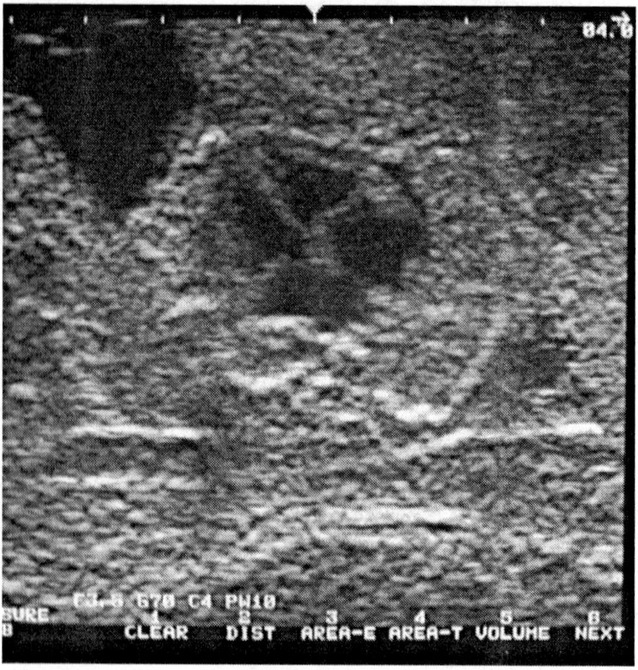

Figure 36-12
Transabdominal scan, fetal heart, four chamber view.

(1) On the right side of the umbilical vein, the gallbladder is visible with its typical pear-shaped appearance.
(2) The fetal stomach is seen as a C-shaped fluid-filled structure caudal to the fetal heart.
(3) Sometimes, fluid-filled loops and nondilated bowel are seen in the normal fetus.
(4) At term, the bowel may contain meconium, causing the bowel to be more echogenic and prominent.

c. It is very important to visualize the fetal kidneys because many congenital anomalies involve the urogenital system.
(1) The kidneys are best visualized in a transverse scan, below the liver, as two relatively sonolucent circular structures on either side of the fetal spine (Fig. 36-13).
(2) The central part of each kidney is hypoechoic (renal pelvis filled with fetal urine).
(3) In a longitudinal section, kidneys appear as bean-shaped structures, very close to the each side of the lumbar spine.

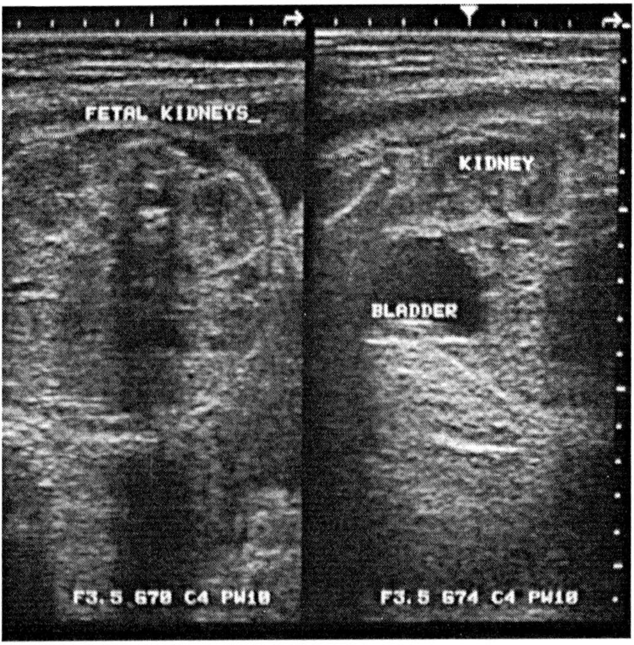

Figure 36-13
Transabdominal scan, 37 weeks of gestational age. Fetal kidneys in longitudinal (*right*) and transverse (*left*) scan. Full bladder is visible in longitudinal scan.

d. In the lower portion of the fetal abdomen (fetal pelvis), a hypoechoic structure is visible (see Fig. 36-13); this is the fetal urinary bladder.
   (1) This is a fluid-filled structure that should not be confused with amniotic fluid that is between the fetal thighs.
   (2) Visualization of a full fetal bladder is important to document renal function.

4. Fetal skeleton
   a. The fetal spine is visible from the first trimester on by transvaginal probe, but detailed examination is possible after the 16th week.
      (1) In longitudinal planes, the spine appears in the form of two echogenic parallel lines.
      (2) On the transverse section three ossification centers in triangular formation are seen.
         (a) The anterior one is within the vertebral body, and two posterior centers represent the pars interarticularis.
   b. Examination of the fetal limbs should include documentation of four extremities, limb movements, and the length of the long bones.

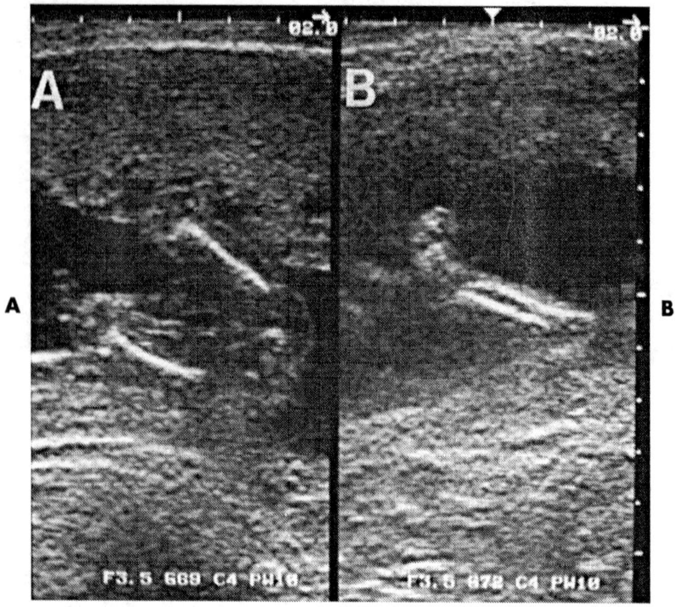

Figure 36-14
Transabdominal scan, 16 weeks gestational age. Fetal long bones of extremities: **A,** Both of the femurs. **B,** Tibia and fibula.

(1) Fetal extremities are visible during the first trimester; moreover fingers and toes can be imaged by high-frequency vaginal scan from the 12th week onward.
(2) The best visible and measurable part of each extremity is the ossified diaphysis of the long bone (Fig. 36-14).
(3) The length of the humerus and femur are approximately identical before 22 weeks gestation.
(4) The length and shape of the long bones of extremities are important regarding the excluding of skeletal malformations.

5. Amniotic fluid
   a. Amniotic fluid volume estimation is very important in fetal biophysical scoring.
   b. Experienced ultrasonographists can estimate the amniotic fluid volume by visual inspection scanning of the entire uterine cavity.
      (1) A large amount of fluid is polyhydramnios (Fig. 36-15).
         (a) Overall, 1% of pregnancies are complicated by hydramnios, whereas 20% of problem pregnancies result from anomalous fetuses.
         (b) Some malformations commonly associated with polyhydramnios are listed in the box on p. 890.

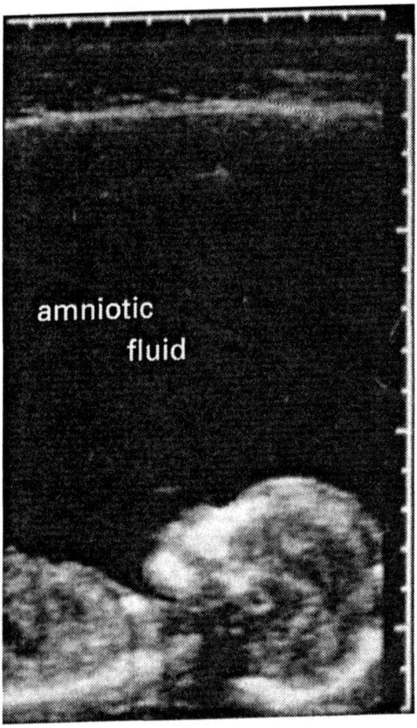

Figure 36-15
Transabdominal scan, 19 weeks of gestational age. Polyhydramnios.

(2) Oligohydramnios is present if it is very difficult to find any "pocket" of fluid without the umbilical cord in the space.
   (a) Conditions and malformations associated with oligohydramnios are IUGR, urinary tract malformation, ruptured membranes, and postdate pregnancy.
   (b) Objective evaluation is possible calculating the amniotic fluid index (AFI).
      i. The AFI is obtained by dividing the uterus into four quadrants, separating the top and the bottom by the mother's umbilicus and side to side by the linea alba/nigra.
      ii. The AFI is calculated as a total sum of measurements obtained for the largest vertical pocket in each quadrant.
      iii. Normal values during pregnancy are depicted in Fig. 36-16.

6. Umbilical cord
   a. The umbilical cord is usually seen very easily as two small arteries surrounding the large umbilical vein when the cord is seen in cross section (Fig. 36-17).

Fetal Malformations Commonly Associated with Polyhydramnios

NEURAL TUBE DEFECTS

Anencephaly
- Hydrocephaly
- Encephalocele

GASTROINTESTINAL SYSTEM

Gastroschisis
- Omphalocele
- Duodenal atresia
- Tracheoesophageal fistula

RESPIRATORY TRACT

Pulmonary hypoplasia
- Chylothorax

FETAL CHROMOSOMAL ABNORMALITIES

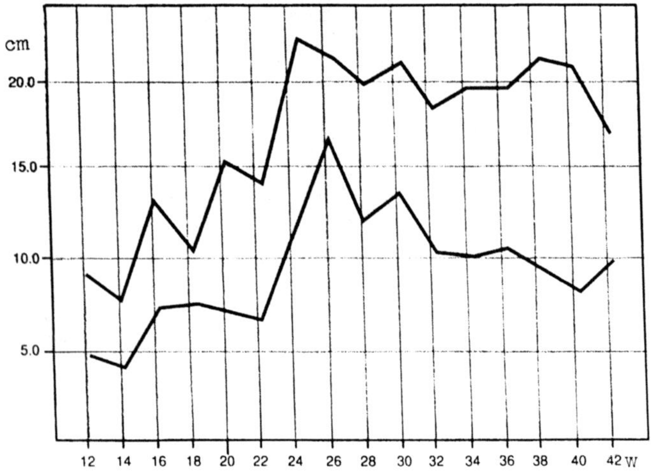

Figure 36-16
Amniotic fluid index (AFI) rate vs. gestational age. AFI represents a sum of four pockets of amniotic fluid obtained from each quadrant of intrauterine volume in a longitudinal scan.

b. A two-vessel cord (single umbilical artery syndrome) may be associated with various fetal malformations, maternal diabetes, or twin gestation.

7. Placental morphology
   a. Placenta previa and placental abruptio are the most important placental disorders obligatorily recognizable by transabdominal or transvaginal scanning.

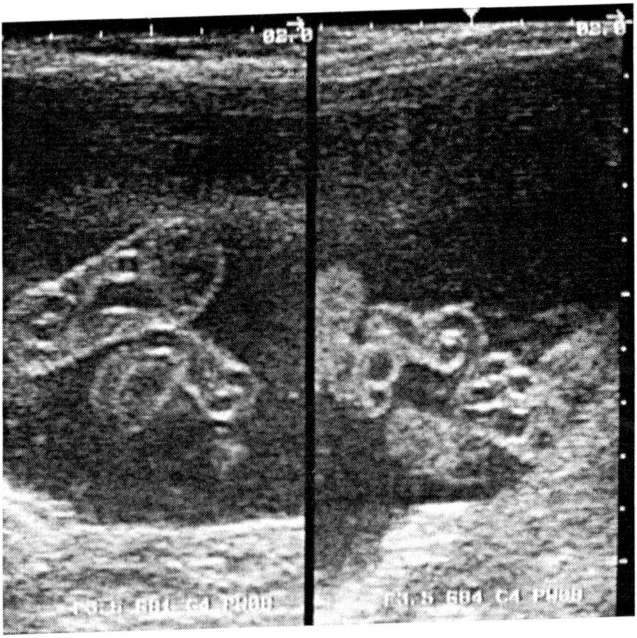

Figure 36-17
Normal appearance of umbilical cord. Umbilical vein is rounded with double-piped echo of umbilical arteries.

(1) Placenta previa
   (a) Placental tissue is covering uterine internal ostium completely (placenta previa totalis) or partially (placenta previa partialis).
(2) Placenta abruptio
   (a) The most common findings are increased echogenicity of one placental part caused by fresh bleeding, placental separation because of retroplacental bleeding, or clotted blood adjacent to the placenta.
(3) Color Doppler technique can be helpful in the diagnosis of placenta succenturiata, placenta bipartita, and vasa previa, enabling easier detection and visualization of blood vessels.

Ultrasonographic diagnosis of fetal malformations

1. Screening of fetal malformations is a basic part of ultrasonographic practice in obstetrics.
2. Sensitivity (false negatives) and specificity (false positives) of ultrasonography for the detection of fetal anomalies is relatively high, ranging from 75% to 95% each, influenced by the training of the operator and the quality of the equipment.

3. In a high-risk population (prevalence of more than 20%), use of ultrasound for the diagnosis of some malformations is corroborated by the excellent sensitivity (89% to 99%) and specificity (99% to 100%) obtained, even when excluding cardiovascular malformations, which have one of the highest prevalences.
4. However, the validity of ultrasound as a screening test for fetal malformation in the general population can be partly compromised because of the operator's experience and equipment quality.
5. Very few congenital anomalies are heralded by maternal history; therefore, every prenatal examination with ultrasound should include a systemic search for anomalies.

Neural tube defects (NTDs)

1. Hydrocephaly
   a. Sonographic landmarks are hypoechoic dilated cerebral ventricles, BPD greater than expected, and abnormal intracranial anatomy.
   b. The disorder is recognizable by dilation of the cerebral lateral ventricles, particularly by dilation of their frontal and occipital horns.

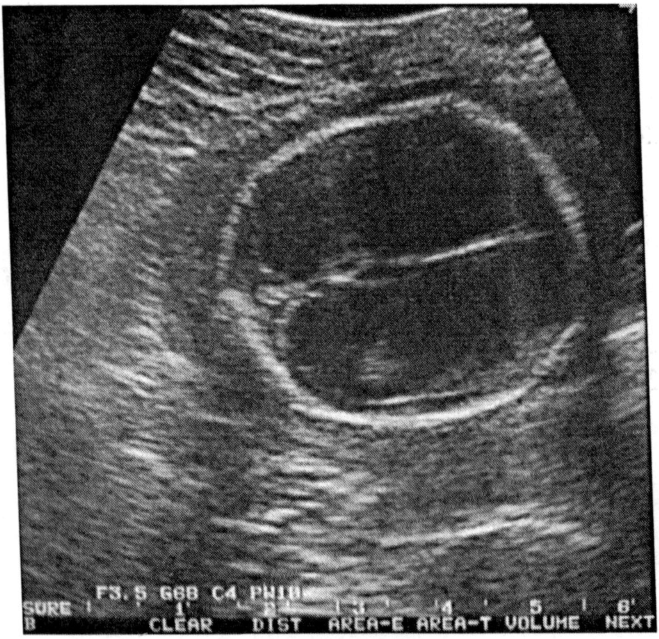

Figure 36-18
Transabdominal scan, 21 weeks of gestational age. Hydrocephaly; brain tissue is pressed adjacent to the inner skull.

(1) The hypoechoic dilated ventricles, filled with cerebrospinal fluid are the dominant sign of disorder (Fig. 36-18).
(2) It is very difficult to establish the diagnosis before the 18th week of gestation because of the physiologic, relative enlargement of cerebral ventricles fulfilled with hyperechogenic choroid plexuses.
(3) After the 18th to 20th week, the ratio between cerebral lateral ventricles and cerebral hemispheres (V/H ratio) has to be constantly lower than 0.3 (Fig. 36-19).
(4) Measurement of the V/H ratio has to be performed from the midline echo to the lateral border of the frontal horn and compared with the hemispheric width in the same section, measured from the midline echo to the inner table of the skull.
(5) Brain tissue is reduced and compressed to the skull.
(6) The ventricles begin to dilate before the biparietal diameter becomes abnormally large; therefore, the enlargement of the head BPD will be latter marker of disease.

c. Differential diagnosis includes primarily hydranencephaly and holoprosencephaly.

2. Hydranencephaly
   a. Hydranencephaly results from the occlusion of internal carotid arteries with consequent necrosis, liquefaction, and absence of cerebral hemisphere.
3. Holoprosencephaly
   a. Holoprosencephaly is a developmental abnormality of midline cranial structures.
   b. The head is of smaller or normal size, marked with the absence of midline falx echo.

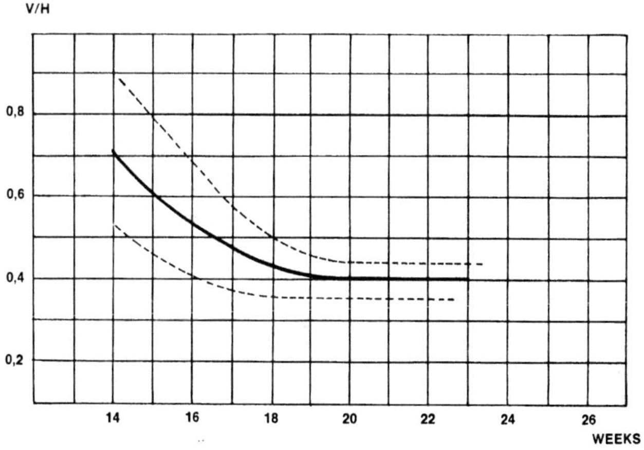

Figure 36-19
Ventriculohemispheric ratio vs. gestational age.

c. Facial anomalies, including cleft lip and cyclopia, are usually associated with holoprosencephaly.

4. Microcephaly
   a. This condition is defined as an abnormally small head, measuring more than three standard deviations below the normal.
   b. It is usually diagnosed after the 24th week in a fetus that had demonstrated normal growth but in which the head to abdomen ratio is too low.
   c. The etiology is unknown, but it is associated with chromosomal abnormalities, *in utero* infections, or fetal alcohol syndrome.
5. Anencephaly
   a. Anencephaly is one of the most common anomalies of the fetal central nervous system.
   b. The main sonographic landmark is an absence of cranial vault and brain clearly visible by transvaginal sonography even from the 12th week onward.
   c. Later in pregnancy, in a longitudinal section, the cervical spine ends with a dysmorphic fetal head that lacks cranial vault (Fig. 36-20).
   d. Only the structures of the brain stem and cerebellum can be seen.

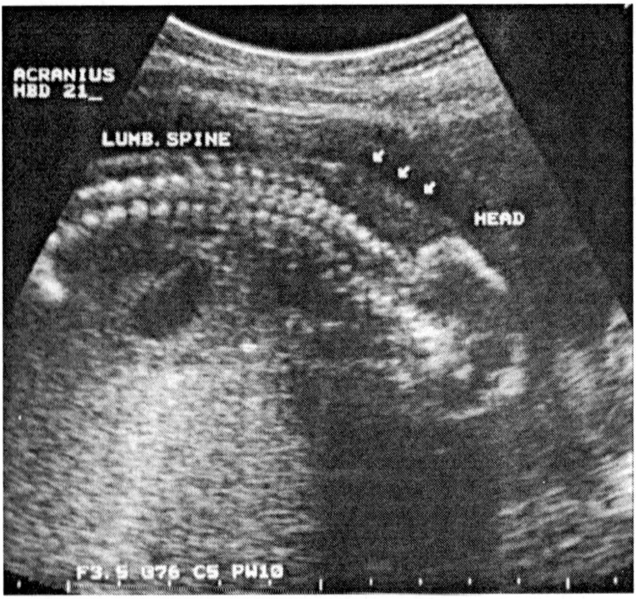

Figure 36-20
Transabdominal scan, 21 weeks of gestational age. Acranius or anencephalus; cervical spine (*arrows*) ends with abnormally shaped fetal head; flat bones of fetal skull are missing.

e. Some central functions are always preserved so that the vital functions can be present even after delivery.
f. Acrania is a constant finding and the calvarium remains collapsed on the base of the skull.
g. The defect is never covered by skin or bone.
h. The most prominent finding is the fetal eyes protruded on the base of the skull, causing a froglike appearance of the fetal head.

6. Encephaloceles
   a. Sacular structures protruding from the bony calvarium in a frontal or occipital portion help identify encephaloceles.
   b. It should be distinguished from the cystic hygromas of fetal neck.
7. Spinal abnormalities
   a. The most common defect is spina bifida.
      (1) It is a fusional defect marked with a separation of posterior ossification centers.
      (2) Ultrasound findings include:
         (a) The posterior centers display a U-shape in transverse scan (Fig. 36-21).
         (b) In a longitudinal section, the defect should be registered according to the finding of spinal "divergention" (Fig. 36-22).

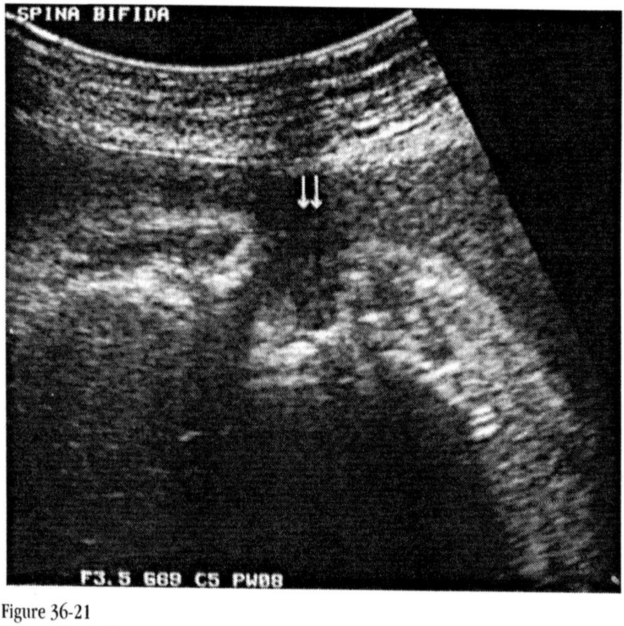

Figure 36-21
Transabdominal scan, 32 weeks of gestational age. Spina bifida: transverse section of U-shaped defect of fetal spine (*arrows*).

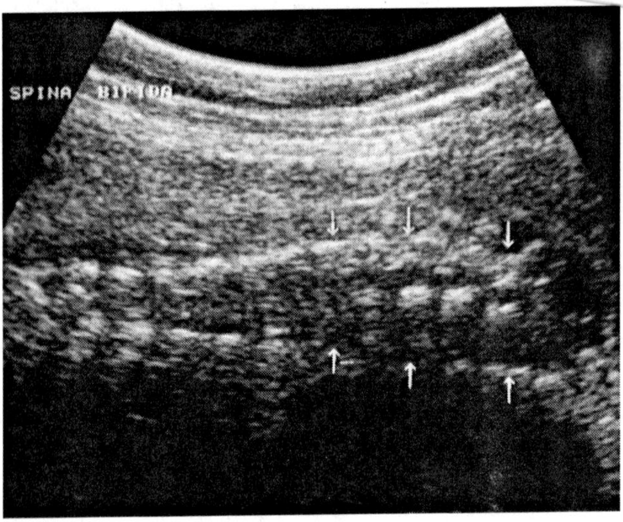

Figure 36-22
Transabdominal scan, 32 weeks of gestational age. Spina bifida: longitudinal section, divergention of spinal tapering is depicted (*arrows*).

(c) The parts of fetal brain or spinal cord can herniate through the defect (Fig. 36-23).

b. Common findings could be an abnormal configuration of the cerebellum with flattening of the posterior aspect caused by the obliteration of the cisterna magna (banana sign) and frontal bossing of the skull, which gives the parietal bones a pointed appearance (lemon sign).

8. Myelomeningocele (spina bifida cystica)
   a. This is seen as a cystic mass projecting posteriorly from the spine (see Fig. 36-23).
   b. If spontaneous rupture occurs there is no visible sac, but only a spinal fusional defect.
   c. It may be associated with other types of NTD such as hydrocephaly or encephalocele.

Abnormalities of the fetal thorax

1. The fetal chest can be demonstrated by ultrasound even during the end of the first trimester by transvaginal high-frequency probes.
   a. FHR is the main landmark.
   b. However, abnormalities of the fetal thorax, mainly connected to skeletal dysplasias or oligohydramnios, are clearly visible after 16 to 18 weeks.
2. Skeletal dysplasias are the group of systemic disorders involving also the fetal ribs and thoracic spine.

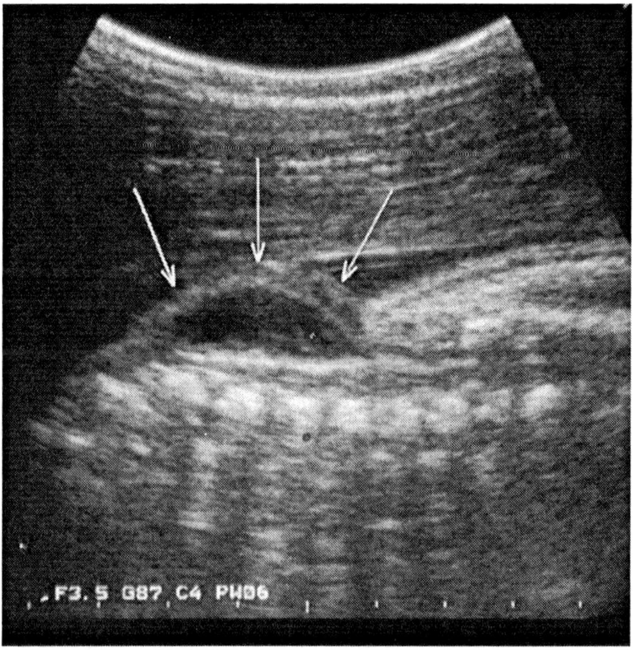

Figure 36-23
Transabdominal scan, 32 weeks of gestational age. Protruded myelomeningocele (*arrows*) in longitudinal section.

a. The most common skeletal disorder involving the fetal chest is the group of skeletal dysplasias associated with "bell-shaped" or narrow thorax (Fig. 36-24).
b. Rib fractures are visible in prenatal osteogenesis imperfecta.
c. Thoracic malformation associated with pulmonary hypoplasia is visible in oligohydramnios caused by renal dysplasia.

3. Fetal heart abnormalities
   a. Fetal echocardiography is the most difficult task in sonographic practice.
   b. Despite the technical and educational problems, the successful diagnosis of a congenital heart defect is possible even during the second trimester.
   c. In 30% of cases, heart anomalies are associated with chromosomal abnormalities.
   d. Fetal echocardiography should be the matter of specially educated staff on the third-level of ultrasound expertise.
4. Hydrothorax (collection of fluid within chest compressing the lungs)
   a. Hydrothorax may be associated with heart failure, Rh immunization, or nonimmune fetal hydrops.

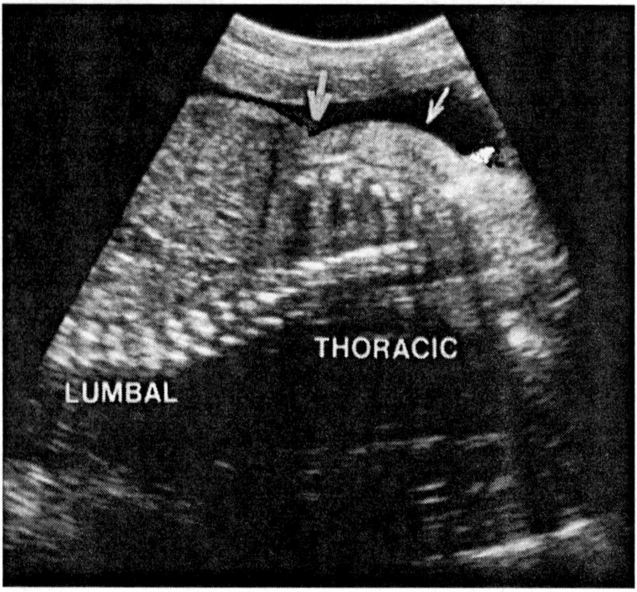

Figure 36-24
Skeletal dysplasia with narrowed thorax detected in 32nd week of gestational age. Note the small thoracal diameter compared to the abdominal (*bold arrow*), and relatively edematous soft tissue of the chest (*arrow*).

b. Elevation of intrathoracic pressure may result in pulmonary hypoplasia and abnormal lung maturation secondary to compression of normal lung tissue (Fig. 36-25).

Abnormalities of the fetal abdomen

1. Diaphragmatic hernia
   a. Usually, it is a defect of the posterolateral region of the diaphragm.
   b. Sonographic diagnosis includes three characteristic signs: hydramnios, mediastinal shift, and an inability to visualize a normal abdominal anatomy.
   c. The most often herniated organ is the small bowel, the loops of which can be visualized within the thoracic cavity.
   d. The mediastinal structure and heart can be dislocated, depending on the size of the defect.
2. Intestinal obstruction
   a. Duodenal atresia is the most common type of obstruction.
   b. A characteristic sonographic sign is "double-bubble" sign, consisting of two round, hypoechoic, cystic structures, positioned very close to each other, in the upper abdomen.

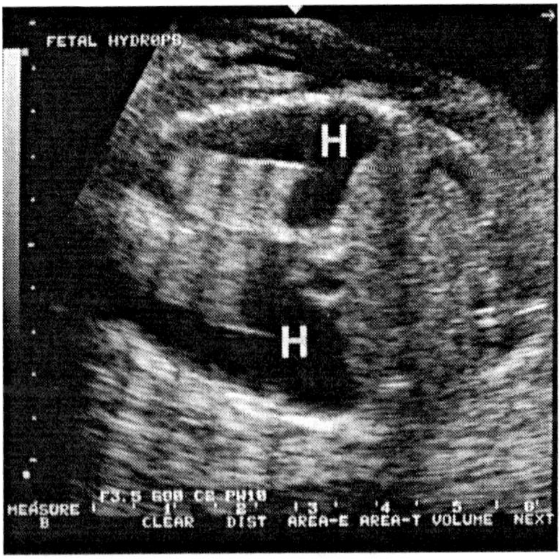

Figure 36-25
Transabdominal scan, 30 weeks of gestational age. Bilateral fetal hydrothorax (*H*); fetal lungs are hypoplastic.

(1) The left cyst represents the dilated stomach, the right one is obstructed duodenum, and a thin communication between them may be visible representing the pyloric narrowing.

c. Hydramnios is present in 50% of cases with duodenal atresia.
d. The situation is similar in other intestinal obstructions, located lower in the abdomen.
e. Jejunal or ileal atresias are characterized by several cystic structures representing dilated bowel loops.
f. It should be emphasized that a normal finding in early pregnancy does not imply the possibility for developing later gastrointestinal obstruction.
g. Because duodenal atresia is associated in almost 50% of cases with other malformations or chromosomal defects, the fetus should be examined carefully and karyotypinig is indicated.

3. Abdominal wall defects: omphalocele, gastroschisis
   a. Omphalocele
      (1) Omphalocele is the result of the failure of four embryonic disc folds to fuse into a primitive pleuroperitoneal cavity.
      (2) The result of fusion failure is a midline abdominal wall defect (Fig. 36-26).
      (3) The herniated sac, located on the abdominal cord insertion site, may contain intestinal loops, liver, stomach, or spleen.
      (4) The herniated sac is covered by a membrane consisting of amnion externally and peritoneum internally.

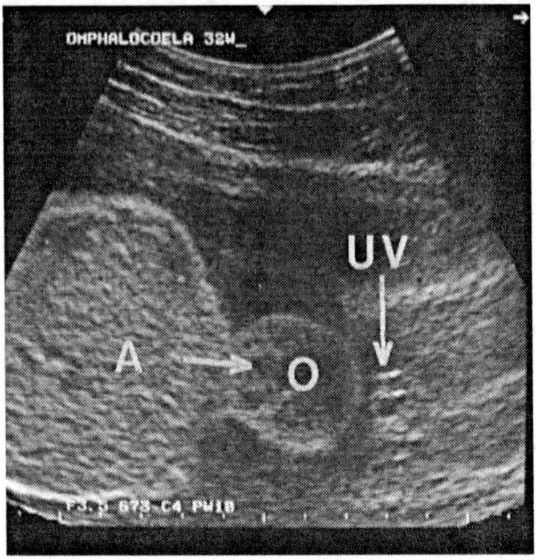

Figure 36-26
Omphalocele detected in 32nd week of gestational age. Few intestinal loops are protruded throughout abdominal cavity (*A*) into herniated umbilical sac (*O*)

(5) The umbilical cord insertion has to be located on the top of the hernited sac with the umbilical vessels spreading within the sac wall.
(6) Ten percent to 20% of fetuses with omphalocele are chromosomally abnormal.
(7) It should be emphasized that very early diagnosis of omphalocele is possible by transvaginal sonography, even during the early second trimester.
(8) Moreover, later confirmation of this diagnosis should be established because the physiologic herniation of the midgut during the first trimester may be prolonged and may mimic the ventral wall defect.

b. Gastroschisis
(1) Gastroschisis is an abdominal wall defect mainly located in the right paraumbilical region.
(2) The defect is caused by an abnormal development of the umbilical coelom and may be associated with other abnormalities.
(3) As compared with omphalocele, only the bowel herniates through the defect, and there is no covering membrane.
(4) The ultrasonic finding of bowel loops floating in the amniotic fluid, throughout the opened abdominal wall, is usually characteristic.
(5) Because the defect is located paraumbilically, the umbilical cord inserts normally.

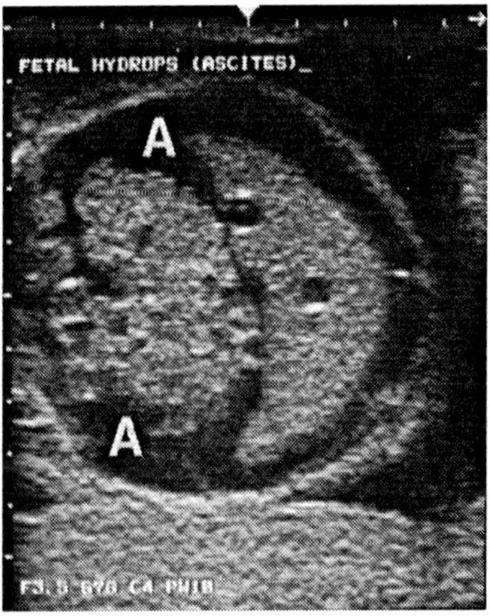

Figure 36-27
Transabdominal scan, 28 weeks gestational age. Free fluid collected in fetal abdomen, ascites (*A*); visceral organs are floating within the transudated liquid.

4. Fetal ascites
   a. Fetal ascites is marked by the finding of free fluid in abdominal cavity.
   b. Ultrasonically, free fluid is visualized as an anechoic area surrounding fetal viscera (Fig. 36-27).
   c. Fetal ascites is of varying etiology (e.g., Rh immunization, nonimmune fetal hydrops, cardiac anomalies, perinatal infections).
   d. It is commonly associated with a general collection of fluid, including even soft tissues (Fig. 36-28).

Genitourinary malformations

1. Two kidneys and a bladder should be clearly recognized in every fetus after 16 weeks gestation, or a renal disorder should be suspected.
2. The most common anomalies are urinary obstructive disorders, multicystic kidneys, polycystic kidneys, and renal dysplasias (agenesis).
3. Several obstructive disorders have been recognized on ultrasound according to the following findings.
   a. Obstruction at the ureteropelvic junction is usually unilateral and associated with retrograde dilation of the renal calyx and pelvis (unilateral hydronephrosis consequented).
   b. Obstruction originating from a posterior urethral valve, found only in males, sometimes produces massive dilation of the bladder and bilateral hydroureters and hydronephrosis, visible as hypoechoic, irregulary shaped areas within the entire abdomen and pelvis.

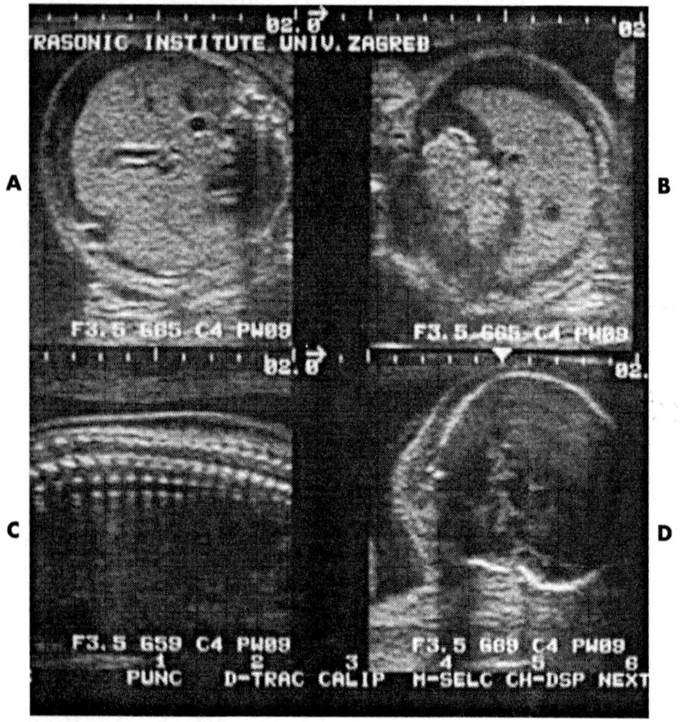

Figure 36-28
Nonimmune fetal hydrops: **A,** Ascites. **B,** Ascites. **C,** Edematous skin of lumbal part. **D,** Scalp edema surrounding fetal head.

4. The multicystic kidney is the most common of all neonatal abdominal masses.
   a. The affected kidney is poorly organized and enlarged, with absent appearance of normal parenchymal structure.
   b. The diagnosis is suggested by the presence of multiple cysts separated by well-defined septa.
   c. The cysts are commonly greater than 1 cm in diameter but may be even larger, filling the greater part of the abdominal cavity (Fig. 36-29).
5. Fetal hydronephrosis
   a. The entire kidney will be dilated by a single large anechoic cyst.
   b. This cyst could be composed of a few dilated communicating spaces representing the extremely dilated renal pelvis and calices.
   c. Greater or lesser amounts of renal parenchyma border the lateral margins of the cyst (Fig. 36-30).

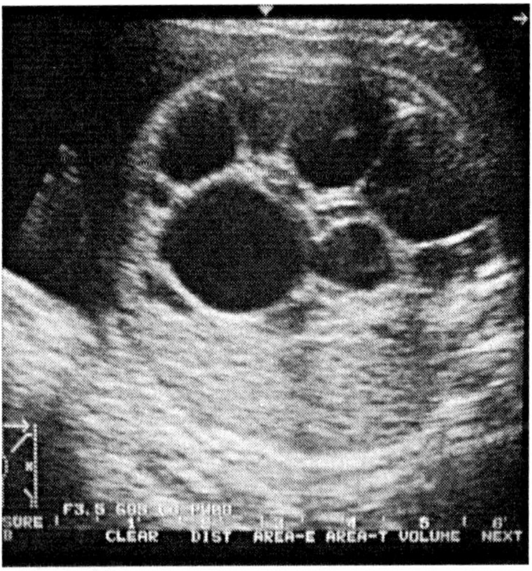

Figure 36-29
Multicystic kidney in transverse section of fetal abdomen. One half of the abdominal section is occupied with rounded cystic structures representing dysplastic, enlarged kidney.

6. Infantile polycystic kidneys disease (Potter type I)
   a. This disease is caused by the dilation and hyperplasia of collecting tubules caused by developmental dysplastic disorders.
   b. Recent investigations confirm the genetic etiology of the disorder.
   c. It is invariably bilateral and characterized by symmetric massive enlargement of kidneys, which are hyperechoic with the maintenance of normal reniform structure (Fig. 36-31).
   d. Medullary ductal ectasia and countless radially distributed ductal cysts replace normal renal tissue.
   e. Most microcysts, which lend a "spongy" appearance to the polycystic kidney, are difficult to discern.
   f. Ultrasonographic appearance is that of large and hyperechogenic, homogeneously solid kidneys.
   g. Renal function is always compromised, the bladder is usually small, but associated oligohydramnios is a relatively common complication.
   h. Although renal function is variable, it is generally incompatible with life beyond the neonatal period.
7. Renal agenesis or dysplasia
   a. Renal agenesis should be suspected when visualization of fetal kidneys is missing and an extremly decreased volume of amniotic fluid is present.

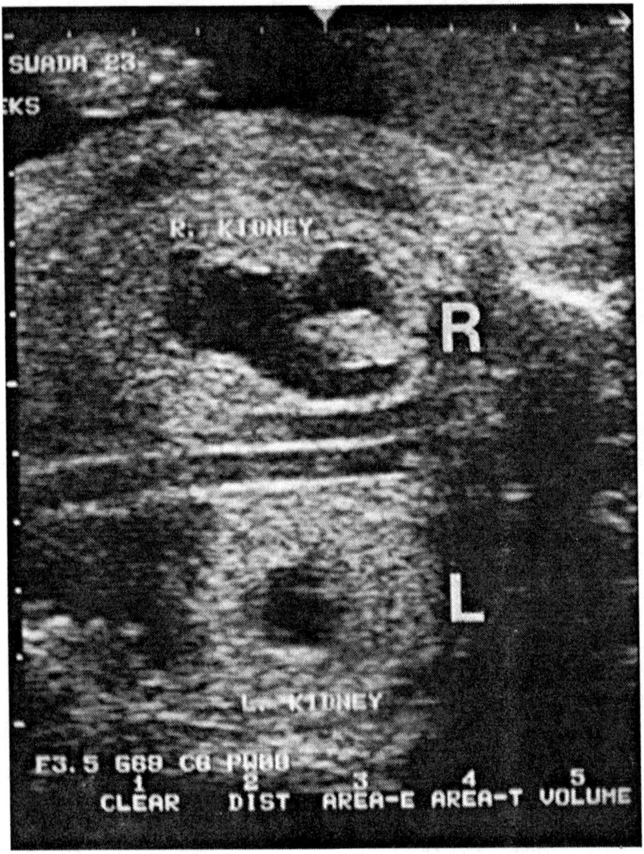

Figure 36-30
Hydronephrosis, longitudinal section of fetal abdomen; renal calices are dilated irregularly, involving right (*R*) and left (*L*) kidneys.

b. Decreased or completely reduced urine production and urinary output is the mechanicm of anhydramnios.

Skeletal abnormalities

1. The fetal skeleton is one of the earliest visible structures in sonoembryology.
2. A complete examination of the fetal skeleton and limbs is possible from the early second trimester, after the ossification of primary ossification centers in the flat and long bones (Figs. 36-32 and 36-33).

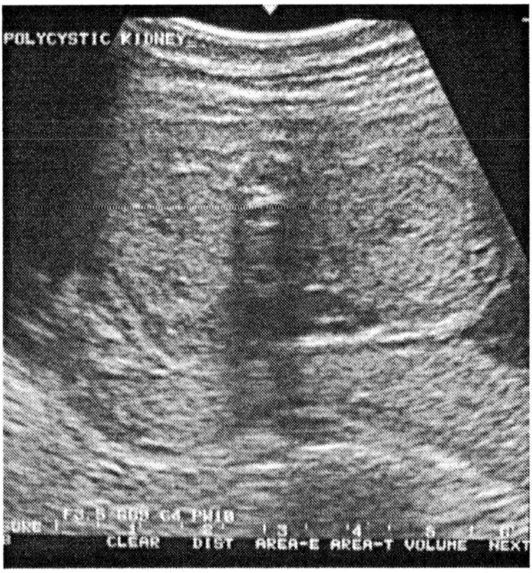

Figure 36-31
Polycystic kidneys; bilateral hyperechoic masses represent enlarged fetal kidneys, commonly associated with oligohydramnios.

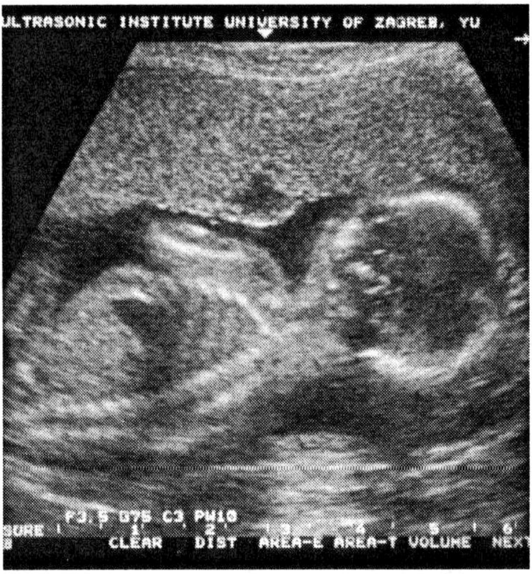

Figure 36-32
Transabdominal scan, 22 weeks of gestational age. Panoramic view of fetal skeleton, ossified parts of skeleton are visible, including long bones, ribs, spine, and skull.

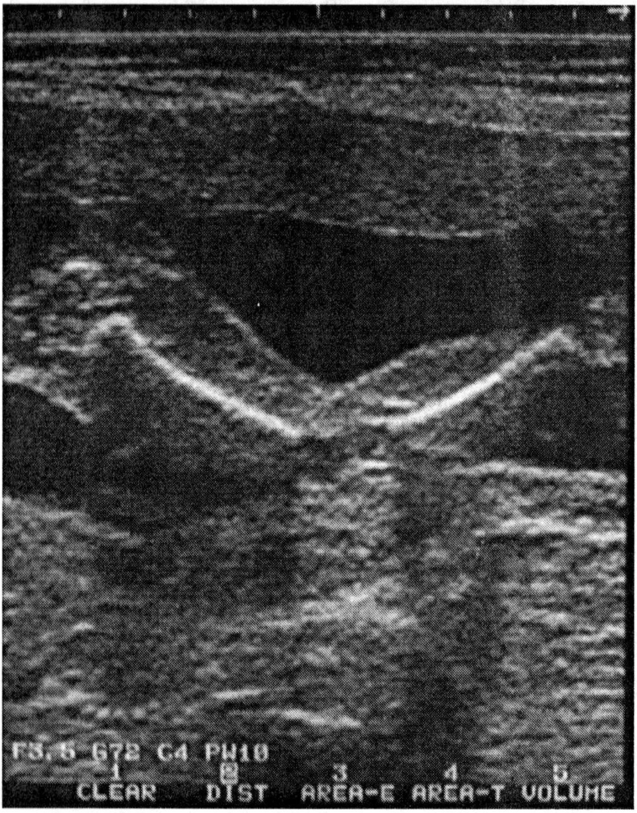

Figure 36-33
Transabdominal scan, 21 weeks of gestational age. Long bones of fetal leg. Ossified diaphyses of femur and tibia are visible and measureable.

3. A complete examination of fetal limbs and skeleton in a fetus at risk of having skeletal dysplasias should include all long bone measurements and morphologic examination of each skeletal part.
4. Skeletal abnormalities are subdivided in the following three groups:
   a. Systemic skeletal dysplasias with consequent short limbed dwarfism
   b. Disorders associated with hypomineralization of the skeleton and consequent intrauterine fractures of ribs and long bones (perinatal type of osteogenesis imperfecta)
   c. Isolated limb reduction abnormalities and minor defects (amelia, hemimelia, polydactyly, syndactyly)

5. Clinically, it is very important to exclude the group of systemic skeletal dysplasias with hypoplastic or narrow thorax (see Fig. 36-24).
   a. In these cases cardiopulmonary insufficiency and decompensation are obligatory complications during the neonatal period, compromising postnatal viability.
6. Biochemical screening is a helpful complementary tool in screening for structural defects.
   a. A significant linear correlation has been confirmed between high rates of MSAFP and fetal anomalies.
   b. This correlation, which was once thought to be only for NTDs, has now been confirmed for other congenital defects, and even found to be valid for unsatisfactory gestational evolutions.
   c. Situations associated with high levels of MSAFP are as follows:
      (1) NTDs (including the high AFP levels in amniotic fluid because of transudation from exposed neural tissue)
      (2) Abdominal wall defects
      (3) Cystic hygromas
      (4) Sacrococcygeal teratomas
      (5) Gastrointestinal obstructions
      (6) Renal anomalies
      (7) Cystadenomatoid tumor of the lungs
      (8) Some chromosomal abnormalities
         (a) Fetal chromosomal disorders are more frequently associated with lower levels of MSAFP, but a consensus has not been reached concerning this screening in an unselected population.
         (b) Additional biochemical markers have been studied, such as beta-HCG, estriol E3, and the Papp-A test.
      (9) Fetal demise
   d. False-positive results can be obtained from multiple gestation.

Color Doppler velocimetry in obstetrics

Basic physics

1. Doppler ultrasound provides the ability to detect blood flow using the Doppler shift frequency.
2. The Doppler shift is the difference between the transmitted and received frequencies.
3. Only moving reflectors, such as blood cells or a vessel wall, can produce Doppler shift.
4. Doppler ultrasound equipment is capable of detecting the Doppler shift signal and can distinguish those signals from echoes returning from static interfaces such as soft tissue.
5. Spectral analysis of the Doppler signals provides the ability to display flow waveforms throughout a heart cycle, between systole and diastole.
6. According to displayed spectral analysis, an operator can characterize normal and abnormal arterial and venous flow patterns and determine the direction and velocity characteristics of blood flow.

7. Doppler flow assessment is greatly facilitated by the use of color Doppler imaging, which allows the simultaneous overlayed display of anatomic (gray scale) and flow (color) information.
8. Because a gray scale format is used to display echoes from tissue, colors are assigned to display the flow data.
9. Two basic colors are used to differentiate flow direction.
   a. Blood flow toward the transducer is displayed in red
   b. Blood flowing away from transducer is displayed in blue.
10. Turbulent flow in color Doppler imaging is typically represented as a mosaic pattern with spectral mixture of basic colors.
11. The great advantage of color display is that it permits rapid identification of vascular structures, both large and small, and typically results in reduced examination times.

The use of color Doppler ultrasound in fetal monitoring

1. Using the advanced technologies of pulsed or continuous-wave Doppler ultrasound, we are able to evaluate blood flow on several levels within the fetoplacental unit, obtaining signals from different vessels.
2. Displayed spectral analysis, the so-called sonogram, is available for quantitative and semiquantitative analysis.
3. Doppler waveforms of vessels have been described in a variety of ways, but all are based on the relationship between systole and diastole.
4. Numeric indices of blood flow, obtained from the displayed sonogram, are indicators of vascular resistance in each vessel.
5. They have been developed as useful, but indirect, criteria for the oxygenation of the fetoplacental unit.
6. Perhaps the most simple of these indices to compute are as follows:
   a. Systolic to diastolic ratio [S/D (A/B)]
   b. Resistance index (RI)
   c. Pulsatility index (PI)
7. The vessels studied to estimate fetal well-being and oxygenation include uterine arteries, umbilical arteries, fetal descending aorta, and middle cerebral artery.
   a. Representative artery waveforms for each level of the fetoplacental unit are depicted in Figs. 36-34 through 36-37.
8. During a normal pregnancy, development of a normal placenta includes a secondary wave of trophoblastic invasion into uterine vessels during the early second trimester.
   a. The result is maximal dilation of the spiral arteries that are out of maternal autoregulation.
   b. The placental blood pool is developing into a low-resistance blood flow system with extensive diastolic flow.
   c. Uterine blood flow increases approximately 10-fold from conception to term.
9. During the advance of pregnancy, the amount of diastolic flow increases.
   a. Placental insufficiency causing IUGR and fetal hypoxemia has been found in cases when diastolic flow fails to increase as a pregnancy progresses.

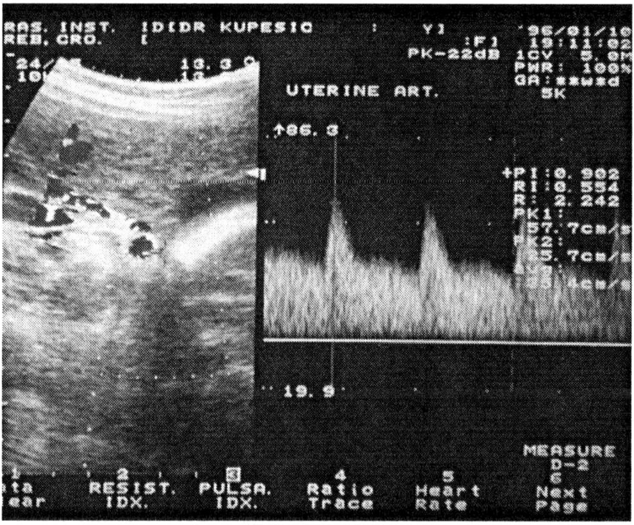

Figure 36-34
Normal sonogram of uterine artery blood flow obtained by color Doppler technique.

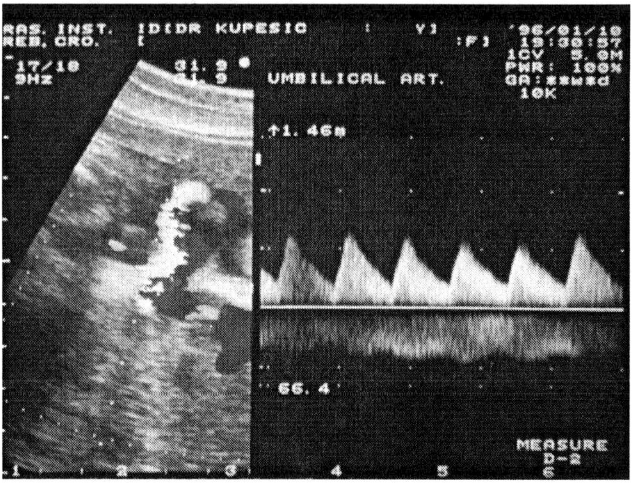

Figure 36-35
Normal sonogram of umbilical artery blood flow obtained by transabdominal color Doppler technique.

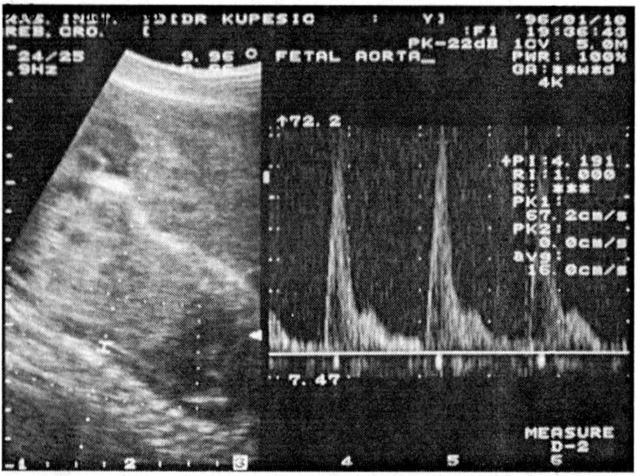

Figure 36-36

Sonogram of aortic blood flow represented with higher resistance index and relatively lower diastolic flow, consecutively.

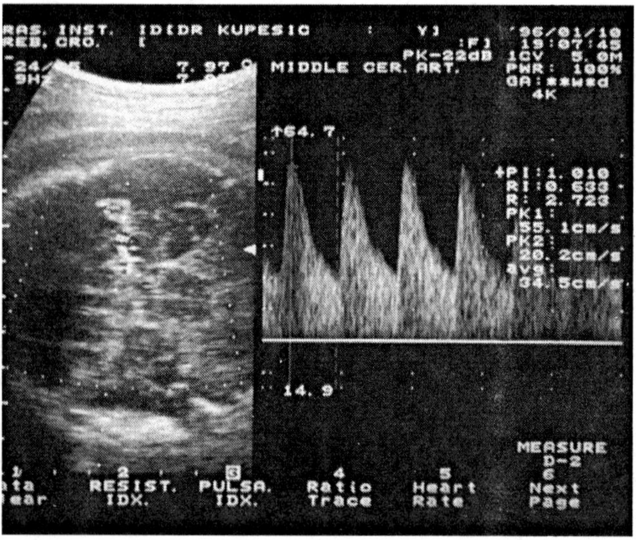

Figure 36-37

Middle cerebral artery depicted at 36 weeks of gestational age, followed by blood flow sonogram.

10. Prenatal color Doppler studies provide the most information in cases with compromised fetal condition.
   a. The main indications for color imaging followed by Doppler measurements during pregnancy are as follows:
      (1) Early pregnancy failure (blood flow changes in uteroplacental circulation because of missed abortion and intrauterine hematomas)
      (2) Pregnancy-induced hypertension, with consecutive maternal, fetal, and placental pathology
      (3) IUGR: changes in the resistance index or pulsatility index in the fetal vessels finally reflect centralization of flow in response to fetal hypoxemia
      (4) Early detection of fetal distress (hypoxia) regardless of its etiology
      (5) Fetal echocardiography: morphologic color-coded examination of cardiac structure and malformations; Doppler evaluation of cardiac output
      (6) Twin-to-twin transfusion syndrome
      (7) Placental circulatory pathology (placenta previa, placenta succenturiata, vasa previa)
      (8) Rh immunization: progressive fetal anemia characterized by an increase in the mean blood velocity in all the fetal vessels investigated
   b. Doppler ultrasound investigation should start as soon as the pathologic condition is recognized.
      (1) The umbilical artery is the vessel of choice, representing the vascular resistance on placental level.
      (2) The investigations of vascular resistance in the fetal descending aorta and arteria cerebri media will indicate the level of fetal compensatory abilities and early signs of blood flow centralization (brain sparing effect) caused by fetal hypoxia.
   c. The values recorded and the index calculated should be compared with charts of standard values for the equipment used, and the gestational age.
   d. Increased peripheral resistance in the umbilical artery and descending aorta is frequently associated with fetal hypoxemia and an abnormal cardiotocographic pattern.
      (1) Consecutive IUGR has been detected 60% to 80% of the time in cases where the umbilical artery waveforms are abnormal.
      (2) In the umbilical circulation, when there is increased resistance in the placental vessels, there is such great back pressure during diastole that forward flow (from fetus to placenta) ceases.
      (3) When placental resistance is most severe, the direction of flow in the umbilical artery may actually be reversed.
      (4) Absence in diastole, reverse diastolic flow, or notching of the waveform at the end of systole are abnormal findings and are clear indicators for intensive fetal surveillance because there is a strong association with fetal death in utero.

e. In other vessels, such as the uterine artery, absent diastolic flow may occur because of vasospasm.
   (1) This is commonly associated with maternal hypertension.
f. Increased blood flow (decreased vascular resistance) in the circle of Willis and middle cerebral artery is found in moderate to severe fetal growth retardation associated with fetal hypoxemia.
   (1) It is the compensatory mechanism of brain sparing when the fetus adjusts to placental insufficiency and shunts more blood to its brain.

Assessment of fetal biophysical profile (BPP)

1. A combination of biophysical variables was first introduced by Manning in 1980. It is a combination of nonstress CTG testing and real-time ultrasonography used to study the dynamic, intrauterine behavior of the fetus.
2. The most important factor in the sensitivity of this testing method is the combination of acute (FHR reactivity, fetal movement, fetal breathing movement, and fetal tone) and chronic (amniotic fluid volume) markers of fetal condition.
3. The variables of BPP are scored either 0 or 2.
4. The maximal score for a BPP is 10, and the minimal score is 0.
5. In general, a score of 6 or more is acceptable.
6. A score of 2 points each is given for each of the following criteria that are met:
   a. Fetal breathing movements: 30 seconds of sustained breathing during a 30-minute observation
   b. Fetal movement: Three or more gross body movements in a 30-minute observation
   c. Fetal tone: At least one episode of motion of a limb from a position of flexion to extension and rapid return to flexion
   d. Fetal reactivity: Two or more FHR accelerations of at least 15 beats per minute (bpm), lasting at least 15 seconds, and associated with fetal movement in a 10 to 20 minute observation
   e. Qualitative amniotic fluid volume: The presence of a pocket of amniotic fluid that measures at least 2 cm in two perpendicular planes with fluid evident throughout the uterine cavity
7. A fetal BPP score of 8 or more is reassuring of fetal well-being; however, a BPP score less than 8 is nonreassuring and repeat testing or delivery is indicated.

Suggested reading

Carrera JM, Di Renzo GC, editors: *Recommendations and protocols for prenatal diagnosis,* pp. 32-35, Report of the European Study Group on Prenatal Diagnosis 1993, EAPM

Chervenak FA, Isaacson GC, Campbell S: *Ultrasound in obstetrics and gynecology,* Boston, 1993, Little, Brown.

Fleischer C, Romero R, Manning FA, et al: *The principles and practice of ultrasonography in obstetrics and gynecology,* ed 4, Norwalk, CT, 1991, Appleton & Lange.

Jurkoviae D, Jeauniaux E: *Ultrasound and early pregnancy,* New York, 1996, Parthenon.
Kurjak A, editor: *Atlas of ultrasonography in obstetrics and gynecology,* Zagreb, 1986, Mladost.
Kurjak A: *Transvaginal color Doppler,* Lancs, NJ, 1991, Parthenon.
Levi S, Hyjazi Y, Schaaps JP, et al: *Sensitivity and specificity of routine ultrasound screening for congenital anomalies by ultrasound,* the Belgian Multicentric study, *Ultrasound Obstet Gynecol* 1:102-110, 1991.
Meisner I, Bar-Ziv J: *In utero diagnosis of skeletal disorders. An atlas of prenatal sonographic and postnatal radiologic correlation,* Boca Raton, FL, 1993, CRC Press.
Roberts NS: Ultrasound in pregnancy. In Beck W, editor: *Obstetrics and gynecology,* ed 3, Philadelphia, 1993, Harwal Publishing, pp. 127-143.
Romero R, Pilu G, Jeanty P, et al: *Prenatal diagnosis of congenital anomalies,* Norwalk, CT, 1988, Appleton & Lange.
Rottem S, Bronshtein M: Transvaginal sonographic diagnosis of congenital anomalies between 9 weeks and 16 weeks menstrual age, *J Clin Ultrasound* 18:307-314, 1990.
Sabbagha R: *Diagnostic ultrasound,* ed 3, Philadelphia, 1994, JB Lippincott.
Timor-Tritsch IE, Peisner DB, Raju S: Sonoembriology: an organ oriented approach using a high frequency vaginal probe, *J Clin Ultrasound* 18:286-289, 1990.

37 Formulary

Tamara S. Evans, Pharm.D., B.C.P.S.

37.1 PREGNANCY RISK CATEGORIES

The Food and Drug Administration has established five categories (A, B, C, D, and X) to indicate a drug's potential for causing birth defects or risks to the fetus. It should be noted that even if placed in the lowest risk category (category A), a drug should not be used in pregnancy unless clearly needed.

Category A: Controlled studies in women fail to demonstrate a risk to the fetus in the first trimester, and the possibility of fetal harm appears remote.
Category B: Animal studies do not demonstrate a fetal risk and there are no controlled studies in pregnant women, or animal studies have shown an adverse effect on the fetus but well-controlled studies in women have failed to demonstrate a risk to the fetus.
Category C: Studies in animals have shown teratogenic or embryocidal effects but there are no controlled studies in women, or studies in women and animals are not available.
Category D: Positive evidence of human fetal risk exists, but the benefits from use in pregnant women may be acceptable despite the risk (e.g., life-threatening situations or serious diseases for which safer drugs cannot be used or are ineffective).
Category X: Studies in animals or humans have demonstrated fetal abnormalities or there is evidence of fetal risk based on human experience or both, and the risk of using the drug clearly outweighs any possible benefit.

37.2 FORMULARY

Acetaminophen (Tylenol, Panadol)

How supplied: Tabs, 80, 160, 325, 500, 650 mg; caps, 500 mg; suppositories, 120, 125, 300, 325, 650 mg; granules, 80 mg; elixir, 130, 160, 325, 500 mg/15 ml; solution, 100 mg/ml, 120 mg/2.5 ml

Indications: For use as an analgesic or antipyretic
Adult dosage: 325 to 650 mg q4-6h; maximum dose, 4 g/day
Contraindications and precautions: Hypersensitivity to acetaminophen, hepatic function impairment, pregnancy category B
Adverse effects: Acetaminophen rarely causes severe toxicity or side effects when used as directed.

Acetaminophen and codeine (Tylenol with Codeine) [T&C]

How supplied: Tabs, T&C No.1 = 7.5 mg codeine + 300 mg APAP, T&C No.2 = 15 mg codeine + 300 mg APAP, T&C No.3 = 30 mg codeine + 300 mg APAP, T&C No.4 = 60 mg codeine + 300 mg APAP; elixir, 12 mg codeine + 120 mg APAP/5 ml.
Indications: Relief of mild to moderate pain
Adult dosage:
- Elixir: 15 ml, PO, q4h prn; not to exceed 4 g APAP/day
- Tabs: 1 to 2 tabs q4-6h prn; not to exceed 4 g APAP/day

Contraindications and precautions: Hypersensitivity to codeine or acetaminophen, pregnancy category C, head injury and increased ICP, acute abdominal conditions, hepatic dysfunction, concomitant use of CNS depressants

Acetaminophen and hydrocodone (Lortab, Co-Gesic, Vicodin)

How supplied: Tabs, Vicodin, Co-Gesic, Lortab 5/500 = 5 mg hydrocodone + 500 mg APAP; solution, 2.5 mg hydrocodone + 120 mg APAP/5 ml
Indications: Relief of moderate to severe pain
Adult dosage: One tab or 5 ml; PO, q4-6h prn; maximum dose, 4 g APAP/day
Contraindications and precautions: Hypersensitivity to hydrocodone or acetaminophen, pregnancy category C, head injury and increased intracranial pressure (ICP), acute abdominal conditions, hepatic dysfunction, concomitant use of central nervous system (CNS) depressants

Acetaminophen and oxycodone (Tylox, Percocet)

How supplied: Tabs, Percocet = 5 mg oxycodone + 325 mg APAP, Tylox = 5 mg oxycodone + 500 mg APAP; solution, 5 mg oxycodone + 325 mg APAP/5 ml.
Indications: Relief of moderate to severe pain
Adult dosage: 1 tab or 5 ml, PO, q6h prn; maximum dose, 4 g APAP/day.
Contraindications and precautions: Hypersensitivity to oxycodone or acetaminophen, pregnancy category C, head injury and increased ICP, acute abdominal conditions, hepatic dysfunction, concomitant use of CNS depressants

Acetaminophen and propoxyphene (Darvocet, Propacet, Wygesic)

How supplied: Tabs, Darvocet-N 50 = 50 mg propoxyphene + 325 mg APAP, Darvocet-N 100 and Propacet 100 = 100 mg propoxyphene + 650 mg APAP, Wygesic = 65 mg propoxyphene + 650 mg APAP.

Indications: Relief of mild to moderate pain
Adult dosage: 1 to 2 tablets, PO, q4-6h prn; not to exceed 4 g APAP/day
Contraindications and precautions: Reducing total daily dosage should be considered in hepatic or renal impairment; alcohol and other sedative or drowsiness-producing drugs should be avoided; pregnancy category C.

Acetylsalicylic acid, Aspirin, ASA

How supplied: Tabs, 81, 165, 227.5, 325, 500, 650, 975 mg; suppositories, 120, 200, 300, 600 mg
Indications: Mild to moderate pain; fever; various inflammatory conditions such as rheumatic fever, rheumatoid arthritis, and osteoarthritis
Unlabeled uses: Low-dose aspirin may be useful in preventing toxemia of pregnancy.
Adult dosage
- Prevention of preeclampsia in high-risk patients: 60 to 150 mg qd beginning at 28 to 30 weeks of gestation
- Minor aches and pains: 325 to 650 mg q4h prn
- Arthritis and other rheumatic conditions: 3.2 to 6 g/day in divided doses

Contraindications and precautions: Hypersensitivity to salicylates or nonsteroidal antiinflammatory drugs; risks associated with long-term aspirin use in pregnancy include maternal antepartum and postpartum bleeding, prolonged gestation, prolonged labor, neonatal bleeding, premature closure of the ductus arteriosus, and neonatal pulmonary hypertension.
Adverse effects: Nausea, dyspepsia, heartburn, hives, rash, angioedema, tinnitus, reversible hepatic dysfunction, prolongation of bleeding time, thrombocytopenia, bronchospasm, and anaphylaxis

Acyclovir (Zovirax)

How supplied: Tabs, 200, 800 mg; suspension, 200 mg/5 ml; injection, 500 mg/10 ml vial; ointment, 5%
Indications: Treatment of initial and recurrent HSV-1, HSV-2, and varicella–zoster infections
Adult dosage
- Initial genital herpes: 200 mg, PO, q4h five times daily × 10 days
- Chronic suppressive therapy for recurrent disease: 400 mg, PO, bid for up to 12 months
- Intermittent therapy: 200 mg, PO, q4h five times daily × 5 days. Therapy should be initiated at the earliest sign or symptom of recurrence.
- Genital or mucocutaneous herpes (ointment): Applied to affected areas q3h six times daily × 7 days; a finger cot or rubber glove is used to prevent spread of infection.
- Acute treatment of herpes zoster: 800 mg, PO, q4h five times daily × 7 to 10 days
- Herpes simplex infections in immunocompromised patients: 5 mg/kg, IV, q8h × 7 days
- Severe initial clinical episodes of herpes genitalis: 5 mg/kg, IV, q8h × 5 days
- Varicella–zoster infections in immunocompromised patients: 10 mg/kg, IV, q8h × 7 days
- Herpes simplex encephalitis: 10 mg/kg, IV, q8h × 10 days

Elimination: Renal excretion; dosage should be adjusted in renal impairment.

Contraindications and precautions: Hypersensitivity to acyclovir or any component of the formulation; pregnancy category C

Adverse effects: Transient elevations of serum creatinine or blood urea nitrogen (BUN), nausea, vomiting, itching, rash, hives, transaminase elevations, lethargy

Amantadine (Symmetrel)

How supplied: Caps, 100 mg; syrup, 50 mg/5 ml

Indications and adult dosage

- Prophylaxis and treatment of influenza A: 200 mg qd or 100 mg bid
- Parkinson's disease: 100 mg/day initially, may be increased gradually to a maximum of 400 mg/day in divided doses.
- Drug-induced extrapyramidal reactions: 100 mg bid; may be increased to 300 mg/day in divided doses.

Elimination: Excreted in the urine; dose should be adjusted in renal impairment.

Contraindications and precautions: Pregnancy category C

Adverse effects: Nausea, dizziness, light-headedness, and insomnia

Amikacin (Amikin)

How supplied: Injection, 50 mg/ml, 250 mg/ml

Indications: Reserved for the treatment of microorganisms resistant to other antibiotics; particularly useful in hospitals with a high incidence of gentamicin-resistant or tobramycin-resistant gram negative organisms (see Appendix XI).

Adult dosage (IV/IM)

- Loading dose: 7.5 mg/kg
- Maintenance dose: 5 mg/kg q8h or 7.5 mg/kg q12h or dose adjustment based on patient's calculated creatinine clearance (Cr Cl).

$$\text{Cr Cl} = \frac{(140 - \text{age})(\text{ideal body weight})}{72 \times \text{serum creatinine}} \times 0.85 \text{ for females}$$

Cr Cl (ml/min)	Percentage of loading dose
70	88 q12h
50	79 q12h
25	81 q24-36h
10	60 q48h

- After 24 hours of therapy a serum peak level should be obtained 30 minutes after IV administration of the drug (60 minutes after IM administration) and a trough level just before the next dose: Therapeutic peak concentration is 20 to 30 μg/ml, therapeutic trough concentration is <5 μg/ml; serum creatinine should be monitored qd to qod while the patient is receiving amikacin.

Elimination: Excreted by glomerular filtration; dosage should be adjusted in renal impairment and based on serum concentrations.

Contraindications and precautions: Pregnancy category D; hypersensitivity to aminoglycosides; use with other nephrotoxic agents should be avoided.

Adverse effects: Renal toxicity characterized by decreased Cr Cl, cells or casts in the urine, decreased urine specific gravity, or increasing BUN or serum creatinine; ototoxicity manifested as both auditory and vestibular toxicity; neuromuscular blockade

Amoxicillin (Amoxil, Biomox, Polymox, Trimox)

How supplied: Tabs, 125, 250 mg; caps, 250, 500 mg; oral suspension, 50 mg/ml, 125 mg/5 ml, 250 mg/5 ml

Indications: Treatment and prophylaxis of infections caused by susceptible microorganisms (see Appendix XI)

Adult dosage

- *Chlamydia trachomatis* (alternative in pregnancy): 500 mg, PO, tid × 7 to 10 days
- Respiratory, genitounary (GU) tract, skin, and soft tissue infections: 250 to 500 mg, PO, tid

Contraindications and precautions: Hypersensitivity to any penicillin (PCN)

Amoxicillin/Clavulanate (Augmentin)

How supplied: Tabs, 250, 500 mg; chewable tabs, 125, 250 mg; oral suspension, 125, 250 mg/5 ml

Indications: Treatment of infections caused by susceptible microorganisms including β-lactamase-producing strains (see Appendix XI)

Adult dosage

- Chancroid (alternative regimen): 500 mg, PO, tid × 7 days
- Usual treatment regimens: 250 to 500 mg, PO, tid

Contraindications and precautions: Hypersensitivity to any PCN

Ampicillin (Omnipen, Polycillin, Principen)

How supplied: Caps, 250, 500 mg; oral suspension, 100 mg/ml, 125 mg/5 ml, 250 mg/5 ml, 500 mg/5 ml; injection, 125, 250, 500 mg, 1, 2 g

Indications: Treatment of infections caused by susceptible microorganisms (see Appendix XI)

Adult dosage

- Respiratory tract and soft tissue infections
  1. PO: 250 to 500 mg q6h
  2. IM/IV: 500 to 1000 mg q6h
- Bacterial meningitis or septicemia: 1 to 2 g, IV, q4-6h

Elimination: Excreted by kidneys; dosage should be adjusted in renal impairment.

Contraindications and precautions: Hypersensitivity to any PCN

Adverse effects: Maculopapular rash, pruritus, urticaria, nausea, vomiting, diarrhea, eosinophilia.

Patient information: Patient should take oral ampicillin on an empty stomach 1 hour before or 2 hours after meals.

Ampicillin and sulbactam (Unasyn)

How supplied: Injection, 1.5 g (1 g ampicillin + 0.5 g sulbactam), 3.0 g (2 g ampicillin + 1 g sulbactam)

Indications: Treatment of infections caused by susceptible microorganisms. Especially useful for treating intra-abdominal or gynecologic infections caused by β-lactamase-producing strains of *Staphylococcus aureus, Escherichia coli,* and *Bacteroides* (including *B. fragilis*) (see Appendix XI).
Adult dosage: 1.5 to 3 g, IV/IM,q6h; not to exceed 4 g/day sulbactam
Elimination: Excreted by kidneys; dosage should be adjusted in renal impairment.
Contraindications and precautions: Hypersensitivity to any PCN
Adverse effects: Pain at injection site, thrombophlebitis, diarrhea, rash, nausea, and vomiting

Atenolol (Tenormin)

How supplied: Tabs, 25, 50, 100 mg; injection, 5 mg/10 ml
Actions: Beta-adrenergic blocker
Indications: Hypertension; angina pectoris; acute myocardial infarction (MI)
Adult dosage

- Oral: 50 to 100 mg qd
- IV (acute MI): 5 mg IV over 5 minutes followed by 5 mg, IV, 10 minutes later

Contraindications and precautions: Sinus bradycardia; pregnancy category C (use should be avoided during the first trimester; lowest possible dose should be used).
Adverse effects: Bradycardia, hypotension, dizziness, fatigue, nausea, vomiting, and diarrhea

Azithromycin (Zithromax)

How supplied: Caps, 250 mg
Indications: Treatment of individuals ≥16 years old with infections caused by susceptible microorganisms (see Appendix XI)
Adult dosage

- *Chlamydia trachomatis* (urethritis, cervicitis, conjunctivitis, or proctitis): 1 g orally as a single dose
- Chancroid: 1 g orally as a single dose
- Chronic obstructive pulmonary disease (COPD), pneumonia, pharyngitis or tonsillitis, and uncomplicated skin infections: 500 mg as a single dose on the first day followed by 250 mg qd on days 2 through 5 for a 1.5-g total dose

Elimination: Primarily excreted unchanged in bile.
Contraindications and precautions: Pregnancy category B; hypersensitivity to azithromycin, erythromycin, or any macrolide antibiotic
Adverse effects: Nausea, vomiting, diarrhea, and elevated liver function tests
Interactions: Patients receiving concomitant theophylline or warfarin should be monitored.
Patient information: This medication should be taken at least 1 hour before a meal or at least 2 hours after a meal; not to be taken with aluminum-containing and magnesium-containing antacids.

Aztreonam (Azactam)

How supplied: Injection, 500 mg, 1 g, 2 g
Indications: Treatment of infections caused by susceptible gram negative microorganisms (see Appendix XI)

Adult dosage (IM/IV)
- Urinary tract infection: 500 mg to 1 g q8-12h
- Moderately severe systemic infections: 1 to 2 g q8-12h
- Severe systemic or life-threatening infections: 2 g q6-8h (maximum dose 8 g/day)

Elimination: Excreted by kidneys; dosage should be adjusted in renal impairment.

Contraindications and precautions: Hypersensitivity to aztreonam; pregnancy category B; patients who have had anaphylactic or urticarial reactions to penicillins or cephalosporins should be monitored carefully.

Adverse effects: Phlebitis, rash, nausea, vomiting, diarrhea, and liver enzyme elevations

Benzquinamide (Emete-Con)

How supplied: Injection, 50 mg/vial

Indications: Prevention and treatment of nausea and vomiting associated with anesthesia and surgery; prophylactic use should be restricted to those patients in whom emesis would endanger the surgical outcome or result in harm to the patient.

Adult dosage
- IM: 50 mg (0.5 to 1 mg/kg). First dose should be repeated in 1 hour, then q3-4h prn; to prevent nausea and vomiting, should be given IM at least 15 minutes before emergence from anesthesia.
- IV: 25 mg (0.2 to 0.4 mg/kg as a single dose) slowly; subsequent doses should be IM.

Contraindications and precautions: Safety for use during pregnancy has not been established; sudden increase in blood pressure (BP) and transient arrhythmias have occurred following IV administration.

Adverse effects: Drowsiness, dry mouth, shivering, sweating, hypertension, and arrhythmias

Bromocriptine (Parlodel)

How supplied: Tabs, 2.5 mg; caps, 5 mg

Indications and adult dosage
- Hyperprolactinemia-associated dysfunctions: Initially, 1.25 to 2.5 mg qd with meals; 2.5 mg may be added as tolerated q3-7d until optimal therapeutic response is achieved (usually 5 to 7.5 mg per day).
- Prevention of physiologic lactation: 2.5 mg bid × 14 days; treatment should not be started sooner than 4 hours after delivery.
- Parkinsonism: Initial dose is 1.25 mg bid; may be increased q2wk by 2.5 mg/day.
- Acromegaly: 1.25 to 2.5 mg qhs for initial 3 days; increase by 1.25 to 2.5 mg as tolerated every 3 to 7 days.

Contraindications and precautions: Not to be used in pregnancy

Adverse effects: Nausea, vomiting, anorexia, headache, dizziness, drowsiness, and hypotension.

Buprenorphine (Buprenex)

How supplied: Injection, 0.324 mg (equivalent to 0.3 mg buprenorphine)/ml

Indications: Relief of moderate to severe pain

Adult dosage: 0.3 mg, IM or slow IV, q6h prn. If required, may be repeated once up to 0.3 mg, 30 to 60 minutes after initial dose.

Contraindications and precautions: Hypersensitivity to buprenorphine, pregnancy category C, head injury and increased ICP, hepatic function impairment, respiratory depression, dizziness or drowsiness

Butoconazole (Femstat)

How supplied: Vaginal cream, 2%

Indications: Local treatment of vulvovaginal candidiasis

Adult dosage

- Pregnant patients (second and third trimesters only): one applicator full (5 g) intravaginally qhs × 6 days
- Nonpregnant patients: one applicator full (5 g) intravaginally qhs × 3 days; may repeat × 3 days, if necessary.

Butorphanol (Stadol)

How supplied: Injection, 1, 2 mg/ml; nasal spray, 10 mg/ml

Indications

- Parenteral and nasal: Management of pain, including postoperative analgesia
- Parenteral: For preoperative or preanesthetic medication, to supplement balanced anesthesia, for relief of pain during labor

Adult dosage

- Pain
  1. IV: 0.5 to 2 mg q3-4h prn
  2. IM: 1 to 4 mg q3-4h prn; not to exceed single doses of 4 mg.
  3. Nasal: 1 mg (one spray in one nostril). An additional 1-mg dose may be given within 60 to 90 minutes if adequate pain relief is not achieved. The initial two-dose sequence may be repeated in 3 to 4 hours prn.
- Preoperative or preanesthetic use: Usual dose is 2 mg, IM, 60 to 90 minutes before surgery.
- Balanced anesthesia: 2 mg IV shortly before induction or 0.5 to 1 mg IV in increments during anesthesia
- Labor: 1 to 2 mg IV/IM in full-term patients in early labor; repeated after 4 hours

Contraindications and precautions: Hypersensitivity to butorphanol, pregnancy category C, head injury and increased ICP, renal or hepatic function impairment, respiratory depression

Adverse effects: Nausea, vomiting, hypotension, dry mouth, and somnolence

Calcium carbonate (Os-Cal, Os-Cal + D)

How supplied: Os-Cal 250 = 625 mg calcium carbonate (each tab contains 250 mg of elemental calcium); Os-Cal 500 = 1250 mg calcium carbonate (each tab contains 500 mg of elemental calcium); + D products provide additional 125 USP units of vitamin D; Os-Cal Fortified tablets and Os-Cal Plus tablets = 250 mg elemental calcium plus vitamins and minerals.

Indications: Calcium replacement therapy

Adult dosage: 500 mg to 2 g bid-qid

Contraindications and precautions: Renal caculi, hypophosphatemia, hypercalcemia, and vitamin D intoxication

Captopril (Capoten)

How supplied: Tabs, 12.5, 25, 50, 100 mg
Actions: ACE inhibitor
Indications: Hypertension, heart failure
Adult dosage

- Hypertension: Initially, 25 mg, PO, bid to tid; maintenance dose is 25 to 150 mg bid to tid; not to exceed a daily dose of 450 mg.
- Heart failure: Initially, 6.25 to 12.5 mg tid; may be increased as tolerated; not to exceed a daily dose of 450 mg.

Contraindications and precautions: Use during pregnancy should be avoided because of fetal and neonatal associated morbidities and mortalities; bilateral or unilateral renal artery stenosis; electrolytes should be monitored.

Adverse effects: Rash, cough, hyperkalemia, proteinuria, nausea, vomiting, and dysgeusia

Carbenicillin (Geocillin)

How supplied: Tabs, 382 mg
Indications: The treatment of acute and chronic urinary tract infections in asymptomatic bacteriuria caused by susceptible microorganisms (see Appendix XI).
Adult dosage: 382 to 764 mg, PO, qid
Elimination: Excreted by kidneys; dosage should be adjusted in renal impairment.
Contraindications, precautions and adverse effects: See Penicillin.

Carboprost tromethamine (Hemabate)

How supplied: Injection, 250 μg carboprost and 83 μg tromethamine per ml
Indications: For the termination of pregnancy between 13 and 20 gestational weeks as calculated from the first day of the last normal menstrual period; postpartum hemorrhage caused by uterine atony, which has not responded to conventional management (prior treatment should include use of IV oxytocin, manipulative techniques such as uterine massage and, unless contraindicated, IM ergot preparations)
Adult dosage

- Abortion: For IM use only. Initial dose 250 μg (1 ml) by deep IM injection. Subsequent doses of 250 μg at 1.5- to 3.5-hour intervals, depending on uterine response. Dose may be increased to 500 μg if uterine contractility is inadequate after several 250-μg doses. Not to exceed a 12-mg total dose or continuous administration for >2 days.
- Refractory postpartum uterine bleeding: Initial dose 250 μg by deep IM injection. In some cases, multiple dosing at 15- to 90-minute intervals may be necessary for successful outcome. Not to exceed a total dose of 2 mg (eight doses).

Contraindications and precautions: Hypersensitivity to any of these agents; acute pelvic inflammatory disease; active cardiac, pulmonary, renal or hepatic disease. To be used cautiously in patients with a history of asthma, hypotension, or hypertension; cardiovascular, adrenal, renal, or hepatic disease; anemia; jaundice; diabetes; epilepsy; or a scarred uterus.

Adverse effects: Nausea, vomiting, diarrhea, headache, flushing, anxiety or tension, hot flashes, arrhythmias, and dyspnea or wheezing

Cefaclor (Ceclor)

How supplied: Caps, 250, 500 mg; oral suspension, 125, 187, 250, 375 mg/5 ml

Indications: Treatment of infections caused by susceptible microorganisms (see Appendix XI)

Adult dosage: 250 to 500 mg, PO, q8h

Elimination: Excreted by kidneys; dosage should be adjusted in renal impairment.

Contraindications and precautions: Hypersensitivity to cephalosporins, pregnancy category B

Adverse effects: See Cephalexin.

Cefadroxil (Duricef, Ultracef)

How supplied: Caps, 500 mg; tabs, 1 g; oral suspension, 125, 250, 500 mg/5 ml

Indications: Treatment of infections caused by susceptible microorganisms (see Appendix XI)

Adult dosage: 500 mg to 1 g, PO, q12h (maximum dose 2 g/day)

Elimination: Excreted by kidneys; dosage should be adjusted in renal impairment.

Contraindications and precautions: Hypersensitivity to cephalosporins, pregnancy category B

Adverse effects: See Cephalexin.

Cefamandole (Mandol)

How supplied: Injection, 500 mg, 1 g, 2 g

Indications: Treatment of infections caused by susceptible microorganisms (see Appendix XI)

Adult dosage: 500 mg to 2 g, IV/IM, q4-8h (maximum dose 12 g/day)

Elimination: Excreted by kidneys; dosage should be adjusted in renal impairment.

Contraindications and precautions: Hypersensitivity to cephalosporins, pregnancy category B

Adverse effects: See cefotetan; vitamin K reversible coagulopathy, disulfiram-like reaction with alcohol ingestion

Cefazolin (Ancef, Kefzol)

How supplied: Injection, 250 mg, 500 mg, 1 g

Indications: Treatment of infections caused by susceptible microorganisms and for surgical prophylaxis (see Appendix XI)

Adult dosage

- Treatment of infections: 250 mg to 2 g, IV/IM, q8h (maximum dose 12 g/day)
- Surgical prophylaxis: 1 g, IV/IM, 30 to 60 minutes before surgery (vaginal or abdominal hysterectomy; cesarean section, second-trimester abortion). Postoperative doses of prophylactic drugs are generally unnecessary but may continue cefazolin, 500 mg to 1 g, IV/IM, q6-8h $\times$ 24 hours.

Elimination: Excreted by kidneys; dosage should be adjusted in renal impairment.
Contraindications and precautions: Hypersensitivity to cephalosporins, pregnancy category B
Adverse effects: Nausea, vomiting, diarrhea, local phlebitis at injection site, eosinophilia, and elevation in liver enzymes

Cefepime (Maxipime)

How supplied: Injection, 1 g, 2 g
Indications: A fourth-generation cephalosporin used for the treatment of susceptible gram positive and gram negative microorganisms (see Appendix XI)
Adult dosage: 500 mg to 2 g, IV/IM, q8-12h
Elimination: Excreted by kidneys; dosage should be adjusted in renal impairment.
Contraindications and precautions: Hypersensitivity to cephalosporins
Adverse effects: Headache, nausea, rash, and diarrhea

Cefixime (Suprax)

How supplied: Tabs, 200, 400 mg; oral suspension, 100 mg/5 ml
Indications: Treatment of infections caused by susceptible microorganisms (see Appendix XI)
Adult dosage: 200 mg q12h or 400 mg single dose for uncomplicated gonorrhea (limited data on effectiveness for pharyngeal infection)
Elimination: Excreted by kidneys; dosage should be adjusted in renal impairment.
Adverse effects: See Cephalexin.

Cefonicid (Monocid)

How supplied: Injection, 500 mg, 1 g
Indications: Treatment of infections caused by susceptible microorganisms and for surgical prophylaxis (see Appendix XI)
Adult dosage
- Treatment of infections: 1 g, IV/IM, q24h (maximum 2 g/day)
- Prophylaxis: Single 1-g dose 60 minutes before surgery (or after umbilical cord is clamped in cesarean section)

Elimination: Excreted by kidneys; dosage should be adjusted in renal impairment.
Contraindications and precautions: Hypersensitivity to cephalosporins, pregnancy category B
Adverse effects: See Cefotetan.

Cefoperazone (Cefobid)

How supplied: Injection, 1 g, 2 g
Indications: Treatment of infections caused by susceptible microorganisms (see Appendix XI)
Adult dosage: 1 to 2 g, IV/IM, q12h (doses of 6 to 12 g daily have been used)
Elimination: Excreted extensively in bile; accumulation may occur in patients with hepatic disease or biliary obstruction; no dosage adjustment required in renal impairment.

Contraindications and precautions: Hypersensitivity to cephalosporins; pregnancy category B
Adverse effects: See Cefamandole.

Cefotaxime (Claforan)

How supplied: Injection, 1, 2 g
Indications: Treatment of infections caused by susceptible microorganisms and for surgical prophylaxis (see table)
Adult dosage
- Treatment of infection: 1 to 2 g, IV/IM, q4-12h (maximum dose 12 g/day).
- Uncomplicated gonorrhea: Single dose 500 mg IM
- Disseminated gonococcal infection: 1 g, IV, q8h for 2 to 3 days or until improved, followed by cefixime 400 mg, PO, bid or ciprofloxacin, 500 mg, PO, bid to complete 7 to 10 days total therapy
- Surgical prophylaxis: 1 g, IV/IM, 30 to 90 minutes before surgery
- Cesarean section: 1 g, IV, as soon as the umbilical cord is clamped then 1 g, IV/IM, at 6 and 12 hours later

Elimination: Excreted by kidneys; dosage should be adjusted in renal impairment.
Contraindications and precautions: Hypersensitivity to cephalosporins, pregnancy category B
Adverse effects: See Cefazolin.

Cefotetan (Cefotan)

How supplied: Injection, 1, 2 g
Indications: Management of intraabdominal and gynecologic infections caused by susceptible gram positive cocci and gram negative rods; especially useful for treatment of certain anaerobic and mixed aerobic–anaerobic infections; prophylaxis for postoperative infection following gastrointestinal (GI), obstetric, and gynecologic surgical procedures. Active against *Bacteroides fragilis* but not the DOT group of *Bacteroides,* which occur in pelvic infections (see Appendix XI).
Adult dosage
- Treatment of infections: 500 mg to 2 g, IV/IM, q12h to maximum of 6 g/day.
- Uncomplicated gonorrhea: Single 1-g IM dose.
- Pelvic inflammatory disease (PID) (inpatient): 2 g, IV, q12h × 48 hours or until substantial clinical improvement is demonstrated plus doxycycline, 100 mg, IV/PO, q12h × 14 days total
- Prophylactic use, surgery: To prevent postoperative infection in clean contaminated or potentially contaminated surgery, a single 1- or 2-g IV dose is administered 30 to 60 minutes before surgery.
- Prophylactic use, cesarean section: 1 or 2 g IV as soon as the umbilical cord is clamped

Elimination: Excreted by kidneys; dosage should be adjusted in renal impairment.
Contraindications and precautions: Hypersensitivity to cephalosporins, pregnancy category B
Adverse effects: Most frequently, nausea or diarrhea; local phlebitis at injection site, rash, pruritus, fever, eosinophilia, and elevation in liver enzymes

Cefoxitin (Mefoxin)

How supplied: Injection, 1, 2 g

Indications: Treatment of infections caused by susceptible microorganisms and for surgical prophylaxis; active vs. DOT group of *Bacteroides* (see Appendix XI)

Adult dosage:

- Treatment of infections: 1 to 2 g, IV/IM, q6-8h to maximum of 12 g/day
- Uncomplicated gonorrhea: 2 g, IM, in a single dose
- PID
  1. Inpatient: 2 g, IV, q6h × 48 hours or until substantial clinical improvement is demonstrated plus doxycycline 100 mg, IV/PO, q12h × 14 days total
  2. Outpatient: 2 g IM + probenecid, 1 g, PO, in a single dose concurrently plus doxycycline, 100 mg, PO, q12h × 14 days
- Prophylactic use, surgery: For contaminated or potentially contaminated surgeries, 2 g, IV/IM, 30 to 60 minutes before surgery followed by 2 g q6h after the first dose for no more than 24 hours.
- Prophylactic use, cesarean section: 2 g IV as soon as the umbilical cord is clamped. The second and third 2-g doses are given IV, 4 and 8 hours after the first dose if a three-dose regimen is used.

Elimination: Excreted by kidneys; dosage should be adjusted in renal impairment.

Contraindications and precautions: Hypersensitivity to cephalosporins, pregnancy category B

Adverse effects: See Cefotetan.

Cefpodoxime (Vantin)

How supplied: Tabs, 100, 200 mg; oral suspension, 50, 100 mg/5 ml

Indications: Treatment of infections caused by susceptible microorganisms (see Appendix XI)

Adult dosage: 100 to 400 mg q12h (maximum dose 800 mg/day) *or* single 200-mg dose in uncomplicated gonorrhea and rectal gonococcal infections (no efficacy in pharyngeal gonococcal infections)

Elimination: Excreted by kidneys; dosage should be adjusted in renal impairment.

Contraindications and precautions: Hypersensitivity to cephalosporins, pregnancy category B

Adverse effects: See Cephalexin.

Ceftazidime (Fortaz, Tazicef, Tazidime)

How supplied: Injection, 500 mg, 1 g, 2 g

Indications: Treatment of infections caused by susceptible microorganisms, including activity against *Pseudomonas aeruginosa* (see Appendix XI)

Adult dosage: 1 to 2 g, IV/IM, q8-12h (maximum dose 6 g/day)

Elimination: Excreted by kidneys; dosage should be adjusted in renal impairment.

Contraindications and precautions: Hypersensitivity to cephalosporins, pregnancy category B

Adverse effects: See Cefazolin.

Ceftizoxime (Cefizox)

How supplied: Injection, 500 mg, 1 g, 2 g

Indications: Treatment of infections caused by susceptible microorganisms (see Appendix XI)

Adult dosage

- Treatment of infection: 500 mg to 2 g, IV/IM, q8-12h (maximum dose 12 g/day)
- Uncomplicated gonorrhea (anal or genital): Single dose 500 mg IM
- Disseminated gonococcal infection: See Cefotaxime.

Elimination: Excreted by kidneys; dosage should be adjusted in renal impairment.

Contraindications and precautions: Hypersensitivity to cephalosporins, pregnancy category B

Adverse effects: See Cefazolin.

Ceftriaxone (Rocephin)

How supplied: Injection, 250 mg, 500 mg, 1 g, 2 g

Indications: Treatment of infections caused by susceptible microorganisms (see Appendix XI)

Adult dosage: 1 to 2 g, IV/IM, q12-24h (maximum dose 4 g/day)

- Chancroid (*Hemophilus ducreyi* infection): Single dose 250 mg IM
- Gonococcal infections
  1. Uncomplicated urethral, cervical, rectal, or pharyngeal: 125 mg IM in a single dose
  2. Dessiminated: 1 g, IV/IM, q24h × 2 to 3 days or until improved, followed by cefixime, 400 mg, PO, bid or ciprofloxacin, 500 mg, PO, bid to complete 7 to 10 days total.
  3. Ophthalmia: 1 g IM once, plus saline irrigation.
  4. Neonatal ophthalmia: 25 to 50 mg/kg, IV/IM, in a single dose, not to exceed 125 mg
- PID (outpatient): 250 mg, IM, once plus doxycycline, 100 mg, PO, bid × 14 days

Elimination: Both renal elimination and biliary secretion; no dosage adjustment required in renal impairment.

Contraindications and precautions: Hypersensitivity to cephalosorins, pregnancy category B

Adverse effects: See Cefazolin.

Cefuroxime (Ceftin, Kefurox, Zinacef)

How supplied: Tabs, 125, 250, 500 mg; injection, 750 mg, 1.5 g

Indications: Treatment of infections caused by susceptible microorganisms (see Appendix XI)

Adult dosage

- Oral: 125 to 500 mg q12h or a single 1-g dose in uncomplicated gonorrhea (no efficacy in pharyngeal)
- Parenteral: 750 mg to 1.5 g, IV/IM, q8h (maximum dose 9 g/day)

Elimination: Excreted by kidneys; dosage should be adjusted in renal impairment.

Contraindications and precautions: Hypersensitivity to cephalosporins, pregnancy category B

Adverse effects: See Cefotetan.

Cephalexin (Keflex, Keflet, Keftab)

How supplied: Caps, 250, 500 mg; tabs, 250 mg, 500 mg, 1 g; suspension, 100 mg/ml, 125 mg/5 ml, 250 mg/5 ml

Indications: Treatment of infections caused by susceptible microorganisms (see Appendix XI)

Adult dosage: 250 mg to 1 g, PO, q6h depending on severity of infection. If dose is >4 g/day, parenteral drugs should be used.

Elimination: Excreted by kidneys; dosage should be adjusted in renal impairment.

Contraindications and precautions: Hypersensitivity to cephalosporins, pregnancy category B

Adverse effects: Nausea, vomiting, diarrhea, eosinophilia, and elevation in liver enzymes

Cephalothin (Keflin)

How supplied: Injection, 1, 2 g

Indications: Treatment of infections caused by susceptible microorganisms (see Appendix XI)

Adult dosage: 500 mg to 2 g, IM/IV, q4-6h (maximum dose 12 g/day)

Elimination: Excreted by kidneys; dosage should be adjusted in renal impairment.

Contraindications and precautions: Hypersensitivity to cephalosporins, pregnancy category B

Adverse effects: See Cefazolin.

Cephapirin (Cefadyl)

How supplied: Injection, 500 mg, 1 g, 2 g

Indications: Treatment of infections caused by susceptible microorganisms (see Appendix XI)

Adult dosage: 500 mg to 2 g, IV/IM, q4-6h (maximum dose 12 g/day).

Elimination: Excreted by kidneys; dosage should be adjusted in renal impairment.

Contraindications and precautions: Hypersensitivity to cephalosporins, pregnancy category B

Adverse effects: See Cefazolin.

Cephradine (Velosef)

How supplied: Caps, 250, 500 mg; oral suspension, 125, 250 mg/5 ml; injection, 250 mg, 500 mg, 1 g, 2 g

Indications: Treatment of infections caused by susceptible microorganisms (see Appendix XI)

Adult dosage: 250 mg to 1 g q6h

Elimination: Excreted by kidneys; dosage should be adjusted in renal impairment.

Contraindications and precautions: Hypersensitivity to cephalosporins, pregnancy category B

Adverse effects: See Cefazolin.

Chloramphenicol (Chloromycetin)

How supplied: Caps, 250 mg; oral suspension, 150 mg/5 ml; injection, 100 mg/ml

Indications: Treatment of serious infections in which less potentially dangerous drugs are ineffective or contraindicated (see Appendix XI)
Adult dosage: 50 mg/kg/day in divided doses q6h (maximum 100 mg/kg/day or 4 g/day). To be administered IV only in severe, life-threatening infections (ineffective when given IM) and switched to PO as soon as clinically possible.
Elimination: Metabolized in liver to inactive metabolite; dosage should be adjusted in patients with impaired hepatic function.
Contraindications and precautions: History of hypersensitivity to, or toxicity from, chloramphenicol. Should be monitored with baseline and serial hematologic studies; concomitant therapy with other potential bone marrow depressant agents should be avoided. Use during pregnancy at term or during labor and use during lactation should be avoided.
Adverse effects: Aplastic anemia, thrombocytopenia, granulocytopenia, nausea, vomiting, diarrhea, fever, rash, and gray baby syndrome

Chlorotrianisene (Tace)

How supplied: Caps, 12, 25 mg
Action: Estrogen
Adult dosage

- Moderate to severe vasomotor symptoms associated with menopause: 12 to 25 mg/day given cyclically × 30 days
- Atrophic vaginitis and kraurosis vulvae: 12 to 25 mg/day cyclically × 30 to 60 days
- Female hypogonadism: 12 to 25 mg/day given cyclically × 21 days
- Postpartum breast engorgement: 12 mg, PO, qid × 7 days or 50 mg, PO, q6h × six doses; first dose to be given within 8 hours after delivery.
- **Contraindications and adverse effects:** See Estrogenic substances, conjugated.

Chlorpromazine (Thorazine)

How supplied: Tabs, 10, 25, 50, 100, 200 mg; sustained release (SR) caps, 30, 75, 150, 200, 300 mg; syrup, 10 mg/5 ml, 30 mg/ml, 100 mg/ml; suppositories, 25, 100 mg; injection, 25 mg/ml
Indications: Management of psychotic disorders, control of nausea and vomiting and relief of intractable hiccoughs
Adult dosage

- Psychosis: 10 to 25 mg, PO, tid; may be increased by 20 to 50 mg semiweekly until patient becomes calm and cooperative.
- Nausea or vomiting
  1. Oral: 10 to 25 mg q4-6h prn; may be increased if necessary.
  2. Rectal: 50 to 100 mg q6-8h prn
  3. IM: 25 mg; if no hypotension occurs, 25 to 50 mg q3-4h may be given prn until vomiting stops then switched to PO.
  4. IV: Diluted to 1 mg/ml with saline; may be given 2 mg q2m (do not exceed 25 mg)
- Intractable hiccoughs: 25 to 50 mg, PO, tid to qid; if symptoms persist may be given 25 to 50 mg IM.

Contraindications and precautions: Comatose or severely depressed states, presence of large amounts of other CNS depressants, pregnancy category C

Adverse effects: Sedation, extrapyramidal symptoms, anticholinergic effects, orthostatic hypotension, and jaundice.

Chorionic gonadotropin, human (HCG) (A.P.L., Glukor, Chorex-5, Chorex-10, Profasi HP, Follutein)

How supplied: Injection, 200 U, 500 U, 1000 U, 2000 U/ml

Indications: Induction of ovulation in the anovulatory, infertile woman in whom the cause of anovulation is secondary and not a result of primary ovarian failure, and who has been appropriately pretreated with human menotropins

Adult dosage: 5000 to 10,000 USP units 1 day following the last dose of menotropins

Contraindications and precautions: Precocious puberty, androgen-dependent neoplasm, prior allergic reaction to chorionic gonadotropin, pregnancy category C

Adverse effects: Ovarian hyperstimulation, a syndrome of sudden ovarian enlargement; ascites with or without pain and pleural effusion; rupture of ovarian cysts with resultant hemoperitoneum; multiple births; arterial thromboembolism; headache, irritability, restlessness, depression, fatigue, edema, precocious puberty, gynecomastia, and pain at injection site

Ciprogloxacin (Cipro)

How supplied: Tabs, 250, 500, 750 mg; injection, 200, 400 mg

Indications: Primarily used for the treatment of susceptible gram negative microorganisms (see Appendix XI)

Adult dosage

- Oral: 250 to 750 mg q12h
- Parenteral: 200 to 400 mg, IV, q12h
- Chancroid (alternative regimen): 500 mg, PO, bid × 3 days
- Uncomplicated gonoccocal infection: 500 mg, PO, in a single dose plus doxycycline
- Disseminated gonococcal infection: 500 mg, PO, bid to complete a full week of therapy after treatment with initial regimen (ceftriaxone, 1 g, IV/IM, q24h for 24 to 48 hours after improvement begins

Elimination: Excreted by kidneys; dosage should be adjusted in renal impairment.

Contraindications and precautions: Hypersensitivity to fluoroquinolones or the quinolone group of antibacterial agents (cinoxacin and nalidixic acid); not to be used during pregnancy or lactation

Adverse effects: Nausea, vomiting, diarrhea, headache, rash, photosensitivity, elevated alanine and aspartate aminotransferases (SGOT/SGPT), dizziness

Patient information: Administration with magnesium-containing or aluminum-containing antacids, or products containing iron or zinc is to be avoided because of interference with bioavailability.

Cisapride (Propulsid)

How supplied: Tabs, 10 mg

Indications: Symptomatic treatment of patients with nocturnal heartburn resulting from gastroesophageal reflux disease (GERD)

Adult dosage: 10 mg qid 15 minutes before meals and at hs
Contraindications and precautions: Patients in whom an increase in GI motility could be harmful, pregnancy category C
Adverse effects: Diarrhea, abdominal pain, nausea, headache, and flatulence

Clarithromycin (Biaxin)

How supplied: Tabs, 250, 500 mg; oral suspension, 125, 250 mg/5 ml
Indications: Treatment of infections caused by susceptible microorganisms (see Appendix XI)
Adult dosage: 250 to 500 mg, PO, q12h
Elimination: Excreted via the liver and kidneys; dosage should be adjusted in severe renal impairment.
Contraindications and precautions: Pregnancy category C; hypersensitivity to clarithromycin, erythromycin, or any of the macrolide antibiotics
Adverse effects: Diarrhea, nausea, taste disturbances, dyspepsia, abdominal pain, and headache
Drug interactions: See Erythromycin.
Patient information: May be given without regard to meals.

Clindamycin (Cleocin)

How supplied: Caps, 75, 150, 300 mg: oral solution, 75 mg/5 ml; injection, 150 mg/ml; vaginal cream, 2%
Indications: Management of infections caused by gram positive cocci and anaerobic organisms. Particularly useful in the treatment of peritonitis and intra-abdominal abscess (typically resulting from anaerobic organisms resident in the normal GI tract), infections of the female pelvis and genital tract such as endometritis, nongonococcal tuboovarian abscess, pelvic cellulitis, and postsurgical vaginal cuff infection. Also used for treatment of bacterial vaginosis (*Gardnerella* vaginitis) (see Appendix XI).
Adult dosage
- Oral: 150 to 300 mg q6h. More severe infections: 300 to 450 mg q6h (max. 450 mg q6h).
- Parenteral (IV/IM): Serious infections by aerobic gram positive cocci and the more sensitive anaerobes: 600 to 1200 mg/day in two to four divided doses. More severe infections, particularly those from *Bacteroides fragilis, Peptococcus* species, or *Clostridium* species (not *C. perfringens*): 1200 to 2700 mg/day in two to four divided doses. Maximum dose not to exceed 4800 mg/day. Single IM injections >600 mg are not recommended.
- Bacterial vaginosis:
  1. Oral: 300 mg, bid × 7 days
  2. Vaginal: One applicator full 2% cream qhs × 7 days
- Pelvic inflammatory disease (PID):
  1. Inpatient alternative: 900 mg, IV, q8h plus gentamicin for at least 48 hours after demonstrated clinical improvement, then followed with doxycycline, 100 mg, PO, bid or clindamycin, 450 mg, PO, qid to complete 14 days of total therapy
  2. Outpatient alternative: 450 mg, PO, qid plus ofloxacin, 400 mg, PO bid × 14 days

Elimination: Metabolized in liver. No adjustment required for renal impairment.

Contraindications and precautions: Hypersensitivity to lincosamides, safety during pregnancy has not been established.

Adverse effects: Nausea, vomiting, diarrhea, pseudomembranous colitis with bloody mucoid diarrhea, rash, and transient elevation in alanine aminotransforase (ALT) or aspartate aminotransferase (AST)

Clomiphene (Clomid, Serophene)

How supplied: Tabs, 50 mg

Indications: Treatment of ovulatory failure in patients desiring pregnancy whose partners are fertile and potent. The following criteria must be met: (1) normal liver function, (2) normal levels of endogenous estrogen as estimated from vaginal smears, endometrial biopsy, assay of urinary estrogen, or from bleeding in response to progesterone. Therapy is ineffective in patients with primary pituitary or ovarian failure.

Unlabeled use: Clomiphene has been used to treat male infertility, either in doses of 25 mg daily × 25 days with 5 days rest, or at doses of 100 mg every Mon, Wed, and Fri

Adult dosage

- Initial therapy: First course is 50 mg/day × 5 days starting around the fifth day of the cycle.
- Second course of therapy: Increase of the dosage in patients not responding to the first course. If ovulation has not occurred after the first course, a second course should be administered of 100 mg/day × 5 days. This course may be started 30 days after the previous one.
- Third course of therapy: The majority of patients responding will respond to the first course of therapy; three courses are an adequate therapeutic trial.

Contraindications and precautions: Liver disease, history of hepatic dysfunction or abnormal bleeding of undetermined origin. Not to be administered in cases of suspected pregnancy, in presence of abnormal uterine bleeding, or before a complete pelvic examination. Multiple pregnancy is possible and poses potential hazards.

Adverse effects: Vasomotor flushes, abdominal discomfort, distension, bloating, abnormal uterine bleeding, nausea, vomiting, abnormal ovarian enlargement, and ophthalmologic symptoms usually described as "blurring" spots or flashes

Clonidine (Catapres, Catapres-TTS)

How supplied: Tabs, 0.1, 0.2, 0.3 mg; transdermal, 0.1, 0.2, 0.3 mg/24 hours

Actions: Stimulates central inhibitory alpha-adrenergic receptors.

Indications: Hypertension

Adult dosage

- Oral: 0.1 to 0.8 mg/day in divided doses bid (maximum dose = 2.4 mg/day)
- Transdermal: Initially, 0.1 mg system q7d; may increase after 1 to 2 weeks; maximum dose = two 0.3-mg systems.

Contraindications and precautions: Rebound hypertension may result if discontinued abruptly. Pregnancy category C: Not currently recommend during pregnancy because of reports of embryotoxicity.

Adverse effects: Dry mouth, drowsiness, dizziness, constipation, postural hypotension

Clotrimazole (Gyne-Lotrimin, Mycelex, Lotrimin)

How supplied: Vaginal tabs, 100, 500 mg; vaginal cream, 1%; topical cream, solution, or lotion, 1%; troches, 10 mg

Indications: Treatment of local fungal infections

Adult dosage

- Vulvovaginal candidiasis
  1. One 100-mg tablet inserted intravaginally qhs × 7 nights recommended regimen during pregnancy
  2. Two 100-mg tablets inserted intravaginally qhs × 3 nights
  3. One 500-mg tablet inserted intravaginally, one time only, preferably at bedtime
  4. One applicator full (5 g) vaginal cream qhs × 7 to 14 days
- Oropharyngeal candidiasis: One troche slowly dissolved five times daily × 14 days.
- Cutaneous fungal infection: Topical application bid

Cloxacillin (Cloxapen, Tegopen)

How supplied: Caps, 250, 500 mg; oral solution, 125 mg/5 ml

Indications: Treatment of infections caused by penicillinase-producing staphylococci (see Appendix XI)

Adult dosage: 250 mg to 1 g, PO, q6h

Contraindications and precautions: Hypersensitivity to any PCN

Codeine

How supplied: Tabs, 15, 30, 60 mg; injection, 30, 60 mg/ml

Indications: Relief of mild to moderate pain and for coughing induced by chemical or mechanical irritation of the respiratory system

Adult dosage

- Analgesic: 15 to 60 mg, PO/IM/IV/SC, q4-6h prn. Maximum dose = 360 mg/24 hours.
- Antitussive: 10 to 20 mg q4-6h. Maximum dose = 120 mg/24 hours.

Contraindications and precautions: See Morphine.

Cyclizine (Marezine)

How supplied: Tabs, 50 mg; injection, 50 mg/ml

Indications: Prevention and treatment of nausea, vomiting, and dizziness of motion sickness

Adult dosage

- Oral: 50 mg taken 30 minutes before departure and q4-6h prn; maximum dose = 200 mg daily.
- Parenteral: 50 mg, IM, q4-6h prn

Contraindications and precautions: Pregnancy category B; patients must use caution while driving or performing other tasks requiring alertness.

Adverse effects: Drowsiness, nervousness, anorexia, dry nose and throat, and cholestatic jaundice

Danazol (Danocrine)

How supplied: Caps, 50, 100, 200 mg

Actions: A synthetic androgen, danazol suppresses the pituitary–ovarian axis by inhibiting the output of pituitary gonadotropins.

Indications and Adult dosage

- Endometriosis amenable to hormonal management: 800 mg/day in two divided doses to best achieve amenorrhea and rapid response to painful symptoms; therapy to begin during menstruation or it must be made sure that the patient is not pregnant; maintenance dose individualized to 200 to 400 mg in two divided doses; therapy to be continued uninterrupted for 3 to 6 months; may be extended to 9 months.
- Fibrocystic breast disease: Dosage ranges from 100 to 400 mg/day in two divided doses; therapy to begin during menstruation or it must be made sure that patient is not pregnant; breast pain and tenderness are usually relieved by the first month and eliminated in 2 to 3 months; elimination of nodularity requires 4 to 6 months of uninterrupted therapy.

Contraindications and precautions: Undiagnosed abnormal genital bleeding; markedly impaired hepatic, renal, or cardiac function; pregnancy and lactation

Adverse effects: Acne, edema, mild hirsutism, decrease in breast size, deepening of the voice, oily skin or hair, weight gain, flushing, sweating, vaginitis, nervousness, emotional lability, elevated liver function tests (LFTs), and jaundice

Diazepam (Valium)

How supplied: Tabs, 2, 5, 10 mg; SR capsules, 15 mg; oral solution, 5 mg/5 ml, 5 mg/ml; injection, 5 mg/ml

Indications: Management of anxiety disorders or short-term relief of the symptoms of anxiety, acute alcohol withdrawal, muscle relaxant, anticonvulsant

Adult dosage

- Anxiety disorders and relief of symptoms of anxiety: 2 to 10 mg, PO, bid to qid; 2 to 10 mg IV/IM, may be repeated in 3 to 4 hours if necessary.
- Muscle spasm: 2 to 10 mg, PO, tid or qid; 5 to 10 mg, IM/IV, initially, then 5 to 10 mg in 3 to 4 hours if necessary
- Preoperative: 5 to 15 mg, IV, 5 to 10 minutes before procedure
- Status epilepticus: 5 to 10 mg, IV, initially; may be repeated in 10 to 15 minute intervals up to total maximum dose of 30 mg.
- Note: Use lower doses in elderly and debilitated patients; the IM route is painful and provides erratic absorption.

Contraindications and precautions: Hypersensitivity to benzodiazepines, concomitant ingestion of alcohol or other CNS depressants, pregnancy category D

Adverse effects: Sedation, drowsiness, memory impairment, bradycardia, and hypotension

Diazoxide (Hyperstat)

How supplied: Injection, 15 mg/ml

Actions: Relaxes smooth muscle in the peripheral arterioles.

Indications: Emergency reduction of blood pressure

Adult dosage: 30 mg, IV, q1-2m for hypertensive emergencies in the course of preeclampsia or eclampsia

Contraindications and precautions: Pregnancy category C, neonatal hyperglycemia following intrapartum administration of diazoxide has occurred.

Adverse effects: Nausea, vomiting, tachycardia, fluid retention, and hyperglycemia

Diclofenac (Cataflam, Voltaren)

How supplied: Tabs, 50 mg (as potassium); delayed release tablets, 25, 50, 75 mg

Indications: Acute and chronic treatment of the signs and symptoms of rheumatoid arthritis, osteoarthritis, and ankylosing spondylitis

Diclofenac potassium: Management of pain and primary dysmenorrhea

Adult dosage: Maximum dose = 200 mg/day; if GI upset occurs, should be taken with food or milk.

- Primary dysmenorrhea and analgesia: 50 mg tid
- Osteoarthritis: 100 to 150 mg/day in divided doses
- Rheumatoid arthritis: 150 to 200 mg/day in divided doses
- Ankylosing spondylitis: 100 to 125 mg/day as 25 mg qid, with an extra 25-mg dose at bedtime, if necessary

Contraindications and adverse effects: See Ibuprofen.

Dicloxacillin (Dynapen, Dycill, Pathocil)

How supplied: Caps, 125, 250, 500 mg; oral suspension, 62.5 mg/5 ml

Indications: Treatment of infections caused by penicillinase-producing staphylococci (see Appendix XI)

Adult dosage: 125 to 500 mg, PO, q6h

Contraindications and precautions: Hypersensitivity to any PCN

Didanosine, ddI, dideoxyinosine (Videx)

How supplied: Tabs, 25, 50, 100, 150 mg; powder for oral solution, 100, 167, 250, 375 mg

Indications: For the treatment of human immunodeficiency virus (HIV) patients with advanced disease who have demonstrated intolerance or significant clinical or immunologic deterioration during zidovudine therapy or who have received prolonged prior zidovudine therapy

Adult dosage:

- Patient weight ≥60 kg: tabs, 200 mg, bid; buffered powder, 250 mg, bid
- Patient weight <60 kg: tabs, 125 mg, bid; buffered powder, 167 mg bid

Elimination: Dose reduction may be necessary in patients with renal or hepatic impairment.

Contraindications and precautions: Pregnancy category B; to be used during pregnancy only if clearly needed

Adverse effects: Peripheral neuropathy, pancreatitis, diarrhea, chills, and fever

Dienestrol (Ortho Dienestrol, DV)

How supplied: Vaginal cream, 0.01% dienestrol in a 30- or 78-g tube

Adult dosage:

- Treatment of atrophic vaginitis, kraurosis vulvae associated with menopause: Usual dosage is one applicator full once or twice daily × 1 to 2 weeks, then reduce to one-half initial dosage for a similar period. A maintenance dosage is one applicator full one to two times a week after achievement of vaginal mucosa restoration.

Contraindications and adverse effects: See Estrogenic substances, conjugated.

Diethylstilbestrol (DES)

How supplied: Tabs, 1, 5 mg

Adult dosage:

- Emergency postcoital contraception: 25 mg, PO, bid × 5 days started no later than 72 hours after intercourse
- Inoperable, progressing breast cancer: 15 mg/day chronically

Contraindications and adverse effects: See Estrogenic substances, conjugated.

Diflunisal (Dolobid)

How supplied: Tabs, 250, 500 mg

Indications: Acute or long-term symptomatic treatment of mild to moderate pain, rheumatoid arthritis, and osteoarthritis

Adult dosage:

- Mild to moderate pain: Initially, 500 mg to 1 g, followed by 250 to 500 mg q8-12h
- Osteoarthritis or rheumatoid arthritis: 500 mg to 1 g daily in two divided doses; maximum dose = 1.5 g/day.

Contraindications and precautions: Hypersensitivity to diflunisal; patients in whom acute asthmatic attacks, urticaria, or rhinitis are precipitated by aspirin or other nonsteroidal antiinflammatory drugs; pregnancy category C

Adverse effects: Nausea, dyspepsia, diarrhea, vomiting, hepatitis, dysuria, interstitial nephritis, headache, dizziness, and rash

Dimenhydrinate (Dramamine)

How supplied: Tabs, 50 mg; caps, 50 mg; injection, 50 mg/ml; liquid, 12.5 mg/4 ml, 15.62 mg/5 ml

Indications: For the prevention and treatment of nausea, vomiting, dizziness, or vertigo of motion sickness

Adult dosage:

- Oral: 50 to 100 mg q4-6h; not to exceed 400 mg/24 hours
- IM: 50 mg prn
- IV: 50 mg diluted in 10 ml NaCl injection, given over 2 minutes

Contraindications and precautions: Pregnancy category B; to be used with caution in conditions that may be aggravated by anticholinergic therapy; use with other CNS depressants is to be avoided.

Adverse effects: Drowsiness, confusion, nervousness, blurring of vision, hypotension, and tachycardia

Dinoprostone, Prostaglandin E_2, PGE_2 (Prostin E2, Prepidil)

How supplied: Vaginal suppository, 20 mg; gel, 0.5 mg

Indications:

- For the termination of pregnancy between 12 and 20 weeks gestation as calculated from the first day of the last normal menstrual period
- Management of nonmetastatic gestational trophoblastic disease (benign hydatidiform mole)

- For ripening an unfavorable cervix in pregnant women at or near term with a medical or obstetrical need for labor induction

Adult dosage:

- Abortion, hydatidiform mole: One 20-mg suppository intravaginally q3-5h until desired effect; not to be administered for >2 days
- Cervical ripening: 0.5 mg gel inserted into the cervical canal just below the level of the internal os; may be repeated 0.5 mg q6h. The maximum recommended cumulative dose for a 24-hour period is 1.5 mg.

Contraindications and precautions: Hypersensitivity to any of these agents; acute pelvic inflammatory disease; active cardiac, pulmonary, renal, or hepatic disease; obstetric emergencies where the benefit to risk ratio for either the fetus or the mother favors surgical intervention

Adverse effects:

- Suppository: Nausea, vomiting, diarrhea, headache, flushing, anxiety or tension, chills or shivering
- Gel
  1. Maternal: Uterine contractile abnormality, nausea, vomiting, diarrhea, back pain
  2. Fetal: Any heart rate abnormality, bradycardia, deceleration

Diphenhydramine (Benadryl, Benylin Cough)

How supplied: Caps, 25, 50 mg; tabs, 25, 50 mg; syrup, 12.5 mg/5 ml; injection, 10, 50 mg/ml

Indications: Allergic manifestations; active and prophylactic treatment of motion sickness; nighttime sleep aid; parkinsonism; nonnarcotic cough suppressant (syrup)

Adult dosage:

- PO: 25 to 50 mg q6-8h; for sleep 25 to 50 mg qhs given
- IM/IV: 10 to 50 mg q6-8h; maximum dose = 400 mg/day.

Contraindications and precautions: Pregnancy category B; concomitant use of monoamine oxidase (MAO) inhibitors, alcohol, or other CNS depressants is to be avoided.

Adverse effects: Drowsiness, sedation, postural hypotension, and anorexia

Diphenoxylate with atropine (Lomotil)

How supplied: Tabs, 2.5 mg diphenoxylate and 0.025 mg atropine; liquid, 2.5 mg diphenoxylate and 0.025 mg atropine/5 ml

Indications: Adjunctive therapy in the management of diarrhea

Adult dosage: Initial dose is 5 mg qid

Contraindications and precautions: Diarrhea associated with pseudomembranous enterocolitis or enterotoxin-producing bacteria, pregnancy category C

Adverse effects: Pruritus, dizziness, drowsiness, headache, anorexia, nausea, vomiting, and flushing

Doxycycline (Vibramycin, Doryx)

How supplied: Caps, 50, 100 mg; tabs, 50, 100 mg; oral suspension, 25 mg/5 ml; syrup, 50 mg/5 ml; injection, 100, 200 mg

Indications: Treatment of infections caused by susceptible organisms including *Chlamydia trachomatis, Mycoplasma pneumoniae,* and rickettsial infections (see Appendix XI)

Adult dosage:
- Usual oral dose: 200 mg on the first day of treatment (100 mg q12h); followed with a maintenance dose of 100 mg/day (given as a single dose or 50 mg bid). Maximum daily dose is 200 mg/day.
- Uncomplicated urethral, endocervical, or rectal infections caused by *Chlamydia trachomatis:* 100 mg, PO, bid × 7 days
- Lymphogranuloma venereum: 100 mg, PO, bid × 21 days
- Primary and secondary syphilis (nonpregnant penicillin-allergic patients): 100 mg, PO, bid × 14 days (continued for 4 weeks in late syphilis)
- Endometritis, salpingitis, parametritis, or peritonitis: Doxycycline, 100 mg, IV, bid and cefoxitin or cefotetan until 48 hours after documented clinical improvement; then continued doxycycline, 100 mg, PO, bid × 14 days.

Elimination: Enterohepatic circulation in bile and secreted in an inactive form into the feces; no dosage adjustment necessary for renal impairment

Contraindications and precautions: Hypersensitivity to any of the tetracyclines. Not to be used during pregnancy (category D). Tetracyclines cross the placenta and can cause retardation of skeletal development in the developing fetus. The use of tetracyclines during the period of tooth development may cause permanent discoloration of deciduous and permanent teeth.

Adverse effects: Anorexia, nausea, vomiting, photosensitivity reactions, and maculopapular and erythematous rashes

Patient information: Unlike other tetracyclines, doxycycline may be taken with food or milk. Patients should avoid prolonged exposure to sunlight or sunlamps.

Enalapril (Vasotec)

How supplied: Tabs, 2.5, 5, 10, 20 mg; injection, 1.25 mg/ml

Actions: ACE inhibitor

Indications: Hypertension, heart failure

Adult dosage:
- Hypertension
  1. Oral: 5 mg qd initially; maintenance dose is 10 to 40 mg/day as a single dose or two divided doses
  2. IV: 1.25 mg, IV, q6h over 5 minutes
- Heart failure: 2.5 mg, PO, once or twice daily, initially; maintenance dose is 5 to 20 mg per day given in two divided doses

Contraindications and precautions: Use during pregnancy is to be avoided because of fetal and neonatal associated morbidities and mortalities; bilateral or unilateral renal artery stenosis; electrolytes should be monitored.

Adverse effects: Hypotension, dizziness, cough, rash, hyperkalemia, nausea, and vomiting

Enoxacin (Penetrex)

How supplied: Tabs, 200, 400 mg

Indications: Treatment of infections caused by susceptible microorganisms (see Appendix XI)

Adult dosage:
- Treatment of UTI: 200 to 400 mg, PO, q12h
- Uncomplicated gonorrhea: Single dose 400 mg, PO

Contraindications and precautions and adverse effects: See Ciprofloxacin.
Patient information: To be taken at least 1 hour before or 2 hours after a meal

Ergonovine maleate

How supplied: Tabs, 0.2 mg; injection, 0.2 mg/ml
Indications: Prevention and treatment of postpartum and postabortal hemorrhage caused by uterine atony
Adult dosage:
- Parenteral: The usual IM (or emergency IV) dose is 0.2 mg. IM injection usually produces a firm contraction of the uterus within a few minutes.
- Oral (or sublingual): One or two tablets to minimize late postpartum bleeding may be given every 6 to 12 hours until danger of uterine atony has passed, usually 48 hours. Severe cramping is evidence of effectiveness but may justify reduction in dosage.

Contraindications and precautions: Induction of labor; cases of threatened spontaneous abortion; previous allergic or idiosyncratic reactions to the drug; to be used cautiously in patients with hypertension, heart disease, venoatrial shunts, mitral valve stenosis, obliterative vascular disease, sepsis, and hepatic or renal impairment
Adverse effects: Nausea, vomiting, ergotism, blood pressure elevation, headache, ringing in ears, chest pain, and shortness of breath

Erythromycin

How supplied:
- Base (E-Mycin, Ery-Tab, Eryc, PCE): Tabs, 250, 333, 500 mg; caps, 250 mg
- Estolate (Ilosone): Tabs, 500 mg; caps, 250 mg; suspension, 125, 250 mg/5 ml
- Stearate (Eramycin, Erythrocin Stearate): Tabs, 250, 500 mg
- Ethylsuccinate (EryPed, E.E.S.): Tabs, 200, 400 mg; suspension, 200, 400 mg/5 ml
- Lactobionate: Injection, 500 mg, 1 g
- Ophthalmic ointment: 5 mg/g ointment

Indications: Treatment of infections caused by susceptible microorganisms (see Appendix XI)
Adult dosage:
- Usual dose: 250 mg to 1 g bid-qid (maximum dose 4 g/day)
- Nongonococcal urethritis (alternative regimen)
- Base: 500 mg, PO, qid × 7 days, *or* 250 mg, PO, qid × 14 days
  1. Ethylsuccinate: 800 mg, PO, qid × 7 days, *or* 400 mg, PO, qid × 14 days
  2. *Chlamydia trachomatis* infection in pregnancy or in nonpregnant patients intolerant of tetracyclines: 500 mg, PO, qid × 7 days, *or* 800 mg, PO, qid × 7 days
- Lymphogranuloma venereum (alternative regimen): 500 mg, PO, qid × 21 days

- *Hemophilus ducreyi* (chancroid): 500 mg, PO, qid × 7 days
- Gonococcal infections (uncomplicated urethral, endocervical, or rectal) or in pregnancy: 500 mg, PO, qid × 7 days
- Ophthalmia neonatorum prophylaxis: For prevention of gonococcal or chlamydial conjunctivitis, a thin line of ointment approximately 0.5 to 1 cm long should be instilled into each conjunctival sac. Prophylaxis should be administered to infants born by cesarean section as well as those delivered vaginally.

Elimination: In normal hepatic function the drug is concentrated in the liver and excreted via the bile. No dosage adjustment is necessary in renal impairment.

Contraindications and precautions: Hypersensitivity to erythromycin; erythromycin estolate not to be used in pregnancy or preexisting liver disease

Adverse effects: Rash, phlebitis (with IV administration), abdominal cramps, anorexia, nausea, vomiting, diarrhea, and hepatotoxicity (most commonly associated with estolate salt)

Drug interactions: Can increase serum levels and potentiate effects of warfarin, carbamazepine, digoxin, theophylline, certain antihistamines, and other hepatically eliminated drugs.

Esterified estrogens (Estratab, Menest)

How supplied: Tabs, 0.3, 0.625, 1.25, 2.5 mg

Adult dosage:

- Moderate to severe vasomotor symptoms, atrophic vaginitis or kraurosis vulvae associated with menopause: 0.3 to 1.25 mg, PO, qd cyclically (3 weeks on, 1 week off)
- Female hypogonadism: 2.5 to 7.5 mg, PO, qd in divided doses for 20 days followed by a 10-day rest period
- Female castration and primary ovarian failure: 1.25 mg, PO, qd cyclically.
- Inoperable, progressing breast cancer: 10 mg, PO, tid for at least 3 months

Contraindications and adverse effects: See Estrogenic substances, conjugated.

Estradiol (Estrace, Estraderm)

How supplied: Tabs, 0.5, 1, 2 mg; transdermal system, 0.05 mg/24 hours, 0.1 mg/24 hours, vaginal cream, 0.1 mg estradiol/g

Adult dosage:

- Moderate to severe vasomotor symptoms, vulvar or vaginal atrophy associated with menopause, female hypogonadism, female castration, primary ovarian failure
  1. Oral: Treatment initiated with 1 or 2 mg/day. For maintenance therapy, must be titrated to determine the minimal effective dose; cyclic therapy is recommended.
  2. Transdermal: Initially the 0.05-mg system applied to the skin twice weekly. Dose should be adjusted as necessary to control symptoms, using the lowest dose possible. Attempts should be made to taper or discontinue the drug at 3 to 6 month intervals. Therapy may be given continuously in patients who do not have an intact uterus. In patients with

an intact uterus, therapy may be given on a cyclic schedule (3 weeks on, 1 week off).

3. Vaginal cream (atrophic vaginitis and kraurosis vulvae): 2 to 4 g qd × 2 weeks. Gradually reduce to one-half initial dosage for a similar period. A maintenance dose of 1 g one to three times per week may be used after restoration of the vaginal mucosa has been achieved.

- Inoperable, progressing breast cancer: Usual dose is 10 mg, PO, tid for at least 3 months in appropriately selected patients.
- Prevention of osteoporosis:
  1. Oral: 0.5 mg, PO, qd cyclically (3 weeks on, 1 week off) as soon as possible after menopause. Dosage may be adjusted if necessary to control concurrent menopause symptoms.
  2. Transdermal: Initiated with 0.05-mg system twice weekly as soon as possible after menopause. Discontinuation may reestablish natural rate of bone loss.

Contraindications and adverse effects: See Estrogenic substances, conjugated.

Estradiol cypionate in oil (depGynogen, Depogen, Dura-Estrin)

How supplied: Injection, 5 mg/ml

Adult dosage:

- Moderate to severe vasomotor symptoms associated with menopause: Usual dosage range is 1 to 5 mg, IM, q3-4wk
- Female hypogonadism: 1.5 to 2 mg, IM, at monthly intervals.

Contraindications and adverse effects: See Estrogenic substances, conjugated.

Estradiol valerate in oil (Delestrogen, Valergen, Duragen, Gynogen L.A.)

How supplied: Injection, 10, 20, 40 mg/ml

Adult dosage:

- Moderate to severe vasomotor symptoms, atrophic vaginitis or kraurosis vulvae associated with menopause, female hypogonadism, female castration or primary ovarian failure: 10 to 20 mg q4wk
- Prevention of postpartum breast engorgement: 10 to 25 mg as a single injection at the end of the first stage of labor

Contraindications and adverse effects: See Estrogenic substances, conjugated.

Estrogenic substances, conjugated (Premarin)

How supplied: Tabs, 0.3, 0.625, 0.9, 1.25, 2.5 mg; injection, 25 mg; vaginal cream, 0.625 mg conjugated estrogens/g

Adult dosage:

- Moderate to severe vasomotor symptoms associated with menopause: 1.25 mg, PO, qd cyclically (3 weeks on, 1 week off).
- Atrophic vaginitis and kraurosis vulvae:
  1. Oral: 0.3 to 1.25 mg or more qd cyclically
  2. Vaginal cream: 2 to 4 g, intravaginally, qd cyclically

- Female hypogonadism: 2.5 to 7.5 mg, PO, qd, in divided doses for 20 days, followed by a rest period of 10 days
- Female castration and primary ovarian failure: 1.25 mg, PO, qd cyclically; should be adjusted to lowest effective level according to severity of symptoms and patient response.
- Osteoporosis: 0.625 mg, PO, qd cyclically
- Inoperable progressing breast cancer: 10 mg, PO, tid for at least 3 months
- Prevention of postpartum breast engorgement: 3.75 mg, PO, q4h × five doses or 1.25 mg, PO, q4h × 5 days
- Dysfunctional uterine bleeding: 25 mg IV/IM; may repeat in 6 to 12 hours if necessary.

Contraindications: Known or suspected pregnancy, estrogen-dependent neoplasia, breast cancer (except in appropriately selected patients being treated for metastatic disease), undiagnosed abnormal genital bleeding, active thrombophlebitis or thromboembolic disorders, history of thrombophlebitis, thrombosis or thromboembolic disorders associated with previous estrogen use

Adverse effects: Breakthrough bleeding; spotting, change in menstrual flow; dysmenorrhea; amenorrhea during and after treatment; nausea; vomiting; abdominal cramps; bloating; headache; migraine; dizziness; and mental depression

Estrone (Estronol Theelin Aqueous, Estrone 5, Kestrone 5)

How supplied: Injection, 2, 5 mg/ml

Adult dosage:

- Replacement therapy of estrogen deficiency-associated conditions: Initial relief of symptoms may be obtained by the administration of 0.1 to 1 mg of estrone weekly in single or divided doses. Some patients may require up to 0.5 to 2 mg weekly.
- Senile vaginitis and kraurosis vulvae: Usually 0.1 to 0.5 mg estrone two or three times per week
- Abnormal uterine bleeding caused by hormone imbalance: May respond to brief courses of intensive estrogen therapy. Usual dose range is 2 to 5 mg qd × several days.
- Inoperable progressing breast cancer in appropriately selected postmenopausal women: Usual dose is 5 mg three or more times weekly according to severity of pain.

Contraindications and adverse effects: See Estrogenic substances, conjugated.

Estropipate (Ogen, Ortho-Est)

How supplied: Tabs, 0.625, 1.25, 2.5, 5 mg; vaginal cream, 1.5 mg estropipate/g

Adult dosage:

- Moderate to severe vasomotor symptoms, atrophic vaginitis, or kraurosis vulvae associated with menopause
  1. Oral: 0.625 to 5 mg, PO, qd, cyclically (3 weeks on, 1 week off)
  2. Vaginal cream: 2 to 4 g, intravaginally, qd cyclically

- Female hypogonadism, castration, or primary ovarian failure: To be administered cyclically, 1.25 to 7.5 mg/day for the first 3 weeks, followed by an 8 to 10 day rest period
- Osteoporosis prevention: 0.625 mg, PO, qd for 25 days of a 31-day cycle per month

Contraindications and adverse effects: See Estrogenic substances, conjugated.

Ethinyl estradiol (Estinyl)

How supplied: Tabs, 0.02, 0.05, 0.5 mg

Adult dosage:

- Moderate to severe vasomotor symptoms associated with menopause: 0.02 to 1.5 mg, PO, qd cyclically (3 weeks on, 1 week off)
- Female hypogonadism: 0.05 mg one to three times daily during the first 2 weeks of a theoretical menstrual cycle; during the last half of the arbitrary cycle followed with progesterone; continued for 3 to 6 months
- Inoperable, progressing breast cancer: 1 mg, PO, tid chronically for palliation
- Emergency postcoital contraception: 2.5 mg, PO, bid, starting within 72 hours of intercourse and continued × 5 days.

Contraindications and adverse effects: See Estrogenic substances, conjugated.

Etodolac (Lodine)

How supplied: Caps, 200, 300 mg

Indications: Management of pain; acute and long-term use in the management of signs and symptoms of osteoarthritis

Adult dosage: Maximum dose = 1200 mg/day or 20 mg/kg in patients ≤60 kg.

- Analgesia: 200 to 400 mg q6-8h prn
- Osteoarthritis: 200 to 400 mg, PO, bid-qid

Contraindications and adverse effects: See Ibuprofen.

Fenoprofen (Nalfon)

How supplied: Caps, 200, 300 mg; tabs, 600 mg

Indications: Relief of mild to moderate pain; relief of the signs and symptoms of rheumatoid arthritis and osteoarthritis

Adult dosage: Maximum dose = 3.2 g/day; if GI upset occurs, should be taken with food or milk

- Mild to moderate pain: 200 mg q4-6h prn
- Rheumatoid arthritis and osteoarthritis: 300 to 600 mg tid to qid

Contraindications and adverse effects: See Ibuprofen.

Ferrous sulfate (Feratab, Fer-in-Sol, Feosol)

How supplied: Tabs, 195 (39 mg iron), 250 (50 mg iron), 300 (60 mg iron), 324 mg (65 mg iron); caps, 250 mg (50 mg iron); syrup, 90 mg (18 mg iron) per 5 ml; elixir, 220 mg (44 mg iron) per 5 ml; drops, 75 mg (15 mg iron) per 0.6 ml, 125 mg (25 mg iron) per 1 ml

Indications: For the prevention and treatment of iron-deficiency anemias

Adult dosage

- Recommended daily allowances (elemental iron)
  1. Adult females (11 to 50 years old): 15 mg; ≥51 years old: 10 mg
  2. Pregnancy: 30 mg
  3. Lactation: 15 mg
- Iron replacement therapy in deficiency states: Adults, 100 to 200 mg (2 to 3 mg/kg) elemental iron daily in three divided doses

Contraindications and precautions: Hemochromatosis, hemosiderosis, hemolytic anemias

Adverse effects: GI upset, anorexia, nausea, vomiting, constipation, and diarrhea

Patient information: To be taken on an empty stomach; if GI upset occurs, to be taken after meals or with food; coadministration with antacids, tetracyclines, or fluoroquinolones should be avoided.

Fluconazole (Diflucan)

How supplied: Tabs, 50, 100, 200 mg; oral suspension, 10 mg/ml; injection, 200, 400 mg

Indications: Vulvovaginal, oropharyngeal, esophageal, systemic candidiasis; cryptococcal meningitis

Adult dosage

- Vulvovaginal candidiasis: 150 mg, PO, once
- Oropharyngeal candidiasis: 200 mg on day 1, then 100 mg qd × 2 weeks
- Esophageal candidiasis: 200 mg on day 1, then 100 mg qd × 3 weeks; treated for at least 2 weeks after symptoms resolve; maximum daily dose 400 mg
- Systemic candidiasis: 400 mg on day 1, then 200 mg qd for a minimum of 4 weeks; treated for at least 2 weeks after symptoms resolve
- Cryptococcal meningitis: 400 mg on day 1, then 200 to 400 mg qd for 10 to 12 weeks after CSF is negative; 200 mg qd used to suppress relapse in AIDS patients.

Elimination: Renal excretion; dosage adjustment required in renal impairment.

Contraindications and precautions: Hypersensitivity to fluconazole; pregnancy category C

Adverse effects: Nausea, headache, skin rash, increased LFTs

Drug interactions: Nonsedating antihistamines, theophylline, sulfonylureas, warfarin, zidovudine

Flurbiprofen (Ansaid)

How supplied: Tabs, 50, 100 mg

Indications: Acute or long-term treatment of the signs and symptoms of rheumatoid arthritis and osteoarthritis

Adult dosage: 50 to 100 mg tid to qid. Maximum dose = 300 mg/day; if GI upset occurs, should be taken with food or milk.

Contraindications and adverse effects: See Ibuprofen.

Folic acid

How supplied: Tabs, 0.4, 0.8, 1 mg; injection, 5 mg/ml

Indications: Megaloblastic anemia from folic acid deficiency

Adult dosage: 1 mg, PO, qd

Contraindications and precautions: Not to be used for treatment of vitamin B_{12} deficiency

Furosemide (Lasix)

How supplied: Tabs, 20, 40, 80 mg; solution, 10 mg/ml, 40 mg/5 ml; injection, 10 mg/ml

Actions: Loop diuretic

Indications: Hypertension; edema

Adult dosage

- Hypertension: 40 mg bid, adjusted according to response
- Edema: 20 to 80 mg/day as a single dose

Contraindications and precautions: Anuria; hypersensitivity to loop diuretics or sulfonylureas; pregnancy category C (Diuretics decrease plasma volume and can decrease placental perfusion.)

Adverse effects: Anorexia, nausea, vomiting, diarrhea, dizziness, paresthesia, photosensitivity, orthostatic hypotension, and electrolyte disturbances

Gentamicin (Garamycin, Jenamicin)

How supplied: Injection, 2, 10, 40 mg/ml

Indications: Treatment of infections caused by susceptible microorganisms (see Appendix XI)

Adult dosage (IV/IM)

- Loading dose: 2 mg/kg
- Maintenance dose: 3 to 5 mg/kg/day divided q8-12h or adjusted dose based upon patient's calculated creatinine clearance (Cr Cl). See Amikacin for Cr Cl calculation.

Cr Cl (ml/min)	Percentage of loading dose
70	88% q12h
50	79% q12h
25	81% q24-36h
10	60% q48h

- After 24 hours of therapy a serum peak level should be obtained 30 minutes after IV administration of the drug (60 minutes after IM administration) and a trough level just before the next dose: Therapeutic peak concentration is 4 to 10 μg/ml; therapeutic trough concentration is <2 μg/ml; serum creatinine should be monitored qd to qod while the patient is receiving gentamicin.

Elimination: Excreted by glomerular filtration; dosage should be adjusted in renal impairment and based on serum concentrations.

Contraindications and precautions: Pregnancy category D; hypersensitivity to aminoglycosides; use with other nephrotoxic agents should be avoided.

Adverse effects: See Amikacin.

Granisetron (Kytril)

How supplied: Injection, 1 mg/ml

Indications: Prevention of nausea and vomiting associated with initial and repeat courses of emetogenic cancer therapy

Adult dosage: 10 μg/kg infused IV over 5 minutes beginning within 30 minutes before initiation of chemotherapy, and only on the day(s) chemotherapy is given.
Contraindications and precautions: Pregnancy category B
Adverse effects: Headache, asthenia, somnolence, diarrhea, constipation, AST and ALT elevations

Hepatitis B vaccine (Recombivax HB, Engerix-B)

How supplied: Injection, 10 μg/0.5 ml, 10 μg/ml, 20 μg/ml, 40 μg/ml
Indications: For immunizations against infections caused by all known subtypes of hepatitis B virus
Dosage
- Infants (Engerix-B pediatric formulation 10 μg/0.5 ml): 0.5 ml IM at birth, 1 month, and 6 months to infants born of HBsAg-negative mothers. For infants born of hepatitis B-infected mothers, Engerix-B should be given 0.5 ml IM at birth, 1 month, 2 months, and 12 months.
- Adults: three-dose schedule of 1 ml IM initially, at 1 month and 6 months

Contraindications and precautions: Hypersensitivity to yeast or any component of the vaccines, acute hypersensitivity reactions, pregnancy category C
Adverse effects: Injection site soreness, erythema, swelling, nausea, vomiting, headache, vertigo, arthralgia, pruritus, and rash

Hydralazine (Apresoline)

How supplied: Tabs, 10, 25, 50, 100 mg; injection, 20 mg/ml
Actions: Direct acting arteriolar vasodilator
Indications
- Oral: Second-line agent for maternal hypertension; can be used alone or in combination with other agents.
- Parenteral: Drug of choice for eclampsia; severe essential hypertension when the drug cannot be given orally or when the need to lower BP is urgent

Adult dosage
- Oral: 10 to 50 mg, bid to qid; maximum dose = 300 mg/day.
- Parenteral: 5 to 10 mg, IV/IM, q20-40m or 0.5 to 10 mg/hr constant IV infusion (20 mg/50 ml normal saline [NS])

Contraindications and precautions: Pregnancy category C; to be used only when the potential benefits outweigh potential hazards to the fetus.
Adverse effects: Headache, anorexia, nausea, vomiting, diarrhea, tachycardia, paresthesia, rash, and blood dyscrasias

Hydrochlorothiazide (HydroDIURIL, Oretic, Esidrix)

How supplied: Tabs, 25, 50, 100 mg; solution, 50 mg/5 ml, 100 mg/ml
Actions: Thiazide diuretic
Indications: Hypertension, edema
Adult dosage
- Hypertension: 25 mg, PO, qd; may be increased to 50 mg daily as a single or two divided doses.
- Edema: 25 to 200 mg qd × several days, or until dry weight is attained; maintenance dose is 25 to 100 mg qd or intermittently; refractory patients may require up to 200 mg qd.

Contraindications and precautions: Anuria; renal decompensation; pregnancy category B; diuretics decrease plasma volume and can decrease placental perfusion. Diuretics do not prevent development of toxemia, nor are they useful in the treatment of toxemia.

Adverse effects: Hypovolemia, nausea, vomiting, hyperuricemia, and electrolyte disturbances

Hydromorphone (Dilaudid)

How supplied: Tabs, 1, 2, 3, 4 mg; injection, 1, 2, 3, 4, 10 mg/ml; suppository, 3 mg

Indications: Relief of moderate to severe pain

Adult dosage

- PO: 2 to 4 mg q4-6h prn
- SC/IM: 1 to 4 mg q4-6h prn
- IV: 1 to 4 mg by slow IV injection over 2 to 5 minutes q4-6h prn
- PR: 3 mg q6-8h prn

Contraindications and precautions: Hypersensitivity to hydromorphone, pregnancy category C, head injury and increased ICP, acute abdominal conditions, hepatic dysfunction, concomitant use of CNS depressants

Hydroxyprogesterone caproate (Duralutin, Gesterol L.A. 250, Hylutin, Hyprogest 250)

How supplied: Injection, 125, 250 mg/ml

Action: This long-acting progestin has a 9- to 17-day duration of action.

Adult dosage

- Amenorrhea (primary and secondary), dysfunctional uterine bleeding, metrorrhagia: 375 mg IM
- Production of secretory endometrium and desquamation: Physician should test for continuous endogenous estrogen production (medical D and C); 125 to 250 mg on day 10 of cycle; repeated q7d until suppression is no longer desired.

Contraindications and adverse effects: See Medroxyprogesterone.

Ibuprofen (Advil, Excedrin IB, Medipren, Motrin, Nuprin, Rufen)

How supplied: Tabs, 200, 300, 400, 600, 800 mg; suspension, 100 mg/5 ml

Indications: Treatment of primary dysmenorrhea; relief of signs and symptoms of rheumatoid arthritis and osteoarthritis; relief of mild to moderate pain; reduction of fever

Adult dosage: Maximum dose = 3.2 g/day; if GI upset occurs may be taken with food or milk.

- Primary dysmenorrhea: 400 mg, PO, q4h prn
- Rheumatoid arthritis and osteoarthritis: 400 to 800 mg, PO, tid-qid
- Mild to moderate pain: 400 mg PO, q4-6h prn
- Fever reduction: 200 to 400 mg, PO, q4-6h

Contraindications and precautions

- Nonsteroidal antiinflammatory drugs should be avoided during pregnancy, especially in the third trimester.
- Syndrome of nasal polyps, bronchospastic activity, angioedema, and other symptoms of allergic or anaphylactoid reactions following ingestion of aspirin and other nonsteroidal antiinflammatory drugs

- To be used with caution in patients with a history of GI bleeding, cardiac decompensation, hypertension, impaired renal function, or bleeding disorders
- Concomitant administration of coumarin-type anticoagulants may result in potentiation of their effects.

Adverse effects: Nausea, vomiting, diarrhea, GI bleeding, elevated liver enzymes, and renal impairment

Imipenem–cilastatin (Primaxin)

How supplied: Injection, 250 mg imipenem + 250 mg cilastatin, 500 mg imipenem + 500 mg cilastatin, 750 mg imipenem + 750 mg cilastatin

Indications: Reserved for the treatment of serious infections caused by susceptible microorganisms. Excellent activity against streptococci, enterococci, staphylococci, *Listeria,* most strains of *Pseudomonas* and *Acinetobacter,* and anaerobes such as *B. fragilis* and *Clostridium perfringens* (see Appendix XI)

Adult dosage: 250 to 1000 mg, IV/IM, q6-8h (not to exceed 50 mg/kg/day or 4 g/day; IM total daily doses should not exceed 1500 mg/day)

Elimination: Excreted by kidneys; dosage should be adjusted in renal impairment.

Contraindications and precautions: Patients with a history of PCN hypersensitivity may exhibit cross-reactivity with this medication; pregnancy category C.

Adverse effects: Phlebitis, nausea, vomiting, diarrhea, fever, seizures (in high doses or preexisting renal impairment), tremor, confusion, increased LFTs

Indomethacin (Indocin)

How supplied: Caps, 25, 50 mg; SR caps, 75 mg; oral suspension, 25 mg/5 ml; suppository, 50 mg

Indications: For active stages of moderate to severe rheumatoid arthritis, ankylosing spondylitis, and osteoarthritis; acute bursitis and tendinitis; acute gouty arthritis

Adult dosage: Maximum dose = 200 mg/day; oral formulations administered with food or antacids to minimize gastric irritation

- Moderate to severe rheumatoid arthritis, ankylosing spondylitis, and osteoarthritis: 25 mg, PO, bid tid, increasing at weekly intervals to maximum of 150 to 200 mg/day
- Shoulder bursitis or tendinitis: 25 to 50 mg, PO, tid; usual course of therapy is 7 to 14 days.
- Acute gouty arthritis: 50 mg, PO, tid, then tapered rapidly

Contraindications and precautions: Suppositories not to be administered in patients with rectal bleeding or proctitis. See Ibuprofen.

Ketoconazole (Nizoral)

How supplied: Tabs, 200 mg

Indications: Treatment of systemic fungal infections

Adult dosage: 200 mg, PO, qd; 400 mg, PO, qd in severe infections

Elimination: Hepatic metabolism

Contraindications and precautions: Hypersensitivity to ketoconazole. Not to be used for the treatment of fungal meningitis because of poor CSF penetration. Pregnancy category C. Ketoconazole requires acidity for dissolution and absorption. Interacts with other hepatically metabolized drugs.

Adverse effects: Nausea, vomiting, diarrhea, hepatotoxicity, headache, and dizziness

Ketoprofen (Orudis, Oruvail)

How supplied: Caps, 25, 50, 75 mg; SR caps, 200 mg

Indications: Primary dysmenorrhea; mild to moderate pain; acute or long-term treatment of the signs and symptoms of rheumatoid arthritis and osteoarthritis

Adult dosage: Maximum dose = 300 mg/day; may be taken with food, milk, or antacids to minimize GI adverse effects.

- Primary dysmenorrhea, mild to moderate pain: 25 to 50 mg q6-8h prn
- Rheumatoid arthritis and osteoarthritis: 50 to 75 mg tid-qid

Contraindications and adverse effects: See Ibuprofen.

Ketorolac (Toradol)

How supplied: Tabs, 10 mg; injection, 15 mg/ml, 30 mg/ml, 60 mg/2 ml

Indications: Short-term management of pain

Adult dosage

- Parenteral: 30 to 60 mg, IM, loading dose followed by half of the loading dose (15 to 30 mg) q6h. The recommended maximum total daily dose is 150 mg for the first day and 120 mg/day thereafter; limited to short-term therapy (not >5 days). The lower end of the recommended dosage range is recommended for patients <50 kg, for patients >65 years old, and for patients with reduced renal function.
- Oral: 10 mg, PO, q4-6h prn, for limited duration; maximum dose = 40 mg/day.

Contraindications and adverse effects: See Ibuprofen.

Labetalol (Normodyne, Trandate)

How supplied: Tabs, 100, 200, 300 mg; injection, 5 mg/ml

Action: Alpha-adrenergic and beta-adrenergic blocking agent

Indications: Hypertension

Adult dosage

- Oral: Initially, 100 mg bid; increased by 100 mg, bid, q3d; usual maintenance dose is 200 to 400 mg, bid (maximum dose = 2400 mg/day).
- Parenteral: 20 mg, IV, over 2 minutes, followed by 20 to 80 mg, IV, q10-20m until desired supine BP is achieved or a total of 300 mg has been injected.
- Constant IV infusion method: 200 mg/250 ml D_5W or 0.9% NaCl infused at 1 to 2 mg/min, adjusting for BP response

Contraindications and precautions: Bronchial asthma, severe bradycardia; pregnancy category C; use only if the potential benefits outweigh the potential hazards to the fetus; drug metabolism may be diminished with impaired hepatic function

Adverse effects: Fatigue, headache, drowsiness, nausea, vomiting, bradycardia, heart failure, and bronchostenosis

Levonorgestrel implants (Norplant System)

How supplied: Kit, set of six capsules each containing 36 mg of progestin levonorgestrel

Adult dosage

- Prevention of pregnancy: The implant system is a long-term (up to 5 years) reversible contraceptive system.
  1. Implantation of all six capsules performed during the first 7 days of the onset of menses.
  2. Insertion is subdermal in the midportion of the upper arm about 8 to 10 cm above the elbow crease.
  3. Capsules removed by the end of the fifth year; new capsules may be inserted at that time if continued contraception is desired.

Contraindications: Active thrombophlebitis or thromboembolic disorders; undiagnosed abnormal genital bleeding; pregnancy; acute hepatic disease; liver tumors; breast cancer

Adverse effects: Prolonged bleeding, spotting, amenorrhea, headache, nervousness, nausea, dizziness

Levothyroxine; T_4 (Synthroid, Levoxine, Levothroid)

How supplied: Tabs, 0.025, 0.05, 0.075, 0.088, 0.1, 0.112, 0.125, 0.15, 0.175, 0.2, 0.3 mg; injection, 200, 500 g/vial

Indications: Hypothyroidism

Adult dosage: Individualized dosage

- Usual starting dose is 0.05 mg, with increments of 0.025 mg q2-3wk.

Contraindications and precautions: Acute MI and thyrotoxicosis uncomplicated by hypothyroidism, pregnancy category A, laboratory monitoring necessary.

Adverse effects: Palpitations, tachycardia, cardiac arrhythmias, chest pain, tremors, headache, nervousness, and insomnia

Lomefloxacin (Maxaquin)

How supplied: Tabs, 400 mg

Indications: Treatment of infections caused by susceptible microorganisms (see Appendix XI)

Adult dosage

- Usual dose: 400 mg, PO, qd
- Uncomplicated gonococcal infection: 400 mg, PO, once

Elimination: See Ciprofloxacin.

Contraindications, precautions, and adverse effects: See Ciprofloxacin.

Patient information: Lomefloxacin may be taken without regard to meals.

Loperamide (Imodium)

How supplied: Tabs, 2 mg; caps, 2 mg; liquid, 1 mg/5 ml

Indications: Control and symptomatic relief of acute nonspecific diarrhea and of chronic diarrhea associated with inflammatory bowel disease

Adult dosage: 4 mg followed by 2 mg after each unformed stool; maximum dose = 16 mg/day.

Contraindications and precautions: Pregnancy category B

Adverse effects: Abdominal pain, constipation, dry mouth, nausea, and vomiting

Loracarbef (Lorabid)

How supplied: Caps, 200 mg; oral suspension, 100 mg/5 ml
Indications: Treatment of infections caused by susceptible microorganisms (see Appendix XI)
Adult dosage: 200 to 400 mg q12h
Elimination: Excreted by the kidneys; dosage should be adjusted in renal impairment.
Contraindications and precautions: Hypersensitivity to cephalosporins, pregnancy category B
Adverse effects: See Cephalexin.
Patient information: Should be administered at least 1 hour before or 2 hours after a meal.

Magnesium salts

How supplied: $MgSO_4$ = 12.5% (1 mEq/ml), 50% (4 mEq/ml) injection; magnesium oxide = 140 caps, 400-mg tabs; magnesium gluconate = 500-mg tabs, 54 mg/5 ml liquid; chelated magnesium = 500-mg tabs; magnesium chloride hexahydrate = 535-mg tabs.
Indications: Seizure prevention and control in severe preeclampsia or eclampsia and in convulsions associated with abnormally low levels of plasma magnesium as a contributing factor.
Unlabeled use: Magnesium has demonstrated some effectiveness as an agent to inhibit premature labor (tocolytic).
Adult dosage

- Eclamptic seizure control or prevention
  1. $MgSO_4$, 4 g, IV, dose over 4 to 5 minutes, followed immediately by 10 g IM and then by 5 g, IM, q4h in alternating buttocks, *or*
  2. $MgSO_4$, 4 g/250 ml D_5W or 0.9% NaCl, IV, over 15 minutes, followed by a maintenance infusion of 1 to 2 g/hr by controlled infusion pump
- Tocolytic
  1. $MgSO_4$, 4 to 6 g/250 ml D_5W or 0.9% NaCl IV loading dose over 20 minutes, followed by a maintenance infusion of 2 to 3 g/hr (20 to 40 g in 500 to 1000 ml diluent) and continued for 12 to 24 hours if it is successful
  2. Once contractions have stopped, begin magnesium oxide or gluconate at 250 to 500 mg, PO, q3h

Contraindications and precautions: Not to be given in toxemia of pregnancy during the 2 hours preceding delivery. Serum magnesium levels and clinical status should be monitored to avoid overdosage. Normal serum concentration = 1.5 to 3 mEq/L; "therapeutic" level for preeclampsia, eclampsia, or convulsions = 4 to 7 mEq/L. Deep tendon reflexes, respiratory rate, and urine output should be monitored. Calcium gluconate is the preferred antidote for hypermagnesemia, and a 10-ml ampule of 10% solution should be kept at the bedside of any patient receiving $MgSO_4$.
Adverse effects: Flushing, sweating, hypotension, depressed reflexes, flaccid paralysis, hypothermia, circulatory collapse, and cardiac and CNS depression proceeding to respiratory paralysis

Meclizine (Antivert, Bonine)

How supplied: Tabs, 12.5, 25, 50 mg; caps, 25 mg
Indications: Prevention and treatment of nausea, vomiting, and dizziness of motion sickness; possibly effective for the management of vertigo
Adult dosage
- Motion sickness: Initial dose of 25 to 50 mg, 1 hour before travel; may be repeated q24h prn for the journey's duration
- Vertigo: 25 to 100 mg daily in divided doses

Contraindications and precautions: Pregnancy category B; caution should be used while driving or performing other tasks requiring alertness.
Adverse effects: Drowsiness, restlessness, dry mouth, anorexia

Meclofenamate (Meclomen)

How supplied: Caps, 50, 100 mg
Indications: Treatment of primary dysmenorrhea, treatment of idiopathic heavy menstrual blood loss, relief of mild to moderate pain, acute and chronic rheumatoid arthritis and osteoarthritis
Adult dosage: Maximum dose = 400 mg/day; if GI upset occurs, take with food or milk
- Excessive menstrual blood loss and primary dysmenorrhea: 100 mg tid for up to 6 days, starting at the onset of menstrual flow
- Mild to moderate pain: 50 to 100 mg, PO, q4-6h
- Rheumatoid arthritis and osteoarthritis: 50 to 100 mg, PO, tid-qid

Contraindications and adverse effects: See Ibuprofen.

Medroxyprogesterone (Provera, Amen, Curretab, Depo-Provera, Cycrin)

How supplied: Tabs, 2.5, 5, 10 mg; injection, 100, 150, 400 mg/ml
Adult dosage
- Secondary amenorrhea: 5 to 10 mg, PO, qd × 5 to 10 days: withdrawal bleeding usually occurs 3 to 7 days after therapy ends.
- Abnormal uterine bleeding: 5 to 10 mg, PO, qd × 5 to 10 days, beginning on the 16th or 21st day of the menstrual cycle
- Endometrial or renal carcinoma: Initially, 400 mg to 1000 mg, IM, per week; maintenance dose = 400 mg/month.
- Contraception: 150 mg, IM, q12wk

Contraindications: Hypersensitivity to progestins; thrombophlebitis, thromboembolic disorders, cerebral hemorrhage, or patients with a history of these conditions; impaired hepatic function or disease; breast cancer; undiagnosed vaginal bleeding; missed abortion; as a diagnostic test for pregnancy
Adverse effects: Breakthrough bleeding, spotting, change in menstrual flow, amenorrhea, cervical secretion changes, breast tenderness, masculinization of the female fetus, edema, weight changes, cholestatic jaundice, rash with or without pruritus, acne, melasma or chloasma, and mental depression

Mefenamic acid (Ponstel)

How supplied: Caps, 250 mg
Indications: Primary dysmenorrhea; relief of moderate pain if therapy will be <1 week

Adult dosage: Given with food

- Primary dysmenorrhea: 500 mg, then 250 mg, q6h. Started with onset of bleeding and associated symptoms; treatment >2 to 3 days should not be necessary.
- Acute pain: 500 mg, then 250 mg q6h prn, usually not to exceed 1 week

Contraindications and adverse effects: See Ibuprofen.

Megestrol (Megace)

How supplied: Tabs, 20, 40 mg; suspension, 40 mg/ml

Adult dosage

- Treatment of anorexia, cachexia, or an unexplained significant weight loss in patients with acquired immunodeficiency syndrome (AIDS): (suspension) 200 mg, PO, qid
- Palliative treatment of advanced carcinoma of the breast: 40 mg, PO, qid
- Palliative treatment of advanced carcinoma of the endometrium: 40 to 320 mg/day in divided doses

Contraindications and precautions: As a diagnostic test for pregnancy; prophylactic use to avoid weight loss. To be used with caution in patients with a history of thromboembolic disease.

Adverse effects: Nausea, vomiting, edema, breakthrough bleeding, dyspnea, hyperglycemia, alopecia

Menotropins (Pergonal)

How supplied: Injection, 75 IU follicle stimulating hormone (FSH) activity and 75 IU luteinizing hormones (LH) activity per 2-ml ampule, 150 IU FSH activity and 150 IU LH activity per 2-ml ampule

Actions and indications: Menotropins is biologically standardized for FSH and LH activities to produce ovarian follicular growth in women who do not have primary ovarian failure. Menotropins and HCG given sequentially are indicated for induction of ovulation and pregnancy in the anovulatory fertile patient in whom the cause of anovulation is functional.

Adult dosage

- Initial dosage: Individualized dosage. Initial IM dose is 75 IU FSH/75 IU LH (1 ampule) per day × 9 to 12 days; followed by 10,000 IU HCG 1 day after the last dose of menotropins.
- Repeat dosage: If there is evidence of ovulation but no pregnancy, the regimen may be repeated for at least two more courses before the dose is increased to 150 IU FSH/150 IU LH (2 ampules) per day × 9 to 12 days; followed by 10,000 IU HCG 1 day after the last dose of menotropins.
- The same dose may be repeated for two more courses; larger doses are not recommended.

Contraindications and precautions: High gonadotropin level indicating primary ovarian failure; overt thyroid and adrenal dysfunction; any cause of infertility other than anovulation; abnormal bleeding of undetermined origin; ovarian cysts or enlargement not caused by polycystic ovary syndrome; organic intracranial lesion; pregnancy. Mild to moderate uncomplicated ovarian enlargement, with or without abdominal distension or abdominal pain, occurs in approximately 20% of those treated with HCG and menotropins and generally regresses without treatment in 2 to 3 weeks. Multiple pregnancy may occur.

Adverse effects: Ovarian enlargement, hyperstimulation syndrome, hemoperitoneum, arterial thromboembolism, hypersensitivity, febrile reactions

Meperidine (Demerol)

How supplied: Tabs, 50, 100 mg; syrup, 50 mg/5 ml; injection, 10, 25, 50, 75, 100 mg/ml

Indications and adult dosage

- Relief of moderate to severe pain: 50 to 150 mg, IM/SC/PO, q3-4h prn
- Preoperative medication: 50 to 100 mg, IM/SC, 30 to 90 minutes before beginning anesthesia
- Anesthesia support: May be administered in repeated doses diluted to 10 mg/ml by slow IV injection, or by continuous IV infusion of solution diluted to 1 mg/ml
- Obstetrical analgesia: When pains become regular, 50 to 100 mg, IM/SC, administered q1-3h

Contraindications and precautions: Current or recent use of MAO inhibitors; head injury, increased intracranial pressure; concomitant use of CNS depressants; acute abdominal conditions; convulsive disorders; pregnancy category C

Mestranol/norethynodrel (Enovid 10 mg, Enovid 5 mg)

How supplied: Tabs, 10 mg = 150 µg mestranol + 9.85 mg norethynodrel, 5 mg = 75 µg mestranol + 5 mg norethynodrel

Adult dosage

- Endometriosis: 5 to 10 mg, PO qd × 2 weeks, beginning on day 5 of menstrual cycle; may be increased by 5- or 10-mg increments at 2-week intervals, up to 20 mg/day; this dose continued for 6 to 9 months.
- Hypermenorrhea (for emergency control of severe cases): 20 to 30 mg/day until bleeding is controlled, then reduced to 10 mg and continued through day 24 of cycle

Methyldopa (Aldomet, Amodopa)

How supplied: Tabs, 125, 250, 500 mg; suspension, 250 mg/5 ml; injection, 250 mg/5 ml

Actions: Stimulates central inhibitory alpha-adrenergic receptors.

Indications: Hypertension

Adult dosage

- Oral: 250 to 500 mg, PO, bid-qid; maximum dose = 3 g/day.
- Parenteral: 250 to 500 mg, IV, q6h; administered over 30 to 60 minutes; maximum dose = 1 g q6h.

Contraindications and precautions: Active hepatic disease, pregnancy category B

Adverse effects: Sedation, headache, fatigue, bradycardia, nausea, and vomiting

Methylergonovine maleate (Methergine)

How supplied: Injection, 0.2 mg/ml; tabs, 0.2 mg

Indications: Routine management after delivery of the placenta; postpartum atony and hemorrhage; subinvolution. Under full obstetric supervision, it may be given in the second stage of labor following delivery of the anterior shoulder.

Adult dosage:
- IM: 0.2 mg after delivery of the placenta, after delivery of the anterior shoulder, or during the puerperium; repeated as required, at intervals of 2 to 4 hours. IV administration may induce sudden hypertension and cerebrovascular accidents. If IV administration is considered essential, should be given slowly over no less than 60 seconds, with careful blood pressure monitoring.
- Oral: 0.2 mg three or four times per day in the puerperium for a maximum of 1 week

Contraindications and precautions: Hypertension, toxemia, pregnancy, hypersensitivity; caution should be exercised in the presence of sepsis, obliterative vascular disease, hepatic or renal involvement

Adverse effects: Nausea, vomiting, hypertension, dizziness, headache, tinnitus, diaphoresis, palpitations, temporary chest pain, and dyspnea

Metoclopramide (Reglan)

How supplied: Tabs, 5, 10 mg; syrup, 5 mg/5 ml; injection, 5 mg/ml

Indications and adult dosage
- Prevention of postoperative nausea and vomiting: 10 to 20 mg IM injected near the end of surgery
- Prevention of chemotherapy-induced emesis: 1 to 2 mg/kg, IV, given slowly over 15 minutes, 30 minutes before beginning cancer chemotherapy and repeated q2h × two doses, then q3h × three doses
- GERD: 10 to 15 mg, PO, 30 minutes before each meal and at hs; maximum duration of therapy is 12 weeks.
- Diabetic gastroparesis: 10 mg, PO, 30 minutes before each meal and at hs × 2 to 8 weeks

Contraindications and precautions: When stimulation of GI motility may be dangerous; pregnancy category B

Adverse effects: Extrapyramidal symptoms, drowsiness, fatigue, confusion, diarrhea, galactorrhea, amenorrhea, gynecomastia

Metoprolol (Lopressor, Toprol XL)

How supplied: Tabs, 50, 100 mg; extended release tabs, 50, 100, 200 mg; injection, 1 mg/ml

Action: Beta-adrenergic blocker

Indications: Hypertension, angina pectoris, acute myocardial infarction

Adult dosage
- PO: Initially, 50 to 100 mg/day; maintenance dose = 100 to 450 mg/day qd-bid
- IV (acute MI): 5 mg IV bolus q2m × three doses

Contraindications and precautions: Sinus bradycardia; pregnancy category C (use during the first trimester should be avoided; lowest possible dose should be used).

Adverse effects: Bradycardia, dizziness, fatigue, nausea, vomiting, diarrhea

Metronidazole (Flagyl, Protostat, MetroGel-Vaginal)

How supplied: Tabs, 250, 500 mg; injection, 500 mg; vaginal gel, 0.75%

Indications: Treatment of trichomoniasis, amebiasis, and bacterial vaginosis, as well as serious infections caused by susceptible anaerobic bacteria;

especially useful in infections caused by *Bacteroides fragilis* resistant to clindamycin, chloramphenicol, and penicillin

Adult dosage

- Trichomoniasis: 2 g, PO, once or 500 mg, PO, bid × 7 days
- Bacterial vaginosis (*Gardnerella vaginalis*): 500 mg, PO, bid × 7 days
  1. Alternative regimens: 2 g, PO, once or metronidazole gel, 0.75%, one applicator full (5 g) intravaginally bid × 5 days
- Anaerobic infections: Loading dose 15 mg/kg, IV, over 1 hour (approximately 1 g for 70 kg adult) followed by 7.5 mg/kg, IV, q8h; maximum 4 g/24 hours
- Pseudomembranous colitis: 250 mg, PO, qid or 500 mg, PO, bid × 7 to 10 days
- Giardiasis: 250 mg, PO, tid × 7 days

Elimination: Hepatic metabolism; dose should be reduced in patients with liver impairment.

Contraindications and precautions: Hypersensitivity to metronidazole or other nitroimidazole derivatives; pregnancy category B; not to be used to treat pregnant patients during the first trimester. May enhance the activity of other hepatically metabolized drugs.

Adverse effects: Seizures, peripheral neuropathy, nausea, vomiting, headache, diarrhea, leukopenia

Patient information: Alcohol should be avoided during treatment with metronidazole and for 24 hours thereafter. May be taken with food to avoid GI upset. May cause an unpleasant metallic taste.

Mezlocillin (Mezlin)

How supplied: Injection, 1, 2, 3, 4 g

Indications: Extended spectrum penicillin used for the treatment of infections caused by susceptible microorganisms (see Appendix XI)

Adult dosage: 1.5 to 4 g, IM/IV, q4-6h; maximum daily dose 24 g; maximum single IM dose 2 g

Elimination: Excreted by kidneys; dosage should be adjusted in renal impairment.

Contraindications, precautions, and adverse effects: See Penicillin.

Miconazole (Monistat 3, Monistat 7, Monistat Dual-Pak)

How supplied: Vaginal suppositories, 100, 200 mg; vaginal cream, 2%

Indications: Local treatment of vulvovaginal candidiasis

Adult dosage

- Monistat 3: One suppository inserted intravaginally qhs × 3 days
- Monistat 7: One applicator full cream or one suppository intravaginally qhs × 7 days

Minocycline (Minocin)

How supplied: Caps, 50, 100 mg; tabs, 50, 100 mg; oral suspension, 50 mg/5 ml; injection, 100 mg

Indications: See Doxycycline (see Appendix XI).

Adult dosage

- Oral: 200 mg initially, then 100 mg bid
- Parenteral: 200 mg initially, then 100 mg bid (maximum 400 mg/day)

Elimination: Metabolized in liver and excreted largely by nonrenal routes
Contraindications, precautions, and adverse effects: See Doxycycline.
Patient information: Unlike other tetracyclines, minocycline may be taken with food or milk. Prolonged exposure to sunlight or sunlamps should be avoided.

Morphine

How supplied: Injection, 0.5, 1, 2, 3, 4, 5, 8, 10, 15 mg/ml; tabs, 10, 15, 30 mg; SR tab (MS Contin), 30, 60 mg; solution, 10, 20 mg/5 ml, 20 mg/ml; suppositories, 5, 10, 20, 30 mg
Indications: Relief of moderate to severe acute and chronic pain; preoperatively to sedate patient and allay apprehension, facilitate induction of anesthesia, and reduce anesthetic dosage
Adult dosage

- Oral administration is one third to one sixth as effective as parenteral administration.
- PO: 10 to 30 mg q4h, *or* SR, 30 to 60 mg q8-12h
- SC/IM: 5 to 20 mg q4h
- IV: 2.5 to 15 mg, diluted in 5 ml of water for injection and administered over 5 minutes
- Rectal: 10 to 20 mg q4h
- Epidural: Initial injection of 5 mg in the lumbar region may provide satisfactory pain relief for up to 24 hours. If relief is not achieved within 1 hour, incremental doses of 1 to 2 mg may be administered at intervals sufficient to assess effectiveness. Maximum dose = 10 mg/24 hours.
- For continuous infusion, an initial dose of 2 to 4 mg/24 hours is recommended. If pain relief is not achieved initially, further doses of 1 to 2 mg may be given.

Contraindications and precautions: Hypersensitivity to morphine, pregnancy category C, head injury and increased ICP, acute abdominal conditions, hepatic dysfunction, concomitant use of CNS depressants

Nabumetone (Relafen)

How supplied: Tab, 500, 750 mg
Indications: For acute and chronic treatment of signs and symptoms of osteoarthritis and rheumatoid arthritis
Adult dosage 1000 to 2000 mg daily, divided qd-bid; maximum dose = 2000 mg/day; if GI upset occurs, may be taken with food or milk.
Contraindications and adverse effects: See Ibuprofen.

Nafarelin acetate (Synarel)

How supplied: Nasal solution, 2 mg/ml
Indications: Endometriosis, including pain relief and reduction of endometriotic lesions.

- Experience has been limited to women ≥18 years of age treated for 6 months.

Adult dosage: 400 μg/day. One spray (200 μg) into one nostril in the morning and one spray into the other nostril in the evening. Treatment should start between days 2 and 4 of the menstrual cycle. Maximum dose = 800 μg/day.

Contraindications and precautions: Hypersensitivity GnRH, GnRH-agonist analogs, or any of the excipients in the product; undiagnosed abnormal vaginal bleeding; pregnancy and lactation (pregnancy category X). Ovarian cysts may develop; loss of bone density; menstruation should stop with effective doses of nafarelin.

Adverse effects: Hot flashes, libido decrease, vaginal dryness, headaches, emotional lability, insomnia, acne, myalgia, edema, weight gain, and nasal irritation

Nafcillin (Unipen, Nafcil, Nallpen)

How supplied: Tabs, 500 mg; caps, 250 mg; injection, 500 mg, 1 g, 2 g

Indications: The treatment of infections from penicillinase-producing staphylococci (see Appendix XI)

Adult dosage

- Oral: 250 to 500 mg q4-6h (maximum daily dose is 1 g q4h). NOTE: Oral administration produces low and unpredictable serum levels.
- IM: 500 mg q4-6h
- IV: 500 mg to 2 g q4-6h (maximum daily dose 12 g)

Elimination: Significant hepatic elimination in bile

Contraindications and precautions: Hypersensitivity to any penicillin

Adverse effects: Thrombophlebitis with parenteral administration, nausea, diarrhea, and hypersensitivity reactions

Nalbuphine (Nubain)

How supplied: Injection, 10, 20 mg/ml

Indications: Relief of moderate to severe pain; for preoperative analgesia, as a supplement to balanced analgesia, to surgical and postsurgical anesthesia, and for obstetric analgesia during labor and delivery

Adult dosage: Individualized dosage; usual dose is 10 mg, SC/IM/IV, q3-6h prn. In intolerant individuals, the maximum recommended single dose is 20 mg, with a maximum total daily dose of 160 mg.

Contraindications and precautions: Hypersensitivity to nalbuphine, head injury and increased ICP, renal or hepatic function impairment, respiratory depression; caution should be observed while driving or performing other tasks requiring alertness; patients dependent on narcotics may experience withdrawal symptoms on the administration of nalbuphine.

Naproxen (Aleve, Anaprox, Anaprox DS, Naprosyn)

How supplied: Tabs, 200, 250, 375, 500 mg; suspension, 125 mg/5 ml

Indications: Treatment of primary dysmenorrhea, rheumatoid arthritis, osteoarthritis, ankylosing spondylitis, tendinitis, bursitis, acute gout; relief of mild to moderate pain

Adult dosage: Maximum dose = 1.25 g (1.375 g naproxen sodium) per day; if GI upset occurs, should be taken with food or milk.

- Primary dysmenorrhea, mild to moderate pain, acute tendinitis and bursitis: 500 mg, followed by 250 mg q6-8h
- Rheumatoid arthritis, osteoarthritis, ankylosing spondylitis: 250 to 500 mg bid

• Acute gout: 750 mg, followed by 250 mg q8h until the attack subsides
Contraindications and adverse effects: See Ibuprofen.

Nifedipine (Procardia, Adalat)

How supplied: Caps, 10, 20 mg; SR tabs, 30, 60, 90 mg
Actions: Calcium channel blocker
Indications: Vasospastic angina; chronic stable angina; hypertension
Adult dosage: 10 to 20 mg, PO, tid or sustained release 30 to 90 mg, PO, qd; maximum dose = 120 mg/day. Nifedipine caps may be given SL for hypertensive emergencies.
Contraindications and precautions: Pregnancy category C; to be used only when clearly needed and when potential benefits outweigh potential hazards to the fetus.

Nitrofurantoin (Furadantin, Macrodantin, Macrobid)

How supplied: Tabs, 50, 100 mg; caps, 50, 100 mg; SR caps, 100 mg; oral suspension, 25 mg/5 ml
Indications: Treatment of urinary tract infections (UTI) caused by susceptible microorganisms (see Appendix XI)
Adult dosage
• Treatment: 50 to 100 mg, PO, qid with meals and at bedtime × 7 days; SR caps, 100 mg, PO, q12h × 7 days
• Suppressive therapy: 50 to 100 mg, PO, qhs
Elimination: Renal excretion; not to be used in patients with Cr Cl <40 ml/min
Contraindications and precautions: Hypersensitivity to nitrofurantoin; pregnant women at term because of possibility of hemolysis in the infant
Adverse effects: Anorexia, nausea, emesis, hepatotoxicity, dyspnea, chest pain, cough, pruritus, and urticaria

Nitroprusside (Nipride, Nitropress)

How supplied: Injection, 50 mg/5 ml
Actions: Dilates peripheral arteries and veins through relaxation of vascular smooth muscle.
Indications: Hypertensive crises
Adult dosage: 50 mg/250 to 1000 ml D_5W infused IV at 0.3 to 10 μg/kg/min
Contraindications and precautions: Pregnancy category C (given only if clearly needed); to be discontinued as quickly as possible to avoid cyanide toxicity
Adverse effects: Precipitous drops in BP, nausea, vomiting, tachycardia, and cyanide toxicity

Norethindrone (Norlutin)

How supplied: Tabs, 5 mg
Adult dosage
• Amenorrhea; abnormal uterine bleeding caused by hormonal imbalance in the absence of organic pathology: 5 to 20 mg qd days 5 to 25 of menstruation
• Endometriosis: Initially, 10 mg/day × 2 weeks; increased in increments of 5 mg/day q2wk until 30 mg/day is reached
Contraindications and adverse effects: See Medroxyprogesterone.

Norethindrone acetate (Norlutate, Aygestin)

How supplied: Tabs, 5 mg

- Norethindrone acetate differs from norethindrone only in potency; the acetate is approximately twice as potent.

Adult dosage

- Amenorrhea; abnormal uterine bleeding caused by hormonal imbalance in the absence of organic pathology: 2.5 to 10 mg, qd, days 5 to 25 of the menstrual cycle
- Endometriosis: Initially, 5 mg/day × 2 weeks; increased in increments of 2.5 mg/day q2wk until 15 mg/day is reached

Contraindications and adverse effects: See Medroxyprogesterone.

Norfloxacin (Noroxin)

How supplied: Tabs, 400 mg

Indications: Treatment of infections caused by susceptible microorganisms (see Appendix XI)

Adult dosage

- UTI: 400 mg, PO, q12h
- Uncomplicated gonorrhea: Single dose 800 mg PO

Elimination: See Ciprofloxacin.

Contraindications, precautions, and adverse effects: See Ciprofloxacin.

Patient information: To be taken 1 hour before or 2 hours after meals with a glass of water

Nystatin (Mycostatin, Nilstat)

How supplied: Tabs, 500,000 U; suspension, 100,000 U/ml; troche, 200,000 U; cream, ointment, powder, 100,000 U/g; vaginal tabs, 100,000 U

Indications: Cutaneous or mucocutaneous candidiasis, oral candidiasis, intestinal candidiasis, and vulvovaginal candidiasis

Adult dosage

- Vulvovaginal candidiasis: One tab (100,000 units) inserted intravaginally qhs × 2 weeks
  1. During pregnancy, use of a vaginal applicator may be contraindicated; manual insertion of tablets may be preferred.
- Cutaneous or mucocutaneous candidiasis: Cream, ointment, or powder applied to affected area two to three times daily.
- Intestinal candidiasis: 500,000 to 1,000,000 U (1 to 2 tabs), PO, tid
- Oral candidiasis: 4 to 6 ml, PO, qid (retained in mouth as long as possible before swallowing) *or* 1 to 2 troches 4 to 5 times daily; not to be chewed or swallowed

Contraindications and precautions: Hypersensitivity to nystatin. Vaginal preparation, pregnancy category A

Adverse effects: Nausea, vomiting, diarrhea are observed rarely after oral administration; local irritation.

Ofloxacin (Floxin)

How supplied: Tabs, 200, 300, 400 mg; injection, 200, 400 mg

Indications: Treatment of infections caused by susceptible microorganisms (see Appendix XI)

Adult dosage
- Usual treatment of infection: 200 to 400 mg, PO/IV, q12h
- Acute uncomplicated gonorrhea: Single dose, 400 mg, PO
- *Chlamydia trachomatis* cervicitis or urethritis: 300 mg, PO, q12h × 7 days
- PID (outpatient): 400 mg, PO, bid × 14 days plus clindamycin or metronidazole

Elimination: See Ciprofloxacin.
Contraindications, precautions, and adverse effects: See Ciprofloxacin.
Patient information: Not to be taken with food

Ondansetron (Zofran)

How supplied: Tabs, 4, 8 mg; injection, 2 mg/ml
Indications: Prevention of nausea and vomiting associated with initial and repeat courses of emetogenic cancer chemotherapy; prevention of postoperative nausea or vomiting
Adult dosage
- Prevention of nausea or vomiting associated with cancer chemotherapy
  1. IV: 0.15 mg/kg infused over 15 minutes beginning 30 minutes before the start of emetogenic chemotherapy; repeated 4 and 8 hours after the first dose; *or* a single 32-mg dose infused over 15 minutes beginning 30 minutes before emetogenic chemotherapy
  2. PO: 8 mg, tid; first dose administered 30 minutes before chemotherapy and repeated 4 and 8 hours later; administered 8 mg, PO, q8h for 1 to 2 days after completion of chemotherapy
- Prevention of postoperative nausea or vomiting: Administered 4 mg IV undiluted in not less than 30 seconds (preferably over 2 to 5 minutes) immediately before induction of anesthesia, or postoperatively if the patient experiences nausea or vomiting occurring shortly after surgery.

Contraindications and precautions: Pregnancy category B; not to exceed an 8-mg oral dose in patients with hepatic function impairment
Adverse effects: Diarrhea, headache, fever, abdominal pain, weakness, drowsiness, and shivers

Oxaprozin (Daypro)

How supplied: Tabs, 600 mg
Indications: Acute and long-term use in the management of signs and symptoms of rheumatoid arthritis and osteoarthritis
Adult dosage: 600 to 1200 mg, qd; maximum dose = 1800 mg/day (or 26 mg/kg, whichever is lower) in divided doses
Contraindications and adverse effects: See Ibuprofen.

Oxytocin (Pitocin, Syntocinon)

How supplied: Injection, 10 U/ml; nasal spray, 40 U/ml
Indications:
- Parenteral:
  1. Antepartum: To initiate or improve uterine contractions to achieve early vaginal delivery, for fetal or maternal reasons
  2. Postpartum: To produce uterine contractions during the third stage of labor and to control postpartum bleeding or hemorrhage

- Nasal: For initial milk letdown

Adult dosage

- Induction or stimulation of labor: Administered by IV infusion; initial dose should be no more than 1 to 2 mU/min (0.001 to 0.002 U/min); the dose should be gradually increased in increments of no more than 1 to 2 mU/min at 15- to 30-minute intervals until a contraction pattern has been established that is similar to normal labor. Maximum doses should rarely exceed 20 mU/min. The oxytocin infusion should be discontinued immediately in the event of uterine hyperactivity or fetal distress and oxygen administered to the mother.
- Control of postpartum uterine bleeding
  1. IV infusion: 10 to 40 U to a maximum of 40 U added to 1 L of a nonhydrating diluent and run at a rate necessary to control uterine atony
  2. IM: 10 U administered after delivery of the placenta
- Treatment of incomplete or inevitable abortion: IV infusion of 10 U of oxytocin with 500 ml 0.9% NaCl or D_5W/0.9% NaCl infused at a rate of 10 to 20 mU (20 to 40 drops) per minute
- Initial milk letdown: Nasal spray, one spray into one or both nostrils 2 to 3 minutes before nursing or pumping of breasts.

Contraindications and precautions: Significant cephalopelvic disproportion; unfavorable fetal positions or presentations that are undeliverable without conversion before delivery; benefit to risk ratio in obstetrical emergencies for either the fetus or the mother favors surgical intervention; hypersensitivity to the drug. Oxytocin (nasal) is contraindicated in pregnancy.

Adverse effects

- Maternal: Anaphylactic reaction, postpartum hemorrhage, cardiac arrhythmia, fatal afibrinogenemia, nausea, vomiting, premature ventricular contractions (PVCs), increased blood loss, and pelvic hematoma. Uterine hypertonicity, spasm, tetanic contraction, or rupture of the uterus may occur as a result of excessive dosage or hypersensitivity to the drug. A slow oxytocin infusion over a 24-hour period was associated with severe water intoxication with convulsions and coma. Maternal death caused by oxytocin-induced water intoxication has occurred.
- Fetal: Bradycardia, PVCs, and other arrhythmias; permanent CNS or brain damage and death. Low Apgar scores at 5 minutes and neonatal jaundice and retinal hemorrhage have occurred because of use of oxytocin in the mother.

Penicillin G benzathine (Bicillin L-A, Permapen)

How supplied: Injection, 300,000 U, 600,000 U/ml

Indications: A long-acting parenteral PCN used in the treatment of moderately severe infections caused by penicillin G-sensitive microorganisms

Adult dosage: Administered by deep IM injection into the upper outer quadrant of the buttock.

- Early syphilis (primary, secondary, or latent syphilis of <1 year's duration): 2.4 million units IM once (Some practitioners recommend repeating this regimen after 7 days, especially in HIV-infected patients.)

- Late syphilis (>1 year's duration, cardiovascular, gumma, late-latent): 2.4 million units IM once weekly × 3 weeks
- Group A streptococcal infection (prevention of recurrent rheumatic fever): 1.2 million units q4wk

Contraindications, precautions, and adverse effects: See Penicillin.

Penicillin G benzathine and procaine combined (Bicillin C-R, Bicillin C-R 900/300)

How supplied: Injection, 300,000 (150,000 U each PCN G benzathine and PCN G procaine), 600,000 U/ml (300,000 units each PCN G benzathine and PCN G procaine)

Adult dosage

- Streptococcal infections: 2.4 million units IM × 1.
- Pneumococcal infections (except pneumococcal meningitis): 1.2 million units IM q2-3d until afebrile × 48 hours

Penicillin G procaine (Crysticillin, Wycillin)

How supplied: Injection, 300,000 U/ml, 600,000 U/ml, 1,200,000 U/2 ml, 2,400,000 U/4 ml

Indications: A long-acting parenteral penicillin used in the treatment of moderately severe infections caused by penicillin G-sensitive microorganisms

Adult dosage: Administered by deep IM injection into the upper outer quadrant of the buttock

- Neurosyphilis: 2.4 million units, IM, daily plus probenecid, 500 mg, PO, qid, both × 10 to 14 days
- Congenital syphilis: 50,000 U/kg, IM, daily for 10 to 14 days
- Pneumococcal infections: 600,000 to 1.2 million units/day

Contraindications, precautions, and adverse effects: See Penicillin. Also, injection site sterile abscess or local sterile inflammatory reaction may occur. Each 300,000 U contains 120 mg procaine, which may cause CNS effects such as tinnitus, headache, hallucinations, or, rarely, seizures.

Penicillin V (V-Cillin K, Beepen-VK, Pen-V, Pen-Vee K, Veetids '250', Veetids '500')

How supplied: Tabs, 125, 250, 500 mg; solution, 125, 250 mg/5 ml

Penicillin G Potassium, Penicillin G Sodium (Pfizerpen, Pentids '400', Pentids '800')

How supplied: Injection, 1, 2, 3, 5, 10, 20 million U/vial; tabs, 200,000 U (125 mg), 250,000 U, 400,000 U (250 mg), 500,000 U, 800,000 U (500 mg); syrup, 400,000 U/5 ml

Indications: Treatment of infections caused by susceptible microorganisms (see Appendix XI).

Adult dosage:

- Parenteral: 1 to 24 million units/day divided q4-6h
- Oral: 125 to 500 mg, PO, qid
- Neurosyphilis: 2 to 4 million units, IV, q4h × 10 to 14 days (Patients allergic to penicillin should be desensitized.)

• Congenital syphilis: 50,000 U/kg, IV, q8-12h × 10 to 14 days

Elimination: Excreted by kidneys; dosage should be adjusted in renal impairment.

Contraindications and precautions: History of hypersensitivity to penicillins, cephalosporins, or imipenem; pregnancy category B; use may cause diarrhea, candidiasis, or allergic responses in the nursing infant.

Adverse effects: Hypersensitivity reactions such as maculopapular or urticarial rash, fever, bronchospasm, eosinophilia; nausea, vomiting, diarrhea, and phlebitis

Patient information: Penicillin G to be taken on an empty stomach 1 hour before or 2 hours after meals. Absorption of penicillin V is not significantly affected by food.

Pentazocine (Talwin, Talwin NX)

How supplied: Injection, 30 mg/ml; tabs, 50 mg + 0.5 mg naloxone

Indications

- Oral and parenteral: Relief of moderate to severe pain
- Parenteral: For preoperative or preanesthetic medication; supplement to surgical anesthesia

Adult dosage

- Oral: Initially, 50 mg q3-4h; increased to 100 mg if necessary; maximum dose = 600 mg/day.
- Parenteral: 30 mg, IM/SC/IV, q3-4h; maximum dose = 360 mg/day.

Contraindications and precautions: Hypersensitivity to pentazocine; head injury and increased intracranial pressure; renal or hepatic function impairment; respiratory depression; caution should be observed while driving or performing other tasks requiring alertness, coordination, or physical dexterity.

Phenytoin (Dilantin)

How supplied: Injection, 50 mg/ml; chewable tabs, 50 mg; caps, 30, 100 mg; oral suspension, 30 mg, 125 mg/5 ml

Indications: Control of grand mal and psychomotor seizures

- Parenteral: Control of status epilepticus

Adult dosage

- Usual PO dose is 4 to 6 mg/kg/day.
  1. This can be given in divided doses (100 mg, PO, tid) or as one daily dose (300 mg, PO, qd) of extended phenytoin sodium capsules (Dilantin Kapseals) when patient compliance is a problem.
  2. If an oral loading dose is necessary, patient should be given a total of 1 g divided into three doses (400, 300, 300 mg) and administered at 2 hour intervals; maintenance dose is then instituted 24 hours after the loading dose; periodical serum levels should be obtained (therapeutic range is 10 to 20 mg/L).
- Status epilepticus: Loading dose of 10 to 15 mg/kg by slow IV injection (≤50 mg/min) followed by 100 mg, PO/IV, q6-8h

Contraindications and precautions: Sinus bradycardia, atrioventricular (AV) block greater than first degree; not to be used for seizures secondary to hypoglycemia or other metabolic causes; phenytoin should be discontinued if patient develops skin rash; to be used with caution in elderly patients and in patients with impaired liver function; continuous monitoring of ECG and BP is necessary when administering IV phenytoin loading dose; phenytoin is associated with many drug interactions.

Adverse effects: Nystagmus, ataxia, dysarthria, slurred speech, dizziness, CNS depression, nausea, vomiting, diarrhea, hepatitis, and rash

Piperacillin (Pipracil)

How supplied: Injection, 2, 3, 4 g

Indications: Extended spectrum penicillin used for the treatment of infections caused by susceptible microorganisms; especially useful against gram negative organisms such as *Pseudomonas aeruginosa* (see Appendix XI)

Adult dosage: 2 to 4 g, IV/IM, q4-6h; maximum daily dose 24 g; maximum single IM dose 2 g

Elimination: Excreted by kidneys; dosage should be adjusted in renal impairment.

Contraindications, precautions, and adverse effects: See Penicillin.

Piperacillin/Tazobactam (Zosyn)

How supplied: Injection, 2.25, 3.375, 4.5 g

Indications: See Piperacillin. Addition of tazobactam extends spectrum to include infections caused by β-lactamase-producing organisms.

Adult dosage: Usual dose is 3.375 g, IV, q6h × 7 to 10 days

Elimination: Excreted by kidneys; dosage should be adjusted in renal impairment.

Contraindications and precautions: Hypersensitivity to any PCN

Adverse effects: Diarrhea, headache, constipation, nausea, insomnia, and rash

Piroxicam (Feldene)

How supplied: Caps, 10, 20 mg

Indications: For acute or long-term use in relief of signs and symptoms of osteoarthritis and rheumatoid arthritis

Adult dosage: 20 mg daily divided qd to bid; maximum dose = 20 mg/day; if GI upset occurs, should be taken with food or milk.

Contraindications and adverse effects: See Ibuprofen.

Prochlorperazine (Compazine)

How supplied: Tabs, 5, 10, 25 mg; SR caps, 10, 15, 30 mg; suppositories, 2.5, 5, 25 mg; syrup, 5 mg/5 ml; injection, 5 mg/ml

Indications: Control of nausea and vomiting

Adult dosage

- Oral: 5 to 10 mg, tid-qid; or SR capsule, 15 mg qm or 10 mg bid
- Rectal: 25 mg, bid
- IM: 5 to 10 mg, q3-4h prn; not to exceed 40 mg/day
- IV: 5 to 10 mg, 15 to 30 minutes before induction of anesthesia, or to control acute symptoms during and after surgery

Contraindications and precautions: Comatose or severely depressed states, presence of large amounts of other CNS depressants, pregnancy category C

Adverse effects: Sedation, extrapyramidal symptoms, anticholinergic effects, orthostatic hypotension, and jaundice

Progesterone (Gesterol 50, Progestaject)

How supplied: Injection, 50 mg/ml

Adult dosage

- Amenorrhea: 5 to 10 mg, IM, qd × 6 to 8 consecutive days. Withdrawal bleeding can be expected 48 to 72 hours after the last injection if ovarian activity has produced a proliferative endometrium.
- Functional uterine bleeding: 5 to 10 mg, IM, qd × six doses. Bleeding should cease within 6 days. When estrogen is also given, progesterone should be given after 2 weeks of estrogen therapy. Injections should be discontinued when menstrual flow begins.

Contraindications and adverse effects: See Medroxyprogesterone.

Progesterone intrauterine system (Progestasert)

How supplied: Intrauterine system, T-shaped unit containing a reservoir of 38 mg progesterone

Indications: Intrauterine contraception in women who have had at least one child; are in a stable, mutually monogamous relationship; and have no history of PID

Adult dosage: A single system inserted into the uterine cavity. Contraceptive effectiveness is retained for 1 year, and the system must be replaced 1 year after insertion.

Contraindications: Pregnancy or suspected pregnancy, previous ectopic pregnancy, presence or history of PID, patient or partner has multiple sexual partners, sexually transmitted disease, postpartum endometritis or infected abortion, pelvic surgery, uterine distortion, uterine or cervical malignancy, genital bleeding of unknown etiology, incomplete involution of the uterus following abortion or childbirth, previously inserted intrauterine device (IUD) still in place, genital actinomycosis, susceptibility to microorganism infections, and IV drug abuse

Promethazine (Phenergan)

How supplied: Tabs, 12.5, 25, 50 mg; syrup, 6.25, 25 mg/5 ml; suppositories, 12.5, 25, 50 mg; injection, 25, 50 mg/ml

Indications: Active and prophylactic treatment of motion sickness, prevention and control of nausea and vomiting associated with anesthesia and surgery, antiemetic in postoperative patients

Adult dosage

- Nausea and vomiting
  1. PO/PR: 12.5 to 25 mg q6h prn
  2. IM: 12.5 to 25 mg q4h prn
- Motion sickness: 25 mg, PO/PR, bid
- Sedation: 25 to 50 mg, PO/PR, at hs
- Preoperative use: 50 mg, PO/PR, the night before surgery

Propoxyphene (Darvon, Darvon-N)

How supplied: Caps, 32, 65 mg; tabs, 100 mg; suspension, 10 mg/ml

Indications: Relief of mild to moderate pain

Adult dosage

- Propoxyphene HCl: 65 mg, PO, q4h prn; not to exceed 390 mg/day
- Propoxyphene napsylate: 100 mg, PO, q4h prn; not to exceed 600 mg/day

Contraindications and precautions: Reduction of total daily dosage should be considered in hepatic or renal impairment. Alcohol and other sedative or drowsiness-producing drugs should be avoided.

Propranolol (Inderal, Inderal LA)

How supplied: Tabs, 10, 20, 40, 60, 80, 90 mg; SR caps, 60, 80, 120, 160 mg; oral solution, 4, 8, 80 mg/ml; Injection, 1 mg/ml

Actions: Nonselective beta-adrenergic blocker

Indications: Hypertension, angina pectoris, acute MI, migraine prophylaxis, essential tremor

Adult dosage

- Hypertension: Initially, 40 mg, PO, bid; usual maintenance dose = 120 to 240 mg/day bid-tid or 120 to 160 mg qd (SR).
- Migraine prophylaxis: Initially, 80 mg/day (SR) or divided; maintenance dose = 160 to 240 mg/day in divided doses

Contraindications and precautions: Sinus bradycardia; bronchial asthma or COPD; pregnancy category C (use to be avoided during the first trimester; lowest possible dose to be used).

Adverse effects: Bronchospasm, bradycardia, dizziness, depression, fatigue, nausea, and vomiting; may blunt signs and symptoms of hypoglycemia.

Quinestrol (Estrovis)

How supplied: Tabs, 100 μg

Adult dosage

- Moderate to severe vasomotor symptoms associated with menopause, atrophic vaginitis, kraurosis vulvae, female hypogonadism, female castration and primary ovarian failure: 100 μg, PO, qd for 7 days, initially; followed with 100 μg once weekly for maintenance starting 2 weeks after treatment begins. May be increased to 200 μg per week to optimize therapeutic response.

Contraindications and adverse effects: See Estrogenic substances, conjugated.

RH_O (D) immune globulin (Gamulin Rh, HypRho-D, Rhesonativ, RhoGAM)

How supplied: Single-use vials

Indications and adult dosage

- Full term delivery: To prevent sensitization to the Rh_O (D) factor and to prevent hemolytic disease of the newborn in a subsequent pregnancy, one vial administered IM, preferably within 72 hours of delivery.
- Antepartum prophylaxis: One vial (approx. 300 μg) injected IM at 26 to 28 weeks gestation and one vial within 72 hours after an Rh-incompatible delivery to prevent Rh isoimmunization during pregnancy.
- Following amniocentesis, miscarriage, abortion, or ectopic pregnancy at or beyond 13 weeks' gestation: One vial IM

Contraindications and precautions: Not to be given IV; not to be given to the postpartum infant, to a Rh_O (D)-positive individual, or to a Rh_O (D)-negative individual previously sensitized to the Rh_O (D) antigen.

Rimantadine (Flumadine)

How supplied: Tabs, 100 mg; syrup, 50 mg/5 ml

Indications: Prophylaxis and treatment of illness caused by various strains of influenza A virus

Adult dosage

- Prophylaxis: 100 mg, PO, bid; dose reduced to 100 mg qd in patients with severe hepatic dysfunction or renal failure (Cr Cl ≤10 ml/min) and elderly nursing home patients.
- Treatment: Same as above; therapy should be continued for 7 days from the initial onset of symptoms

Contraindications and precautions: Hypersensitivity to rimantadine and amantadine; pregnancy category C

Adverse effects: Insomnia, dizziness, headache, nausea, vomiting

Ritodrine (Yutopar)

How supplied: Injection, 10 mg/ml, 15 mg/ml; tabs, 10 mg

Indications: Management of preterm labor in suitable patients. Therapy should be instituted as soon as the diagnosis of preterm labor is established and contraindications are ruled out in pregnancies of 20 or more weeks gestation.

Adult dosage: The initial IV treatment is usually followed by oral therapy. The optimum dose of the drug is determined by a balance of adverse effects and uterine response. Recurrences of unwanted preterm labor should be treated with IV infusion of ritodrine.

- IV: 150 mg ritodrine/500 ml fluid. The initial dose is 0.1 mg/min to be gradually increased by 0.05 mg/min every 10 minutes until the desired result is attained. The usual effective dosage is between 0.15 and 0.35 mg/min, continued for at least 12 hours after uterine contractions cease. Alternative regimen = 0.05 mg/min initially, increased 0.05/mg/min every 20 minutes to a maximum of 0.35 mg/min. If the maternal heart rate >140 beats/min, the dosage of ritodrine should not be increased further.
- Oral maintenance: 10 mg approximately 30 minutes before the termination of IV therapy, then 10 mg q2h for the first 24 hours; thereafter, 10 to 20 mg q4-6h, depending on uterine activity and unwanted effects; maximum dose = 120 mg/day. Treatment should be continued as long as it is desirable to prolong pregnancy.

Contraindications and precautions: Before the 20th week of pregnancy and in those conditions in which continuation of pregnancy is hazardous to the mother or fetus, pregnancy category B

Adverse effects: Palpitations, tremor, nausea, vomiting, headache, erythema, nervousness, jitteriness, restlessness, emotional upset, and anxiety; neonatal effects may include increased heart rate, hypoglycemia, and ileus.

Scopolamine, transdermal (Transderm-Scop)

How supplied: Transdermal therapeutic system, 1.5 mg scopolamine delivers 0.5 mg scopolamine *in vivo* over 3 days.

Indications: Prevention of nausea and vomiting associated with motion sickness in adults.

Adult dosage: One system applied behind the ear at least 4 hours before the antiemetic effect is required. Scopolamine 0.5 mg will be delivered over 3 days

Contraindications and precautions: Glaucoma; pregnancy category C; to be used with caution in patients with pyloric obstruction or urinary bladder neck obstruction and in patients suspected of having intestinal obstruction

Adverse effects: Dry mouth, dizziness, blurred vision, dilation of the pupils, drowsiness, disorientation, and confusion

Spectinomycin (Trobicin)

How supplied: Injection, 400 mg/ml

Indications: Acute gonorrheal cervicitis, urethritis, and procitis in the female caused by susceptible strains of *Neisseria gonorrhea.* In pregnancy to be used only in patients allergic to beta-lactams.

Adult dosage: 2 g, IM, once

Contraindications and precautions: Hypersensitivity to spectinomycin. Not effective for gonococcal pharyngeal infection.

Adverse effects: Injection site soreness, urticaria, chills, fever, dizziness, and nausea

Sulfanilamide (Vagitrol, AVC)

How supplied: Vaginal cream, vaginal suppositories

Indications: For the treatment of *Candida albicans* vulvovaginitis only

Adult dosage: One applicator full or one suppository intravaginally once or twice daily continued through one complete menstrual cycle

Contraindications and precautions: Hypersensitivity to any component, kidney disease, pregnancy at term, lactation

Adverse effects: Local irritations and, rarely, allergic reactions, pruritus, and urticaria

Sulfisoxazole (Gantrisin)

How supplied: Tabs, 500 mg; syrup, 500 mg/5 ml

Indications: Treatment of infections caused by susceptible microorganisms (see Appendix XI)

Adult dosage

- *Chlamydia trachomatis:* 500 mg, PO, qid × 10 days (inferior efficacy to other regimens)
- Lymphogranuloma venereum: 500 mg, PO, qid × 21 days
- Usual dose: 4 to 8 g/day divided q4-6h

Contraindications and precautions: Hypersensitivity to sulfonamides or chemically related drugs. Safety for use during pregnancy has not been established; not to be used during pregnancy at term. May potentiate effects of warfarin, sulfonylureas, or hydantoins.

Adverse effects: Photosensitivity, agranulocytosis, aplastic anemia, leukopenia, thrombocytopenia, generalized skin eruptions, nausea, vomiting, diarrhea, and crystalluria

Sulindac (Clinoril)

How supplied: Tabs, 150, 200 mg

Indications: For acute or long-term use in the relief of signs and symptoms of osteoarthritis, rheumatoid arthritis, ankylosing spondylitis, acute painful shoulder, and acute gouty arthritis

Adult dosage: Maximum dose = 400 mg/day; administered 150 to 200 mg, PO, bid with food

Contraindications and adverse effects: See Ibuprofen.

Terbutaline (Brethine, Bricanyl, Brethaire)

How supplied: Tabs, 2.5, 5 mg; aerosol, 0.2 mg/actuation; injection, 1 mg/ml

Indications: A bronchodilator for bronchial asthma and for reversible bronchospasm from other causes

Unlabeled use: Oral and IV terbutaline have successfully inhibited premature labor.

Adult dosage:

- Bronchodilatory effects
  1. Inhalation: Two inhalations separated by 60 seconds q4-6h
  2. Oral: 2.5 to 5 mg q6h, three times daily during waking hours; maximum dose = 15 mg/24 hr
  3. Parenteral: 0.25 mg SC; may repeat 0.25 mg in 15 to 30 minutes if significant improvement does not occur. Do not exceed a total dose of 0.5 mg in 4 hours.
- Inhibition of premature labor
  1. IV: Diluted to 20 to 50 μg/ml for continuous infusion. Initiated at 5 to 10 μg/min; titrated upward q10-15m to a maximum of 80 μg/min. IV dosage should be maintained at the minimum effective dose for 4 hours.
  2. Oral: Usually initiated 12 to 24 hours after an intravenous infusion is started. The maintenance dosage ranges from 2.5 to 5 mg q4-6h.
  3. SC: May be administered after IV infusions before switching to oral treatment, or as an initial treatment before initiating long-term oral therapy.
     a. Transitional: 0.25 mg q4-6h
     b. Initial: 0.25 mg q30-60m effectively inhibits uterine contractions. Maximum dose = 1 mg.

Contraindications: Preexisting maternal medical conditions that would be seriously affected by the pharmacologic properties of a betamimetic drug.

Adverse effects: Tachycardia, tremor, palpitations, shortness of breath, and dizziness

Terconazole (Terazol 7, Terazol 3)

How supplied: Vaginal cream, 0.4%, 0.8%; vaginal suppository, 80 mg

Indications: Local treatment of vulvovaginal candidiasis

Adult dosage

- Cream
  1. 0.4%: One applicator full (5 g) intravaginally qhs × 7 days
  2. 0.8%: One applicator full (5 g) intravaginally qhs × 3 days
- Suppositories: One suppository intravaginally qhs × 3 days

Tetracycline (Achromycin V, Panmycin, Robitet Robicaps, Sumycin)

How supplied: Caps, 100, 250, 500 mg; tabs, 250, 500 mg; oral suspension, 125 mg/5 ml; injection, 100, 250, 500 mg

Indications: See Doxycycline; see Appendix XI.

Adult dosage

- Oral: 250 to 500 mg qid
  1. Early syphilis (nonpregnant penicillin-allergic patient): 500 mg qid × 14 days (Continued × 30 days for late syphilis.)
  2. Chlamydia trachomatis (uncomplicated urethral, endocervical, or rectal): 500 mg, PO, qid × 7 days.
- Parenteral
  1. 250 to 300 mg, IM, qd, or divided q8-12h
  2. 250 to 500 mg, IV, q6-12h (maximum 2 g/day); physician should change to PO therapy as soon as clinically indicated.

Elimination: Renal excretion; dosage adjustment necessary in renal impairment.

Contraindications, precautions, and adverse effects: See Doxycycline.

Patient information: Given 1 hour before or 2 hours after meals; administration with dairy products, antacids, laxatives, or iron-containing products should be avoided. Prolonged exposure to sunlight or sunlamps should be avoided.

Thiethylperazine (Torecan)

How supplied: Tabs, 10 mg; suppository, 10 mg; injection, 5 mg/ml

Indications: Relief of nausea and vomiting

Adult dosage

- PO/PR: 10 to 30 mg daily in divided doses
- IM: 10 mg qd-tid; not to be used IV since severe hypotension may result.

Ticarcillin (Ticar)

How supplied: Injection, 1, 3, 6 g

Indications: Extended spectrum penicillin used for the treatment of infections caused by susceptible microorganisms; especially useful against gram negative organisms such as *Pseudomonas aeruginosa* (see Appendix XI)

Adult dosage: (IM/IV) 1 to 4 g q4-6h. Maximum daily dose = 24 g; maximum single IM dose = 2 g.

Elimination: Excreted by kidneys; dosage should be adjusted in renal impairment.

Contraindications, precautions, and adverse effects: See Penicillin.

Ticarcillin/clavulanate (Timentin)

How supplied: Injection, 3.1 g (3 g ticarcillin + 0.1 g clavulanic acid)

Indications: See Ticarcillin. Addition of clavulanic acid extends spectrum to include infections caused by β-lactamase-producing organisms

Adult dosage: 3.1 g, IV, q4-6h

Elimination: Excreted by kidneys; dosage should be adjusted in renal impairment.

Contraindications, precautions, and adverse effects: See Penicillin.

Tioconazole (Vagistat-1)

How supplied: Vaginal ointment, 6.5%

Indications: Local treatment of vulvovaginal candidiasis

Adult dosage: Single dose; one applicator full (4.6 g) inserted intravaginally just before bedtime
Contraindications and precautions: Pregnancy category C

Tobramycin (Nebcin)

How supplied: Injection, 10, 40 mg/ml vials
Indications: Used for the treatment of infections caused by susceptible microorganisms. Superior to gentamicin for *Pseudomonas aeruginosa* infections (see Appendix XI).
Adult dosage: See Gentamicin.
Contraindications, precautions, and adverse effects: See Amikacin.

Tolmetin (Tolectin)

How supplied: Tabs, 200, 600 mg; caps, 400 mg
Indications: Treatment of acute flares and long-term management of rheumatoid arthritis and osteoarthritis; treatment of juvenile rheumatoid arthritis
Adult dosage: 400 to 600 mg, PO, tid; maximum dose = 1800 mg/day; should be given with antacids, other than sodium bicarbonate, if GI upset occurs
Contraindications and adverse effects: See Ibuprofen.

Trimethobenzamide (Tigan)

How supplied: Caps, 100, 250 mg; suppositories 100, 200 mg; injection, 100 mg/ml
Indications: Control of nausea and vomiting
Adult dosage
- Oral: 250 mg tid to qid
- Rectal: 200 mg tid to qid
- IM: 200 mg tid to qid

Contraindications and precautions: Hypersensitivity to trimethobenzamide, benzocaine, or similar local anesthetics; safety for use during pregnancy has not been established.
Adverse effects: Hypersensitivity reactions, parkinson-like symptoms, hypotension or pain following IM injections, blurred vision, coma, convulsions, depression, diarrhea

Trimethoprim (TMP) and sulfamethoxazole (SMZ) (Co-Trimoxazole, Bactrim, Septra)

How supplied: Tabs, 80 mg TMP/400 mg SMZ, 160 mg TMP/800 mg SMZ; suspension, 40 mg TMP–200 mg SMZ/5 ml; parenteral, 80 mg TMP–400 mg SMZ/5 ml
Indications: Treatment of infections caused by susceptible microorganisms including UTIs, respiratory and gastrointestinal infections, and *Pneumocystis carinii* pneumonia (PCP) (see Appendix XI)
Adult dosage
- UTIs, shigellosis, and acute otitis media: 160 mg TMP/800 mg SMZ q12h × 10 to 14 days (5 days for shigellosis)
- Acute exacerbations of chronic bronchitis: 160 mg TMP/800 mg SMZ q12h × 14 days

- Traveler's diarrhea: 160 mg TMP/800 mg SMZ q12h × 5 days
- *Pneumocystis carinii* pneumonia
  1. Treatment: 15 to 20 mg/kg/day (based on TMP) in four divided doses × 21 days
  2. Prophylaxis: 160 mg TMP/800 mg SMZ (one double-strength tablet) PO three times per week

Elimination: Renal excretion; dosage should be adjusted in renal impairment.

Contraindications and precautions: Hypersensitivity to trimethoprim or sulfonamides; not to be used during pregnancy at term or during lactation

Adverse effects: Nausea; vomiting; anorexia; rash; urticaria; agranulocytosis; aplastic, hemolytic, or megaloblastic anemia; thrombocytopenia; and BUN and serum creatinine elevation

Triple sulfa (Sultrin Triple Sulfa, Trysul, V.V.S., Gyne-Sulf)

How supplied: Vaginal tablets (172.5 mg sulfathiazole, 143.75 mg sulfacetamide, 184 mg sulfabenzamide, and urea); vaginal cream (3.42% sulfathiazole, 2.86% sulfacetamide, 3.7% sulfabenzamide)

Indications: Treatment of *Gardnerella vaginalis* vaginitis

Adult dosage

- One tablet intravaginally AM and PM × 10 days, repeated if necessary
- One applicator full intravaginally, bid, × 4 to 6 days; treatment may then be reduced 25% to 50%; repeated if necessary

Contraindications and precautions: Hypersensitivity to any components; kidney disease; pregnancy at term; lactation

Adverse effects: Local irritation and, rarely, allergic reactions, pruritus, and urticaria

Urofollitropin (Metrodin)

How supplied: Injection, 0.83 mg (75 IU FSH activity) per ampule

Actions and indications: Urofollitropin stimulates ovarian follicular growth in women who do not have primary ovarian failure. Urofollitropin and HCG given sequentially are indicated for the induction of ovulation in patients with polycystic ovarian disease who have an elevated LH/FSH ratio and who have failed to respond to clomiphene therapy.

Adult dosage

- Initial dose: 75 IU/day IM urofollitropin × 7 to 12 days followed by 5000 to 10,000 U of HCG, 1 day after the last urofollitropin dose.
- If there is evidence of ovulation but no pregnancy, this dosage regimen may be repeated for at least two more courses before the dose is increased to 150 IU of FSH qd × 7 to 12 days.
- This dose should be followed with 5000 to 10,000 U of HCG 1 day after the urofollitropin dose.
- If evidence of ovulation is present, but pregnancy does not ensue, the same dose should be repeated for two more courses. Larger doses are not recommended.

Contraindications and precautions: High levels of both LH and FSH indicating primary ovarian failure; overt thyroid or adrenal dysfunction; an organic intracranial lesion such as a pituitary tumor; the presence of any cause of infertility other than anovulation; abnormal bleeding of undetermined origin; ovarian cysts or enlargement not caused by polycystic ovary syndrome. Reports of multiple births have been associated with urofollitropin. Contraindicated in pregnancy.

Adverse effects: Hyperstimulation syndrome characterized by sudden ovarian enlargement accompanied by ascites with or without pain or pleural effusion, mild to moderate ovarian enlargement, abdominal pain, pain, rash, swelling, or irritation at injection site, arterial thromboembolism, and hemoperitoneum

Vancomycin (Vancocin, Lyphocin, Vancoled)

How supplied: Caps, 125, 250 mg; oral solution, 1, 10 g; injection, 500 mg, 1 g

Indications: Orally for the treatment of pseudomembranous colitis caused by *Clostridium difficile.* Parenteral use is for the treatment of infections caused by susceptible gram positive organisms including methicillin-resistant staphylococci (see Appendix XI).

Adult dosage

- Pseudomembranous colitis: 125 to 500 mg, PO, qid × 7 to 10 days
- Parenteral: 500 mg to 1 g IV q12h
  1. Doses should be adjusted to achieve peak serum levels 20 to 40 μg/ml and trough concentrations 5 to 10 μg/ml. Drug should be infused over at least 60 minutes to avoid hypotension and "red man syndrome."

Elimination: Excreted by kidneys; dosage adjustment required for renal impairment; not removed by dialysis.

Contraindications and precautions: Hypersensitivity to vancomycin, pregnancy category C

Adverse effects: "Red man syndrome" (upper body flushing, hypotension, maculopapular rash), increased serum creatinine or BUN concentrations, hearing loss, vertigo, and neutropenia

Zalcitabine, ddC, dideoxycytidine (Hivid)

How supplied: Tabs, 0.375, 0.75 mg

Indications: Used in combination with zidovudine in patients with advanced HIV infections (CD4 cell count ≤300/mm^3) who have demonstrated significant clinical or immunologic deterioration.

Adult dosage: 0.75 mg, PO, q8h concomitantly with zidovudine, 200 mg, PO, q8h

Elimination: Renal excretion; dosage should be adjusted in renal impairment.

Contraindications and precautions: Hypersensitivity to zalcitabine or any components of the product; pregnancy category C

Adverse effects: Peripheral neuropathy, pancreatitis, esophageal ulcers, nausea, rash, and pruritus

Zidovudine, AZT, ZDV (Retrovir)

How supplied: Caps, 100 mg; syrup, 50 mg/5 ml; injection, 10 mg/ml

Indications: Management of patients with HIV infection with evidence of impaired immunity (CD4 cell count of ≤500/mm^3)

Adult dosage: Initial, 200 mg, PO, q4h (1200 mg/day) × 1 month, then reduced to 100 mg, PO, q4h while awake (500 mg/day) or 200 mg, PO, q8h

Contraindications and precautions: Pregnancy category C; administered to a pregnant woman only if clearly needed

Adverse effects: Anemia, granulocytopenia, headache, nausea, insomnia, and myalgia

Suggested reading

American hospital formulary service 1994, American Society of Hospital Pharmacists, Bethesda, MD 20814.

Briggs GG, Freeman RK, Yaffe SJ: *Drugs in pregnancy and lactation,* ed 2, Baltimore, 1986, Williams & Wilkins.

CDC 1993 sexually transmitted treatment guidelines, *MMWR* 42(RR-14):1-102, 1993.

Choice of contraceptives, *Med Lett Drugs Ther* 34:111, 1992.

Drug facts and comparisons, Facts and Comparisons, Inc., St Louis, MO 63146.

McCombs J: Treatment of preeclampsia and eclampsia, *Clin Pharm* 11:236-45, 1992.

Remuzzi G, Ruggenenti P: Prevention and treatment of pregnancy-associated hypertension: What have we learned in the last 10 years? *Am J Kidney Dis* 18:285-305, 1991.

Travis BE, McCullough JM: Pharmacotherapy of preterm labor, *Pharmacotherapy* 13(1):28-36, 1993.

Appendices

Tamara S. Evans, Pharm.D., B.C.P.S.

APPENDIX I. ANTIEMETICS

Agent	Preparations	Usual Adult Dosage
Chlorpromazine (Thorazine)	Tabs: 10, 25, 50, 100, 200 mg Spansules: 30, 75, 150, 200, 300 mg Syrup: 10 mg/5 ml Supp.: 25, 100 mg Inj.: 25 mg/ml	PO: 10 mg q4h IM: 25 mg q4h until vomiting stops PR: 50 mg q6h
Hydroxyzine (Vistaril)	Tabs/caps: 10, 25, 50, 100 mg Syrup: 25 mg/5 ml, 10 mg/5 ml Inj.: 25 mg/ml	PO: 25-50 mg q6-8h IM: 50 mg q6-8h
Metoclopramide (Reglan)	Tabs: 5, 10 mg Syrup: 5 mg/5 ml Inj.: 5 mg/ml	PO: 10 mg q8h IM/IV: 10 mg q6-8h
Prochlorperazine (Compazine)	Tabs: 5, 10, 25 mg Spansules: 10, 15, 30 mg Syrup: 5 mg/5 ml Supp.: 2.5, 5, 25 mg Inj.: 10 mg/2 ml	PO: 5-10 mg q6-8h PR: 25 mg bid IM: 5-10 mg q3-4h (not to exceed 40 mg/day) IV: 5-10 mg by slow IV injection (≤5 mg/min; not to exceed 40 mg/day)
Thiethylperazine (Torecan)	Tabs: 10 mg Supp.: 10 mg Inj.: 10 mg/2 ml	PO/PR/IM: 10 mg q8h
Trimethobenzamide (Tigan)	Caps: 100, 250 mg Supp.: 200 mg Inj.: 100 mg/ml	PO: 250 mg q6-8h PR: 200 mg q6-8h IM: 200 mg q6-8h

Tabs, Tablets; *supp.*, suppositories; *inj.*, injection; *caps*, capsules.

APPENDIX II. BENZODIAZEPINES*†

Drug	How Supplied	Dosage	Half-Life (Hours)	Indications
Alprazolam (Xanax)	Tabs: 0.25, 0.5, 1, 2 mg	0.25-0.5 mg tid	12-15	Anxiety
Chlordiazepoxide (Librium)	Tabs, caps: 5, 10, 25 mg Inj.: 100 mg/5 ml	5-25 mg qid	48-96	Anxiety
Clonazepam (Klonopin)	Tabs: 0.5, 1, 2 mg	0.5-2 mg tid	18-50	Anticonvulsant
Clorazepate (Tranxene)	Tabs, caps: 3.75, 7.5, 15 mg Long-acting (Tranxene SD): 11.25, 22.5 mg	3.75-15 mg tid, *or* 11.25-22.5 mg qd	30-96	Anxiety
Diazepam (Valium)	Tabs: 2, 5, 10 mg Soln: 5 mg/ml, 5 mg/5 ml Inj.: 5 mg/ml	2-10 mg bid-qid	20-80	Anxiety, anticonvulsant; muscle relaxant
Estazolam (ProSom)	Tabs: 1, 2 mg	1-2 mg hs	10-24	Insomnia
Flurazepam (Dalmane)	Caps: 15, 30 mg	15-30 mg hs	48-96	Insomnia
Halazepam (Paxipam)	Tabs: 20, 40 mg	20-40 mg tid-qid	14	Anxiety
Lorazepam (Ativan)	Tabs: 0.5, 1, 2 mg Inj.: 2, 4 mg/ml	1-2 mg bid-tid	10-20	Anxiety
Oxazepam (Serax)	Caps: 10, 15, 30 mg Tabs: 15 mg	10-15 mg tid-qid	5-20	Anxiety
Prazepam (Centrax)	Tabs: 10 mg Caps: 5, 10, 20 mg	10 mg bid-qid	48-96	Anxiety
Quazepam (Doral)	Tabs: 7.5, 15 mg	7.5-15 mg hs	39	Insomnia
Temazepam (Restoril)	Caps: 15, 30 mg	15-30 mg hs	10-20	Insomnia
Triazolam (Halcion)	Tabs: 0.125, 0.25 mg	0.125-0.25 mg hs	2-5	Insomnia

*Warnings: Pregnancy category D; benzodiazepines and their metabolites freely cross the placenta and accumulate in the fetal circulation.
†Adverse effects: Sedation, drowsiness, depression, confusion, constipation, diarrhea, dry mouth, bradycardia, and hypotension.
Tabs, Tablets; *supp.,* suppositories; *inj.,* injection; *caps,* capsules.

APPENDIX III. CORTICOSTEROIDS

Drug	Approximate Equivalent Dose (mg)	Glucocorticoid Potency	Mineralocorticoid Potency	How Supplied
Short Acting				
Cortisone	25	0.8	2	Tabs: 5, 10, 25 mg
Hydrocortisone	20	1	2	Tabs: 5, 10, 20 mg Susp.: 10 mg/5 ml Inj.: 100, 250, 500, 1000 mg vials
Intermediate Acting				
Prednisone	5	4	1	Tabs: 1, 2.5, 5, 10, 20, 50 mg Soln.: 5 mg/5 ml, 5 mg/ml
Prednisolone	5	4	1	Tabs: 5 mg Soln.: 15 mg/5 ml, 5 mg/5 ml Inj.: 20 mg/ml, 25 mg/ml, 50 mg/ml
Triamcinolone	4	5	0	Tabs: 1, 2, 4, 8 mg Soln.: 4 mg/5 ml Inj.: 3, 5, 10, 20, 25, 40 mg/ml
Methylprednisolone	4	5	0	Tabs: 2, 4, 8, 16, 24, 32 mg Inj.: 40, 125, 500 mg/vial; 1, 2 g/vial
Long Acting				
Dexamethasone	0.75	20-30	0	Tabs: 0.25, 0.5, 0.75, 1, 1.5, 2, 4, 6 mg Soln.: 0.5 mg/5 ml, 0.5 mg/0.5 ml Inj.: 4, 8, 10, 16, 20, 24 mg/ml
Betamethasone	0.6-0.75	20-30	0	Tab: 0.6 mg Soln.: 0.6 mg/5 ml Inj.: 4 mg/ml

Tabs, Tablets; *susp.*, suspension; *inj.*, injection; *soln.*, solution.

APPENDIX IV. DRUG THERAPY OF CHRONIC HYPERTENSION IN PREGNANCY

Drug/Dose	Maternal Adverse Effects	Fetal and Neonatal Adverse Effects	Comments
Atenolol 50-100 mg/day	Bradycardia, dizziness, fatigue, nausea, vomiting, diarrhea	Fetal and neonatal bradycardia and hypoglycemia, impaired fetal response to hypoxia, intrauterine growth retardation	Avoid in early pregnancy
Captopril 50-100 mg/day (bid)	Rash, taste impairment, neutropenia, proteinuria	Spontaneous abortion, growth retardation, oligohydramnios, skull hypoplasia, anuria	Do not use in pregnancy
Clonidine 0.1-0.8 mg/day (bid)	Postural hypotension, drowsiness, dry mouth, rebound hypertension	Experimental evidence of embryotoxicity	Limited data in pregnancy; not currently recommended
Enalapril 5-10 mg/day	Rash, taste impairment, neutropenia, proteinuria	Spontaneous abortion, growth retardation, oligohydramnios, skull hypoplasia anuria	Do not use in pregnancy
Furosemide 20-40 mg/day (qd or bid)	Hypovolemia, hyperuricemia, pancreatitis	Neonatal bleeding and thrombocytopenia (?)	Use to treat heart failure and refractoriness to beta-antagonists and vasodilators
Hydralazine 50-200 mg/day (bid or tid)	Tachycardia, dizziness, headache	Thrombocytopenia (?)	Second-line agent; can be added to methyldopa or beta-blockers
Hydrochlorothiazide 25-50 mg/day	Hypovolemia, hyperuricemia, pancreatitis	Neonatal bleeding and thrombocytopenia (?)	Use to treat heart failure and refractoriness to beta-antagonists and vasodilators

Labetalol 200-400 mg/day (bid)	Nausea, vomiting, bradycardia, heart failure, bronchostenosis	Fetal distress, neonatal bradycardia, possibly reduced response to hypoxia	More experience is needed
Methyldopa 0.5-3 g/day (bid-qid)	Sedation, fatigue, positive Coombs' tests	Neonatal tremors	Agent of choice because of the well-documented safety for the mother and the fetus
Metoprolol 50-225 mg/day (bid)	Bradycardia, dizziness, fatigue, nausea, vomiting, diarrhea	Fetal and neonatal bradycardia and hypoglycemia, impaired fetal response to hypoxia, intrauterine growth retardation	Avoid in early pregnancy
Nifedipine 30-120 mg/day (tid)	Tachycardia, headache, flushing, ankle edema	Limited data; teratogenic (?)	Extensive testing in progress; not currently recommended
Propranolol 40-240 mg/day (bid-tid)	Dizziness, depression, bronchospasm, nausea, vomiting, diarrhea, constipation, heart failure, bradycardia	Fetal and neonatal bradycardia and hypoglycemia, impaired response to hypoxia, intrauterine growth retardation	Avoid in early pregnancy

From Remuzzi G, Ruggenenti P: Prevention and treatment of pregnancy-associated hypertension: What have we learned in the last 10 years? *Am J Kidney Dis* 18:285-305, 1991.

APPENDIX V. DRUG THERAPY OF PREECLAMPSIA OR ECLAMPSIA

Drug/Dose/Route	Maternal Adverse Effects	Fetoplacental Adverse Effects	Comments
Preeclampsia			
Hydralazine 5 mg IV/IM, then 5-10 mg q20-40min or 0.5-10 mg/hr, IV, constant infusion	Headache, flushing, nausea, vomiting, tachycardia	Uteroplacental hypoperfusion or vasoconstriction, fetal distress	Relatively safe if carefully titrated
Nifedipine 10 mg, SL/PO, q20-30min	Headache, flushing, nausea, tachycardia	Uterine atony and hemorrhage, inhibition of labor	Limited experience
Eclampsia			
Magnesium sulfate 4-6 g IV/IM in ~10 minutes, then 1 g/hr IV or 4 g IV in ~5 minutes, then 10 g IM and 5 g, IM, q4h	Respiratory or cardiac depression	Fetal or neonatal depression	Monitor blood levels (goal = 4-7 mEq/L) and deep tendon reflexes, continue for 12-24 hr after delivery
Hypertensive Emergencies in the Course of Preeclampsia/Eclampsia			
Labetalol 50 mg, IV, slow inj., then 1-2 mg/min	Nausea, vomiting, bradycardia, heart failure, bronchostenosis	Fetal distress, neonatal bradycardia, reduced response to hypoxia (?)	Limited experience second-line agent
Diazoxide 30 mg, IV q1-2min	Nausea, vomiting, tachycardia, fluid retention, hyperglycemia	Inhibition of labor, neonatal hyperglycemia	Administer under strict medical control; avoid large boluses
Nitroprusside 0.3-10 μg/kg/min, IV, constant infusion	Nausea, vomiting, tachycardia, cyanide toxicity	Fetal cyanide toxicity	Administer only in ICUs for life-threatening HTN

From Remuzzi G, Ruggenenti P: Prevention and treatment of pregnancy-associated hypertension: What have we learned in the last 10 years? *Am J Kidney Dis* 18:285-305, 1991.
Inj., Injection; *ICU*, intensive care unit; *HTN*, hypertension.

APPENDIX VI. HISTAMINE H_2 RECEPTOR ANTAGONISTS

Agent	Preparations	Dosage
Cimetidine* (Tagamet)	Tabs: 200, 300, 400, 800 mg Liq.: 300 mg/5 ml Inj.: 300 mg/2 ml	Active peptic ulcer disease: 800 mg qhs, 300 mg qid, or 400 mg bid Maintenance: 400 mg qhs IV: 300 mg q6-8h or total dose administered as continuous infusion over 24 hr
Famotidine* (Pepcid)	Tabs: 20, 40 mg Oral susp.: 40 mg/5 ml Inj.: 10 mg/ml	Active peptic ulcer disease: 40 mg qhs, or 20 mg bid Maintenance: 20 mg qhs IV: 20 mg q12h or total dose administered as continuous infusion over 24 hr
Nizatidine† (Axid)	Pulvules: 150, 300 mg	Active peptic ulcer disease: 300 mg qhs, 150 mg bid Maintenance: 150 mg qhs
Ranitidine* (Zantac)	Tabs: 150, 300 mg Susp.: 15 mg/ml Inj.: 25 mg/ml, 0.5 mg/ml	Active peptic ulcer disease: 300 mg qhs or 150 mg bid Maintenance: 150 mg qhs IV: 50 mg q6-8h or total dose administered as continuous infusion over 24 hr

*Pregnancy category B.
†Pregnancy category C.
Tabs, tablets; *liq.*, liquid; *inj.*, injection; *susp.*, suspension.

APPENDIX VII. INSULIN PREPARATIONS

Preparation	Onset (hr)	Peak (hr)	Duration (hr)
Rapid Acting			
Regular (crystalline zinc)	½-1		6-8
Semilente	1-1½	5-10	12-16
Intermediate Acting			
NPH	1-1½	4-12	24
Lente	1-2½	7-15	24
Long Acting			
Protamine zinc insulin (PZI)	4-8	14-24	36
Ultralente	4-8	10-30	>36

APPENDIX VIII. LAXATIVES

Class	Agent	Dosage
Bulk-forming agents	Calcium polycarbophil (Fibercon)	2 tabs qd-qid with 8 oz of liquid after each dose
	High-fiber supplement (Fibermed)	2 biscuits qd
	Psyllium hydrophilic mucilloid (Metamucil)	1 tbsp or packet qd-tid with 8 oz of liquid with each dose
	Psyllium, senna (Perdiem)	1 tbsp qd-bid with 8 oz of liquid with each dose
	Methylcellulose (Citrucel)	1 tbsp qd-tid with 8 oz cold water with each dose
Osmotic agents	Lactulose (Chronulac, Cephulac)	1-2 tbsp qd-bid
	Sorbitol (30%-70%)	30 ml qd
	Glycerin suppository	1-2 qd
Stimulants	Castor oil	30-60 ml qd
	Bisacodyl (Dulcolax)	5-15 mg PO, qd 10 mg, PR, qd
	Phenolphthalein (Ex Lax)	1-2 qd
Emollients	Casanthranol docusate sodium (Pericolace)	100 mg, PO, bid
Salts	Milk of Magnesia	30 ml qd
	Magnesium citrate	240 ml prn

APPENDIX IX. ORAL CONTRACEPTIVES

Brand Name and Regimen	Estrogen	Amount (µg)	Progestin	Amount (mg)
Monophasic*				
Loestrin 1/20, 21, 28Fe	EE	20	NETA	1.0
Loestrin 1.5/30, 21, 28Fe	EE	30	NETA	1.5
Nordette-21, -28	EE	30	LNG	0.15
Lo/Ovral, 21, 28	EE	30	NG	0.3
Levlen, 21, 28	EE	30	LNG	0.15
Levora, 21, 28	EE	30	LNG	0.15
Desogen, 28	EE	30	DSG	0.15
Ortho-Cept, 21, 28	EE	30	DSG	0.15
Genora 1/35, 21, 28	EE	35	NET	1.0
Genora 0.5/35, 21, 28	EE	35	NET	0.5
N.E.E. 1/35, 21, 28	EE	35	NET	1.0
Nelova 1/35E, 21, 28	EE	35	NET	1.0
Nelova 0.5/35E, 21, 28	EE	35	NET	0.5
Norethin 1/35E, 21, 28	EE	35	NET	1.0
Norinyl 1+35, 21, 28	EE	35	NET	1.0
Ortho-Novum 1/35, 21, 28	EE	35	NET	1.0
Brevicon, 21, 28	EE	35	NET	0.5
Modicon, 21, 28	EE	35	NET	0.5
Ovcon-35, 21, 28	EE	35	NET	0.4
Demulen 1/35, 21, 28	EE	35	EDDA	1.0
Ortho-Cyclen, 21, 28	EE	35	NGS	0.25
Genora 1/50, 21, 28	ME	50	NET	1.0
Nelova 1/50M, 21, 28	ME	50	NET	1.0
Norethin 1/50M, 21, 28	ME	50	NET	1.0
Norinyl 1+50, 21, 28	ME	50	NET	1.0
Ortho-Novum 1/50, 21, 28	ME	50	NET	1.0
Ovcon-50, 21, 28	EE	50	NET	1.0
Demulen 1/50, 21, 28	EE	50	EDDA	1.0
Ovral, 21, 28	EE	50	NG	0.5
Biphasic†				
Jenest-28	7-EE	35	7-NET	0.5
	14-EE	35	14-NET	1.0
Nelova 10/11, 21, 28	10-EE	35	10-NET	0.5
	11-EE	35	11-NET	1.0
Ortho-Novum 10/11, 21, 28	10-EE	35	10-NET	0.5
	11-EE	35	11-NET	1.0

*Monophasic: Provides a fixed dosage of estrogen to progestin throughout the cycle.

†Biphasic: Estrogen amount remains the same throughout the cycle. In first half of cycle decreased progestin/estrogen ratio allows endometrial proliferation. In second half of cycle increased ratio provides adequate secretory development.

EE, Ethinyl estradiol; *ME*, mestranol; *NET*, norethindrone; *NETA*, norethindrone acetate; *EDDA*, ethynodiol diacetate; *NG*, norgestrel; *LNG*, levonorgestrel; *DSG*, desogestrel; *NGS*, norgestimate.

Continued.

APPENDIX IX. ORAL CONTRACEPTIVES—cont'd

Brand Name and Regimen	Estrogen	Amount (μg)	Progestin	Amount (mg)
Triphasic‡				
Tri-Norinyl, 21, 28	7-EE	35	7-NET	0.5
	9-EE	35	9-NET	1.0
	5-EE	35	5-NET	0.5
Ortho-Novum 7/7/7, 21, 28	7-EE	35	7-NET	0.5
	7-EE	35	7-NET	0.75
	7-EE	35	7-NET	1.0
Tri-Levlen, 21, 28	6-EE	30	6-LNG	0.05
	5-EE	40	5-LNG	0.075
	10-EE	30	10-LNG	0.125
Triphasil, 21, 28	6-EE	30	6-LNG	0.05
	5-EE	40	5-LNG	0.075
	10-EE	30	10-LNG	0.125
Ortho Tri-Cyclen	7-EE	35	7-NGS	0.180
	7-EE	35	7-NGS	0.215
	7-EE	35	7-NGS	0.250
Progestin Only (Minipill)				
Micronor			NET	0.35
Nor-Q.D.			NET	0.35
Ovrette			NG	0.075

‡Triphasic: Estrogen amount remains the same or varies and progestin amount varies throughout cycle.

Administration and Dosage

- Prevention of pregnancy
  1. Sunday-start: If the manufacturer's instructions recommend starting the regimen on Sunday, the first tablet is taken on the first Sunday after menstruation begins. If menstruation begins on Sunday, the first tablet is taken on that day.
  2. 21-day regimen. The first day of menstrual bleeding is day 1 of the cycle. Beginning on day 5 of cycle, one tablet is taken daily for 21 days, according to number of tablets supplied for one cycle. No tablets are taken for 7 days; a new course of 21 days is started, whether bleeding has stopped or not. Withdrawal flow will normally occur 2 or 3 days after the last tablet is taken.
  3. 28-day regimen: Same as 21-day regimen, except some products contain seven inert or iron-containing products to permit continuous daily dosage during the entire 28-day cycle. The seven inert or iron tablets are taken on the last 7 days of the cycle.
  4. Progestin-only products: Starting on the first day of menstruation, one tablet is taken daily at the same time each day, every day of the year.

- Postpartum administration of estrogen–progestin-containing contraceptives in nonnursing mothers may begin at the first postpartum examination (4 to 6 weeks), regardless of whether spontaneous menstruation has occurred.
  1. An increased risk of thromboembolism is associated with immediate postpartum use.
  2. Postpartum administration of progestin-only products may be initiated 2 weeks postpartum; however, the increased risk of thromboembolic disease associated with the postpartum period must be considered.
- Postcoital contraception (within 72 hours of unprotected intercourse)
  1. Ovral: Two tablets to start and two tablets 12 hours later
  2. Ethinyl estradiol: 2.5 mg bid × 5 days

Contraindications: Thrombophlebitis; thromboembolic disorders; history of deep vein thrombophlebitis; cerebral vascular disorders; myocardial infarction, coronary artery disease, or angina pectoris; breast carcinoma or estrogen-dependent neoplasia; undiagnosed abnormal uterine bleeding; past or present liver tumors that developed during use of estrogen-containing products; known or suspected pregnancy; and cholestatic jaundice of pregnancy or jaundice with prior pill use

Adverse effects

- Minor: Breakthrough bleeding or spotting, nausea, vomiting, breast tenderness, weight gain, fluid retention, psychic changes, sleep disturbances, and melasma
- Serious: Thrombophlebitis and thrombosis, pulmonary embolism, cerebrovascular disorders, myocardial infarction, optic neuritis, hepatic adenoma, hypertension, migraine headache, psychic depression, and cervical dysplasia
- Warnings: Women who use oral contraceptives (OCs) should not smoke. An increased risk of cardiovascular side effects is associated with smoking. This risk increases with age and with heavy smoking and is quite significant in women >35 years of age.

Patient information

- Take OCs exactly as directed at intervals not exceeding 24 hours to achieve maximum contraceptive effectiveness.
  1. Take tablets with a meal or at bedtime.
  2. Efficacy depends on strict adherence to the dosage schedule.
- May cause breakthrough bleeding or spotting during the first few months of therapy; notify physician if it continues past the second month.
- Use an additional method of birth control until after the first week of administration in the initial cycle.
- Missed doses: The possibility of spotting or bleeding is increased if only one tablet is missed.
  1. The possibility of ovulation occurring increases with each successive day that scheduled tablets are missed.
  2. Any time ≥ 1 active tablet has been missed, use another method of contraception until tablets have been taken for 7 consecutive days.
  3. The following is suggested if one or more tablets are forgotten:
     a. One tablet: Take it as soon as remembered, or take two tablets the next day; alternatively take one tablet, discard the other missed tablet,

continue as scheduled and use another form of contraception until menses.

b. Two consecutive tablets: Take two tablets as soon as remembered with the next pill at the usual time, or take two tablets daily for the next 2 days, then resume the regular schedule. Use an additional form of contraception for the remainder of the cycle.
c. Three consecutive tablets: Begin a new compact of tablets, starting on day 1 of the cycle after the last pill was taken or starting 7 days after the last tablet was taken. Use an additional form of birth control until pills have been taken for 7 days.

APPENDIX X. ORAL HYPOGLYCEMICS

Drug	How Supplied (Tablets, mg)	Equivalent Dose (mg)	Doses/day	Maximum Daily Dose	Duration (Hours)
First Generation					
Acetohexamide* (Dymelor)	250, 500	500	1-2	1.5 g	12-24
Chlorpropamide* (Diabinese)	100, 250	250	1	750 mg	Up to 60
Tolazamide* (Tolinase)	100, 250, 500	250	1	1.0 g	12-24
Tolbutamide* (Orinase)	250, 500	1000	2-3	3.0 g	6-12
Second Generation					
Glipizide* (Glucotrol)	5, 10	10	1-2	40 mg	10-16
Glyburide†					
(Nonmicronized (DiaBeta, Micronase)	1.25, 2.5, 5	5	1-2	20 mg	24
Micronized (Glynase PresTab)	1.5, 3	3	1-2	12 mg	24

*Pregnancy category C.
†Pregnancy category B.

APPENDIX XI. PENICILLINS AND RELATED ANTIBIOTICS

Organisms	Penicillin G/V	Amoxicillin	Ampicillin	Antistaphy-lococcal Penicillin*	Extended Spectrum Penicillin†	Amp/Sulb Amox/Clav	Ticar/Clav Pip/Tazo-bactam	Aztreonam	Imipenem
Staphylococcus aureus	+‡	+‡	+‡	+	+‡	+	+		+
Staphylococcus epidermidis	+‡	+‡	+‡	+	+‡	+	+		+
Streptococcus pneumoniae	+	+	+	+	+	+	+		+
Streptococcus faecalis	+	+	+		+	+	+		+
Streptococcus viridans	+	+	+	+	+	+	+		
Corynebacterium diphtheriae	+								
Listeria monocytogenes	+		+			+			
Moraxella (Branhamella) catarrhalis						+	+		+
Neisseria gonorrhoeae	+‡	+	+		+	+	+	+	+
Citrobacter sp.					+		+	+	+
Enterobacter sp.					+		+	+	+
Escherichia coli		+	+		+	+	+	+	+
Klebsiella pneumoniae					+	+	+	+	+
Morganella morganii					+		+	+	+
Proteus mirabilis		+	+		+	+	+	+	+
Proteus vulgaris					+		+	+	+
Salmonella sp.		+	+		+	+	+	+	+
Serratia sp.					+		+	+	+
Shigella sp.			+						
Gardnerella vaginalis		+	+			+			
Hemophilus influenzae		+	+		+	+	+	+	+
Pseudomonas aeruginosa					+		+	+	+
Clostridium perfringens	+	+	+		+	+	+		+
Peptococcus and *Peptostreptococcus*	+	+	+		+	+	+		+
Bacteroides fragilis					+	+	+		+
Bacteroides sp.	+				+	+	+		+
Treponema pallidum	+								

+, Generally susceptible. *Antistaphylococcal penicillin = oxacillin, nafcillin, methicillin, dicloxacillin, cloxacillin. †Extended spectrum penicillin = ticarcillin, piperacillin, mezlocillin, azlocillin. ‡Non-penicillinase producing.

Organisms	Cefadroxil	Cefazolin	Cephalexin	Cephalothin	Cephapirin	Cephradine	Cefaclor	Cefamandole	Cefmetazole	Cefonicid	Cefotetan	Cefoxitin	Cefuroxime	Cefixime	Cefoperazone	Cefotaxime	Cefpodoxime	Cefprozil	Ceftazidime	Ceftizoxime	Ceftriaxone	Loracarbef	Cefepime
Staphylococcus aureus	+	+	+	+	+	+	+	+	+	+	+	+	+		+	+	+	+	+	+	+	+	+
Staphylococcus epidermidis	+	+	+	+	+	+	+	+	+	+	+	+	+		+	+	+	+	+	+	+	+	+
Streptococcus pneumoniae	+	+	+	+	+	+	+	+	+	+	+	+	+	+	+	+	+	+	+	+	+	+	+
Streptococcus faecalis																							
Streptococcus viridans	+	+	+	+	+	+	+	+	+	+	+	+	+	+	+	+	+	+	+	+	+	+	+
Corynebacterium diphtheriae																							
Listeria monocytogenes																							
Moraxella (Branhamella) catarrhalis							+	+	+	+	+	+	+	+	+	+	+	+	+	+	+	+	+
Neisseria gonorrhoeae							+	+	+	+	+	+	+	+		+	+	+		+	+	+	+
Citrobacter sp.															+	+			+	+	+		+
Enterobacter sp.															+	+			+	+	+		+
Escherichia coli	+	+	+	+	+	+	+	+	+	+	+	+	+	+	+	+	+	+	+	+	+	+	+
Klebsiella pneumoniae	+	+	+	+	+	+	+	+	+	+	+	+	+	+	+	+	+	+	+	+	+	+	+
Morganella morganii									+		+	+		+	+	+			+	+	+		+
Proteus mirabilis	+	+	+	+	+	+	+	+	+	+	+	+	+	+	+	+	+	+	+	+	+	+	+
Proteus vulgaris									+		+	+		+	+	+			+	+	+		+
Salmonella sp.																							+
Serratia sp.									+		+	+		+	+	+			+	+	+		+
Shigella sp.																							+
Gardnerella vaginalis																							+
Hemophilus influenzae	+	+	+	+	+	+	+	+	+	+	+	+	+	+	+	+	+	+	+	+	+	+	+
Pseudomonas aeruginosa															+				+				
Clostridium perfringens									+		+	+	+		+	+			+	+			
Peptococcus and *Peptostreptoccus*		+							+		+	+	+		+	+			+	+			+
Bacteroides fragilis									+		+	+			+	+				+			
Bacteroides sp.									+		+	+			+	+				+			
Treponema pallidum																					+		

Continued.

APPENDIX XI. PENICILLINS AND RELATED ANTIBIOTICS—cont'd

Organisms	Amikacin	Gentamicin	Tobramycin	Azithromycin	Clarithromycin	Erythromycin	Lomefloxacin	Ciprofloxacin	Norfloxacin	Ofloxacin	Chloram-phenicol	Clindamycin	Metronidazole	Sulfonamides	Tetracyclines	TMP-SMZ	Vancomycin	Nitrofurantoin
Staphylococcus aureus		+	+	+	+	+	+	+	+	+		+			+	+	+	+
Staphylococcus epidermidis							+	+	+	+		+				+	+	
Streptococcus pneumoniae				+	+	+	+	+		+	+	+			+	+	+	
Streptococcus faecalis		+															+	+
Streptococcus viridans				+	+	+	+	+		+		+			+		+	
Listeria monocytogenes	+	+	+	+	+	+					+				+	+		
Moraxella (Branhamella) catarrhalis				+	+	+	+	+		+					+	+		
Neisseria gonorrhoeae				+	+	+	+	+	+	+					+			
Citrobacter sp.	+	+	+				+	+	+	+						+		+
Enterobacter sp.	+	+	+				+	+	+	+				+		+		+
Escherichia coli	+	+	+				+	+	+	+				+	+	+		+
Klebsiella pneumoniae	+	+	+				+	+	+	+				+		+		+
Morganella morganii	+	+	+				+	+	+	+				+	+	+		
Proteus mirabilis	+	+	+				+	+	+	+				+	+	+		
Serratia sp.	+	+	+				+	+	+	+						+		
Gardnerella vaginalis							+	+		+		+	+					
Hemophilus influenzae				+	+		+	+		+	+				+	+		
Legionella pneumophila				+	+	+		+		+								
Pseudomonas aeruginosa	+	+	+				+	+	+	+								
Clostridium difficile													+				+	
Clostridium perfringens				+	+	+					+	+	+		+			
Peptococcus and *Peptostreptococcus*				+	+	+					+	+	+		+			
Bacteroides fragilis											+	+	+		+			
Bacteroides sp.											+	+	+		+			
Chlamydia trachomatis				+	+	+	+	+		+				+	+			
Mycoplasma pneumoniae				+	+	+	+	+		+					+			
Borrelia burgdorferi (Lyme disease)				+		+									+			
Treponema pallidum				+	+	+									+			

Index

Page numbers in *italics* indicate figures; page numbers followed by a *t* indicate tables.

F

P

W